THIRD EDITION

Cancer of the Breast

WILLIAM L. DONEGAN, M.D., F.A.C.S.
Professor of Surgery
Medical College of Wisconsin
Chief, Department of Surgery
Mt. Sinai Medical Center
Milwaukee, Wisconsin

JOHN S. SPRATT, M.S.P.H., M.D., F.A.C.S.
Professor of Surgery (Surgical Oncology)
Professor of Community Health
Head, Division of Health Systems
The James Graham Brown Cancer Center
  of the University of Louisville School of Medicine
Louisville, Kentucky
Clinical Professor of Surgery
Uniformed Services University of the Health Sciences
Bethesda, Maryland

1988
W. B. SAUNDERS COMPANY
Harcourt Brace Jovanovich, Inc.
Philadelphia □ London □ Toronto
Montreal □ Sydney □ Tokyo

W. B. SAUNDERS COMPANY
Harcourt Brace Jovanovich, Inc.

The Curtis Center
Independence Square West
Philadelphia, PA 19106

Library of Congress Cataloging-in-Publication Data

Cancer of the breast.

Rev. ed. of: Cancer of the breast / William L. Donegan and John S. Spratt. 2nd ed. 1979.

Includes bibliographies and index.

1. Breast—Cancer.   I. Donegan, William L., 1932–
   II. Spratt, John S. (John Stricklin), 1929–
   [DNLM: 1. Breast Neoplasms. WP 870 C2155]
RC280.B8C316 1988   616.99′449   87-16691
ISBN 0-7216-1819-7

Editor: Edward H. Wickland, Jr.
Developmental Editor: David Kilmer
Designer: Karen O'Keefe
Production Manager: Carolyn Naylor
Manuscript Editor: Catherine Fix
Illustration Coordinator: Walt Verbitski
Indexer: Dorothy Stade

Listed here is the latest translated edition of this book together with the language of the translation and the publisher.

Spanish (1st Edition)—Editorial Cientifico—Medica, Barcelona, Spain

Cancer of the Breast   ISBN 0-7216-1819-7

© 1988 by W. B. Saunders Company. Copyright 1967 and 1979 by W. B. Saunders Company. Copyright under the Uniform Copyright Convention. Simultaneously published in Canada. All rights reserved. This book is protected by copyright. No part of it may be reproduced, stored in a retrieval system, or transmitted in any form or by any means, electronic, mechanical, photocopying, recording, or otherwise, without written permission from the publisher. Made in the United States of America. Library of Congress catalog card number 87-16691.

Last digit is the print number: 9   8   7   6   5   4   3   2

Contributors

JOSEPH C. ALLEGRA, M.D.
Professor and Chairman, Department of Medicine, University of Louisville, Louisville, Kentucky
Chemotherapy of Breast Cancer

E. JOY ARPIN, M.D., F.R.C.S.(C)
Assistant Professor, Division of Neurological Surgery, Department of Surgery, University of Louisville School of Medicine; Staff, Norton-Kosair Children's Hospitals, Humana Hospital (University), Veterans Administration Medical Center, Louisville, Kentucky
Neurologic Aspects of Breast Cancer

RICKY J. BALLOU, M.S., Ph.D., M.D.
Associate in Anatomy, University of Louisville School of Medicine, Louisville, Kentucky
Chemosensitivity of Cultured Human Breast Cancer Cells

JERRY A. BASH, Ph.D.
Associate Professor, Department of Microbiology and Immunology, University of Miami School of Medicine; Director, Surgical Cancer Research Laboratory, Miami Beach, Florida
Immunology and Immunotherapy of Mammary Tumors

SHARLEEN JOHNSON BIRKIMER, Ph.D., R.D.
Professor, Department of Health, Physical Education and Recreation, and Director of Dietetic Program, University of Louisville, Louisville, Kentucky
Nutrition and Breast Disease

JAMES D. COX, M.D.
Professor and Chairman, Department of Radiation Oncology, College of Physicians and Surgeons, Columbia University; Director, Radiation Oncology Service, Presbyterian Hospital, New York, New York
Definitive, Adjuvant, and Palliative Radiation Therapy for Mammary Cancer

WILLIAM L. DONEGAN, M.D., F.A.C.S.
Professor of Surgery, Medical College of Wisconsin; Chief, Department of Surgery, Mt. Sinai Campus, Sinai Samaritan Medical Center, Milwaukee, Wisconsin
Introduction to the History of Breast Cancer; Epidemiology and Etiology; Diagnosis; Staging and Primary Treatment; Surgical Management; Screening and Follow-up; Multiple Primary Cancers in Mammary and Extramammary Sites and Cancers Metastatic to the Breast; Local and Regional Recurrence; Mammary Carcinoma and Pregnancy; Sarcomas of the Breast; Cancer of the Male Breast

JOHN W. GAMEL, M.D.
Associate Professor, Department of Ophthalmology, University of Louisville School of Medicine; Staff, Humana Hospital (University), Veterans Administration Medical Center, Louisville, Kentucky
Metastasis to the Eye and Ocular Adnexa

RICHARD A. GREENBERG, Ph.D., M.P.H., F.A.C.E.
Professor of Epidemiology and Biostatistics, University of Louisville, Louisville, Kentucky
Epidemiology and Etiology; Screening and Follow-up; Statistical Methods in Cancer Research

M. J. JURKIEWICZ, M.D., F.A.C.S.
Professor of Surgery, Emory University School of Medicine; Chief, Plastic Surgery, Emory Affiliated Hospitals, Atlanta, Georgia
Breast Reconstruction

CARL G. KARDINAL, M.D., F.A.C.P.
Associate Professor of Clinical Medicine, Louisiana State University School of Medicine; Co-Director, Ochsner Cancer Institute and Ochsner Clinic, New Orleans, Louisiana
Endocrine Therapy of Breast Cancer

ARTHUR H. KEENEY, M.D., D.Sc.
Distinguished Professor of Ophthalmology, University of Louisville School of Medicine; Staff, Humana Hospital (University), Norton-Kosair Children's Hospitals, Veterans Administration Medical Center, Louisville, Kentucky
Metastasis to the Eye and Ocular Adnexa

SHARON KRUMM, R.N., M.S.N.
Adjunct Clinical Associate, University of Missouri-Columbia, School of Nursing; Director of Nursing, Ellis Fischel State Cancer Center, Columbia, Missouri
Nursing Care

JOHN STRAUCH MEYER, M.D.
Visiting Professor of Pathology, Washington University School of Medicine, St. Louis; Chief Pathologist and Director of Laboratories, St. Luke's Hospital, Chesterfield, Missouri
Cell Kinetics of Breast and Breast Tumors

JOHN PETER MINTON, M.D., M.Msc., Ph.D., F.A.C.S.
Professor of Surgery and American Cancer Society Professor of Clinical Oncology, Ohio State University; Staff, The Ohio State University Hospitals, Columbus, Ohio
Physiology of the Breast

MYRON MOSKOWITZ, M.D., F.A.C.R.
Professor of Radiology, University of Cincinnati; Director of Breast Imaging, University Hospital, Cincinnati, Ohio
Breast Imaging

CHRISTIAN PALETTA, M.D.
Assistant Professor of Surgery, Division of Plastic and Reconstructive Surgery, St. Louis University School of Medicine; Surgical Staff, St. Louis University Hospital, Cardinal Glennon Children's Hospital, St. Mary's Medical Center, John Cochran Veterans Administration Center; Director, Cleft Palate Clinic, Cardinal Glennon Children's Hospital, St. Louis, Missouri
Breast Reconstruction

CARLOS M. PEREZ-MESA, M.D.
Professor in Pathology, University of Missouri Medical School; Director of Pathology, Department of Laboratories, Ellis Fischel State Cancer Center, Columbia, Missouri
Gross and Microscopic Pathology

JANELL SEEGER, M.D.
Assistant Professor of Medicine, The James Graham Brown Cancer Center of the University of Louisville School of Medicine, Louisville, Kentucky
Chemotherapy of Breast Cancer

CHRISTOPHER B. SHIELDS, M.D., F.R.C.S.(C)
Professor, Division of Neurological Surgery, Department of Surgery, University of Louisville School of Medicine; Staff, Norton-Kosair Children's Hospitals, Humana Hospital (University), Veterans Administration Medical Center, Louisville, Kentucky
Neurologic Aspects of Breast Cancer

JOHN A. SPRATT, M.S., M.D.
Senior Assistant Resident, Department of Surgery, Duke University Medical Center, Durham, North Carolina
Growth Rates

JOHN S. SPRATT, M.S.P.H., M.D., F.A.C.S.
Professor of Surgery (Surgical Oncology), Professor of Community Health, and Head, Division of Health Systems, The James Graham Brown Cancer Center of the University of Louisville School of Medicine, Louisville, Kentucky; Clinical Professor of Surgery, Uniform Services University of the Health Sciences, Bethesda, Maryland
Anatomy of the Breast; Epidemiology and Etiology; Growth Rates; Chemosensitivity of Cultured Human Breast Cancer Cells; Screening and Follow-up; Multiple Primary Cancers in Mammary and Extramammary Sites and Cancers Metastatic to the Breast; Statistical Methods in Cancer Research; Surgical Management

GORDON R. TOBIN, M.D., F.A.C.S.
Professor of Surgery, University of Louisville School of Medicine; Staff, Humana Hospital (University), Norton-Kosair Children's Hospitals, Louisville Veterans Administration Medical Center, Jewish Hospital, Louisville, Kentucky
Anatomy of the Breast

MICHAEL T. TSENG, Ph.D.
Professor of Anatomy, and Director, Tumor Evaluation Laboratory, University of Louisville School of Medicine, Louisville, Kentucky
Chemosensitivity of Cultured Human Breast Cancer Cells

DANIELLE TURNS, M.D.
Professor of Psychiatry, University of Louisville School of Medicine; Chief, Psychiatry Service, Veterans Administration Medical Center, Louisville, Kentucky
Psychosocial Factors

MARC K. WALLACK, M.D.
Associate Professor of Clinical Surgery, The Mount Sinai Medical Center, New York, New York; Chairman, Department of General Surgery, Mount Sinai Medical Center, Miami Beach, Florida
Immunology and Immunotherapy of Mammary Tumors

JOHN A. WATERS, M.D.
Surgical Staff, St. Luke's Hospital, Saginaw, Michigan
Metastasis to the Eye and Ocular Adnexa

FRANCIS R. WATSON, Ph.D.
Private Consultant, Lakeland, Florida
Statistical Methods in Cancer Research

J. FRANK WILSON, M.D.
Professor and Chairman, Department of Radiation Oncology, Medical College of Wisconsin; Active Staff, Milwaukee County Medical Complex, Froedert Memorial Lutheran Hospital, West Allis Memorial Hospital; Consulting Staff, Community Memorial Hospital, Zablocki Veterans Administration Medical Center, Mount Sinai Medical Center, Milwaukee, Wisconsin
Definitive, Adjuvant, and Palliative Radiation Therapy for Mammary Cancer

JAMES L. WITTLIFF, Ph.D., F.A.C.B.
Professor of Biochemistry, University of Louisville School of Medicine, and Director, Hormone Receptor Laboratory, The James Graham Brown Cancer Center of the University of Louisville, Louisville, Kentucky
Steroid Receptor Analyses, Quality Control, and Clinical Significance

JAMES W. YATES, Ph.D.
Associate Professor, Exercise Physiology, Exercise Physiology Laboratory, University of Louisville, Louisville, Kentucky
Physical Fitness and Weight Control

Preface
To the Third Edition

This third edition of *Cancer of the Breast* in many ways represents a new book. Nearly all chapters of the second edition have been expanded and edited to bring it up to date. New chapters have been added, and some of the older chapters have been rewritten with new authors. The complex issues associated with preventing breast cancer and the panorama of benign disorders of the breast have led to new chapters on nutrition and on the physiology of the breast.

Throughout we have sought to maintain a book of immediate relevance to the clinician dealing with breast cancer and to retain the greatest possible degree of scientific credibility. That effort in previous editions has often made this book of value to the basic scientist interested in breast cancer as well. Toward this latter end, the book contains much new data.

There will not be found a unanimity of conclusions. Where differences of opinion exist, we have sought to display alternative arguments openly. For example, one of us (JSS) remains a skeptic that mammography can be expected to bring about a sustained or publicly affordable reduction in the risk of dying of breast cancer. These concerns are aired in the chapter on screening and follow-up; the alternative position by Moskowitz is in the chapter on breast imaging.

There remain many areas of uncertainty where questions on the control of breast cancer have not been studied with the scientific exactness necessary. Thus, much work remains to be done, and research in the control of breast cancer remains an ongoing public health challenge.

We are deeply indebted to our many contributors. Collectively, we hope we have presented a text that will be well received and useful. The fine staff at the W. B. Saunders Company have done their usual superb job, as have our secretaries, Susan Albertin, Betsy Hagan, Pam Greer, and Rhonda Hawley.

WILLIAM L. DONEGAN
JOHN S. SPRATT

Contents

CHAPTER 1
Introduction to the History of Breast Cancer 1
    William L. Donegan

CHAPTER 2
Anatomy of the Breast 16
    John S. Spratt and Gordon R. Tobin

CHAPTER 3
Physiology of the Breast.. 34
    John Peter Minton

CHAPTER 4
Epidemiology and Etiology 46
    John S. Spratt, William L. Donegan, and Richard A. Greenberg

CHAPTER 5
Nutrition and Breast Disease 74
    Sharleen Johnson Birkimer

CHAPTER 6
Diagnosis 125
    William L. Donegan

CHAPTER 7
Breast Imaging 167
    Myron Moskowitz

CHAPTER 8
Gross and Microscopic Pathology... 206
    Carlos M. Perez-Mesa

CHAPTER 9
Cell Kinetics of Breast and Breast Tumors 250
    John Strauch Meyer

CHAPTER 10
Growth Rates 270
    John S. Spratt and John A. Spratt

CHAPTER 11
Steroid Receptor Analyses, Quality Control, and
Clinical Significance... 303
    James L. Wittliff

CHAPTER 12
Staging and Primary Treatment.. 336
    William L. Donegan

CHAPTER 13
Surgical Management.. 403
    John S. Spratt and William L. Donegan

CHAPTER 14
Definitive, Adjuvant, and Palliative Radiation Therapy for
Mammary Cancer.. 462
    J. Frank Wilson and James D. Cox

CHAPTER 15
Chemotherapy of Breast Cancer... 475
    J. Seeger and J. C. Allegra

CHAPTER 16
Chemosensitivity of Cultured Human Breast Cancer Cells............... 492
    Ricky J. Ballou, Michael T. Tseng, and John S. Spratt

CHAPTER 17
Endocrine Therapy of Breast Cancer...................................... 501
    Carl G. Kardinal

CHAPTER 18
Immunology and Immunotherapy of Mammary Tumors 541
    Marc K. Wallack and Jerry A. Bash

CHAPTER 19
Screening and Follow-up 558
    John S. Spratt, William L. Donegan, and Richard A. Greenberg

CHAPTER 20
Nursing Care 591
Sharon Krumm

CHAPTER 21
Breast Reconstruction 614
Christian Paletta and M. J. Jurkiewicz

CHAPTER 22
Multiple Primary Cancers in Mammary and Extramammary Sites and
Cancers Metastatic to the Breast 632
William L. Donegan and John S. Spratt

CHAPTER 23
Local and Regional Recurrence.. 648
William L. Donegan

CHAPTER 24
Metastasis to the Eye and Ocular Adnexa 664
John A. Waters, John W. Gamel, and Arthur H. Keeney

CHAPTER 25
Neurologic Aspects of Breast Cancer..................................... 670
Christopher B. Shields and E. Joy Arpin

CHAPTER 26
Mammary Carcinoma and Pregnancy..................................... 679
William L. Donegan

CHAPTER 27
Sarcomas of the Breast 689
William L. Donegan

CHAPTER 28
Cancer of the Male Breast 716
William L. Donegan

CHAPTER 29
Psychosocial Factors 728
Danielle M. Turns

CHAPTER 30
Statistical Methods in Cancer Research 739
  Francis R. Watson, Richard A. Greenberg, and John S. Spratt

CHAPTER 31
Physical Fitness and Weight Control 768
  James W. Yates

Index 779

CHAPTER 1

WILLIAM L. DONEGAN

Introduction to the History of Breast Cancer

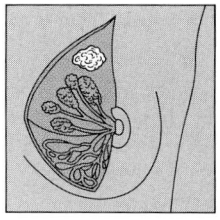

This brief history is dedicated to R. S. Handley, who died June 16, 1984. He was a life-long student of breast cancer and a dedicated surgeon and teacher. He encouraged the author's studies and demonstrated through his example the wise and humane practice of surgery.

Physicians who share an interest in breast cancer know that it is an ancient disease. Breast tumors were described by the Egyptians 3000 years before Christ. Subsequently, Greek and Roman physicians wrote about it, and the record continued through the Middle Ages and into modern times. The excellent histories of Cooper (1941), Lewison (1953), Ackerknecht (1965), Power (1934–1935), and Mansfield (1976) are valuable resources for this account.

Surgery is the oldest means of treating breast cancer. It has been used in every age, yet enthusiasm for it has waxed and waned. Operations have been devised, discarded, rediscovered, changed, and abandoned again in seemingly endless fashion as physicians sought to employ the science and technology of their times. It is in the growth of knowledge about this disease that the story of surgery for breast cancer takes on meaning and continuity. The course of events permits four periods to be identified. The earliest period can be characterized as empiric, and treatment was discouraged. Experience had taught that some tumors of the breast were aggravated by operations. These were best recognized and left undisturbed. Next, cancers were considered a systemic disease. Removal of a breast tumor might give temporary relief, but it could not be expected to cure. The third period was one of growing optimism, based on the thesis that breast cancer began as a local disease, and if found early was curable with proper local treatment. Finally, in the modern era, the problem has been recognized as being more complex than previously appreciated, and new principles of treatment are evolving.

The Early Period

Surgery was not performed for breast cancer in ancient Egypt. The Edwin Smith surgical papyrus, which dates from the Egyptian pyramid age around 3000–2500 B.C., describes eight cases of tumors or ulcers of the breast. Tumors that were hard, were cool to the touch, and contained fluid were distinguished from inflammations and abscesses; for the former, the writer admits "there is no treatment." Reference is made to one case treated by cauterization with a fire stick. The later Ebber's papyrus (1600–1500 B.C.) makes no reference to cancer of the breast.

Indian writings dating to 2000 B.C. mention the treatment of tumorous growths with surgical extirpation, cautery, and arsenic compounds. Cuneiform tablets of Assyria, with writings that date to this same period, only mention the occurrence of breast cancer.

In an isolated account, Herodotus (484–425 B.C.) gives Democedes, a Persian physician who lived in Greece at that time, credit for curing the wife of King Darius of a "tumor" of the breast that had ulcerated and spread.

The most famous of Greek physicians, Hippocrates (460–370 B.C.), mentioned breast cancer only twice and both times darkly. He stated, "A woman in Abdera had a carcinoma of the breast and bloody fluid ran from the nipple. When the discharge stopped, she died." Later, he described what must have been a typical course in a patient: "and hard tumors appear in the breast, some large and some smaller, these do not suppurate, but continually grow harder and harder. From these grow hidden cancers . . . and everything [the patients] eat tastes bitter, and if you give them more to eat, they refuse it, and shut their mouths. They become delirious, their eyes are hard, and they do not see clearly, and pains dart from the breast to the neck and beneath the shoulder blades, thirst seizes upon them, the nipples are dry, and the whole body becomes emaciated . . . When they have gone as far as this, they do not recover, but die of this disease." From his experience he counseled, "It is better not to apply any treatment in cases of occult cancer; for if treated, the patients die quickly, but if not treated they hold out for a long time."

Interestingly, the early Romans performed extensive surgery for cancer of the breast, including removal of the pectoral muscles. The Roman scholar Aulus Cornelius Celsus (42 B.C.–37 A.D.) advised against this practice as well as against caustic medicines, cautery, and excision. He described the evolution from a benign tumor, which the Greeks called a "cacoethes," to a carcinoma without ulceration, to an ulcer, and, finally, to a "thymium," and counseled that "none of these can be removed but the cacoethes; the rest are irritated by every method of cure." To distinguish a cacoethes from a carcinoma, he advised first treating with caustics and, if the symptoms grew milder, proceeding to incision and the cautery. If the disease was irritated, however, the transition to carcinoma had already occurred, and only mild medicines were appropriate.

Cancer as a Systemic Disease

In the second century Galen (131–203 A.D.) dominated medicine. The prestige of this famous Greek physician who worked among the Romans was such that his teachings were perpetuated for 1000 years. Hippocrates earlier had taught that disease was caused "by the particular humor that prevails in the body." Galen expanded and refined this humoral theory of disease. He attributed cancer to an excess of black bile in the body, calling it a local manifestation of the constitutional disturbance "melancholia." "Cancerous tumors develop with greatest frequency in the breast of women," he said. "Such unnatural tumors have their source in the black bile, a superfluous residue of the body." This systemic concept must have corresponded well with what appeared to be the prospects for cure at that time. It was Galen who likened the appearance of cancers to that of a crab, with the large veins extending from all sides giving the appearance of legs.

Nevertheless, Galen excised those tumors that were removable, and, apparently appreciating the value of wide removal, recommended excision through the healthy surrounding tissues. "Make accurate incisions surrounding the whole tumor so as not to leave a single root," he counseled. "Let the blood flow and do not check it at once but make pressure on the surrounding veins so as to squeeze out the thick blood." Galen insisted that ligatures invited recurrence in the surrounding tissues and avoided them.

Leonidus of the Alexandrian school (180 A.D.) had also learned to place his incisions through normal tissues wide of the tumor but was more concerned than Galen about controlling hemorrhage. Aetius quotes Leonidus, "placing the patient in a recumbent position, I make an incision into the sound part of the breast, above the cancer, and immediately apply the cautery until an eschar is produced to stop the bleeding." He then proceeded to alternately cut and cauterize until the breast was removed, with a final cauterization intended to eradicate any residual tumor. The use of knife and cautery, as described by Leonidus, persisted for more than 1000 years, as did the avoidance of ligatures.

Little surgical progress was made during the Dark Ages. Most medical historians attribute this to the humoral theory of disease taught by Hippocrates and by Galen, the slavish adherence to Galen as the ultimate authority on things medical, and the strong pervasive influence of the church. The Council of Tours in 1162 discouraged surgery as treatment for cancer of the breast. The cruel persecution of St. Agatha, canonized by the early church and invoked as the patron saint of women with breast disease, included amputation of the breasts, and this was often depicted in art with the surgical instruments of the day. In consequence, cautery and caustics became the predominant methods of treatment even though it continued to be widely accepted that breast cancer was an incurable disease. Perhaps the blurred distinction between malignant and benign tumors permitted sufficient successes to keep hope alive. Albucasis (1013–1106 A.D.), an Arabian surgeon who produced the first illustrated treatise on cautery, doubted the value of surgery and knew of no case of breast cancer that had been cured. Other notables perpetuated earlier techniques. Lanfrank (A.D. 1296) in France used the 1100 year old cut and cauterize technique of Leonidus. Ambrose Paré (1510–1590) excised small breast tumors but substituted sulfuric acid for the hot cautery. Large tumors were treated with milk, ointment, and vinegar. Henri D'Mondeville (1260–1320) and Guy D'Chauliac (1300–1367) both operated on breast cancers that could be widely excised, but the former preferred arsenic and zinc chloride caustic pastes for large tumors. Unorthodox treatments temporarily employed during this time included bisection of the affected breast with an attempt to dissolve the tumor by means of a ligature, practiced by Francisco Araceo (1493–1571) in Spain. Compression of the breast with lead plates was used by Lenard Fuchs (1501–1566).

The end of the Dark Ages was marked by extremes. In the 16th century, William Clowes (1560–1634), Queen Elizabeth's physician, advocated the laying on of hands, and for a time royal persons were solicited to touch the afflicted in hopes of healing them. Peter Lower (1597) applied goat's dung, and later James Cook (1614–1688) practiced bleeding from the basilic vein. Some applied frogs, bisected chickens, or fresh parts of other animals to the affected breast with results that remain obscure.

At the same time, innovators began to loosen the bonds of tradition. Andreas Vesalius (1514–1564), the father of modern anatomy, published De Humani Corporis Fabrica in 1543, which corrected the errors of Galen's anatomy, and substituted ligatures for the hot cautery when excising breast cancers. Jacques Guillemeau (1550–1601) reinstituted removal of the pectoralis major muscle along with the breast. At the school in Salerno, Italy, Marcus Aurelius Severinus (1580–1659) began to remove axillary lymph nodes along with the breast. He, as well as Ambrose Paré earlier, was among the first to appreciate that they were a part of the tumorous process.

The 16th century initiated a resurgence of surgery, and the next two centuries were noteworthy for techniques of mastectomy that were both thorough and efficient in their execution.

In a time without anesthesia, the motivation was a mercifully swift amputation of the breast. Scultetus (1595–1645) accomplished this by passing two large needles attached to heavy cords through the base of the breast in opposite directions, and while pulling up on the cords, swiftly amputated the breast with a knife, following which hemostasis was achieved with a cauterizing iron. Wilhelm Fabry (1560–1634), a German barber surgeon who was a pupil of Vesalius, accomplished the same end with large metal tongs, which, when closed, encompassed the base of the breast with an iron ring. Traction on the instrument then stretched the breast away from the chest wall, permitting it to be amputated swiftly and accurately with a knife. Godefrides Bidloo illustrated in 1708 his own special instruments for swift amputation, consisting of a knife, a one-pronged fork, and a two-pronged fork. One or both forks were thrust through the base of the breast to transfix it and provide traction before using the knife (Fig. 1–1). The evolution of this method culminated in 1721 with the technique of Gerard Tabor. Tabor employed a hinged instrument composed of two semicircles with handles that could be clamped around the base of the breast. A curved knife blade hinged at the same fulcrum could be swept through the ring in one stroke, completing the operation in perhaps no more than 1 or 2 seconds. The breast was removed more completely by these procedures than with any earlier technique, and many later ones,

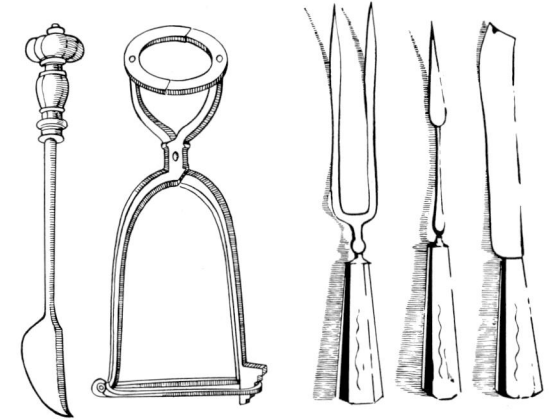

Figure 1–1. Mastectomy instruments used by Fabricus Hildanus (left) and by Godefridus Bidloo (right) in the 17th century. In each case the breast was either transfixed with a metal ring on tongs or with forks and then quickly cut away with a knife. (Redrawn from Cooper, W. A.: The history of radical mastectomy. Ann. Med. Hist. 3:36, 1941.)

but because the resulting wound was large and required many months to heal, they were abandoned in favor of less complete procedures that permitted closure of the skin.

In 1662 Reverend John Ward described an operation that he observed in which after the skin was cut, the tumor was bluntly separated from surrounding tissues with the hands. On each of the succeeding 2 days the wound was opened and additional portions of the tumor cut out. The patient died several months later with cancer still present in the breast. It was to discourage piecemeal operations that Jean Louis Petit (1674–1750), the foremost French surgeon of the period, wrote in his Traite des Operations concerning carcinoma of the breast that all tissues should be removed in one piece. Although his excision of the breast was less complete than that of Scultetus before him, he urged the removal of all enlarged axillary lymph nodes and of the pectoralis fascia and pectoralis muscle if they appeared to be involved.

During this period, cancer remained conceptually a systemic disease. After discovery of the lymphatic system, which resulted from Ascelli's description of lacteals in 1622 and the description of the thoracic duct by Pecquet, Bartholinus, and Rud Beck in 1651, René Descartes (1596–1650) substituted a lymph theory of the origin of breast cancer for Galen's black bile theory, and this was perpetuated by John Hunter (1728–1793) in the 18th century. Hunter taught that a defect existed in the lymph and, where it coagulated, breast cancer made its appearance. This represented little improvement over Galen's black bile theory, but it may have had the effect of fostering the removal of enlarged axillary lymph nodes.

Breast Cancer as a Local Disease

In the 18th century a concept was introduced that provided hope for surgical cure. In 1757, a French surgeon, Henry François LeDran, advanced the theory that cancer began in its earliest stages as a local disease. It spread first by lymphatics to regional nodes and subsequently entered the general circulation (LeDran, 1757). LeDran's theory offered the possibility that if surgery were performed sufficiently early it could encompass and cure the disease. Bernard Peyrilhe (1773), as well as other notables of the day, embraced this pivotal concept and, during the next century, it gradually replaced the humoral theory of cancer.

The constitutional theory did not die easily. More than a century later Henry Arnott of St. Thomas Hospital in London still felt obliged to argue for the local origin of cancer and the value of early surgery (Arnott, 1871). He likened cancer to a thistle in a cornfield. "If this weed be allowed to remain until the flowerhead has passed to its stage of ripe, feathery seeds, these are wafted hither and thither, and, taking root, become so intimately and largely mingled with the corn that the complete removal of the nuisance is impossible without greatly endangering the whole crop. But if the original plant be removed at once all this danger is avoided." "Our problem," he said, prescient of future mass screening, "is to discover these tumors before the afflicted one can do so."

With the acceptance of the local theory, the principles of curative surgery sanctioned wide en bloc operations and surgical resection at the earliest possible moment. These principles guided efforts for the next 100 years and kindled unparalleled optimism for surgical cure. In the words of LeDran, "Every cancer begins by the obstruction of one or more glands," and "we may hope for a perfect cure." As early as 1773, Peyrilhe advised an operation that removed the cancerous breast along with the axillary contents and the pectoralis major muscle, the same operation introduced by Halsted more than 100 years later. Jean Louis Petit warned against cutting through the mammary gland and urged removal of the axillary nodes as well as the pectoral fascia and pectoralis muscle if necessitated by the extent of involvement. His contemporary, Lorensius Heister (1683–1758), removed not only the pectoralis major muscle but ribs as well if necessary to remove all the tumor.

Advances in science and medicine in the 19th century included the introduction of general anesthesia in 1846, of antisepsis in 1867, and of microscopic pathology. These advances accrued to the benefit of all surgery. Specific to the treatment of breast cancer, the period was noted for the development of radical surgery and for the discovery that breast cancer was hormonally dependent. In the closing decade of the 19th century, x-rays and radium were discovered, and radiotherapy made its debut.

During most of the 19th century operations for cancer of the breast were still dangerous, and surgeons continued to be pessimistic about the results. Overwhelming infection was the major cause of operative mortality, being as high as 20 per cent in some series. The selection of obvious cancers for surgery and poor postoperative care contributed to the dismal results. Alexander Monroe (1773–1859) reviewed 60 cases of surgically treated breast cancer at this time and found only four patients free of disease at the end of 2 years. Sir James Paget in 1853 confessed to having never seen a cure and advised that "in deciding for or against the removal of a cancerous breast, in any single case, we may, I think, dismiss all hope that the operation will be a final remedy for the disease." Equally pessimistic, Hayes Agnew (1818–1892) wrote, "I do not despair of carcinoma being cured somewhat in the future, but this blessed achievement will never be wrought of the knife of the surgeon." Robert Liston's opinion in 1840 was that "recourse may be had to the knife in some cases, but the circumstances must be very favorable indeed to induce a surgeon to recommend or warrant him in undertaking any operation for removal of malignant disease of the breast."

In these years no consistent practice can be found with respect to the amount of skin and breast removed or the removal of enlarged axillary lymph nodes. The ominous nature of the latter was fully appreciated. In Scotland, James Sime observed in 1842, "it appears that the result of operations for carcinoma when the glands are affected is almost always unsatisfactory, however perfectly they may seem to have been taken away. The reason for this probably is that the glands do not participate in the disease unless the system is strongly disposed to it and consequently their removal, however freely and effectually executed, cannot prevent the patient's relapse."

Two forces pushed radical surgery forward, however: the theory of local origin and the practical effort to eliminate local recurrence. Ultimately these two forces reinforced each other. The former culminated in the permeation theory of Sampson Handley and the latter in operations to routinely remove the entire breast, the axillary contents, and finally, the pectoral muscles—in sum, the radical mastectomy of William Halsted.

In 1867 the case for local origin was given renewed impetus by Charles H. Moore at the Middlesex Hospital in London (Fig. 1–2) (Moore, 1867). In a publication entitled "On the Influence of Inadequate Operations on the Theory of Cancer" Moore observed that recurrences after limited operations for breast cancer were generally near the scar and that their pattern suggested centrifugal spread from the original site (Fig. 1–3). He concluded that surgical failure was due not to a systemic diathesis but to failure of the surgeon to remove all local extensions of the disease. His principles of surgical cure are classic:

1. "It is not sufficient to remove the cancer or any portion only of the breast in which it is situated; mammary cancer requires the careful extirpation of the entire organ. The attempt to save skin which is in any degree unsound is

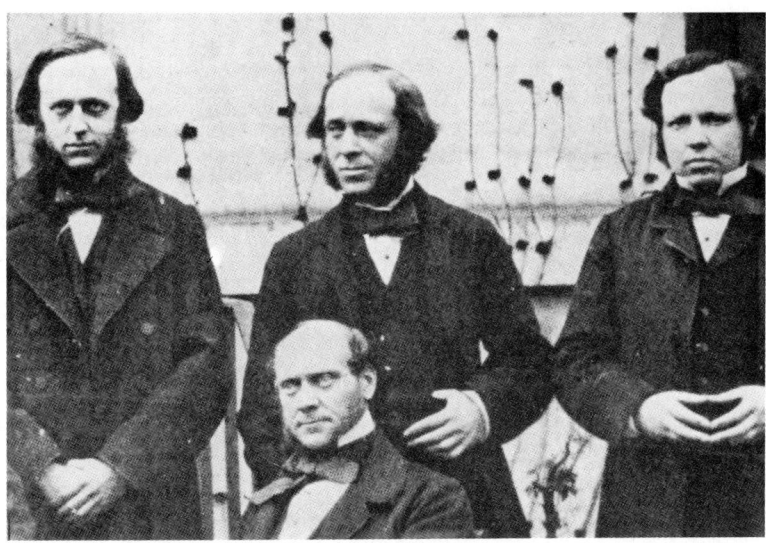

Figure 1–2. Charles Moore (top center) supported the local origin of breast cancer and authored a classic paper in 1867 advocating routine total en bloc removal of the breast. He is pictured with associates outside of the Middlesex Hospital in London, England. (From archives of Middlesex Hospital.)

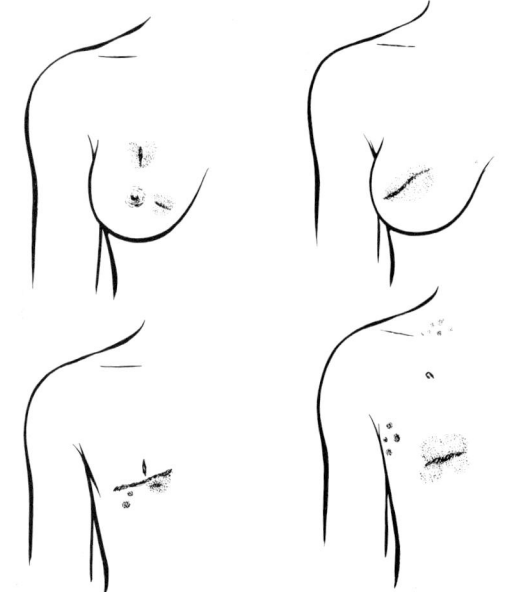

Figure 1–3. Four examples of cases illustrated by C. H. Moore in 1867 show local recurrence of breast cancer after "inadequate operations." The local origin of breast cancer was supported by this evidence and it provided the foundation for wide en bloc removal of the entire breast as appropriate initial treatment. Dark lines indicate excisional scars and gray areas recurrent carcinoma. (Redrawn from Moore, C. H.: On the influence of inadequate operations on the theory of cancer. Med. Clin. Trans. [Lond.], 32:245, 1867.)

of all errors perhaps the most pernicious, and whenever its condition is doubtful, that texture should be freely removed."

2. "In the performance of the operation, it is desirable to avoid, not only cutting into the tumor, but also seeing it. No actually morbid texture should be exposed, lest the active microscopic elements in it be set free and lodge in the wound."

3. "Diseased axillary glands should be taken away by the same dissection as the breast itself, without dividing the intervening lymphatics."

The importance of Moore's paper lies in its evidence for the local origin of breast cancer and for supporting wide removal en bloc of all diseased and suspected tissues as a principle of cure. Moore's operation was widely adopted. Joseph Lister (1837–1912) supported his concept and was perhaps the first to expose the axilla by division of the pectoral muscles. Samuel W. Gross, professor of surgery at Jefferson Medical College in Philadelphia and in Louisville, enlarged it to include removal of the pectoral fascia.

Routine removal of the entire breast is clearly traceable to Moore, and routine removal of the axillary nodes is possibly so. Although originally he referred only to removal of "diseased axillary glands," Moore subsequently stated that they can never be assumed to be healthy (Power, 1934–1935). Surgeons became increasingly aware of the difficulty of determining by palpation whether or not axillary lymph nodes were involved, and impressed with the frequency of axillary recurrence when they were not included, they began to remove them routinely. In Britain, William M. Banks of Liverpool pioneered this practice. In a paper read before the British Medical Association at Worcester, in 1882, entitled "Free Removal of Mammary Cancer with Extirpation of the Axillary Glands as a Necessary Accompaniment," he reported 46 cases and said, "In the present paper the principal object is to advocate the removal of the axillary glands as well as the breast in all cases. . . . I have been quietly practicing this for 3-4 years" (Banks, 1902). As early as 1871 Küster of Berlin included axillary dissection as an essential part of mastectomy, whether or not lymph nodes could be felt in the axilla during the operation, and Halsted later gave Küster credit for being the first to advocate systematic cleaning out of the axilla (Küster, 1883). Routine axillary dissection dramatically reduced recurrences at that site. Schmid (1887) reported that among 95 cases of recurrence in Küster's series only one occurred in the axilla.

The pectoralis fascia and its underlying muscle were the next tissues to become suspect, largely through the microscopic research of vonVolkman and Heidenhain. The microscope had become a powerful tool in the 19th century (Schlumberger, 1944). By midcentury, the cell, as the unit structure of plant and animal life, had been identified by Schleiden (1838) and Schwann (1839, tr. 1847). The pioneering work of Johannes Müller was to identify the cellular nature of cancers in his 1838 landmark publication, "On the fine structure and form of morbid tumors." Virchow deduced that all cells came from previous cells and revolutionized pathologic anatomy with his "Die Cellular Pathologie," considered one of the most important medical books of all time. Joseph Claude Recamier had introduced the concept of metastasis in 1829 and this was further refined by the German school. Wilder credits the microscopic research of Thiersch (1822–1895) and of Waldeyer (1872) with the concept that metastases originate from transplanted cancer cells rather than by the spread of tumor "juices" and, further, that the cells were liberated from the primary tumor into the lymph and blood by both continuous growth and embolization (Wilder, 1956). To explain the distribution of metastases, researchers became divided between those who considered it an impartial process determined by mechanical entrapment of cells and those who, with Steven Paget (1889), believed in the theory of "seed and soil" (i.e., cancer cells lodge and grow selectively only at favorable locations).

Germany led in this era of histologic discovery. VonVolkman was one of the first to supplement removal of the breast and axillary contents with routine removal of the fascia of the pectoralis major muscle. In 1875, he explained, "I was led to adopt this procedure because on microscopical examination I repeatedly found when I had not expected it that the fascia was already carcinomatous whereas the muscle was certainly not involved" (Halsted, 1894–1895). Heidenhain's observations went further (Heidenhain, 1889). He reported that he had examined 18 of Küster's mastectomy specimens in which the pectoralis muscle was removed and found unsuspected microscopic invasion of the muscle in three cases. Heidenhain believed that in such cases contraction of the muscle could spread cancer cells throughout the lymphatics of its entire substance. Thus, Heidenhain concluded, "Removal of a piece of the muscle with the tumor is not enough." He recommended that, in cases when the cancer had grown into the pectoralis major muscle or was adherent to its fascia, the muscle be removed in its entirety.

This thought was extended by William Stewart Halsted, Professor of Surgery at the Johns Hopkins Hospital. Halsted was particularly aware of developments in Germany. His contribution to the progress of surgery lay in advocating routine removal of the pectoralis major muscle and in reinforcing the principle of en bloc resection. Said Halsted in 1894, "The pectoralis major muscle, entire or all except its clavicular portion, should be excised in every case of cancer of the breast, because the operator is enabled thereby to remove in one piece all of the suspected tissues. The suspected tissue should be removed in one piece, (1) lest the wound become infected by the division of tissues invaded by the disease, or of lymphatic vessels containing cancer cells, and (2) because shreds or pieces of cancerous tissue might readily be overlooked in a piecemeal extirpation" (Halsted, 1894–1895).

Halsted's operation removed the entire breast with its overlying skin, the pectoralis major muscle, and the axillary contents; it was initially known as the "complete operation" and ultimately as "radical mastectomy." It was used by Halsted in 1883 in "almost every case" and was mentioned in a publication by him in 1891 entitled "The Treatment of Wounds with a Special Reference to the Value of the Blood Clot in the Management of Dead Spaces" (Halsted, 1891). In 1894 he published in the Johns Hopkins Hospital Reports the results of 50 cases treated since 1889 in this manner. Halsted emphasized the dramatic reduction in local recurrences (only 6 per cent in his series) compared with the 56 to 81 per cent reported by surgeons in Europe. By present definitions, 18 per cent of the 50 cases had recurrence in and around the wound at that time. Nevertheless, after 37 years, Lewis and Rienhoff (1932) at Johns Hopkins reported that the recurrence locally had risen in the original cases to only 31.5 per cent, still a distinct improvement over previous results.

The radical mastectomy was an idea whose time had arrived. In the same year as Halsted's 1894 report, Willie Meyer, Professor of Surgery at the New York Postgraduate Medical School, reported a similar operation independently conceived but motivated by the same rationale that Halsted had expressed (Meyer, 1894). As Meyer performed his first operation on September 19, 1894, Halsted preceded him by several years. Only details of the operation varied. Meyer used a diagonal incision, which ultimately became more popular than Halsted's tear drop incision, excised the pectoralis minor muscle rather than dividing it as Halsted had done (a modification later adopted by Halsted), and dissected the axilla before dividing the breast and muscles from the chest wall, rather than afterwards, as in the Halsted procedure. Both surgeons emphasized the necessity of removing a large amount of skin sufficient to require split-thickness skin grafting, a procedure that had recently been developed by Thiersch in 1886.

Was Meyer's method preceded by another's? *The Lancet* of February 4, 1893, relates that Arbuthnot Lane in Britain discussed an operation in which he "took away the whole of the pectoral muscles with the subjacent breast, and then carefully dissected from the vessels and nerves of the axilla every bit of areolar tissue together with the lymphatic vessels and glands" (Clinical Society of London, 1893). He then "urged the advisability of removing the pectoral muscles and fascia forming the anterior wall of the axilla with the lymphatic vessels in relation to it. By these means not only were the primary growth and the cancerous glands removed, but, also, all the lymphatic channels along which infection had extended."

The radical mastectomy received conceptual support in the permeation theory of W. Sampson Handley of London, which, at the close of the 19th century, epitomized the biology of breast cancer (Handley and Thackray, 1969). Handley's theory, based on autopsy studies, was that cancers originated at one focus and spread from it exclusively through lymphatics. The lymphatic spread was by growth in continuity (permeation) rather than embolic and occurred equally in all directions. Regional lymph nodes, which were perfect filters of cancer cells, halted the progess of permeation until the tumor was able to grow through them, and only then were the cells capable of reaching the bloodstream for embolic spread. Hematogenous dissemination happened only very late in the preterminal phase of the disease. Lymphatic permeation occurred principally in deep fascial planes, and seemingly discontinuous metastases were an illusion created by a process of obliterative lymphangitis, which erased the continuity.

Handley's permeation theory was endorsed by Halsted, and the two surgeons gave an enormous impetus to radical extirpative surgery. Theoretically, it was possible even in advanced stages of the disease for a surgeon who was sufficiently aggressive to encompass the cancer and all of its extensions. Said Halsted, "We believe, with Handley, that cancer of the breast in spreading centrifugally preserves in the main continuity with the original growth," and again, "Though the area of disease extend from cranium to knee, breast cancer in the broad sense is a local affection, and there comes to the surgeon an encouragement to greater endeavor with the cognition that the metastases to bone, to pleura, to liver are probably parts of the whole, and that the involvements are almost invariably by process of lymphatic permeation, and not embolic by way of the blood" (Halsted, 1907).

Another of Halsted's practices that became firmly entrenched was biopsy followed by immediate mastectomy. Increasingly aware of the need for accurate diagnosis, he made incisions for biopsy with increasing frequency. Being also aware of the implantability of cancer, he said, "The excision of a specimen for macroscopic or microscopic examination is never resorted to except just before operation" (Halsted, 1907).

The wide scope of Halsted's operation greatly reduced the frequency of recurrence in the surgical area, but it is difficult to establish that it improved the chances of cure. Some of Halsted's cases were not cancers; others were obviously advanced. Bloodgood described one of Halsted's early cases as follows: "The tumor now occupies the entire breast and is adherent to the pectoral muscle. The nipple is retracted. There is a large abscess in the axilla" (Halsted, 1894–1895). In an actuarial analysis, only 8 per cent of Halsted's first 50 cases were alive and free of disease at the end of 4 years. Greenough at the Massachusetts General Hospital reported better results with incomplete operations (Greenough et al., 1907). Henderson and Canellos (1980) compared Halsted's cases with earlier untreated cases from Middlesex Hospital and estimated no more than 12 per cent improvement in survival. Aware of the complexity of the lymphatic system, Rudolph Metas criticized the "complete" operation as not being a complete removal. Nevertheless, Halsted's prestige and his influence as a teacher resulted in wide acceptance of his operation in the United States and abroad (Rutkow, 1978). After a period of indiscriminate use, the contraindications to radical mastectomy were defined through the scholarly work of Cushman Haagensen in New York, and improved results understandably proceeded pari passu with more careful case selection and earlier diagnosis (Haagensen, 1971).

In the 20th century, radical surgery reached its zenith. It soon became evident to Halsted that his operation was incomplete, and he extended it by dividing the clavicle and removing the supraclavicular nodes. Occasionally enlarged internal mammary nodes were removed as well. Halsted abandoned these modifications because removing the supraclavicular nodes seldom cured a patient if metastases were present (10 per cent of cases at 3 years) and the internal mammary nodes could not readily be removed en bloc. With this demonstration that little could be gained by enlarging the operation, radical mastectomy in its original form was accepted as the ultimate surgery for cancer of the breast for the next 40 years.

It was not long (1922), however, until W.

Sampson Handley refocused attention on internal mammary metastases with parasternal biopsies and advocated their treatment with interstitial radium (Handley, 1922). This work was extended by his son, Richard S. Handley (1952), who routinely biopsied internal mammary nodes during radical mastectomy in a series of 119 patients and found metastases in 34 per cent of the cases (Fig. 1–4). The implications were clear; spread of tumor to these nodes doomed fully one third of all radical mastectomies to failure. In response to this information, the radical mastectomy was extended by a number of surgeons to include the removal of these nodes, an operation which became known as "extended radical mastectomy." Margottini in Italy was the first to do this routinely in 1948 (Margottini, 1952). In keeping with the radical concept, Urban, Sugarbaker, and others in the United States advocated the removal of the internal mammary nodes en bloc with the remainder of the specimen (Sugarbaker, 1953; Urban, 1964). Because of its logic, feasibility, and safety, this operation was adopted at many centers. Dahl-Iverson and associates in Denmark went further, removing the supraclavicular as well as the internal mammary nodes at the time of mastectomy, but not as an en bloc dissection (Dahl-Iversen and Tobiassen, 1969). Prudente amputated the upper extremity en bloc with mastectomy in an attempt to cure relatively advanced cases, and Wangensteen culminated this progression with "super radical" mastectomy, in which Halsted's procedure was extended to include supraclavicular, internal mammary, and mediastinal lymph nodes, first in two stages and later in one (Prudente, 1949; Wangensteen et al., 1956). Although Wangensteen and colleagues found that 57.8 per cent of 64 patients with clinically operable breast cancer had nodal metastases beyond the limits of the standard radical mastectomy, they abandoned the procedure because of high operative mortality (12.5 per cent) and the lack of a significant improvement in results.

Radiation therapists in the 20th century inherited and applied the concept of radical en bloc ablation. After Roentgen's discovery of x-rays in 1875 and Emil Grubbe's demonstra-

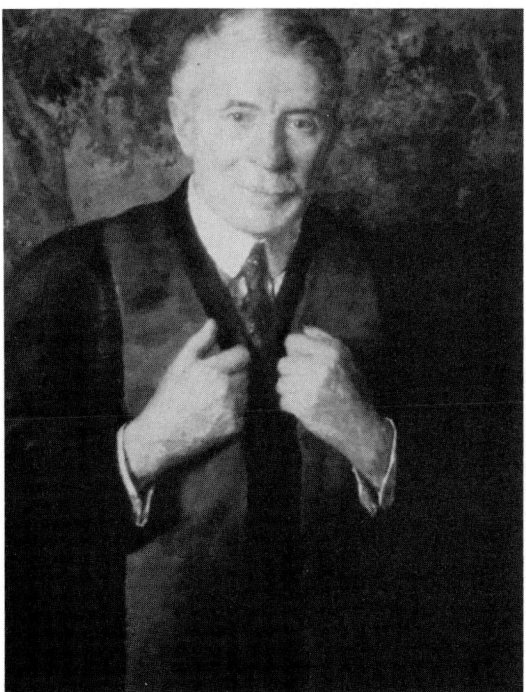
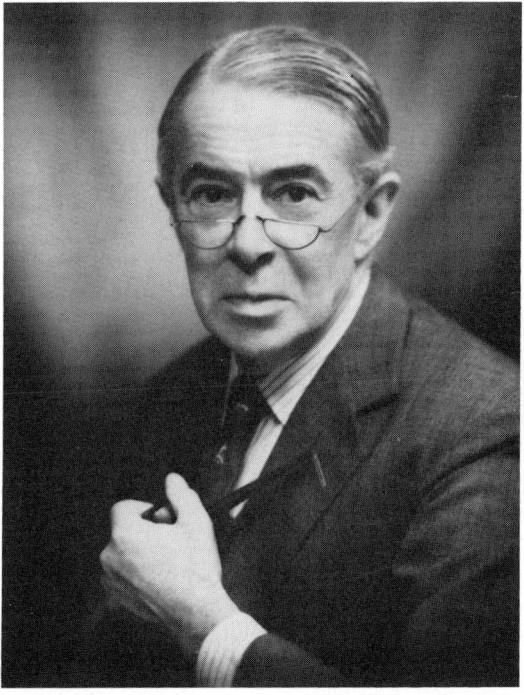

Figure 1–4. *A*, William Sampson Handley (left) (April 10, 1872–March 18, 1962) formulated the permeation theory of breast cancer spread, which supported the radical mastectomy. *B*, Richard S. Handley, O.B.E. (right) (May 2, 1909–June 16, 1984), surgeon to the Middlesex Hospital, London, who demonstrated the frequency of metastases to internal mammary lymph nodes in operable cases of breast cancer and popularized the modified radical mastectomy. The latter wryly confided to the author of this chapter that some American surgeons apparently thought there was a single Handley who had published for 80 years. The photographs were very kindly supplied by Mrs. R. S. Handley.

tion the following year in Chicago that they were useful to treat breast cancer (Grubbe, 1933), the story of radiotherapy is one of progressively improving technology, precision, and interst in two questions: Could irradiation improve the results of radical surgery, and could radical irradiation be substituted for radical surgery? Ionizing irradiation was initially focused on inoperable cases but soon was used to supplement radical operations. Irradiation of the internal mammary and supraclavicular lymph nodes proved more acceptable to surgeons than extended mastectomies, and the practice of supplementing surgery with irradiation when metastases were found in axillary lymph nodes or when the primary tumor lay medially in the breast became widespread.

The few advocates of simple mastectomy found a champion at midcentury in Robert McWhirter of Edinburgh, who challenged the status quo by reporting that 757 patients with operable breast cancer treated with simple mastectomy and irradiation of the supraclavicular, internal mammary, and axillary lymph nodes had a 5 year survival rate (62 per cent), comparable to that being achieved with radical surgery (McWhirter, 1948). McWhirter's work implied that irradiation was effective treatment not only for the internal mammary and supraclavicular lymph nodes but for the axillary nodes as well. The question then remained whether cancer could be controlled in the breast itself, a question of great cosmetic interest. Early work by Keynes in England and Baclesse in France indicated that this might be so (Keynes, 1937; Baclesse, 1965). Preliminary efforts in this direction produced 5 year survival rates in operable cases comparable to those treated surgically, but local morbidity was prohibitive (Hochman and Robinson, 1960). High energy sources introduced in the mid-1950s reduced cutaneous morbidity, and the attractive prospect of breast preservation led inevitably to studies in several centers in which radical irradiation constituted the primary mode of treatment (Prosnitz et al., 1977). Surgery was relegated to local removal of the primary tumor for diagnosis and biochemical analysis and removal of axillary nodes for staging purposes and to determine the need for adjuvant chemotherapy. The issues of irradiation carcinogenesis, long-term tumor control, and long-term morbidity remained to be answered, but early survival results indicated that irradiation had become a possible alternative to mastectomy for the treatment of breast cancer (Harris et al., 1983).

A final heritage from the 19th century was the discovery that breast cancer was hormone dependent. Sir Astley Cooper had noted earlier (1836) that the growth of breast cancers sometimes fluctuated with the menstrual cycle, and Schinzinger noted that the disease grew more slowly in postmenopausal women. Schinzinger even suggested castration as a means for artificially producing this change. Finally, in 1896, Thomas Beatson of Scotland reported that surgical castration of two patients with advanced breast cancer produced temporary tumor regression, and for the first time a systemic treatment was available for patients with this disease (Beatson, 1896). It was subsequently shown that irradiation ablation of the ovaries was equally effective. In 1942, Farrow and Adair demonstrated the beneficial effects of castration in men. In rapid succession, Huggins and Bergenstal (1951) demonstrated benefit from adrenalectomy, and Luft and Olivecrona (1953) from hypophysectomy. Not all benefited, but in the one third of patients who did, estrogen deletion was generally conceded to be the salient mechanism. Patient selection remained an inexact process until the discovery of estrogen receptors in the 1960s. Estrogen-dependent tumors contained a specific protein in the cellular cytoplasm that selectively bound estradiol (Jensen et al., 1967; McGuire et al., 1975), and its absence in significant quantities identified patients who would not respond to endocrine ablation, sparing them the morbidity of useless treatment.

Recent Concepts

The acceptance of radical mastectomy was virtually complete in the first half of the 20th century. Surgeons generally were convinced that it could not be improved; Halsted had tried to do so and failed. Standard management for breast tumors became hospital admission with biopsy under general anesthesia, frozen section for diagnosis, and immediate radical mastectomy. Deformity of the chest, lymphedema of the arm in many cases, and occasional irradiation-induced sarcomas were small prices to pay for an optimum chance of cure The feature that most marked developments of the later 20th century was a turbulent reevaluation of these concepts.

The stimulus for reassessment had a dual origin. First, it became increasingly apparent that the limits of radical surgery had been reached without achieving cure in at least one third of cases. Despite the fact that radical mastectomy, or its extensions, was taught in every medical school and was widely practiced, death rates from breast cancer remained undiminished. A constant 21 to 25 women per 100,000 population continued to die of this disease each year. Second, accumulating knowledge about the biology of breast cancer changed the understanding of this disease, and the new insights explained the therapeutic stalemate. It became evident, for example, that the tumor frequently arose in multiple sites throughout the breast and often spread so early in its course that the period of local confinement had come to an end long before its presence was discovered. Early diagnosis, advocated by physicians through the centuries, became a greater challenge than previously imagined.

The permeation theory of tumor spread was an early casualty. In 1931, Gray massaged contrast material into mastectomy specimens and demonstrated that the lymphatics around the primary tumor, even when axillary nodes contained metastases, were neither obliterated nor filled with cancer cells (Gray, 1938–1939). Thus, in early cases, embolism rather than permeation was the principal method of lymphatic spread. Gray's discovery weakened the en bloc principle of radical surgery and contributed to the rationale for the modern modified mastectomy (i.e., removal of the breast and axillary contents while preserving the pectoralis major muscle). The modified mastectomy, essentially the same operation used by Küster and by Banks 70 years earlier, was reintroduced in England in the 1930s by Patey, championed by R.S. Handley, and subsequently pioneered in the United States by Auchincloss and by Madden (Patey and Dyson, 1948; Madden, 1965; Patey, 1967; Handley and Thackray, 1969; Auchincloss, 1970). Because of its cosmetic superiority and equivalent results, it had replaced Halsted's radical mastectomy in the United States by 1975 as the operation most often performed for operable breast cancer (Lazaro et al., 1978; NIH Consensus Development Conference Summary, 1979).

Another blow to the permeation theory was delivered in 1955 by Engell, who demonstrated venous dissemination of cancer cells from early operable tumors. It was evident that early spread was not solely through lymphatics and that venous embolization frequently, if not always, preceded attempts to surgically encompass the diseased tissues. Cure evidently depended on events other than the removal of every tumor cell.

Only a few years later, Fisher and Fisher's investigations (1967) refuted the belief that regional lymph nodes served as filters of cancer cells. They demonstrated in rabbits that living tumor cells easily passed through lymph nodes into efferent lymphatics and also probably into veins through lymphaticovenous connections. Not only were lymph nodes poor filters, but in addition cancer cells seemed to pass easily back and forth between the blood vessel and lymphatic systems (Fisher and Fisher, 1966).

Tumor kinetics received increasing scrutiny. Observed gross rates of growth of breast cancers studied by Gershon-Cohen and others permitted theoretical calculations that suggested that breast cancers existed for several years before they reached clinically detectable size (Gershon-Cohen et al., 1963; Bond, 1968). The ample opportunity to metastasize widely during this protracted period of occult growth obviously placed a limit on the absolute curability of breast cancer (Park and Lees, 1951). In the minds of some investigators, the question of whether invasive breast cancer was ever cured remained open (Mueller and Jeffries, 1975).

The concept of immunological resistance against tumors also grew and was credited with limited success. As early as 1922, W.S. Handley observed, "There is a considerable body of evidence that lymphatic glands are able to deal with cancer cells in limited doses; Williams especially has drawn attention to the fact that, in days when the axillary glands were not removed with the breast, axillary recurrence was not so frequent as with our present microscopical knowledge of axillary gland invasion we should expect to find it." This observation was confirmed 55 years later by Fisher in a controlled clinical trial (Fisher, 1977). At midcentury the immunology of cancer was placed on a firmer basis with the demonstration of tumor-related antigens and a host response (Foley, 1953). The intense subsequent research in cancer immunology generated the concept of a dynamic tumor-host interaction that could be influenced by biological events in favor of one or the other. Circumstantial support for strong host resistance could be found in occasional spontaneous regressions of cancer, long delayed recurrences, and surgical cure in circumstances when this seemed highly unlikely, possibly through the body's ability to destroy small numbers of residual tumor cells. Rapid tumor growth and early death implied poor host resistance. Conceptually, surgery for neoplasia became less akin to the excision of a foreign body than to a means of conducting biological warfare.

As the initial immune response was vested in regional lymph nodes, the routine removal, or irradiation, of clinically normal nodes came into question. George Crile, Jr., was prominent among those who opposed radical surgery (Crile, 1971). Impressed both with the morbidity of axillary node dissection and his favorable experience with limited operations at the Cleveland Clinic, Crile maintained that there was no advantage to prophylactic dissection of clinically normal nodes even if they contained occult cancer. Said he, "It is just as effective to defer treatment until the nodes become palpably involved." Bond suggested that prophylactic node dissections might even be detrimental (Bond, 1968). Fisher speculated that if host resistance were reflected in destruction of metastases within nodes, normal nodes might well represent strong host resistance rather than the absence of metastatic spread (Fisher, 1976).

The uncertain biology of the exceptionally small breast cancers being detected raised questions about the need for routine mastectomy. The rationale for total mastectomy was based not only on the effort to remove all local extensions of cancer but also the observation that even in early cases breast cancer arose as a multifocal change throughout the mammary parenchyma. Many foci of in situ or microinvasive cancer could be identified in at least 50 per cent of mastectomy specimens (Gallager and Martin, 1969; Schwartz et al., 1980). Nevertheless, the frequency with which these microscopic tumors became clinical cancers during the patient's remaining lifetime was unknown.

These questions about radical surgery fortunately coincided with the emergence of new scientific tools: the prospective randomized clinical trial and modern statistical analysis. These exercises in clinical discipline, which served to reduce the biases of patient selection that plagued earlier studies, were used initially in England in the 1950s to evaluate adjuvant irradiation. In a climate of rising controversy about local treatment, they were widely adopted by concerned physicians.

Early trials focused on treatment of regional nodes. Within a relatively short period, they compared radical mastectomy plus postoperative irradiation with simple mastectomy plus postoperative irradiation (Brinkley and Haybittle 1966; Bergdahl, 1978), radical mastectomy with radical mastectomy plus postoperative irradiation (Patterson and Russell, 1959), simple mastectomy plus postoperative irradiation with radical mastectomy (Bruce, 1971), simple mastectomy plus postoperative irradiation with mastectomy extended to the supraclavicular and internal mammary lymph nodes (Kaae and Johansen, 1969), simple mastectomy with simple mastectomy plus postoperative irradiation (Murray et al., 1977), radical mastectomy with radical mastectomy plus internal mammary node dissection (Lacour et al., 1976; Veronesi and Valagussa, 1981), and simple mastectomy with radical mastectomy (Fisher et al., 1977). The results were as follows:

1. The stage of disease had a decided influence on survival, whereas variations of treatment did not.

2. The presence or absence of metastases in regional nodes was of prime prognostic importance, as was the absolute number of nodes involved.

3. Postoperative irradiation improved local and regional control of the tumor without improving survival.

4. Routine removal of axillary lymph nodes or of internal mammary lymph nodes reduced tumor recurrence at these sites without improving survival.

5. Irradiation controlled metastases in regional lymph nodes as well as did surgical removal.

6. Removal of axillary lymph nodes often resulted in lymphedema of the arm, which was increased further by use of irradiation.

These studies established what Halsted and other surgeons of his time observed almost 100 years earlier (i.e., that radical local treatment resulted in improved local and regional control of tumor). The routine removal of regional lymph nodes helped prevent progressive growth of nodal metastases and provided prognostic information, without influencing survival.

Other clinical trials focused on management of the breast itself. At Guy's Hospital, London, patients were randomized for treatment between local tumor excision or radical mastectomy, each followed by postoperative irradiation. Low doses of irradiation resulted in a high frequency of recurrence in the breast and nodes after the more limited surgical procedure (Hayward, 1977). Studies in Italy and the United States subsequently determined that high doses of irradiation could largely prevent recurrence in the breast after local tumor removal (Veronesi, 1977; Fisher, 1977).

It is apparent that the two concepts that had advanced radical surgery had reached their limits. The concept of local origin provides a basis for cure only if diagnosis can be made before dissemination occurs, which means while the disease is still occult, and this remains an imperfect attainment. The effort to prevent local-regional failures through enlarging the field of operation reached anatomic limits without eliminating mortality. Recognition that failures were likely to result from early occult dissemination initiated the present era of systemic adjuvant chemotherapy.

The story of mammography, which permits breast cancer to be discovered when only millimeters in diameter, is a chapter in this effort too important not to mention but too lengthy to be related here. Detection has become focused on screening asymptomatic individuals and on widespread public education.

Conclusion

After 5000 years the cause of breast cancer remains unknown, and a practical means of prevention is not at hand. Progress lies principally in maximizing the results of local treatment through detection of the disease while it is still localized.

Surgeons who treat breast cancer now seek principles based on new concepts. In this pursuit, Bernard Fisher has been most instrumental in laying old concepts to rest and defining new ones. The elements on which a new biologic basis for surgery must be founded, according to Fisher, are contrasted with Halstedian concepts in Table 1–1. The thoughtful but enigmatic statement of Fisher and Gebhardt (1978) comes as close as any to a new biologic basis for cancer surgery: "The primary aim of oncologic surgery (with or without aid of radiation therapy) at present seems to be directed toward reducing the tumor burden to a number of viable cells that are entirely destroyable by: (1) host immunologic (and possibly other) factors alone, (2) systemically administered anti-cancer agents, or (3) a combination of both." Unfortunately, the critical reduction and the extent of surgery required to reach it remain obscure. Hayward was more specific. He identified four current obligations of the surgeon: (1) to provide local tumor control, (2) to determine the pathologic status of axillary lymph nodes, (3) to provide tumor tissue for diagnosis and biologic markers, and (4) to provide local treatment that is compatible with systemic adjuvant therapy (Hayward, 1981).

Table 1–1. ALTERNATIVE HYPOTHESES OF TUMOR BIOLOGY

Halstedian	Alternative
Tumors spread in an orderly defined manner based upon mechanical considerations	There is no orderly pattern of tumor cell dissemination
Tumor cells traverse lymphatics to lymph nodes by direct extension, supporting en bloc dissection	Tumor cells traverse lymphatics by embolization, challenging the merit of en bloc dissection
The positive lymph node is an indicator of tumor spread and is the instigator of disease	The positive lymph node is an indicator of a host-tumor relationship, which permits development of metastases rather than being the instigator of distant disease
Regional lymph nodes (RLN) are barriers to the passage of tumor cells	RLN are ineffective as barriers to tumor cell spread
RLN are of anatomic importance	RLN are of biological importance
The bloodstream is of little significance as a route of tumor dissemination	The bloodstream is of considerable importance in tumor dissemination
A tumor is autonomous of its host	Complex host-tumor interrelationships affect every facet of the disease
Operable breast cancer is a local-regional disease	Operable breast cancer is a systemic disease
The extent and nuances of operation are the dominant factors influencing patient outcome	Variations in local-regional therapy are unlikely to substantially affect survival

(From Fisher, B.: A commentary on the role of the surgeon in primary breast cancer. Breast Cancer Res. Treat., 1:17, 1981. Reprinted with permission.)

The long evolution to radical surgery was based principally on the clear demonstration that it controlled the local tumor more effectively than limited operations. This benefit cannot be discarded without an equally effective substitute. If the conceptual base was faulty, it must be appreciated that the biology of breast cancer is still imperfectly understood. Much depends on developments in radiation therapy and systemic therapy. Surgery and radiation are both effective local treatments, and a choice between the two may be a matter simply of relative morbidities. If in the unlikely event that cancers can be routinely discovered in their earliest phases, this choice may be the only decision that is necessary. If systemic therapy proves capable of curing only when the tumor burden is reduced to a minimum, then surgery, or radiation, or some combination may prove the best means of accomplishing this end. If a totally effective systemic therapy is eventually found, local treatment may become unnecessary altogether.

REFERENCES

Ackerknecht, E. H.: History and geography of the most important diseases. New York, Hafner, 1965, p 162.

Arnott, H.: On the therapeutical importance of recent views of the nature and structure of cancer. St. Thomas Hosp. Rep., 2:103, 1871.

Auchincloss, H.: Modified radical mastectomy: Why not? Am. J. Surg., 119:506, 1970.

Baclesse, F.: Five-year results in 431 breast cancers treated solely by roentgen rays. Ann. Surg., 161:103, 1965.

Banks, W. M.: A brief history of the operations practiced for cancer of the breast. Br. Med. J., 1:5, 1902.

Beatson, G. T: On the treatment of inoperable cases of carcinoma of the mamma: Suggestions for a new treatment with illustrative cases. Lancet, 2:104, 1896.

Bergdahl, L.: Simple and radical mastectomy with postoperative irradiation: A controlled trial. Am. Surg., 44:369, 1978.

Bond, W. H.: The influence of various treatments on survival rates in cancer of the breast. In Jarrett, A. S. (ed.): The Treatment of Carcinoma of the Breast. Amsterdam, Excerpta Medical Foundation, 1968.

Brinkley, D., and Haybittle, J. L.: Treatment of stage II carcinoma of the female breast. Lancet, 2:291, 1966.

Bruce, J.: Operable cancer of the breast. A controlled clinical trial. Cancer, 28:1443, 1971.

Clinical Society of London: Effectual method of operating for cancer of the breast. Lancet, 1:248, 1893.

Cooper, W. A.: The history of the radical mastectomy. Ann. Med. Hist., 3:36, 1941.

Crile, G., Jr.: Treatment of cancer of the breast: Past, present, and future. Cleve. Clin. Q., 38:47, 1971.

Dahl-Iversen, E., and Tobiassen, T.: Radical mastectomy with parasternal and supraclavicular dissection for mammary carcinoma. Ann. Surg., 170:889, 1969.

Engell, H. C.: Cancer cells in the circulating blood. Acta Chir. Scand. (Suppl. 201), 1955.

Farrow, J. H., and Adair, F. E.: Effect of orchiectomy on skeletal metastases from cancer of the male breast. Science, 95:654, 1942.

Fisher, B.: Some thoughts concerning the primary therapy of breast cancer. Recent Results Cancer Res., 57:150, 1976.

Fisher, B.: United States trials of conservative surgery. World J. Surg., 1:327, 1977.

Fisher, B.: A commentary on the role of the surgeon in primary breast cancer. Breast Cancer Res. Treat., 1:17, 1981.

Fisher, B., and Fisher, E. R.: The interrelationship of hematogenous and lymphatic tumor cell dissemination. Surg. Gynecol. Obstet., 122:791, 1966.

Fisher, B., and Fisher, E. R.: Barrier function of lymph node to tumor cells and erythrocytes. I. Normal nodes. Cancer, 20:1907, 1967.

Fisher, B., and Gebhardt, M. C.: The evolution of breast cancer surgery: Past, present, and future. Semin. Oncol., 5:385, 1978.

Fisher, B., Montague, E., Redmond, C., et al.: Comparison of radical mastectomy with alternative treatments for primary breast cancer. Cancer, 39:2827, 1977.

Foley, E. J.: Antigenic properties of methyl-cholanthrene-induced tumors in mice of the strain of origin. Cancer Res., 13:835, 1953.

Gallager, H. S., and Martin, J. E.: Early phases in the development of breast cancer. Cancer, 24:1170, 1969.

Gershon-Cohen, J., Berger, S. M., and Klickstein, H. S.: Roentgenography of breast cancer moderating concept of "biologic predeterminism." Cancer, 16:961, 1963.

Gray, J. H.: The relation of lymphatic vessels to the spread of cancer. Br. J. Surg., 26:462, 1938–1939.

Greenough, R. B., Simmons, C. C., and Barney, J. D.: The results of operations for cancer of the breast at the Massachusetts General Hospital from 1894 to 1904. Trans. Am. Surg. Assoc., 25:80, 1907.

Grubbe, E. H.: Priority in the therapeutic use of x-rays. Radiology, 21:156, 1933.

Haagensen, C. D.: Diseases of the Breast. 2nd Ed. Philadelphia, W. B. Saunders, 1971, p. 622.

Halsted, W. S.: The treatment of wounds with especial reference to the value of the blood clot in the management of dead spaces. Johns Hopkins Hosp. Rep., 2:255, 1891.

Halsted, W. S. : The results of operations for the cure of cancer of the breast performed at the Johns Hopkins Hospital from June, 1889 to January, 1894. Johns Hopkins Hosp. Rep., 4:297, 1894–1895.

Halsted, W. S.: The results of radical operations for the cure of cancer of the breast. Trans. Am. Surg. Assoc., 25:61, 1907.

Handley, R. S., and Thackray, A. C.: Conservative radical mastectomy (Patey's operation). Ann. Surg., 170:880, 1969.

Handley, W. S.: Cancer of the Breast and its Treatment. 2nd Ed. London, John Murray, 1922, p. 256.

Harris, J. R., Hellman, S., and Silen, W.: Conservative Management of Breast Cancer. New Surgical and Radiotherapeutic Techniques. Philadelphia, J. B. Lippincott, 1983.

Hayward, J. L.: The surgeon's role in primary breast cancer. Breast Cancer Res. Treat., 1:27, 1981.

Hayward, J. L.: The Guy's trial of treatments of "early" breast cancer. World J. Surg., 1:314, 1977.

Heidenhain, L.: Ueber die Ursachen der localen Krebsrecidive nach Amputation mammae. Berlin, Verhandlungen der Deutschen Gesellschaft fur Chirurgie, Achtzehnter Congress, 1889.

Henderson, I. C., and Canellos, G. P.: Cancer of the breast: The past decade. N. Engl. J. Med., *302*:17 (Part I); *302*:787, (Part II), 1980.

Hochman, A., and Robinson, E.: Eighty two cases of mammary cancer treated exclusively with roentgen therapy. Cancer, *15*:670, 1960.

Huggins, C., and Bergenstal, D. M.: Influence of bilateral adrenalectomy, adrenocorticotrophin, and cortisone acetate on certain human tumors. Science, *144*:482, 1951.

Jensen, E. V., DeSombre, E. R., and Junglblut, P. W.: Estrogen receptors in hormone responsive tissues and tumors. In Wissler, R. W., Dao, T. L., and Wood, S. (Eds.): Endogenous Factors Influencing Host-Tumor Balance. Chicago, University of Chicago Press, 1967, p 15.

Kaae, S., and Johansen, H.: Simple mastectomy plus postoperative irradiation by the method of McWhirter for mammary carcinoma. Ann. Surg., *170*:895, 1969.

Keynes, G.: Conservative treatment of cancer of the breast. Br. Med. J., *2*:643, 1937.

Küster, E.: Zur Behandlung des Brustkrebses. Arch. Clin. Chir., *29*:723, 1883.

Lacour, J., Bucalossi, P., Cacers, E., et al.: Radical mastectomy versus radical mastectomy plus internal mammary dissection. Cancer, *37*:206, 1976.

Lazaro, E. J., Rush, B. F., Jr., and Swaminathan, A. P.: Changing attitudes in the management of cancer of the breast. Surgery, *84*:441, 1978.

LeDran, H. F.: Memoire avec un précis de plusieurs observations sur le cancer. Mem. Acad. Roy. Chir., *3*:1, 1757.

Lewis, D., and Rienhoff, W. F., Jr.: A study of the results of operations for the cure of cancer of the breast. Ann. Surg., *95*:336–400, 1932.

Lewison, E. F.: The surgical treatment of breast cancer: An historical and collective review. Surgery, *34*:904, 1953.

Luft, R., and Olivecrona, H.: Experiences with hypophysectomy in man. J. Neurosurg., *10*:301, 1953.

Madden, J. L.: Modified radical mastectomy. Surg. Gynecol. Obstet., *121*:1221, 1965.

Mansfield, C.: Early breast cancer. Its history and results of treatment. In Wolsky, A. (Ed.): Experimental Biology and Medicine. Monographs on Interdisciplinary Topics. Vol. 5. New York, S. Karger, 1976, p. 2.

Margottini, M.: Recent developments in the surgical treatment of breast cancer. Acta Unio Int. Contra Cancrum, *8*:176, 1952.

McGuire, W. L., Carbone, P. P., and Vollmer, E. P.: Estrogen Receptors in Human Breast Cancer. New York, Raven Press, 1975.

McWhirter, R.: The value of simple mastectomy and radiotherapy in the treatment of cancer of the breast. Br. J. Radiol., *21*:599, 1948.

Meyer, W.: An improved method of the radical operation for carcinoma of the breast. Med. Rec., *46*:746, 1894.

Moore, C. H.: On the influence of inadequate operations on the theory of cancer. Med. Chir. Trans., *32*:245, 1867.

Mueller, C. B., and Jeffries, W.: Cancer of the breast: Its outcome as measured by the rate of dying and causes of death. Ann. Surg., *182*:334, 1975.

Müller, J.: Ueber den feinern Bau und die Formen der krankhaften Geshwulste. Berlin, G. Rehner, 1838.

Murray, J. G., MacIntyre, J., Simpson, J. S., et al.: Cancer research campaign study of the management of "early" breast cancer. World J. Surg., *1*:317, 1977.

NIH Consensus Development Conference Summary: The treatment of primary breast cancer: Management of local disease. Vol. 2, No. 5, June 5, 1979.

Park, W. W., and Lees, J. C.: The absolute curability of cancer of the breast. Surg. Gynecol. Obstet., *93*:129, 1951.

Patey, D. H.: A review of 146 cases of carcinoma of the breast operated on between 1930 and 1943. Br. J. Cancer, *21*:260, 1967.

Patey, D. H., and Dyson, W. H.: The prognosis of carcinoma of the breast in relation to the type of operation performed. Br. J. Cancer, *2*:7, 1948.

Patterson, R., and Russell, M. H.: Clinical trials in malignant disease. Part III. Breast cancer: Evaluation of postoperative radiotherapy. J. Fac. Radiologists, *10*:175, 1959.

Power, D.: The history of the amputation of the breast to 1904. Liverpool Med.-Chir. J., *42/43*:29, 1934–1935.

Prosnitz, L. R., Goldenberg, I. S., Packard, R. A., et al.: Radiation therapy as initial treatment for early stage cancer of the breast without mastectomy. Cancer, *39*:917, 1977.

Prudente, A.: L'amputation inter-scapulo-mammothoracique (technique et resultats). J. Chir., *65*:729, 1949.

Rutkow, I. M.: William Stewart Halsted and the Germanic influence on education and training programs in surgery. Surg. Gynecol. Obstet., *146*:602, 1978.

Schleiden, M. J.: Beitrag zur Phytogenesis. Arch. Anat. Physiol., *5*:137, 1838.

Schlumberger, H. G.: Origins of the cell concept in pathology. Arch. Pathol., *37*:396, 1944.

Schmid, H.: Zue Statistick der Mammacarcinome und deren Heilung. Deutsche Zeitschrift fur Chirurgie, *26*:139, 1887.

Schwann, T.: Microscopical Researches into the Accordance in the Structure and Growth of Animals and Plants, translated from German by H. Smith. London, Sydenham Society, 1847.

Schwartz, G. F., Patchefsky, A. S., Feig, S. A., et al.: Multicentricity of non-palpable breast cancer. Cancer, *45*:2913, 1980.

Sugarbaker, E. D.: Radical mastectomy combined with in-continuity resection of the homolateral internal mammary node chain. Cancer, *6*:969, 1953.

Urban, J. A.: Surgical excision of internal mammary nodes for breast cancer. Br. J. Surg., *51*:209, 1964.

Veronesi, U., and Valagussa, P.: Inefficacy of internal mammary nodes dissection in breast cancer surgery. Cancer, *47*:170, 1981.

Veronesi, U.: Conservative treatment of breast cancer: A trial in progress at the cancer institute of Milan. World J. Surg., *1*:324, 1977.

Virchow, R.: Die Cellularpathologie. Berlin, A. Hirschwald, 1858.

Wangensteen, O. H., Lewis, F. J., and Arhelger, S. W.: The extended or super-radical mastectomy for carcinoma of the breast. Surg. Clin. North Am., *36*:1051, 1956.

Wilder, R. J.: The historical development of the concept of metastasis. J. Mt. Sinai Hosp., New York, *23*:728, 1956.

CHAPTER 2

JOHN S. SPRATT
GORDON R. TOBIN

Anatomy of the Breast

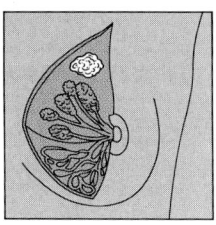

Ablative cure of mammary carcinoma by surgical or radiation therapy is based on the assumption that viable cancer is limited to the mamma or to the mamma and the regional lymph nodes. Confinement of cancer to the lymph nodes further requires that the cancer cells have arrived in the nodes via afferent lymphatics, that the nodal sinuses have retained the cancer cells, and that some of these cells have survived and are engaged in metastatic growth and replication.

If the metastatic foci in the lymph nodes are not removed or destroyed, sustained cancerous growth will result in increasing morbidity from uninhibited local progression and generalized dissemination. Resection of the lymph nodes, therefore, is pertinent to the surgical management of mammary cancer and local control of cancer on the chest wall. Knowledge of the presence or absence of metastases in the lymph nodes is essential in prognostication.

The design of surgical and radiation therapy has been based largely on an empirical knowledge of the location of the mamma and regional lymph node anatomy. Of equal importance is a consideration of functional lymphatic anatomy as studied by injection and by statistics of the distribution of lymph node metastases, and the dissemination of cancer beyond its locoregional confines.

This chapter reviews the pertinent parts of the developmental, topographic, fascial, muscular, neural, lymphatic, and vascular anatomy of the breast and mammary region. Emphasis is placed on the functional anatomy of lymphatics.

Developmental Anatomy

Embryologically, the human breast develops in the pectoral portion of an ectodermal thickening extending from the axilla to the vulva bilaterally. This "milk streak" is present by the sixth week of fetal life. By the ninth week, most of the line has atrophied except in the pectoral region. Here the nipple bud appears as a proliferating mass of basal cells.

By the end of the third month of gestation, squamous cells from the surface begin to invade the nipple bud. The mammary ducts develop as downgrowths from this, terminating in lobular buds that proliferate into acini with sexual maturity.

The entire gland develops as a large dermal and subcutaneous organ from a single focus on the skin. This point is pertinent to the lymphatic drainage of the breast, as discussed subsequently. As is true of all embryonal organogenesis, anomalous development can occur at any phase of the ontogeny (Geschickter, 1943).

Topographic Anatomy

The adult mammary gland is situated principally between the superficial and deep layers of the superficial pectoral fascia of the anterior chest wall, extending roughly from the second to the sixth or seventh anterior intercostal space. This cephalocaudal dimension is 10 to 12 cm on the average, and the gland generally has a maximum thickness of 3 to 5 cm.

The nonlactating breast weighs 150 to 200 g; the lactating gland may weigh as much as

400 to 500 g. The gland is divided into 15 to 20 lobes, each with an excretory duct passing centrally to the nipple. The nipple, located at about the fourth interspace in youth, contains 15 to 20 orifices of the excretory ducts.

Passing from the deep layer of superficial fascia on the deep surface of the breast up between the lobes to the corium of the mammary skin are the suspensory ligaments of the breast (Cooper's ligaments). The deep layer of the superficial fascia on the undersurface of the breast is separated from the deep fascia by a fascial cleft. The presence of this cleft allows for considerable mobility of the breast.

Fascial Anatomy

The mammary gland is contained principally within the superficial pectoral fascia. This layer of fatty areolar tissue is continuous below with Camper's superficial abdominal fascia and above with superficial cervical fascia.

Superiorly, the lower fibers of the platysma muscle separate the superficial fascia from the deep pectoral fascia. The deep pectoral fascia covers the pectoralis major muscle.

The mammary gland is attached to the sternum and superolaterally to the clavicle and axillary fascia. Inferiorly, it is continuous with the deep fascia of the abdominal wall.

As the breast ducts and lobules arborize through the layers of superficial fascia, they maintain an intimate relation to the skin, and the peripheral extent of the arborization is frequently indistinct. The intimate relation of breast parenchyma to dermis has been used as the basis for justifying the elevation of very thin skin flaps and the performance of a wide dissection, as discussed later under total mastectomy.

The anatomy of breast parenchyma is relevant to the desire by some to do a "prophylactic" or "preventive" mastectomy in the hope that breast cancer may be prevented. Goldman and Goldwyn (1973) explored this proposition and confirmed that breast tissue remains after these mastectomies. They performed subcutaneous mastectomies in cadavers with no known breast pathology according to the promoted surgical technique. Then they sampled the subareolar breast tissue remaining. They found five cadavers had breast tissue at other sites, and in only one of the 12 cadavers was no residual breast tissue found by their sampling technique. They cautioned that mastectomy cannot be considered completely prophylactic, as subcutaneous mastectomy does not remove all breast tissue. Although they recommended multiple biopsies before the insertion of implants, such a small sample of the total area of resection could be expected to present a considerable sampling error.

The reduction of breast tissue volume cannot be assumed to bring about a proportional reduction in cancer risk for a wide variety of reasons. Two of these reasons are the cancer promoting effects of surgery and the increased concentration of the effect on residual breast tissue by humoral promoters. The failure of Klamer and colleagues (1983) to prevent breast cancer in a rat model dosed with a potent breast carcinogen by resecting the entire mammary fold is further evidence of the anatomic extent of the breast in mammals and the difficulties associated with efforts to remove it totally. This position is also supported by Jackson and associates (1984). In fact, development of breast cancer has been reported after subcutaneous mastectomies that were performed for benign disease (Goodnight et al., 1984; Bowers and Radlauer, 1969). Goodnight and coworkers pointed out that when valid reasons for doing a preventive mastectomy can be identified, a total mastectomy is the minimal operation. They contend that subcutaneous mastectomy as a cancer-preventing procedure must be regarded as an experimental treatment. Since no surgical techique of mastectomy predictably removes all breast tissue (Hicken, 1940), prophylactic mastectomy remains a valid concern as it is based on unproved assumptions. The possibility that these assumptions are valid strongly endorses the need for appropriately designed clinical studies.

FASCIA DEEP TO THE PECTORALIS MAJOR MUSCLE

The deep surface of the pectoralis major muscle is covered by the clavipectoral fascia, which envelops the pectoralis minor muscle. Superficial to the pectoralis minor muscle, it forms a thickened layer of fascia attached to the clavicle. This thickened clavipectoral fascia superior to the pectoralis minor is pierced by the anterior thoracic vessels and nerve and by the cephalic vein with variations as discussed below.

The pectoralis fascia thickens to form the roof of the axillary space. Below and lateral to the pectoralis minor muscle it fuses with the deep fascia of the anterior surface of the pectoralis major muscle. This fascia continues as a thin cover for the serratus anterior muscle, and it also envelops the axillary vessels, forming the vascular sheath.

The fatty areolar tissue lying between the clavipectoral fascial layers anteriorly, the axillary vascular sheath superiorly, and the thin fascia on the chest wall and deep muscles (intercostal muscles, serratus anterior muscle, coracobrachialis muscle, and subclavius muscle) envelops the axillary lymph cord containing large valvular lymphatics from the upper extremity and the axillary lymph nodes in proximity to the branches of the great veins in the axilla surrounded by fatty areolar tissue (Figs. 2–1 and 2–2) (Singer, 1935).

Muscular and Neural Anatomy

The principal muscles encountered in the surgery of the breast include (1) pectoralis major, (2) pectoralis minor, (3) serratus anterior, (4) latissimus dorsi, (5) subscapularis, and (6) the aponeurosis of the external oblique and rectus abdominis. The lower fibers of the platysma muscle crossing the clavicle in the superficial fascia, the subclavius, and the coracobrachialis are viewed in the periphery of the surgical field but require no comment.

The pectoralis major muscle, deep to the fascial cleft behind the breast and invested by the deep fascia, has its origin from the medial half of the clavicle, the lateral sternum, the cartilage of the sixth and seventh ribs, and the aponeurosis of the external oblique muscle.

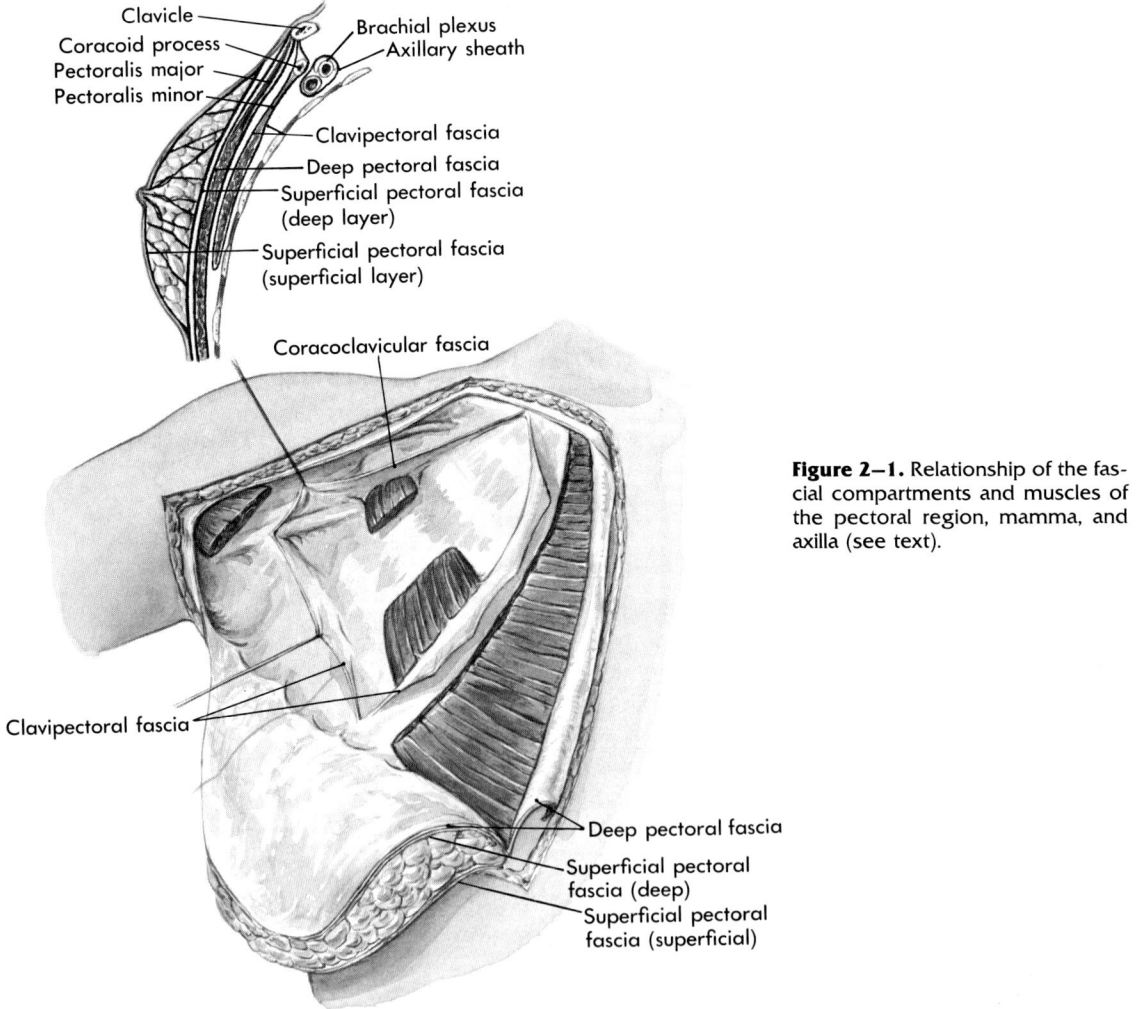

Figure 2–1. Relationship of the fascial compartments and muscles of the pectoral region, mamma, and axilla (see text).

2 • Anatomy of the Breast   19

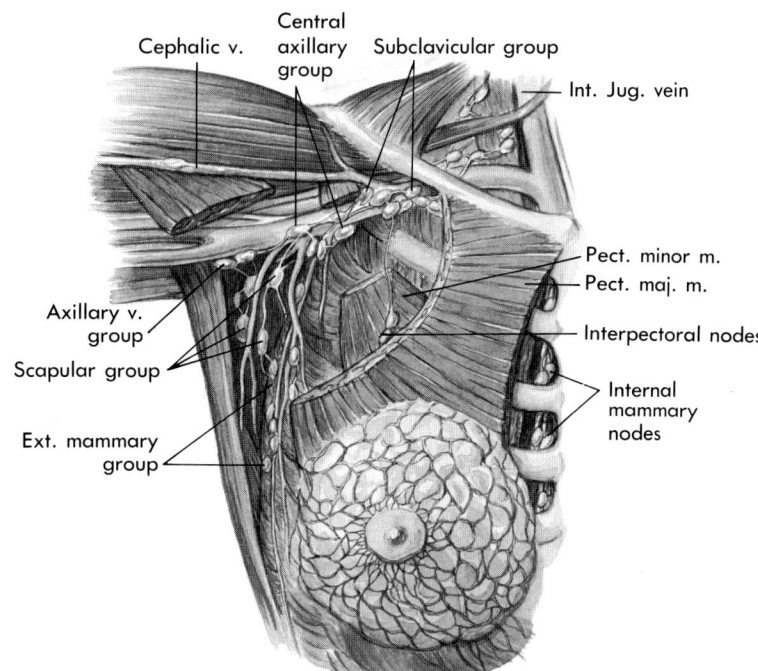

Figure 2–2. Principal lymph node groups tend to parallel the major veins. A coarse labyrinth of valvular lymphatics lying on the deep layer of the superficial fascia constitutes the major afferent lymphatics to these lymph nodes. The deep fascia and muscles have few lymphatics and little relation to the plexus in the superficial fascia that drains the mamma. The lymphatics from the plexus in the superficial fascia probably penetrate the muscles only in the few loci penetrated by veins, as for example, the acromiothoracic artery and vein perforating the pectoralis major muscle.

From this broad origin it converges to an insertion on the greater tubercle of the humerus.

The muscle is composed of many segments, which are a phylogenetically preserved expression of internal metamerism in the pectoral girdle. The segments can be separated surgically, as they have independent neurovascular supplies (Tobin, 1985). This has clinical significance for reconstructive surgery using flaps from this muscle (Tobin et al., 1982) and for the technique of modified mastectomy described later in this chapter and in the chapter on surgical technique.

The authors have studied the natural cleavage between the clavicular and sternocostal portions of the muscle by fresh cadaver dissections and now routinely use this cleavage for exposure in the performance of mastectomies to preserve the pectoralis major muscle innervation. These dissections are illustrated in Figures 2–3 to 2–9 and will be referred to again in the chapter on surgical technique. The dissections confirm that the cleavage is quite visible when the deep pectoral fascia has been dissected laterally, as for a Patey mastectomy. At this point, the cleavage may be opened throughout its length to expose the axillary fascia and axillary fat pad under the deep surface of the pectoralis major muscle. The pectoralis minor muscle is seen beneath this deep fascia. This exposure permits easy, direct

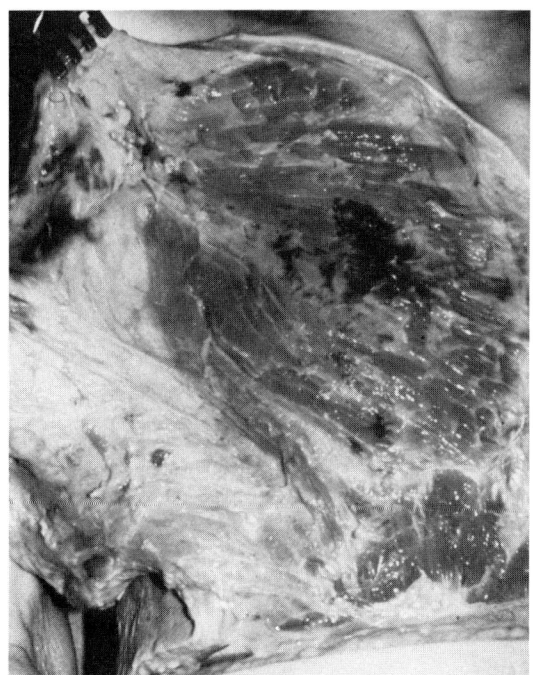

Figure 2–3. The deep pectoral fascia has been resected laterally to the edge of the pectoralis major muscle. The mamma is superficial to the deep pectoral fascia and has been reflected laterally. This fascia may be partially reflected from the deep surface of the pectoralis major, taking care not to transect nerves or vessels going to this muscle. This dissection is the same as that followed in modified radical mastectomy to the point where a retractor can be placed under the free edge of the muscle in order to pull it anteromedially and expose the axilla.

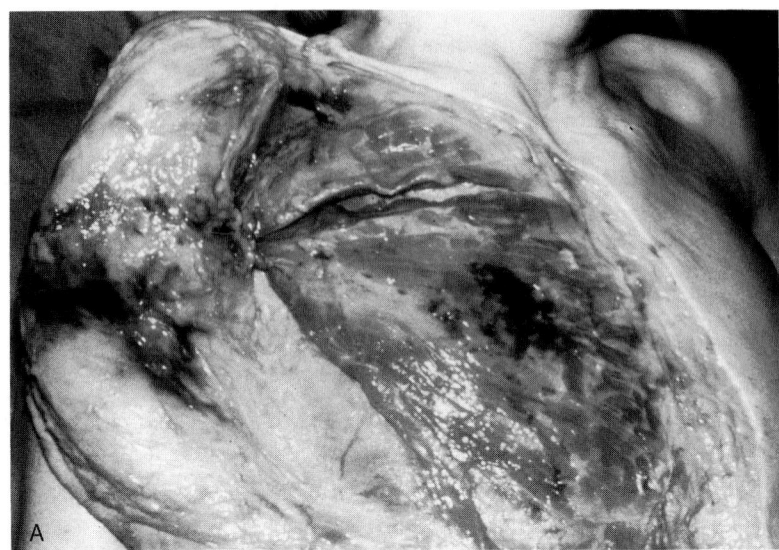
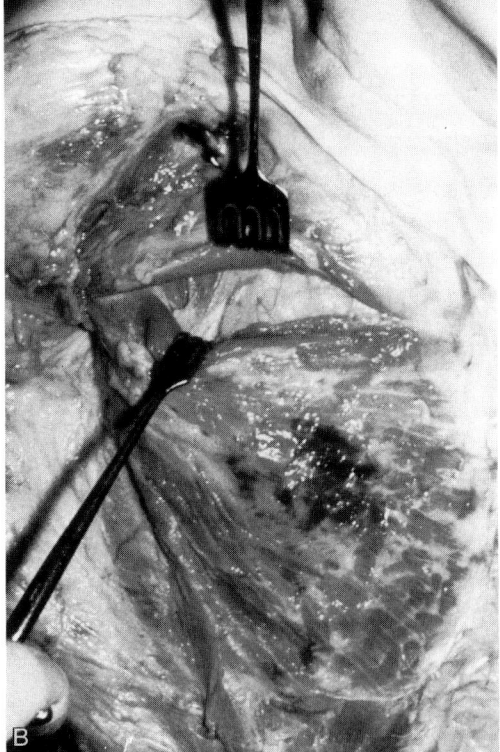

Figure 2–4. The natural cleavage between the clavicular and sternocostal origins of the pectoralis major muscle has been opened (*A*) and is separated by retractors (*B*). The pectoralis minor muscle shows through the axillary fascia laterally, and the lymph node–bearing axillary fat pad can be seen in *B* medial to the pectoralis minor. At this point, the contents of the axillary fat pad may be palpated with considerable accuracy for firm lymph nodes. When they are numerous and high, it may not be possible to preserve the nerve and blood supply to the pectoralis major without exposing cancer-containing lymph nodes and lymphatics. A decision can be made at this point as to whether an effort should be made to dissect the nerves out and preserve them.

2 • Anatomy of the Breast   21

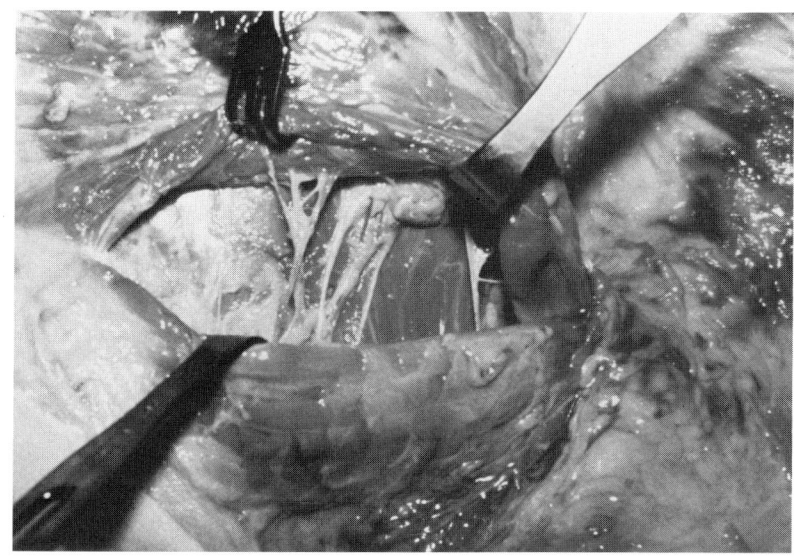

Figure 2–5. By retracting the sternal portion of the pectoralis major muscle inferiorly, the variable number and distribution of nerve branches, and their relation to the pectoralis minor muscle, can be seen. The removal of the pectoralis minor must now be planned in a way that preserves these branches. When a branch transgresses the body of the pectoralis minor, this muscle may have to be dissected away in pieces to preserve it. Any areolar tissue lying between the pectoral muscles that might contain intrapectoral lymph nodes may be removed with this dissection.

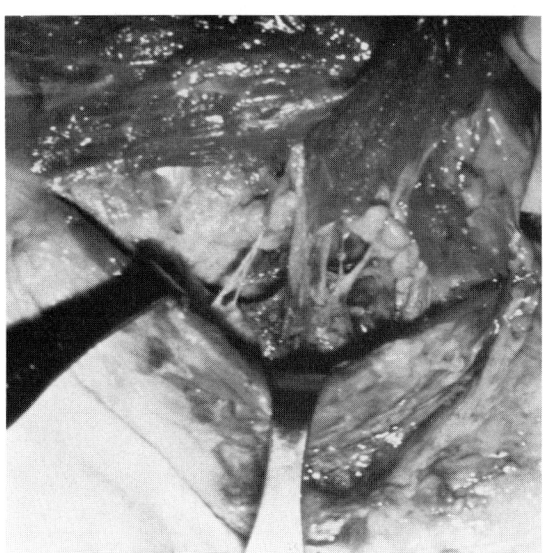

Figure 2–6. The pectoralis minor muscle has been transected at its insertion and is being dissected away from the nerves down to the pectoralis major. The pectoralis minor is enveloped by axillary fascia, which may be followed to its origin on the thorax. The origin is divided, and the muscle is removed from the field to expose the axillary fat pad for complete high dissection, including the sheath of the axillary vein.

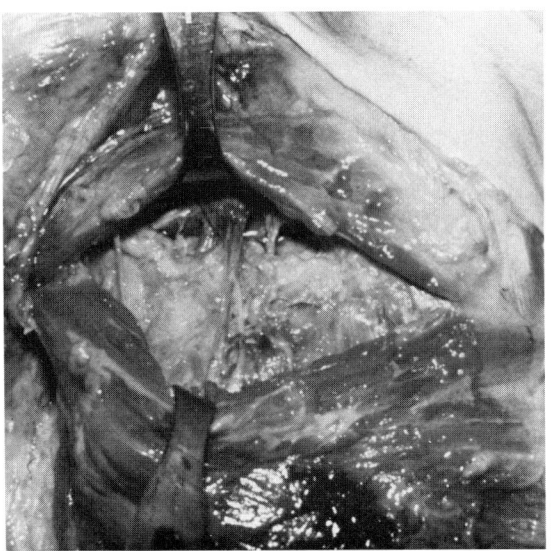

Figure 2–7. The pectoralis minor muscle has now been removed, and the intact branches of the nerves to the pectoralis major are exposed. From this point, the axillary vein may be demonstrated, and the axillary fat pad may be dissected away from the nerve branches. Any remaining attachments of fascia to the deep surface of the pectoralis major may be divided, avoiding injury to nerves. The remaining axillary dissection can then be carried out, preserving the nerves to the latissimus dorsi muscle and the serratus anterior nerves that usually lie just beneath the lateral and medial layers of axillary fascia.

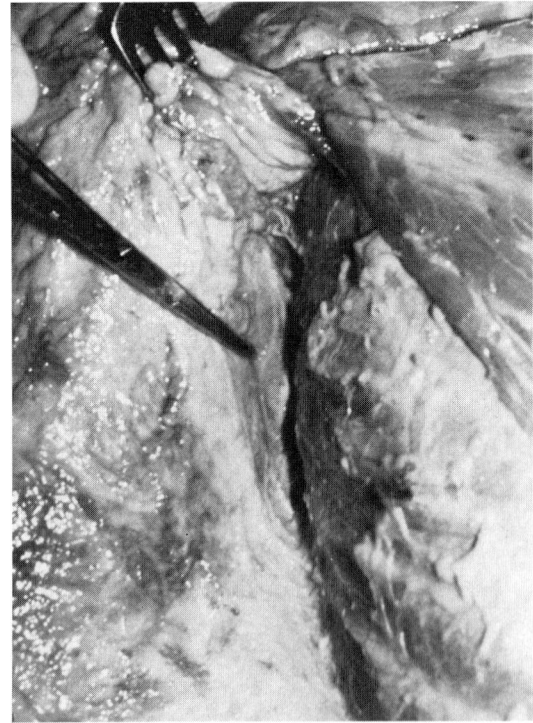

Figure 2–8. The clamp points to the nerve of the serratus anterior muscle just under the axillary fascia adjacent to the chest wall. For this nerve to be preserved, it must be dissected out of the fascia and be mobilized from its site of appearance below the axillary vein to its muscular insertion.

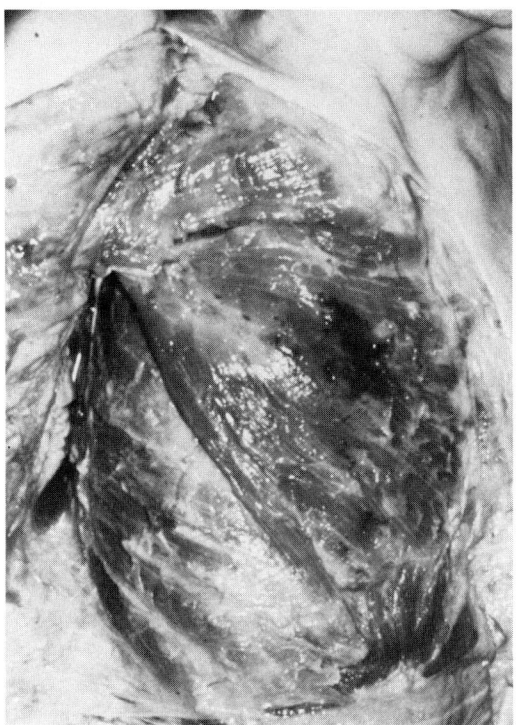

Figure 2–9. The entire breast, axillary fat pad, pectoralis minor muscle with intrapectoral lymph nodes, and the axillary fat pads have now been removed, leaving an intact, innervated, and vascularized pectoralis major muscle. If the patient so desires, a mammary prosthesis or tissue expander may be placed deep to the pectoralis major at this time, or either can be placed at a later procedure. The intact nerves to the serratus anterior and latissimus dorsi muscles are seen.

visualization of the pectoralis major innervation and permits the surgeon to palpate the axillary fat pad directly for enlarged lymph nodes. If unresectable nodal involvement is not found, the surgeon may then proceed to perform the dissection of the axillary fat pad with excellent exposure and preserve the muscular innervation and vascularization. The surgeon needs a clear understanding of the variability of the innervation to do this. This is appreciated in our dissections (Figs. 2–3 to 2–9). Moreover, Serra and colleagues (1984) have quantified the variations in innervation. They stress the importance of preserving the nerves to the pectoralis major that innervate the lower third of the muscle (the costoabdominal insertions or the external segments of the muscle). A schematic drawing of the innervation is provided in Figures 2–10 and 2–11. In Figure 2–12 the distribution of nerves in the dissections of Serra and colleagues are compared with those of Moosman (1980). Without preservation of these nerves, the denervated portions of the pectoralis major muscle become flaccid and atrophic. Nerve sacrifice becomes essential only when dissection of the axillary fat pad so requires.

The relation of the branches of the lateral pectoral nerve to the pectoralis minor muscle is quite intimate, as is shown in Figure 2–13. The various divisions of the nerve may decussate on either side of the muscle and through its body. The body of the muscle may be dissected away from the nerve when the nerve passes through the body of the pectoralis minor muscle. It should be noted that the number of nerve branches is highly variable. Preservation of one or two branches does not necessarily completely free the patient from risk of pectoralis major denervation, nor does it free the surgeon from the need for careful dissection throughout the procedure.

The pectoralis major muscle is dominantly innervated by the lateral anterior thoracic nerves arising from the lateral cord of the brachial plexus. The nerve passes over the first part of the axillary vein, and its branches pierce the clavipectoral fascia to enter the deep surface of the muscle.

The pectoralis minor muscle arises from the anterior and medial surfaces of the third, fourth, and fifth ribs and inserts as a tendon into the coracoid process of the scapula. Innervation is into the deep surface via the medial anterior thoracic nerve. Except for the loss of soft tissue on the anterior thoracic wall, no measurable disability attends the loss of function of the pectoralis minor muscle. The functional loss following removal of the pectoralis major muscle is readily measurable, but the degree of disability produced is small and is well tolerated by most individuals.

The serratus anterior muscle is important in stabilization of the scapula on the thorax. Its denervation results in a winged scapula, and this palsy, alone or in conjunction with the loss of the latissimus dorsi and the pectoralis muscles, can be a source of significant morbidity. For this reason, the nerve to the serratus anterior muscle is usually preserved in mammary surgery. The muscle arises from the upper nine ribs as a thin sheet with fibers passing superiorly and posteriorly to an insertion into the ventromedial angle and along the ventrovertebral border of the scapula. The lower four points of origin interdigitate with the external oblique muscle.

The nerve to the serratus anterior muscle (the long thoracic nerve or the external respi-

Text continued on page 28

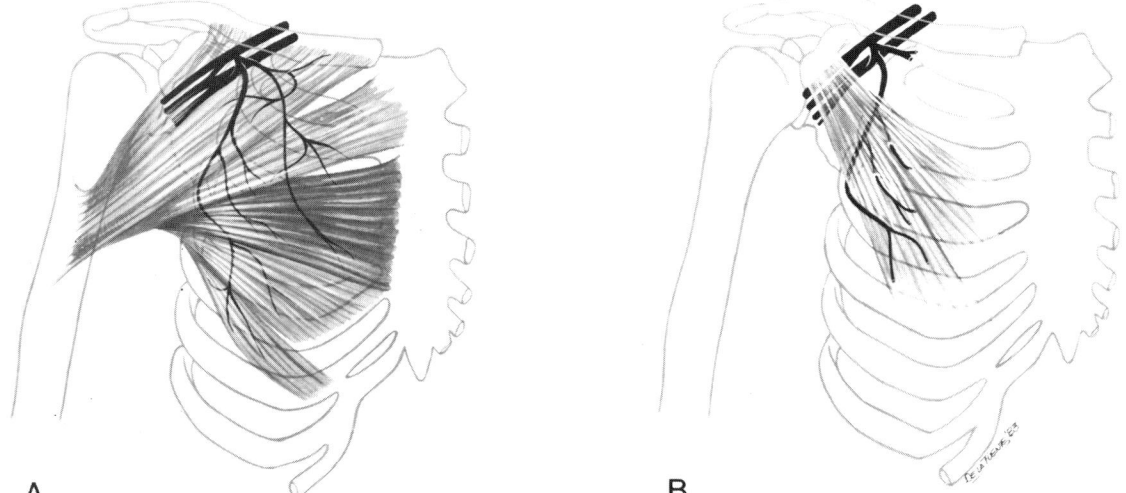

Figure 2–10. *A*, The medial pectoralis nerve innervates the clavicular and sternal origins of the pectoralis major muscle. *B*, The lateral pectoralis nerve descends along the edge of the pectoralis minor muscle, crossing it, and courses between the two pectoral muscles to supply the innervation of the lower third and the costoabdominal insertions of the pectoralis major muscle. (From Serra, G. E., et al.: Lateral pectoralis muscle: The need to preserve it in the modified radical mastectomy. J. Surg. Oncol., 26:278, 1984. Reprinted with permission.)

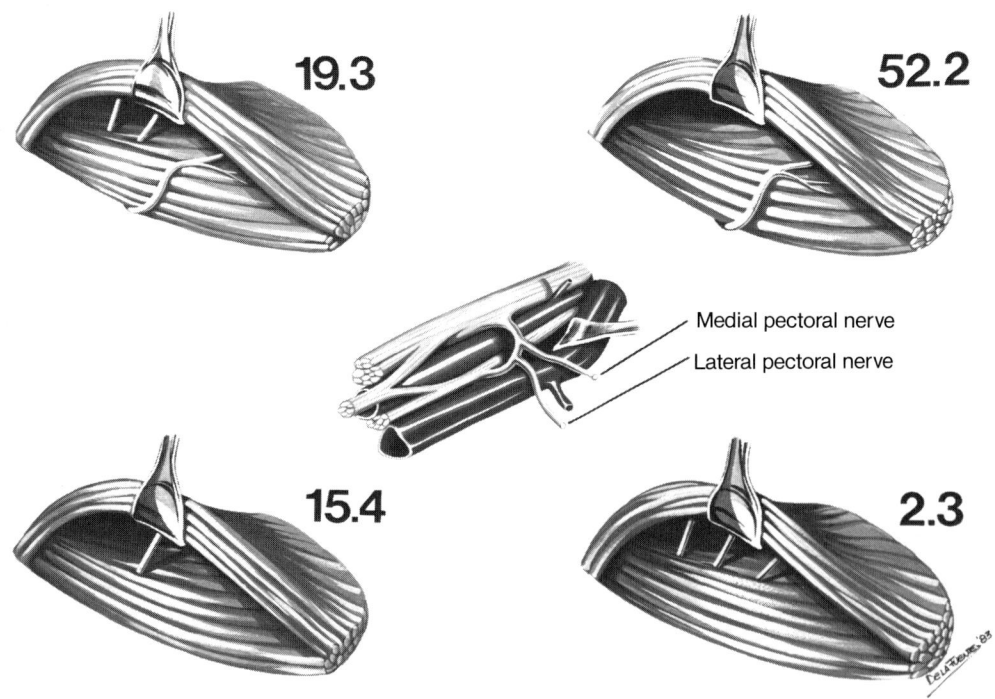

Figure 2–11. Relationships of the lateral thoracic nerve to the pectoralis minor muscle. (From Serra, G. E., et al.: Lateral pectoralis muscle: The need to preserve it in the modified radical mastectomy. J. Surg. Oncol., 26:278, 1984. Reprinted with permission.)

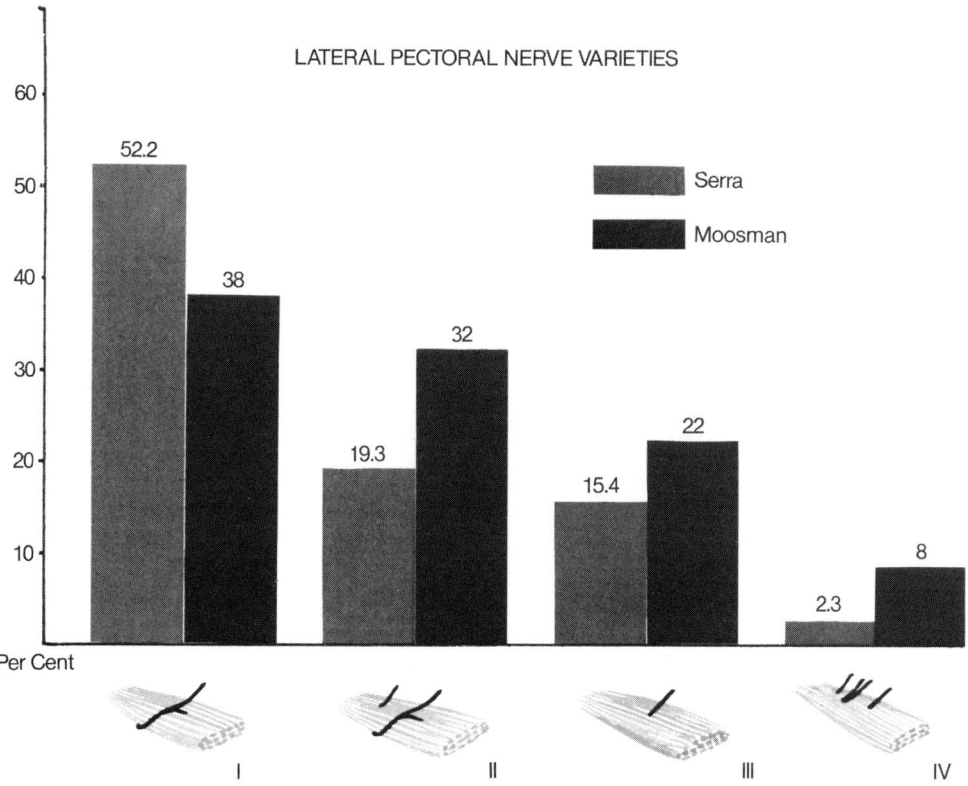

Figure 2–12. Comparison of the dissections of Serra and Moosman quantifying the relationship of the lateral pectoral nerve to the pectoralis minor muscle. Numbers indicate percentages. (From Serra, G. E., et al.: Lateral pectoralis muscle: The need to preserve it in the modified radical mastectomy. J. Surg. Oncol., 26:278, 1984. Reprinted with permission.)

26　2 • Anatomy of the Breast

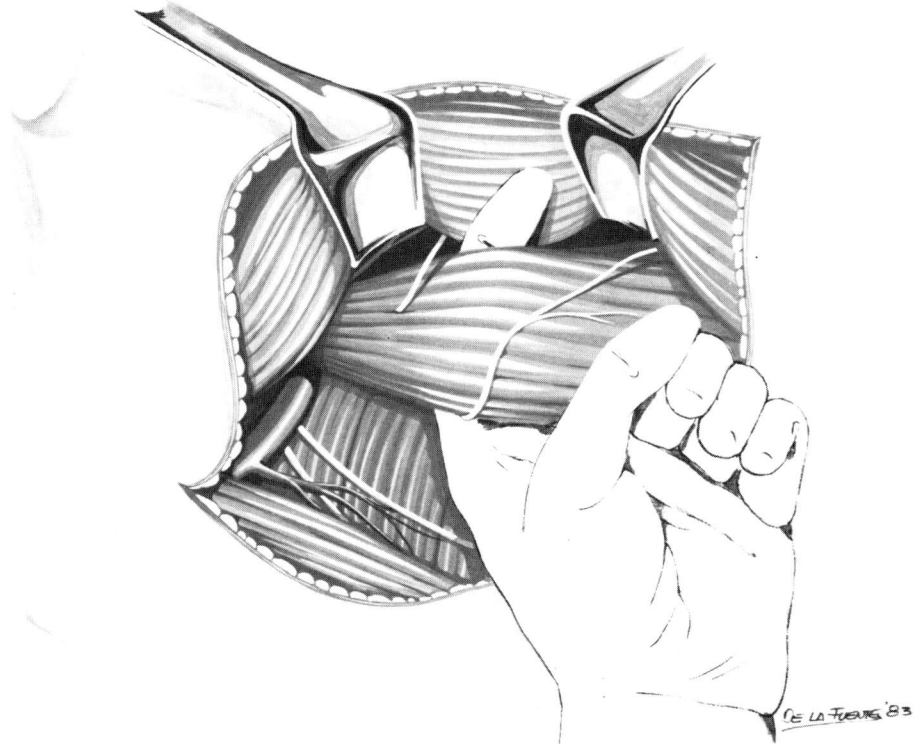

A

Figure 2–13. *A*, The surgical anatomy of the relationship of various nerves to the pectoralis minor muscle after incision of fascia. *B*, The exposure of the axilla is obtained by dividing the origin of the pectoralis minor on the chest wall. *C*, The transected but still innervated pectoralis minor muscle may be sutured to its origin on the thorax at the completion of the axillary dissection. (From Serra, G. E., et al.: Modified radical mastectomy technique of E. Scanlon. Int. J. Breast Mammary Pathol., 1985. Reprinted with permission.)

Illustration continued on opposite page

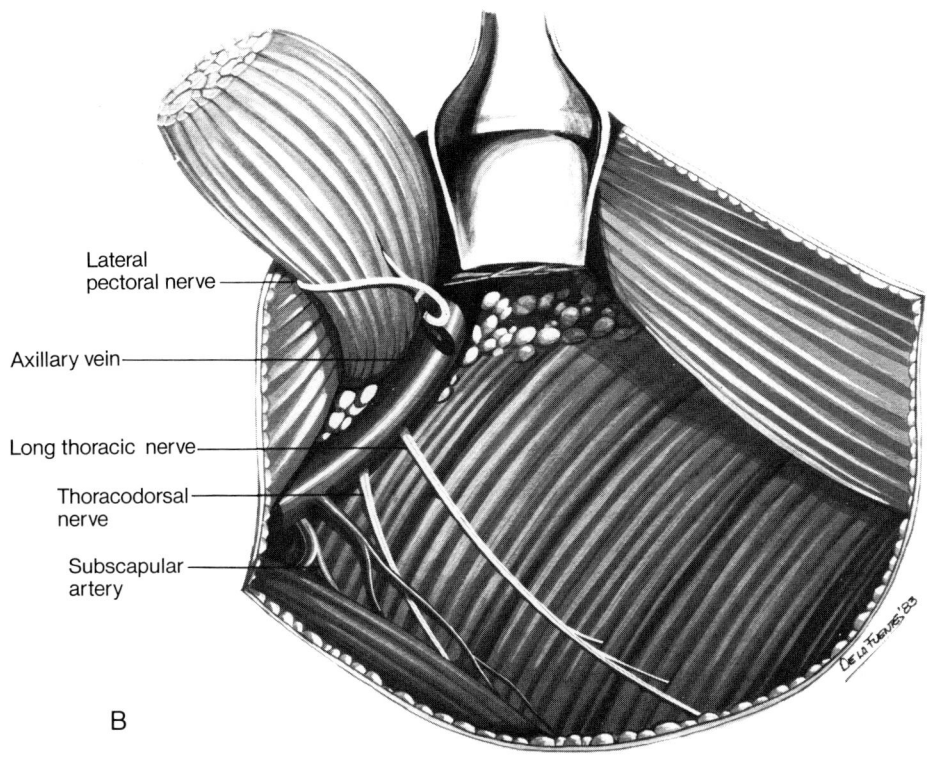

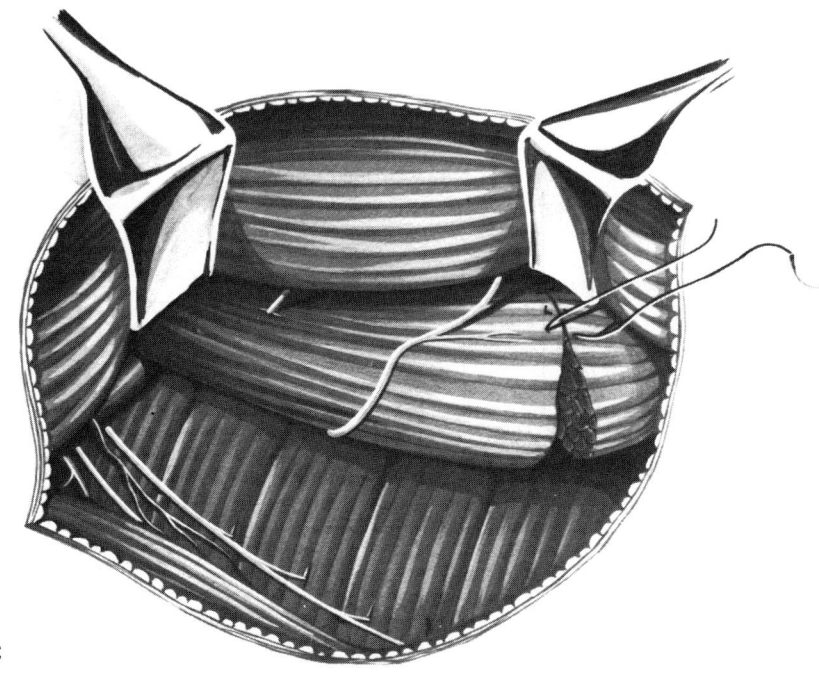

Figure 2–13 Continued

ratory nerve of Bell) arises above the clavicle and the mammary surgical field and passes deep to the axillary artery, staying close to the thoracic wall. As it passes caudally, it gives branches to the serratus anterior muscle.

The long thoracic nerve is superficial to the deep fascia investing the serratus anterior muscle. When the fascia is stripped away from the serratus anterior during the deep portion of the axillary dissection, the nerve can easily be seen. The fascia adjacent to the nerve must be divided so that the nerve can be isolated from the axillary contents throughout its length.

The latissimus dorsi muscle is of importance in mammary surgery because the deep fascia investing the muscle is continuous anteriorly with the axillary fascia and because the nerve to the muscle traverses the axillary contents. The muscle has a broad origin on the back and sweeps forward and superiorly to insert into the intertubercular groove of the humerus.

The anterior edge of the latissimus dorsi muscle is almost vertical in the midaxillary line. This edge marks the dorsal extent of a total mastectomy with or without preservation of the pectoralis major muscle. Detachment of the investing fascia of the muscle at this edge is equivalent to the detachment of the axillary fascia from its dorsal attachment.

The nerve to the latissimus dorsi muscle (thoracodorsal nerve) arises from the posterior cord of the brachial plexus, appears beneath or dorsal to the axillary vein along the posterior axillary wall, and passes through the lymph node–bearing areolar tissue of the axilla to the upper portion of the muscle. When necessary for adequate removal of axillary nodal metastases, the latissimus dorsi neurovascular supply must be removed; the functional loss is measurable but is tolerated well by most individuals (Tobin et al., 1980). When possible, however, the latissimus dorsi neurovascular supply should be preserved by careful dissection, as this both lessens functional loss and preserves the muscle for reconstructive purposes.

The deep axillary fascia is stripped laterally from the subscapularis muscle. The muscle passing between the subscapular fossa and the lesser tubercle of the humerus forms the lateral wall of the axilla just inferior or caudal to the axillary vein. In dissecting the fascia from the muscle, it is pertinent to look for and preserve the nerve to the subscapularis muscle, lying on the muscle's upper anterior surface. This muscle produces medial rotation of the arm and assists in flexion, extension, abduction, and adduction of the arm. It helps stabilize the humerus in the glenoid fossa. A subscapularis palsy can produce significant morbidity.

The external oblique muscle is of consequence because its upper slips of origin interdigitate with the origins of the pectoralis minor and serratus anterior muscles. Medially, its aponeurosis forms the anterior rectus sheath and marks the lower extent of a radical mastectomy. Also, this muscle is of value in chest wall reconstruction, if local recurrence requires anterior chest wall resection.

Lymphatic and Blood Vascular Anatomy

Certain general principles regarding lymphatic anatomy of any site are applicable to the breast. The subepithelial plexus of lymphatics is valveless and is confluent with the subepithelial plexus over the entire body surface. Lymph can flow in any direction in this plexus but does so sluggishly. This subepithelial plexus (sometimes called the papillary plexus because of its tuftlike extensions into the connective tissue of the epidermal papillae) is connected by vertical lymphatics to a coarse valvular labyrinth of subdermal lymphatics. This was well demonstrated by Gray (1939) when he injected mammary skin with Thorotrast.

Centrally the subepithelial and subdermal plexuses are confluent with the subareolar plexus, which in turn communicates with fine lymphatics of the lactiferous ducts. These lymphatics lie in the loose connective tissue just outside the myoepithelial layer of the duct wall (Bonser et al., 1961). The subareolar plexus also receives lymphatics from the areola and nipple.

The lymphatics paralleling the lactiferous ducts are equivalent to the vertical lymphatics that connect the subepithelial and subdermal lymphatics elsewhere in the body with the deep subcutaneous plexus (Spratt et al., 1965).

The breast is a specialized dermal organ that undergoes most of its growth during puberty. Growth probably occurs within the ducts and lobules by lengthening of existing lymphatics rather than development of new ones. If lactiferous duct lymphatics are equivalent to the vertical connecting lymphatics, their valve structure would be equivalent, and a unidirectional lymph flow from superficial to deep would exist. Thus, the lymph should flow from the subareolar plexus via the lactiferous duct lymphatics to the perilobular and deep subcutaneous lymphatic plexus. Injection studies refute the older concept that lymph flows centripetally to the subareolar plexus (Turner-Warwick, 1959; Halsell et al., 1965). Rather, lymph flows unidirectionally in valvular lymphatics from superficial to deep and toward the regional lymph nodes.

The functional anatomy of the lymphatics is the most important determinant of the direction of lymph flow. The valvular lymphatics undergo wavelike contractures that "milk" the lymph toward the regional lymph nodes. As a result, intralymphatic cancer cell emboli are rarely seen in unobstructed valvular lymphatics. Reverse flow in valvular lymphatics is possible only in the presence of the dilation that accompanies obstruction to flow. The valvular lymphatics frequently will rupture before permitting reverse flow.

These valvular lymphatics must be regarded as a continuum interconnected as a coarse labyrinth of anastomotic channels. The lymphatics roughly follow the major veins, and the volume of lymph flow is roughly proportional to the volume of blood flow to a particular organ. Normally, lymph can bypass obstructed lymph nodes through the anastomotic channels. Thus, lower nodes can be missed, and the first metastasis may appear at a higher node.

Two other anatomic situations can make lymph nodes ineffective filters. Lymphatics have been observed to empty directly into veins without passing through nodes (Wallace, 1965), and lymph can pass directly into the efferent veins of lymph nodes instead of into efferent lymphatics (Pressman and Simon, 1961). Neither phenomenon has been demonstrated for the fine lymphatics of the breast.

The lymphatics lying within the deep fascia about muscular compartments (i.e., within the fascia of the pectoralis major muscle) are fine in size and communicate little with the subcutaneous plexus. Studies have shown these lymphatics to be of little or no significance in the spread of mammary cancer (Turner-Warwick, 1959; Auchincloss, 1963).

The principal blood supply to the breast is from (1) branches of the axillary artery, including the thoracoacromial branches that supply and perforate the pectoralis major muscle; (2) the anterior perforating branches of the intercostal arteries; (3) the lateral perforating branches of the intercostal arteries; and (4) the lateral thoracic artery, which comes around the lateral muscle border and supplies and perforates the lateral muscle segment, emerging as myocutaneous perforators to the overlying breast and skin. Valvular lymphatics of the subcutaneous and intramammary plexi assure unidirectional flow toward lymph nodes in the axilla, to the internal mammary chain, and to intercostal lymphatic nodes lying posteriorly in a paravertebral position. These lymph nodes tend to lie in the fat pad around the bifurcation of major veins.

The proportion of lymph flowing to the paravertebral glands and their significance as a site for primary metastasis from mammary cancer have never, to the author's knowledge, been investigated. However, they certainly would be a suspected source of the posterior mediastinal and pleural metastases and the associated pleural effusion that is often seen late in the course of mammary cancer.

Lymphatics that follow the lateral perforating intercostal vessels perhaps are the cause of the ipsilateral predilection of malignant pleural effusions. Vital dye injected into the mammary parenchyma has been demonstrated in these lymphatics on occasion during mastectomy (Donegan, unpublished data).

On the basis of the proportion of radioactivity in lymph nodes after intramammary injection with gold (^{198}Au), Hultborn and associates (1955) estimated that only 1 to 3 per cent of the lymph flow from the breast entered the internal mammary lymph nodes. However, colloidal gold went to the internal mammary lymph nodes in small amounts *regardless* of the portion of the mammary gland injected (Fig. 2–14). Supraclavicular nodes were also examined, and radioactivity was found. Some radioactivity was present in the liver as well.

The studies by Fisher and Fisher (1972) on the pathophysiology of cancer metastases have greatly broadened insight into the complex interrelationships between lymphatic and hematogenous spread and the receptivity of tissues to the establishment of metastatic growths. The unifying concept derived from their studies is shown in Figure 2–15.

The studies of Fisher and Fisher support the concept that tumor cells that are primarily lymph-borne may reach the blood vascular system, through which they become further dispersed. These same cells freely circulating in the blood may reenter the lymphatics and appear in the thoracic duct lymph. In this situation, the two vascular systems are unified.

Cancer cells may be entrapped in regional

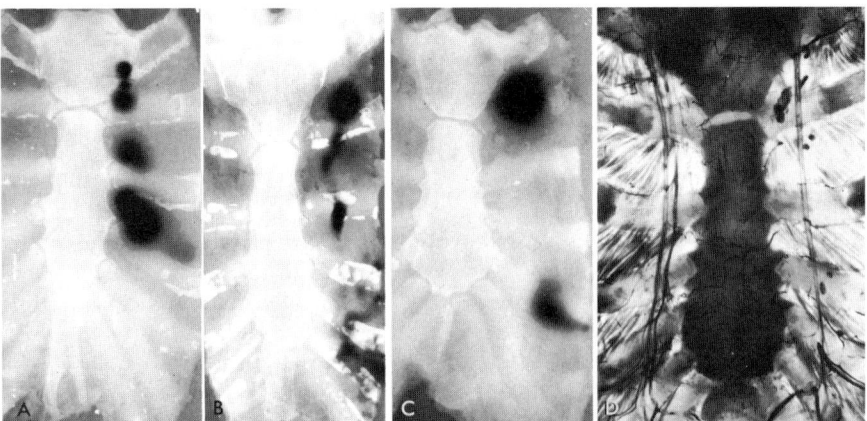

Figure 2–14. Anatomy of the internal mammary lymph node chain as demonstrated by the accumulation of ^{198}Au in the lymph nodes following intramammary injection of a colloidal suspension of the isotope (A–C) and in a cleared sternal specimen (D). (From Turner-Warwick, R. T.: The lymphatics of the breast. Br. J. Surg., 46:574, 1959. Reprinted with permission.)

lymph nodes. They may also enter the blood vascular system within lymph nodes, or they may completely bypass nodes via collateral lymphatics, disseminating by means of the thoracic duct directly into the bloodstream. The ability of tissues to accommodate the entrapment and allow growth of cancer cells arriving in the capillary beds of the tissues is determined by many variables, both humoral and local.

The conclusion to be drawn from many studies is that local ablative therapy with or without the inclusion of regional lymph nodes is not enough to adequately treat many cancers. The ease with which cancer cells can spread through lymph and blood vascular conduits as a consequence of the anastomoses between these systems makes many former concepts about the progression of cancer obsolete. Localization at the site of origin and spread to no more than first order regional lymph nodes are functions of the biologic characteristics of specific cancers, not limitations imposed by the anatomy of the lymph vascular system. Detailed descriptions of nonanatomic tumor-host relationships as variations in immune response and the contact inhibition of cells that may affect their behavior do not belong in a chapter on anatomy, however.

In the study by Hultborn and colleagues (1955), about 97 to 99 per cent of the radioactivity in the lymph nodes was found in the axillary nodes. This lymph node concentration represented only about 10.5 per cent of the ^{198}Au injected because most radioactivity remained at the site of the injection. No assessment of the radioactivity in the posterior intercostal lymph nodes was made. Also, the proportion of flow can vary widely when principal pathways are obstructed, as may be the case in metastatic mammary cancer.

Other potential routes of spread from the lower and medial glands might be via the lymphatic plexus on the rectus sheath to the subperitoneal areolar plexus. When metastatic cancer is so obstructive as to produce extensive reflux into the valveless subepithelial plexus, the cancer cells may go to the skin in any direction through this plexus. The major, and generally the primary, group of lymph nodes acquiring lymphatic metastases remains the axillary group.

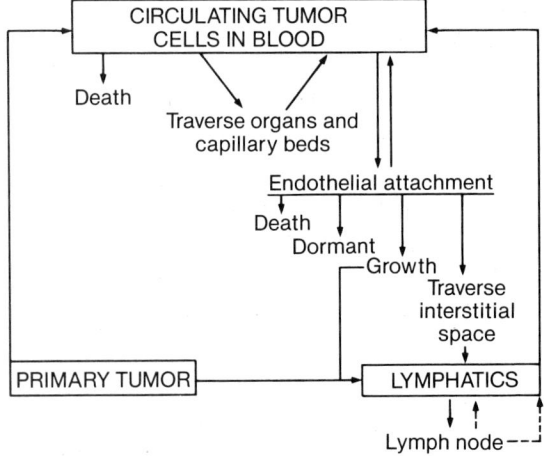

Figure 2–15. A unifying concept of tumor cell dissemination.

The axillary lymph nodes have been divided into several subgroups by anatomists. Pickren and coworkers (1965), in clearing axillary lymph nodes for studying the pathologic anatomy of metastases, subdivided the nodes as follows: (1) the highest nodes, including the subclavicular or higher axillary vein group from the apex of the axilla (from beneath the clavicle to the lower border of the pectoralis minor muscle); (2) interpectoral nodes, lying between the pectoralis major and pectoralis minor muscles; (3) the lower axillary vein group, from the border of the pectoralis minor muscle to the lateral limits of dissection; and (4) the central group, including the external mammary, paramammary, and scapular nodes (Auchincloss, 1963).

The lymphatics from the posterior breast that accompany the thoracoacromial vessels pass through the interpectoral group en route to the upper axillary chain. Most lymphatics arise in the lobules and pass through the substance of the breast and through the axillary fascia to the external mammary lymph nodes. These lymphatics lie approximately parallel to the lateral thoracic vessels (Fig. 2–2).

The internal mammary lymph nodes accompany the internal mammary artery and vein (Fig. 2–14). The lymph nodes are found in the intercostal spaces and posterior to the costal cartilages close to the sternum. Variable numbers of lymph nodes exist, but they can usually be removed entirely by ligation of the internal mammary vessels in the first and fifth interspaces, resecting the second through the fifth costal cartilages along with a margin (about 1 cm) of the sternum and the subjacent areolar tissue and pleura. Most of the nodes are in the upper parasternal area near bifurcations of the intercostal and internal mammary veins.

Afferent lymph vessels are received from the upper abdominal wall and the anterior thoracic wall, and efferent vessels from the anterior diaphragmatic nodes are also received into the internal mammary lymph drainage channels. Efferent lymphatics connect the nodes and terminate above in the various lymphatics that enter the jugular veins. Cross anastomosis of lymphatics in the retrosternal area between these chains is the rule (Fig. 2–16) (Turner-Warwick, 1959; Rouviere, 1938).

If the axillary lymph node filter is involved extensively or "clogged" with metastases, the chance for surgical cure drops precipitously, and both the lymphatic fluid and the metastasizing cancer cells increasingly follow the alternate pathways. When the axillary nodes are involved with cancer, the frequency of internal mammary lymph node metastases rises and intramammary edema (causing peau d'orange) is increasingly likely to occur.

Cells traversing lymphatics in all directions are likely to be entrapped by the cessation and alteration of lymph flow that follows radical mastectomy. These entrapped cells and the

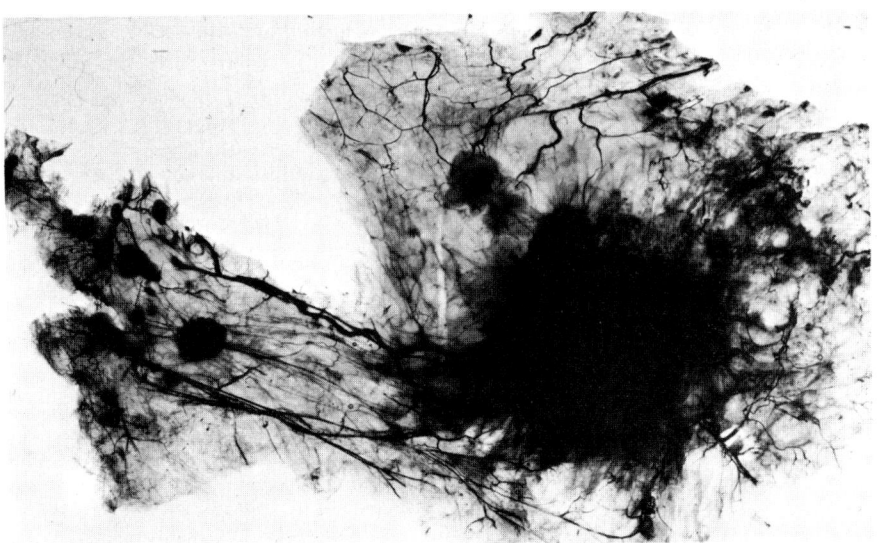

Figure 2–16. A cleared mastectomy specimen injected preoperatively with iron–prussian blue. The coarse labyrinth of blood vessels and the less distinct lymphatics accompanying them toward the regional nodes can be seen. (From Turner-Warwick, R. T.: The lymphatics of the breast. Br. J. Surg., 46:574, 1959. Reprinted with permission.)

occult metastases in lesser lymph nodes then account for some chest wall recurrences and treatment failures. Other chest wall recurrences probably originate from systemically circulating tumor cells entrapped in the healing wound. At this point, the indications for therapy can no longer be based on the routine and empirical application of an operative procedure designed to ablate the disease in a relatively early phase. Rather, the treatment plan must now be based on the probabilities of affecting the natural history of the cancer favorably or unfavorably.

Alterations in Lymphatic Anatomy Following Axillary Dissection or Radiotherapy

The lymphatics play a vital role in clearing tissue of protein and cellular debris. Their role in removing fluid is secondary, as most fluid that leaks into tissue spaces from arterial capillaries as a result of high arteriolar pressure and capillary permeability is reabsorbed on the capillary venular side by osmotic pressure. Most tissue nourishment occurs by diffusion in parallel with this process. When lymphatics are inadequate to sustain the egress of proteins, the osmotic gradient shifts toward the tissue side, and edema occurs. The protein-rich edematous fluids stimulate the development of fibrosis, which leads to fibrokeratotic lymphedema. Inadequate lymph drainage from the upper extremity occurs with the ablation of axillary lymphatics by surgery, high-dose irradiation, persistent neoplasm, or repetitive infection with lymphangitis. Although new lymphatics will partially bridge the defect, the drainage of lymph from the upper extremity will never return to normal. This anatomic change is permanent, and the risk of incipient fibrokeratotic lymph edema is lifelong, requiring special considerations in patient education and management (discussed under appropriate sections of the text) (Kinmouth, 1982).

REFERENCES

Auchincloss, H.: Significance of location and number of axillary metastases in carcinoma of the breast; a justification for a conservative operation. Ann. Surg., *158*:37, 1963.

Bonser, G. M., Dossett, J. A., and Jull, J. W.: Human and Experimental Breast Cancer. Springfield, Ill., Charles C Thomas, 1961.

Bowers, D. G., Jr., and Radlauer, C. B.: Breast cancer of prophylactic subcutaneous mastectomies and reconstruction with Silastic protheses. Plast. Reconstr. Surg., *44*:541, 1969.

Fisher, B., and Fisher, E. R.: The interrelationship of hematogenous and lymphatic tumor cell dissemination. Surg. Gynecol. Obstet., *122*:791, 1966.

Fisher, B.: Prospects for the control of metastases. Cancer, *24*:1263, 1969.

Fisher, E. R., and Fisher, B.: Experimental studies of factors influencing development of hepatic metastases. XVII. Role of thyroid. Cancer Res., *26*:2248, 1966.

Fisher, E. R., and Fisher, B.: Effects of x-irradiation of parameters of tumor growth, histology, and ultrastructure. Cancer, *24*:39, 1969.

Fisher, E. R., and Fisher, B.: Local lymphoid response as an index of tumor immunity. Arch. Path., *94*:137, 1972.

Geschickter, C. F.: Diseases of the Breast. Philadelphia, JB Lippincott Co, 1943.

Goldman, L. D., and Goldwyn, R. M.: Some anatomical considerations of subcutaneous mastectomy. Plast. Reconstr. Surg., *51*:501, 1973.

Goodnight, J. E., Jr., Quagliana, J. M., and Morton, D. L.: Failure of subcutaneous mastectomy to prevent the development of cancer. J. Surg. Oncol., *26*:198, 1984.

Gray, J. H.: The relation of lymphatic vessels to the spread of cancer. Br. J. Surg., *26*:462, 1939.

Halsell, J. T., Smith, J. R., Bentlage, C. R., et al.: Lymphatic drainage of the breast demonstrated by vital dye staining and radiography. Ann. Surg., *162*:221, 1965.

Hicken, N. F.: Mastectomy. Clinical pathologic study demonstrating why most mastectomies result in incomplete removal of the mammary gland. Arch. Surg., *40*:6, 1940.

Hultborn, K. A., Larsen, K. G., and Raghnult, I.: The lymph drainage from the breast to the axillary and parasternal lymph nodes: Studied with the aid of colloidal Au[198]. Acta Radiol. (Stockh.), *43*:52, 1955.

Jackson, C. F., Palmquist M., Swanson, J., et al.: The effectiveness of prophylactic subcutaneous mastectomy in Sprague-Dawley rats induced with 7, 12-dimethylbenz anthraeene. Plast. Reconstr. Surg., *73*:249–255, 1984.

Kinmouth, J. B.: The Lymphatics. Surgery, Lymphography and Diseases of the Chyle and Lymph System. London, Edward Arnold, 1982.

Klamer, T. W., Donegan, W. L., and Max, M. H.: Breast tumor incidence in rats after partial mastectomy resection. Arch. Surg., *118*:933, 1983.

Moosman, D. A.: Anatomy of the pectoral nerves and their preservation in modified mastectomy. Am. J. Surg., *139*:883, 1980.

Peacock, E. E., Jr.: Biological basis for management of benign disease of the breast—case against subcutaneous mastectomy. Plast. Reconstr. Surg., *55*:14, 1975.

Pickren, J. W., Rube, J., and Auchincloss, H.: Modification of conventional radical mastectomy: A detailed study of lymph node involvement and follow-up information to show its practicality. Cancer, *18*:942, 1965.

Pressman, J. J., and Simon, M. B.: Experimental evidence of direct communications between lymph nodes and veins. Surg. Gynecol. Obstet., *113*:537, 1961.

Rouviere, J.: Anatomie des Lymphatiques de l'Homme (Transl. MJ Tobias). Ann Arbor, Mich., Edwards Bros., 1938.

Serra, G. E., Maccarone, G. B., Ibarra, P. E., et al.: Lateral pectoralis nerve: The need to preserve it in the modified radical mastectomy. J. Surg. Oncol., 26:278, 1984.

Singer, E.: Fasciae of the Human Body and Their Relations to the Organs They Envelop. Baltimore, Williams & Wilkins, 1935.

Spratt, J. S., Shieber, W., and Dillard, B.: Anatomy and Surgical Technique of Groin Dissection. St. Louis, C. V. Mosby, 1965.

Tobin, G. R.: Pectoralis major segmental anatomy and segmentally split pectoralis major flaps. Plast. Reconstr. Surg., 75:814, 1985.

Tobin, G. R., Gordon, J. A., Smith, B., et al.: Preserving motor function by splitting muscle and myocutaneous pedicles. Plast. Surg. Forum, 31:559, 1980.

Tobin, G. R., Spratt, J. S., Bland, K. I., et al.: One-stage pharyngoesophageal and oral myocutaneous reconstruction with two segments of one musculocutaneous flap. Am. J. Surg., 144:489, 1982.

Turner-Warwick, R. T.: The lymphatics of the breast. Br. J. Surg., 46:574, 1959.

Wallace, S.: Direct communication between a lymph channel in neck and external jugular vein visualized by lymphography and x-ray obtained. In Spratt, J. S., Shieber, W., and Dillard, B. (Eds): Anatomy and Surgical Technique of Groin Dissection. St. Louis, C. V. Mosby, 1965.

CHAPTER 3

JOHN PETER MINTON

Physiology of the Breast

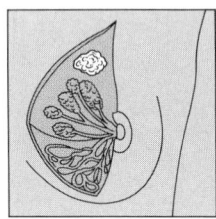

Breasts change. The structure, size, form, and function of breast tissue result from an intricate combination of hormone signals and ratios that permit breast epithelial cells to produce and secrete milk for the nourishment and sustenance of infants.

Breasts develop from an ectodermally derived plaque of cells inconspicuously located in the abdominal region that regresses soon after its appearance at 6 weeks postfertilization except in the anterior thoracic portion of the embryo. The anlage of the lactiferous ducts has invaded the mesodermal connective tissue by 16 to 24 weeks. By 8 months of gestation, the nipple and areola have developed. Breasts of the newborn may secrete a fluid (witches' milk), showing the responsiveness of these tissues to hormone stimulation.

The breast is a tubuloalveolar gland. By puberty, 15 to 20 ducts are formed, and the arborization develops into 10 to 15 lobes, which are separate glands embedded within the breast's fatty stroma. The drainage mechanism is a separate excretory lactiferous duct that expands beneath the nipple into a collecting sinus. The cellular surface area in these duct systems is immense because of the many branches. Lobes are separated by dense connective tissue septa. Each septum carries its cadre of blood vessels, nerves, and lymphatics. The connective tissue normally divides the lobes into lobules, each with its own interlobular ducts. The lactiferous ducts are lined with a stratified squamous epithelium near the nipple. Deeper into the breast parenchyma the lining cells are cuboidal, and then become columnar.

The secretory units of the breast are the alveoli or saccular invaginations of the lactiferous ducts. It is these secretory units that are so responsive to hormone modulations that promote growth or regression of the breast tissue. Surrounding each alveolus are the myoepithelial cells. These cells form a web around the alveolar structure and along the outside of the interlobular channels. Contraction of the myoepithelial cells is responsible for the emptying ("let-down") or ejection of milk from the lobules into the lactiferous ducts.

The postpubertal breast may be mature but inactive. A proliferative phase occurs during pregnancy, followed by a lactating stage for milk production after parturition, after which regression takes place. An involutional or atrophic phase occurs after lactation ceases and when menopause occurs. Minor physical changes also occur in some women's breasts during the menstrual cycle (Halban, 1905). The premenstrual enlargement is not well understood but is speculated to be due to hyperemia and edema.

In the inactive or resting stage prior to pregnancy, the breast lobules consist of tubules or ducts separated by connective and adipose tissue. Bud-like sacculations arise from the ducts, and the gland becomes mostly a lactiferous unit with interlobar and intralobular ducts.

The proliferative phase occurring in pregnancy is associated with major changes. Breast growth early in pregnancy is a hyperplasia of the ductal and secretory elements. Later in pregnancy, hypertrophy of alveolar cells and secretory elements is coupled with decreases in fat and fibrous connective tissue.

During lactation, the lining cells in the alveolar sacculations become columnar and look like exocrine cells. These cells deposit their lipids, fluids, carbohydrates, and proteinaceous products into the alveolar lumen. Protein products leave the cells by exocytosis from the cell's apex without loss of cytoplasm. Lipids are transported out with a significant decrease in cell cytoplasm. Contractions of the myoepithelial cells force the fluid from the alveolar sacculus into alveolar ducts and on into the lactiferous ducts and sinuses. The hormonal and neurologic trigger for these myoepithelial contractions is the suckling stimulation from the infant.

Regression, involution, and atrophy follow when the infant's suckling no longer stimulates the breast. Residual alveolar milk products are reabsorbed, and the breast parenchyma involutes and is replaced with increased fat and connective tissue. Macrophages and histocytes are active during this involutional process in the ducts and alveoli.

Near the menopause, involution results in the disappearance of alveoli and intralobular ducts and the hyalinization of these structures.

The process of lactation is controlled by a series of complex hormonal and biochemical events. The levels of progesterone, estrone, estradiol, estriol, prolactin, and placental lactogen all increase during the 40 weeks of gestation (Rigg et al., 1977; Del Pozo and Brownell, 1979; Carr et al., 1981; Tulchinsky et al., 1985). However, estrogen by itself may not be as important in breast growth as it was initially assumed to be. Progesterone appears to stimulate the growth of the lobuloalveolar segments of the breast while inhibiting secretory activity by blocking the terminal differentiation, which is later induced by prolactin (Davis et al., 1972). Cortisol appears to potentiate the action of prolactin on breast differentiation. The induction of lactation may occasionally occur in nulliparous women as well as in men by a regular suckling stimulus (Brown, 1978; Rosner, 1979). Lactogenesis is triggered by a fall in the plasma progesterone levels when plasma prolactin and breast development are adequate to promote milk secretion (Kuhn, 1969, 1977). At parturition the levels of placental lactogen disappear rapidly (hours). Progesterone levels fall more slowly (several days); estrogens fall over the first week post partum. Prolactin falls slowly (longer than 14 days) in the non-nursing mother. In nursing mothers, prolactin falls much more slowly, with the fall usually being dependent on the time the infant nurses (Delvoye et al., 1977; Hiba et al., 1977). Although placental hormonal influences have long been suspected of being a significant inhibitor of lactation, and retained placental fragments have been shown to delay lactation, prolactin appears to be the most necessary hormone for lactation, and use of an inhibitor, bromocriptine, can suppress lactation (Brun del Re et al., 1973; Kuhn, 1977). Occasionally lactation has occurred in women with low prolactin levels. The real trigger preparing for lactation is now suspected to be the post partum decline in progesterone along with the long hormonal preparation for lactation that is completed at childbirth (Franks et al., 1877). Nipple neurosensory reflexes to the brain must be triggered to stimulate the secretion of the hormones, oxytoxin and prolactin. Oxytocin stimulates the contraction of the myoepithelial cells, producing milk ejection or "let-down." Prolactin drives the synthesis and secretion of milk into the alveolar spaces. Milk production seems to be regulated by infant demand, and prolactin appears to be important in milk volume production (Brun del Re et al., 1973; Aono et al., 1977; Gross and Eastman, 1979; Kauppila et al., 1981).

Once the stimulus of breast feeding stops, involution begins nearly immediately. Milk composition changes rapidly following weaning, with increases in protein, sodium, and chloride concentrations and a decrease in potassium, lactose, and citrate (Hartman and Kulski, 1978). Both IgA and lactoferrin increase, and this is believed to be related to a deterioration of the blood-milk barriers, permitting plasma to enter alveolar lumina. Breast blood flow decreases with involution, and a decline in the enzymes necessary for milk production occurs. Alveolar distention is believed to be a major factor inducing cessation of lactation.

The Hormones

Oxytocin is synthesized in pure form in the magnocellular neurons in the supraoptic and paraventricular nucleus of the hypothalamus (du Vigneaud et al., 1954; Morris et al., 1977; Zimmerman and Defendini, 1977). The fibers of the paraventricular nucleus pass to the supraoptic nucleus, where they join fibers from the latter nucleus, which travel to the median eminence of the posterior pituitary. Oxytocin, a 10,000 dalton (D) protein, is released by exocytosis of secretory granules (Robinson et al., 1977; Theodosin and Dreifuss, 1977; Amico et al., 1981). Its action is mediated through an electrical potential–producing nerve depolarization prior to milk ejection in experimental animals (Poulain et al., 1977).

Oxytocin release may be a conditioned reflex in response to an infant's cry, and nonrelease may occur under conditions of pain or emotional stress (Barowicz, 1978; Clarke and Merrick, 1978; Moos and Richard, 1979). Oxytocin release can be stimulated by catecholamines when epinephrine and dopamine are injected into the intracerebral ventricle. In contrast, alpha-adrenergic blocking agents and dopamine antagonists will inhibit the milk ejection response. Beta-adrenergic agonists and antiagonists block milk ejection. These activities appear to be mediated by the central nervous system. Morphine blocks milk ejection by preventing the release of oxytocin from the nerve terminals in the posterior pituitary. Beta-endorphins of pituitary origin modulate oxytocin release within the pituitary.

Oxytocin interacts with the myoepithelial cells located in the basement membrane of the alveolus and along the intralobular ducts. Oxytocin binding sites have been localized, and oxytocin receptors are believed to increase in the breast and uterus at parturition. Oxytocin apparently acts by phosphorylation of myosin, producing the contraction of the myoepithelial cells (Bremel and Shaw, 1978). This contraction is best accomplished by intermittent releases of oxytocin rather than a continuous secretion, emphasizing the relationship with intermittent suckling of the nipple as a stimulus for milk ejection.

The interrelationship of a variety of hormones is very important in understanding breast function. A review of these hormones and their interactions follows.

Lactogenic hormones are single-chain polypeptides with molecular weights of 21,000 to 23,000 D and include prolactin and growth hormone, both pituitary hormones, and placental lactogen or chorionic somatomammotropin. Prolactin is probably the most important hormone secreted in response to suckling, and combining with receptors on the milk-secreting cells, it stimulates milk production. Prolactin also stimulates mammary growth and differentiation.

The role of placental lactogens and growth hormone roles is less clear. The genes for the production of placental lactogen and growth hormone are located on chromosome 17 (Owerbach et al., 1980). The similarity of the primary and intervening sequences of these genes suggests gene reduplication as the origin of these hormones.

Prolactin is synthesized on membrane-bound ribosomes, processed in the Golgi membranes, stored in secretory granules, and secreted by exocytosis. Prolactin inhibitory factor (dopamine), estrogens, thyrotropin releasing hormone, and endorphins are involved in the control of prolactin production. Prolactin release is controlled by prolactin inhibitory factor (PIF), which is secreted into the pituitary portal blood system by the tubuloinfundibular neurons of the hypothalamus (De Hertogh et al., 1975; Del Pozo and Brownell, 1979). PIF is dopamine, and this suppresses the production and release of prolactin by interacting with the dopamine receptor sites on prolactin-producing cells. L-Dopa, which is converted to dopamine, and bromocriptine, a dopamine agonist, interfere with prolactin release. Prolactin mRNA transcription is inhibited by dopaminergic compounds (Minton and Dickey, 1973; Morris et al., 1977; Moos and Richard, 1979). Long-term administration of estrogen increases both pituitary and plasma prolactin levels. This results from an increase in the number and activity of pituitary prolactin cells (Lloyd et al., 1975). Chronic elevated estrogen response appears to block the effect of dopamine on prolactin production and produces hypertrophy of pituitary cells, an accumulation of intracellular prolactin-containing granules, and an increase in the content of prolactin transcription–specific mRNA. Estrogen treatment appears to decrease the inhibitory effects of dopamine on prolactin release (Raymond et al., 1978; Antakly et al., 1980). Estrogen has also been shown to augment prolactin release at the hypothalamus (De Hertogh et al., 1975; Labrie et al., 1980). Thyrotropin releasing hormone (TRH) is not thought to be important in prolactin release, although a TRH infusion can be used to determine prolactin reserve. Both calcium and TRH are important for inducing electrical activity in prolactin cells and releasing prolactin (Sand et al., 1980; Vincent et al., 1980). TRH does augment prolactin mRNA transcription, however (Raymond et al., 1978; Potter et al., 1981).

Prolactin release has been enhanced by stress, possibly by hypothalamic opiates. The morphine agonist naloxone decreases prolactin secretion and oxytocin release (Nicoll and Bern, 1972). The dopamine agonist bromocriptine blocks prolactin release, whereas phenothiazine stimulates milk secretion by blocking dopamine synthesis (De Hertogh et al., 1975; Del Pozo et al., 1977; Fluckiger, 1978; Del Pozo and Brownell, 1979).

Prolactin increases the production of the milk protein casein and increases synthesis of casein mRNA (Guyette et al., 1979; Teyssot and Houdebine, 1980). Prolactin increases the rate of fatty acid production and synthesis in breast tissues and also shifts the synthesis to medium chain fatty acids, which are characteristic of lactating breast tissue (Strong et al., 1972; Wang et al., 1972). Lipoprotein production is not clearly defined at this time.

Prolactin binds to mammary cell surface prolactin membrane receptors. Changes in the number of prolactin receptors on mammary cells correlate with the level of serum prolactin and the period of early lactation (Bohnet et al., 1977; McNeilly and Friesen, 1977). Ergot alkaloids block this increase in receptors, and an increase in receptors can be produced by injecting prolactin into the system (Djiane and Durande, 1977). Because progesterone blocks the increase in receptors, the ratio between serum prolactin and progesterone levels seems important in modulating receptor increases. Prolactin plasma membrane receptor levels appear to be variably dependent on a variety of hormonal concentrations and ratios. Increases or decreases in receptor concentrations change the sensitivity of the cell for milk production. These variations in receptor concentrations imply receptor internalization and processing of hormone receptor complexes.

Prolactin appears to be internalized in the cell to promote a secretory signal for cellular milk production (Nolin and Witorsch, 1976; Nolin, 1978; Shiu, 1980). Current studies support the concept that prolactin is involved in transduction via microtubules to activate casein mRNA and promote casein synthesis (Houdebine et al., 1979; Houdebine and Djiane 1980).

Human placental lactogen (HPL) levels rise continually throughout pregnancy. Hypoglycemia and the mass of the placenta are the only factors that have been proved to change placental lactogen (Bigazzi et al., 1979). Bromocriptine does not. HPL seems to have a role in lactation not dissimilar to prolactin, but HPL's major role must be related to breast growth and differentiation during pregnancy, as its decrease is rapid after the placenta is delivered at parturition.

Estrogen, progesterone, and adrenocortical hormones play a role in the modulation of the lactogenous hormones. Estrogens seem to stimulate mammary growth and development but inhibit milk secretion, yet they promote prolactin secretion by the anterior pituitary gland (McManus and Welsch, 1980).

Estrogens are responsible for the proliferation of mammary epithelium, especially the ductile portions in the gland. Nearly all studies show a relationship between estrogen and intact pituitary function for satisfactory mammary growth (Edwards et al., 1979; Leclerg and Heuson, 1979). A correlation between these hormones has been made with plasma estradiol-17β levels and prolactin at puberty, pregnancy, and menarche, and in association with oral contraceptive use (Robyn et al., 1977; Hertz et al., 1978).

Estrogens in breast tissue bind with the estrogen receptors in the cytosol, and this bound receptor then moves to the nucleus (Shyamala and Nandi, 1972). Estrogen receptors are specific and do not cross react with other hormones. There is strong evidence that estrogens in combination with prolactin can produce and promote a galactorrhea syndrome (Antunes et al., 1977). Interestingly, estrogen is believed to be produced in normal breast tissues as well as breast cancer tissue (Edwards et al., 1979). Excessive estrogen does stop lactation and is associated with a decrease of prolactin in the mammary epithelial cells, suggesting interference with prolactin binding to the mammary epithelial cell by the internalizing or modulating of prolactin receptor sites (Lemarchand-Beraud et al., 1977).

Progesterone appears to synergize with estrogen and prolactin to produce full lobuloalveolar development of the gland. Progesterone's inhibitory effect on the initiation of milk secretion during pregnancy has been mentioned. Progesterone prevents an accumulation of enzymes necessary for the terminal differentiation of breast cells for lactation but actively promotes breast growth. Progesterone in combination with estrogen is responsible for lobuloalveolar development during pregnancy and prevents an increase of lactose content in breast tissue in pregnancy (Folley and Malpress, 1948; Kuhn, 1977; Cowie, 1978; Topper and Freeman, 1980). In addition, progesterone inhibits the prolactin-induced rise of alpha-lactalbumin in breast tissue during pregnancy (Turkington and Hill, 1969; Speake et al., 1976). Progesterone also decreases prolactin-induced rises in casein and casein mRNA and inhibits glucose oxidation and conversion to lipids (De Hertogh et al., 1975; Greenbaum et al., 1978; Rosen et al., 1978; Teyssot and Houdebine, 1980). It is speculated that progesterone inhibits the process of breast epithelial differentiation by inhibiting cortisol binding and preventing glucocorticoid potentiation of prolactin action (Ganguly et al., 1982). In addition, progesterone may modify ribosomal RNA and casein mRNA synthesis (Teyssot and Houdebine, 1980). Progesterone binding sites appear to decrease significantly during lactation, accounting for a lack of progesterone effect on the breasts during lactation.

Lactation cannot be initiated or sustained in the absence of glucocorticoids. Current speculation suggests that progesterone withdrawal at parturition allow cortisol to exert a stimulus for lactation. Glucocorticoid receptors bound with glucocorticoids translate to the nucleus after binding, but progesterone can bind this receptor and this prevents translocation and blocks glucocorticoid action (Shyamala, 1975; Shyamala and Dickson, 1976). Glucocorticoids increase the accumulation of casein and casein mRNA when breast tissue is exposed to prolactin (Mills and Topper, 1970; Devinoy and Houdebine, 1977; Bolander and Topper, 1979). When prolactin is absent, there is little activity (Devinoy and Houdebine, 1977).

Insulin is an important tissue culture requirement for mammary epithelial cell growth, but aside from its importance in the regulation of nutrients stored in the liver, fat, and muscle, it does not seem to play an important role in breast tissue development. Insulin is important in breast lipid synthesis, regulating the transport of glucose into the acinar cells (Robinson et al., 1978). Not only is the availability of glucose affected by insulin, but glucose metabolites such as lactate and pyruvate also influence the fatty acid production of lactating epithelial cells (Bartley and Abraham, 1976).

Thyroid hormone is involved in the promotion of mammary growth and lactation, but its role is believed to be more permissive than regulatory (Lyons, 1958). For example, in the presence of low concentrations of prolactin, thyroxine promotes satisfactory lobulovalveolar development (Singh and Bern, 1969). High doses of thyroxine shut the system down (Vonderhaar, 1979). Prostaglandins are thought to act as one of the factors in preparturition inhibition of secretion.

Cyclic adenosine monophosphate (cAMP) appears to shift the balance between growth and differentiation toward growth. When breast tissue is stimulated by progesterone, cAMP will maintain inhibition of the terminal changes leading to lactogenesis (Sapag-Hagar and Greenbaum, 1974; Yang et al., 1980).

The mechanisms of milk production involve five different pathways. The first four are transcellular pathways: (1) Protein, citrate, calcium, phosphate, and lactose all leave their cells of origin through exocytosis in Golgi-derived secretory vesicles. (2) Milk fat is secreted in the form of milk fat globules. (3) Water, sodium, potassium, and chloride are secreted across the cell membranes. (4) Immunoglobulins such as IgA and other plasma proteins exit by pinocytosis or exocytosis. (5) Leukocytes, sodium, and plasma protein may enter the milk by a paracellular route or between the membranes of the cells of lactation from the surrounding capillary nutritional source. Each alveolar unit creates about 1 or 2 ml of milk per gram of tissue per day. Milk is stored adjacent to the cells that produce it, and on myoepithelial cell contraction the milk passes rapidly through the duct system and out of the breast. Little of the milk product is reabsorbed in transit. Exocytosis is the process by which most milk components are packaged into secretory vesicles and leave the cells. The amino acid sequence of milk proteins is coded in nuclear DNA, which is transcribed into messenger RNA (mRNA) that passes to the cytoplasm, where the messenger RNA translates to ribosomes bound to the rough endoplasmic reticulum. As proteins are synthesized, amino acids are inserted into the sequence across the endoplasmic reticular membrane. Carbohydrate groups are added according to the appropriate sequence. The product is then transferred to a Golgi system for sorting and storage. Calcium, phosphates, and citrate enter the Golgi vesicles from the cytoplasm. Inside the Golgi vesicles, calcium and phosphates combine with caseins and phosphoproteins and form aggregates or micelles. Lactose is formed in the Golgi system from an interaction of the membrane-bound galactosyl transference and alpha-lactalbumin. Lactose osmotically attracts water into the Golgi vesicles. The vesicles containing lactose, water, milk protein, calcium, phosphates, and citrates pass to the apical membrane of the cell, fuse, and are released into the lumina.

Triglycerides are synthesized in the cytoplasm and smooth endoplasmic reticulum of alveolar cells and coalesce into large droplets, which become enveloped in apical plasma membranes and separate as fat globules. Sodium, potassium, and water move into the secretory vesicle in response to osmotic gradients. Chloride and bicarbonates may have active transport systems at the apical membranes to account for the electrolyte disequilibrium (Peaker, 1977, 1978; White et al., 1981).

Milk composition changes dramatically in the first 5 days of lactation. Initially, in pregnancy, breasts secret precolostrum, which has high sodium chloride, lactoferrin, and immunoglobulin concentrations. Colostrum, which is high in immunoglobulin, is secreted for the first 5 days after delivery. Finally, a milk product high in lactose is secreted. Milk proteins are alpha-lactalbumin (30 per cent) lactoferrin (10 to 20 per cent), casein (40 per cent), and immunoglobulin A (IgA) 10 per cent). Other proteins include IgG, IgM, lysozyme, and serum albumin. Less concentrated proteins found in milk include a variety of binding proteins, hormones, and epidermal growth factor (corticosterone-binding protein), vitamin B_{12} binding protein, folate-binding protein, prolactin, and milk fat globule membrane protein. In addition, over 30 enzymes have been identified in human milk. Most of these enzymes are part of the Golgi apparatus secretion (Jenness, 1974; Mather and Keenan, 1975; Waxman and Schreiber, 1975; Payne et al., 1976; Bezkorovainy, 1977; Carpenter, 1980; Mather et al., 1980; Samson et al., 1980; Sandberg et al., 1981; Anderson et al., 1982).

Casein accounts for 40 per cent of the protein secreted by the human breast (Jenness, 1979). Alpha and beta caseins contain proline residues and a carboxyl and phosphate negatively charged end group that commonly interacts with calcium. The opposite end is hydrophobic. Alpha-lactalbumin derived from lysozyme is a cofactor in lactose synthesis and a major source of lactose production. Lactoferrin is an iron-binding protein resembling transferrin. It is concentrated in colostrum and is bacteriostatic and bacteriocidal by binding available iron necessary for bacterial replication (Weinberg, 1978). IgA is present early in lactation, but IgG and IgM are less concentrated in human milk. Serum albumin is present, at a concentration of 2 mg/ml in colostrum, but this changes to 0.5 mg/ml in later stages (Phillippy and McCarthy, 1979). Milk fat globule membranes are enveloped by apical plasma membrane. Xanthine oxidase and butyrophilin are proteins associated with this fat globule membrane. This protein has been found only in the apical surface of mammary epithelium (Franke et al., 1981).

The author of this chapter began physiologic studies of breast tissue in 1972 with an attempt to clinically decrease circulating prolactin levels in women with breast cancer. Twenty per cent of the women with breast cancer metastatic to the bones who had bone pain were given L-dopa (250 mg every 4 hours) and experienced dramatic relief from bone pain and a subsequent long-term clinical benefit from endocrine ablative surgery (Dickey and Minton, 1972 a, b; Minton and Dickey, 1973; Ferrar et al., 1981). These studies implied that in some women with metastatic breast cancer, bone pain could be controlled by serum prolactin suppression using L-dopa as a prolactin inhibiting factor (Minton, 1974, 1976). It was speculated that the decrease in bone pain was due to a lowered cellular metabolism of hormone-sensitive breast cancer cells, reducing the production of the pain-producing prostaglandin E_2 (Kibbey et al., 1979). Studies in experimental animals subjected to hormonal manipulation and prolactin suppression demonstrated significant changes in intratumor prostaglandin levels, which correlated with tumor regression (Foecking et al., 1982, 1983).

The measurement of cAMP levels in normal breast tissue, fibrocystic breast tissue, and breast cancer tissue showed suggestion of a significant increase in cancer tissue (Minton et al., 1979, Ferrar et al., 1981). The cAMP increase in these tissues was not due to an increase in phosphodiesterase, which allegedly inhibits the breakdown of cAMP and results in its build-up. A significant rise occurred in adenylate cyclase activity, suggesting a promotional effect on cAMP production (Foecking et al., 1980; Elliott et al., 1981; Minton et al., 1981a). The observations that the adenylate cyclase level was elevated pointed to the possibility of an endogenous hormonal influence on the activation of the cAMP system, but an analysis of serum estrogen levels did not show a significant difference. Because painful, swollen, and lumpy breasts were associated with elevated cAMP levels and associated protein kinase activities, which led to fibrosis and "fibrocystic disease," a program aimed at abstention from consumption of cAMP activating agents was undertaken (Minton et al., 1979).

Women with "fibrocystic breast disease" were asked to abstain from consumption of methylxanthine-containing products, such as coffee, tea, colas, and chocolate. In a few months (less in younger women), both pain and lumps began to resolve and improvement persisted as long as the patients abstained from methylxanthine consumption (Minton et al.,

1981a). In some women, even after total abstention from caffeine products and after resolution for benign breast disease problems, breast symptoms began to recur. In other women no clear improvement was seen (Minton and Abou-Issa, 1986). Analysis of a careful diet diary of everything these women ate and drank showed that women in whom disease had resolved had made subtle changes in their eating patterns. Women in whom inactive disease was reactivated had begun to consume an increased proportion of tyramine-containing food products. In some cases these were foods that they had neither liked nor eaten frequently prior to abstaining from methylxanthines. Most women could not explain their new preference for these food products. Some noted they experienced a "high" or "kick" from tyramine-containing food products. Tyramine-containing foods include cheese, wine, beer, spices, nuts, mushrooms, bananas, and other, less commonly consumed products, such as pickled herring. In general, these are the food products people with high blood pressure are asked to avoid because of their adverse effects on hypertension.

Other factors, such as nicotine use and emotional and physical stresses, were also found to reactivate fibrocystic breast disease (Fig. 3–1). The changes in breasts after consumption of tyramine food product led the author to measure serum catecholamine levels in women. Methylxanthines, nicotine, and tyramine consumption can elevate serum catecholamines and increase catecholamine release in humans. Methylxanthine and catecholamine levels were measured in women with no breast disease, fibrocystic breast disease, and breast cancer. The results showed that women with benign and malignant breast disease had a higher level of circulating catecholamines than women without breast disease when the circulating levels of methylxanthines were the same (Minton and Abou-Issa, submitted for publication, b) (Table 3–1). This observation suggests a different sensitivity to caffeine for catecholamine release in women with breast disease. Dopamine, the prolactin inhibiting factor, was lower in patients with higher catecholamine levels, implying a reason for the higher prolactin levels in the breast cancer patients observed by Malarkey and colleagues (1977, 1983). Methylxanthine-stimulated increased release of catecholamines and increased circulating catecholamines would have no clinical importance unless receptor activity in the breast tissue for these hormones could be demonstrated. An analysis of the beta-adrenergic receptor sites in normal and benign breast conditions was done to determine if the receptor concentrations were the same in women with benign fibrocystic breast disease and normal breast tissue. A significant increase was demonstrated in fibrocystic breast tissue compared with normal breast tissue. In addition, there appeared to be a supersensitivity to the interaction of catecholamines with beta-adrenergic receptors that induced an avalanche of adenylate cyclase activity and hence increased cAMP and ultimately produced the excess of fluid and fibrosis in breasts deemed to be affected by fibrocystic breast disease (Minton and Abou-Issa, submitted for publication, b) (Fig. 3–2). The possibility that a predisposition for increased beta-receptor concentrations is genetic rather than induced needs further clarification, as does the possibility that the supersensitivity may vary significantly depending on other hormone concentrations (e.g., estrogens) during the menstrual cycle.

Animal studies pointed out a cancer-promoting relationship between fat consumption

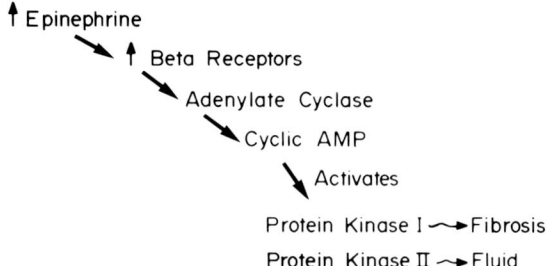

Figure 3–2. Graphic presentation of the response of fibrocystic breast tissue to beta-receptor activation.

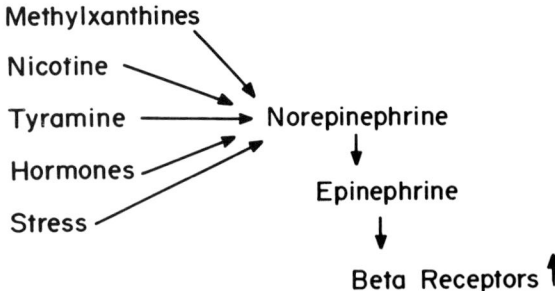

Figure 3–1. Graphic presentation of the factors that may promote fibrocystic disease.

Table 3–1. SERUM METHYLXANTHINES (NG/ML) AND CATECHOLAMINES (PG/ML) IN CONTROLS COMPARED WITH WOMEN WITH MASTALGIA AND BREAST CANCER

	Control	Cyclic Mastalgia	Noncyclic Mastalgia	Breast Cancer
Age	30.4 ± 2.0	33 ± 1.6	42.6 ± 2.8	60.8 ± 3.3
Number	17	30	6	7
Caffeine	2567.8 ± 490	2256.7 ± 327.9 NS	3341 ± 934.5 NS	4949 ± 1016.8S (193%)
Theobromine	413.6 ± 36.4	588.8 ± 89.8 NS	850.2 ± 246.5 S (205%)	819.3 ± 132.2 SSS (198%)
Total methylxanthines	3294.9 ± 517.2	3184.4 ± 412.2 NS	4728.8 ± 907.9 NS	6321.6 ± 1189.4 SS (192%)
Epinephrine	275.6 ± 54.6	1121.2 ± 222.1 SSS (406%)	1623.6 ± 291.1 SSS (589%)	991.5 ± 695.2 NS
Norepinephrine	403.7 ± 61.2	511.9 ± 49.4 S (127%)	907.5 ± 313.2 S (224%)	514.2 ± 55.5 NS
Dopamine	1250.6 ± 265.1	588.8 ± 64.2 SSS (47%)	577 ± 77.1 S (46%)	342.6 ± 60 SSS (27%)
Dopa	267.5 ± 66.4	267.3 ± 31.8 NS	340.5 ± 38 NS	540.0 ± 84 S

NS (not significant): $p > 0.05$
S: $p < 0.05$
SS: $p < 0.01$
SSS: $p < 0.005$

at 40 to 45 per cent of total calorie intake per day and early breast cancer production when animals consuming caffeine were also exposed to a carcinogen (Minton et al., 1981a). A series of animal studies evaluating beta-glucuronidase activity as a carrier of potential carcinogens, as well as cancer promotional agents, such as unbound estrogens, led to the observation that endogenous serum beta-glucuronidase can be lowered in rats with D-glucaric acid, and the anticipated effects of known carcinogens were significantly reduced (Walaszek et al., 1986).

Women with fibrocystic breast disease have been found to have concentrations of beta-glucuronidase in cystic fluid that vary tenfold in different breast cysts. In addition, current studies show that women with breast disease fall into two major categories, those with high serum beta-glucuronidase and those with low serum beta-glucuronidase (Minton et al., submitted for publication, a, b) (Fig. 3–3).

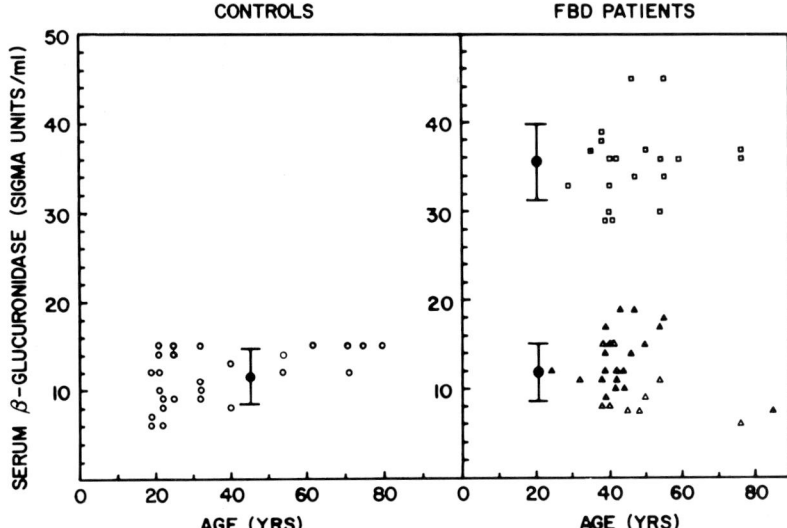

Figure 3–3. Distribution of serum β-glucuronidase levels in Sigma units/ml in patients with fibrocystic breast disease (FBD) and controls.

Women with breast disease fit the stress profile (Bammer and Newberry, 1981). If these women have a genetic mechanism that promotes secretory activity in breast tissue as a result of endogenous catecholamine stimulation of adenylate cyclase and its cascade (Fig. 3–1), and if a subset of these women have a high circulating beta-glucuronidase level and can concentrate exogenous carcinogens consumed in an American diet of high fats, nitrates, and transformed hydrocarbons, it is possible that carcinogenic agents are transported to the breast ductal system, where cancer is known to develop. There is then reasonable probability that over an extended period and after repeated exposures to carcinogenic agents, certain cells will undergo malignant transformation. In addition, caffeines or the other agents that may be consumed by unsuspecting but sensitive individuals who release excessive catecholamines may cause a double effect, decreasing immune surveillance by NK, T, and B cells involved in cancer surveillance (Tonneson et al., 1985; Blazar et al., 1986). Then, cancer cells may propagate unchallenged by the individual's immune defense mechanisms. The end result will be a situation in which the growth of malignant cells may be promoted in a susceptible individual.

Acknowledgments

Studies are supported by funds from The Ohio State University Research Development Fund No. 532809; the Grand Chapter of the Ohio Order of the Eastern Star; National Chapter of the Phi Beta Psi Sorority; National Cancer Institute, American Cancer Society Grant CP-25A, Project 716385.

REFERENCES

Amico, J. A., Seif, S. M., and Robinson, A. G.: Oxytocin in human plasma: Correlation with neurophysin and stimulation with estrogen. J. Clin. Endocrinol. Metab., 52:988, 1981.

Anderson, N. G., Powers, M. T., and Tollaksen, S. L.: Proteins of human milk. I. Identification of major components. Clin. Chem. N.Y., 28:1045, 1982.

Antakly, T., Pelletier, G., Zeytinoglu, F., and Labrie, F.: Changes of cell morphology and prolactin secretion induced by 2-Br-x-ergocyptine, estradiol, and thyrotropin-releasing hormone in rat anterior pituitary cells in culture. J. Cell. Biol., 86:377, 1980.

Antunes, J. L., Housepian, E. M., Frantz, A. B., et al.: Prolactin-secreting pituitary tumors. Ann. Neurol., 2:148, 1977.

Aono, T., Shioji, T., Shoda, T., et al.: The initiation of human lactation and prolactin response to suckling. J. Clin. Endocrinol. Metab., 44:1101, 1977.

Bammer, K., and Newberry B. H. (Eds.): Stress and Cancer. Toronto, C. J. Hogrefe, 1981.

Barowicz, T.: Inhibitory effect of adrenaline on oxytocin release in the ewe during the milk-ejection reflex. J. Dairy Res., 46:41, 1978.

Bartley, J. C., and Abraham, S.: The absolute rate of fatty acid synthesis by mammary gland slices from lactating rats. J. Lipid Res., 17:467, 1976.

Bezkorovainy, A.: Human milk and colostrum proteins: A review. J. Dairy Sci., 60:1023, 1977.

Bigazzi, M., Ronga, R., Lancranjan, I., et al.: Pregnancy in an acromegalic woman during bromocriptine treatment: Effects on growth hormone and prolactin in the maternal, fetal and amniotic compartments. J. Clin. Endocrinol. Metab., 48:9, 1979.

Blazar, B. A., Rodrick, M. L., O'Mahony, J. B., et al.: Suppression of natural killer-cell function in humans following thermal and traumatic injury. J. Clin. Immunol., 6:26, 1986.

Bohnet, H. G., Gomez, F., and Friesen, H. G.: PRL and estrogen binding sites in the mammary gland of the lactating and non-lactating rat. Endocrinology, 101:1111, 1977.

Bolander, F. F., Jr., and Topper, Y. J.: Relationships between spermidine, glucocorticoid and milk proteins in different mammalian species. Biochem. Biophys. Res. Commun., 90:1131, 1979.

Bremel, R. D., and Shaw, M. E.: Actomyosin from mammary myoepithelial cells and phosphorylation by myosin light chain kinase. J. Dairy Sci., 61:1561, 1978.

Brown, R. E.: Relactation with reference to application in developing countries. Clin. Pediatr., 17:333, 1978.

Brun del Re, R., del Pozo, E., de Grandi, P., et al.: Prolactin inhibition and suppression of puerperal lactation by Br-ergo cryptine (CB154). A comparison with estrogen. Obstet. Gynecol., 41:884, 1973.

Carpenter, G.: Epidermal growth factor is a major growth promoting agent in human milk. Science, 210:198, 1980.

Carr, B. R., Parker, C. R., Jr., Madden, J. D., et al.: Maternal plasma adrenocorticotropin and cortisol relationships throughout human pregnancy. Am. J. Obstet. Gynecol., 139:416, 1981.

Clarke, G., and Merrick, L. P.: A tentative identification of the synaptic transmitters involved in the neural regulation of oxytocin release. J. Physiol., 277:19, 1978.

Cowie, A. T.: Backward glances. In Yokoyama, A., Mizuno, H., and Nagasawa, H. (Eds.): Physiology of Mammary Glands. Baltimore, University Park Press, 1978, p. 43.

Davis, J. W., Wilkman-Coffelt, J., and Eddington, C. L.: The effect of progesterone on biosynthetic pathways in mammary tissue. Endocrinology, 91:1011, 1972.

De Hertogh, R., Thomas, K., Bietlot, Y., et al.: Plasma levels of unconjugated estrone, estradiol and estriol and of HCS throughout pregnancy in normal women. J. Clin. Endocrinol. Metab., 40:93, 1975.

Del Pozo, E., Hiba, J., Lancranjan, I., et al.: Prolactin measurements throughout the life cycle. In Crosignani, P.G., and Robyn, C. (Eds.): Prolactin and Human Reproduction. London, Academic Press, 1977, p. 61.

Del Pozo, E., and Brownell, J.: Prolactin: I. Mechanisms of control, peripheral actions and modification by drugs. Horm. Res., 10:143, 1979.

Delvoye, P., Demaegd, M., Delogne-Desnoeck, Jr., et al.: The influence of the frequency of nursing and of previous lactation experience on serum prolactin in lactating mothers. J. Biosoc. Sci., 9:447, 1977.

Devinoy, E., and Houdebine, L.-M.: Effects of glucocorticoids on casein gene expression in the rabbit. Eur. J. Biochem., 75:411, 1977.

Dickey, R. P., and Minton, J. P.: Levodopa relief of bone pain from breast cancer. N. Engl. J. Med., 286:843, 1972a.

Dickey, R. P., and Minton, J. P.: L-Dopa effect on prolactin, follicle-stimulating hormone, and luteinizing hormone in women with advanced breast cancer: A preliminary report. Am. J. Obstet. Gynecol., 114:266, 1972b.

Djiane, J., and Durand, P.: Prolactin-progesterone antagonism in self-regulation of prolactin receptors in the mammary gland. Nature, 266:641, 1977.

du Vigneaud, V., Ressler, C., Swan, J. M., et al.: The synthesis of oxytocin. J. Am. Chem. Soc., 76:3115, 1954.

Edwards, D. P., Chamness, G. C., and McGuire, W. L.: Estrogen and progesterone receptor proteins in breast cancer. Biochim. Biophys. Acta, 560:457, 1979.

Elliot, J., Abou-Issa, H., Foecking, M. K., et al.: Cyclic nucleotides as predictors of benign to malignant progression of breast disease. Breast, 7:6, 1981.

Ferrar, J. J., Reiches, N. A., and Minton, J. P.: Endocrine ablation in breast cancer patients who have failed cytotoxic therapy. J. Surg. Oncol., 18:231, 1981.

Fluckiger, E. W.: Lactation inhibition by ergot drugs. In Yokoyama, A., Mizuno, H., and Nagasawa, H. (Eds.): Physiology of Mammary Gland. Baltimore, University Park Press, 1978, p. 71.

Foecking, M. K., Minton, J. P., and Matthews, R. H.: Progressive patterns in breast diseases. Med. Hypotheses, 6:659, 1980.

Foecking, M. K., Kibbey, W. E., Abou-Issa, H., et al.: Hormone dependence of dimethylbenz(a)anthracene-induced mammary tumor growth; correlation with prostaglandin E2 content. J. Natl. Cancer Inst., 69:443, 1982.

Foecking, M. K., Abou-Issa, H., Webb, T., et al.: Concurrent changes in growth-related biochemical parameters during regression of hormone dependent rat mammary tumors. J. Natl. Cancer Inst. 71:773, 1983.

Folley, S. J., and Malpress, F. H.: Hormonal control of lactation. In Pincus, G. (Ed.): The Hormones. Vol. 1. New York, Academic Press, 1948, p. 745.

Franke, W. W., Heid, H. W., Grund, C., et al.: Antibodies in the major insoluble milk fat globule membrane-associated protein: Specific location in apical regions of lactating epithelial cells. J. Cell. Biol., 89:485, 1981.

Franks, S., Kiwi, R., and Nabarro, J. D. N.: Pregnancy and lactation after pituitary surgery. Br. Med. J., 1:882, 1977.

Ganguly, R., Majumder, P. K., Ganguly, N., et al.: The mechanism of progesterone-glucocorticoid interaction in regulation of casein gene expression. J. Biol. Chem., 257:2182, 1982.

Greenbaum, A. L., Sochor, M., and McLean, P.: Regulation of mammary gland metabolism, pathways of glucose utilization, metabolic profile and hormone response of a modified mammary gland cell preparation. Eur. J. Biochem., 878:505, 1978.

Gross, B. A., and Eastman, C. J.: Prolactin secretion during prolonged lactational amenorrhoea. Aust. N.Z.J. Obstet. Gynaecol., 19:95, 1979.

Guyette, W. A., Matusik, R. J., and Rosen, J. M.: Prolactin-mediated transcriptional and post-transcriptional control of casein gene expression. Cell, 17:1013, 1979.

Halban, J.: Die innere Secretion von Ovarium und Placenta und ihre Bedeutung fur die Function der Milchdruse. Arch. Gynaek., 75:353, 1905.

Hartmann, P. E., and Kulski, J. K.: Changes in the composition of the mammary secretion of women after abrupt termination of breast feeding. J. Physiol., 275:1, 1978.

Hertz, J., Anderson, A. N., and Larsen, J. F.: Correlation between prolactin and progesterone, oestradiol 17B and oestriol during early human pregnancy. Clin. Endocrinol., 9:97, 1978.

Hiba, J., Del Pozo, E., Genazzani, A., et al.: Hormonal mechanism of milk secretion in the newborn. J. Clin. Endocrinol. Metab., 44:973, 1977.

Houdebine, L.-M., Djiane, J., and Clauser, H.: Endocrinologie—rôle des lysosomes, des micro-tubules, et des microfilaments dans le mécanisme de l'action lactogène de la prolactine sur la glande mammaire de lapine. C. R. Acad. Sci. Ser. D., 289:679, 1979.

Houdebine, L.-M., and Djiane, J.: Effects of lysomotropic agents, and of microfilament- and microtubule-disrupting drugs on the activation of casein-gene expression by prolactin in the mammary gland. Mol. Cell. Endocrinol., 17:1, 1980.

Jenness, R.: The composition of milk. In Larson, B. L., and Smith, V. R. (Eds.): Lactation: A Comprehensive Treatise. Vol. III. New York, Academic Press, 1974, p. 3.

Jenness, R.: The composition of human milk. Semin. Perinatol., 3:225, 1979.

Kauppila, A., Kivinen, S., and Ylikorkala, O.: Metoclopramide increases prolactin release and milk secretion in puerperium without stimulating the secretion of thyrotropin and thyroid hormones. J. Clin. Endocrinol. Metab., 52:436, 1981.

Kibbey, W. E., Bronn, D. G., and Minton, J. P.: Prostaglandin synthetase and prostaglandin E2 levels in human breast carcinoma. Prostaglandins and Medicine, 2:133, 1979.

Kuhn, N. J.: Progesterone withdrawal as the lactogenic trigger in the rat. J. Endocrinol., 44:39, 1969.

Kuhn, N. J.: Lactogenesis: The search for trigger mechanisms in different species. Symp. Zool. Soc. (Lond.), 41:165, 1977.

Labrie, F., Ferland, L., Di Paolo, T., et al.: Modulation of prolactin secretion by sex steroids and thyroid hormones. In MacLeod, R., and Scapagnini, U. (Eds.): Central and Peripheral Regulation of Prolactin Function. New York, Raven Press, 1980, p. 97.

Leclerg, G., and Heuson, J. C.: Physiological and pharmacological effects of estrogens in breast cancer. Biochim. Biophys. Acta, 560:427, 1979.

Lemarchand-Beraud, T., Reymond, M., Berthier, C., et al.: Effects of oestrogens on prolactin and TSHA secretion in women. In Crosignant, P. G., and Robyn, C. (Eds.): Prolactin and Human Reproduction. London, Academic Press, 1977, p. 135.

Lloyd, H. M., Meares, J. D., and Jacobi, J.: Effects of oestrogen and bromocryptine on in vivo secretion and mitosis in prolactin cells. Nature, 255:497, 1975.

Lyons, W. R.: Hormonal synergism in mammary growth. Proc. R. Soc. Lond. Ser. B, 149:303, 1958.

McManus, M. J., and Welsch, C. W.: DNA synthesis of benign human breast tumors in the untreated athymic "nude" mouse. Cancer, 45:2160, 1980.

McNeilly, A. S., and Friesen, H. G.: Binding of prolactin to the rabbit mammary gland during pregnancy. J. Endocrinol., 74:507, 1977.

Malarkey, W. B., Schroeder, L. L., Stevens, V. C., et al.: Disordered nocturnal prolactin regulation in women with breast cancer. Cancer Res., 37:4650, 1977.

Malarkey W. B., Kennedy, M., Allred, L. E., et al.: Physiologic concentrations of prolactin can promote growth of human breast tumor cells in culture, J. Clin Endocrinol. Metabol., 56:673, 1983.

Mather, I. H., and Keenan, T. W.: Studies on the structure of milk fat globule membrane. J. Membr. Biol., 21:65, 1975.

Mather, I. H., Tamplin, C. B., and Irving, M. G.: Separation of the proteins of bovine milk-fat-globule membrane by electrofocusing with retention of enzymatic and immunological activity. Eur. J. Biochem., 110:327, 1980.

Mills, E. S., and Topper, Y. J.: Some ultrastructural effects of insulin, hydrocortisone, and prolactin on mammary gland explants. J. Cell Biol., 44:310, 1970.

Minton, J. P.: Prolactin and human breast cancer. Am. J. Surg., 128:628, 1974.

Minton, J. P.: Precise selection of breast cancer patients with bone metastasis for endocrine ablation. Surgery, 80:513, 1976.

Minton, J. P., and Abou-Issa, H.: Fibrocystic breast disease—its management and explanation. In Najarian, J. S., and Delaney, J. P. (Eds.): Advances in Breast and Endocrine Surgery. Chicago, Year Book Medical Publishers, 1986, p. 15.

Minton, J. P., and Abou-Issa, H.: Increased β-adrenergic adenylate cyclase activity in human fibrocystic breast disease. Surgery (submitted for publication, b).

Minton, J. P., and Dickey, R. R.: Levodopa test to predict response of carcinoma of the breast to surgical ablation of endocrine glands. Surg. Gynecol. Obstet., 136:971, 1973.

Minton, J. P., Abou-Issa, H., Elliot, J. B., et al.: Biochemical subgrouping of benign breast disease to define premalignant potential. Surgery, 90:652, 1981a.

Minton, J. P., Foecking, M. K., Webster, D. J. T., et al.: Response of fibrocystic disease to caffeine withdrawal and correlation of cyclic nucleotides with breast disease. Am. J. Obstet. Gynecol., 135:157, 1979.

Minton, J. P., Walaszek, Z., Schooley, W., et al.: β-Glucuronidase levels in patients with fibrocystic breast disease. Br. Cancer Res. Treat. (submitted for publication, a).

Moos, F., and Richard, P.: The inhibitory role of β-adrenergic receptors in oxytocin release during suckling. Brain Res., 169:595, 1979.

Morris, J. F., Sokol, H. W., and Valtin, H.: One neuron-one hormone. Recent evidence from Brattleboro rats. In Moses, A. M., and Share, L. (Eds.): International Conference on the Neurohypophysis. New York, Karger, 1977, p. 58.

Nicoll, C. S., and Bern, H. A.: On the actions of prolactin among the vertebrates: Is there a common denominator? In Wolstenholme, G. E. N. and Knight, J. (Eds.): Lactogenic Hormones, Ciba Foundation Symposium. Edinburgh, Churchill Livingstone, 1972, p. 299.

Nolin, J. M.: Target cell prolactin. In McKerns, K. W. (Ed.): Structure and Function of the Gonadotropins. New York, Plenum Press, 1978, p. 151.

Nolin, J. M., and Witorsch, R. J.: Detection of endogenous immunoreactive prolactin in rat mammary epithelial cells during lactation. Endocrinology, 99:949, 1976.

Owerbach, D., Rutter, W. J., Martial, J. A., et al.: Genes for growth hormone, chorionic somatomammotropin and growth hormone-like gene are on chromosome 17 in humans. Science 209: 289, 1980.

Payne, D. W., Peng, L.-H., Pearlman, W. H., et al.: Corticosteroid-binding proteins in human colostrum and milk and rat milk. J. Biol. Chem., 251:5272, 1976.

Peaker, M.: The aqueous phase of milk; Ion and water transport. In Peaker, M. (Ed.): Comparative Aspects of Lactation. New York, Academic Press, 1977, p. 113.

Peaker, M.: Ion and water transport in the mammary gland. In Peaker, M. (Ed.): Lactation: A Comprehensive Treatise. New York, Academic Press, 1978, p. 437.

Phillippy, B. O., and McCarthy, R. D.: Multi-origins of milk serum albumin in the lactating goat. Biochim. Biophys. Acta, 584:298, 1979.

Potter, E., Nicolaisen, A. K., Ong, E. S., et al.: Thyrotropin-releasing hormone exerts rapid nuclear effects to increase production of the primary prolactin mRNA transcript. Proc. Natl. Acad. Sci. USA, 78:6662, 1981.

Poulain, D. A., Wakerly, J. B., and Dyball, R. E. J.: Electrophysiological differentiation of oxytocin and vasopressin-secreting neurons. Proc. R. Soc. Lond., Ser. B, 196:367, 1977.

Raymond, V., Beaulieu, M., Labrie, F., et al.: Potent antidopaminergic activity of estradiol at the pituitary level on prolactin release. Science, 200:1173, 1978.

Rigg, L. A., Lein, A., and Yen, S. S. C.: Pattern of increase in circulating prolactin levels during human gestation. Am. J. Obstet. Gynecol., 129:454, 1977.

Robinson, A. G., Seif, S. M., Huellmantel, A. B., et al.: Physiologic and pathologic secretion of neurphysins in the rat. In Moses, A. M., and Share, L. (Eds.): International Conference on the Neurohypophysis. New York, S. Karger, 1977, p. 136.

Robinson, A. M., Girard, J. R., and Williamson, D. H.: Evidence for a role of insulin in the regulation of lipogenesis in lactating rat mammary gland. Biochem. J., 176:343, 1978.

Robyn, C., Delvoye, P., Van Exter, C., et al.: Physiological and pharmacological factors influencing prolactin secretion and their relation to human reproduction. In Crosignani, P. G., and Robyn, C. (Eds.): Prolactin and Human Reproduction. London, Academic Press, 1977, p. 17.

Rosner, M. D.: Galactorrhea in men. J.A.M.A., 1:1327, 1979.

Rosen, J. M., O'Neal, D. L., McHugh, J. E., et al.: Progesterone-mediated inhibition of casein mRNA and polysomal casein synthesis in the rat mammary gland during pregnancy. Biochemistry, 17:290, 1978.

Samson, R., Mirtle, C., and McClelland, D. B. L.: The effect of digestive enzymes on the binding and bacteriostatic properties of lactoferrin and vitamin B_{12} binder in human milk. Acta Paediatr. Scand., 59:517, 1980.

Sand, O., Haug, E., and Gautvik, K. M.: Effects of thyroliberin and H-aminopyridine in action potentials and prolactin release and synthesis in rat pituitary cells in culture. Acta Physiol. Scand., 108:247, 1980.

Sandberg, D. P., Begley, J. A., and Hall, C. A.: The content, binding, and forms of vitamin B_{12} in milk. Am. J. Clin. Nutr., 34:1717, 1981.

Sapag-Hagar, M., and Greenbaum, A. L.: Adenosine 3':5'-monophosphate and hormone interrelationships in the mammary gland of the rat during pregnancy and lactation. Eur. J. Biochem., 47:303, 1974.

Shiu, R. P. C.: Processing of prolactin by human breast cancer cells in long term tissue culture. J. Biol. Chem., 255:4278, 1980.

Shyamala, G., and Nandi, S.: Interactions of 6,7-^{3}H-17β estradiol with the mouse lactating mammary tissue in vivo and in vitro. Endocrinology, 91:861, 1972.

Shyamala, G.: Glucocorticoid receptors in mouse mammary tumors: Specific binding to nuclear components. Biochemistry, 14:437, 1975.

Shyamala, G., and Dickson, C.: Relationship between receptor and mammary tumor virus production after stimulation by glucocorticoid. Nature, 262:107, 1976.

Singh, D. V., and Bern, H. A.: Interaction between prolactin and thyroxine in mouse mammary gland lobulo-alveolar development in vitro. J. Endocrinol., 45:579, 1969.

Speake, B. K., Dils, R., and Mayer, R. J.: Regulation of enzyme turnover during tissue differentiation. Interactions of insulin, prolactin and cortisol in controlling the turnover of fatty acid synthetase in rabbit mammary gland in organ culture. Biochem. J., 154:359, 1976.

Strong, C. R., Forsyth, I., and Dils, R.: The effects of hormones on milk-fat synthesis in mammary explants from pseudo-pregnant rabbits. Biochem. J., 128:509, 1972.

Teyssot, B., and Houdebine, L.-M.: Role of PRL in the transcription of B-casein and 28S ribosomal genes in the rabbit mammary gland. Eur. J. Biochem., 110:236, 1980.

Teyssot, B., and Houdebine, L.-M.: Role of progesterone and glucocorticoids in the transcription of the B-casein and 28-S ribosomal genes in the rabbit mammary gland. Eur. J. Biochem., 114:597, 1981.

Theodosin, D. T., and Dreifus, J. J.: Ultrastructural evidence for exo-endocytosis in the neurohypophysis. In Moses, A. M., and Share, L. (Eds.): International Conference on the Neurohypophysis. New York, S. Karger, 1977, p. 88.

Tonnesen, E., Brinklov, M. D., Schou, O. A., et al.: Natural killer cell activity in a patient undergoing open-heart surgery complicated by an acute myocardial infarction. Acta Pathol. Microbiol. Immunol. Scand. [C], 93: 229, 1985.

Topper, Y. J., and Freeman, C. S.: Multiple hormone interactions in the developmental biology of the mammary gland. Physiol. Rev., 60:1049, 1980.

Tulchinsky, D., Hobel, C. J., Yeager, E., et al.: Plasma estrone, estradiol, progesterone, and 17-hydroxyprogesterone in human pregnancy. Am. J. Obstet. Gynecol., 112:1095, 1972.

Turkington, R. W., and Hill, R. L.: Lactose synthetase: Progesterone inhibition of the induction of x-lactalbumin. Science, 163:1458, 1969.

Vincent, J. D., Dufy, B., Gourdji, D., et al.: Electrical correlates of prolactin secretion in cloned pituitary cells. In MacLeod, R., and Scapagnini, U. (Eds.): Central and Peripheral Regulation of Prolactin Function. New York, Raven Press, 1980, p. 141.

Vonderhaar, B. K.: Lactose synthetase activity in mouse mammary glands is controlled by thyroid hormones. J. Cell Biol., 82:675, 1979.

Walaszek, Z., Hanausek-Walaszek, M., Minton, J. P., et al.: Dietary glucarate as anti-promoter of 7,12-dimethylbenz(a)anthracene-induced mammary tumorigenesis. Carcinogenesis, 7:1464, 1986.

Wang, D. Y., Hallowes, R. C., Bealing, J., et al.: The effect of prolactin and growth hormone on fatty acid synthesis by pregnant mouse mammary gland in organ culture. J. Endocrinol., 53:311, 1972.

Waxman, S., and Schreiber, C.: The purification and characterization of the low molecular weight human folate binding protein using affinity chromatography. Biochemistry, 14:5422, 1975.

Weinberg, E. D.: Iron and infection. Microbiol. Rev., 42:45, 1978.

White, M. D., Ward, S., and Kuhn, N. J.: Composition, stability and electrolyte permeability of Golgi membranes from lactating rat mammary gland. Biochem. J., 200:663, 1981.

Yang, J., Guzman, R., Richards, J., et al.: Growth factor- and cyclic nucleotide-induced proliferation of normal and malignant mammary epithelial cells in primary culture. Endocrinology, 107:35, 1980.

Zimmerman, E. A., and Defendini, R.: Hypothalamic pathways containing oxytocin, vasopressin and associated neurophysins. In Moses, A. M., and Share, L. (Eds.): International Conference on the Neurohypophysis. New York, S. Karger, 1977, p. 22.

CHAPTER 4

JOHN S. SPRATT
WILLIAM L. DONEGAN
RICHARD A. GREENBERG

Epidemiology and Etiology

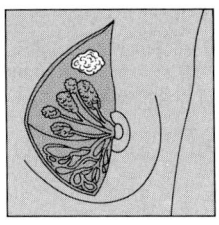

Cancer of the breast occurs most frequently in mice, rats, dogs, and humans, and almost exclusively affects the females of the species. Among humans it is widely distributed throughout the world. Few diseases have had the intense epidemiologic study accorded mammary cancer; as a result, much information is available from the United States as well as from numerous other countries. Beyond simply defining the magnitude of the problem, epidemiologic studies have identified characteristics that place individuals at high risk for this cancer and have provided clues to its etiology.

Mortality

Breast lumps were described by the Egyptians several thousand years before Christ; after 400 B.C., Greek and Roman physicians accurately described lethal tumors of the breast, but their frequency is unknown (Farrow, 1971). Cancer of the breast led cancer deaths in women from 1948 until 1985, when it was exceeded by cancer of the lung. It is now the third leading cause of cancer death in the United States, exceeded only by cancer of the lung and of the colorectum.

The estimated number of newly diagnosed invasive carcinomas in the breast in the United States in 1987 was 900 males and 130,000 females. The estimated number of deaths attributable to breast cancer in the United States in 1987 was 300 males and 41,000 females (ACS, 1987).

This results in an age-adjusted death rate of 27.1 per 100,000 women, placing the United States fourteenth among 48 nations. The highest death rate is 33.8 per 100,000 women in England and Wales, and the lowest is Nicaragua, with a rate of 0.4 per 100,000 women. In the United States there has been no significant change in this rate since 1930.

Silverberg (1985) concluded that 26 per cent of all new cancer cases and 18 per cent of cancer deaths in women in 1985 would be related to breast cancer. Citing the actual number of breast cancer–related deaths in the United States in 1981, he concluded that there would be 36,483 deaths with strong age dependence—15 to 34 years (665), 35 to 54 years (7947), 55 to 74 years (18,645), and 75+ years (9219). The estimated lifelong probability for eventually developing a breast cancer among girls born in 1987 is 10 per cent and of eventually dying of breast cancer is 3 per cent. However, this risk varies with both age and race (Table 4–1).

Readers interested in the history and current status of various sources of vital statistics on the incidence, mortality, and distribution of cancer in the United States and around the world are referred to Guinee (1985).

As already stated, the annual death rate for women, adjusted on the 1940 United States Census population, has not diminished since 1930. Rather, it has risen slightly, from 21 to 27.1 deaths per 100,000 women. In 1948, breast cancer exceeded cancer of the uterus as the leading cause of cancer deaths in women and remained the predominant cause until 1985 (Fig. 4–1). Except at the extremes of age it maintains preeminence, surpassed only in girls under 15 years of age by leukemia and in

Table 4-1. PROBABILITY OF DYING OF CANCER OF THE FEMALE BREAST WITHIN SPECIFIED PERIODS OF TIME FOR WOMEN AT SELECTED AGES WITH PREVIOUSLY UNDIAGNOSED CANCER OF THE BREAST*

Period of Time	White Women	Black Women
Age 20		
Within 10 years	0.00	0.02
Within 20 years	0.09	0.15
Eventually	3.05	3.11
Age 35		
Within 10 years	0.14	0.21
Within 20 years	0.56	0.72
Eventually	3.56	2.98
Age 50		
Within 10 years	0.33	0.35
Within 20 years	1.04	0.93
Eventually	2.75	2.14
Age 65		
Within 10 years	0.43	0.26
Within 20 years	1.01	0.78
Eventually	1.53	1.14

*Adapted from Seidman, H., et al.: Probabilities of eventually developing or dying of cancer—United States, 1985. CA, 35:36, 1985. Used with permission.

women over 74 years of age by colorectal cancer. Its ravages are such that among women 40 to 44 years of age it exceeds all other causes of death, interrupting many otherwise vigorous and healthy lives.

Age-specific death rates generally mirror the curves of incidence, showing a steady rise during the premenopausal years beginning in the third decade of life and continuing to rise after menopause, but at a diminished rate (Fig. 4-2). At age 80 years, approximately 130 breast cancer deaths are recorded annually per 100,000 females. Age-specific death rates have not changed significantly for any one age group during the last four decades. In men, deaths are negligible before age 40 years, but rise thereafter parallel to, but far below, the postmenopausal slope for women.

Mortality rates in the nonwhite United States population are similar to those for the white population. Ninety-two per cent of the nonwhite United States population is black, and the 7000 new cases of breast cancer estimated yearly in this population constitute 22.6 per cent of all cancers in black females, a figure only slightly less than the 26.6 per cent in white females. Statistics for 1978 reflect a death rate of 27.1 per 100,000, with little difference in mortality rates between white and nonwhite women in the United States (Silverberg, 1985). The gap that previously existed, showing low rates for the nonwhite population, has been closed, probably a result, in part, of more complete reporting. In view of the low breast cancer mortality rates generally reported from black nations and the association of breast cancer with high socioeconomic status, however, it is interesting to speculate that some of this increase may reflect environmental influences or increasing affluence of the black population in the United States. The increase has been noted in almost all age groups.

In 1975 the Epidemiology Branch of the National Cancer Institute published an atlas of death rates from breast cancer for the white population by county of residence for the continental United States, which clearly demonstrated a remarkable concentration of mortality in the northeastern part of the country, particularly in urban areas (Fig. 4-3). The geographic tie with urbanization and indus-

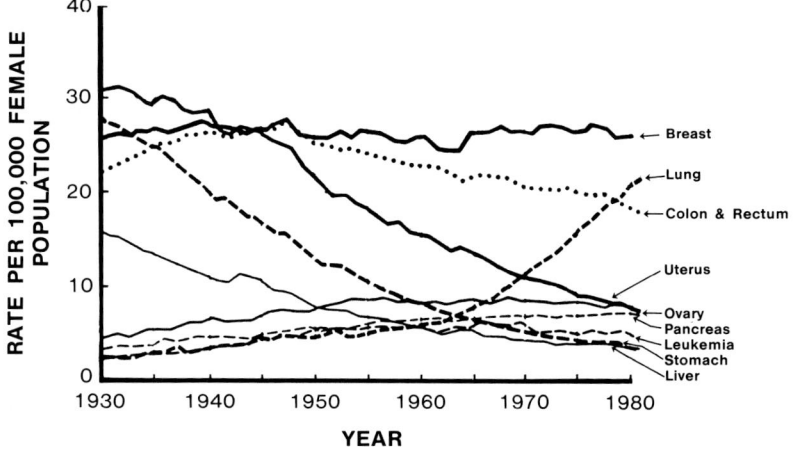

Figure 4-1. Age-adjusted cancer death rates for the female population, United States, 1930–1981. (From Silverberg, E.: Cancer Statistics—1985. CA 35:19, 1985. Used with permission.)

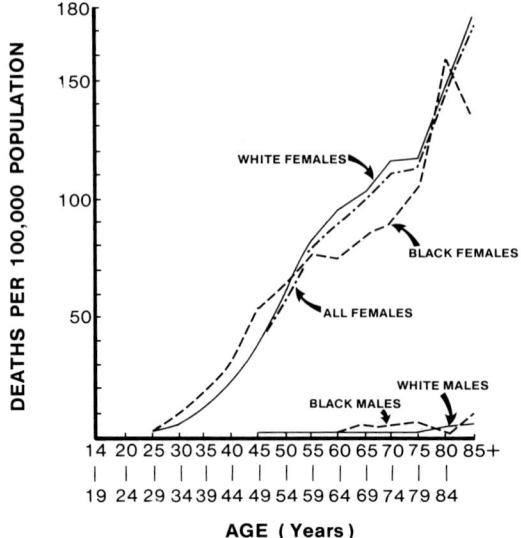

*SEER; Cancer Incidence and Mortality in the United States 1973-81
NIH Publication No. 85-1837

Figure 4–2. Age-specific average death rate from breast cancer in the United States.

trialization suggests environmental causes for this disease. Although exposure to carcinogens might be inferred from the association, it should be noted that Japan is a highly urban and industrialized nation, yet it has a remarkably low national death rate from breast cancer.

Striking differences are evident in international breast cancer death rates. Figure 4–4 shows rates for 42 countries. Notable are the highest rate in Denmark and the low rates in Japan and Honduras, which are respectively only one fifth and one fiftieth that in Denmark. Mortality rates are steady or rising in most countries.

Changing mortality in migrant populations strengthens the inferences that environments or life styles are important determinants of breast cancer risk. Japanese living in the continental United States or Hawaii have higher mortality rates from breast cancer than do Japanese living in Japan, and the rates are higher for Japanese born in the United States (Nisei) than for immigrants who were born in Japan (Issei) (Seidman, 1972).

Moolgavkar and colleagues (1979, 1980, 1984), using data from various sources, concluded that whereas the incidence rates of female breast cancer vary in different parts of the world, the "shapes of the age-specific incidence curves were remarkably similar."

These curves show a steady increase in the age-specific incidence rates from first appearance in the young adult to the end of life. A transient dip in incidence might occur at menopause. In the Japanese, there is an unexplained decrease after menopause (see Fig. 4–6).

Fox (1979) made the interesting observation that the reported incidence of breast cancer increased by 18 per cent between 1935 and 1965 but increased by 50 per cent between 1965 and 1975. The mortality rate, however, remained unchanged and constant over 40 years. In breaking these data down he observed that only about 40 per cent of the women afflicted with breast cancer had a fatal illness. The other 60 per cent had a much more benign disease with a relative mortality rate only moderately different from women of the same age without cancer. He observed that the "increasing detection of an entity that is histologically defined as malignant but biologically relatively benign could account for the observed increase in incidence." Evidence continues to be accumulated that supports this conclusion, as discussed in the chapter on screening and follow-up and that on growth rates. Manton and Stallard (1980) developed a model to include time from tumor initiation to death, the competing risk effects of other disease, and differential susceptibility to disease components. They observed that the age distribution from premenopausal breast cancer deaths was similar to the patterns in non-Western countries. However, the incidence of postmenopausal disease in non-Western countries was lower, and they hypothesized that the difference could be due to nutritional factors.

Incidence

At present, an estimated 130,900 new cases of breast cancer occur in the United States annually for both sexes combined. Breast cancers are exceeded only by cancer of the skin, colorectum, and lung. Women accounted for 130,000 of the new cases, for an annual rate of 75.5 cases per 100,000 females. Since 1947 the incidence has increased 3.6 per cent, to 26.6 per cent for white women and 22.6 per cent for black women. A woman's lifetime risk of developing this cancer is at present 1 in 10.

Risk for the disease is strongly age-related. The age-specific incidence (i.e., the number of

4 • Epidemiology and Etiology   49

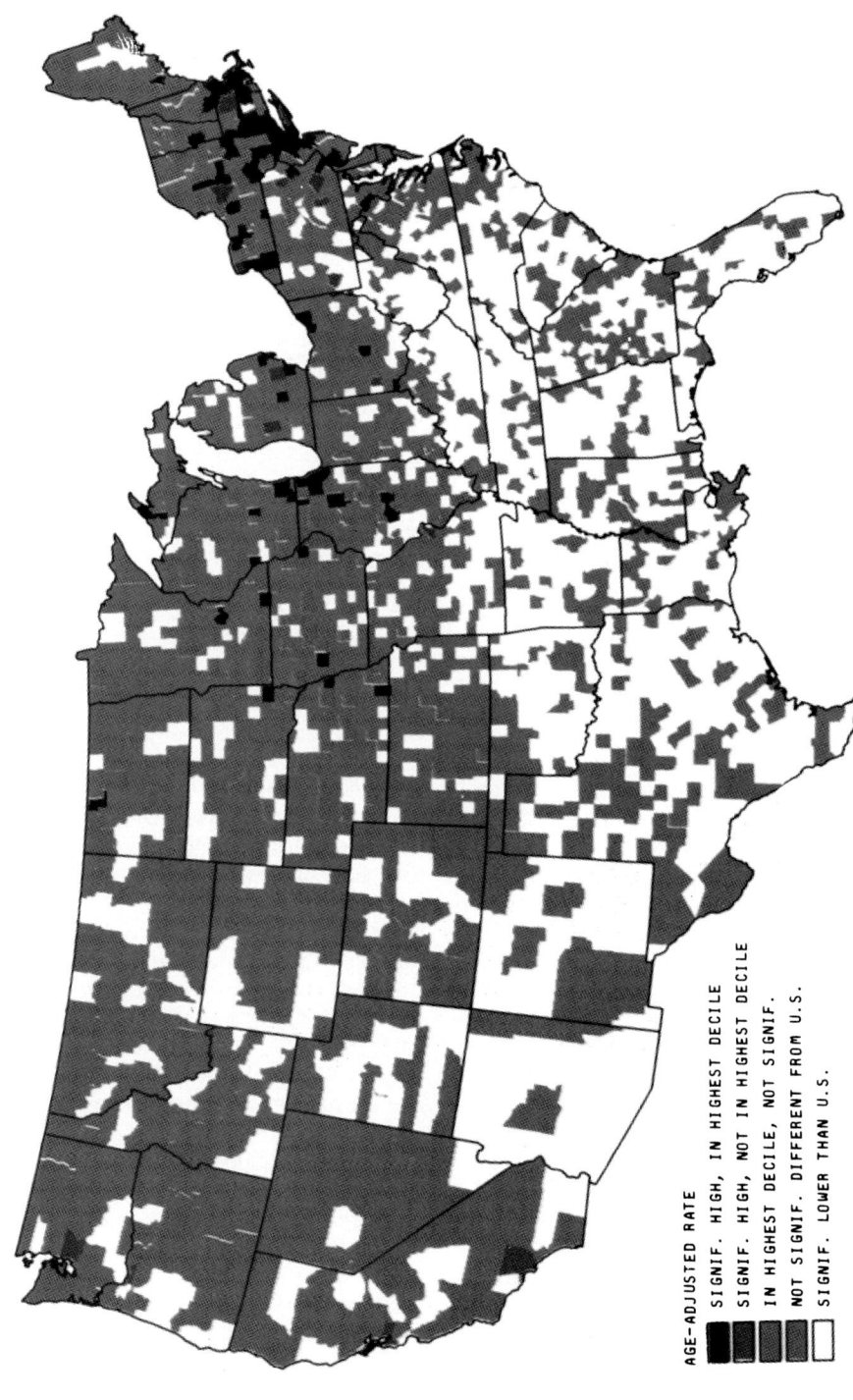

Figure 4–3. Breast cancer mortality rates for white women, 1950 to 1969, by county. (Department of Health, Education and Welfare.)

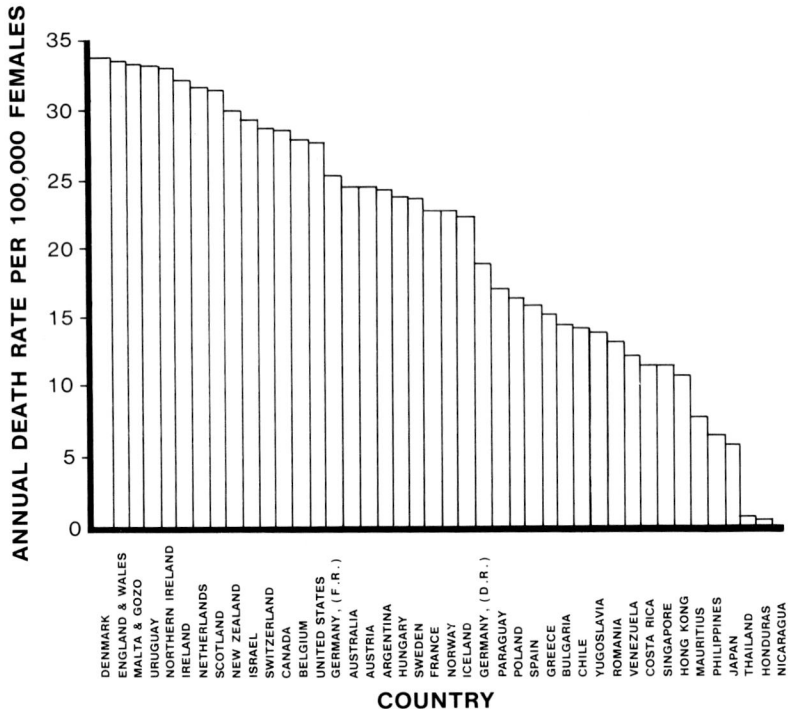

Figure 4–4. Age-standardized female breast cancer death rates for 42 countries, 1976 to 1977. (Redrawn after Seidman, H., and Mushinski, M. H.: In Feig, S. A., and McLelland, R. [Eds.]: Breast Carcinoma: Current Diagnosis and Treatment. New York, Masson, 1983, p. 9.)

cases per year per 100,000 women in each age group), displays a progressive rise with increasing age. Characteristic of the curve is a rapid climb during reproductive years after age 30 years, an abrupt and temporary dip at the time of menopause (Clemmesen's hook), and a continued rise at a slower rate during the postmenopausal years. The change in the slope of the curve at menopause suggests an underlying age-related incidence on which is superimposed an accelerated rate during the hormonally active reproductive years. DeWaard (1969) interpreted the peculiarities of the curve as evidence of a bimodal age distribution caused by a change from ovarian to adrenal hormonal predominance at menopause. The observation that most patients with cancer of the breast are in the sixth and seventh decades of life is not inconsistent with the progressive rise of risk with age. The elderly represent a relatively small segment of the total population, with the result that younger age groups contribute a greater absolute number of cases. During the years 1967 to 1979, 68 per cent of 961 breast cancer patients at the Medical College of Wisconsin affiliated hospitals were between 40 and 70 years of age, with those over 80 years old representing only 7 per cent of the total. The average age was 60 years (Fig. 4–5).

As illustrated in Figure 4–6, the major differences in international incidence and death rates occurred in postmenopausal women. In the United States, the age-specific mortality continues to rise after menopause at only a slightly reduced rate, whereas among Japanese the incidence declines after menopause and continues to do so as age advances.

Bailar and Smith (1985) analyzed trends in various reports of incidence and mortality data on cancer. With respect to breast cancer, they made the following observations: The incidence rates of breast cancer showed a sharp increase in 1974, but a lower rise in subsequent years. The 1974 spike coincided with the "public disclosure that the wives of the President and Vice President had breast cancer," following which a major public effort to screen for breast cancer was promoted. Because this was associated with no impact on country-wide

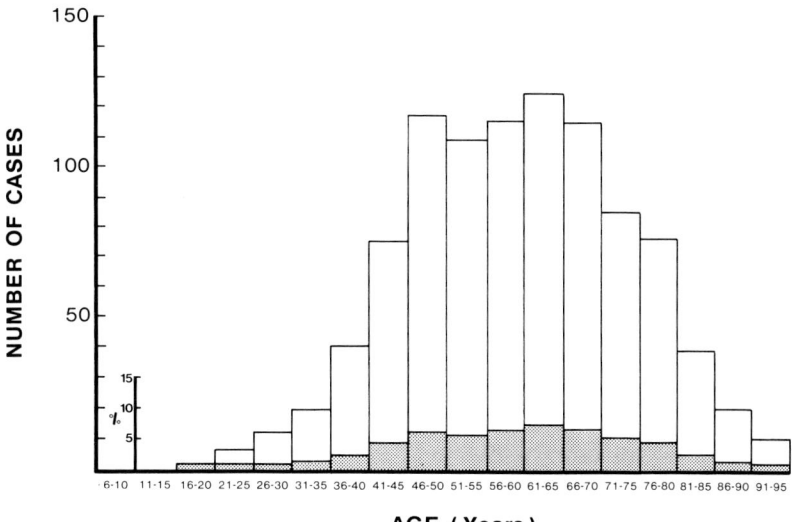

Figure 4–5. Age distribution of 961 patients with breast cancer, 1967–1979, Milwaukee, Wisconsin.

breast cancer mortality rates or in case survival rates, a shift in diagnostic criteria is strongly suggested. The possibility that such a shift in diagnostic criteria might occur with very early breast cancer is discussed in the chapter on screening.

Possible Etiologic Factors

GENETIC AND FAMILIAL ASPECTS

Indications that breast cancer risk is genetically influenced are found in its association with genetically determined traits and medical conditions, racial predispositions, and familial tendencies. In many instances, environmental factors cannot be excluded in accounting for some or all of the observed phenomena.

The high frequency of breast cancer in men with Klinefelter's syndrome (with eunuchoidism, gynecomastia, testicular atrophy, and aspermia) is associated with the extra X chromosome that characterizes these individuals (i.e., XXY). The incidence of breast cancer in Klinefelter's syndrome is said to be 66 times the usual rate in men, approaching the frequency in women. Possibly 3.3 per cent of men with breast cancer have this syndrome (Mulvihill, 1975). Rather than constituting a specific marker for breast cancer, however, the extra X chromosome in these individuals probably serves to increase the risk of female-related diseases generally.

Other genetic associations are known. Breast cancer may appear as one component of a symptom complex associated with an autosomal dominant single gene trait, the multiple hamartoma syndrome (Cowden's disease). Lipomas, fibromas, angiomas, gastrointestinal polyps, thyroid tumors, fibrocystic

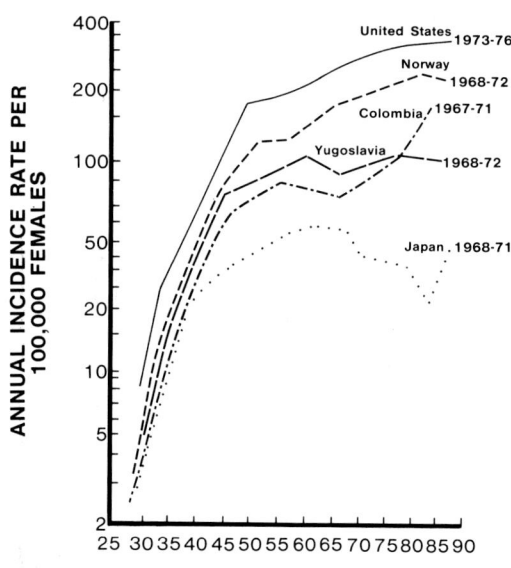

Figure 4–6. International breast cancer incidence rates by age. (Modified from Seidman, H., and Mushinski, M. H.: In Feig, S. A., and McLelland, R. [Eds.]: Breast Carcinoma: Current Diagnosis and Treatment. New York, Masson, 1983, p. 9. Used with permission.)

disease of the breast, nervous system abnormalities, and mucocutaneous warts characterize this disease, and it affects both men and women (Gentry et al., 1974). Susceptibility to breast cancer has been associated genetically with the allele for wet as opposed to dry ear wax, not a frivolous observation as ceruminous glands and mammary glands are both of the aprocine type (Petrakis, 1971). The dominant allele (wet), which may occur homozygously or heterozygously, is the rule in Western populations, in whom breast cancer incidence is high, whereas the recessive allele for dry cerumen is prevalent in Orientals, who have a low rate of breast cancer. Japanese women with breast cancer appear to have a higher frequency of the wet type of cerumen than Japanese cancer-free controls. This association is of limited value for defining a high-risk population in the United States, however, as 99 per cent of both white and black women have wet type cerumen.

Another potential genetic link is suggested by Lemon (1974). Breast cancer patients are observed to have low estriol excretion rates and low renal clearances of estriol as well as deficiencies of estradiol hydroxylating activity in leukocytes in 58 per cent of cases. Lemon postulated a genetic impairment of 16-alpha-hydroxylase, which converts estradiol to estriol and possibly is an expression of a mutant allele.

The wide disparity in international breast cancer mortality rates, particularly between Oriental and Western women, suggests genetically determined racial differences in susceptibility. If genetic factors are involved, it is necessary to postulate environmental influences to explain the changes that occur in immigrant populations. For example, Japanese immigrants to the United States largely maintain their low risk of breast cancer, but they do display a rise toward the higher risk observed in the United States (Seidman, 1972). Obviously, concomitant changes in diet, environmental contacts, and social habits accompany the change of domicile. The rising incidence of breast cancer in black women in the United States may not be due entirely to improved reporting and similarly suggests environmental determinants.

Repeated demonstrations of strong familial tendencies for mammary cancer provide suspicion for an inherited factor. The majority of investigations on this subject have shown that female relatives of women with cancer of the breast have a higher rate of the disease than would be expected in the general population. These familial associations can, however, occur through common dietary habits or similar environmental exposure.

Jacobsen (1946) reviewed early reports, among which was the personal genealogy of Broca in 1866, in which 10 of 24 female relatives died of breast cancer. In 1963 Lilienfeld summarized eight studies, six of which reported a familial tendency to breast cancer. Adding to these the report of Wynder and colleagues (1976), it is evident from the resulting table (Table 4–2) that the probability of breast cancer for mothers of probands is approximately double that of the general population and for sisters it is almost 2.5 times the expected risk.

A well-controlled study by Macklin in Ohio (1959) showed that not only mothers and sisters but also grandmothers, female cousins, and aunts of probands manifested an increased risk, which was present in both the maternal and the paternal lines. The risk was significantly greater than in relatives of individuals

Table 4–2. STUDIES OF THE FAMILIAL AGGREGATION OF BREAST CANCER

| | | | Prevalence or Mortality of Breast Cancer | | | | | |
| | | | Mothers of Cases | | | Sisters of Cases | | |
Author	Year	Cases Studied	Observed	Expected	Ratio	Observed	Expected	Ratio
Jacobsen	1946	200	21	7.0	3.0	13	5	2.6
Penrose et al.	1948	300	25	11.0	2.3	23	7	3.3
Passey et al.	1952	585	23	20.0	1.1	—	—	—
Smithers et al.	1952	556	29	13.9	2.1	—	—	—
Woolf	1955	200	4	2.1	1.9	8	3.2	2.5
Anderson et al.	1958	544	9	7.7	1.2	28	12.4	2.3
Murphy and Abbey	1959	200	7	3.0	2.3	2	6	0.3
Macklin	1959	295	11	5.6	2.0	14	5	2.8
Wynder et al.	1976	134	4	2.0	2.0	11	4	2.8
					Overall = 1.8			Overall = 2.3

(From Lilienfeld, A. M.: The epidemiology of breast cancer. Cancer Res., 23:1503, 1963. Reprinted with permission.)

without cancer or in those of patients with cancer of sites other than the breast. The fact that unmarried relatives of breast cancer patients were affected more frequently than married ones suggests enhancement of a genetic factor among the unmarried.

Risk among relatives is not uniform. The study of Anderson (1974) confirmed a breast cancer frequency twice as high in first degree relatives of probands as in relatives of controls with other types of cancer. Risk was highest for daughters: mothers, 0.8; sisters, 2.7; daughters, 4.6 (Anderson, 1974). Interestingly, risk was not increased in relatives of postmenopausal patients, but rose to 3.1 for relatives of premenopausal patients. A fivefold excess was observed in the families of patients with bilateral disease, and a ninefold excess was seen if the disease occurred both premenopausally and bilaterally. Furthermore, if the proband's cancer was bilateral, first degree relatives had a risk of bilateral cancer nine times higher than would be expected. A young woman whose mother and sister had premenopausal breast cancer, especially if it was bilateral in either case, had an estimated 50 per cent risk of developing breast cancer. Anderson (1974) found patients with family histories of breast cancer to be younger and to have a higher frequency of bilaterality than others. Blood type O, benign breast disease, and ovarian cysts and tumors tended to be more frequent among young patients with positive family histories.

Some studies have shown a tendency for breast cancer to maintain the same laterality in affected female relatives, and for earlier development of the disease in patients whose mothers were affected (Busk and Clemmeson, 1947; Bucalossi and Veronesi, 1957). Haagensen (1971) found that daughters developed breast cancer an average of 12 years earlier than their mothers and maternal aunts. A practical guide for estimating familial risk has been published by Ottman and coworkers (1983). Selected risks are shown in Figure 4–7A, B.

Knudsen's model for heritable and nonheritable tumors provides a logical explanation for some observations implicating inheritance in breast cancer (Knudsen et al., 1976). It presumes that tumors are derived from a single cell and are the product of two mutational events. The first event may be either prezygotic or postzygotic, and the second is always postzygotic. When the first event is prezygotic, it will be inherited and conferred to every cell. Subsequently, since all cells are potentiated and may be triggered by only one additional event, tumors would be expected to be multiple and occur relatively early in life. If both mutational events were postzygotic, convergence in the same cell would be required. Such a convergence would be relatively unlikely and, as a consequence, noninherited tumors would tend to be single and occur later in life. On the basis of this model, the age distribution and bilaterality of breast cancer suggest that about 30 per cent of the cases are of an inherited type.

The extent of linkage between genetic factors and the development of breast cancer remains incompletely defined. The great natural prevalence of breast cancer often creates difficulty in differentiating between environmental and genetic associations. If a cancer is genetically predisposed to occur, biomarkers consistent with genetic aberration should be discoverable. Lynch and coworkers (1984), in analyzing the pedigree of breast cancer patients, concluded that only 5 per cent of the breast cancer patients reported family pedigrees compatible with hereditary (autosomal dominant) breast cancer syndromes. An additional 13 per cent reported family aggregations that failed to meet the criteria as being hereditary. They concluded that among 112,000 new breast cancers occurring in the United States in 1982, between 2410 and 8790 (95 per cent confidence) patients would have met the criteria of hereditary association. Associated factors included younger age at onset, bilaterality, vertical transmission, and specific tumor associations consistent with genetic heterogeneity. Lynch's group observed that monolayer tissue cultures of dermal biopsy specimens from patients and high risk relatives was associated with hyperdiploidy. The enzyme glutamate-pyruvate transaminase (GPT) was found associated with a "breast cancer susceptibility gene." Both low urinary estrone and estradiol glucuronides were reported in association with hereditary breast cancer. "Morphologic stigmata" of hereditary breast cancer were not found. The prognosis with hereditary breast cancer was actually better than for breast cancers in general (Albano et al., 1982).

The problem in putting this information to practical use is the need for differentiating between phenotypic (environmental) and genetic heredity and the ability to test the efficacy of an intervention strategy of proven value in reducing risk of dying from breast cancer.

Case identification is attained with a high

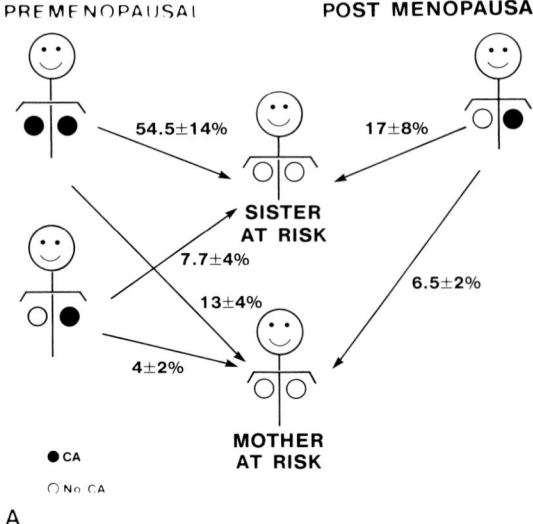

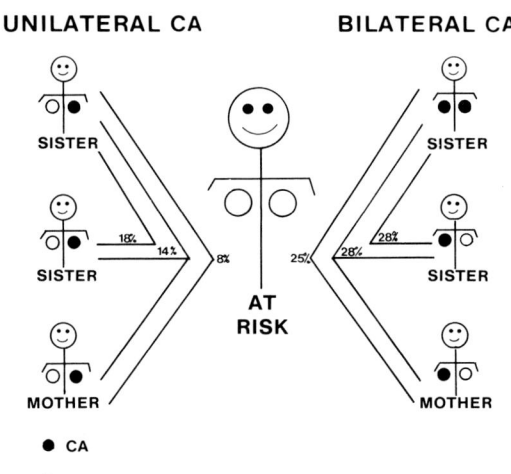

Figure 4-7. *A,* Percentage risk of breast cancer for premenopausal and postmenopausal women to age 70 years. (Based on data from Ottman, R., et al.: Practical guide for estimating risk for familial breast cancer. Lancet, 2:556, 1983). *B,* Percentage risk for unilateral and bilateral breast cancer to age 70 years. (Based on data of Anderson, D. E., and Badzioch, M. D.: Risk of familial breast cancer. Cancer, 56:383, 1985.)

false positive rate (Lynch et al., 1978). No controlled data yet exist to show that any pattern of prophylactic intervention enhances survivorship. Such a control would be essential, as Lynch's own group has shown that survivorship is better with breast cancers occurring in a genetically familial way. Patient anxiety with even an unconfirmed family history can reach psychologically serious states, and caution has to be exercised in concluding that genetically familial breast cancer is a risk in a particular woman.

Using data from the Danish Twin Register, Holm and colleagues (1980) observed that the number of breast cancers developing in co-twins after the first breast cancer diagnosis was increased by a factor of nearly 6 in monozygotic co-twins and by a factor of 2 in dizygotic co-twins. For cancers at other sites, the observed and expected number of cancers was about the same in both groups. There was no significant difference in the mean age at diagnosis. Among 40 monozygotic co-twins with only one twin affected, a greater association with breast cancer was seen in unmarried and nulliparous women. A tendency of the cancerous twin to have her first child at a later age than her co-twin was not significant.

Fishman and coworkers (1979) reported that women with a familial risk had lower urinary estrone and estradiol levels than matched controls. The difference was highly significant. Lynch and colleagues (1981) reported consistently lower levels of plasma prolactin, gonadotropin, estrone, and estradiol for familial high risk groups, but the differences were not significant. They also observed that familial cancers occurred at an earlier age, were frequently bilateral, exhibited vertical transmission, and had a survivorship greater than that associated with the nonfamilial cancers.

Cairns (1981) concluded that there really is no satisfactory evidence for a familial influence on the risk for breast cancer. Furthermore, familial influence is unstable, and many synergistic factors may affect the level of risk. Cairns concluded that the familial influence is not the deciding factor.

Moore and colleagues (1983) provided a comprehensive review of factors associated with or suspected of being associated with the causes of breast cancer, covering heritage, menses, marital state, parity, nursing, contraceptives, benign epithelial disorders of the breast, hormonal factors, cancer, iatrogenic factors, immunologic factors, viral aspects, diet, and psychosomatic factors. A major problem they identified was the difficulty in stratifying the degree of relevance to the many factors implicated. Often they seem to relate in synergistic ways. No factor seems of great importance when considered singly. Predisposition, carcinogens, promoters, and inhibitors all interact in the individual in unique ways. Moore and coworkers concluded that the role of diet is of great importance but has been studied inadequately. The influences begin to assume importance in the very early years of life. Using discriminant analysis of risk factors in various studies, they provided the rankings given in Table 4–3.

Other factors implicated in the increased risk of breast cancer include elevated blood prolactin and corpus luteum hormone levels and a lowered progesterone concentration. Excessive consumption of alcohol, use of hair dyes, and a variety of synthetic chemicals may contribute to risk. Co-risk factors for breast cancer associated with a family history (Macera et al., 1982) include 12 years or more from menarche to first birth, use of thyroid medication, and, for postmenopausal women, a Quetelet index score greater than 3.35. With a negative family history, an increased risk for breast cancer was associated with large breasts and a childhood spent in urban areas (Fishman et al., 1978).

VIRUSES

Viruses are known to cause a number of benign and malignant neoplasms in animals. Of particular interest with regard to the possible viral etiology of human breast cancer is the mouse mammary tumor virus (MMTV). The observation by Bittner in 1936 that mice with a high incidence of spontaneous mammary cancer passed this disease to their offspring through nursing led to the discovery of a "milk factor," which proved to be a virus with a ribonucleic acid (RNA) core and a type B virion morphology. Further research demonstrated that the virus could be transmitted not only in milk but also in tissues and at the time of fertilization in the gametes. Expression of the oncogenic potential of the virus was modified by genetic as well as by hormonal influences.

Although evidence now exists that viruses may cause mammary cancer in the monkey (Mason-Pfizer monkey virus) and in the rat (R-35 virus), the MMTV has proved the most promising model for investigation with electron microscopy, immunologic techniques, and molecular hybridization providing the tools of research. The case for a viral role in human mammary cancer may be summarized as follows:

1. Type B particles morphologically similar to MMTV, as well as particles of other types, can often be found in human breast milk and in some human mammary cancers.

2. An enzyme characteristic of RNA-type oncogenic viruses, RNA-directed DNA polymerase (RDDP), can be found in human milk, and is associated with particles having the same density as MMTV.

3. On migration inhibition testing, human leukocytes that are immunologically sensitive to human in situ breast cancer are also sensitive to MMTV.

4. The sera of some patients with breast cancer react immunologically with both MMTV virions and with mouse tumors rich in MMTV.

5. Molecular hybridization studies using MMTV-generated deoxyribonucleic acid

Table 4–3. FACTORS SELECTED BY STEPWISE LINEAR DISCRIMINANT ANALYSIS

Rank	Rural Zulu Versus Urban Zulu	Urban Zulu Breast Cancer Versus No Cancer	South Africa (White) Breast Cancer Versus No Cancer	Philadelphia Breast Cancer Versus No Cancer
1	Menarche to first delivery	Lamb + goat in diet	Worry	Menarche to first delivery
2	Fat in diet	Breast stimulation	Age at marriage	Breast stimulation
3	Grains in diet	Age at first delivery	Express emotions	Age at frequent sex
4	Breast stimulation	Age at menopause	Breast-feed children	
5	Lamb + goat in diet	Grains in diet	Vegetables in diet	
6	Period length	Home big enough		
7	Number of children			
8	Enough money			
9	Like home environment			
10	Home big enough			
		Correct classifications		
No breast cancer	86% (59/64)	82% (62/76)	97% (35/36)	63% (83/126)
Breast cancer	91% (69/76)*	86% (18/21)	85% (11/13)	58% (30/52)

*Numbers for urban Zulu without cancer.
(From Moore, D. H., et al.: Breast carcinoma etiological factors. Adv. Cancer Res., 40:189, 1983. Reprinted with permission.)

probes demonstrate a relationship between the RNA in human breast cancers and the RNA of MMTV. Thus, oncogenic virus–related information can be found in human breast cancer.

6. Based on viral dynamics associated with high and low cancer strains, the mouse model suggests that viral expression in humans would be expected late in life and could be variable, an expectation consistent with human experience (MacMahon et al., 1973; Moore, 1974; Papaioannou, 1974).

Although the evidence is highly suggestive that MMTV, or a similar virus, is instrumental in the genesis of human breast cancer, it is not conclusive. Infectivity and oncogenicity of the particles found in human breast milk have not been demonstrated. Furthermore, mouse mammary cancer, which seldom metastasizes and is promoted rather than reduced by early pregnancy, is less akin to the human form than is mammary cancer in the rat, for which evidence for a viral cause is tenuous. The mode by which a human virus might be transmitted remains obscure; clinical studies have not been able to correlate breast feeding with increased cancer risk, and in the United States, where breast feeding has declined, the incidence of breast cancer has risen. Despite these inconsistencies, the search for a human mammary tumor virus is spurred by the example of a viral agent in the mouse and by the fact that identification of an etiologic virus might lead to effective methods of preventing the disease.

ENDOCRINE FACTORS

Mammary cancers arise in an endocrine-dependent organ and are often responsive to hormones. It is tempting, therefore, to link the genesis of breast cancer with disturbed hormone metabolism. Among the possibilities suggested by current research are excessive estrogen production, subnormal androgen production, and prolactin abnormalities.

Estrogen Metabolism. Lemon (1965) found that patients with breast cancer tend to excrete a smaller portion of estriol (E_3) in the urine compared with the two other major estrogen fractions, estrone (E_1) and estradiol (E_2). The significance of this observation lies in the fact that estradiol and estrone are carcinogens for mice and rats, whereas estriol shares little of this activity. On the contrary, estriol is known to impede the action of some mammary carcinogens (dimethylbenzanthracene, or DMBA) and may in fact inhibit the other two estrogens (Villee and Hagerman, 1957; Pullinger, 1961). Subnormal production of estriol could, therefore, create a carcinogenic environment as a result of the relatively unantagonized remaining estrogens. Lemon found an estriol quotient expressed as

$$\frac{(E_3) \text{ mg/24 hr}}{(E_1) + (E_2) \text{ mg/24 hr}}$$

to be low in 71 per cent of patients with breast cancer but in only 30 per cent of controls. Patients with "premalignant" mastopathy shared a low quotient with the majority of breast cancer patients. Further support for this thesis is found in the low urinary estriol quotient of Oriental women, who have a low risk of breast cancer compared with that of North American women. The quotient tends to decline with increasing risk when Orientals migrate to Hawaii (Dickinson et al., 1974).

Weighing against the estriol hypothesis are the failure of the quotient to be uniformly decreased in patients with breast cancer, the lack of correlation of circulating levels of estriol to which body tissues are exposed with levels of urinary estriol, and the fact that the absolute quantity of estriol produced may not differ in women with high and low urinary fractions (Zumoff et al., 1975). In normal metabolism, E_1 and E_2 are interconvertible, but E_3 is formed irreversibly from E_2. If an abnormality of estrogen metabolism is involved in the genesis of breast cancer, its locus might be in processes controlling conversion of estradiol to estriol. It is of interest that Fishman and associates (1962) reported estriol excretion closely dependent on the level of thyroid hormone–mediated tissue oxygenation. If estriol is important in blocking carcinogens, this suggests a mechanism associating thyroid disease with cancer of the breast.

Androgen Metabolism. Investigations by Bulbrook and associates possibly implicate androgen metabolism in mammary carcinoma (Bulbrook et al., 1964; Bulbrook, 1973). This work began with studies of steroid excretion before and after adrenalectomy and hypophysectomy. Urinary etiocholanolone and 17-hydroxycorticosteroids were among the excretory products measured, and a formula involving these two agents, 80–80(17-OHCS)mg/24 hr + etiocholanolone (micrograms/24 hr), evolved as a discriminant. When etiocholanolone excretion was high and 17-hydroxycorticosteroids low, a positive discriminant resulted, and when the reverse was true, a negative discriminant resulted. Normal women almost all showed positive discriminants. More than half of patients with carcinoma of the breast had negative discriminants. In patients with early cancer, a positive discriminant indicated a relatively good prognosis after radical mastectomy, with improved chance of survival and of having a long free interval; in advanced disease, it indicated a good chance of responding to endocrine ablative procedures.

Etiocholanolone and its precursor dehydroepiandrosterone (DHEA) are products of androgen metabolism; low levels and a negative discriminant could result from subnormal androgen production, suggesting that reduced androgen stimulation might carry the same carcinogenic potential as overstimulation from high levels of estrogen. To clarify whether this unfavorable excretion pattern predisposes to or results from the disease, urine specimens were collected from 5000 normal women between the ages of 25 and 55 years on the island of Guernsey in the English Channel. The steroid pattern of approximately 60 women who have subsequently developed carcinoma of the breast supports the case for cancer developing more frequently in women with a low level of etiocholanolone compared with controls. Awkward aspects of this investigation are that etiocholanolone has no known biologic function and that Japanese women have a low, rather than the expected high, excretion (Cole, 1974). Although the significance of this pattern in English women is not clear, it could possibly serve to identify a high risk group.

Prolactin. A number of observations suggest that prolactin, the pituitary hormone important for milk production, may have a role in the genesis of human breast cancer (Wilson et al., 1973). Prolactin stimulates the growth of DMBA-induced breast cancers in rodents. Hypophysectomy, which eliminates the source of prolactin, not only prevents normal breast development but also often causes regression of both rodent and human mammary cancers. In tissue culture, 31 per cent of human breast cancers have been demonstrated to be prolactin dependent (Hobbs et al., 1973). Hypothyroidism, which increases prolactin secretion, is suspected of being associated with breast cancer. Furthermore, patients with painful osseous metastases often experience marked transient reduction of bone pain after prolactin suppression (Minton and Dickey, 1973; Sasaki et al., 1976).

Nevertheless, significant differences in serum prolactin levels have not been demonstrated consistently between breast cancer patients and controls, and prolactin suppressors such as levodopa and CB154 (2-bromo-α-ergocryptine) have proved of little therapeutic value in treatment of the human disease (Wilson et al., 1973; Kwa et al., 1974). Contrary to expectations, objective tumor regressions have been observed in response to hormone therapy that increased prolactin levels (Wilson et al., 1973). Reports that reserpine-containing medications, which raise prolactin levels, promote breast cancer have not been confirmed.

Thyroid Function. Evidence for an association between thyroid disease and breast cancer is largely based on inference. Similar frequencies of mammary cancer and goiter in certain regions of the world are evident in demographic data (World Health Organization, 1952; Humphrey and Swerdlow, 1964). The relatively high incidence of the two in Denmark, England, Wales, the Netherlands, Switzerland, Mexico, and Thailand and the low incidence in Japan, Chile, and Iceland are notable (Finley and Bogardus, 1960). Clinical statistics also suggest a higher than expected incidence of thyroid disease in breast cancer patients (Levy and Levy, 1951; Repert, 1952). Of 2545 patients with breast cancer at Ellis Fischel State Cancer Hospital (EFSCH), Columbia, Missouri, 2.7 per cent had a thyroid operation prior to or subsequent to the diagnosis of their cancer (1960–1979 data).

Animal experiments provide some support for an association with hypothyroidism. Proliferative histologic changes are observed in breasts of thyroidectomized rats, and thyroid feedings can inhibit carcinogenic agents and tumor transplants in animals (Smithcors and Leonard, 1942; Spencer, 1954). Primary hypothyroidism is known to increase prolactin in humans; the latter promotes murine breast cancer (Buckman and Peake, 1976). Further evidence derives from clinical studies in which thyroid is given varying credit for arrest of recurrent mammary carcinoma or prophylaxis against recurrence in humans (Loeser, 1954; Lemon, 1955). Kapdi and Wolfe (1976) reported a higher than expected frequency of breast cancer among women taking thyroid medications and speculated that underlying hypothyroidism or the thyroid medication itself might be responsible.

Although a body of evidence suggests that the hypothyroid state may be conducive to the development of malignant disease of the breast, evidence of a clear relationship remains elusive. Breast cancer is not notably frequent among patients who are clinically thyroid deficient. Wilkins and Morton (1963) were unable to demonstrate significant alteration of tumor incidence, time of tumor appearance, tumor growth rate, incidence of mortality, or time of mortality in mice with transplanted mammary adenocarcinoma treated with L-thyroxine or any of three other thyroid hormone analogues. This parallels the clinical experience of Emery and Trotter (1963) with advanced human breast cancer. Moreover, Cappelli and Margottini (1964) were unable to detect a decrease in thyroid function in 43 patients with cancer of the breast by measuring ^{131}I uptake, total plasma iodine levels, or protein-bound iodine (PBI). Thus, a significant relationship between human breast cancer and thyroid function remains to be established.

REPRODUCTIVE FUNCTION

In 1700, Ramazinni of Padua noted that breast cancer was frequent among nuns and attributed their susceptibility to a celibate life (Shimkin, 1973). More than a century later (1844), Rigoni-Stern in Verona associated the disease with aging; again noting the high frequency among single women as well as four cases in priests, he advocated an investigation of religious orders. Links between breast cancer and reproductive function have now been well established. Compared to controls, women with breast cancer are more likely to be unmarried, to have married later in life, to have become pregnant for the first time at an older age, and to have fewer children. Furthermore, they are less likely to have had an artificial menopause and more likely to have had a late menopause (Herrell, 1937; Lilienfeld, 1956).

A great improvement over retrospective studies was that of Shapiro and associates (1968), who were able to analyze prospective risk factors in 20,211 women interviewed at their initial visit to a breast screening project in New York City. In this population, 111 cancers were diagnosed during a mean follow-up period of 1.5 years, and the ratio of observed to expected cancers was computed for various characteristics (Table 4–4). An excess of breast cancers occurred in women who had never been married (2.3 times), in those who had no more than two pregnancies (2 times), in those with an early menarche (1.7 times), and in those with 30 or more aggregate years of menstrual activity (1.4 times). In addition, high risks were confirmed in connection with benign breast disease and a family history of breast cancer. A minor increase was associated with high educational attainment, and Jewish women appeared more susceptible than the average. A protective effect of breast feeding and prolonged lactation found in earlier, less well controlled studies was not found. On the basis of this and other recent studies, it now appears that whatever else might recommend breast feeding, reduction of breast cancer risk is not included (Lowe and MacMahon, 1970; Kalache et al., 1980).

A factor of considerable importance, and one that integrates a number of observations, is the reduced risk that accrues from full-term pregnancy at an early age (Fig. 4–8). MacMahon and colleagues (1973) found that women who gave birth to their first child at or after the age of 35 years had a twofold higher risk of breast cancer than women who had their first child when less than 20 years of age. A pregnancy late in life increased the risk above that of nulliparous women. This observation explains the association of reduced risk with early marriage and with multiparity. Early marriage provides no protection to nonparous women, and multiparity is important only in-

Table 4–4. COMPARISON OF RELATIVE RISKS FOR BREAST CANCER AND SELECTED CHARACTERISTICS

Characteristics	Ratio of Relative Risk
Never married versus married	2.3*
1 or 2 pregnancies versus 3 or more pregnancies	2.0*
Age at menarche, under 12 versus 15 or older	1.7
Aggregate years menstrual activity, 30 years or more versus less than 30 years	1.4
Breast conditions, 1 or more versus none	3.1*
Sisters, 1 or more with breast cancer versus none	1.9

*Statistically significant increase.
(Adapted from Shapiro, S., et al.: The search for risk factors in breast cancer. Am. J. Public Health, 58:820, 1968. Used with permission.)

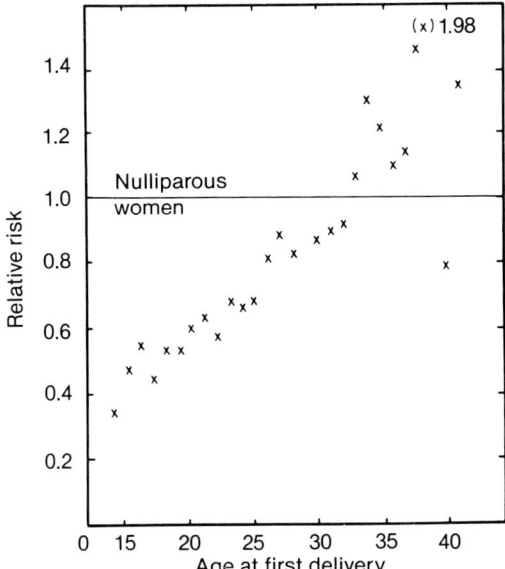

Figure 4–8. Relative risk of breast cancer related to age at first delivery. (From MacMahon, B., et al.: Etiology of human breast cancer: A review. JNCI, 50:21, 1980. Used with permission.)

sofar as the first full-term pregnancy occurs at an early age. The importance of early pregnancy infers that endocrinologic events early in life determine eventual risk, possibly through a maturing influence that is protective to mammary epithelium. Through analogy with the rat model, it also suggests that initial carcinogenic exposure occurs early in life. Pregnancy in the rat protects against a mammary carcinogen if it precedes exposure but promotes cancer formation if it follows exposure. The protective effect of early pregnancy in humans and the promoting influence of a late first pregnancy suggest that exposure of humans occurs as early as the second decade of life.

The obvious predilection of breast cancer for females relates it to ovarian function, but specifics of ovarian function also seem to influence risk. Prolonged duration of cyclic ovarian activity through early menarche, late menopause, or both, is associated with higher than average lifetime risk. Interruption of ovarian activity markedly reduces this risk. Bilateral oophorectomy before age 40 reduces the incidence of breast cancer by 75 per cent in both parous and nulliparous women (Feinleib, 1968). After the fourth decade, surgical castration provides no significant protection. Pelvic irradiation sufficient to produce artificial menopause similarly protects against the disease. The fact that castration is protective and interrupts the cyclic interplay between estrogens and progesterone further implicates these two hormones in the problem of breast cancer.

ESTROGENS AND ORAL CONTRACEPTIVES

Physiologic effects of estrogens on the breast include stimulation of ductal growth, promotion of stromal development, accretion of fat, and pigmentation of the areola. It is uncertain whether estrogens can cause cancer of mammary tissues. Concern stems from the fact that estrogens can accelerate breast cancer development in strains of mice predisposed to this disease and can stimulate, as well as retard, the growth of established breast cancers in humans (Kennedy, 1962). Both synthetic and natural estrogens are widely consumed by women in the United States for prevention of postmenopausal changes and for contraception; for this reason, any evidence of carcinogenicity is of considerable importance.

Mammary parenchyma removed in biopsies of women on estrogen replacement or oral contraceptives displays no distinctive changes when compared with tissues from others not taking these medications, nor does the nature of the lesions removed differ (Vessey et al., 1971; Fechner, 1972; Ariel, 1973). In an unpublished review by Pakalns at the Medical College of Wisconsin, 75 per cent of benign tumors removed from the breasts of 28 oral contraceptive users proved to be fibroadenomas, a frequency no greater than that in age-matched controls not taking oral contraceptives.

Burch and Byrd (1971) reported a follow-up of 511 women treated with estrogens, usually Premarin, for prolonged periods after hysterectomy. During a total of 5441 patient-years of observation, 45 benign breast tumors and nine mammary carcinomas were diagnosed. No bilateral or inflammatory cancers were observed, and the frequency of cancers did not exceed the expected age-specific incidence. Breast cancers evolved 10 years later than might be anticipated, and cancers of all types appeared reduced. Arthes and associates (1971) could not document a higher frequency of estrogen use among women with breast cancer than in controls matched for age, race, marital status, hospital, and time of hospital admission. Hoover and associates (1976), however, found evidence for delayed risk. Excess risk of breast cancer among 1891 women given conjugated estrogens for natural or surgical menopause was found only after 10 years of observation and increased thereafter to twice the expected risk after 15 years. Furthermore, risk increased with cyclic use, and the expected protection afforded by castration and multiparity was not evident.

The long-term use of conjugated estrogens has been reported to increase relative risk (RR) in certain categories of women (Glass et al., 1979). It was highest with nulliparity, first parity past age 30 years, and a family history of breast cancer. These RRs are subject to modification by ovarian status. With intact ovaries, the RR was 1.2, varying to 2.2 for women who had undergone bilateral oophorectomy.

Ross and colleagues (1979) reported a significant increase in breast cancer risk among women who had received more than 1500 mg of lifetime conjugated estrogen (3 years at 1.25 mg daily).

Others have failed to find increased risk associated with estrogen replacement. Evidence that the use of estrogen and progesterone combinations in postmenopausal women might reduce the risk of breast cancer was found by Gambrell and coworkers (1983) in a prospective study of 5563 postmenopausal women. After 37,236 patient-years of follow-up, the frequency of breast cancer in estrogen-progesterone users was significantly lower than in the untreated group (67.3 per 100,000 per year versus 342.3) and lower than expected from National Cancer Institute (NCI) Surveillance, Epidemiology, and End Results (SEER) data. Use of combinations with progesterone may be the safest course for women requiring estrogen replacement.

Oral contraceptives ordinarily contain both estrogen and progesterone. In a case control study, Vessey and associates (1971) found a higher use rate among matched controls than among 220 breast cancer patients, suggesting that any influence may be a protective one. Paffenbarger and colleagues (1975) also found no overall greater frequency of use among 425 breast cancer patients than among 872 controls, but a significantly higher use was observed among the former before their first childbirth. This discovery tends to reconfirm that delay of first pregnancy, by oral contraceptives or perhaps by other means, increases breast cancer risk. Further analyses of these data for relative risk revealed that, whereas use of oral contraceptives in general did not increase risk, long-term use (2 to 4 years) was associated with a significantly increased risk of breast cancer (1.9) (Fasal and Paffenbarger, 1975). The risk reached elevenfold among long-term users with previous benign disease. Paradoxically, although oral contraceptives appeared to prevent benign breast disease in this study, their use in its presence substantially increased cancer risk.

Two recent extensive studies, one in England by the Royal College of General Practitioners (1981) and another in the United States by the Centers for Disease Control (CDC) (1983) found no increased risk associated with oral contraceptives, either overall or within specific subgroups at high risk. The CDC report involved a case control study of 689 breast cancers in women 20 to 54 years old and in 1077 controls. Relative risk was 0.9 between users and never-users, and oral contraceptives did not increase risk in women with benign breast disease, in those with a family history of breast cancer, or in those who used them before their first pregnancy. The Royal College of General Practitioners continues to observe 23,000 users and a similar number of nonusers entered in 1968. To date no significant increase of breast cancer has been found in users.

Uncontrolled observations with progestational agents used as contraceptives suggest no increase of breast cancers but also no protective effect (Zanartu et al., 1973).

To date, studies of estrogen use for menopause or contraception are limited in scope and may be premature. Typically, the potential of most carcinogens is not fully expressed until 15 years following exposure. Estrogens have been used to prevent menopausal changes for about 40 years; oral contraceptives have been in widespread use only since 1965. It would appear that continued close surveillance is warranted.

RADIATION CARCINOGENESIS

The potential capacity of ionizing radiation to produce breast cancer has been repeatedly confirmed. The induction of neoplasia is dose and time dependent. The question is not whether breast cancer can be induced by radiation but whether clinical benefits of ionizing radiation for diagnostic purposes can be obtained with minimal risk. The importance of this question has acquired increased relevance with the widescale use of mammographic examination of the breast. Chapter 6 addresses progress in improving the quality of mammographic examination while steadily reducing radiation exposure.

Increasing attention has been given to radiation's carcinogenicity for breast tissue. In 1950, Lorenz and associates were able to demonstrate that mice and guinea pigs subjected to chronic whole body gamma irradiation developed an excessive number of breast cancers compared with controls not so exposed. In 1965, Mackenzie reported an increased incidence of breast cancer in women who received high doses of irradiation to the anterior chest during repeated fluoroscopies in conjunction with treatment of pulmonary tuberculosis. The excess of breast cancers began to appear after an average latent period of 16 years, at an earlier age than would be expected in the general population, and in the areas of the breast most heavily irradiated.

The work was confirmed by similar observations elsewhere (Myrden and Hiltz, 1969). A survey of 606 women treated in upstate New York for postpartum mastitis with 75 to 1000 roentgens (R) also revealed more than twice the expected number of breast cancers, invariably located in the treated breast (Mettler et al., 1969). The Atomic Bomb Casualty Commission detected carcinogenic effects among women exposed to whole body irradiation in the bombings of Hiroshima and Nagasaki (Wanebo et al., 1968). Exposure to 90 rad or more was followed by development of breast cancers at a rate two to four times that in comparison groups after a mean latent period of 15 years. The increase was most evident in those exposed at an early age. Cancer of the male breast has been reported to have followed irradiation for prepubertal gynecomastia 35 years earlier (Lowell et al., 1968).

Evidence that repetitive fluoroscopic examination of the chest for tuberculosis as well as with radiotherapy for postpartum mastitis is associated with breast cancer continues to be found (Lowell et al., 1968; Logan et al., 1979; Dvoretsky et al., 1980; Howe et al., 1982).

A review of the Swedish experience with 1115 women treated for benign breast disease by ionizing radiation was reported by Baral and colleagues (1977). With an average follow-up of 31.5 years, the number of breast cancers occurring in the irradiated group was four times the expected value, and this was independent of the age at which radiation was given.

The tragic epidemiologic experiment created by the atomic bomb attacks on Japan has generated considerable data on levels of radiation exposure and the risk of cancer development. Mossman's review (1984) provides a current compilation of opinion and includes consideration of the atomic bomb survival data.

1. Radiation-induced cancers are indistinguishable from naturally occurring cancers. (For the breast this has been confirmed by a pathologic review of breast cancers occurring in atomic bomb victims [Tokuoka et al., 1984]).

2. Radiation-induced cancers appear in almost every tissue of the body. There are some resistant tissues, but the female breast is susceptible.

3. Sensitivity to radiation carcinogenesis varies considerably in various tissues and organs: The highest sensitivity is to be found in the female breast, thyroid gland, and myelogenous tissues.

4. Cancer induction by radiation has a long latent period. Whether this latent period is one of induction or slow subclinical progression is uncertain. For solid neoplasms, as occur in the breast, this period may range for 20 to 30 years, and, for the breast, the period has been estimated to range from 5 to 30 years.

5. Age, sex, and other factors may contribute to cancer induction, complicating the ability to study the true impact of radiation carcinogenesis. Youthful age at exposure and the susceptibility of both thyroid and breast tissue to radiation carcinogenesis contributes to an increased prevalence of radiation-induced solid tumors in women (BEIR III, 1980).

6. The dose-response relationships are different for different cancers. Breast cancer seems to fit a linear, no-threshold dose model (Boice et al., 1978; BEIR III, 1980).

7. Risk estimates of the capacity of radiation to induce cancer are based largely on high dose data. The reason is that the smaller numbers of cancers induced by lower doses lead to statistical uncertainty as to the proportion of breast cancer induced. The dose-response model and the threshold dose required in human models has, therefore, been estimated by extrapolating dose-response curves for higher doses. The prevailing opinion of radiation biologists is that risk of cancer induction is directly related to the dose of radiation, but

there is no threshold dose below which no cancers are induced. Other models of these data and statistical limitations on the methods used leave the question unresolved.

A consensus study holds that 50 to 200 excess breast cancers occur per 1 million persons per lifetime exposure per centigray of radiation, and 10 to 60 excess deaths occur from breast cancer under the same parameters (UNSCEAR, 1977).

More recently, based on modern low-dose techniques in which the mean breast dose for a two-view study is 0.17 rad, Feig estimated that one mammogram theoretically would cause one excess breast cancer per two million women examined per year after a latent period of 10 years (Feig, 1983).

The potential danger of excessive irradiation to the whole body or breast seems clear. The fact that no threshold dose is acknowledged below which danger is nonexistent justifies concern about cumulative exposures for diagnostic purposes as well as for therapy. Perhaps the single greatest source of mammary irradiation at present is mammography. The capacity of mammography to detect small breast cancers is undisputed, but with poor technique, poorly calibrated equipment, and repetitive examinations without clear indications, this valuable diagnostic tool could enhance the problem it was designed to help eliminate. An exposure of one rad per examination will increase a woman's lifetime risk of breast cancer 1 per cent (Upton, 1976). One hundred examinations would double the lifetime risk. Midbreast dose per examination is now as low as 80 millirad. With proper technique and indications and with dose-reducing technologic improvements, the biologic price of mammography can be kept low; nevertheless, it should be paid only by those who, on the basis of reliable information, can be expected to obtain a net benefit. In view of the long latency of radiation carcinogenesis, the ultimate consequences of both diagnostic and therapeutic irradiation of the breast must remain under continuing evaluation.

DIET AND OBESITY

Much attention has been given to qualitative and quantitative aspects of diet as promoters of breast cancer. Ingested foods are recognized as potential vehicles for small amounts of carcinogens, such as nitrosamines, aflatoxins, and polycyclic hydrocarbons, that may be introduced during food processing or storage. Although none of the former have been linked to breast cancer in humans, the potential of contamination can be appreciated by the fact that a single exposure to a potent agent may be sufficient to induce cancer in susceptible individuals. One 10 mg dose of the polycyclic hydrocarbon dimethylbenzanthracene (DMBA) is sufficient to produce breast cancer in rats.

More intriguing are the quantity and composition of diet. Both overfeeding and underfeeding can affect tumor genesis in the laboratory animal (Carroll, 1975). Chronic, continuous underfeeding and caloric restriction without producing inanition can inhibit the appearance of spontaneous and induced mammary tumors in mice. Slowing of cellular activity, a consequence of undernutrition, may account for this effect. Conversely, mice made artificially obese evolve spontaneous mammary cancers faster than do controls.

An excessively fatty diet may also be influential. Diets high in fat regularly increase the incidence of mammary tumors in both mice and rats and appear to promote tumor development when fed to rats after exposure to DMBA. Epidemiologic correlations with these laboratory observations include associations between dietary fat intake and mortality for cancer of the breast, intestinal cancer, and prostatic cancer. Carroll (1975) demonstrated a particularly striking direct correlation between per capita consumption of dietary fat in 39 countries and the age-adjusted mortality rate from breast cancer (Fig. 4–9). An age-adjusted mortality rate from breast cancer exists in countries with a per capita fat intake of 140 to 150 gm per day, that is 5 to 10 times higher than in those with an intake of 50 gm per day or less, and the association pertains primarily to animal rather than vegetable fats.

In support of these observations is the work of deWaard (1975), relating body weight to increased risk for breast cancer in postmenopausal women. It is known that with cessation of estrogen function at the time of menopause, estradiol is replaced by estrone as the major circulating estrogenic steroid; the latter is produced predominantly by the brain, liver, and peripheral fatty tissues from androstenedione generated in the adrenal gland (Poortman et al., 1973; Siiteri et al., 1973). Obesity is associated not only with increases in the output of androstenedione by the adrenal but also with

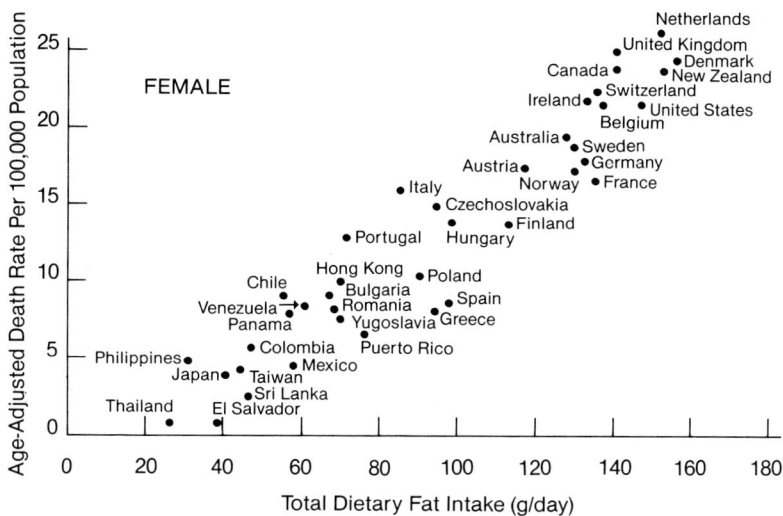

Figure 4–9. Correlation between per capita consumption of dietary fat and age-adjusted mortality from breast cancer in different countries. (From Carroll, K. K.: Experimental evidence of dietary factors and hormone-dependent cancers. Cancer Res. 35:3374, 1975. Used with permission.)

its conversion to estrone. The biologic effect of this excess was demonstrated by deWaard (1969), who was able to correlate estrogenic stimulation of vaginal epithelium with obesity in postmenopausal women. By this mechanism, obesity could serve to promote the growth of hormone-sensitive tumors, such as breast cancer. High fat diets also increase prolactin production in the rat, a fact that led Wynder (1976) to suggest that a disturbed prolactin-to-estrogen ratio might be a determinant of breast cancer risk. The indirect evidence linking breast cancer and uterine cancer to estrogens and both to obesity suggests a common promotor, possibly altered steroid metabolism. Complex associations identified between diet (qualitatively and quantitatively) and the induction and lethality of breast cancer are addressed in Chapter 5. The appendix to Chapter 5 provides an approach toward dietary analysis intended to help women to avoid foods associated with a higher incidence of both benign and malignant breast diseases.

The focus of the early literature was on reliable and valid ways to contribute information on dietary intake to nutritional status studies designed to prevent the development of the classic nutritional deficiency diseases, such as scurvy and pellagra. Since the 1960s, the emphasis has changed. Now dietary intake data in epidemiologic studies are designed to establish any possible influence on the development of cardiovascular disease and cancer.

The role of diet in carcinogenesis has emerged because of the growing awareness that dietary excesses, deficiencies, and various imbalances can play a role in the etiology of various neoplastic diseases.

The incidence and mortality rates for breast cancer are higher in industrialized nations, with the exception of Japan, than in developing countries. Using epidemiologic data, researchers have attempted to explain much of the variation of dietary factors, especially lipid intake. For example, Gray and associates (1979) compared the incidence and mortality rates of breast cancer in women from 34 countries. They found the breast cancer incidence and mortality rates were correlated with the height, weight, and age at menarche of the women. Even after controlling for height, weight, and menarche age, significant correlations of breast cancer with per capita total dietary fat and animal protein consumption were found. Knox (1977) found a similar association between total fat intake and cancer of the breast when he examined the nutrient intakes and breast cancer mortality rates in many of the same countries.

Hems (1978) and Drasar and Irving (1973) used dietary data from the United Kingdom to study possible correlations between dietary intake and breast cancer rates in developed and developing countries. They both found breast cancer rates were positively correlated with total fat intake, animal protein, and animal fat. Hems also found a positive correlation with refined sugar. Drasar and Irving reported a positive, but nonsignificant, correlation between sugar and breast cancer rates.

In a later study, Hems (1980) examined the changes in breast cancer mortality rates for all women in England and Wales between 1911 and 1975. He found the changes in mortality were associated with changes in consumption of dietary fat, sugar, and animal protein one to two decades earlier.

Kolonel and associates (1981) at the Cancer Center of Hawaii used a food frequency consumption questionnaire with 4657 adults over 45 years of age from various ethnic groups in Hawaii to determine the subjects' usual weekly intake of 85 food items. The foods were selected to cover the main sources of dietary fat and protein, and, to a lesser extent, the intake of other dietary components. The nutrient components examined were the following: total fat; vegetable, meat, fish, and dairy fat; saturated and unsaturated fatty acids; dietary cholesterol; carbohydrate; and vitamins A and C. These investigators examined the incidence of cancer at 15 different sites in relation to the nutrient information. They found a significant positive association between breast cancer and fat (total fat, saturated and unsaturated fat, and animal fat) and animal protein. Gray and coworkers (1979) have reviewed the epidemiologic nutritional correlations with breast cancer incidence.

TRAUMA

The appearance of malignant neoplasms at the site of old burn scars (Marjolin's ulcer), chronic osteomyelitic sinuses, and chronic anal fistulas is believed by many to incriminate chronic trauma as a factor in carcinogenesis. Two patients who developed mammary carcinoma in chronic burn scars of the breast were reported by Peden in 1947. The authors are aware of a 56 year old man who had adenocarcinoma of the breast in a chronic scar that resulted from total avulsion of the areola at 16 years of age.

The frequency with which patients trace the onset of cancer to a single injury raises the question of acute trauma as an initiating factor. It is generally believed that this association is a function of the psychologic need to find an explanation for the illness and that the trauma served to draw the individual's attention to a preexistent lesion. Only 11.3 per cent of 2529 patients with breast cancer at EFSCH gave a history of antecedent trauma to the involved breast. Wynder (1976) gave a similar figure (9.0 per cent) in 632 American patients.

Postulates on this subject formulated at the Second International Conference on Cancer, Paris, 1910, endorsed by Dr. James Ewing, and published for medicolegal application in 1926, are as follows:

1. Reasonable proof of authenticity and adequacy of the trauma.
2. Previous integrity of the wounded part.
3. Origin of tumor at the exact point of injury.
4. Reasonable time limit between injury and tumor appearance (3 weeks to 3 years).
5. Positive diagnosis of presence and nature of the tumor.

The lack of evidence that carcinoma occurs at sites of acute trauma more frequently than by chance calls into question the merit of legal causality. In acknowledging the possibility of a relationship, modern concepts of tumor growth have placed the "reasonable time limit" into better perspective. The growth rates of mammary carcinoma observed clinically range widely (see Chapter 10). Furthermore, about 30 doublings are required for a single dividing cell to produce a clinically detectable tumor mass 1.0 cm in diameter (10^9 cells) (MacDonald, 1965). Thus, if a neoplasm originates as a single cell, if the time required to double its volume is constant, and if a cancer were to be initiated by acute trauma, it can be speculated that the most rapidly growing tumor would require no less than 3 months after the episode to become detectable (3 days times 30 doublings = 90 days). Only with exceptionally rapid growth, detection at an unusually small size, or the malignant transformation of more than one cell might it be expected earlier. The induction of neoplasia by acute mechanical trauma is an extremely unlikely or even nonexistent event. Ewing's conditions for causality do not fit current statistical and cytokinetic knowledge and are best ignored.

It should be noted that the work of Klamer and Donegan (1983) and that of Jackson and colleagues (1984) provide some evidence that direct trauma may promote mammary tumor development in certain circumstances. Rats were exposed to the carcinogen DMBA, and breast tissue was surgically resected to various extents up to 75 per cent. Animals with resections developed as many tumors as did intact animals with a full complement of breast tissue, suggesting that the effect of carcinogenesis was not reduced by partial removal of the breast. Whether an enhancement secondary to ablative trauma occurred in residual breast tissue remains to be resolved.

CANCER IN ASSOCIATION WITH A FOREIGN BODY

Carcinoma of the breast has been reported adjacent to implanted cardiac pacemakers (Biran et al., 1979). The observation of two such cancers led the authors to change the placement of pacemakers to a position not likely to be in breast tissue.

The mastitis induced by silicone in breast tissue, resulting from both leaking protheses and injected silicone, renders the interpretation of both the findings of physical and mammographic examination inexact. This obscured early diagnosis of cancers developing in these breasts, according to Morgenstern and coworkers (1985), who reported a series of 12 women with this association. Causation of cancer was not implied but also could not be excluded on the basis of the data reported. Inflammatory breast cancer has been reported in breasts injected with silicone. These cases have often been misdiagnosed at first as "silicone mastitis" (Lewis, 1980).

INFLAMMATORY CANCER

The unique nature and lethality of inflammatory breast cancer (IBC) merited a targeted epidemiologic study of this cancer using SEER data (Levine et al., 1985). The study addressed data from 1975 through 1981 in the nine geographic areas covered by the SEER program. Cases were divided as to the method of diagnosis—both clinical and pathologic, clinical only, and pathologic only. The IBCs occurred in younger patients independently of race. All categories had similar frequency of metastatic disease at the time of diagnosis. At 3 years posttreatment, survival for the three groups was 34, 60, and 52 per cent, respectively. Comparatively, the survivorship of all patients with breast cancer at 3 years was 90 per cent. The national patterns of treatment were found to be considerably more variable than for non-IBCs. The conclusion was that the importance of this entity, though relatively infrequent among all breast cancers seen, merited more systematic assessment of the presence of dermal lymphatic involvement associated with breast cancer. This lymphatic involvement is not an essential histopathologic criterion of IBC, as confirmed by Lucas and Perez-Mesa (1978).

EXTRAMAMMARY CANCERS

Appreciating associations between cancers can suggest common causes and lead to early detection of second cancers. A predilection of patients with breast cancers for second mammary cancers is widely accepted, but evidence for excess risk of cancers at nonmammary sites is elusive. Mider and associates (1952) in Rochester, New York, found no increase of second cancers among 941 patients with carcinoma of the breast when the New York State Tumor Registry was used as a reference. Summarizing reports on multiple cancers, Cook (1966) found a higher than expected association between breast and endometrial cancer. On the other hand, among 19,394 patients with breast cancer in Connecticut, Schoenberg and associates (1969) found excess second cancers of the ovary, corpus uteri, and large intestine. With further studies on the New York State Tumor Registry data, however, Schottenfeld and Berg (1971) found 9792 patients with breast cancer in New York City at greater than expected risk for cancers of the ovary (2.1 times the expected) as well as the larynx (6.8 times), the thyroid (4 times), soft tissues (4.5 times), and bones (6.4 times). Cancers of the large bowel occurred no more often than expected, whereas those of the endometrium were significantly reduced.

In most instances, no rationale for the associations observed is evident; in others, a common causality is suggested. A higher than expected incidence of mammary cancers among women with endometrial cancers has been noted in several reports, raising the possibility of a common hormonal etiology between these two endocrine hormone–sensitive tumors. On the other hand, a predisposition to endometrial cancer following an initial breast cancer is not observed consistently. Excessive soft tissue sarcomas among Schottenfeld and Berg's cases of breast cancer appeared to be a consequence of treatment, the majority having occurred in irradiated tissues or edematous arms.

Skepticism is justified regarding statistical associations between neoplasms. Registry data used for estimating cancer risk vary in completeness. Misleading information is particularly likely when the reference registry is not in the same region as the observed population. Cancer incidence rates vary in different regions of the United States and from country to country, as do mortality data. The interpretation of the experience at the EFSCH with second nonmammary cancers depends on the particular registry from which estimated risk is derived. During prolonged follow-up of 406 patients treated with radical mastectomy for cancer of the breast during the years 1944–1945, 1947–1950, and 1953–1958, 16 extramammary primaries were observed, 14 of which were diagnosed subsequent to the breast cancer and two simultaneously. As might be expected in this rural population, skin cancers predominated, followed in order of frequency by cancer of the colorectum, cancer of the uterus, and a single melanoma (Table 4–5). The observed incidence for most of these cancers fell within the range expected according to age-specific data from five tumor registries located in the United States. Only the single melanoma exceeded the range.

These data failed to establish that women treated for operable cancer of the breast as their first neoplasm were any more prone than others to develop cancer subsequently at extramammary sites. Using a local control population and Connecticut State Tumor Registry data, Spratt and Hoag (1966) similarly were unable to demonstrate an excess of second cancers among 710 patients treated initially for breast cancer at EFSCH and observed for up to 20 years. This evidence, in conjunction with the inconsistencies displayed in other studies, suggests that the follow-up examination of such women needs no modification from that indicated to detect new cancers in women of comparable age in the general population. Women treated for cancer of the breast are not immune to independent cancers at other sites, and suspicious symptoms should prompt appropriate diagnostic procedures. Further discussion on multiple primary cancers is to be found in Chapter 22.

CHRONIC CYSTIC MASTOPATHY

Symptomatic chronic cystic mastopathy (CCM), also known as fibrocystic disease, chronic cystic changes, cystic disease, chronic cystic disease, chronic cystic mastitis, Schimmelbusch's disease, Reclus's disease, and by a number of other synonyms, is an affliction of the reproductive years.

Among the types of chronic cystic mastopathy, proliferative changes have constituted the major risk for the ultimate development of breast cancer. Sandison's examination in 1962 of 1300 breasts at autopsy permits construction of age-specific incidences of various cystic and proliferative changes that associate epithelial proliferation, or "epitheliosis," with mammary cancer (Fig. 4–10). Pathologists have reported the association of ductal hyperplasia and infiltrating cancer in the same breast, suggesting an evolution from hypoplasia to cancer. Gallagher and Martin (1969) postulated induction and promotion phases in this transition, the first being a reversible

Table 4–5. NONMAMMARY CANCERS DIAGNOSED SIMULTANEOUSLY WITH OR SUBSEQUENT TO THE TREATMENT OF 406 PATIENTS WITH MAMMARY CARCINOMA (EFSCH)

Cancer Site	Number Observed*	Number Expected†				
		N.Y.	Conn.	Nevada	El Paso	Alameda
Skin	8	2.2	—	3.3	10.6	—
Basal cell = 6						
Epidermoid = 2						
Colorectum	4	4.0	5.8	3.2	3.2	5.0
Colon = 3						
Rectum = 1						
Uterus	3	3.9	2.5	3.3	3.0	3.0
Cervix = 2						
Corpus = 1						
Melanoma	1	0.1	0.2	0.2	0.2	0.2

*16 cancers developed in 15 patients (3.7 per cent) during 2591 patient-years of followup.
†Number of cancers expected during age- and sex-specific followup of identical period according to five tumor registries in the United States (Doll et al., 1970).

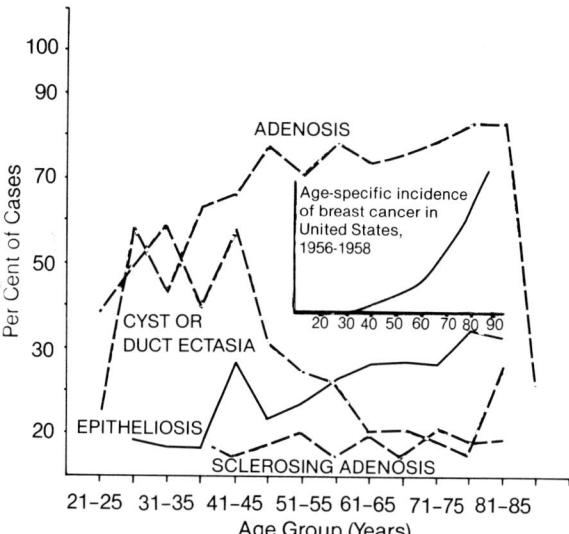

Figure 4–10. Age-specific incidence of various manifestations of fibrocystic changes in breasts of 800 females at autopsy. (Chart compiled from data in Sandison, 1962.)

change from normal ductal epithelium to hyperplasia, followed by an irreversible change to carcinoma or permanent hyperplasia.

Foote (1945) implicated atypical ductal papillomatosis as leading to cancer of the breast. In a large study, an equal incidence of ductal papillomatosis was found in carcinomatous and noncarcinomatous breasts, but atypical cellular changes were evident five times more frequently in the former.

Davis (1964) considered solid hyperplasia even more dangerous than papillomatosis because 6.2 per cent of women with solid hyperplasia subsequently developed breast cancer, compared with only 3.8 per cent of those with papillomatosis. Fully 50 per cent of carcinomas developed in the breast opposite that in which the diagnosis of cystic change was established, an observation in support of the "field" theory of mammary carcinogenesis and one that discourages ipsilateral mastectomy for this condition as a prophylactic measure against cancer.

Humphrey and Swerdlow (1968) considered hyperplasia in large ducts more dangerous than similar changes in small ducts. Carcinoma developed in 6 of 18 patients with large duct hyperplasia within 1 to 13 years of diagnosis. Cancer developed under skin flaps in residual breast tissue in 2 of these 18 cases after simple mastectomy, emphasizing the point that operations that fail to remove all breast tissue do not provide effective prophylaxis against mammary cancer.

In a second longitudinal study, Spratt and colleagues (1985) reported the experience with chronic cystic mastopathy confirmed by biopsy after discovery in a breast screening program for 10,128 women between 35 and 70 years of age in the Breast Cancer Demonstration and Detection Project at the University of Louisville, Kentucky. In this period, 1396 breast biopsies were recommended, with results as shown in Figure 4–11. After 6 to 10 years of follow-up, only four cancers developed during 2443.5 woman-years of follow-up, giving an incidence of cancers of 0.00164 per woman year, entirely within the range of the expected.

Both the cases in which some type of chronic cystic mastopathy was found synchronous with a cancer and cases in which only CCM and no synchronous cancer were found were sorted in matrices. Tables 4–6, 4–7, and 4–8 show the association of the histologic type of CCM,

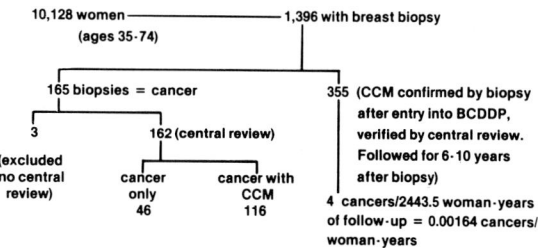

Figure 4–11. Stratification flow diagram for patients on whom biopsy was performed as a result of recommendations originating from screening in the Breast Cancer Demonstration and Detection Project, University of Louisville (BCDDP), according to histopathologic diagnoses. (From Spratt, J. S., et al.: Association of chronic cystic mastopathy, xeromammographic patterns and cancer. Cancer, 55:1372, 1985. Used with permission.)

Table 4-6. MATRIX ASSOCIATION OF TYPES OF CHRONIC CYSTIC MASTOPATHY (CCM), WOLFE'S PARENCHYMAL MAMMOGRAPHIC PATTERNS (XM), AND CANCERS DIAGNOSED IN FOLLOW-UP AFTER DIAGNOSIS OF CCM AND XM

Type of Chronic Cystic Mastopathy	Wolfe's Parenchymal Patterns						Cancers/ Category
	D_y	N_1	P_1	P_2C	P_2L	P_2N	
Lobular hyperplasia	10	12	15	26	66*	27	1/156
Sclerosing adenosis	7	11	15	17*	45	22*	2/117
Ductal papillary hyperplasia	13	16	19	26*	60	25*	2/159
Ductal papillary hyperplasia with apocrine metaplasia	3	9	6	8	26	8	0/60
Ductal nonpapillary hyperplasia	2	1	11	5	9	4	0/32
Ductal nonpapillary hyperplasia with apocrine metaplasia	1	0	0	1	1	4*	1/7
Cyst, epithelial	12*	14	37	45*	90*	38	3/246
Cyst, epithelial, with apocrine metaplasia	13	21	21	34*	79*	30	2/198
Lobular hyperplasia with atypia	0	0	0	0	1	1	0/2
Ductal hyperplasia with atypia	2	2	4	4*	8	2	1/22
Cancers/category	1/63	0/06	0/178	1/166	1/385	1/161	4/355

*Cancer (1) in subset.
(From Spratt, J. S., et al.: Association of chronic cystic mastopathy, xeromammographic patterns and cancer. Cancer, 55:1372, 1985. Reprinted with permission.)

Wolfe's parenchymal mammographic patterns, and cancers diagnosed in follow-up. Clearly there is no clustering in these matrices, implicating either a xeromammographic pattern or histologic type of chronic cystic mastopathy as being precancerous. As the authors noted, a much larger series followed for longer periods of time might produce a trend of association of greater significance. Certainly, the majority of women develop the changes of chronic cystic mastopathy with no strongly cancerous predisposition. These women need reassurance to alleviate anxiety.

Two significant studies with long-term follow-up have given better definition to what might and might not be precancerous. Dupont and Page (1985) followed 10,366 women undergoing breast biopsies consecutively in Nashville, Tennessee, hospitals. The median duration of follow-up was 17 years among 3303 patients selected for follow-up. They observed that women with proliferative disease but without atypical hyperplasia had a risk of cancer 1.9 times the risk of women with nonproliferative lesions. With atypical hyperplasia this risk rose to 5.3 times (3.1 to 8.8 with 95 per cent confidence). Family history associated with nonproliferative disease had little risk. When family history was combined with atypia, the breast cancer risk was 11 times greater (5.5 to 24 with 95 per cent confidence) than the risk of cancer in women with nonpro-

Table 4-7. ASSOCIATION OF CANCERS CONFIRMED AT FIRST BIOPSY WITH CHRONIC CYSTIC MASTOPATHY

Type of Chronic Cystic Mastopathy	Number with Cancer at First Biopsy	Number with No Cancer at First Biopsy	Number with No Cancer at First Biopsy in Whom Cancer Developed During Follow-up
Lobular hyperplasia	29	156	1
Sclerosing adenosis	43	117	2
Ductal papillary hyperplasia	63	159	2
Ductal papillary hyperplasia with apocrine metaplasia	23	60	0
Ductal nonpapillary hyperplasia	22	32	0
Ductal nonpapillary hyperplasia with apocrine metaplasia	5	7	1
Cyst, epithelial	72	246	3
Epithelial cyst with apocrine metaplasia	41	198	2
Lobular hyperplasia with atypia	10	2	0
Ductal hyperplasia with atypia	35	22	1
Total number of patients	116	355	4

(From Spratt, J. S., et al.: Association of chronic cystic mastopathy, xeromammographic patterns and cancer. Cancer, 55:1372, 1985. Reprinted with permission.)

Table 4-8. MAMMARY CANCER SUBSEQUENT TO CYSTIC DISEASE

Reference	Number of Patients	Lesion	Follow-up (Years)	Observed Cancers	Excess Cancer Risk	Breast With Subsequent Cancer Ipsi: Contralateral‡
Davis, 1964	284	Cystic disease	13 mean	7	1.7	4:2
	86	Ductal hyperplasia	12 mean	3	2.5	1:1
Potter, 1968	100	Benign	16–20	10	4.8	
Veronesi, 1968	1009	Cystic disease	8.8 mean	25	2.0	18:7
Haagensen, 1971	1693	Gross cysts	1+	72	4.1	28:25
Donnelly, 1975	370	All benign	13.5 median	14	1.6	7:7
	96	CCM*		9	2.9†	

*Chronic cystic mastitis.
†In patients 40–49 years old observed cancers = 10 times the expected.
‡In some cases the preceding benign lesion was bilateral.

liferative lesions and a negative family history. The presence of calcification in association with proliferative disease increased the cancer risk. Benign cysts alone did not increase cancer risk. However, when combined with a family history, the risk rose to 2.7 times greater than in women without these factors. Of great significance was the observation that the majority (70 per cent) of all women who undergo breast biopsy are not at greater risk. They suggested that breast biopsies might be considered in women with family histories of breast cancer to reassure women with no proliferative histologic changes in the breast. More effective surveillance might then be explored for women with a combination of family history and atypia, and they should follow a life style associated with the least probability of promoting breast cancer. (See Chapter 5.)

A source of confusion in assessing the precancerous implications of various types of mastopathy has been variable nomenclature. A consensus conference sponsored by the College of American Pathologists has recommended a clarifying simplification of nomenclature (1986). Slight increased cancer risk (1.5 to 2 times) was considered to exist with moderate to florid hyperplasia, either solid or papillary, and when papillomas were present with a fibrovascular core. A moderate increased risk (5 times) was considered to exist with borderline lesions of atypical hyperplasia, either ductal or lobular. Other histopathologic patterns were not considered to be associated with an increased risk of cancer.

Whether there is a causative or aggravating association between the widespread use of oral contraceptives and chronic cystic mastopathy is an important question that has been the subject of a number of studies with mostly negative but still contradictory results. The contradictions are easily attributable to the hospital-based nature of most studies, with biases attributable to this select population and to the relatively small number of cases followed for variable and possibly inadequate time periods. From these studies it may be concluded that, if a relation exists, it is not a strong one. Two recent studies were consistent in their refutation of a protective effect from oral contraceptives in reducing the prevalence of CCM (Berkowitz et al., 1984; Franceschi et al., 1984).

Berkowitz and coworkers (1984) revealed a trend toward an increase in CCM in postmenopausal women who had been oral contraceptive users. However, even a strong association would not establish a cause and effect relation. Numerous covariables would have to be considered before even implying that a causative relation exists.

EPIDEMIOLOGIC ASPECTS OF MALE BREAST CANCER

Breast cancer in males is infrequent but not rare. The Third National Cancer Survey for 1969–1971 placed the annual incidence rate at 0.6 per 100,000 men. It accounts for 0.2 per cent of all cancers in boys and men. The 900 cases that occur in the United States each year constitute slightly less than 1 per cent of the total newly diagnosed breast cancers. It is tempting to relate the relative risk to the obvious difference in breast size between the sexes. As in women, the incidence increases with age, but onset is generally later in life, and men who develop cancer average 10 years older; occasional cases, nevertheless, occur as early as the third decade.

Although a defect in estrogen metabolism is suspected, no definite hormonal abnormality is regularly identified with male breast cancer. Some aspects of the disease are reminiscent of the rat model. In high incidence rat lines, males share little of the risk unless they are feminized with exogenous estrogens, in which case breast development occurs and breast cancers make their appearance. Similarly, signs of feminization are often present in men with breast cancer. Gynecomastia is associated in 5 per cent to 18 per cent of cases, and ductal hyperplasia is seen. Men with Klinefelter's syndrome, which includes breast development, have a risk of breast cancer that is 66 times normal. Breast cancer also has been reported in male transsexuals taking maintenance estrogens (Symmers, 1968). Cancer in the breasts of men taking estrogens for prostatic cancer occurs, but it is not common and is usually metastatic carcinoma from the prostate. Schottenfeld and associates (1963) found a higher incidence of past orchitis and previous orchiectomy among males with breast cancer than among matched controls. Associations were also found with exposure to x-rays, benign breast disease, and family history of breast cancer. Everson and associates (1976) provided evidence for a familial susceptibility specifically for men, having observed a total of six cases in two families. Elevated estrogen excretion was detected in three of the male family members.

Summary

Although the cause of mammary cancer in humans remains obscure, epidemiologic data, animal models, and in-depth studies of patient populations are providing insights. The rapid progress and sophistication of these investigations promise to clarify with increasing precision the genetic and environmental determinants of risk, if not the fundamental cause. The importance of this information cannot be overestimated; inherent in it lies the possibility of prevention.

REFERENCES

Albano, W. A., Recabaren, J. A., and Lynch, H. T.: Natural history of hereditary cancer of the breast and colon. Cancer, *50*:360, 1982.

American Cancer Society: 1978 Cancer Facts and Figures. New York, American Cancer Society, 1978.

American Cancer Society: 1987 Cancer Facts and Figures. New York, American Cancer Society, 1987.

Anderson, D. E.: Genetic study of breast cancer. Identification of a high risk group. Cancer, *34*:1090, 1974.

Anderson, D. E., and Badzioch, M. D.: Risk of familial breast cancer. Cancer, *56*:383, 1985.

Ariel, I. M.: Enovid therapy (norethynodrel with mestranol) for fibrocystic disease. Am. J. Obstet. Gynecol., *117*:453, 1973.

Arthes, F. G., Sartwell, P. E., and Lewison, E. F.: The pill, estrogens, and the breast. Cancer, *28*:1391, 1971.

Bailar, J. C., and Smith, E. M.: Progress against cancer? Presented at annual meeting of the American Association for the Advancement of Science, 1985.

Baral, E., Larsson, L.-E., and Mattsson, B.: Breast cancer following irradiation of the breast. Cancer, *40*:2905, 1977.

BEIR III (Advisory Committee on the Biological Effects of Ionizing Radiation): The effects on populations of exposure of low levels of ionizing radiation. Washington, D. C., Division of Medical Sciences, National Research Council, National Academy of Science Press, 1980.

Berkowitz, G. S., Kelsey, J. L., LiVolsi, V. A., et al.: Oral contraceptive use among pre- and postmenopausal women. Am. J. Epidemiol., *120*:82, 1984.

Biran, S., Keren, A., Farkas, T., et al.: Development of carcinoma of the breast at the site of implanted pacemakers in two patients. J. Surg. Oncol., *11*:7, 1979.

Bittner, J. J.: Some possible effects of nursing on the mammary gland tumor incidence in mice. Science, *84*:162, 1936.

Boice, J. D., Rosenstein, M., and Trout, E. D.: Estimation of breast doses and breast cancer risk associated with repeated fluoroscopic chest examinations of women with tuberculosis. Radiat. Res., *73*:373, 1978.

Bucalossi, P., and Veronesi, U.: Some observations on cancer of the breast in mothers and daughters. Br. J. Cancer, *11*:337, 1957.

Buckman, M. T., and Peake, G. T.: Prolactin in clinical practice. J.A.M.A., *236*:871, 1976.

Bulbrook, R. D., Deshpande, N., and Ellis, F. G.: Androgens in human breast cancer. Proc. R. Soc. Med., *57*:523, 1964.

Bulbrook, R. D.: Prediction of response of breast cancer to treatment. *In* Holland, J. F., and Frei, E. (Eds.): Cancer Medicine. Philadelphia, Lea & Febiger, 1973, p. 907.

Burch, J. C., and Byrd, B. F.: Effects of long-term administration of estrogen on the occurrence of mammary cancer in women. Ann. Surg., *174*:414, 1971.

Busk, T., and Clemmesen, J.: Frequencies of left- and right-sided breast cancer. Br. J. Cancer, *1*:345, 1947.

Cairns, J.: The origin of human cancers. Nature (Lond.), *289*:353, 1981.

Cappelli, L., and Margottini, M.: Thyroid function in cancer patients. Acta Un. Int. Cancer, *20*:1493, 1964.

Carroll, K. K.: Experimental evidence of dietary factors and hormone-dependent cancers. Cancer Res., *35*:3374, 1975.

Centers for Disease Control: Cancer and hormone study. Long-term oral contraceptive use and the risk of breast cancer. J.A.M.A., *249*:1591, 1983.

Cole, P.: Epidemiology of breast cancer: An overview. Report to the Profession, Breast Cancer. U.S. Department of Health, Education and Welfare, September 30, 1974, p. 11.

Consensus Meeting, Oct. 3 to 5, 1985, New York: Is 'Fibrocystic Disease' of the Breast Precancerous? Convened by the Cancer Committee of the College of American Pathologists, Arch. Pathol. Lab. Med., 110:171–173, 1986.

Cook, G. B.: A comparison of single and multiple primary cancers. Cancer, 19:959, 1966.

Davis, H. H., Simons, M., and Davis, J. B.: Cystic disease of the breast. Relationship to carcinoma. Cancer, 17:957, 1964.

deWaard, F.: The epidemiology of breast cancer—review and projects. Int. J. Cancer, 4:577, 1969.

deWaard, F.: Breast cancer incidence and nutritional status with particular reference to body weight and height. Cancer Res., 35:3351, 1975.

Dickinson, L. E., MacMahon, B., Cole, P., et al.: Estrogen profiles of Oriental and Caucasian women in Hawaii. N. Engl. J. Med., 291:1211, 1974.

Doll, R., Muir, C., and Waterhouse, J. (Eds.): International Union Against Cancer (UICC) Incidence in Five Continents. Vol. 2. Berlin, Springer-Verlag, 1970.

Drasar, B. S., and Irving, D.: Environmental factors and cancer of the colon and breast. Br. J. Cancer, 27:167, 1973.

Dupont, W. D., and Page, D. L.: Risk factors for breast cancer in women with proliferative breast disease. N. Engl. J. Med., 312:146, 1985.

Dvoretsky, P. M., Woodard, E., Bonfiglio, T. A., et al.: The pathology of breast cancer in women irradiated for acute postpartum mastitis. Cancer, 46:2257, 1980.

Emery, E. W., and Trotter, W. R.: Triiodothyronine in advanced breast cancer. Lancet, 1:358, 1963.

Everson, R. B., Fraumeni, J. F., Wisson, R. E., et al.: Familial male breast cancer. Lancet, 1:9, 1976.

Farrow, J. H.: Antiquity of breast cancer. Cancer, 28:1369, 1971.

Fasal, E., and Paffenbarger, R. S., Jr.: Oral contraceptives as related to cancer and benign lesions of the breast. JNCI, 55:767, 1975.

Fechner, R. E.: Benign breast disease in women on estrogen therapy. Cancer, 29:273, 1972.

Feig, S. A.: Low-dose mammography: Assessment of theoretical risk. In Feig, S. A. and McLelland, R. (Eds.): Breast Carcinoma, Current Diagnosis and Treatment. New York, Masson, 1983, pp. 69–76.

Feinleib, M.: Breast cancer and artificial menopause. A cohort study. JNCI, 41:315, 1968.

Finley, J. W., and Bogardus, G. M.: Breast cancer and thyroid disease. Q. Rev. Surg. Obstet. Gynecol., 17:139, 1960.

Fishman, J., Hellman, L., Zumoff, B., et al.: Influence of thyroid hormone on estrogen metabolism in man. J. Clin. Endocrinol., 22:389, 1962.

Fishman, J., Fukushima, D., O'Connor, J., et al.: Plasma hormone profiles of young women at risk for familial breast cancer. Cancer Res., 38:4006, 1978.

Fishman, J., Fukushima, D. K., O'Connor, J., et al.: Low urinary estrogen glucuronides in women at risk for familial breast cancer. Science, 204:1089, 1979.

Foote, F. W., and Stewart, F. W.: Comparative studies of cancerous versus noncancerous breasts. Ann. Surg., 121:197, 1945.

Fox, M. S.: On the diagnosis and treatment of breast cancer. J.A.M.A., 241:489, 1979.

Franceschi, S., LaVecchia, C., Parazzini, F., et al.: Oral contraceptives and benign breast disease: a case control study. Am. J. Obstet. Gynecol., 149:602, 1984.

Gallagher, H. S., and Martin, J. E.: Early phases in the development of breast cancer. Cancer, 24:1170, 1969.

Gambrell, R. D., Jr., Maier, R. C., and Sanders, B. I.: Decreased incidence of breast cancer in post-menopausal estrogen-progesterone users. Obstet. Gynecol., 62:435, 1983.

Gentry, W. C., Jr., Eskrit, N. R., and Gorland, R. J.: Multiple hamartoma syndrome (Cowden's disease). Arch. Dermatol., 109:521, 1974.

Glass, A., Hoover, R., Finkle, W., et al.: Conjugated estrogen (CE) use and the risk of breast cancer. Cancer Treat. Rep., 63:1209, 1979.

Gray, G. E., Pike, N. C., and Henderson, B. E.: Breast cancer incidence and mortality rates in different countries in relation to known risk factors and dietary practices. Br. J. Cancer, 39:1, 1979.

Guinee, V.: Cancer data systems. Curr. Probl. Cancer, 9:1, 1985.

Haagensen, C. D.: Diseases of the Breast. Philadelphia, W.B. Saunders, 1971, p. 364.

Hems, G.: Associations between breast-cancer mortality rates, child-bearing, and diet in the United Kingdom. Br. J. Cancer, 41:429, 1980.

Hems, G.: The contributions of diet and childbearing to breast cancer rates. Br. J. Cancer, 37:974, 1978.

Herrell, W. E.: Relative incidence of oophorectomy in women with or without carcinoma of the breast. Am. J. Cancer, 29:659, 1937.

Hobbs, J. R., Salih, H., Flax, H., et al.: Prolactin dependence in human breast cancer. Proc. R. Soc. Med., 66:866, 1973.

Holm, N. V., Hauge, M., and Harvald, B.: Etiologic factors of breast cancer elucidated by a study of unselected twins. JNCI, 65:285, 1980.

Hoover, R., Gray, L. A., Sr., Cole, P., et al.: Menopausal estrogens and breast cancer. N. Engl. J. Med., 295:401, 1976.

Howe, G. R., Miller, A. B., and Sherman, G. J.: Breast cancer mortality following fluoroscopic irradiation in a cohort of tuberculosis patients. Cancer Detect. Prev., 5:175, 1982.

Humphrey, L. J., and Swerdlow, M. A.: The relationship of breast disease to thyroid disease. Cancer, 17:1170, 1964.

Humphrey, L. J., and Swerdlow, M. A.: A large duct epithelial hyperplasia and carcinoma of the breast. Arch. Surg., 97:592, 1968.

Jackson, C. F., Palmquist, M., Swanson, J., et al.: Effectiveness of prophylactic subcutaneous mastectomy in Sprague-Dawley rats induced with 7,12-dimethylbenzanthracene. Plast. Reconstr. Surg., 73:249, 1984.

Jacobsen, C. O.: Heredity in breast cancer: A genetic and clinical study of 200 probands. Copenhagen, Nyt Nordirk Forlag, 1946.

Kalache, A., Vessey, M. P., and McPherson, K.: Lactation and breast cancer. Br. J. Med., 280:223, 1980.

Kapdi, C. C., and Wolfe, J. N.: Breast cancer-relationship to thyroid supplements for hypothyroidism. J.A.M.A., 236:1124, 1976.

Kennedy, B. J.: Massive estrogen administration in premenopausal women with metastatic breast cancer. Cancer, 15:641, 1962.

Klamer, T. W., Donegan, W. L., and Max, M. H.: Breast tumor incidence in rats after partial mammary resection. Arch. Surg., 118:933, 1983.

Knox, E. G.: Foods and diseases. Br. J. Prev. Soc. Med., 31:71, 1977.

Knudsen, A. G., Strong, L. C., and Anderson, D. E.: Heredity and cancer in man. Prog. Med. Genet., 9:113, 1976.

Kolonel, L. N., Hankin, J. H., Lee, J., et al.: Nutrient

intakes in relation to cancer incidence in Hawaii. Br. J. Cancer, 44:332, 1981.
Kwa, H. G., Engelsman, E., De Jong-Bakker, M., et al.: Plasma-prolactin in human breast cancer. Lancet, 1:433, 1974.
Lemon, H. M.: Arrest of metastatic mammary carcinoma by cortisone and thyroid therapy. Forum, 6:414, 1955.
Lemon, H. M.: Estrogens. In Holland, J. F., and Frei, E., III (Eds.): Cancer Medicine. Philadelphia, Lea & Febiger, 1974, p. 911.
Lemon, H. M., and Westfall, R. H.: Abnormal estrogen metabolism in human breast cancer. Scientific Exhibit No. 305, 114th AMA Annual Convention, New York, June 20–24, 1965.
Levine, P. H., Steinhorn, S. C., Ries, L. G., et al.: Inflammatory breast cancer: the experience of the Surveillance, Epidemiology, and End Results (SEER) program. JNCI, 74:291, 1985.
Levy, J., and Levy, J. A.: The role of the hypometabolic state in cancer. Am. Pract. Digest. Treat., 2:522, 1951.
Lewis, C. M.: Inflammatory carcinoma of the breast following silicone injections. Plast. Reconstr. Surg., 66:134, 1980.
Lilienfeld, A. M.: The relationship of cancer of the female breast to artificial menopause and marital status. Cancer, 9:927, 1956.
Lilienfeld, A. M.: The epidemiology of breast cancer. Cancer Res., 23:1503, 1963.
Loeser, A. A.: A new therapy for prevention of postoperative recurrences in genital and breast cancer: Six years' study of prophylactic thyroid treatment. Br. Med. J., 2:1380, 1954.
Logan, W. W., Plansur, P. S., Cullinan, A., et al.: Increased incidence of breast carcinoma in patients with irradiation for post-partum mastitis: A screening situation. J. Surg. Oncol., 11:239, 1979.
Lorenz, E.: Some biologic effects of long continued irradiation. Am. J. Roentgenol., 63:176, 1950.
Lowe, C. R., and MacMahon, B.: Breast cancer and reproductive history of women in South Wales. Lancet, 1:153, 1970.
Lowell, D. M., Martineau, R. G., and Luria, S. B.: Carcinoma of the male breast following radiation. Report of a case 35 years after radiation therapy of unilateral prepubertal gynecomastia. Cancer, 22:581, 1968.
Lucas, F. V., and Perez-Mesa, C.: Inflammatory carcinoma of the breast. Cancer, 41:1595, 1978.
Lynch, H. T., Albano, W. A., Danes, B. S., et al.: Genetic predisposition to breast cancer. Cancer, 53:612, 1984.
Lynch, H. T., Albano, W. A., Organ, C. H., et al.: Surveillance and management of hereditary breast cancer. Breast, 7:2, 1981.
Lynch, H. T., Harris, R. E., Organ, C. H., Jr., et al.: Management of familial breast cancer. I. Biostatistical-genetic aspects and their limitations as derived from a familial breast cancer resource. Arch. Surg., 113:1053, 1978.
MacDonald, I.: The breast. In Nealon, T. F., Jr. (Ed.): Management of the Patient with Cancer. Philadelphia, W.B. Saunders, 1965, p. 440.
Macera, C., Leung, R., and King, M. C.: Comparison of risk factors associated with familial and non-familial breast cancer (Abstract). Am. J. Epidemiol., 116:563, 1982.
Mackenzie, I.: Breast cancer following multiple fluoroscopies. Br. J. Cancer, 19:1, 1965.
Macklin, M. T.: Comparison of the number of breast cancer deaths observed in relatives of breast cancer patients and the number expected on the basis of mortality rates. JNCI, 22:927, 1959.
MacMahon, B., Cole, P., and Brown, J.: Etiology of human breast cancer: A review. JNCI, 50:21, 1973.
Manton, K. G., and Stallard, E.: A two-disease model of female breast cancer: Mortality in 1969 among white females in the United States. JNCI, 64:9, 1980.
Mettler, F. A., Hempelmann, L. H., Dutton, A. M., et al.: Breast neoplasms in women treated with x-rays for acute postpartum mastitis. A pilot study. JNCI, 43:803, 1969.
Mider, G. B., Schilling, J. A., Donovan, J. C., et al.: Multiple cancer—a study of other cancers arising in patients with primary malignant neoplasms of the stomach, uterus, breast, large intestine, or hematopoietic system. Cancer, 5:1104, 1952.
Ministry of Health Reports on Public Health and Medical Subjects, No. 32. London, His Majesty's Stationery Office, 1926.
Minton, J. P., and Dickey, R. P.: Levodopa test to predict response of carcinoma of the breast to surgical ablation of endocrine glands. Surg. Gynecol. Obstet., 136:971, 1973.
Moolgavkar, S. H., Day, N. E., and Stevens, R. G.: Two-stage model of carcinogenesis: Epidemiology of breast cancer in females. JNCI, 65:559, 1980.
Moolgavkar, S. H., Stevens, R. G., and Lee, J. A. H.: Effect of age on the incidence of breast cancer in females. JNCI, 62:493, 1979.
Moolgavkar, S. H., Stevens, R. G., and Lee, J. A. H.: Age and breast cancer incidence. Eur. J. Cancer Clin. Oncol., 20:1453, 1984.
Moore, D. H.: Evidence in favor of the existence of human breast cancer virus. Cancer Res., 34:2322, 1974.
Moore, D. H., Moore, D. H., II, and Moore, C. T.: Breast carcinoma etiological factors. Adv. Cancer Res., 40:189, 1983.
Morgenstern, L., Gleischman, S. H., Michel, S. L., et al.: Relation of free silicone to human breast carcinoma. Arch. Surg., 120:573, 1985.
Mossman, K. L.: Ionizing radiation and cancer. Cancer Invest., 2:301, 1984.
Mulvihill, J. J.: Congenital and genetic diseases. In Fraumeni, J. F., Jr. (Ed.): Persons at High Risk of Cancer. New York, Academic Press, 1975, p. 11.
Myrden, J. A., and Hiltz, J. E.: Breast cancer following multiple fluoroscopies during artificial pneumothorax treatment of pulmonary tuberculosis. Can. Med. Assoc. J., 100:1032, 1969.
National Research Council: Diet, nutrition, and cancer. Washington, D. C.: National Academy Press, 1982.
Ottman, R., King, M., Pike, M. C., et al.: Practical guide for estimating risk for familial breast cancer. Lancet, 2:556, 1983.
Paffenbarger, R. S., Jr., Fasal, E., Simmons, M. E., et al.: Cancer risk as related to use of oral contraceptives during fertile years. Presented at symposium on Cancer Epidemiology and the Clinician, October 23–25, 1975, Boston.
Papaioannou, A. N.: Etiologic factors in cancer of the breast in humans. Surg. Gynecol. Obstet., 138:257, 1974.
Peden, J. G., Jr.: Carcinoma of the breast following burn. Am. J. Surg., 73:519, 1947.
Petrakis, N. L.: Cerumen genetics in human breast cancer. Science, 173:347, 1971.
Poortman, J., Thyssen, J. H. H., and Schwarz, F.: Androgen production and conversion to estrogens in nor-

mal postmenopausal women and in selected breast cancer patients. J. Clin. Endocrinol. Metab. *37*:101, 1973.

Pullinger, B. D.: Increase in mammary carcinoma and adenoma and incidences of other tumors in C₃Hf virgin females after ovariectomy and high dosage with some estrogens. Br. J. Cancer, *15*:574, 1961.

Repert, R. W.: Breast carcinoma study: Relation to thyroid disease and diabetes. J. Michigan Med. Soc., *51*:1315, 1952.

Ross, R. K., Gerkins, V. R., Paganini-Hill, A., et al.: Menopausal estrogen use and breast cancer. Cancer Treat. Rep., *63*:1209, 1979.

Royal College of General Practitioners: Breast cancer and oral contraceptives: Findings in Royal College of General Practitioners' Study. Br. Med. J., *282*:208, 1981.

Sandison, A. T.: Autopsy study of adult human breast. National Cancer Institute Monograph No. 8. U.S. Dept. of Health Education and Welfare, 1962.

Sasaki, G. H., Leung, B. S., and Fletcher, W. S.: Levodopa test and estrogen receptor assay in prognosticating response of patients with advanced cancer of the breast to endocrine therapy. Ann. Surg., *183*:341, 1976.

Schoenberg, B. S., Greenberg, R. A., and Eisenberg, H.: Occurrence of certain multiple primary cancers in females. JNCI, *43*:15, 1969.

Schottenfeld, D., and Berg, J.: Incidence of multiple primary cancers. IV. Cancers of the female breast and genital organs. JNCI, *46*:161, 1971.

Schottenfeld, D., Lilienfeld, A. M., and Diamond, H.: Some observations on the epidemiology of breast cancer among males. Am. J. Public Health, *53*:890, 1963.

Seidman, H.: Cancer of the Breast. Statistical and Epidemiological Data. New York, American Cancer Society, 1972.

Seidman, H., Silverberg, E., and Holleb, A.: Cancer statistics, 1976. A comparison of white and black populations. New York, American Cancer Society, 1972.

Seidman, H., and Mushinski, M. H.: Breast cancer: Incidence, mortality, survival, and prognosis. *In* Feig, S.A., and McLelland, R. (Eds.): Breast Carcinoma—Current Diagnosis and Treatment. New York: Masson Publishing, 1983, p. 9.

Shapiro, S., Strax, P., Venet, L., et al.: The search for risk factors in breast cancer. Am. J. Public Health, *58*:820, 1968.

Shimkin, M. B.: Epidemiology of breast cancer in recent results of cancer research. New York, Springer-Verlag, 1973, p. 6.

Siiteri, P. K., Hemsell, D. L., Edwards, C. L., et al.: Estrogen and endometrial carcinoma. *In* Scow, R. O. (Ed.): Proceedings of the Fourth International Congress on Endocrinology, Washington, D. C. Amsterdam: Excerpta Medica, 1973, p. 1237.

Silverberg, E.: Cancer statistics. CA *35*:19, 1985.

Smithcors, J. F., and Leonard, S. L.: Relation of thyroid to mammary gland structure in the rat with special reference to the male. Endocrinology, *31*:454, 1942.

Spencer, J. G.: The influence of thyroid in malignant disease. Br. J. Cancer, *8*:393, 1954.

Spratt, J. S., Jr., and Hoag, M. G.: Incidence of multiple primary cancers per man-year of follow-up. Ann. Surg., *164*:775, 1966.

Spratt, J. S., Alagia, D. P., Greenberg, R. A., et al.: Association of chronic cystic mastopathy, xeromammographic patterns and cancer. Cancer, *55*:1372, 1985.

Symmers, W.: Carcinoma of breast in transsexual individuals after surgical and hormonal interference with the primary and secondary sex characteristics. Br. Med. J., *2*:83, 1968.

Tokuoka, S., Asano, M., Yamamoto, T., et al.: Histologic review of breast cancer cases in survivors of atomic bombs in Hiroshima and Nagasaki, Japan. Cancer, *54*:849, 1984.

UNSCEAR (United Nations Scientific Committee on the Effects of Atomic Radiation): Sources and effects of ionizing radiation. UNSCEAR 1977 Report to the General Assembly, with Annexes. New York, United Nations, 1977.

Upton, A. C.: Critics, defenders express views about routine mammography. J.A.M.A., *236*:541, 1976.

Vessey, M. P., Doll, R., and Sutton, P. M.: Investigation of the possible relationship between oral contraceptives and benign and malignant breast disease. Cancer, *28*:1395, 1971.

Villee, C. A., and Hagerman, D. D.: Compounds with antiestrogenic activity in vitro. Endocrinology, *60*:552, 1957.

Wanebo, C. K., Johnson, K. G., Sato, K., et al.: Breast cancer after exposure to the atomic bombings of Hiroshima and Nagasaki. N. Engl. J. Med., *279*:667, 1968.

Warren, S.: A radiation-induced breast cancer. Cancer, *32*:921, 1973.

Wilkins, R. H., and Morton, D. L.: The influence of thyroid hormone analogues on an isotransplanted spontaneous mammary adenocarcinoma in mice. Cancer, *16*:558, 1963.

Wilson, R. G., Buchan, R., Roberts, M. M., et al.: Prolactin and breast cancer. Proc. R. Soc. Med., *66*:865, 1973.

World Health Organization: Evolution of mortality in Europe during 20th century: Cancer mortality. Annex: Non-European countries. Epid Vital Statistics Report *5*:1, 1952.

Wynder, E. L., Chan, P., Cohen, L., et al: Overview-nutrition and breast cancer. Breast, *2*:11, 1976.

Zanartu, J., Onetto, E., Medina, E., et al.: Mammary gland nodules in women under continuous exposure to progestagens. Contraception, *7*:203, 1973.

Zumoff, B., Fishman, J., Bradlow, H. L., et al.: Hormone profiles in hormone-dependent cancers. Cancer Res., *35*:3365, 1975.

CHAPTER 5

SHARLEEN JOHNSON BIRKIMER

Nutrition and Breast Disease

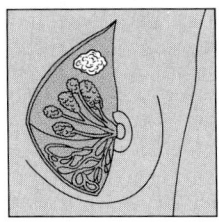

The notion that what a person eats may be involved in the development of cancer is not a new idea; it was discussed in the Middle Ages. In the past decade the public and scientific community have become much interested in probing the relationship between dietary components and cancer. An understanding of the role of nutrients in the initiation and promotion of oncogenic cells is important in preventing and managing cancer in humans.

In investigating possible dietary causes of cancer, research has taken two basic forms: epidemiologic investigations into the association between various dietary components and several types of malignancies in humans; and laboratory experiments with neoplastic induction in animal models. Research indicates that a wide variety of nutrients are capable of developing a wide variety of tumors. The level of nutrient intake needed to cause tumor development is frequently well within the typical human intake. This may mean that dietary studies on cancer should focus less on the role of traditional chemical carcinogens, which are needed in larger than normal amounts to induce cancer, and more on establishing relationships that may exist between the usual human intake and the development of oncogenic tissue (National Research Council, 1982; Rivlin, 1982; Campbell, 1983).

For women in most Western countries, breast cancer is the leading type of cancer. Epidemiologic and experimental evidence indicates that dietary factors are a major etiologic factor, especially after menopause. Most of the research, done since 1975, has focused on dietary fat and total kcalorie intake (Miller, 1977; Moore et al., 1983; Wynder and Rose, 1984). However, the possible roles of protein (Lubin et al., 1981), various vitamins (Graham, 1983; King and McCay, 1983) and minerals (Ip and Sinha, 1981), and methylxanthines (Minton et al., 1979a; Lubin et al., 1985a) have been investigated.

Epidemiologic Studies

Epidemiologic researchers try to associate individual dietary risk factors over a long period of time with the occurrence of breast disease in a defined population group (National Research Council, 1982). Owing to the complex nature of diet, these studies have been called the most challenging and controversial in cancer epidemiology (Lyon et al., 1983).

Epidemiologic studies can be used to circumvent two limitations of laboratory research in which animal models are used. First, the results can be applied directly to humans; the findings need not be extrapolated from one species to another. Second, because the levels and patterns of exposure to the dietary components reported in the studies occurred in women, there is no need to interpolate from the artificially high levels frequently used in laboratory animal models (National Research Council, 1982).

Some problems occur with epidemiologic studies, however. Ethical issues are foremost. The scientist, relying primarily on subject observation, cannot have any major intervention in the diet. Bias can enter into the study's selection of participants. The women being studied may not be representative of the female population. However, the major difficulty is the long latency period between the person's first exposure to the offending dietary component and the actual development of breast disease (National Research Council, 1982).

Methods of Dietary Information Intake

Epidemiologists and nutritionists have developed several methods for collecting dietary information. Some, based on government production and disappearance statistics, involve no personal contact between the researcher and the population studied. Other methods assess the nutrient intake of individuals through client interviews or by collecting the data from questionnaires (National Research Council, 1982; Guthrie, 1986).

GROUP DATA

The primary method of collecting group data indirectly involves calculating the national per capita food consumption information by using food balance sheets or food disappearance data that are based on governmental data of agricultural productivity, food imported and exported, and estimates of food consumed by animals or destroyed in storage. The researcher compares the rate of various types of cancer with the national per capita disappearance of a particular nutrient, such as fat.

This method has problems, too. The researcher must first assume that there is an equal distribution of food among the population. Data developed from this method are also based on the amount of food that has disappeared within the country, not the actual food consumed. In addition, the quality of the data used varies from country to country (Armstrong and Doll, 1975; Miller, 1977; National Research Council, 1982).

The household food inventory is a more direct method of collecting group dietary data. At the beginning of the weekly or monthly study period, the researcher or someone in the household records the type and amount of all food in the house. During the study, a record is kept of food purchased for consumption within the household as well as food consumed away from the home. At the end of the study period, another inventory is taken of the food within the home.

An estimate is made of food consumed by animals, lost in storage, and placed in the garbage. The average amount of nutrients consumed per day is calculated by dividing the total household intake of each food by the number of days in the study and then the number of persons in the family. The limitations of this method include the assumption of an even distribution of food among family members; the possibility that the members of the household may modify their food purchases because they know they are participants in a research project; and the possibility of incorrectly kept records (National Research Council, 1982; Guthrie, 1986).

INDIVIDUAL ASSESSMENT

Most investigations into a possible relationship between dietary components and breast cancer use individual dietary data because the information obtained will be a more valid representation of the food actually consumed by the subject. No universal agreement exists on the terminology used in naming the various methods of collecting individual dietary data, but the following are commonly used terms: diet recall, food records or diaries, and diet history (National Research Council, 1982; Lyon et al., 1983; Russell-Briefel et al., 1985; Guthrie, 1986).

The strengths and weaknesses of each method have been discussed in a number of review articles (Becker et al., 1960; Houser and Bebb, 1981; Krantzler et al., 1982; Sorenson, 1982; Lyon et al., 1983). One major concern when using any of these methods is the ability and willingness of the subjects to state their usual food consumption correctly. Methods that require the ability to read and write will limit the subjects to older children and adults. Some adults are not suitable because they are functionally illiterate or do not have the mental capacity to complete a simple form requesting dietary information.

A common problem is the subject's inability to state correctly the portion sizes of food consumed. Guthrie (1984) found that some type of aid was necessary in estimating portion sizes. When she studied the ability of 147 young adults to describe the amount of food presented to them, she found they could state accurately the amount of some foods, such as orange juice, but for others error rates were very high. Over 70 per cent of the subjects had more than 70 per cent errors in estimating the amount of salad dressing and butter used.

Nutritionists frequently use plastic food models, measuring cups, and measuring spoons to assist the subjects in stating the amount of food they consumed (Moore et al., 1967; Lyon et al., 1983; Guthrie, 1986). Other tools used have been colored photographs of food (Kolonel et al., 1983) and geometric models (Russell-Briefel et al., 1985).

A *dietary recall* is usually done for the 24 or 48 hours before the interview. It can be given orally to the investigator or written down by the subject. A faulty memory or intentional falsification is a potential problem, but as this is a retrospective method, the subject cannot change the food consumed the day of the recall. Other advantages are the relatively short amount of time needed to determine food intake compared with other methods, and the researcher's opportunity to probe for missing or incomplete data.

A disadvantage with recall is its limited usefulness in determining the nutrient intake of specific individuals because of the wide day-by-day variations in food consumption. Recalls may, however, be a reliable source of group data (Gersovitz et al., 1978; Graham, 1983; Samet et al., 1984; Guthrie, 1986).

Since breast cancer has a long latency period, 24 hour recalls have validity only if the immediate past eating habits are representative of long-term eating patterns. Few studies have appeared comparing past and current eating patterns. Ohlson and Harper (1976) followed the food habits of 158 educated women in 1935 and attempted to recontact each one in 1944, 1955, and 1973. They received responses from 87 women in 1973. There was a reduction in kcalorie intake as the women grew older. They had reduced their consumption of desserts, had decreased their use of table fat and fat used in food preparation, and had replaced whole milk with low fat milk. The study did not attempt to determine the statistical significance of the nutrient changes shown.

Other reports (Jensen et al., 1984; Rohan and Potter, 1984) show that the recall of diet consumed up to 37 years ago is strongly influenced by current dietary habits and, therefore, information on the current diet, supplemented by information on changes, can provide useful information on the dietary causes of disease with a long latency period. Dietary recall is also an appropriate method of assessing nutrient intake for a woman when a nutrition counselor needs to suggest changes in food consumption as part of the breast cancer prevention programs (Zeman, 1983).

The *dietary record* or *diary* requires that the subject maintain an accurate record of all food consumed at home and away from home for a specific period of time. The period of the record may vary from a few days to 1 year, but the most common length of time is from 3 to 7 days. The diary may be recorded on paper, on a tape recorder, or by telephone to the research center. The major advantage of this method, as opposed to recall, is that it reduces errors due to daily variations in food intake. However, subjects may become tired of recording their food intake if the record period is longer than 1 week.

Additional disadvantages are the possibility of the subjects' altering their intake during the investigation period or being inaccurate in their recording (Gersovitz et al., 1978; National Research Council, 1982; Kim et al., 1984a,b; Samet et al., 1984; Guthrie, 1986). The Beltsville 1 year dietary intake study is an example of one in which subjects were given training (Mertz and Kelsay, 1984). The subjects attended a training session and completed a 7 day practice record to assess their ability to follow the researcher's instructions.

Some nutrition researchers do not consider this method suitable for large scale studies because of the time needed for subject training, follow-up contacts, and coding data for computerized analysis. Nonetheless, it frequently is used to validate other methods of dietary intake in the same study population (Balogh et al., 1968; Nomura et al., 1976; Mahalko et al., 1985). It may be used by a nutritionist during counseling to determine dietary changes.

Seasonal variations in intake can be a problem in the recall and record methods. If the study period is long enough, data can be collected for each of the four major seasons (Kim et al., 1984a,b). If not, the subjects may be asked about seasonal variations in intake, and the study should state the possibility of seasonal bias.

One-day records may not be adequate in determining intake for specific individuals owing to day-by-day and weekday versus weekend intake differences (Houser and Bebb, 1981; Guthrie and Crocetti, 1985). Using data from the 1977 USDA Nationwide Food Consumption Survey, Pao and colleagues (1985) reported few statistical differences between 3 day and 1 day mean intakes in their subsample of 8779 individuals. If group, rather than individual, data are needed and the sample size is large enough, 1 day recalls or records seem to be adequate for most nutrients (Lyon et al., 1983).

Dietary histories, another method of assessing individual intake, differ from recall and record. Owing to the long latency period of cancer, the dietary history is commonly used to relate diet and cancer in epidemiology studies by determining past food intake. It is sometimes combined with a recall or record of the current intake (Morgan et al., 1978; Lyon et al., 1983; Willett et al., 1985).

During interviews or through questionnaires, subjects are asked about their past eating habits, including the number and type of meals commonly consumed each day, food likes and dislikes, seasonal variations in types and amount of food consumed, and the frequency per week or month of the consumption of various food groups (e.g., milk, green vegetables, and citrus fruit). A typical interview, which runs from 45 to 60 minutes, requires well-trained interviewers (or well-trained subjects if using self-administered questionnaires), standardized forms, and visual aids to assist the subject in estimating portion sizes (National Research Council, 1982; Guthrie, 1986).

Owing to the ease, speed, and lower cost of data collection, cancer epidemiologists often use a *food frequency inventory or questionnaire* and do not do a true diet history (Samet et al., 1984; Russell-Briefel et al., 1985). Food frequency inventories or questionnaires ask the subjects how often they consume various individual foods or food groups. Standards do not exist for the number of foods used on a questionnaire or for the number of frequency categories offered. Rohan and Potter (1984) assessed the frequency of consumption of 141 foods in a case-control study of bowel cancer; they did not state the number of frequency categories offered. Samet and colleagues (1984) used nine frequency categories for 55 foods in a case-control study of lung cancer; Russell-Briefel and coworkers (1985) used only five categories for 40 foods.

Byers and associates (1985) examined how many foods are needed on a food frequency questionnaire to assess specific nutrient intake for epidemiologic purposes. They found that most of the variability of nutrient intake in their western New York state population could be accounted for by using only 15 to 20 carefully chosen foods. The purpose of the study needs to be considered when selecting the number of foods to be listed. If a point estimate of actual nutrient or energy intake is needed, more foods will be needed than for a study determining the relative variation in intake between two populations. Assessments of only one nutrient may require fewer foods, whereas studies for the frequency of foods high in several nutrients or total energy intake will need more. Studies of cultures that have a wide variety of foods available will require more foods than studies of cultures with less variety.

Not all studies determine the portion sizes or assume subjects consume usual serving sizes (Rohan and Potter, 1984; Russell-Briefel et al., 1985). Research at University of Pennsylvania (Guthrie, 1984; Krebs-Smith and Smiciklas-Wright, 1985) shows that the subjects considered a wide variety of portion sizes to be their typical servings. Thus, frequency alone may be adequate for case-controlled or cohort studies that compare subjects' relative intakes. This would make data acquisition from self-administered questionnaires or telephone interviews easier (Samet et al., 1984).

VALIDITY OF METHODS

The validity of diet intake methods generally is assessed by comparing two or more methods. Russell-Briefel and coworkers (1985) compared the vitamin A intake of middle-aged men with three methods: 24 hour recall, 3 day food record, and a food frequency inventory. Considerable variability was found in the estimated vitamin A content.

The food frequency interview gave the highest estimates and the food record the lowest. Since the authors assumed standard portions on the food frequency interview, some of the differences shown are probably due to the differences in portion sizes actually consumed and reported on the recalls and records.

When Mahalko and associates (1985) compared diet histories and 7 day food records in 54 older adults, they found that the two methods provided estimates of intake that were close enough for use in epidemiologic studies with a large enough sample. They found significant mean differences for several nutrients, however. Mean total fat, saturated fatty acids, oleate, linoleate, and cholesterol values were significantly higher in the food record method, whereas ascorbic acid and potassium were significantly higher in the dietary history method. Vitamin A showed only a Pearson's correlation of 0.22.

Because the food records were completed by the subjects in the week following the dietary history interview, seasonal variations in intake probably did not account for the differences reported. The authors also used visual aids to assist in determining portion sizes. Thus, the differences in nutrient intake reported in the two methods are not readily explained. Better methods of validating dietary intake data are needed. Caution is also required in comparing data obtained by two different methods.

RELIABILITY OF DIETARY DATA

The reliability of dietary information is usually evaluated by attempting to reproduce the information originally obtained at a later time. A major limitation is that food habits may have changed between the two assessment times. This occurred in one study designed to reproduce a diet history questionnaire in breast cancer cases and controls. White controls showed less reproducibility than the white patients or Japanese cases or controls. The authors suspect that the poorer agreement in the white controls may be due to greater variability in their diets (Hankin et al., 1983).

Van Staveren and colleagues (1985) found good reproducibility of dietary histories 1 month later. Weekend days had poorer reproducibility than did the weekdays. With the exception of the white controls mentioned earlier, a study done with Hawaiian women showed good reproducibility within 3 months of the original interview (Hankin et al., 1983). Other researchers (Jain et al., 1980; Willett et al., 1985) have also found good reproducibility of diet history questionnaires, diet records, and food frequency questionnaires up to 1 year after the original study.

ANALYSIS OF DATA

Regardless of the method chosen, most studies translate food intake into an estimation of food nutrients and energy. The nutrients evaluated depend on the objectives. For total fat, the investigator does not need to determine the linoleic acid and saturated fat in a diet. A study reporting any differences between vegetarians and nonvegetarians must distinguish between animal and vegetable sources of protein.

Quantitative assessments of nutrient intake relying on food composition tables may not reflect the specific composition of the food consumed by the subjects owing to differences in nutrient content from the soil in which the food was grown, food processing, and storage conditions (National Research Council, 1982; Lyon et al., 1983). This has led to the interest in recent years in establishing a national data base that would serve as a standard for professionals in evaluating nutrient intakes for research purposes (Shanklin et al., 1985).

CONCLUSIONS

Each method has its advantages and disadvantages. None is universally regarded as the most valid and reliable method for obtaining information. Data obtained by one method should probably not be compared to data obtained by another. Conflicting conclusions of some of the studies may be due to methods that are poorly designed and controlled.

Investigators for methodologic studies and future research need to help subjects accurately recall or record the name, preparation method, and portion size of each food typically consumed. They also need to determine the best way to train individuals for determining the usual food consumed. Researchers need to be familiar with the usual foods and the common food preparation methods used in a study population so they can ask follow-up questions when the information is incomplete or deviates from usual patterns.

Obesity

The National Institute of Health concluded recently that the desire of most Americans to be thin is not just a matter of vanity; any degree of obesity is potentially life-threatening. An obese person is more prone to hypertension, adult-onset diabetes, hypercholesterolemia, hypertriglyceridemia, heart disease, gallstones, arthritis, gout, and complications of elective and emergency surgery of all types.

Obese women have higher death rates for cancers of the gallbladder, biliary passages, and endometrium. Postmenopausal women who are at least 40 per cent above their desirable weight have a higher mortality rate from breast cancer (Burton and Foster, 1985; Kolata, 1985).

CRITERIA FOR OBESITY

Most investigations of the relationship between body weight and breast disease use Quetelet's index or body mass index as the criteria for obesity because obesity can be measured independently of height (Khosla and Lowe, 1967; Adami et al., 1977; Brinton et al., 1981; Berkowitz et al., 1985). This index may be expressed as weight (kg) divided by height (cm) squared, multiplied by 10,000 (Brinton et al., 1981). A 1985 National Institutes of Health consensus conference, however, suggested that using the Metropolitan Life Insurance tables or the calculation of body mass index may be equally valid in large populations (Burton and Foster, 1985).

BENIGN DISEASE

Being thin may increase the risk of developing benign breast disease (Cole et al., 1978; Brinton et al., 1981; Hislop and Elwood, 1981; Soini et al., 1981; Berkowitz et al., 1985; Pastides et al., 1985). Berkowitz and coworkers (1985) found an association between a low Quetelet index and chronic cystic mastopathy in premenopausal and postmenopausal women, but the association was stronger in premenopausal women. Hislop and Elwood (1981) found the association only in women over age 30 years. Although Brinton and associates (1981) did not analyze the data by menopausal status, they reported an association between a low Quetelet index and benign breast disease.

Parazzini and colleagues (1984) were not able to produce evidence of a linear relationship between body mass index and benign breast disease when compared to the control group. The lack of consistency in selection of controls, somewhat different criteria for benign breast disease, and the fact that breast lumps are more difficult to detect in women with more adipose tissue may account for at least some of the lack of agreement (Ernster, 1981; Soini et al., 1981; Parazzini et al., 1984).

BREAST CANCER IN PREMENOPAUSAL VERSUS POSTMENOPAUSAL WOMEN

Epidemiologic research has shown a relationship between total kcalorie availability in a country and the incidence or mortality rate of breast cancer (Armstrong and Doll, 1975; Gray et al., 1979). Since the availability of a large number of calories can lead to obesity, it is not surprising that researchers have reported a correlation between excess body fat and breast cancer in postmenopausal females for several years. Such a relationship may not exist in premenopausal females; obesity may even be protective in women prior to menopause (Mirra et al., 1971; deWaard, 1975; Choi et al., 1978; Helmrich et al., 1983; Willett and MacMahon, 1984b). Brisson and coworkers (1984), however, found body weight and body mass related to breast cancer in premenopausal and postmenopausal women, especially when the mammographic features of the disease were considered. In contrast to most other studies, that of Whittemore and associates (1985) found increased weight-for-height during college years related to breast cancer, but not 20 to 30 years later in a group of University of Pennsylvania alumnae.

In the 1970s, de Waard and coworkers published several studies showing that postmenopausal women with breast cancer weigh more than their cohorts without cancer (de Waard and Baanders–van Halewijn, 1974; de Waard, 1975; de Waard et al., 1977). In one study, de Waard and colleagues (1977) attempted to attribute about one half of the differences in breast cancer incidence between regions in Holland with a high incidence and one in Japan with a low incidence to differences in body height and weight. Much of the correlation is removed if an adjustment is made for the correlation of height and weight. De Waard concluded that being overweight, per se, as defined by the Quetelet index, is not so much a risk factor as is being both overweight and tall. Having a large body surface area increases the relative risk of breast cancer.

Being overweight did not emerge as a risk factor for premenopausal women or early postmenopausal women in a study done by Lubin and colleagues in Israel (1985b), but being overweight, especially if the weight was gained recently, was a risk factor for breast cancer in women 60 years of age and over. The authors determined the weight of the study population at age 18, during "most of adult life," and "recent" weight. The weight *prior to* the illness was used as the "recent weight." This is a better research tool than the use of weight at the time the cancer was diagnosed, which was used by Brisson and coworkers (1984). A potential problem with the Lubin study, however, is that the height and weight data used were the result of self-reported information from the participants. When the subjects were not able to supply the information, interviewers were allowed to estimate height as short, average, or tall, and recent weight as thin, average, or fat.

In the study by Lubin and colleagues (1985b), body size was calculated according to Quetelet's formula and by estimating body surface area. Using 21 as the ideal body mass for a woman with a medium frame, about half of the study population was 20 per cent or more overweight; the incidence of excess weight increased as the population aged. When the study population was considered as a whole, no significant differences were seen between the patients and controls in mean height, weight, or body mass, except that patients had a lower mean body mass index for most of their adult life than did the surgical controls. No significant differences were seen in the patient-neighborhood control comparisons.

When age and menstrual status were taken into consideration, however, the postmenopausal breast cancer population that was 60 years of age and over had a significantly higher recent body mass index (BMI)—that is, they were fatter—than both control groups. They had at least twice the risk of developing breast cancer than did postmenopausal women over 60 years old who had lower BMI. The younger postmenopausal women with breast cancer had a lower recent BMI than the controls, but the difference was significant only when compared to the surgical controls. Premenopausal patients 39 years of age and younger were slighter lighter in weight than the controls, but the difference was not significant. The premenopausal women with breast cancer who were 40 years old had a significantly lower recent BMI than the surgical controls, but not the neighborhood controls.

The study by Lubin and coworkers (1985b) had a large sample size—1065 breast cancer cases and a combined total of 1945 controls—which made it easier to achieve statistical significance. Other studies had smaller sample sizes (Burch et al., 1981) or used controls that may not be representative of the general population (Stavraky and Emmons, 1974; Burch et al., 1981; Brisson et al., 1984). These differences in study design make it difficult to compare results among studies. Other researchers have not been able to find a difference in breast cancer incidence based on the weight or height of the subjects (Ravnihar et al., 1967; Stavraky and Emmons, 1974; Adami et al., 1977; Burch et al., 1981; Kuno et al., 1981). Some of the differences in findings may be attributed to the characteristics of the control groups.

For example, a high percentage of controls in the Stavraky and Emmons study (1974) were from a hospitalized population that had malignant diseases at sites other than the breast. Epidemiologists cannot estimate the degree of bias introduced by using hospitalized patients as controls, but it may be considerable (Adami et al., 1977).

A Swedish study (Adami et al., 1977) used age-matched controls from the general population, but the cases and controls may not have been comparable on socioeconomic status factors and reproductive history. Burch and colleagues (1981) were not able to detect a statistically significant difference in height and weight between 55 newly diagnosed primary breast cancer patients, 65 to 79 years old, and 57 control subjects within the same age group. Unfortunately, however, the control subjects had been matched for age and residence to patients with bowel cancer for a different research study, but they were not specifically matched for age and residence to the breast cancer patients. Since there was a trend for the patients to be heavier and shorter than the control subjects, better matched controls and a larger subject pool might have allowed the difference to reach statistical significance.

Another possible explanation for the differing results is shown in a study done by Zumoff and Dasgupta (1983). They were able to relate obesity to breast cancer only in populations previously known to have a statistically significant amount of obesity. These investigations were done in a variety of countries, which may account for some of the varying results.

BREAST CANCER PROGNOSIS

Factors such as obesity, which may influence the initiation of breast cancer, may also influence prognosis. Several studies have shown a relationship between body weight and breast cancer morbidity. Women in the lowest weight categories, in most of the studies, had the longest survival time (Donegan et al., 1978; Boyd et al., 1981; Tartter et al., 1981; Zumoff et al., 1982; Eberlein et al., 1985). Other researchers have found no relationship (Sohrabi et al., 1980; Heasman et al., 1985).

Tartter and coworkers (1981) found that women who weighed less than 150 pounds prior to a mastectomy had a 5 year disease-free survival rate of 67 per cent, as opposed to a 49 per cent survival rate for women who weighed over 150 pounds. When body weight and presurgery serum cholesterol levels were both considered, women who weighed over 150 pounds and who had a high serum cholesterol level had a significantly shorter survival rate than women who weighed less and had a low serum cholesterol level. In 1981, Boyd and colleagues showed a body weight of 64 kg (140.8 pounds) to be significantly associated with differences in survival; the best survival rate was in women weighing less than 64 kg. For Donegan and coworkers (1978), the cutoff point for a lack of recurrence of cancer was 59 kg (130 pounds) or less, especially if the women did not have axillary lymph node metastases. These latter findings are noteworthy because the authors were able to follow some patients for 24 years after mastectomy.

Based on the Canadian study by Boyd and colleagues (1981), a weight of less than 64 kg (140.8 pounds) was used as the arbitrary separation point for a 15 year study of breast cancer relapse in 316 patients treated at the National Cancer Institute, National Institutes of Health (Eberlein et al., 1985). They reported significantly longer disease-free and survival times in women who weighed less than 64 kg when they first came to the institute. When the number of positive nodes and age of the patients were included in the regression analysis, the effect of weight was reduced to statistically nonsignificant levels. The authors cautioned that the admission weight values used in the statistical equations were not always the premastectomy weight as some of the women were referred following their surgery. It is not possible to know how much this influenced the results.

Because weight alone may not be the significant factor, several studies analyzed the relationship between the Quetelet index and survival rates (Donegan et al., 1978; Boyd et al., 1981; Tartter et al., 1981; Eberlein et al., 1985; Gregorio et al., 1985). All of these investigations indicated that a longer survival time was associated with a low Quetelet index; the relationship was statistically significant in two of the studies (Boyd et al., 1981; Eberlein et al., 1985), but not in the other two (Tartter et al., 1981; Gregorio et al., 1985).

Adding serum cholesterol to the Quetelet index data still did not make the association statistically significant in the study of Tartter and coworkers (1981). When Eberlein and colleagues (1985) adjusted for nodal status and age, the association was still statistically significant, but the significance level dropped from $P = 0.01$ to $P = 0.18$.

In a Canadian study designed primarily to observe changes in body weight during adjuvant chemotherapy for breast cancer, Heasman and coworkers (1985) reported no association between weight gain and disease recurrence. This lack of relationship was also obtained by using the Quetelet index and body surface area as measures of body size, with and without adjustment for other prognostic factors, such as hormonal receptor status and number of axillary nodes involved. Similarly, the patient's body weight, Quetelet index, and body surface area at entry into the institute did not have a lineal relationship to survival.

Sohrabi and colleagues (1980) came to a similar conclusion when they retrospectively studied 106 consecutive women who had undergone a mastectomy in a university-affiliated hospital. They found that recurrence of breast cancer is related to tumor size and to nodal status. Obesity was related to tumor size and nodal status, but no relationship could be found between obesity (defined according to the Quetelet index) and a poor prognosis.

It is not possible to explain completely the conflicting results of studies into the possible association between weight and recurrence of breast cancer because the studies cited did not control for the same variables.

The Quetelet index, which takes the height of the woman into account, is probably a better measure of body mass than is weight alone; a taller woman would be expected to have a higher body weight. Menopausal status, nodal state, pathologic stage, and treatment modality could all influence the survival rate. Although some studies state they controlled for some of these variables, others do not provide this information. The length of time also varied; researchers followed their populations from 5 years (Tartter et al., 1985; Heasman et al., 1981) to 24 years (Donegan et al., 1978). Therefore, the results are not comparable on this dimension either.

CONCLUSIONS

Obesity appears to be a major risk factor for the development of breast cancer in postmenopausal women, but evidence is less clear for the development of breast cancer and benign breast diseases in premenopausal women. Some evidence shows that obesity may actually be protective for benign disease and premenopausal breast cancer, but women who are obese during their premenopausal years are not likely to lose weight when they approach menopause. The opposite—weight gain after menopause—is usually true.

As the data that suggest obesity has a protective effect during the menstruating years are scanty, women should not be encouraged to gain weight during these years as a means of avoiding breast cancer. In addition, obesity is associated with other medical problems, such as hypertension and adult-onset diabetes, and women should be concerned about avoiding these as well.

The ability of obesity to impact unfavorably on breast cancer prognosis requires further study. These studies should control for factors such as age of patient, extent of metastases, type and extent of surgical procedure, and type of chemotherapy. Researchers also should attempt to determine the weight of the woman prior to the development of the cancer rather than use the weight immediately following diagnosis of the cancer or the postsurgery weight.

Finally, research needs to focus on the weight at which a woman actually should be considered obese. The commonly used height and weight tables and Quetelet index may not be the best methods for determining the correct weight for a woman. Many sports medicine research centers are beginning to use the hydrostatic weighing method of determining the percentage of the body's weight that is fat (Katch et al., 1967). Perhaps this would also be a useful tool for breast cancer research. Unfortunately, however, the ideal percentage of body fat has not yet been determined.

Lipids

Of all the dietary components that have been associated with breast cancer in the epidemiologic and experimental literature, lipids have received the most attention and have been extensively reviewed by many authors (Carroll, 1975; Rivlin, 1982; National Research Council, 1982; Moore et al., 1983; Rogers, 1983; Willett and MacMahon, 1984b; Wynder and Rose, 1984). The relationship between a diet high in the simple lipids (commonly called dietary fat), especially the polyunsaturated fatty acids, and mammary carcinogenesis has been known since the 1940s (Tannenbaum, 1942; Tannenbaum and Silverstone, 1949). However, the positive relationship between polyunsaturated fatty acids and breast cancer is not as clear in human studies as it is in animal work (Hems, 1978). In recent years, a possible relationship has been established between the derived lipid, cholesterol, and breast disease (Hems, 1978; Dyer et al., 1981).

EPIDEMIOLOGIC EVIDENCE

Breast cancer is a disease whose cause is probably multifactorial. Dietary fat is only one of the factors. Armstrong (1976) was not able to relate the increase in breast cancer incidence and mortality rate in the United States, England, and Wales between 1950 and 1973 to any of the epidemiologic factors studied, including fat consumption. Based on epidemiologic evidence and case-control studies, Kolonel and associates (1983) suggested that dietary fat was probably only a weak risk factor in breast disease in Hawaii, but one that required further study with better research methods and tools.

Several international correlation studies have shown an association between per capita fat disappearance and breast cancer incidence or mortality (Lea, 1966; Carroll et al., 1968; Armstrong and Doll, 1975; Gray et al., 1979). The data are frequently called food consumption data, but, as was discussed in the *Methods of Dietary Intake* section of this chapter, they actually represent food disappearance within the country. These studies are of interest, but they must be interpreted cautiously because they assume equal distribution of food within the population (men, women, and children), and the data quality varies from country to country (Armstrong and Doll, 1975; National Research Council, 1982).

In the 1960s, Lea (1966) developed the concept that the international differences in breast cancer incidence might be influenced by differences in environmental temperature. Because environmental temperature influences the foods grown and consumed in a country, he examined the consumption of various dietary components in 23 countries in an attempt to provide support for this theory. Instead, he found a high correlation between dietary fat disappearance data and age-adjusted death rate from malignant breast neoplasms. Armstrong and Doll (1975) determined the correlation between per capita fat consumption and breast cancer incidence in 23 countries and breast cancer mortality in 32 countries. Both breast cancer incidence ($r = 0.79$) and mortality ($r = 0.89$) had a positive correlation with total fat consumption. The gross national product also had a positive correlation with fat consumption and breast cancer incidence, which indicates that other factors, such as level of economic development, have an effect. Based on the methods of standardization used by Armstrong and Doll (1975), Gray and coworkers (1979) published a paper showing a positive correlation between the incidence of breast cancer and total fat of 0.78 and a correlation of 0.93 for mortality rates.

Generally, epidemiologic studies report animal fat intake does not correlate as well as total dietary fat with breast cancer, and intake of vegetable fat has little, if any, relationship (Food Balance Sheets, 1971; Carroll, 1975). Using Food and Agriculture per capita food disappearance data, Hems (1978) calculated correlation coefficients between dietary components in the years 1964–1966 and breast cancer mortality in 1970–1971 in 41 countries. Large and positive correlations were found between mortality and the following dietary variables: total kcalories, fat, and protein; animal calories, fat, and protein; and sugar. Total fat, animal protein, and animal kcalories correlated so highly with one another that Hems could not state if one of these components had a role independent of the others. Vegetable calories, vegetable fat, starch, and total carbohydrate had smaller positive, or even negative, relationships to breast cancer mortality.

Hems concluded that "breast-cancer rates were significantly correlated with the 'animal' component, but the correlation with the 'vegetable' component, independently of the 'animal' component, was negligibly small." The dietary factors did not correlate with obesity, height, or estrogen levels, so Hems believes the dietary relationships were not just the result of an association with other factors believed to be related to breast cancer mortality. He stated that food consumption had been stable enough in these countries so that dietary data from 1964 to 1966 could be used to calculate correlation coefficients with mortality rates in 1970–1971. Based on the epidemiologic evidence, therefore, the possible enhancing effect of unsaturated fatty acids on breast tumorigenesis shown in animal studies must be viewed with caution and requires further study.

Women who emigrate from a country with a low incidence of breast cancer to one with a higher incidence gradually approach the risk level in the new country. Several studies have suggested that one of the factors involved in the change in risk is altered dietary habits (Buell, 1973; Bjarnason et al., 1974; Modan et al., 1975; Miller, 1977; Wynder, 1980; Kolonel et al., 1983; Mettlin, 1984). Japan has one of the lowest rates of breast cancer mortality, and the United States one of the highest; the second and third generations of Japanese women who emigrated to the United States have displayed a higher breast cancer mortality rate than the original generation who emigrated. The incidence rate is now similar to that of United States born women (Buell, 1973). Women who emigrated from Asia and Africa to Israel showed a similar rise in the incidence of breast cancer as they moved from a low risk to a high risk area. In this group of women, even the original generation that emigrated showed a rise in breast cancer rates. Perhaps this is because they adopted the lifestyle patterns, including eating habits, of their new country faster than did the Japanese women (Modan et al., 1975; Kakar and Henderson, 1985).

Other authors have studied breast cancer mortality trends within a fairly small geographic area. The British wartime experience provided a time of reverse Westernization of the diet. During World War II, the content of the diet in England and Wales decreased in fat, sugar, and meat. These changes correlated with a reduction in breast cancer mortality rates two decades later. In contrast, correlations with diet were poor when analyzed on a region by region or urban versus rural basis. Perhaps this was due to a small range of variations in eating habits between regions (Hems, 1980).

Within the United States, age-adjusted breast cancer mortality rates have been positively associated with dairy products and negatively associated with egg consumption (Gaskill et al., 1979). The data used in this report came from two different sources; the regional figures were compiled from the 1965–1966 Household Food Consumption Survey conducted by the United States Department of Agriculture using individual interviews (United States Department of Agriculture,

1970, 1974); the state-by-state data were compiled from per capita food demand estimates published between 1969 and 1973 (Raunikar et al., 1969–1973). The cancer death rates were from the period 1969–1971. The latency period of breast cancer is not known, but it must be assumed that eating habits were stable to relate dietary components from the mid-1960s to early 1970s to cancer death rates in 1969–1971. An additional concern about this study is the absence of potentially useful data. For example, the state food demand figures do not include estimates for butter because it was pooled with margarine data. Demand estimates likewise are not available for alcohol, vegetable fat, complex carbohydrates, and bread.

ANIMAL EXPERIMENTAL WORK

Laboratory experimental work on mice and rats is useful in an attempt to relate dietary fat to breast carcinogenesis. Animal models allow the researcher to overcome the ethical issues involved in working with humans. Also, the environment can be controlled and simplified to a greater extent than in human experiments. However, animals are not human, and the results of animal experiments may not be directly generalized to humans (National Research Council, 1982). As early as 1942, Tannenbaum reported the role of dietary fat as contrasted with total energy intake per se in enhancing mammary tumor development in mice. A year later, Lavik and Baumann (1943) published a report that differed somewhat from that of Tannenbaum in that total caloric intake was found to be more important in the chemically induced skin tumors of mice. This early work on the role of lipids in carcinogenesis, including breast tumors, has been thoroughly reviewed by Carroll and Khor (1975).

Some investigators have used mammary tumors that developed spontaneously (Abraham et al., 1984) and others have used tumors that have been induced by various carcinogenic agents (Carroll and Khor, 1971; King and McCay, 1983; Minton et al., 1983; Cave and Jurkowski, 1984). On the basis of these studies, dietary fat is believed to affect primarily the developmental stage of tumor formation by altering the tumor latency period rather than having an effect on initiation of the tumor (Carroll and Khor, 1975; Hopkins et al., 1976; National Research Council, 1982; Aylsworth et al., 1984; Cave and Jurkowski, 1984; Erickson et al., 1985).

The theory concerning the stage of tumorigenesis in which lipid is involved may need to be modified, however. Kritchevsky and associates (1984) showed that high fat and high calorie diets can initiate carcinogenesis, not merely exhibit promotional characteristics. Abraham and coworkers (1984) found a discontinuity in the sequence of events from normal to neoplastic tissue. Both normal and neoplastic mammary tissues responded to the addition of corn oil to the diet by enhanced growth of the tissues, but preneoplastic, hyperplastic alveolar nodule cells did not respond to corn oil with enhanced growth.

The other major finding of animal research is the role of total dietary fat, especially unsaturated fat, in enhancing mammary tumor development (Carroll et al., 1968; Carroll and Khor, 1971; Minton et al., 1983; Abraham et al., 1984; Garbor et al., 1985). The work of King and McCay (1983) is representative of many studies that have shown that animals fed a diet high in polyunsaturated fat have a higher incidence of mammary tumors than animals fed an isocaloric diet high in saturated fat. Animals fed a 20 per cent by weight corn oil diet developed tumors at an incidence rate of 95 to 100 per cent. There was only a 60 to 70 per cent incidence rate when they were fed a 20 per cent by weight diet containing 18 per cent coconut oil plus 2 per cent linoleic acid esters. A low fat diet containing 2 per cent corn oil yielded only a 30 to 40 per cent mammary tumor incidence rate, however, which shows the role of total fat in the diet.

Some unsaturated fatty acids many have a beneficial effect. Karmali and associates (1984) were able to inhibit tumor growth in rats who were administered marine oil that was rich in omega-3 fatty acids. They postulated the inhibition of mammary tumorigenesis was linked, in part, to the inhibitory effect of the omega-3 fatty acids on arachidonic acid metabolism. Arachidonic acid is a precursor of prostaglandins, which are present in large amounts in human and experimental tumors (Karmali, 1980).

Other investigators have been impressed with the role of total lipid in the diet, as opposed to the source of the lipid, in the promotion of tumors (Cave and Jurkowski, 1984; Boissoneault et al., 1985). When the polyunsaturated fat component (corn oil) exceeded 3 per cent of the weight of the diet of the rats, total lipid, not type of fat, best correlated with a reduction in tumor latency period. A 100 per cent tumor incidence rate was shown in rats fed a diet containing either 20 per cent corn oil or 3 per cent corn oil and 17 per cent tallow. Corn oil diets below 3 per cent showed a low tumor incidence rate and an increase in the latency period.

The type of fat in the diet may have an influence even at high levels, as was shown in a report by Jurkowski and Cave the following year (1985). When each rat was fed at the 20 per cent level, menhaden oil, a polyunsaturated marine oil, produced fewer tumors and a longer tumor latency period than did corn oil (Jurkowski and Cave, 1985).

CASE-CONTROL STUDIES

Compared to the number of animal experiments reported, few case-control studies involving women with breast cancer appear in the literature. The expense of a large scale case-control study, the difficulty in controlling variables, and ethical issues all undoubtedly contribute to the sparsity.

A study done at four Canadian sites produced evidence that total fat intake is a significant risk factor for breast cancer (Miller et al., 1978). There were 400 breast cancer patients and 400 well-matched controls. The subjects were interviewed about 5 months after surgery with three different methods: diet history method, a food frequency questionnaire, and a 24 hour recall, which was used as a training aid for a 4 day diet record. Visual aids were used to assist the subjects in estimating portion sizes of food.

The mean intakes of total kcalories and nutrients varied, according to dietary intake methodology used, but generally, irrespective of menopausal status, the subjects consumed more total kcalories, total fat, saturated fat, oleic acid, linoleic acid, and cholesterol than did the controls. The authors believed the diet history method the most representative of the true energy and nutrient intake because many women failed to return their diet record; responses on a 24 hour recall may not be typical of usual eating habits. None of the differences in mean energy or nutrient intake shown by the history method, however, were statistically significant.

When risk ratios were calculated for the premenopausal women according to the diet history, total fat, saturated fat, and cholesterol had risk ratios that were significantly above those that were expected. For postmenopausal women, only total fat showed a risk ratio significantly above expected.

Another Canadian study, which involved women from Alberta, Canada, showed higher risk ratio factors associated with fat intake (Lubin et al., 1981). The study compared the diets of a group of 577 women with breast cancer with the diets of 826 control women. The authors used an eight item food consumption questionnaire: beef and other red meat; pork; chicken and other fowl; fish; eggs; cheese; creams; and sweet desserts. The women chose the frequency of intake according to six categories. The women were not asked about the portion sizes commonly consumed or food preparation methods. Questions were asked about the amount and type of milk consumed and whether or not butter was consumed.

When risk ratio factors were calculated, a more frequent consumption of beef, pork, sweet desserts, and butter or margarine, as opposed to vegetable oils, significantly elevated the risk factor. Since the authors did not ask about portion sizes consumed, food preparation methods used, or usual consumption of carbohydrate-rich foods, such as vegetables, fruit, and grain products, they could not translate the food frequency information into precise estimates of protein, fat, and carbohydrate consumed. They did, however, calculate age-adjusted, relative risks of breast cancer for animal fat, animal protein, and cholesterol, based on the assumption that the women consumed usual serving sizes of food.

The risk factors for the consumption of animal fat and animal protein were highly significant; the relationship with dietary cholesterol was not. The data did not allow the authors to calculate the risk factors for saturated versus unsaturated fatty acids. The greater relative risk shown in this study (Lubin et al., 1981) as opposed to the first Canadian study (Miller et al., 1978) may be attributable to the different dietary questions asked and to the use of population controls in the Lubin study and neighborhood controls in the Miller one.

Contrary to the increased relative risk shown by these two studies, a large scale case-control study done by Graham and colleagues (1982), using hospital controls, failed to show an increased risk of breast cancer due to animal fat, vegetable fat, or total fat consumption. Studies using a predominately vegetarian sample of women (Kinlen, 1982; Phillips and Snowdon, 1983) also have failed to show an increased risk for breast cancer due to meat or fat consumption.

An interesting approach to the study of the role of diet in breast cancer was reported by Nomura and colleagues (1978). Assuming that spouses ate similar diets, they studied the diets of 86 Japanese men married to women who had breast cancer and compared their diets to that of 6774 Japanese men married to women without breast cancer. Based on the food frequency method of intake, the spouses of women with breast cancer consumed more meat, butter/margarine/cheese, corn, and wiener than did the control spouses. The meat and butter/margarine/cheese information was based on assumption of usual portion sizes of food. The higher intake of corn and wiener was based on a study also using the food frequency method, but information was obtained about portion sizes consumed. A 24 hour recall of their diets did not show any significant differences in total fat, saturated fat, unsaturated fat, or cholesterol consumed.

SERUM AND DIETARY CHOLESTEROL

Although hypercholesterolemia is a well-recognized risk factor for atherosclerotic disease (McGee and Gordon, 1976), any possible relationship to cancer is less well established. A few studies have shown an inverse relationship between serum cholesterol levels and cancer (Beaglehole et al., 1980; Kark et al., 1980). This relationship, however, may be attributable to undiagnosed cancer patients in the sample who had lower serum cholesterol due to metabolic errors produced by the malignant cells (Rose and Shipley, 1980). Keys and associates (1985) were not able to find any evidence of a cancer–serum cholesterol relationship in a Seven Countries Study, but they stated that "the possibility of such an effect cannot be denied." Contrary to what has been observed by others, Dyer and coworkers (1981) reported a significantly positive relationship (5 per cent level) between serum cholesterol and breast cancer in a large, Chicago-based study of serum cholesterol level and risk of death from many types of cancer. As there were only five breast cancer deaths in this study, these results need to be interpreted cautiously.

Most case-control studies of breast cancer do not report dietary cholesterol values. The studies that do provide this information have yielded inconsistent results. The premenopausal, but not the postmenopausal, subjects in the study by Miller and colleagues (1978) had a risk ratio for dietary cholesterol that was significantly greater than expected. Other studies have not found any significant differences in the diets of women with breast cancer (Lubin et al., 1981) or in the diets of their spouses (Nomura et al., 1978).

MECHANISMS

It is apparent from the many hypotheses that have been proposed to explain the role of dietary fat in mammary carcinogenesis that this phenomenon is not well understood. Several journal articles have reviewed the literature in the area (Smithline et al., 1975; Hankin and Rawlings, 1978; Wynder and Rose, 1984). The most commonly discussed theory is that dietary fats may modify endogenous hormonal status in a woman, and the altered hormones or their metabolites can either enhance or retard tumor development. Dietary lipids may influence prolactin-binding capacity of mammary tumors (Cave and Jurkowski, 1984), estriol to estrone ratio (Dickinson et al., 1974), and serum estrogen levels (Hawkins et al., 1985). The work of Aylsworth and colleagues (1984b), however, suggests that circulating levels of estrogen or prolactin, or both, are not involved. Other research lines include the possible role of lipids in altering cell-mediated cytotoxicity (Thomas and Erickson, 1985), that high levels of polyunsaturated fatty acids may promote tumors by inhibiting mammary intercellular communication (Aylsworth et al., 1984a), and the possibility of using antioxidants to inhibit lipid-induced mammary carcinogenesis (King and McCay, 1983).

CONCLUSIONS

The epidemiologic and experimental data that show a positive relationship between dietary fat intake and the development of breast cancer are quite extensive and fairly impressive. Few case-control studies have been published, and their conclusions are not as definitive as the epidemiologic and experimental work, but they too show a trend for a high level of dietary fat to be associated with breast cancer.

Protein and Carbohydrate

Because nutrients are so interrelated, it is difficult to separate the influence of dietary proteins, carbohydrates, and lipids on breast disease. A diet high in fat will usually be at least moderately high in protein, too, because meat and meat substitutes are excellent sources of both nutrients. Only the macronutrients—proteins, lipids, and carbohydrates—provide kcalories in the diet. Therefore, if the percentage of kcalories in the diet that come from protein and fat is higher than the average, carbohydrate will have to provide a smaller than normal percentage. The reverse is also true.

It is not surprising, then, to find that both dietary protein and lipids are positively correlated with breast cancer in epidemiologic data (Armstrong and Doll, 1975; Hems, 1978; Gray et al., 1979; Lubin et al., 1981). Nor should it be unexpected to find that refined sugar is positively related to breast cancer mortality rates (Hems, 1978; Lubin et al., 1981). The women in industrialized nations who consume diets high in fat and protein also consume diets high in refined sugar products.

Very little of the animal work done has focused on the possible role of protein in breast disease. Carroll (1975) did an extensive review of the animal data from the 1940s to the mid-1970s that attempted to relate diet and hormone-dependent cancers. He concluded that dietary protein had little, if any, effect on the formation of mammary tumors. The conflicting results between the epidemiologic data and Carroll's review of the literature are probably due to the ability of animal researchers to provide rations with a wider range of energy-nutrient content than is normally found in human dietary intake.

Laboratory experiments on cancer at sites on the body other than the breast have shown that chemically induced cancers tend to be suppressed on diets low enough in protein to also suppress growth. High protein diets tend to enhance carcinogenesis (National Research Council, 1982). Perhaps further experimental research will show this is also true of breast cancer, but the small number of studies in the literature makes it difficult to draw even a tentative conclusion.

Vitamins and Minerals

Most of the epidemiologic and animal research relating dietary components to breast disease has focused on the role of lipids and excess body fat, but the role of the micronutrients, vitamins and minerals, has received little attention. The small amount done, however, means definitive conclusions cannot be drawn, and more research definitely is needed. The interrelated nature of nutrients is a factor in micronutrient as well as macronutrient research. Because of the nature of the food sources, diets high in protein and fat tend to be high in different nutrients than diets rich in carbohydrate. Statistical techniques can help to separate out the dependent from the independent variables, but caution is still needed when attempting to separate out the influence of a single dietary component on breast disease.

VITAMIN A

Vitamin A is the general name for a diverse collection of chemical compounds found in animal and plant foods. The forms found predominantly in animal foods are retinol (the alcohol), retinal (the aldehyde), and retinoic acid (the acid form). The precursor forms, the carotenes, are found in plant foods, especially those that are dark green or yellow in color. For example, carrots, broccoli, and acorn squash are all rich in carotenes. The carotenes become biologically active after they are converted to retinol in the intestinal wall (Guthrie, 1986).

The Recommended Dietary Allowance (RDA) of vitamin A for nonpregnant, nonlactating females above 11 years of age is 800 micrograms (μg) of retinol equivalents (RE) per day. One RE equals 1 μg retinol, 6 μg beta-carotene, or 12 μg of other provitamin carotenoids (National Academy of Sciences, 1980). Before 1974, the RDA for vitamin A was measured in International Units (IU), and 800 RE was equivalent to approximately 4000 IU. The advantage of using RE as the unit of measurement is that it takes into account the variations in absorption and metabolism of the various forms of vitamin A. Most food charts still list vitamin A in terms of IU and assume that animal foods contain retinol and plant foods provide the vitamin in the beta-carotene form.

Because vitamin A may be stored in the liver, it is not essential that the RDA level be consumed every day. When consumed in excess, vitamin A is known to be toxic. The daily intake of vitamin A needed and the length of time this level must be consumed before toxic levels are reached vary among persons, but toxic symptoms have been seen with daily intakes of as little as 16,000 RE. Six to 15 months of high intake is usually needed before the symptoms of toxicity appear. Carotene is not known to be toxic if consumed in excessive amounts, probably because the amount is absorbed as the intake increases (Guthrie, 1986).

Most studies attempting to relate vitamin A intake to cancer have involved sites other than the breast. Epidemiologic studies have shown a negative relationship between consumption of green and yellow vegetables and cancer of the lung (MacLennan et al., 1977), gastrointestinal tract (Modan et al., 1981), bladder (Mettlin and Graham, 1979), colon (Graham et al., 1978), and lung, stomach, and prostate (Hirayama, 1979). Using a food frequency questionnaire in a prospective cohort study of 1271 elderly Massachusetts residents, Colditz and associates (1985) reported a significantly decreased cancer risk with an increasing intake on the green and yellow vegetable score of the questionnaire. Since the score for "carrots or squash" and "salads" was not associated with a decreased risk of cancer, their results do not lend support to the role of beta-carotene as the factor in vegetables that decreases the incidence of cancer. The intake of strawberries, tomatoes, dried fruits, and broccoli was associated with a decreased relative risk of cancer death. Of these foods, only broccoli and dried apricots are high in vitamin A. Other studies have not found a relationship between vitamin A and cancer (Graham et al., 1983; Kolonel et al., 1983). Unfortunately, most of the studies do not attempt to distinguish between the forms of vitamin A found in the diet. This may account for some of the differences in results. An additional problem is the use of selected green and yellow vegetables (and sometimes fruit) to estimate the vitamin A intake of the subjects and the assumption that they consume average portion sizes. This may not be an accurate way to estimate vitamin A intake because portion sizes vary from person to person, and foods vary widely in vitamin A; in addition, the food frequency lists may not list the foods rich in vitamin A commonly consumed by the subjects.

Breast Cancer. A large scale, case-control epidemiology study in Buffalo, New York, using a food frequency questionnaire found no large difference in the amount of vitamin A or cruciferous vegetables consumed by the breast cancer cases and the controls per month (Graham et al., 1982; Graham, 1983). The relative risk of breast cancer decreased, however, with increased intake of vitamin A. The difference was significant only for women 55 years of age and over. Women in that age range who consumed little vitamin A had 1.53 times the risk of developing breast cancer compared with those who consumed over 30,100 RE (150,500 IU) per month. The authors assumed usual portion sizes of food were consumed when estimating the vitamin A content of the diet. The results might have been different if actual portion sizes had been estimated.

Experimental work with animals has shown that various retinoids may inhibit the carcinogenic process in mammary cells. McCormick and coworkers (1980) demonstrated an inhibition of mammary cancer when retinyl acetate was fed to rats. Grubbs and colleagues (1977) inhibited the incidence of 7,12-dimethylbenz[a]anthracene-induced benign and cancerous mammary tumors with a synthetic retinoid, retinyl methyl ether. Takahashi and Biempica (1985) have suggested the possibility of using vitamin A to prevent mammary metastasis by inhibiting the production of collagenases, which may facilitate the tumor metastasis. Nagasawa (1984) found a different effect of vitamin A when he treated GRS/A mice with vitamin A for the first 5 days of postnatal life. He reported an increase in the incidence of both pregnancy-dependent and autonomous mammary tumors in the mice that were fed vitamin A. The development of autonomous mammary tumors was especially interesting. All of the experimental mice developed mammary tumors by 13 months of age, compared with 57.9 per cent autonomous tumor development in the control mice.

Benign Disease. Vitamin A may be a useful treatment for the pain of benign breast disease in women who are not responsive to methylxanthine withdrawal or the use of analgesics (Band et al., 1984). When 12 premenopausal women with measurable pain from benign breast disease were treated with 30,000 RE (150,000 IU) vitamin A per day for 3 months, nine patients reported a marked improvement in breast pain, and five had complete or partial decrease in measurable breast mass. Unfortunately, mammographic parenchyma patterns remained unchanged in 11 of the 12 women. Signs of toxicity developed in half the subjects.

Mechanism of Action. The mechanism by which one or more forms of vitamin A may influence breast disease is not known. Some retinoids appear to inhibit the promotion or progression of chemically induced mammary cancer in experimental animals (Moon et al., 1983), but they may also be effective inhibitors during the initiation phase of carcinogenesis (McCormick et al., 1980). Retinol may have a dose-dependent, antiproliferative effect on human mammary cancer cells when studied in vivo and in vitro; the inhibition seen is not due to an alteration in host cell immunity but is solely the result of the influence of retinol on the tumor (Fraker et al., 1984). One study has shown that human mammary cells may have an altered sensitivity to retinoic acid (Ueda et al., 1985), which is consistent with the dose-dependent response noted by Fraker and colleagues (1984).

Conclusions. The epidemiologic and laboratory evidence relating vitamin A to breast disease is promising, but further work obviously needs to be done. Perhaps something other than carotene in green and yellow vegetables is responsible for the decrease in mammary tumors seen in animals and older human females who consume large amounts of vitamin A (Willet and MacMahon, 1984a). The researchers need to use intake methods that give a more precise estimation of the vitamin A content of the diet in case-control studies. Assuming usual serving sizes of fruits and vegetables may result in an estimation of the vitamin A content of the diet that deviates widely from the actual value.

VITAMIN E AND SELENIUM

Vitamin E. The term vitamin E includes a mixture of at least eight compounds, including tocopherols and tocotrienols. The most biologically active tocopherol is d-alpha-tocopherol. Currently RRR-alpha-tocopherol is the standard for measuring the vitamin E value of food. Since 1980, the vitamin E activity in the RDA has been expressed in milligrams of tocopherol equivalents (TE). Tocopherol equivalents take into consideration the potency of the various forms of vitamin E. The RDA for a nonpregnant, nonlactating female 11 years of age and older is 8 mg TE. The amount of vitamin E needed in the diet increases with the intake of polyunsaturated fatty acids. It has not been possible to devise a formula relating vitamin E need to polyunsaturated fatty acid intake. As a result, the RDA is based on the amount needed to support blood levels of vitamin E that are considered adequate.

International units, used prior to the 1980 edition of the RDA, are sometimes used in current literature and food tables. The conversion of IU to milligrams depends on the form of tocopherol being used, but 1 mg of tocopherol is equal to 1 IU of alpha-tocopherol. Unfortunately, most food composition tables only list alpha-tocopherol content of foods, so it is difficult to relate intake to recommendations in terms of TE (National Academy of Sciences, 1980; Guthrie, 1986).

Selenium. No RDA has been established for selenium, but the National Academy of Sciences (1980) considers 50 to 200 µg to be in the adequate and safe range. The selenium content of plant foods depends on the soil in which they were grown. Animals develop selenium poisoning if they graze predominately on plants growing in soil rich in selenium (Guthrie, 1986). Because humans consume food grown on a wide range of soils, they are not likely to develop selenium toxicity unless they supplement their diets with large amounts of the mineral. Only 2.5 to 3.0 mg of selenium may produce harmful effects (Underwood, 1973; Young and Richardson, 1979).

Antioxidant Role. The most well-researched role of vitamin E is as an antioxidant in plant and animal tissue, especially those containing polyunsaturated fatty acids. In the absence of adequate antioxidants, excessive free radicals may form from the oxidation of unsaturated fatty acids and damage the plant or animal tissue (Guthrie, 1986). Selenium is also an endogenous antioxidant because it is an essential component of glutathione peroxidase, one of the major enzymes involved in protecting cells against oxidative tissue damage (Chow, 1979). Vitamins A and C also appear to play a role in the antioxidant process. The higher the level of polyunsaturated fatty acids in the diet, the greater is the need for an antioxidant to prevent tissue damage (Witting, 1969). At least one species of animal (female chickens) appears not to have a requirement for an antioxidant if fed a diet low enough in fat (Bieri et al., 1960).

Vitamin E and Breast Disease. As was discussed in the *Lipids* section of this chapter, experimental animal work and epidemiologic evidence in humans have shown a possible relationship between a diet high in fat and breast cancer. In animals, polyunsaturated fatty acids enhance mammary carcinogenesis more than do saturated fatty acids; the evidence for an effect related to degree of saturation is less clear in human studies. These observations have led several researchers to investigate the ability of the antioxidants vitamin E and selenium to prevent or lessen the development of chemically induced mammary tumors in animals. The roles of selenium and vitamins A, C, and E in the antioxidant process, with special attention to their possible role in prevention of cancer, have been reviewed extensively by several authors (King and McCay, 1983; Rogers, 1983; Combs and Combs, 1984; Willett and MacMahon, 1984b; Kakar and Henderson, 1985; McCay, 1985).

More reports have been published on the possible effect of selenium on mammary tumors than on the influence of vitamin E. Brief reports by Harman (1969) and Lee and Chen (1979) showed at least some reduction in tumors in animals fed vitamin E, but Wattenberg (1972) and King and McCay (1983) were not able to report this effect. King and McCay (1983) fed groups of rats diets known to cause chemically induced mammary gland tumors that varied in the amount of fat, degree of fatty acid saturation, and the presence or absence of an antioxidant. They found the expected increase in percentage of mammary tumors in the rats fed the high polyunsaturated fatty acid diet as contrasted with one high in saturated fat or simply low fat, even without the addition of an antioxidant. However, neither alpha-tocopherol nor butylated hydroxyanisole (BHA) was an effective inhibitor of tumors at any level of fat or degree of fatty acid saturation in the diet. The most effective antioxidants were buylated hydroxytoluene (BHT) and propyl gallate.

No epidemiologic evidence exists associating vitamin E with mammary cancer. Data of this nature will be difficult to obtain because vitamin E is present in such a wide range of foods (vegetable oils, whole grain cereal products, and eggs). Current dietary intake methods do not allow the researcher to define groups with clearly different levels of intake (National Research Council, 1982). Small differences in vegetable oil intake, for example, are difficult to obtain because subjects are not able to clearly state usual portion sizes. Also, food frequency questionnaires, which assume all subjects consume the same portion sizes, will not be useful in obtaining vitamin E intake data. A carefully done food record may possibly be a useful technique.

Several reports exist, however, concerning the use of vitamin E in benign breast disease. In the mid-1960s, Abrams (1965) found vitamin E useful in relieving some of the symptoms of premenopause. Two other groups of investigators (London et al., 1978; Sundaram et al., 1981) reported a positive response to vitamin E in women with mammary dysplasia.

Recently, however, Ernster and coworkers (1985) were not able to find a beneficial effect of vitamin E on benign breast disease in a 2 month, double-blind, randomized clinical trial in which 37 women took 600 IU alpha-tocopherol and 36 women took a placebo. Ernster and colleagues believe the conflicting findings may be due to a lack of adequate controls in the three studies mentioned earlier.

Selenium and Breast Disease. Most of the literature on the possible inhibitory role of selenium in carcinogenesis has been published in the last 15 years. Recent literature is indicative of how tentative many of the conclusions are. Combs and Clark (1985) published a review article that extensively reviewed the animal, cohort, and case-control literature in the area. They concluded that "almost all of these investigations have found high-level Se treatments to cause at least moderate (15 to 35 percent) reductions in tumor incidence." Selenium treatments were ineffective in reducing tumors in only eight studies.

Several authors have observed a decrease in the development of either spontaneously developed (Schrauzer et al., 1978) or carcinogen-induced (Ip, 1981a,b; Ip and Sinha, 1981; Medina et al., 1983; Medina and Shepherd, 1984; Thompson et al., 1984) mammary tumors when animals were fed selenium or when it was added to a selenium-deficient diet (Harr et al., 1972). The addition of selenium is especially beneficial if the animal diet is high in polyunsaturated fat (Ip and Sinha, 1981).

After adding selenium to the high fat diet of rats at various times before and after the administration of the DMBA carcinogen, Ip (1981b) concluded that the element has a prophylactic effect in both the initiation and promotion phases of carcinogenesis, but a continuous intake is necessary to achieve the maximal inhibition. Probably the most interesting finding of his experiment was the ability of selenium to inhibit the reappearance of mammary tumors that had regressed after ovariectomy. Ip's data suggest that selenium not only may function as a chemopreventive to mammary tumors but may also be used as an adjuvant chemotherapeutic agent.

In an investigation involving the addition of both selenium and vitamin E in the diet, Horvath and Ip (1983) found that the vitamin supplementation alone was ineffective in reducing the incidence of tumors and latency period in DMBA-induced carcinogenesis. The addition of selenium, however, significantly reduced tumor incidence and length of the latency period. Selenium supplementation alone significantly reduced the latency period but not the incidence of tumors.

Both Horvath and Ip (1983) and Medina and coworkers (1983) found that the anticarcinogenic action of selenium could not be attributed to the role of selenium in glutathione peroxidase activity. This may be because the enzyme itself is the limiting factor. It is already operating near its maximal capacity, and additional selenium cannot further increase activity (Horvath and Ip, 1983).

Little epidemiologic evidence exists concerning the relationship between dietary or serum selenium and breast cancer. The reports that do exist show conflicting relationships between these variables. Using food disapppearance data, Schrauzer and colleagues (Schrauzer, 1976; Schrauzer et al., 1977a,b) have correlated per capita intake of selenium with cancer mortality rates in 23 countries. They found an inverse relationship between selenium intake and several cancers, including that of the breast. Using pooled blood from healthy donors in the United States and other countries, they found a significant inverse relationship between serum selenium and breast cancer.

In a case-control study involving 35 breast cancer patients and 27 control women, McConnell and colleagues (1980) found that the patients had significantly lower serum selenium levels. Shamberger and coworkers (1973) found no relationship between selenium levels in the blood of breast cancer patients and those of normal subjects.

Conclusions. The evidence showing a relationship between a low vitamin E content of the diet and breast disease is not as adequate as the data relating inadequate selenium and breast disease. Until breast carcinogenesis is better understood, and the precise functions of vitamin E and selenium at the cellular level are determined, it will be difficult to make a dietary recommendation to women with any degree of certainty. At present, however, women should be encouraged to include foods rich in vitamin E and selenium in their diets.

VITAMIN C

Considerable attention has been focused on the possible role of vitamin C in preventing cancer (Cameron et al., 1979), but little research has been reported concerning its possible role in breast cancer. In his case-control study in Buffalo, New York, using the food frequency method of dietary intake, Graham (1983) found no relationship between vitamin C intake and breast cancer. However, since portion sizes of food were not estimated, it can only be said that the breast cancer patients did not differ in their frequency of consuming foods rich in vitamin C.

Alcohol

For the past few years, several large-scale epidemiologic studies have attempted to relate alcohol consumption to breast cancer. The results have been inconsistent. Large case-control studies in Israel and North America (Rosenberg et al., 1982), Italy (La Vecchia et al., 1985a), and France (Le et al., 1984) have shown increases of up to two times in the relative risk of breast cancer for women who drank alcohol as opposed to women who do not drink. This was true even when the usual confounding variables, such as hormonal status, obesity, and number of children, were taken into consideration. Others, however, have found little influence (Begg et al., 1983; Hiatt and Bawol, 1984) or none (Byers and Funch, 1982; Paganini-Hill and Ross, 1983; Webster et al., 1983).

Some of the conflicting results may be attributed to sampling differences. For example, about 5 per cent of the women in the California study (Hiatt and Bawol, 1984) consumed more than three drinks per day. In the Byers and Funch study (1982), the highest level of alcohol consumption reported was an average of less than one drink per day. Le and coworkers (1984) included women with cholelithiasis in their controls (18 per cent of controls), but La Vecchia and colleagues (1985a) considered women with cholelithiasis to be ineligible as controls because of the association of this condition with obesity and multiparity, two factors known to influence breast cancer risk. Other studies (Rosenberg et al., 1982; Hiatt and Bawol, 1984) did not control for other dietary variables, such as fat consumption.

Conclusions. There appears to be no clear-cut body of evidence relating alcohol consumption to breast cancer. However, the presence of case-control studies from different countries showing a positive association between the two factors, when traditional risk factors such as Quetelet index are taken into consideration, indicates that further studies in the area would be useful.

Caffeine

Methylxanthines include the compounds caffeine, theophylline, and theobromine. All are purine-base compounds commonly found in plant foods. Coffee, tea, soft drinks, chocolate, and some over-the-counter drugs contain methylxanthines, either as a natural constituent or as an additive. Caffeine is found in coffee, tea, chocolate, and the kola beans used in soft drinks. Tea also contains theobromine and theophylline. Cocoa contains theobromine in addition to the caffeine (Graham, 1978).

In the past few years, much interest has been generated about the possible role of methylxanthines, especially caffeine, as a risk factor for benign or malignant breast disease, but these studies have yielded inconsistent results (Minton et al., 1981; Odenheimer et al., 1984; Le, 1985; Lubin et al., 1985a; Rosenberg et al., 1985). Extensive reviews of the literature have concluded that there is little scientific basis for associating caffeine intake with chronic cystic mastopathy and other forms of benign breast disease (Curatolo and Robertson, 1983; Pozniak, 1985). There is perhaps a negative correlation between caffeine consumption and breast cancer (Le, 1985; Lubin et al., 1985a).

Caffeine May Influence Breast Disease. An animal experiment using DMBA-induced breast cancer in rats (Minton et al., 1983) concluded that caffeine and unsaturated fatty acids in the diet enhanced the development of mammary tumors by decreasing latency time and increasing the incidence of multiple tumors.

A series of studies by Minton and colleagues at Ohio State University showed that when caffeine and other beverages containing methylxanthine were eliminated from the diet of women who had what they classified as clinical chronic cystic mastopathy, a majority experienced disappearance of the symptoms (Minton et al., 1979a, 1981). Women with and without breast disease did not differ significantly on past methylxanthine exposure, with the exception of chocolate consumption; the percentage of women with chronic cystic mastopathy who had consumed chocolate was slightly more than the control women.

As the result of a questionnaire given to these women seeking information about their family history of benign and malignant breast disease, researchers believe that women with chronic cystic mastopathy may have a genetic predisposition that makes them more sensitive to benign and malignant breast disease. Using graphic stress telethermometry to precisely measure the course of the breast disease, Brooks and coworkers (1981) confirmed Minton's reports of improvement in chronic cystic mastopathy when methylxanthines were restricted in the diet.

An Italian study (La Vecchia et al., 1985b) showed a positive association between methylxanthine consumption and dysplastic disease of the breasts, but not fibroadenomas. The association gained strength with duration of consumption. Coffee drinkers had an increased risk of carcinoma, but not of fibroadenomas (Mansel et al., 1982).

Several case-control studies have shown that there is a possible relationship between caffeine consumption and various forms of benign breast disease (Lawson et al., 1981; Ernster et al., 1982; Boyle et al., 1984; Odenheimer et al., 1984). In two of these studies (Lawson et al., 1981; Ernster et al., 1982), the authors stated that the association was so modest that their data added little support to the claim that caffeine consumption is related to breast disease. Boyle and coworkers (1984) found an association only in women with chronic cystic mastopathy and not in women with fibroadenoma and other forms of benign breast disease.

Using discordant twins in a case-control

study of risk factors for benign breast disease allowed Odenheimer and colleagues (1984) to control for genetic and early environmental factors. They found a significantly positive association between benign breast disease and coffee consumption. The association, stronger in monozygotic than in dizygotic twins, lends support to a possible genetic role in benign disease.

Caffeine May Not Influence Breast Disease. In a well-designed study using 2651 newly diagnosed breast cancer cases and 1501 controls with nonmalignant conditions and 385 controls with cancers at sites other than the breast, Rosenberg and associates (1985) could find no relationship between recent consumption of regular coffee, decaffeinated coffee, or tea and the incidence of breast cancer. The findings were the same in women with and without a history of what they classified as chronic cystic mastopathy and when the cases were compared with either set of controls. They studied recent caffeine consumption because of the animal research that suggests that caffeine may act as a tumor promoter (Mori and Hironi, 1977; Welsch et al., 1983); hence, recent consumption is more relevant than the history of caffeine intake.

An Israeli case-control study showed no relationship between benign breast disease and methylxanthine consumption (Lubin et al., 1985a). The authors were able to use two or more pathology specimens to verify the histologic type and ductal grading. Other studies have relied on palpation methods to verify the existence of benign breast disease.

Lubin and coworkers also controlled for other factors, such as age and ethnic origin, that are believed to influence the incidence of benign disease. The food and beverage information was obtained by the food frequency method of dietary data intake. They also elicited information about past and present methylxanthine intake. In an attempt to assess recall bias, they reinterviewed some of the women 3 to 9 months after the first interview and found a 74 per cent agreement for categories of coffee consumption.

When Le (1985) took into consideration the usual variables believed to influence breast disease in a French study, she found that the risk of breast cancer was inversely associated with coffee consumption. The risk of benign disease was not significantly associated with coffee consumption. Lubin and colleagues (1985a) also found a diminished risk of breast cancer with high, as opposed to low, methylxanthine consumption.

Other reports have not shown an association between caffeine consumption and benign breast disease (Marshall et al., 1982; Heyden and Muhlbaier, 1984; Lubin et al., 1985a) or death from breast cancer (Phillips and Snowdon, 1983).

Concerns About the Literature. Authors and reviewers have expressed reservations about some aspects of the methodologies from these studies. Some investigators did not ask about the use of caffeine-containing pills (Ernster et al., 1982; Boyle et al., 1984; Odenheimer et al., 1984) or about sources of caffeine other than coffee (Odenheimer et al., 1984). Ernster and coworkers (1982) stated observer bias could have been a factor in their study. Other problems Pozniak (1985) mentioned in her review included a lack of randomization, a lack of controlling for variables such as method of birth control or number of pregnancies, and the use of breast palpation as the only measure of improvement.

Many of the studies used the food frequency interview method of information intake and asked the women about cups of coffee consumed each day. They usually assumed a cup was equivalent to 5 or 6 ounces (Bunker and McWilliams, 1979; Lubin et al., 1985a). With the popularity of 12 to 16 ounce coffee mugs, however, the number of cups of coffee drunk daily may not be a good research question. In addition, Boyle and colleagues (1984) and Rosenberg and coworkers (1985) were among the few to ask women to distinguish between caffeinated and decaffeinated coffee and tea consumption. Because other authors had not asked women for this separation, it could explain differences in results.

The brand and method of preparation also influence the caffeine content of coffee and tea. Instant freeze-dried coffee has less than half the caffeine content of automatic drip coffee; the caffeine content of tea has been shown to vary by over 100 per cent depending on brand and length of brewing time (Bunker and McWilliams, 1979). An analysis of the caffeine content of 86 home-prepared beverage samples showed a wide variation in caffeine content per cup of coffee and tea (Gilbert et al., 1976). Few authors state that these variations in caffeine content were considered in the data analysis.

On the basis of current literature, it is not possible to draw any definite conclusions about the nature of the relationship between methylxanthine consumption and breast disease. A recent article by Le (1985) has accurately summed up the literature at this point, "The complex relationships between coffee consumption, benign breast disease and breast cancer need further epidemiologic study to reach definitive conclusions."

Catecholamines

According to Cooper and associates (1978) "the term 'catecholamine' refers, generically, to all organic componds that contain a catechol nucleus (a benzene ring with two adjacent hydroxyl substituents) and an amine group." In practical terms, the word usually refers to dihydroxylphenylethylamine (dopamine) and its products, norepinephrine and epinephrine. The catecholamines may be formed from the amino acid tyrosine in brain cells, sympathetic nerves, adrenal chromaffin cells, and sympathetic ganglia. The primary pathway for formation of catecholamines is believed to be the conversion of tyrosine to dihydroxyphenylalanine (dopa) prior to the formation of the catecholamines, dopamine, norepinephrine, and epinephrine. The rate limiting step is the first one in which tyrosine is converted to dopa. An alternative pathway for tyrosine metabolism is decarboxylation to tyramine which also can produce norepinephrine and epinephrine (Cooper et al., 1978).

One of first steps in the metabolism of the catecholamines in the tissues may be either the addition of a methyl group on the benzene ring by catechol-O-methyltransferase (COMT) or oxidation of amine side chain by the enzyme monoamine oxidase (MAO), although these may not be the primary mechanisms for terminating the action of norepinephrine in sympathetic nerve terminals (Cooper et al., 1978).

Epinephrine can stimulate both alpha- and beta-adrenergic receptors in tissues. The beta-adrenergic effects are associated with an increase in adenylate cylcase activity, the enzyme that forms cyclic adenosine monophosphate (cAMP) from adenosine triphosphate (ATP). The rise in cAMP leads to an activation of protein kinases. It is this activity that accounts for most of the biochemical effects of the hormone (Martin et al., 1985).

CATECHOLAMINES AND BREAST DISEASE

Caffeine stimulates urinary catecholamine release (Bellet et al., 1969). Because caffeine and the catecholamines have similar biochemical functions of elevating cyclic nucleotides (Minton et al., 1979b; Martin et al., 1985), Minton became interested in the role of catecholamines in breast disease.

This interest was stimulated by clinical observations of a group of women who, despite their abstinence from caffeine and nicotine (which also stimulates catecholamines), still had the physical symptoms of benign breast disease. Through the women's use of food diaries, he learned they consumed an abundance of foods high in tyramines. When these foods were eliminated from their diet, many of the symptoms were eliminated (J. P. Minton, personal communication, November, 1985).

Biochemical studies done on women with normal and benign breast tissue has shown that fibrocystic breast tissue contains about twice as much cAMP and cyclic guanosine monophosphate (cGMP) activity. It also has about twice the basal adenylate cyclase activity as normal breast tissue. This probably resulted from increased synthesis as opposed to decreased breakdown of the nucleotide (Foecking et al., 1980; Minton et al., 1981). Levels of cAMP in vivo in malignant lesions are even higher than in benign and normal tissue (Minton et al., 1979a, 1986). One study hypothesizes that these elevated cAMP levels may stimulate the protein-synthesizing capabilities of the cell and indirectly lead to the overproduction of fibrous tissue and cyst fluid found in chronic cystic mastopathy (Minton et al., 1979b).

When Minton determined the levels of circulating catecholamines and caffeine in women with chronic cystic mastopathy, he compared the levels with those found in control women. There were significantly elevated catecholamine values in women with cyclic mastalgia; the difference in mean caffeine concentration was not significant. Women with chronic cystic mastopathy had significantly lower dopamine values than control women (J. P. Minton, personal communication, November, 1985).

If the problem in breast disease is excessive stimulation of beta-adrenergic receptors in breast tissue, perhaps a reduction in tyramine-containing foods and other catecholamine stimulating factors, such as nicotine and stress, will decrease beta-receptor activity, which would lead to a decreased cAMP production and chronic cystic mastopathy.

Vasoactive Amines in Food

The desire to restrict tyramine in the diet is similar to the dietary prescription given to someone who is using one of the drugs known as monoamine oxidase inhibitors (MAOIs). Tyramine, dopamine, and norepinephrine (all phenylalanine derivatives), serotonin (tryptophan derivative), and histamine are all known to cause a marked increase in blood pressure, nausea, vomiting, and severe occipital headaches. This hypertensive crisis can be life-threatening (Blackwell et al., 1967; Lovenberg, 1973; Stockley, 1973). The best-known MAOIs are sometimes used in severely depressed individuals who do not respond to tricyclic antidepressants. Normally, MAO metabolizes the pressor amines before they reach the systemic circulation, but MAOIs inhibit this process, allowing tyramine to reach the systemic circulation and produce the hypertension and other symptoms mentioned (Lovenberg, 1973; Zeman, 1983). Several authors have reviewed the need to restrict tyramine and other amines in the diet of individuals who are using MAOIs (Sjoqvist, 1965; Blackwell et al., 1967; Pettinger and Oates, 1968; Blackwell, 1981a,b; Pare et al., 1982; Sullivan and Shulman, 1984).

Because the role of tyramine in breast disease is still speculative, the amount needed in the daily diet to promote breast disease is not known. The only reference point is the amount needed to produce a reaction in individuals using MAOIs. Obvious pressor effects have been produced with as little as 6 mg of tyramine; 10 mg produced a marked pressor effect, and 25 mg resulted in a severe hypertensive crisis (Horwitz et al., 1964; Blackwell and Marley, 1966). Other dietary factors, such as other foods eaten, amount of fat in the diet, and individual differences in gastric emptying time, probably have an influence on the amount of tyramine needed to elevate blood pressure (Blackwell et al., 1967; Sheehan et al., 1980–1981).

The amines in the food supply may be synthesized by certain plants or they can be the result of microbial contamination or fermentation of foods. The tyramine content of foods has received more research attention than the other amines because of the well-established assay procedures for measuring tyramine content in food. There are also higher amounts of tyramine than of other amines in most foods. For example, some of the organisms used in preparing some cheeses and fermented foods contain tyrosine decarboxylase. Restricting tyramine-rich foods in the diet of individuals who use MAOIs has stimulated research (Lovenberg, 1973; Lieb, 1977).

Reviews on tyramine and other vasoactive amines found in food can be found in several sources (Lovenberg, 1973; Maga, 1978; McCabe and Tsuang, 1982; Zeman, 1983). There is no consensus on dietary restrictions for limiting tyramine. Hospital diet manuals, dietary handbooks, and journal articles vary widely in the number and type of foods not allowed in diets of patients on MAOIs (University of Iowa Hospitals and Clinics, 1979; Sheehan et al; 1980–1981; American Dietetic Association Diet, 1981; Mayo Clinic, 1981; Folks, 1983; Powers and Moore, 1983; Jenike, 1984; Massachusetts General Hospital, 1984; Sullivan and Shulman, 1984).

Some of the variations can be attributed to a lack of comprehensive food tables that list the amounts of tyramine, dopamine, and other pressor agents in foods. Because the tyramine content of food varies from product to product and even between samples of the same food, these tables are difficult to develop. For example, depending on the production process, Sen (1969) found nil to 2170 μg of tyramine per gram in cheese. Brie from Denmark had the least; and Stilton Blue cheese from England the most. The tyramine content of Canadian cheddar cheese varied from 120 to 1530 μg per gram, depending on the aging process. Other researchers have reported tyramine levels similar to those found by Sen (Dahlberg and Kosikowsky, 1948; Voigt et al., 1974).

The content also varies depending on the closeness of the sample assayed to the cheese rind (Price and Smith, 1971). Sour cream and yoghurt may or may not contain tyramine, depending on contamination and production. The only cheeses that do not have detectable tyramine concentrations are cream cheese and cottage cheese (Horwitz et al., 1964; Voigt et al., 1974).

Several meat and fish products contain significant amounts of tyramine. A sample of pickled herring had 3000 μg of tyramine per gram of food (Nuessle et al., 1965). McCabe and Tsuang (1982) calculated that only 3 g (1/10 ounce) of this sample would produce clinical symptoms in an individual using MAOIs. Sen (1969) reported only 470 μg of tyramine per gram of salted dry herring; he speculated that pickled herring may have more than dried herring owing to bacterial contamination. Meat extract preparations, which have a high tyramine content (Sen, 1969), are frequently avoided on a tyramine-restricted diet (Sheehan et al., 1980–1981).

According to Rice and colleagues (1975), semi-dry and dry sausages contain significant amounts of histamine and tyramine. Although histamine content was only slightly higher than would be expected from fresh meat products, the tyramine content was high enough to warrant caution in use of these products in tyramine-restricted dietary plans. Genoa salami averaged 534 μg of tyramine per gram of salami, but the range was from less than 10 μg per gram to 1237 μg per gram. According to Dierick (1974), vasoamine content may actually decrease the longer the dry sausage is allowed to ripen. This further illustrates the wide variation in tyramine content from sample to sample mentioned earlier. Dierick and colleagues were not able to detect any tyramine in the 18 samples of country-cured ham they analyzed, probably because this ham is technically not a fermented meat product.

The tyramine content of food generally increases as the food ages. This is especially true of protein-rich foods, such as tuna fish, liver, ground beef, and cheese (Boulton et al., 1970; McCabe and Tsuang, 1982; Lovenberg, 1973). Using heat in the cooking process apparently does not alter the tyramine content of food (McCabe and Tsuang, 1982).

The fermentation processes used in making beer and wine do not ordinarily produce tyramine, but some imported beers and some red wines (especially Chianti) have tyramine. White wines do not contain tyramine. The grape pulp and seeds are probably the source of amino acids in red wine (Sen, 1969; McCabe and Tsuang, 1982; Powers and Moore, 1983; Jenike, 1983).

Yeast extract, sold as "Marmite" in Britain, contains significant amounts of tyramine (Sen, 1969). It has elevated blood pressure in individuals using MAOIs (Blackwell et al., 1967). Although Marmite is seldom consumed in the United States, brewer's yeast, which contains tyramine and comes in pill and liquid forms, should be restricted on low tyramine diets (McCabe and Tsuang, 1982). The commonly used yeast-leavened breads, however, are generally allowed.

Most fruits and vegetables contain little or no tyramine. Although the banana peel contains 65 μg per gram of peel, the pulp only has 7 μg per gram (Udenfriend et al., 1959). As few people consume peelings, bananas should not constitute a problem on a tyramine-restricted diet. Avocado contains 23 μg of tyramine per gram of food, orange pulp 10 μg per gram, and eggplant 3 μg per gram (Udenfriend et al., 1959); therefore, a woman with breast disease should not eat large portions of avocados and oranges; eggplant probably can be consumed infrequently.

The only vegetable eliminated on all tyramine-restricted diets is fava bean pods, which contain significant amounts of dopamine. This amine is primarily found in the pod of the bean; the seeds have little or no pressor activity (Hodge et al., 1964). These beans, not commonly consumed in the United States, are used in some Mediterranean recipes. They are sometimes known as broad beans, Italian green beans, English bean pods, and Chinese pea pods. Flat, kidney-shaped beans that are pale green in color, the fava beans are at least 0.5 inch in width, much wider than the usual green bean found in United States (Sheehan et al., 1980–1981; McCabe and Tsuang, 1982).

Sheehan and colleagues (1980–1981) list several over-the-counter and prescription drugs that should not be taken by individuals using MAOIs; some contain vasoactive amines. These include some cold medications, narcotics, and amphetamines. A woman who is attempting to limit the amount of tyramine in her diet should check with her physician or pharmacist before taking over-the-counter medications.

As many foods have not been analyzed for tyramine content and the amount of tyramine may vary greatly from sample to sample, it is not possible to be precise in suggesting foods to be allowed and restricted on a low tyramine diet. In addition, the amount of tyramine to be allowed on such diets is not known. Many diet counselors group foods into those not allowed, those allowed occasionally, and those allowed at all times. Unfortunately, these dietary lists vary with these categories (University of Iowa Hospitals and Clinics, 1979; Sheehan et al., 1980–1981; American Dietetic

Association, 1981; Mayo Clinic, 1981; McCabe and Tsuang, 1982; Folks, 1983; Powers and Moore, 1983; Jenike, 1984; Massachusetts General Hospital, 1984; Sullivan and Shulman, 1984). Hospital diet manuals and handbooks tend to be more restrictive; patients using MAOIs who selected the wrong food could have a hypertensive crisis and possibly death. This conservative approach is probably not needed in women with breast disease unless further research shows a definite link between tyramine content of the diet and breast disease.

There is universal agreement on the need to eliminate aged and processed cheeses; fava beans; salted, smoked, or pickled fish; liver; dry fermented and aged sausage products; brewer's yeast, and Marmite on a tyramine- and dopamine-restricted diet. Many authorities also suggest the elimination of all wine, beer, ale, and alcoholic beverages, but all agree on the elimination of red wine, sherry, vermouth, and cognac. Whiskey, gin, and vodka are frequently allowed. Sour cream, avocado, and soy sauce are not allowed on many diet plans and are allowed only in moderation on the others (University of Iowa Hospitals and Clinics, 1979; Sheehan et al., 1980–1981; American Dietetic Association, 1981; Mayo Clinic, 1981; Folks, 1983; Massachusetts General Hospital, 1984; Power and Moore, 1983; Sullivan and Shulman, 1984).

These food restrictions are similar to those reported by Sullivan and Shulman (1984), who examined the frequency with which various foods were restricted on MAOI diets. They reported all diets surveyed restricted wine, aged cheese, and nonfresh fish. Beer, broad bean pods, and yeast extracts were restricted on 75 to 99 per cent of diets surveyed.

According to the references listed earlier, a long list of foods should be consumed only in moderation. These include fruits and vegetables that contain low levels of tyramine, aged dairy products (yoghurt and sour cream), meat extract products (bouillon cubes, for example), and bread products made with a large amount of yeast. A complete list of suggested foods appears in the Appendix to this chapter.

CONCLUSIONS

The tyramine content of the diet may influence breast disease in some women. Future research will need to confirm this hypothesis. Women who have multiple risk factors for breast cancer or currently have chronic cystic mastopathy should be aware of the possible role of tyramine in breast disease and asked to limit their intake of foods containing high amounts of tyramine. The restrictions should not be at the expense of a diet that meets the RDA for the macro- and micronutrients in the diet.

Guide to Food Choices

Diet is only one of many factors that may influence the development of breast disease. There is no research base for suggesting major modifications in the diets of women as a means of preventing breast disease. Sufficient evidence does seem to be available, however, to make the following suggestions:

1. Women should maintain, or attain, their "ideal" weight. Unfortunately, scientists will probably never agree on the ideal weight for an individual woman. The Metropolitan Life Foundation height and weight tables (1983) and the Quetelet index (Khosla and Lowe, 1967) are commonly used guidelines in many of the publications reviewed in this paper. The 1983 edition of the Metropolitan Height and Weight Tables are reproduced in the Appendix to this chapter. These tables present weights based on the lowest mortality for men and women from ages 25 to 50 according to height and body frame, in both English and metric systems. Women who live near a university or sports medicine research center may be able to have the percentage of their body that is fat estimated using the hydrostatic weighing procedure (Katch et al., 1967). This procedure allows the researcher to estimate the amount of body fat and lean body mass and determine a suggested weight for the woman based on the percentage of her body that is fat. Unfortunately, however, the ideal fat percentage of the body is not known.

2. The percentage of kcalories in the diet that comes from fat should be reduced in most women's diets. Thirty per cent of the kcalories coming from fat is a commonly suggested goal (National Research Council, 1982). Scientific data do not provide a strong basis for suggesting a change in the type of fat from saturated fatty acids to polyunsaturated fatty acids, as is commonly suggested for individuals who are attempting to prevent coronary disease (Subcommittee on Diet and Hyperlipidemia, 1973). Animal research data suggest that a diet high

in polyunsaturated fatty acids is correlated with breast cancer (King and McCay, 1983). The human epidemiologic data, however, are less definitive (Hems, 1978).

Some data suggest a reduction in dietary cholesterol would be worthwhile. The diet plan in the Appendix is designed to provide 300 mg or less of dietary cholesterol per day.

3. Women should consume a diet that meets the RDA for protein, vitamins, and minerals (National Academy of Sciences, 1980). This includes the nutrients listed in the table "Estimated Safe and Adequate Daily Dietary Intakes of Selected Vitamins and Minerals" published by the National Academy of Sciences. Because there is not a sufficient amount of data to establish definite recommended daily intakes, the figures presented in the tables give a range of recommended safe intakes.

4. Moderate or no consumption of alcohol and caffeine-containing beverages is advised.

5. Women with multiple risk factors for breast cancer or chronic cystic mastopathy should be asked to consume foods with high tyramine content in moderation, or not at all.

These guidelines are similar to the Dietary Guidelines suggested by the United States Department of Agriculture (1985). In addition to the previous suggestions, these guidelines also advise that individuals consume a diet containing adequate starch and fiber and avoid too much sugar and sodium. The data do not suggest these changes can modify breast disease, but no evidence suggests they would be harmful.

Dietary counseling can help a woman evaluate her current diet and make suggested changes in her eating patterns. Counseling is available from Registered Dietitians and nutritionists at most hospitals and many medical clinics in the United States. Many Registered Dietitians and nutritionists have private dietary counsulting firms; physicians may refer their patients to them. If a Registered Dietitian or nutritionist is not available, the Appendix to this chapter contains dietary plans at several kcalorie levels that may be distributed to women. National and local cancer societies also have resources available.

REFERENCES

Abraham, S., Faulkin, L. J., Hillyard, L. A., et al.: Effect of dietary fat on tumorigenesis in the mouse mammary gland. JNCI, 72:1421, 1984.

Abrams, A. A.: Use of vitamin E in chronic cystic mastitis. N. Engl. J. Med., 272:1080, 1965.

Adami, H. O., Rimsten, A., Stenkvist, B., et al.: Influence of height, weight and obesity on risk of breast cancer in an unselected Swedish population. Br. J. Cancer, 36:787, 1977.

American Dietetic Association Diet. In Handbook of Clinical Dietetics. New York, Yale University Press, 1981, p. C49.

Armstrong, B.: Recent trends in breast-cancer incidence and mortality in relation to changes in possible risk factors. Int. J. Cancer, 17:204, 1976.

Armstrong, B., and Doll, R.: Environmental factors and cancer incidence and mortality in different countries, with special reference to dietary practices. Int. J. Cancer, 15:617, 1975.

Aylsworth, C. F., Jone, C., Trosko, J. E., et al.: Promotion of 7,12-dimethylbenz[a]anthracene-induced mammary tumorigenesis by high dietary fat in the rat: Possible role of intercellular communication. JNCI, 72:637, 1984a.

Aylsworth, C. F., VanVugt, D. A., Sylvester, P. W., et al.: Role of estrogen and prolactin in stimulation of carcinogen-induced mammary tumor development by a high-fat diet. Cancer Res., 44:2835, 1984b.

Balogh, M., Medalie, J. H., Smith, H., et al.: The development of a dietary questionnaire for an ischemic heart disease survey. Israel J. Med. Sci., 4:195–203, 1968.

Band, P. R., Deschamps, M., Falardean, M., et al.: Treatment of benign breast disease with vitamin A. Prev. Med., 13:549, 1984.

Beaglehole, R., Foulkes, M. A., Prior, I. A., et al.: Cholesterol and mortality in New Zealand Maoris. Br. Med. J., 280:285, 1980.

Becker, B. G., Indik, B. P., and Beeuwkes, A. M.: Dietary intake methodologies—a review. Technical Report, University of Michigan, School of Public Health. Ann Arbor, Office of Research Administration, 1960.

Begg, C. B., Walker, A. M., Wessen, B., et al.: Alcohol consumption and breast cancer. Lancet, 1:293, 1983.

Bellet, S., Roman, L., DeCastro, O., et al.: Effect of coffee ingestion on catecholamine release. Metabolism, 18:288, 1969.

Bennett, A.: Prostaglandins and cancer. In Karim, S. M. (Ed.): Practical Applications of Prostaglandins and Their Synthesis Inhibitors. Lancaster, MTP Press, 1979, p. 149.

Berkowitz, G. S., Kelsey, J. L., LiVolsi, V. A., et al.: Risk factors for fibrocystic breast disease and its histopathologic components. JNCI, 75:43, 1985.

Bieri, J. G., Briggs, G. M., Pollard, C. J., et al.: Normal growth and development of female chickens without dietary vitamin E or other antioxidants. J. Nutr., 70:47, 1960.

Bjarnason, O., Day, N., Snaedal, G., et al.: The effect of year of birth on the breast cancer age-incidence curve in Iceland. Br. J. Cancer, 13:689–696, 1974.

Blackwell, B.: Adverse effects of antidepressant drugs. Part 1. Monoamine oxidase inhibitors and tricyclics. Drugs, 21:201, 1981a.

Blackwell, B.: Adverse effects of antidepressant drugs. Part 2. "Second generation" antidepressants and rational decision making in antidepressant therapy. Drugs, 21:273, 1981b.

Blackwell, B., and Marley, E.: Interactions of yeast extracts and their constituents with MAOI inhibitors. Br. J. Pharmacol., 26:142, 1966.

Blackwell, B., Marley, E., Price, J., et al.: Hypertensive interactions between monoamine oxidase inhibitors and foodstuffs. Br. J. Psychiatry, 113:349, 1967.

Boissonneault, G. A., Elson, C. E., and Pariza, M. W.: Enhancement of DMBA-initiated mammary carcinogenesis in rats by dietary fat: The role of net energy. Proc. Natl. Acad. Cancer Res., 26:125, 1985.

Boulton, A. A., Cookson, B., and Paulton, R.: Hypertensive crisis in a patient on MAOI antidepressants following a meal of beef liver. Can. Med. Assoc. J., 102:1394, 1979.

Boyd, N. F., Campbell, N. F., Germanson, T., et al.: Body weight and prognosis in breast cancer. JNCI, 67:785, 1981.

Boyle, C. A., Berkowitz, G. S., LiVolsi, V. A., et al.: Caffeine consumption and fibrocystic breast disease: A case-control epidemiologic study. JNCI, 72:1015, 1984.

Brinton, L. A., Vessey, M. P., Flavel, R., et al.: Risk factors for benign breast disease. Am. J. Epidemiol., 113:203, 1981.

Brisson, J., Morrison, A. S., Kopans, D. B., et al.: Height and weight, mammographic features of breast tissue, and breast cancer risk. Am. J. Epidemiol., 119:371, 1984.

Brooks, P. G., Gart, S., Heldfond, A. J., et al.: Measuring the effect of caffeine restriction on fibrocystic breast disease. The role of graphic stress telethermometry as an objective monitor of disease. J. Reprod. Med., 26:279. 1981.

Buell, P.: Changing incidence of breast cancer in Japanese-American women. JNCI, 51:1479, 1973.

Bunker, M. L., and McWilliams, M.: Caffeine content of common beverages. J. Am. Diet. Assoc., 74:28, 1979.

Burch, J. D., Howe, G. R., and Miller, A. B.: Breast cancer in relation to weight in women aged 65 years and over. Can. Med. Assoc. J., 124:1326, 1981.

Burton, B., and Foster, W. R.: Health implications of obesity: An NIH consensus development conference. J. Am. Diet. Assoc., 85:1117, 1985.

Byers, T., and Funch, D.P.: Alcohol and breast cancer. Lancet, 1:799, 1982.

Byers, T., Marshall, J., Fiedler, R., Zielezny, M., and Graham, S.: Assessing nutrient intake with an abbreviated dietary interview. Am. J. Epidemiol., 122:41–50, 1985.

Cameron, E., Pauling, L., and Leibovitz, B.: Ascorbic acid and cancer: A review. Cancer Res., 39:663, 1979.

Campbell, C.: Opening Remarks for Workshop. In Roe, A. (Ed.): Diet, Nutrition, and Cancer: From Basic Research to Policy Implications. New York, Alan R. Liss, 1983, p. 1.

Carroll, K. K.: Experimental evidence of dietary factors and hormone-dependent cancers. Cancer Res., 35:3374, 1975.

Carroll, K. K., and Khor, H. T.: Effects of level and type of dietary fat on incidence of mammary tumors induced in female Sprague-Dawley rats by 7,12-dimethylbenz[a]anthracene. Lipids, 6:415, 1971.

Carroll, K. K., and Khor, H. T.: Dietary fat in relation to tumorigenesis. Prog. Biochem. Pharmacol., 10:308, 1975.

Carroll, K. K., Gammal, E. B., and Plunkett, E. R.: Dietary fat and mammary cancer. Can. Med. Assoc. J., 98:590, 1968.

Cave, W. T., and Jurkowski, J.: Dietary lipid effects on the growth, membrane composition, and prolactin-binding capacity of rat mammary tumors. JNCI, 73:185, 1984.

Choi, N. W., Howe, G. R., Miller, A. B., et al.: An epidemiologic study of breast cancer. Am. J. Epidemiol., 107:510, 1978.

Chow, C. K.: Nutritional influence on cellular antioxidant defense systems. Am. J. Clin. Nutr., 32:1066, 1979.

Colditz, G. A., Branch, L. G., Lipnick, R. J., et al.: Increased green and yellow vegetable intake and lowered cancer deaths in an elderly population. Am. J. Clin. Nutr., 41:32, 1985.

Cole, P., Elwood, J. M., and Kaplan, S. D.: Incidence rates and risk factors of benign breast neoplasms. Am. J. Epidemiol., 108:112, 1978.

Combs, G. F., Jr., and Combs, S. B.: The nutritional biochemistry of selenium. In Darby, W. J., Broquist, H. P., and Olson, R. E. (Eds.): Annual Review of Nutrition. Palo Alto, Calif., Annual Reviews, 1984, p. 257.

Combs, G. F., and Clark, L. C.: Can dietary selenium modify cancer risk? Nutr. Rev., 43:325, 1985.

Cooper, J. R., Bloom, F. E., and Roth, R. H.: The Biochemical Basis of Neuropharmacology. Fair Lawn, N.J., Oxford University Press, 1978, pp. 102, 120–158.

Curatolo, P. W., and Robertson, D.: The health consequences of caffeine. Ann. Intern. Med., 98:641, 1983.

Dahlberg, A. C., and Kosikowsky, F. V.: The relationship of the amount of tyramine and the numbers of Streptococcus faecalis to the intensity of flavor in American cheddar cheese. J. Dairy Sci., 31:305, 1948.

de Waard, F.: Breast cancer incidence and nutritional status with particular reference to body weight and height. Cancer Res., 35:3351, 1975.

de Waard, F., and Baanders-van Halewijn, E. A.: A prospective study in general practice on breast-cancer risk in postmenopausal women. Int. J. Cancer, 14:153, 1974.

de Waard, F., Cornelis, J. P., Aoki, K., et al.: Breast cancer incidence according to weight and height in two cities of the Netherlands and in Aichi Prefecture, Japan. Cancer, 40:1269, 1977.

Dierick, N., Vandekerckhove, P., and Demeyer, D.: Changes in nonprotein nitrogen compounds during dry sausage ripening. J. Food Sci., 39:301, 1974.

Dickinson, L., MacMahon, B., Cole, P., et al.: Estrogen profiles of Oriental and Caucasian women in Hawaii. N. Engl. J. Med., 291:1211, 1974.

Donegan, W. L., Hartz, A. J., and Rimm, A. A.: The association of body weight with recurrent cancer of the breast. Cancer, 41:1590, 1978.

Dyer, A. R., Stamler, J., Paul, O., et al.: Serum cholesterol and risk of death from cancer and other causes in three Chicago epidemiological studies. J. Chronic Dis., 34:249, 1981.

Eberlein, T., Simon, R., Fisher, S., et al.: Height, weight, and risk of breast cancer relapse. Breast Cancer Res. Treat., 5:81, 1985.

Erickson, K. L., Adams, D. A., and Ross, B.: Dietary fat influences on mammary tumor growth and ^{31}P-nuclear magnetic resonance measurements of metabolic activity. Proc. Natl. Acad. Cancer Res., 26:8, 1985.

Ernster, V. L.: The epidemiology of benign breast disease. Epidemiol. Rev., 3:184, 1981.

Ernster, V., Goodson, W. H., III, Hunt, T. K., et al.: Vitamin E and benign breast "disease": A double-blind, randomized clinical trial. Surgery, 97:490, 1985.

Ernster, V. L., Mason, L., Goodson, W. H., III, et al.: Effects of caffeine-free diet on benign breast disease: A randomized trial. Surgery, 91:263, 1982.

Foecking, M. K., Minton, J. P., and Matthews, R. H.: Progressive patterns in breast disease. Med. Hypotheses, 6:659, 1980.

Folks, D. G.: Monoamine oxidase inhibitors: Reappraisal of dietary considerations. J. Clin. Psychopharmacol., 3:249, 1983.

Food Balance Sheets, 1964–66 Average. Rome, Food and Agriculture Organization of the United Nations, 1971[1]

Fraker, L. D., Halter, S. A., and Forbes, J. T.: Growth inhibition by retinol of a human breast carcinoma cell line in vitro and in athymic mice. Cancer Res., 44:5757, 1984.

Gabor, H., Hillyard, L. A., and Abraham, S.: Effect of dietary fat on growth kinetics of transplantable mammary adenocarcinoma in BALB/c mice. JNCI, 74:1299, 1985.

Gaskill, S. P., McGuire, W. L., Osborne, C. K., et al.: Breast cancer mortality and diet in the United States. Cancer Res., 39:3628, 1979.

Gersovitz, M., Madden, J. P., and Smiciklas-Wright, H.: Validity of the 24-hour dietary recall and seven-day record for group comparisons. J. Am. Diet. Assoc., 73:48, 1978.

Gilbert, R. M., Marshman, J. A., Schwieder, M., et al.: Caffeine content of beverages as consumed. Can. Med. Assoc. J., 114:205, 1976.

Graham, D. M.: Caffeine—its identity, dietary sources, intake and biological effects. Nutr. Rev., 36:97, 1978.

Graham, S.: Results of case-control studies of diet and cancer in Buffalo, New York. Cancer Res., 43(Suppl.):2409, 1983.

Graham, S., Dayal, H., Swanson, M., et al.: Diet in the epidemiology of cancer of the colon and rectum. JNCI, 61:709, 1978.

Graham, S., Haughey, B., and Marshall, J.: Diet in epidemiology of carcinoma of the prostate gland. JNCI, 70:687, 1983.

Graham, S., Marshall, J., Mettlin, C., et al.: Diet in the epidemiology of breast cancer. Am. J. Epidemiol., 116:68, 1982.

Gray, G. E., Pike, M. C., and Henderson, B. E.: Breast-cancer incidence and mortality rates in different countries in relation to known risk factors and dietary practices. Br. J. Cancer, 39:1, 1979.

Gregorio, D. I., Emrich, L. J., Graham, S., et al.: Dietary fat consumption and survival among women with breast cancer. JNCI, 75:37, 1985.

Grubbs, C. J., Moon, R. C., Sporn, M. B., et al.: Inhibition of mammary cancer by retinyl methyl ether. Cancer Res., 37:599, 1977.

Guthrie, H.: Introductory Nutrition. 6th ed. St. Louis, C.V. Mosby, 1986.

Guthrie, H. A.: Selection and quantification of typical food portions by young adults. J. Am. Diet. Assoc., 84:1440, 1984.

Guthrie, H. A., and Crocetti, A.F.: Variability of nutrient intake over a 3-day period. J. Am. Diet. Assoc., 85:325, 1985.

Hankin, J. H., and Rawlings, V.: Diet and breast cancer: A review. Am. J. Clin. Nutr., 31:2005, 1978.

Hankin, J. H., Nomura, A. M., Lee, J., et al.: Reproducibility of a diet history questionnaire in a case-control study of breast cancer. Am. J. Clin. Nutr., 37:981, 1983.

Harman, D.: Dimethylbenzanthracene induced cancer: Inhibiting effect of dietary vitamin E. Clin. Res., 17:125, 1969.

Harr, J. R., Exon, J. H., Whanger, P. D., et al.: Effect of dietary selenium on N-2-fluorenyl-acetamide (FAA)–induced cancer in vitamin E supplemented, selenium depleted rats. Clin. Toxicol., 5:187, 1972.

Hawkins, R. A., Thomson, M. L., and Killen, E.: Oestrone sulphate, adipose tissue and breast cancer. Breast Cancer Res. Treat., 6:75, 1985.

Heasman, K. Z., Sutherland, H. J., Campbell, J. A., et al.: Weight gain during adjuvant chemotherapy for breast cancer. Breast Cancer Res. Treat., 5:195, 1985.

Helmrich, S. P., Shapiro, S., Rosenberg, L., et al.: Risk factors for breast cancer. Am. J. Epidemiol., 117:35, 1983.

Hems, G.: The contributions of diet and childbearing to breast-cancer rates. Br. J. Cancer, 37:974, 1978.

Hems, G.: Associations between breast-cancer mortality rates, child-bearing and diet in the United Kingdom. Br. J. Cancer, 41:429, 1980.

Heyden, S., and Muhlbaier, L. H.: Prospective study of "fibrocystic breast disease" and caffeine consumption. Surgery, 96:479, 1984.

Hiatt, R. A., and Bawol, R.: Alcohol beverage consumption and breast cancer incidence. Am. J. Epidemiol., 120:676, 1984.

Hirayama, T.: Diet and cancer. Nutr. Cancer, 1:67, 1979.

Hislop, T. G., and Elwood, J. M.: Risk factors for benign breast disease: A 30-year cohort study. Can. Med. Assoc. J., 124:283, 1981.

Hodge, J. V., Nye, E. R., and Emerson, G. W.: Monoamine oxidase inhibitors, broad beans, and hypertension crisis. Lancet, 1:1108, 1964.

Hopkins, G. J., West, C. E., and Hard, G. C.: Effect of dietary fats on the incidence of 7,12-dimethylbenz[a]anthracene-induced tumors in rats. Lipids, 11:328, 1976.

Horvath, P. M., and Ip, C.: Synergistic effect of vitamin E and selenium in the chemoprevention of mammary carcinogenesis in rats. Cancer Res., 43:5335, 1983.

Horwitz, D., Lovenberg, W., Engelman, K., et al.: Monoamine oxidase inhibitors, tyramine and cheese. J.A.M.A., 188:1108, 1964.

Houser, H. B., and Bebb, H. T.: Individual variation in intake of nutrients by day, month, and season and relation to meal patterns: Implications for dietary survey methodology. In National Research Council, Committee on Food Consumption Patterns: Assessing Changing Food Consumption Patterns. Washington, National Academy Press, 1981, p. 155.

Ip, C.: Factors influencing the anticarcinogenic efficacy of selenium in dimethylbenz[a]anthracene–induced mammary tumorigenesis in rats. Cancer Res., 41:2683, 1981a.

Ip, C.: Prophylaxis of mammary neoplasia by selenium supplementation in the initiation and promotion phases of chemical carcinogenesis. Cancer Res., 41:4386, 1981b.

Ip, C., and Sinha, D. K.: Enhancement of mammary tumorigenesis by selenium deficiency in rats with a high polyunsaturated fat intake. Cancer Res., 41:31, 1981.

Jain, M., Howe, G. R., Johnson, K. C., et al.: Evaluation of a diet history questionnaire for epidemiologic studies. Am. J. Epidemiol., 111:212, 1980.

Jenike, M. A.: Alcohol and antihistamines not contraindicated with MAOIs? Am. J. Psychiatry, 140:1107, 1983.

Jenike, M. A.: The use of monoamine oxidase inhibitors in the treatment of elderly, depressed patients. J. Am. Geriatr. Soc., 32:571, 1984.

Jensen, O. M., Wahrendorf, J., Rosenquist, A., et al.: The reliability of questionnaire-derived historical dietary information and temporal stability of food habits in individuals. Am. J. Epidemiol., 120:281, 1984.

Jurkowski, J. J., and Cave, W. T.: Dietary effects of menhaden oil on the growth and membrane lipid composition of rat mammary tumors. JNCI, 74:1145, 1985.

Kakar, F., Henderson, M.: Diet and breast cancer. Clin. Nutr., 4:119, 1985.

Kark, J. D., Smith, A. H., and Hames, C. G.: The

relationship of serum cholesterol to the incidence of cancer in Evans County, Georgia. J. Chronic Dis., *33*:311, 1980.

Karmali, R. A.: Review: Prostaglandins and cancer. Prostaglandins Leukotrienes Med., *50*:11, 1980.

Karmali, R. A., Marsh, J., and Fuchs, C.: Effect of omega-3 fatty acids on growth of a rat mammary tumor. JNCI, *73*:457, 1984.

Katch, F., Michael, E., and Horvath, S.: Estimation of body volume by underwater weighing: Description of simple inexpensive method. J. Appl. Physiol., *23*:811, 1967.

Keys, A., Aravanis, C., Blackburn, H., et al.: Serum cholesterol and cancer mortality in the Seven Countries Study. Am. J. Epidemiol., *121*:870, 1985.

Khosla, T., and Lowe, C. R.: Indices of obesity derived from body weight and height. Br. J. Prev. Soc. Med., *21*:122, 1967.

Kim, W. W., Kelsay, J. L., Judd, J. T., et al.: Evaluation of long-term dietary intakes of adults consuming self-selected diets. Am. J. Clin. Nutr., *40*(Suppl.):1327, 1984.

Kim. W.W., Mertz, W., Judd, J. T., et al.: Effect of making duplicate food collections on nutrient intakes calculated from diet records. Am. J. Clin. Nutr., *40*(Suppl.):1333, 1984b.

King, M. M., and McCay, P. B.: Modulation of tumor incidence and possible mechanisms of inhibition of mammary carcinogenesis by dietary antioxidants. Cancer Res., *43*:(Suppl.):2485, 1983.

Kinlen, L. J.: Meat and fat consumption and cancer mortality: A study of strict religious orders in Britain. Lancet, *1*:946, 1982.

Kolata, G.: Obesity declared a disease. Science, *227*:1019, 1985.

Kolonel, L. N., Hankin, J., and Lee, J.: Diet and prostate cancer. Am. J. Epidemiol., *228*:454, 1983.

Kolonel, L. N., Nomura, A. M., Hinds, M. W., et al.: Role of diet in cancer incidence in Hawaii. Cancer Res., *43*:(Suppl.):2397, 1983.

Krantzler, N. J., Mullen, B. J., Comstock, E. M., et al.: Methods of food intake assessment—an annotated bibliography. J. Nutr. Educ., *14*:108, 1982.

Krebs-Smith, S. M., and Smiciklas-Wright, H.: 1985 Typical serving sizes: Implications for food guidance. J. Am. Dietetic Assoc., *85*:1139–1141, 1985.

Kritchevsky, D., Weber, M. W., and Klurfeld, D. M.: Dietary fat versus caloric content in initiation and promotion of 7,12-dimethylbenz[a]anthracene-induced mammary tumorigenesis in rats. Cancer Res., *44*:3174, 1984.

La Vecchia, C., Decarli, A., Franceschi, S., et al.: Alcohol consumption and the risk of breast cancer in women. JNCI, *75*:61, 1985a.

La Vecchia, C., Franceschi, S., Parazzini, F., et al.: Benign breast disease and consumption of beverages containing methylxanthines. JNCI, *74*:995, 1985b.

Lavik, P. S., and Baumann, C. A.: Further studies on tumor-promoting action of fat. Cancer Res., *3*:749, 1943.

Lawson, D., Jick, H., and Rothman, K. J.: Coffee and tea consumption and breast disease. Surgery, *90*:801, 1981.

Le, M. G.: Coffee consumption, benign breast disease, and breast cancer (letter to the editor). Am. J. Epidemiol., *122*:721, 1985.

Le, M. G., Hill, C., Kramar, A., et al.: Alcoholic beverage consumption and breast cancer in a French case-control study. Am. J. Epidemiol., *120*:350, 1984.

Lea, A. J.: Dietary factors associated with death-rates from certain neoplasms in man. Lancet, *2*:332, 1966.

Lee, C., and Chen, C.: Enhancement of mammary tumorigenesis in rats by vitamin E deficiency. Proc. Am. Assoc. Cancer Res. Am. Soc. Clin. Oncol., *20*:132, 1979.

Lieb, J.: Degraded protein-containing foods and monoamine oxidase inhibitors. Am. J. Psychiatry, *134*:1444, 1977.

London, R. S., Solomon, D. M., London, E. D., et al.: Mammary dysplasia: Clinical response and urinary excretion of 11-deoxy-17-ketosteroids and pregnanediol following alpha-tocopherol therapy. Breast, *4*:19 1978.

Lovenberg, W.: Some vaso- and psychoactive substances in food: Amines, stimulants, depressants, and hallucinogens. In Toxicants Occurring Naturally in Foods. 2nd Ed. Washington, D. C., Food and Nutrition Board, National Academy of Sciences, 1973, p. 170.

Lubin, F., Ron, E., Was, Y., et al.: Coffee and methylxanthines and breast cancer: A case-control study. JNCI, *74*:569, 1985a.

Lubin, F., Ruder, A. M., Wax, Y., et al.: Overweight and changes in weight throughout adult life in breast cancer etiology. Am. J. Epidemiol., *122*:579, 1985b.

Lubin, J. H., Burns, P. E., Blot, R. G., et al.: Dietary factors and breast cancer risk. Int. J. Cancer, *28*:685, 1981.

Lyon, J. L., Gardner, J. W., West, D. W., et al.: Methodological issues in epidemiological studies of diet and cancer. Cancer Res., *43*(Suppl.):2392, 1983.

MacLennan, R., Da Costa, J., Day, N. E., et al.: Risk factors for lung cancer in Singapore Chinese, a population with high female incidence rates. Int. J. Cancer, *20*:854, 1977.

Maga, J. A.: Amines in food. Crit. Rev. Food Sci. Nutr., *10*:373, 1978.

Mahalko, J. R., Johnson, L. K., Gallagher, S. K., et al.: Comparison of dietary histories and seven-day food records in a nutritional assessment of older adults. Am. J. Clin. Nutr., *42*:542, 1985.

Mansel, R. E., Webster, D. J. T., Burr, M., et al.: Is there a relationship between coffee consumption and breast disease? Br. J. Surg. *69*:295, 1982.

Marshall, J., Graham, S., and Swanson, M.: Caffeine consumption and benign breast disease: A case-control comparison. Am. J. Public Health, *72*:610, 1982.

Martin, D. W., Jr., Mayes, P. A., and Rodwell, V. W.: Harper's Review of Biochemistry. 20th Ed. Los Altos, Calif., Lange Medical Publications, 1985.

Massachusetts General Hospital: Dietary restrictions during use of monoamine oxidase inhibitors. In Department of Dietetics: Diet Reference Manual. 2nd Ed. Boston, Little, Brown, 1984, p. 103.

Mayo Clinic Tyramine control. In Pemberton, C. M., and Gastineau, C. F. (Eds.): Mayo Clinic Diet Manual. A Handbook of Dietary Practices. Philadelphia, W. B. Saunders, 1981, p. 255.

McCabe, B., and Tsuang, M. T.: Dietary consideration in MAO inhibitor regimens. J. Clin. Psychiatry, *43*:178, 1982.

McCay, P. B.: Vitamin E: Interactions with free radicals and ascorbate. In Olson, R. E., Beutler, E., and Broquist, H. P. (Eds.): Annual Review of Nutrition. Palo Alto, Calif., Annual Reviews, Inc., 1985, p. 323.

McConnell, K. P., Jager, R. M., Bland, K. I., et al.: The relationship of dietary selenium and breast cancer. J. Surg. Oncol., *15*:67, 1980.

McCormick, D. L., Burns, F. J., and Albert, R. E.: Inhibition of rat mammary carcinogenesis by short die-

tary exposure to retinyl acetate. Cancer Res., *40*:1140, 1980.
McGee, D., and Gordon, T.: The results of the Framingham Study applied to four other U.S.-based epidemiologic studies of cardiovascular diseases. *In* Kannel, W. B., Gordon, T. (Eds.): The Framingham Study: An Epidemiological Investigation of Cardiovascular Disease. Section 31. Washington, D. C., DHEW Publication No. (NIH) 76–1083, 1976.
Medina, D., Lane, H. W., and Tracey, C. M.: Selenium and mouse mammary tumorigenesis: An investigation of possible mechanisms. Cancer Res., *43*(Suppl.):2460, 1983.
Medina, D., and Shepherd, F. S.: Selenium inhibition of the neoplastic transformation in preneoplastic mammary cell populations. Cancer Lett., *24*:227, 1984.
Mertz, W., and Kelsay, J. L.: Rationale and design of the Beltsville one-year dietary intake study. Am. J. Clin. Nutr., *40*:1323, 1984.
Metropolitan Life Foundation: Height and weight tables. Statistical Bulletin, *64*:2, 1983.
Mettlin, C.: Diet and the epidemiology of human breast cancer. Cancer, *53*:605, 1984.
Mettlin, C., and Graham, S.: Dietary risk factors in human bladder cancer. Am. J. Epidemiol., *110*:255, 1979.
Miller, A. B.: Role of nutrition in the etiology of breast cancer. Cancer, *39*:2704, 1977.
Miller, A. B., Kelly, A., Choi, N. W., et al.: A study of diet and breast cancer. Am. J. Epidemiol., *107*:499, 1978.
Minton, J. P., Abou-Issa, H., Foecking, M. K., et al.: Caffeine and unsaturated fat diet significantly promotes DMBA-induced breast cancer in rats. Cancer, *51*:1249, 1983.
Minton, J. P., Abou-Issa, H., Reiches, N., et al.: Clinical and biochemical studies on methylxanthine-related fibrocystic breast disease. Surgery, *90*:299, 1981.
Minton, J. P., Foecking, M. K., Webster, D. J., et al.: Response of fibrocystic disease to caffeine withdrawal and correlation of cyclic nucleotides with breast disease. Am. J. Obstet. Gynecol., *135*:157, 1979a.
Minton, J. P., Foecking, M. K., Webster, D. J., et al.: Caffeine, cyclic nucleotides, and breast disease. Surgery, *86*:105, 1979b.
Minton, J. P., Matthews, R. H., and Wisenbaugh, T. W.: Elevated adenosine 3,5'-cyclic monophosphate levels in human and animal tumors in vivo. JNCI, *57*:39, 1976.
Mirra, A. P., Cole, P., and MacMahon, B.: Breast cancer in an area of high parity: Sao Paulo, Brazil. Cancer Res., *31*:77, 1971.
Modan, B., Barell, V., Lubin, F., et al.: Dietary factors and cancer in Israel. Cancer Res., *35*:3503, 1975.
Modan, B., Cuckle, H., and Lubin, F.: A note on the role of dietary retinol and carotene in human gastrointestinal cancer. Int. J. Cancer, *28*:421, 1981.
Moon, R. C., McCormick, D. L., and Mehta, R. G.: Inhibition of carcinogenesis by retinoids. Cancer Res., *43*(Suppl.):2469, 1983.
Moore, D. H., Moore, D. H., II, and Moore, C. T.: Breast carcinoma etiological factors. Adv. Cancer Res., *40*:189, 1983.
Moore, M. C., Judlin, B. C., and Kennemur, P. M.: Using graduated food models in taking dietary histories. J. Am. Diet. Assoc., *51*:447, 1967.
Morgan, R. W., Jain, M., Miller, A. B., et al.: A comparison of dietary methods in epidemiology studies. Am. J. Epidemiol., *107*:488, 1978.
Mori, H., and Hironi, I.: Effect of coffee on carcinogenicity of cycasin. Br. J. Cancer, *35*:369, 1977.
Nagasawa, H.: Stimulation of neonatal treatment with vitamin A of spontaneous mammary tumor development in GRS/A mice. Breast Cancer Res. Treat., *4*:205, 1984.
National Academy of Sciences, Food and Nutrition Board: Recommended Dietary Allowances. 9th Ed. Washington, D. C., National Research Council, 1980.
National Research Council, Committee on Diet, Nutrition and Cancer: Diet, Nutrition and Cancer. Washington, D.C., National Academy Press, 1982.
Nomura, A., Hankin, J. H., and Rhoads, G. G.: The reproducibility of dietary intake data in a prospective study of gastrointestinal cancer. Am. J. Clin. Nutr., *29*:1432, 1976.
Nomura, A., Henderson, B. E., and Lee, J.: Breast cancer and diet among the Japanese in Hawaii. Am. J. Clin. Nutr., *31*:2020, 1978.
Nuessle, W. F., Norman, F. C., and Miller, H. E.: Pickled herring and tranylcypromine reaction. J.A.M.A., *192*:142, 1965.
Odenheimer, D. J., Zunzunegui, M. V., King, M. C., et al.: Risk factors for benign breast disease: A case-control study of discordant twins. Am. J. Epidemiol., *120*:565, 1984.
Ohlson, M. A., and Harper, L. J.: Longitudinal studies of food intake and weight of women from ages 18 to 56 years. J. Am. Diet. Assoc., *69*:626, 1976.
Paganini-Hill, A., and Ross, R. K.: Breast cancer and alcohol consumption. Lancet, *2*:626, 1983.
Pao, E. M., Mickle, S. J., and Burk, M. C.: One-day and 3-day nutrient intakes by individuals—Nationwide Food Consumption Survey findings, spring 1977. J. Am. Diet. Assoc., *85*:313, 1985.
Parazzini, F., La Vecchia, C., Franceschi, S., et al.: Risk factors for pathologically confirmed benign breast disease. Am. J. Epidemiol., *120*:115, 1984.
Pare, C. M. B., Kline, N., Hallstrom, C., et al.: Will amitriptyline prevent the "cheese" reaction of monoamine-oxidase inhibitors? Lancet, *1*:183, 1982.
Pastides, H., Kelsey, J. L., Holford, T. R., et al.: An epidemiologic study of fibrocystic breast disease with reference to ductal epithelial atypia. Am. J. Epidemiol., *121*:440, 1985.
Pettinger, W. A., and Oates, J. A.: Supersensitivity to tyramine during monoamine oxidase inhibition in man. Mechanism at the level of the adrenergic neuron. Clin. Pharmacol. Ther., *9*:341, 1968.
Phillips, R. L., and Snowdon, D. A.: Association of meat and coffee use with cancers of large bowel, breast, and prostate among Seventh-Day Adventists: Preliminary results. Cancer Res., *43*(Suppl.):2403, 1983.
Price, K., and Smith, S. E.: Cheese reaction and tyramine. Lancet, *1*:130, 1971.
Powers, D., and Moore, A. O.: Pressor Agents: Tyramine, dopamine, phenylethylamine in foods and beverages. *In* Food Medication Interactions. 4th Ed. Tempe, Arizona, FMI Publishing, 1983, p. 158.
Pozniak, P. C.: The carcinogenicity of caffeine and coffee: A review. J. Am. Diet. Assoc., *85*:1127, 1985.
Raunikar, R., Purcell, J., Elrod, J. C., et al.: Spatial and temporal aspects of the demand for food in the United States: I-XVII. *In* Research Bulletins Nos. 61, 63, 85, 87, 92, 93, 107, 109, 115, 123, 125, 134, 137-140, and 1943. University of Georgia College of Agriculture Experiment Stations, 1969–1973.
Ravnihar, B., MacMahon, B., and Lindtner, J.: Epidemiology features of breast cancer in Slovenia 1965–1967. Eur. J. Cancer, *7*:295, 1967.
Rice, S., Eitenmiller, R. R., and Koehler, P. E.: Histamine and tyramine content of meat products. J. Milk Food Tech., *38*:256, 1975.
Rivlin, R. S.: Nutrition and cancer: State of the art

relationship of several nutrients to the development of cancer. J. Am. Coll. Nutr., *1*:75, 1982.

Rogers, A. E.: Influence of dietary content of lipids and lipotropic nutrients on chemical carcinogenesis in rats. Cancer Res., *43*(Suppl.):2477, 1983.

Rohan, T. E., and Potter, J. D.: Retrospective assessment of dietary intake. Am. J. Epidemiol., *120*:876, 1984.

Rose, G., and Shipley, M. J.: Plasma lipids and mortality: A source of error. Lancet, *1*:523, 1980.

Rosenberg, L., Miller, D. R., Helmrich, S. P., et al.: Breast cancer and the consumption of coffee. Am. J. Epidemiol., *122*:391, 1985.

Rosenberg, L., Slone, D., Shapiro, S., et al.: Breast cancer and alcoholic-beverage consumption. Lancet, *1*:267, 1982.

Rosenthal, M. B., Barnard, R. J., Rose, D. P., et al.: Effects of a high-complex-carbohydrate, low-fat, low-cholesterol diet on levels of serum lipids and estradiol. Am. J. Med., *78*:23, 1985.

Russell-Briefel, R., Caggiula, A. W., and Kuller, L. H.: A comparison of three dietary methods for estimating vitamin A intake. Am. J. Epidemiol., *122*:628, 1985.

Samet, J. M., Humble, C. G., and Skipper, B. E.: Alternatives in the collection and analysis of food frequency interview data. Am. J. Epidemiol., *120*:572, 1984.

Schrauzer, G. N.: Selenium and cancer; a review. Bioinorg. Chem., *5*:275, 1976.

Schrauzer, G. N., White, D. A., and Schneider, C. J.: Cancer mortality correlation studies. III. Statistical associations with dietary selenium intakes. Bioinorg. Chem., *7*:23, 1977a.

Schrauzer, G. N., White, D. A., and Schneider, C. J.: Cancer mortality correlation studies. IV. Associations with dietary intakes and blood levels of certain trace elements, notably Se-antagonists. Bioinorg. Chem., *7*:35, 1977b.

Schrauzer, G. N., White, D. A., and Schneider, C. J.: Selenium and cancer: Effects of selenium and of the diet on the genesis of spontaneous mammary tumors in virgin inbred female C3H/St mice. Bioinorg. Chem., *8*:387, 1978.

Sen, N. P.: Analysis and significance of tyramine in foods. J. Food Sci., *34*:22, 1969.

Shamberger, R. J., Rukovena, E., Longfield, A. K., et al.: Antioxidants and cancer. I. Selenium in the blood of normals and cancer patients. JNCI, *50*:863, 1973.

Shanklin, D., Endres, J. M., and Sawicki, M.: A comparative study of two nutrient data bases. J. Am. Diet. Assoc., *85*:308, 1985.

Sheehan, D. V., Claycomb, J. B., and Kouretas, N.: Monoamine oxidase inhibitors: Prescription and patient management. Int. J. Psychiatry Med., *10*:99, 1980–1981.

Sjoqvist, F.: Psychotropic drugs. 2. Interaction between monoamine oxidase (MAO) inhibitors and other substances. Proc. R. Soc. Med., *58*:967, 1965.

Smithline, F., Sherman, L., and Kolodny, H. D.: Prolactin and breast carcinoma. N. Engl. J. Med., *292*:784, 1975.

Sohrabi, A., Sandoz, J., Spratt, J. S., et al.: Recurrence of breast cancer. Obesity, tumor size, and axillary lymph node metastases. J.A.M.A., *244*:264, 1980.

Soini, I., Aine, R., Lauslahti, K., et al.: Independent risk factors of benign and malignant breast lesions. Am. J. Epidemiol., *114*:507, 1981.

Sorenson, A. W.: Assessment of nutrition in epidemiologic studies. *In* Schottenfeld, D., and Fraumeni, J. F., Jr. (Eds.): Cancer Epidemiology and Prevention. Philadelphia, W. B. Saunders, 1982. p. 434.

Stavraky, K., and Emmons, S.: Breast cancer in premenopausal and postmenopausal women. JNCI, *53*:647, 1974.

Stockley, I. H.: Monoamine oxidase inhibitors. Part 1. Interactions with sympathomimetic amines. Pharmacol. J., *210*:590, 1973.

Subcommittee on Diet and Hyperlipidemia, Council on Atherosclerosis: A Maximal Approach to the Dietary Treatment of Hyperlipidemias. Diet C. The Low Cholesterol, High Polyunsaturated Fat Diet. New York, American Heart Association, 1973.

Sullivan, E. A., and Shulman, K. I.: Diet and monoamine oxidase inhibitors: A re-examination. Can. J. Psychiatry, *29*:707, 1984.

Sundaram, G. S., London, R., Manimekalai, S., et al.: Alpha-tocopherol and serum lipoproteins. Lipids, *16*:223, 1981.

Takahashi, S., and Biempica, L.: Effects of vitamin A and dexamethasone on collagen degradation in mouse mammary adenocarcinoma. Cancer Res., *45*:3311, 1985.

Tannenbaum, A.: The genesis and growth of tumors. III. Effects of a high fat diet. Cancer Res., *2*:468, 1942.

Tannenbaum, A., and Silverstone, H.: The genesis and growth of tumors. IV. Effects of varying proportion of protein (casein) in the diet. Cancer Res., *9*:162, 1949.

Tartter, P. I., Papatestas, A. E., Ioannovich, J., et al.: Cholesterol and obesity as prognostic factors in breast cancer. Cancer, *47*:2222, 1981.

Thomas, I. K., and Erickson, K. L.: Lipid modulation of mammary tumor cell cytolysis: Direct influence of dietary fats on the effector component of cell-mediated cytotoxicity. JNCI, *74*:675, 1985.

Thompson, H. J., Meeker, L. D., and Kokoska, S.: Effect of an inorganic and organic form of dietary selenium on the promotional stage of mammary carcinogenesis in the rat. Cancer Res., *44*:2803, 1984.

Udenfriend, S., Lovenberg, W., and Sjoerdsma, A.: Physiologically active amines in common fruits and vegetables. Arch. Biochem. and Biophys., *85*:487, 1959.

Ueda, H., Ono, M., Hagino, Y., et al.: Isolation of retinoic acid–resistant clones from human breast cancer cell line MCF-7 with altered activity of cellular retinoic acid–binding proteins. Cancer Res., *45*:3332, 1985.

Underwood, E. J.: Trace Elements. *In* Toxicants Occurring Naturally in Foods. 2nd Ed. Washington, D. C., Food and Nutrition Board, National Academy of Sciences, 1973, p. 43.

United States Department of Agriculture, Agriculture Research Service: Dietary levels of households in the Northeast/North Central Region/South/West, Spring, 1965. *In* Household Food Consumption Survey 1965-1966. Report Nos. 7 to 10. Washington, D. C., U. S. Government Printing Office, January to November, 1970.

United States Department of Agriculture, Agriculture Research Service: Dietary levels of households in the United States, seasons and year 1965–1966. *In* Household Food Consumption Survey 1965–1966. Report No. 18. Washington, D. C., U. S. Government Printing Office, 1974.

United States Department of Agriculture, Agriculture Research Service: Nutritive Value of American Foods. Agriculture Handbook No. 456. Washington, D. C., U.S. Government Printing Office, 1975.

United States Department of Agriculture: Dietary Guidelines for Americans. 2nd Ed. Home and Garden Bulletin 232. Washington, D. C., U. S. Government Printing Office, 1985.

University of Iowa Hospitals and Clinics: Tyramine restricted diet. *In* Recent Advances in Therapeutic Diets. 3rd Ed. Ames, Iowa, The Iowa State University Press, 1979, p. 116.

van Staveren, W. A., de Boer, J. O., and Burema, J.: Validity and reproducibility of a dietary history method estimating the usual food intake during one month. Am. J. Clin. Nutr., *42*:554, 1985.

Voigt, M. N., Eitenmiller, R. R., Koehler, E. H., et al.: Tyramine, histamine and tryptamine content of cheese. J. Milk Food Tech., *37*:377, 1974.

Wattenberg, L. W.: Inhibition of carcinogenic and toxic effects of polycyclic hydrocarbons by phenolic antioxidants and ethoxyquin. JNCI, *48*:1425, 1972.

Webster, L. A., Layde, P. M., Wingo, P. A., et al.: Alcohol consumption and risk of breast cancer. Lancet, *2*:724, 1983.

Welsch, C. W., Scieszka, K. M., Senn, E. R., et al.: Caffeine (1,3,7-trimethylxanthine), a temperature promoter of DMBA-induced rat mammary gland carcinogenesis. Int. J. Cancer, *32*:479, 1983.

Whittemore, A. S., Paffenbarger, R. S., Jr., Anderson, K., et al.: Early precursors of site-specific cancers in college men and women. JNCI, *74*:43, 1985.

Willett, W. C., and MacMahon, B.: Diet and cancer—an overview. N. Engl. J. Med., *310*:633, 1984a.

Willett, W. C., and MacMahon, B.: Diet and cancer—an overview. N. Engl. J. Med., *310*:697, 1984b.

Willett, W. C., Sampson, L., Stampfer, M. J., et al.: Reproducibility and validity of a semiquantitative food frequency questionnaire. Am. J. Epidemiol., *122*:51, 1985.

Witting, L. A.: The oxidation of alpha-tocopherol during the autoxidation of ethyl oleate, linoleate, linolenate, and arachidonate. Arch. Biochem. Biophys., *129*:142, 1969.

Wynder, E. L.: Dietary factors related to breast cancer. Cancer *46*(Suppl.):899, 1980.

Wynder, E. L., and Rose, D. P.: Diet and breast cancer. Hosp. Pract., *19*:73, 1984.

Young, V. R., and Richardson, D. P.: Nutrients, vitamins and minerals in cancer prevention—facts and fallacies. Cancer, *43*(Suppl. 5):2125, 1979.

Zeman, F. J.: Drugs and Nutritional Care. *In* Zeman, F. J. (Ed.): Clinical Nutrition and Dietetics. Lexington, Mass., Collamore Press, 1983, p. 72.

Zumoff, B., and Dasgupta, I.: Relationship between body weight and the incidence of positive axillary nodes at mastectomy for breast cancer. J. Surg. Oncol., *22*:217, 1983.

Zumoff, B., O'Connor, J., Levin, J., et al.: Nonobesity at the time of mastectomy is highly predictive of 10-year disease-free survival in women with breast cancer. Anticancer Res., *2*:59, 1982.

Appendix to Chapter 5

APPENDIX A

Suggestions for Diet Counseling

Diet counseling assists a women in evaluating her current diet and assists her in making changes in her eating patterns. The best is available from a Registered Dietitian (RD) or a nutritionist located in most hospitals and many outpatient clinics. In addition, many Registered Dietitians or nutritionists have private dietary counsulting firms, and physicians may refer their patients to them.

If a referral to a RD is not possible, the following steps may be implemented by someone with a minimal background in nutrition:

1. *Determine whether or not the woman needs to gain or lose weight*

The "ideal" weight for a woman is not known, but the Metropolitan Height and Weight Tables are commonly used guidelines (Metropolitan Life Foundation, 1983). The 1983 edition of this table occurs later in this Appendix.

Another guideline is the Quetelet index (Khosla and Lowe, 1967). This may be expressed several ways, but a common one is weight (kg)/height (cm)^2 × 10,000 (Berkowitz et al., 1985). This index is somewhat difficult to interpret, and researchers use it in different ways. One standard is to use 21 as the "ideal" index for a medium-framed woman, with a normal range of about 19–25 (National Diabetes Data Group, 1979). Guthrie (1986) states that an index above 28 is indicative of obesity. See references in Chapter 5 for more information on interpreting the Quetelet index.

A very quick standard "ideal" weight is 100 pounds plus 5 pounds/inch for height over 60 inches, or 100 pounds minus 5 pounds/inch for a woman under 60 inches (Guthrie, 1986).

If a university or sports medicine research center is available, a woman may be able to have her percentage of body fat determined by hydrostatic weighing (Katch et al., 1967).

2. *Determine the current daily average kcalorie intake of the woman*

The best way to determine the current daily average kcalorie intake of a woman is to have her record her usual food intake for 3 to 4 days on a diet record sheet during a time her weight is relatively stable. A sample set of instructions and diet record form are included later in this Appendix. The average number of kcalories consumed daily may then be determined manually by using one of the three handbooks available from

Superintendent of Documents
U. S. Government Printing Office
Washington, D.C. 20402

1. Calories and Weight: The USDA Pocket Guide
   S/N 001–000–04164–9 $3.75

2. Nutritive Value of Foods
   S/N 001–000–04232–7 $4.50

3. Nutritive Value of American Foods in Common Units
   S/N 001–000–03184–8 $8.50

Software packages are available for computerized analysis of a client's kcalorie and nutrient food intake. Registered dietitians and computer stores can provide more information. Three commonly used computerized nutrition systems are the following:

The Food Processor
ESHA Corporation
P.O. Box 13028
Salem, Oregon 97309

Nutritionist III
N2 N-squared computing
5318 Forest Ridge Road
Silverton, Oregon 97381

Nutri-Calc
PCD Systems, Inc.
P.O. Box 143
Penn Yan, NY 14527

3. *Determine the desired daily kcalorie intake*

A woman maintains her weight when she consumes the same number of kcalories that she expends meeting the combined energy cost of basal metabolic needs, physical activity, and the thermic effect of food. Weight gain occurs when the kcalorie intake exceeds the energy expended; weight loss occurs when energy intake is less than energy expended. The number of kcalories needed for weight maintenance, loss, or gain is not the same for each woman. But a general guideline for weight loss is to subtract 500 to 1000 kcalories a day from the number of kcalories needed for weight maintenance to lose an average of 1 to 5 pounds a week (Guthrie, 1986). Adding 700 to 1000 kcalories a day to those needed to maintain the current weight should allow weight gain.

If it is not possible to calculate the average daily kcalorie intake, the following "rule of thumb" may be used for an estimation of kcalories needed to maintain body weight (Guthrie, 1986):

Energy need = body weight in pounds × 12 for a sedentary woman

= body weight in pounds × 15 for a moderately active woman

= body weight in pounds × 18 for an active woman

4. *Select a weight maintenance, loss, or gain plan for the woman*

The Appendix contains suggested ways to distribute the kcalories among food groups. Diet plans are given for a daily 1000 to 2000 kcalories for women who drink milk and for those who have a lactose intolerance or are allergic to milk. Modifications have been made in the foods allowed so that the plans are low in tyramine and dopamine. A sample day's intake of food is given for an individual on the 1200 kcalorie plan with milk. A registered dietitian should be consulted if additional kcalorie levels are needed or if there are food allergies or intolerances.

5. *Provide the woman with guidelines for a physical activity program*

A well-designed exercise program should be used by all women for whom exercise is medically advisable. See Chapter 31 for further information on exercise programs.

REFERENCES

Berkowitz, G. S., Kelsey, J. L., Li Volsi, V. A., et al.: Risk factors for fibrocystic breast disease and its histopathologic components. JNCI, 75:43, 1985.

Guthrie, H. A.: Introductory Nutrition. 6th Ed. St. Louis, C. V. Mosby, 1986.

Katch, F., Michael, E., and Horvath, S.: Estimation of body volume by underwater weighing: Description of simple inexpensive method. J. Appl. Physiol., 23:811, 1967.

Khosla, T., and Lowe, C. R.: Indices of obesity derived from body weight and height. Br. J. Prev. Soc. Med., 21:122, 1967.

Metropolitan Life Foundation: Height and Weight Tables. Statistical Bulletin, 64:2, 1983.

National Diabetes Data Group: Classification and diagnosis of diabetes mellitus and other categories of glucose intolerance. Diabetes, 28:1039, 1979.

APPENDIX B
Suggested Sources of Additional Information for Diet Counseling

1. Recipe books providing recipes for low-fat menu items:

    The American Heart Association Cookbook, published by Ballantine Books, New York. It is usually available from local heart association offices and bookstores.

    Don't Eat Your Heart Out Cookbook, by Joseph C. Piscatella, published by Workman Publishing, New York.

2. The American Institute for Cancer Research, Washington, D.C., 20069, has information for making good food choices. Write for the list of materials available for the health professional and the breast disease client. The following three booklets are especially useful for women who want to lower the risk of developing cancer:
    - "All About Fat and Cancer Risk"
    - "Dietary Guidelines to Lower Cancer Risk"
    - "Planning Meals That Lower Cancer Risk: A Reference Guide"

3. The Consumer Information Center V, P.O. Box 100, Pueblo, CO 81002, has a catalogue of information on topics of interest to the consumer. There are usually several publications on diet and health.

4. The American Dietetic Association, 430 North Michigan Avenue, Chicago, IL 60611, has a catalogue of publications available. The breast care client may find the cookbooks especially useful.

5. The following book, available at most bookstores, contains basic nutrition information and over 350 recipes to help the breast care client increase the quality of her diet: *Good Food Book: Living the High-Carbohydrate Way,* by Jane Brody, published by W. W. Norton and Company, New York.

APPENDIX C

Instructions for Filling Out the Dietary Record Form

For 4 days, please write down everything you eat and drink that is typical of your eating habits. Try to do the recording when your weight is stable. If you gain or lose weight during the week you are recording your intake, tell your diet counselor so it can be taken into consideration when calculating your suggested daily caloric intake.

Place the food item in the "Name of Food" column. Under "Method of Food Preparation" tell how the food was prepared, such as fried in oil, baked in slightly greased pan, or broiled. In this same column also state whether or not any fruit juice or canned fruit consumed was sweetened or unsweetened, the milk was 2%, 1%, skim, or whole, the soft drinks were dietetic or regular, the coffee or tea was regular or decaffeinated, and what the variety of cheese was, i.e., cheddar, low-fat cottage cheese, or other.

Under the column headed "Portion Size" *state the size portion of food* you consumed. Be as accurate as possible. It can be household measuring cups or ounces, tablespoons, teaspoons, or inches. For example, a meat portion consumed could be 3 inches by 6 inches by ½ inch. If you use sugar or cream in your coffee or tea, state the amount of cream or sugar consumed in this column.

Do not forget to include alcoholic beverages, vitamin and mineral supplements, and all snacks consumed, even if you just took a mouthful of a food item.

Please do not put anything in the column entitled "Coding."

If you have any questions call _____ at the following phone number _____.

APPENDIX C
Diet Record

Name _____ Code _____

Day of Week _____

Name of Food	Method of Preparation	Portion Size	Coding

APPENDIX D

Approximate Composition of Diet Plans

Kcalorie Level	Protein (grams)	Fat (grams)	Carbohydrate (grams)
1000	60	35	110
1200	60	40	150
1500	70	50	195
1800	75	60	240
2000	80	65	270

1200–2000 kcalorie diet plans contain the following percentage distribution of nutrients: 15–20% protein, 30% fat, and 50–55% carbohydrate. The 1000 kcalorie plans have a higher percentage of protein and lower percentage of carbohydrate than the other plans to provide for adequate level of protein intake.

APPENDIX E

Suggested Daily Food Unit Intake Without Milk

Unit List	Kcalories				
	1000	1200	1500	1800	2000
Vegetables	4	4	5	6	6
Fruit	2	4	6	6	7
Bread	5	6	7	10	11
Meat	6	6	6	6	7
Fat	3	4	6	8	9

Nutrient supplements suggested: Vitamin and mineral supplements for 1800 kcalorie diet and below. The supplements should contain the Recommended Dietary Allowance (RDA) level of all vitamins and minerals. Levels above the RDA can produce toxicity. Most multivitamin and mineral supplements do not contain calcium, so 1000–1200 mg of calcium supplements are needed at all kcalorie levels.

APPENDIX F

Suggested Daily Food Unit Intake with Milk

Unit List	Kcalories				
	1000	1200	1500	1800	2000
Milk	2	2	2	2	2
Vegetables	3	4	4	4	6
Fruit	2	3	5	6	7
Bread	4	5	7	9	10
Meat	4	4	5	5	5
Fat	4	5	6	8	9

Nutrient supplements suggested: Vitamin and mineral supplements for 1800 kcalorie diet and below. The supplements should contain the Recommended Dietary Allowance (RDA) level of all vitamins and minerals. Levels above the RDA can produce toxicity. Most multivitamin and mineral supplements do not contain calcium, so 300–500 mg of calcium supplements are needed in addition to diet and other supplements. Calcium should be added to the diet at all kcalorie levels.

APPENDIX G

Sample Menu for 1200 Kilocalories with Milk

Total units allowed per day:
  2 milk units
  4 vegetable units
  3 fruit units
  5 bread units
  4 meat units
  5 fat units

Breakfast
¼ small cantaloupe (1 fruit unit)
1 cup bran flakes (2 bread units)
1 cup skim milk (1 milk unit)

Lunch
Sandwich: 2 slices whole wheat bread (2 bread units)
  2 tablespoons peanut butter (1 meat unit plus 2 fat units)

Salad: 1 cup raw spinach (1 vegetable unit)
  1 tablespoon French dressing made with corn oil (1 fat unit)

1 fresh pear (1 fruit unit)

Dinner
3 ounces broiled halibut (3 meat units)
½ cup cooked macaroni (1 bread unit)
1 cup cooked broccoli (2 vegetable units)
Salad: lettuce, radishes, cucumber slices (all free) with 2 teaspoons corn
  oil (2 fat units) plus vinegar (free) as dressing
12 fresh grapes (1 fruit unit)
1 cup skim milk (1 milk unit)

Snack
½ cup tomato juice (1 vegetable unit)

Plus vitamin and mineral supplements

APPENDIX H

Dietary Fat, Cholesterol, Tyramine, and Dopamine Restricted Diet Plan*

List 1: Milk Unit

One unit of milk contains 12 grams of carbohydrate, 8 grams of protein, a trace of fat, and 80 kcalories.

    Milk is a basic food for your Meal Plan for very good reasons. Milk is the leading source of calcium. It is a good source of phosphorus, protein, some of the B-complex vitamins, including folic acid and vitamin B_{12}, and vitamin A and D. Magnesium is also found in milk.

    Choose _____units of milk from the list each day.

Non-fat Fortified Milk	*Amount in one unit*
Skim or non-fat milk	1 cup
Powdered (non-fat dry, before adding liquid)	⅓ cup
Canned, evaporated-skim milk	½ cup
Buttermilk made from skim milk	1 cup
Yoghurt made from skim milk (*consume in moderation*)	1 cup

Do not use 1% fat, 2% fat or whole milk

*Exchange lists adapted from "Exchange Lists for Meal Planning," American Diabetes Association, Inc. The American Dietetic Association, 1976.

    Tyramine and dopamine modifications are from the references listed in Chapter 5.

List 2: Vegetable Unit

One vegetable unit contains about 5 grams of carbohydrate, 2 grams of protein, and 25 kcalories.

    The generous use of many vegetables, served alone or in other foods, such as casseroles, soups, or salads, contributes to sound health and vitality.

    Dark green, deep yellow, or orange vegetables are among the leading sources of vitamin A. Many of these vegetables are notable sources of vitamin C: asparagus, broccoli, brussels sprouts, cabbage, cauliflower, collards, kale, dandelion, mustard and turnip greens, spinach, rutabagas, tomatoes, and turnips. Particularly good sources of potassium are broccoli, brussels sprouts, beet greens, chard, and tomato juice.

    High folic acid values are found in asparagus, beets, broccoli, brussels sprouts, cauliflower, collards, kale, and lettuce. Moderate amounts of vitamin B_6 are supplied by broccoli, brussels sprouts, cauliflower, collards, spinach, sauerkraut, tomatoes, and tomato juice. Fiber is present in all vegetables.

    Whether you serve them cooked or raw, wash all vegetables even though they look clean. If fat is added in the preparation, omit the equivalent number of fat units.

Do not use any overly ripe vegetables.

Choose _____ units of vegetables from this list each day. One unit is ½ cup cooked or 1 cup raw.

Asparagus	Mustard
Bean sprouts	Spinach
Beets	Turnip
Broccoli	Mushrooms
Brussels sprouts	Okra
Cabbage	Onions
Carrots	Rhubarb
Cauliflower	Rutabaga
Celery	Sauerkraut (*consume in moderation*)
Eggplant (*consume in moderation*)	String beans, green or yellow
Green pepper	Summer squash
Greens:	Tomatoes (*consume in moderation*)
Beets	Tomato juice (*consume in moderation*)
Chard	Turnips
Collards	Vegetable juice cocktail (*consume in moderation*)
Dandelion	
Kale	Zucchini

Do not eat Italian green beans (also called broad bean pods, fava beans, and Chinese pea pods).

The following raw vegetables may be used as desired:

Chicory	Parsley
Chinese cabbage	Radishes
Cucumbers	Watercress
Endive	
Escarole	
Lettuce	

Starchy vegetables are found in the Bread Unit list.

List 3: Fruit Unit

One unit of fruit contains 10 grams of carbohydrate and 40 kcalories.

Most people like to buy fresh fruits when they are in the height of their season. But you can also buy fresh fruits and can or freeze them for off-season use. For variety serve fruit as a salad or in combination with other foods for dessert.

Fruits are valuable for vitamins, minerals, and fiber. Vitamin C, abundant in citrus fruits and juices, is found in raspberries, strawberries, mangoes, cantaloupes, honeydews, and papayas. The better sources of vitamin A include fresh or dried apricots, mangoes, cantaloupes, nectarines, yellow peaches and persimmons. Oranges, orange juice, and cantaloupes provide more folic acid than most of the other fruits in this listing. Many fruits are a valuable source of potassium, especially apricots, bananas, several of the berries, grapefruit, grapefruit juice, mangoes, cantaloupes, honeydews, nectarines, oranges, orange juice, and peaches.

Fruit may be consumed fresh, dried, canned, or raw, as long as no sugar is added. Read the label to see if sugar has been added to the product.

Choose _____ units of fruit from this list each day.

	Amount in one unit
Apple	1 small
Apple juice	⅓ cup
Applesauce (unsweetened)	½ cup
Apricots, fresh	2 medium
Apricots, dried	4 halves
Banana (*consume in moderation*)	½ small (without skin)
Berries	
Blackberries	½ cup
Blueberries	½ cup
Raspberries	½ cup
Strawberries	¾ cup
Cherries	10 large
Cider	⅓ cup
Dates	2
Figs, fresh (*consume in moderation*)	1
Grapefruit	½
Grapefruit juice	½ cup
Grapes	12
Grape juice	¼ cup
Mango	½ small
Melon	
Cantaloupe	¼ small
Honeydew	⅛ medium
Watermelon	1 cup
Nectarine	1 small
Orange (*consume in moderation*)	1 small
Orange juice (*consume in moderation*)	½ cup
Papaya	¾ cup
Peach	1 medium
Pear	1 small
Persimmon, native	1 medium
Pineapple (*consume in moderation*)	½ cup
Pineapple juice (*consume in moderation*)	⅓ cup
Plums, red (*consume in moderation*)	2 medium
Prunes	2 medium
Prune juice	¼ cup
Raisins (*consume in moderation*)	2 tablespoons
Tangerine	1 medium

Cranberries may be used as desired if no sugar is added.

List 4: Bread Unit

One unit of bread contains 15 grams of carbohydrate, 2 grams of protein, and 70 kcalories.

In this list, whole-grain, enriched breads, cereals, germ and bran products, and dried beans and peas are good sources of iron and among the better sources of thiamin. The whole-grain, bran, and germ products have more fiber than products made from refined flours. Dried beans and peas are also good sources of fiber. Wheat germ, bran, dried beans, potatoes, lima beans, parsnips, pumpkin, and winter squash are particularly good sources of potassium.

The better sources of folic acid in this listing include whole-wheat bread, wheat germ, dried beans, corn, lima beans, parsnips, green peas, pumpkin, and sweet potato.

Starchy vegetables are included in this list because they contain the same amount of carbohydrate and protein as one slice of bread.

Choose _____ units of grain products from this list each day.

*Bread**

	Amount in one unit
White (including French and Italian)	1 slice
Whole wheat	1 slice
Rye or pumpernickel	1 slice
Raisin	1 slice
Bagel, small	½
English muffin, small	½
Plain roll, bread	1
Frankfurter roll	½
Hamburger bun	½
Dried bread crumbs	3 tablespoons
Tortilla, 6″	1

*Cereal**

Bran flakes	½ cup
Other ready-to-eat unsweetened cereal	¾ cup
Puffed cereal (unfrosted)	1 cup
Cereal (cooked)	½ cup
Grits (cooked)	½ cup
Rice or barley (cooked)	½ cup
Pasta (cooked), spaghetti, noodles, macaroni	½ cup
Popcorn (popped, no fat added, large kernel)	3 cups
Cornmeal (dry)	2 tablespoons
Flour	2½ tablespoons
Wheat germ	¼ cup

*Crackers**

Arrowroot	3
Graham, 2½ sq.	2
Matzo, 4″ × 6″	½
Oyster	20
Pretzel, 3⅛″ long × ⅛″ dia.	25
Rye wafers, 2″ × 3½″	3
Saltines	6
Soda, 2½″ sq.	4

Dried Beans, Peas and Lentils

Beans, peas, lentils (dried and cooked)	½ cup
Baked beans, no pork (canned)	¼ cup

Starchy Vegetables

	Amount in one unit
Corn	⅓ cup
Corn on cob	1 small
Lima beans	½ cup
Parsnips	⅔ cup
Peas, green (canned or frozen)	½ cup
Potato, white	1 small
Potato (mashed)	½ cup
Pumpkin	½ cup
Winter squash, acorn or butternut	½ cup
Yam or sweet potato	¼ cup

Prepared Foods*

Biscuit 2″ dia. (omit 1 fat unit)	1
Corn bread, 2″ × 2″ × 1″ (omit 1 fat unit)	1
Corn muffin, 2″ dia. (omit 1 fat unit)	1
Crackers, round butter type (omit 1 fat unit)	5
Muffin, plain small (omit 1 fat unit)	1

List 5: Meat Unit (Lean Meat)

One unit of meat contains 7–8 grams of protein, 3–5 grams of fat, and 55–75 kcalories.

All of the foods in the meat unit list are good sources of protein and many are also good sources of iron, zinc, vitamin B_{12} (present only in foods of animal origin), and other vitamins of the vitamin B-complex.

Cholesterol is of animal origin. Eggs and liver are especially rich in cholesterol. Foods of plant origin have no cholesterol.

Oysters are outstanding for their high content of zinc. Crab, trimmed lean meats, the dark muscle meat of turkey, dried beans and peas, and peanut butter all have much less zinc than oysters but are still good sources.

Dried beans, peas, and peanut butter are particularly good sources of magnesium and also potassium.

You may use the meat, fish, or other meat units that are prepared for the family when no fat or flour has been added. If meat is fried, use the fat included in the Meal Plan. Meat juices with the fat removed may be used with your meat or vegetables for added flavor. *Be certain to trim off all visible fat* and measure after it has been cooked. A three-ounce serving of cooked meat is about equal to four ounces of raw meat.

Choose _____units of meat from this list each day. Trim off all visible fat prior to cooking. The amounts stated are for cooked meat. If meat consumed is not very lean, omit one fat unit allowed for that day.

Do not consume any aged or slightly spoiled meat, fish or poultry.

	Amount in one unit
Poultry (without skin)	1 ounce
Beef or veal, very lean	1 ounce
Lamb, very lean	1 ounce
Pork, very lean	1 ounce
Fish, lean, fresh or frozen	1 ounce

---

*Avoid any containing cheese (other than cottage, ricotta, and cream) or larger than normal amounts of yeast.

	Amount in one unit
Canned salmon, tuna, mackerel, crab, or lobster	¼ cup
Clams, oysters, scallops, shrimp	5 or 1 ounce
Drained sardines	3
Low fat cottage cheese*	¼ cup
Skim milk ricotta cheese	¼ cup
Dried beans, peas, or lentils (cooked)†	½ cup
Peanut butter (omit 2 fat units)	2 tablespoons

List 6: Fat Units

One unit of fat contains 5 grams of fat and 45 kcalories.
　　Choose _____ units of fat from this list each day.

	Amount in one unit
Margarine, soft, tub or stick‡	1 teaspoon
Oil (corn, cottonseed, safflower, soy, sunflower)	1 teaspoon
Oil, olive§	1 teaspoon
Oil, peanut§	1 teaspoon
Olives§	5 small
Almonds§	10 whole
Pecans§	2 large whole
Peanuts§	
Spanish	20 whole
Virginia	10 whole
Nuts§	6 small
Mayonnaise‡	1 teaspoon
French dressing or Italian dressing‡	1 tablespoon
Salad dressing, mayonnaise type‡	2 teaspoons
Avocado (4″ diameter)	⅛ (*consume in moderation*)

Select your fat units only from the above list if you want to consume a diet high in polyunsaturated fatty acids and restricted in dietary cholesterol. Individuals with risk factors associated with cardiovascular disease, for example, may want to modify their diet in this manner.

　If cardiovascular disease is not a concern, the fat units may also be selected from the following foods:

	Amount in one unit
Margarine, regular stick	1 teaspoon
Butter	1 teaspoon
Cream, light	2 tablespoons
Cream, heavy	1 tablespoon

---

　*Do not consume any cheese (except low fat cottage cheese or ricotta), smoked fish, pickled fish, liver of any origin, dried and aged sausage, or wild game.
　†Dried beans, peas, and lentils (cooked) may be considered either meat units or bread units.
　‡Made with corn, cottonseed, safflower, soy, and sunflower oil only.
　§Fat content is primarily monounsaturated.

	Amount in one unit
Cream, sour (*consume in moderation*)	2 tablespoons
Cream cheese	1 tablespoon
French or Italian dressing from any oil	1 tablespoon
Lard	1 teaspoon
Mayonnaise from any oil source	1 teaspoon
Salad dressing, mayonnaise type, from any oil source	2 teaspoons

---

The exchange lists from the EXCHANGE LISTS FOR MEAL PLANNING were prepared by committees of the American Diabetes Association, Inc., and the American Dietetic Association in cooperation with the National Institute of Arthritis, Metabolism, and Digestive Disease and the National Heart and Lung Institute, National Institutes of Health, Public Health Service, U.S. Department of Health and Human Services.

*Copyright American Diabetes Association, Inc., The American Dietetic Association, 1976.

APPENDIX I

Tyramine and Dopamine Restricted Diet

Avoid the Following Foods

General: Any aged, fermented or overly ripe food product, including cheese, fish, fruit, vegetable, grain, or beverage

Beverages: Beer, ale, wine, sherry, vermouth, cognac. Very occasionally (three or four times a year, for example), white wine might be consumed. Red wines should never be consumed.

Dairy Products: Aged and processed cheeses. This includes avoiding cheese in mixed-food recipes (for example, pizza, fondue, salad dressings, breads, and crackers). The only cheeses allowed are cottage, ricotta, and cream.

Vegetables: Fava beans (also called English bean pods, Italian green beans, Chinese pea pods, and broad beans). These beans are commonly used in Mediterranean recipes. They are ½ inch or more in width and are kidney shaped. Lima beans, green beans, and wax beans are allowed.

Fruit: Banana peel (for example, in stewed bananas).

Meat Products: Salted, pickled, smoked fish. Some common ones are herring, cod, lox, snail, and caviar. Liver and liverwurst from all origins (beef, pork, and chicken). Dried and aged sausage products. Some examples are salami, pepperoni, summer sausage, and corned beef. Bologna should be consumed soon after purchase.

Miscellaneous: Marmite (also called Bouril). This is a yeast product consumed primarily in England. Brewer's yeast in pill or liquid form. This is a yeast product frequently sold as a vitamin supplement. Medications containing tyramine. Check with a physician or pharmacist before consuming over-the-counter or prescription drugs.

Consume in Moderation or Not at All

Beverages
  Coffee, tea, and caffeine-containing colas
  Gin, whiskey, and vodka

Dairy Products
  Yoghurt
  Sour cream

Vegetables
  Sauerkraut
  Pickles
  Tomatoes
  Eggplant

Fruit
  Figs
  Banana pulp
  Red plums

Fruit Continued
　Raisins
　Avocado, guacomole
　Orange
　Pineapple

Grain Products
　Homemade bread products made with more yeast than used in most recipes

Miscellaneous
　Chocolate
　Bouillon cubes and other meat extract products used to make gravies or soups or add color and flavor to food products
　Soy sauce

APPENDIX J

1983 Metropolitan Height and Weight Tables for Men and Women
(According to Frame, Ages 25–59)

Height (In Shoes)†		Weight in Pounds in Indoor Clothing*		
Feet	Inches	Small Frame	Medium Frame	Large Frame
		Men		
5	2	128–134	131–141	138–150
5	3	130–136	133–143	140–153
5	4	132–138	135–145	142–156
5	5	134–140	137–148	144–160
5	6	136–142	139–151	146–164
5	7	138–145	142–154	149–168
5	8	140–148	145–157	152–172
5	9	142–151	148–160	155–176
5	10	144–154	151–163	158–180
5	11	146–157	154–166	161–184
6	0	149–160	157–170	164–188
6	1	152–164	160–174	168–192
6	2	155–168	164–178	172–197
6	3	158–172	167–182	176–202
6	4	162–176	171–187	181–207
		Women		
4	10	102–111	109–121	118–131
4	11	103–113	111–123	120–134
5	0	104–115	113–126	122–137
5	1	106–118	115–129	125–140
5	2	108–121	118–132	128–143
5	3	111–124	121–135	131–147
5	4	114–127	124–138	134–151
5	5	117–130	127–141	137–155
5	6	120–133	130–144	140–159
5	7	123–136	133–147	143–163
5	8	126–139	136–150	146–167
5	9	129–142	139–153	149–170
5	10	132–145	142–156	152–173
5	11	135–148	145–159	155–176
6	0	138–151	148–162	158–179

*Indoor clothing weighing 5 pounds for men and 3 pounds for women.
†Shoes with 1 inch heels.
Source of basic data: Build Study, 1979, Society of Actuaries and Association of Life Insurance Medical Directors of America, 1980.
Copyright 1983, Metropolitan Life Insurance Company. Reprinted with permission.

APPENDIX K

1983 Metropolitan Height and Weight Tables for Men and Women on Metric Basis
(According to Frame, Ages 25–59)

Height (In Shoes)† Centimeters	MEN Weight in Kilograms (In Indoor Clothing)*			Height (In Shoes)† Centimeters	WOMEN Weight in Kilograms (In Indoor Clothing)*		
	Small Frame	*Medium Frame*	*Large Frame*		*Small Frame*	*Medium Frame*	*Large Frame*
158	58.3–61.0	59.6–64.2	62.8–68.3	148	46.4–50.6	49.6–55.1	53.7–59.8
159	58.6–61.3	59.9–64.5	63.1–68.8	149	46.6–51.0	50.0–55.5	54.1–60.3
160	59.0–61.7	60.3–64.9	63.5–69.4	150	46.7–51.3	50.3–55.9	54.4–60.9
161	59.3–62.0	60.6–65.2	63.8–69.9	151	46.9–51.7	50.7–56.4	54.8–61.4
162	59.7–62.4	61.0–65.6	64.2–70.5	152	47.1–52.1	51.1–57.0	55.2–61.9
163	60.0–62.7	61.3–66.0	64.5–71.1	153	47.4–52.5	51.5–57.5	55.6–62.4
164	60.4–63.1	61.7–66.5	64.9–71.8	154	47.8–53.0	51.9–58.0	56.2–63.0
165	60.8–63.5	62.1–67.0	65.3–72.5	155	48.1–53.6	52.2–58.6	56.8–63.6
166	61.1–63.8	62.4–67.6	65.6–73.2	156	48.5–54.1	52.7–59.1	57.3–64.1
167	61.5–64.2	62.8–68.2	66.0–74.0	157	48.8–54.6	53.2–59.6	57.8–64.6
168	61.8–64.6	63.2–68.7	66.4–74.7	158	49.3–55.2	53.8–60.2	58.4–65.3
169	62.2–65.2	63.8–69.3	67.0–75.4	159	49.8–55.7	54.3–60.7	58.9–66.0
170	62.5–65.7	64.3–69.8	67.5–76.1	160	50.3–56.2	54.9–61.2	59.4–66.7
171	62.9–66.2	64.8–70.3	68.0–76.8	161	50.8–56.7	55.4–61.7	59.9–67.4
172	63.2–66.7	65.4–70.8	68.5–77.5	162	51.4–57.3	55.9–62.3	60.5–68.1
173	63.6–67.3	65.9–71.4	69.1–78.2	163	51.9–57.8	56.4–62.8	61.0–68.8
174	63.9–67.8	66.4–71.9	69.6–78.9	164	52.5–58.4	57.0–63.4	61.5–69.5
175	64.3–68.3	66.9–72.4	70.1–79.6	165	53.0–58.9	57.5–63.9	62.0–70.2
176	64.7–68.9	67.5–73.0	70.7–80.3	166	53.6–59.5	58.1–64.5	62.6–70.9
177	65.0–69.5	68.1–73.5	71.3–81.0	167	54.1–60.0	58.7–65.0	63.2–71.7
178	65.4–70.0	68.6–74.0	71.8–81.8	168	54.6–60.5	59.2–65.5	63.7–72.4
179	65.7–70.5	69.2–74.6	72.3–82.5	169	55.2–61.1	59.7–66.1	64.3–73.1
180	66.1–71.0	69.7–75.1	72.8–83.3	170	55.7–61.6	60.2–66.6	64.8–73.8
181	66.6–71.6	70.2–75.8	73.4–84.0	171	56.2–62.1	60.7–67.1	65.3–74.5
182	67.1–72.1	70.7–76.5	73.9–84.7	172	56.8–62.6	61.3–67.6	65.8–75.2
183	67.7–72.7	71.3–77.2	74.5–85.4	173	57.3–63.2	61.8–68.2	66.4–75.9
184	68.2–73.4	71.8–76.9	75.2–86.1	174	57.8–63.7	62.3–68.7	66.9–76.4
185	68.7–74.1	72.4–78.6	75.9–86.8	175	58.3–64.2	62.8–69.2	67.4–76.9
186	69.2–74.8	73.0–79.3	76.6–87.6	176	58.9–64.8	63.4–69.8	68.0–77.5
187	69.8–75.5	73.7–80.0	77.3–88.5	177	59.5–65.4	64.0–70.4	68.5–78.1
188	70.3–76.2	74.4–80.7	78.0–89.4	178	60.0–65.9	64.5–70.9	69.0–78.6
189	70.9–76.9	74.9–81.5	78.7–90.3	179	60.5–66.4	65.1–71.4	69.6–79.1
190	71.4–77.6	75.4–82.2	79.4–91.2	180	61.0–66.9	65.6–71.9	70.1–79.6
191	72.1–78.4	76.1–83.0	80.3–92.1	181	61.6–67.5	66.1–72.5	70.7–80.2
192	72.8–79.1	76.8–83.9	81.2–93.0	182	62.1–68.0	66.6–73.0	71.2–80.7
193	73.5–79.8	77.6–84.8	82.1–93.9	183	62.6–68.5	67.1–73.5	71.7–81.2

*Indoor clothing weighing 2.3 kilograms for men and 1.4 kilograms for women.
†Shoes with 2.5 cm. heels.
Source of basic data: Build Study, 1979, Society of Actuaries and Association of Life Insurance Medical Directors of America, 1980.
Copyright 1983, Metropolitan Life Insurance Company. Reprinted with permission.

APPENDIX L

How to Determine Your Body Frame By Elbow Breadth

To make a simple approximation of your frame size:

Extend your arm and bend the forearm upwards at a 90-degree angle. Keep the fingers straight and turn the inside of your wrist toward the body. Place the thumb and index finger of your other hand on the two prominent bones on either side of your elbow. Measure the space between your fingers against a ruler or a tape measure. (For the most accurate measurement, have your physician measure your elbow breadth with calipers.) Compare this measure with the measurements shown below.

These tables list the elbow measurements for men and women of medium frame at various heights. Measurements lower than those listed indicate that you have a small frame while higher measurements indicate a large frame.

MEN

Height (In 1-inch Heels)	Elbow Breadth (Inches)	Height (In 2.5 cm. Heels)	Elbow Breadth (Centimeters)
5'2"–5'3"	2½"–2⅞"	158–161	6.4–7.2
5'4"–5'7"	2⅝"–2⅞"	162–171	6.7–7.4
5'8"–5'11"	2¾"–3"	172–181	6.9–7.8
6'0"–6'3"	2¾"–3⅛"	182–191	7.1–7.8
6'4"	2⅞"–3¼"	192–193	7.4–8.1

WOMEN

Height (In 1-inch Heels)	Elbow Breadth (Inches)	Height (In 2.5-cm. Heels)	Elbow Breadth (Centimeters)
4'10"–4'11"	2¼"–2½"	148–151	5.6–6.4
5'0"–5'3"	2¼"–2½"	152–161	5.8–6.5
5'4"–5'7"	2⅜"–2⅝"	162–171	5.9–6.6
5'8"–5'11"	2⅜"–2⅝"	172–181	6.1–6.8
6'0"	2½"–2¾"	182–183	6.2–6.9

Source of basic data: Data tape, HANES I—Anthropometry, goniometry, skeletal age, bone density, and cortical thickness, ages 1–74. National Health and Nutrition Examination Survey, 1971–75, National Center for Health Statistics.

Copyright 1983, Metropolitan Life Insurance Company. Reprinted with permission.

CHAPTER 6

WILLIAM L. DONEGAN

Diagnosis

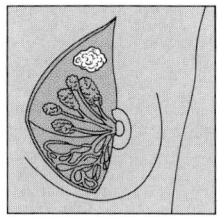

There is only one method of making a definitive diagnosis of breast cancer—histologic examination of tissue. By contrast, there are many techniques for detecting its signs and symptoms. These include medical history, physical examination, mammography, thermography, ultrasonography, and cytologic examination of aspirates and nipple discharge. An accurate diagnosis is fundamental to appropriate staging and treatment.

Most complaints referred to the breasts are not cancer related; benign diseases are far more frequent. In the Breast Clinic of the Medical College of Wisconsin (MCW), cancer ranks low in the overall frequency of diagnoses (Table 6–1), but as it can mimic almost all benign conditions and poses the most important threat to continued well-being, it must always be suspected. The physician must agree with Haagensen (1971, p. 501) that expertise in this field comes with the knowledge that any sign of disease in the breast can be produced by cancer. Its insidiousness and its capacity to spread widely permit the axiom to be carried a step further with the observation that any histologically compatible metastasis in a woman without an obvious source can be generated by occult carcinoma of the breast.

Mammary cancer is primarily a disease of women. Less than 1 per cent of cases occur in men, and it is unusual under the age of 30 years in either sex. In children it is a medical curiosity. Particularly prone are those with a strong family history of the disease, women who are nulliparous or who had a late initial full-term pregnancy, and those who have had a previous biopsy showing atypical hyperplasia. Nevertheless, most cases are not at high risk by the usual standards, and all symptomatic women should be suspect.

The upper outer quadrant of the breast is the most common location for mammary carcinoma. Among 2045 consecutive cases at Ellis Fischel State Cancer Hospital (EFSCH) in which the site of the primary lesion was identified, cancer was located in the upper outer quadrant in 37 per cent (Fig. 6–1). The lower inner quadrant was the least frequently involved (5 per cent of cases), and the upper inner, lower outer, and central areas were intermediate. Twenty per cent of the cancers involved more than one quadrant or were diffuse at the time of diagnosis, and a few could not be allocated to one quadrant or another. The concentration of breast tissue in the upper outer quadrant likely accounts for this particular pattern, as does the slight predominance in the left breast, which averages somewhat larger (Smith et al., 1986). Rarely, carcinomas arise in ectopic mammary tissue along the axillary or abdominal portions of the primitive milk lines (Nicolesco and Velciu, 1968). These cancers serve as a reminder that breast tissue is heir to the same diseases regardless of location (Parikh and Singer, 1983).

A slight but persistent tendency for cancers to occur on the left side has been observed repeatedly, with the difference as great as 11 per cent in some series (Busk and Clemmesen, 1947). At MCW between 1982 and 1987, cancers were located in the left breast in 49 per cent of cases and in the right breast in 47 per cent, with 4 per cent being bilateral and simultaneous.

Signs and Symptoms

The initial signs and symptoms of mammary carcinoma are varied. Table 6–2 lists in order of frequency those reported in 1205 patients (Yorkshire Breast Cancer Group, 1983). More than one may be present at the time of consultation.

125

Table 6–1. BREAST CLINIC CASES, MEDICAL COLLEGE OF WISCONSIN

Fibrocystic disease	197
Fibroadenoma	72
Infections	41
Carcinoma	37
Gynecomastia	16
Lipoma	6
Fat necrosis	5
Duct ectasia	3
Inappropriate lactation	3
Fibrous disease	2
Intraductal papilloma	2
Superficial thrombophlebitis (Mondor's disease)	2
Amastia	2
Polymastia	1

Normal examination, 195; unexplained breast pain, 50; mass, 15; nipple discharge, 23; enlarged axillary node, 4.

Note: Benign diseases far outrank carcinoma as causes of complaints related to the breast.

MASS

By far the most common physical sign of mammary cancer is a mass in the breast (76 per cent of cases). The mass may be tender, but it is more often painless, and in about 73 per cent of cases it is discovered by the patient during bathing or on self-examination. Occasionally a spontaneous sensation of "drawing" or discomfort, or an accidental blow to the breast, leads to its discovery. Husbands sometimes discover such masses. The fact that almost 15 per cent of cancers are painful emphasizes the point that pain or tenderness is no guarantee of innocence. Figure 6–2 diagrams the age distribution of the three most common mass-forming diseases of the breast. In youthful women fibroadenomas predominate, in older ones carcinomas are more prevalent, and between the ages of 25 to 55 years fibrocystic disease is common. Considerable overlap is evident, particularly between ages 35 and 55 years. Thus, a mass in the breast of a woman of any age is suspect until its nature can be established (Fig. 6–3).

NIPPLE DISCHARGE

Nipple discharge is not a frequent complaint or a frequent sign of mammary carcinoma. Only 3 to 5 per cent of consultations (Murad et al., 1982) and only 7.4 per cent of breast operations (Leis et al., 1985) are for discharge. No more than 2 per cent of cancers were associated with discharge in Devitt's series (1985); most that are (80 per cent) also appear as a mass. Only 12 to 20 per cent of cancer-associated discharges are without a mass, and only 10.4 per cent are without a mammographic abnormality (Leis et al., 1985).

Nonspontaneous discharge from multiple ducts of both breasts is generally endocrine- or drug-induced or is symptomatic of diffuse fibrocystic changes. Inappropriate lactation with hyperprolactinemia should suggest the possibility of lactogenic medications, hypothyroidism, or a pituitary tumor (Table 6–3). Appropriate tests for milk and a serum prolactin determination confirm the problem. A careful drug history, determinations of serum TSH,

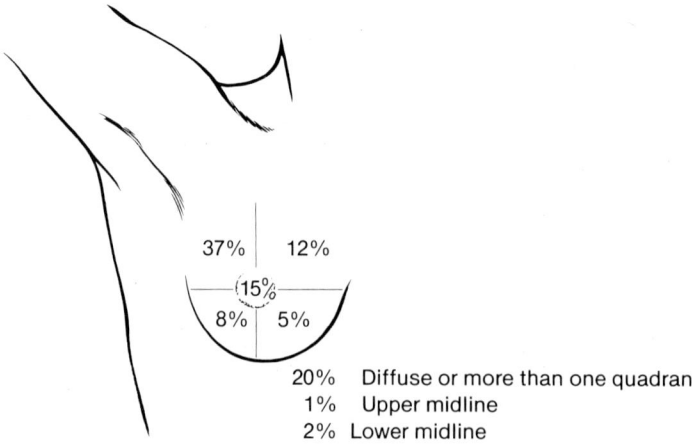

Figure 6–1. The distribution of primary breast carcinoma at Ellis Fischel State Cancer Hospital (EFSCH), 1940 to 196_, in 2045 cases.

Table 6–2. METHOD OF PRESENTATION IN 1205 PATIENTS WITH OPERABLE BREAST CANCER

	Number	Per Cent
Discrete lump	914	76
Swelling	86	8
Pain	58	5
Nipple retraction	43	4
Nipple bleeding, discharge, or crusting	22	2
Skin puckering	15	1
Lump in axilla	15	1
		97

Also bruising, heaviness, tiredness, gallstones, appendicitis, and additional symptoms

From Yorkshire Breast Cancer Group: Symptoms and signs of operable breast cancer, 1976–1981. Br. J. Surg., 70:350, 1983. Reprinted with permission.

T3, and T4, a skull x-ray, and a computed tomographic (CT) scan of the head can all be helpful in evaluating the possibilities. A thin, bloody discharge from both breasts late in pregnancy in the absence of other abnormality is ordinarily of no consequence. It is likely due to epithelial hyperplasia and ceases after parturition (Haagensen, 1971, p. 74).

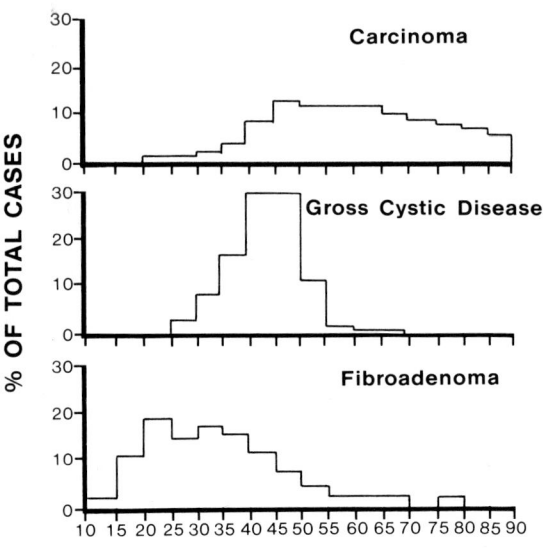

Figure 6–2. The age distributions of the three most common mass-producing breast lesions demonstrate considerable overlap in the 35–55 year age range. Although fibroadenomas predominate in the younger groups, carcinomas in the older ones, and fibrocystic disease during reproductive years, the range for each is wide. (Data on fibroadenoma and gross cystic disease from Haagensen et al., 1981; data on carcinoma from Seidman, 1972.)

Discharges most suggestive of a local lesion, such as cancer, are those that are spontaneous and isolated to one or two ducts of one breast. Persistent discharge is attributable to cancer in 4 to 21 per cent of cases (Murad et al., 1982; Devitt, 1985). In most cases it is due to chronic cystic mestopathy, an intraductal papilloma, or duct ectasia. The characteristics of a discharge cannot be associated invariably with either benign or malignant processes. A thick, grumous material suggests duct ectasia, a milky fluid suggests lactation (the presence of alpha-lactalbumin or lactose proves true milk), and blood suggests duct papilloma. Two thirds of EFSCH patients with mammary carcinoma who reported nipple discharge indicated it was bloody; in the remainder, it was serous or cloudy. In the series of Seltzer and colleagues (1970) bloody discharge was associated with carcinoma about as frequently (25 per cent) as was a serous discharge (21 per cent). Leis and colleagues (1985) found the following types of discharge with cancer: watery, 45.5 per cent; sanguineous, 24 per cent; serosanguineous, 11.9 per cent; and serous, 6.3 per cent.

Both age and the presence of a mass constitute important risk factors. Copeland and Higgins (1960) pointed out that a serosanguineous or bloody discharge was most often benign in patients less than 50 years old and most often attributable to cancer in those older than 50 years. Approximately 12 per cent of Seltzer and associates' patients with discharges but without a mass had cancer, but over the age of 60 years the figure rose to 32 per cent. Among those with a palpable mass the incidence of carcinoma was 31 per cent; beyond the age of 60 years, 65 per cent of patients with both a discharge and a mass had carcinoma. When discharge was not associated with a mass, Chaudary and colleagues (1982) found cancer in 5.9 per cent of cases, and in all instances of cancer the discharge was hemoglobin positive, if not frankly bloody, emphasizing the importance of this test when a mass is not present. Cancer was found in 8 per cent of patients with discharges in the absence of a mass and with a normal mammogram in their small series (Chaudary et al., 1982). In over half of the cases of persistent discharge unassociated with a mass, the source can be localized by palpation (Fig. 6–4). Injection of radiographic contrast material into the duct (galactography) will often demonstrate a filling defect in the duct (Fig. 6–5).

As summarized by Devitt, nipple discharge

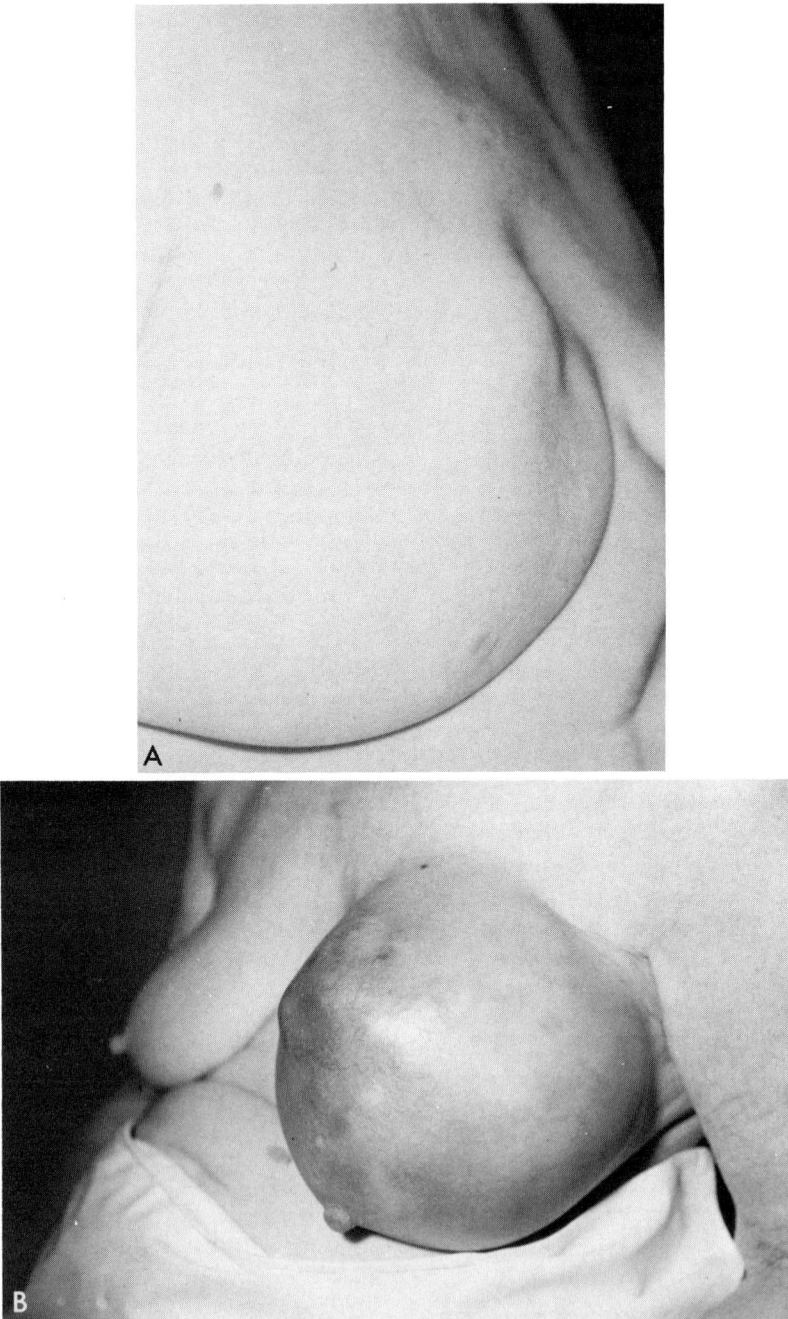

Figure 6–3. A palpable, and sometimes visible, mass is the most frequent presenting sign of mammary carcinoma (*A*). The frequency of metastasis increases progressively with size, emphasizing the importance of prompt detection, but some less frequent histologic types, such as mucinous carcinoma (*B*), may reach impressive size without metastasizing or becoming incurable.

Table 6–3. CAUSES OF CHRONIC HYPERPROLACTINEMIA WITH INAPPROPRIATE LACTATION

Mechanisms	Causes		Diagnosis
Physiologic	Excessive breast manipulation		Discontinue stimulation
Pharmacologic	Category	Brand or Generic Names	Discontinue medication if appropriate
	reserpine, methyldopa	Aldomet	
	chronic opiate use	Morphine, methadone, heroin	
	phenothiazines, chlorpromazine	Thorazine	
	perphenazine	Trilafon	
	thioridazine	Mellaril	
	prochlorperazine	Compazine, Chlorazine	
	fluphenazine	Permitil, Prolixin	
	trifluoperazine	Stelazine	
	thioxanthenes	Taractan	
	butyrophenones	Haldol	
	pimozide	Orap	
	metoclopramide	Reglan	
	dibenzoxazepine antidepressants	Amoxapine (Asendin)	
	cimetidine	Tagamet	
	tricyclic antidepressants	Imipramine, desipramine (Norpramin, Pertofran), amitriptyline, nortriptyline (Aventyl, Pamelor)	
	papaverine derivatives	Verapamil (Calan, Isoptin)	
Pathologic	Primary hypothyroidism		Thyroid function tests
	Hypothalamic disorders, e.g., neoplastic, infectious, vascular, degenerative or granulomatous		
	Pseudocyesis		Pregnancy test
	Pituitary stalk section		History
	Prolactin-secreting adenoma of pituitary		Serum prolactin; CT scan
	Acromegaly		Growth hormone; CT scan
	Cushing's disease		Urinary cortisol; dexamethasone suppression test
	Ectopic production of prolactin (bronchogenic carcinoma, hypernephroma)		Chest x-ray; CT scans
	Chronic renal failure (decreased prolactin clearance)		Renal function tests
	Chest wall lesions, e.g., surgical scars, neoplasms, herpes zoster		Physical examination
Functional	Undiagnosed cases		

Modified from Adashi, E. Y.: Diagnostic evaluation of hyperprolactinemia. Resident & Staff Physician, 31:16PC, 1985. Reprinted with permission.

is not commonly associated with carcinoma, but when it is, it will almost always be accompanied by a palpable mass. When carcinoma is present but not palpable, it will almost always be in an early form (i.e., intraductal, papillary, or lobular carcinoma in situ).

SKIN RETRACTION

Dimpling or retraction of the skin by cancer is produced by shortening of Cooper's ligaments associated with infiltration of cancer. Athough this was once considered virtually diagnostic of mammary cancer (Fig. 6–6), it is now appreciated that some benign lesions can produce this change, notably fat necrosis and plasma cell mastitis. Mondor's disease, originally described by Fiessinger and Mathieu in 1922 and definitively by Mondor in 1939, can also cause retraction of the skin and mimic cancer. Mondor's disease is due to superficial thrombophlebitis of the thoracoepigastric vein. This condi-

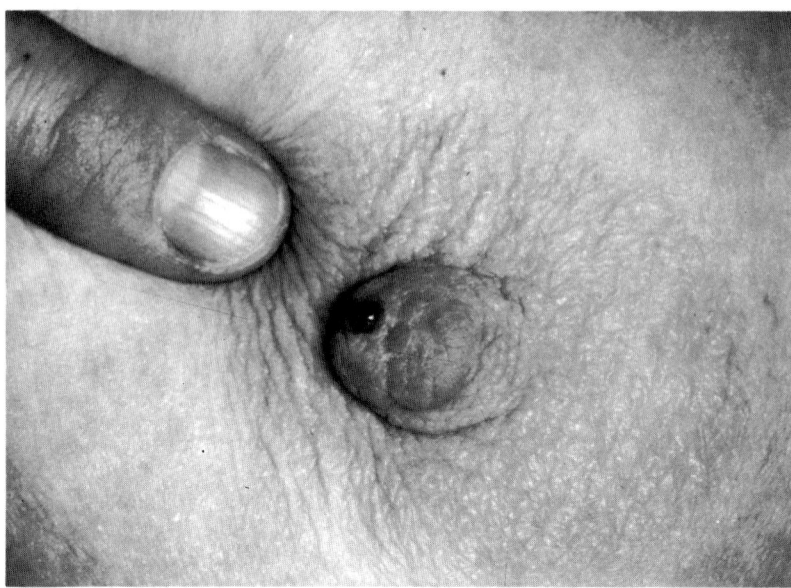

Figure 6–4. Serosanguineous discharge expressed with point pressure from a nonlactating breast. Note that the location of the discharging duct on the nipple corresponds to the involved quadrant of the breast. Palpation with one finger in this manner can localize the diseased duct in the absence of a mass.

tion occurs spontaneously in pendulous breasts or after minor breast operations. It appears as a painful groove in the skin or as a subcutaneous cord on the breast, in the axilla, or on the anterior chest wall, mimicking lymphatic permeation from an occult mammary carcinoma. Histopathologic examination usually demonstrates a sclerosing endophlebitis, but arteries and lymphatics may also be involved (Hatteland and Kluge, 1965). The process is self-limiting and requires only symptomatic treatment. Although the clinical picture is usually diagnostic, a biopsy will resolve the issue when doubt exists.

SKIN CHANGES

Attachment to the overlying dermis with alteration of the normal contour of the breast is sometimes the only visible change produced by carcinoma. Deviation of the affected breast or straightening of its normally curved contour (edge sign) disrupts the two breasts' normal symmetry (Fig. 6–7A). Direct infiltration of the skin may appear as a firm cutaneous plaque. Prominent veins may mark the involved breast (Fig. 6–7B). In advanced cases, marked retraction of the entire breast results (Fig. 6–8), satellite nodules appear (Fig. 6–9), or the skin becomes ulcerated (Fig. 6–10).

AXILLARY ADENOPATHY

As early as 1907, Halsted pointed out that enlarged axillary lymph nodes could be the only sign of occult mammary carcinoma. One per cent or less of all cases first become manifest in this fashion. The Yorkshire Breast

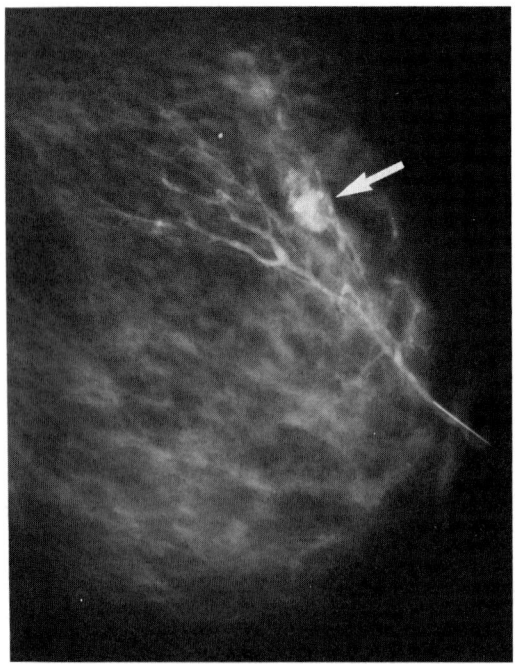

Figure 6–5. A galactogram on a patient with bloody nipple discharge demonstrates an upper ductal system in which a cystic structure (arrow) with a filling defect is seen, representing a papilloma. An injection of the offending duct immediately prior to biopsy with a vital dye (Evans blue) is useful for identifying the tissues to be removed.

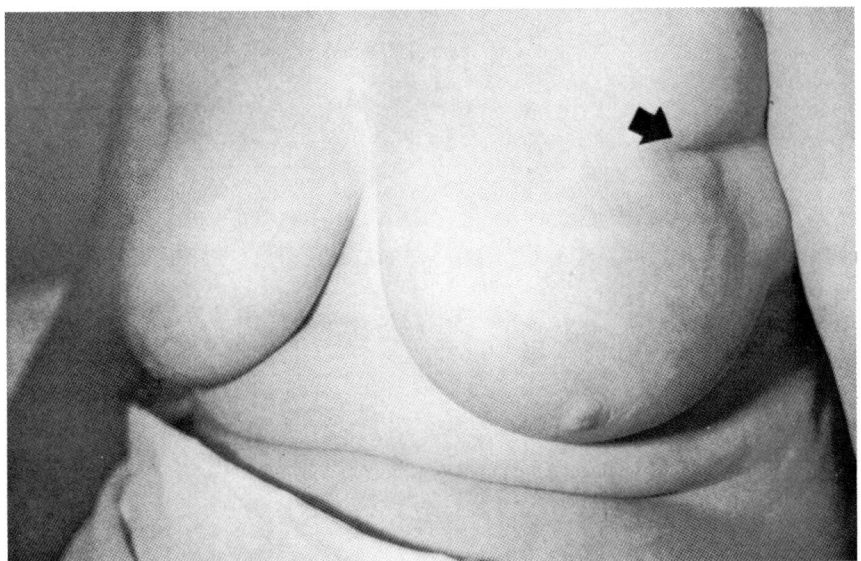

Figure 6–6. Skin dimpling caused by attachment of an underlying carcinoma.

Cancer Group (1983) documented 15 such cases among 1205. Pierce and associates (1957) reviewed 222 biopsies of isolated clinically enlarged axillary lymph nodes and found that 6.9 per cent, or 1 in 14 cases, contained adenocarcinoma.

The list of possible origins for metastatic adenocarcinoma is long and includes liver, lung, ovary, kidney, stomach, pancreas, colon, and breast. When a primary cancer of the gastrointestinal tract or lung can be excluded with appropriate examinations, the ipsilateral breast becomes the most likely source (Copeland and McBride, 1973) (Table 6–4). Estrogen receptors and electron microscopic examination can be helpful (High and Watne, 1985). In the course of evaluation, a mammogram of the breast will reveal an occult primary tumor in 12 to 50 per cent of cases (Ashikari et al., 1976).

If a primary tumor is not found, women with metastatic adenocarcinoma in axillary lymph nodes treated with an ipsilateral mastectomy and axillary dissection are found to have breast cancers in two thirds of the resected breasts, most often in the upper outer quadrant, and the cancers usually prove to be small or minimal (Feuerman et al., 1962; Westbrook and Gallager, 1971; Ashikari et al., 1976). Failure to find a primary tumor does not exclude the breast as the source, as a lesion can be missed by the most industrious pathologist. The survival of individuals with occult carcinoma of the breast who have axillary metastases is consistently more favorable than that of patients with metastases from palpable primaries. Forty-three patients followed by Kaplan and Reinstine (1954) survived an average of 4.8 years. In a small series (29 cases), Patel and coworkers (1981) found survival related to the number of involved axillary nodes. Furthermore, those in whom a primary tumor was not found survived as well as those in whom it was found. Because in many cases a primary tumor will not be found, hormone receptors should be obtained on axillary metastases at the initial biopsy. Rather than performing a mastectomy, Vilcoq and colleagues at the Institute Curie, Paris, treated 11 women with axillary metastases and no clinical or mammographic evidence of a primary breast cancer with primary irradiation to the breast, axillary nodes, and supraclavicular lymph nodes. The doses were between 5000 and 6000 rads. Ten of the 11 patients were alive and free of disease after 5 years. Only three patients with a minimum follow-up of 5 years (27 per cent) had local recurrence in the retained breast and these patients, it was pointed out, could be treated with salvage mastectomy (Vilcoq et al., 1982). Kemeny et al. (1986) found no significant difference in the survival of 11 patients treated with mastectomy and seven patients treated without mastectomy (57% at 5 years), and also concluded that mastectomy was unnecessary for patients with adenocarcinoma in axillary

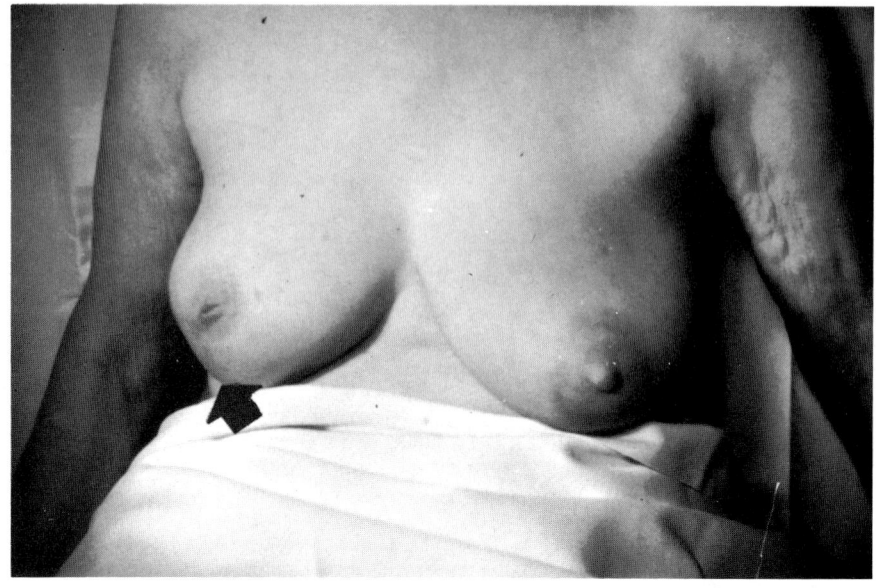

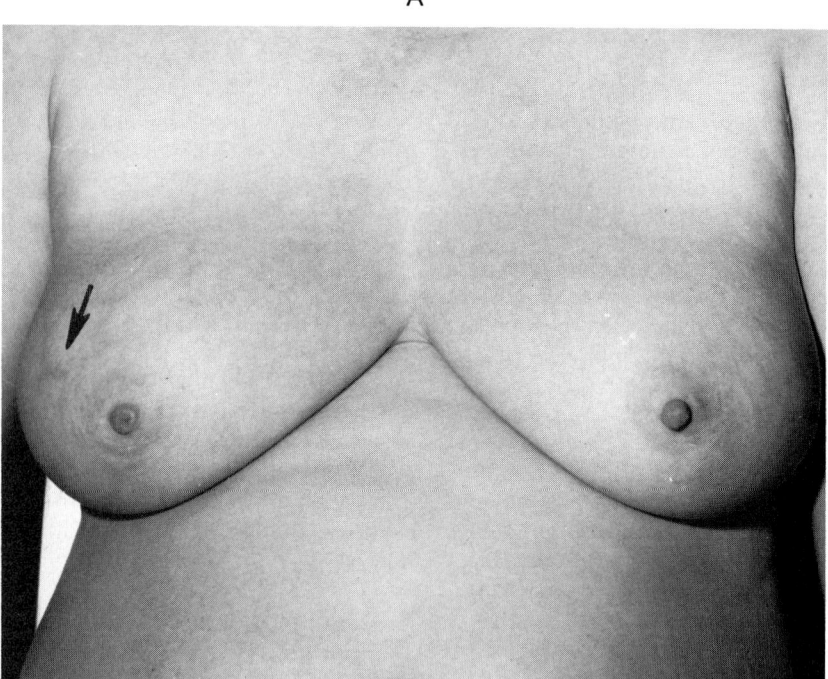

Figure 6–7. *A*, A carcinoma of the right breast producing nipple inversion and a flattened contour. *B*, Prominent veins associated with a carcinoma within the right breast.

nodes and no apparent primary tumor. Axillary dissection and irradiation or chemotherapy were effective treatment.

In the presence of a clinically normal breast and a normal mammogram, such conservative therapy deserves consideration as an alternative to mastectomy.

INFLAMMATORY CARCINOMA

Redness, heat, tenderness, and edema of the skin are the hallmarks of "inflammatory" carcinoma (Fig. 6–11). This dramatic variant so closely mimics an acute infection that the unwary physician may be led into prolonged

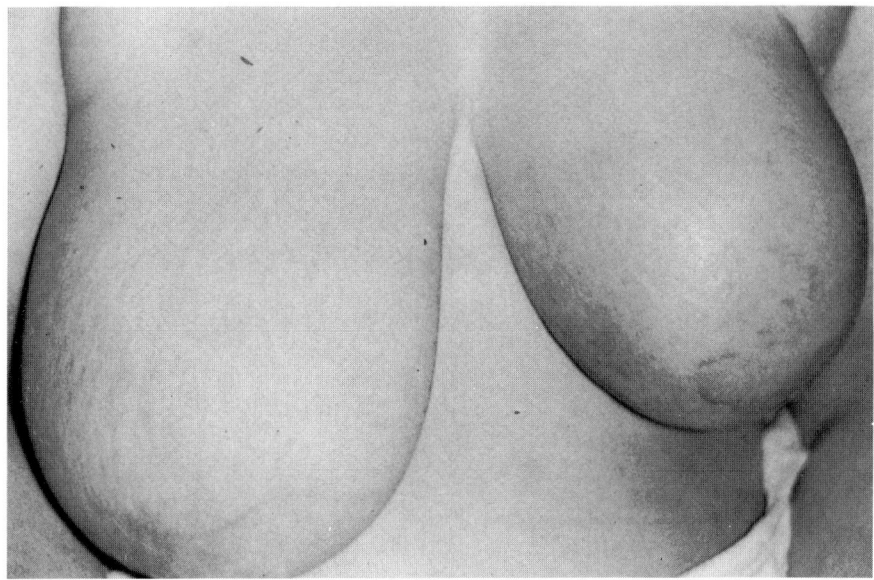

Figure 6–8. Marked retraction of the left breast caused by a large neglected carcinoma.

treatment with antibiotics or an incision and drainage with the mistaken diagnosis of breast abscess. Incision and drainage or antibiotics constituted the initial therapy of 10.5 per cent of 38 consecutive inflammatory carcinomas referred to EFSCH. As early as 1814, the gravity of these signs was recognized by Bell, and a classic report on the subject by Lee and Tannenbaum in 1924 is responsible for establishing the lesion as a clinical entity.

The characteristic signs may initiate the disease (primary inflammatory carcinoma) or may appear later in its course (secondary inflammatory carcinoma), but the latter is less frequent. Both carry the same grave prognosis. Fortunately, inflammatory carcinoma constitutes barely 1.5 to 4 per cent of all cases (Taylor and Meltzer, 1938; Donnelly, 1948; Barber et al., 1961; Richards and Lewison, 1961; Byrd and Stephenson, 1962; Wang and

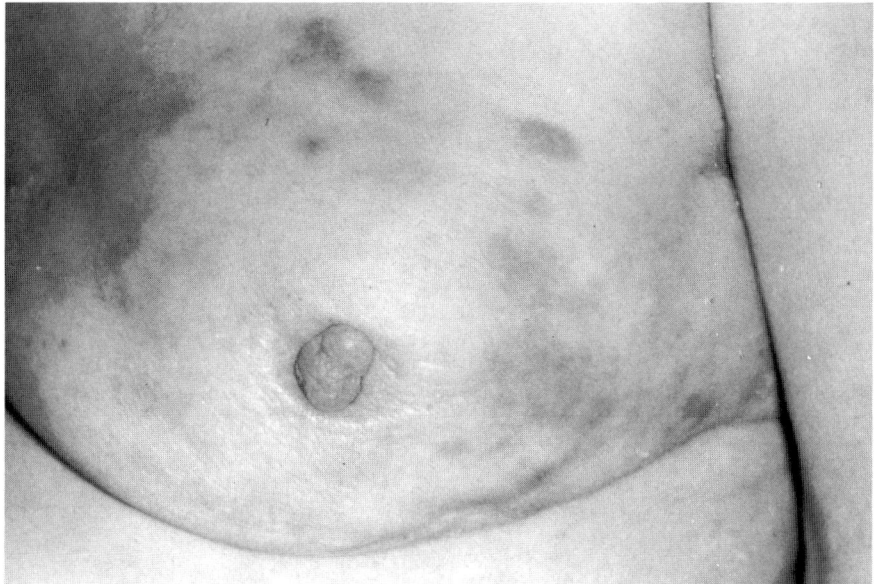

Figure 6–9. Multiple pink satellite nodules in the skin around a locally advanced mammary carcinoma.

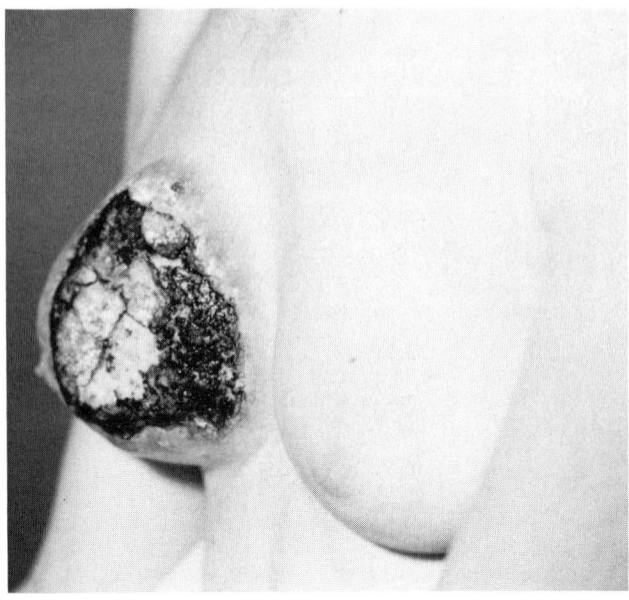

Figure 6–10. Ulceration of the skin in a young woman with locally advanced carcinoma of the right breast. A black, malodorous inflammatory membrane occupies most of the ulcer base.

Griscom, 1964). Only 38 were diagnosed at EFSCH during 18 years. An alleged association with pregnancy and lactation has not been substantiated, but patients do tend to be younger than average.

Inflammatory carcinoma runs a rapid course. The duration of symptoms averages 4 to 6 months. A tumor mass may be noticed first, followed rapidly by enlargement of the breast, swelling, and redness; alternatively, swelling may be the first sign. On examination, generalized induration rather than a discrete tumor is present; ulceration is not common except in very advanced cases. Pain and increased local heat are evident, but systemic signs of infection are infrequent. Only 21 per cent of EFSCH patients with inflammatory carcinoma had a white blood count over 10,000, the highest being 13,900, and fever was observed in only two cases. Metastasis to axillary lymph nodes is early and massive, and patients often have distant dissemination at the time of presentation. Seventy-nine per cent of EFSCH patients had clinically involved axillary lymph nodes, 47 per cent had involved supraclavicular nodes, and 13 per cent had evidence of distant metastases at the initial visit.

The neoplasm has no unique histopathologic characteristics other than permeation of dermal lymphatics, originally described by Bryant in 1889. There is support for dermal lymphatic invasion as a necessary diagnostic feature of inflammatory carcinoma, but it is not always found in clinically typical cases (Manual for Staging of Cancer, 1983; Ellis and Teitelbaum, 1974). Ten of 16 patients with inflammatory carcinoma who had skin biopsies at EFSCH showed this. The fact that this histologic feature can be seen in the absence of the characteristic clinical picture led Saltzstein (1974) to suggest the concept of "occult inflammatory carcinoma." Lucas and Perez-Mesa (1978) divided cases into those with clinical signs only, those without clinical signs but with dermal lymphatic invasion, and those with both. All three groups had an equally poor prognosis. The absence of a palpable mass, the presence of involved axillary nodes, and age less than 50 years are each associated with especially

Table 6–4. AXILLARY METASTASES FROM OCCULT CANCER

Primary determined:	
Breast	19 (32%)
Stomach	2
Lung	1
Pharynx	1
Hodgkin's disease	1
Rhabdomyosarcoma	1
Fibrosarcoma	1
Neurogenic sarcoma	1
Dead, primary not determined:	24
Still surviving without disease:	9

Note: In the absence of an obvious primary site, the breast remains the most likely source for adenocarcinoma in axillary lymph nodes of women.

From Copeland, E. M., and McBride, C. M.: Axillary metastases from unknown primary sites. Ann Surg., 178:25, 1973. Reprinted with permission.

poor survival. The deceptive nature of this neoplasm provides the rationale for biopsying any persistent "mastitis." A biopsy of the skin is necessary to demonstrate dermal lymphatic invasion.

NIPPLE CHANGES

Breasts removed for cancer often show extension of tumor to the nipple histologically (Smith et al., 1976). Lagios and colleagues (1979) found nipple involvement in 30 per cent of mastectomy specimens. Such involvement was particularly likely if primary tumors were within 2.5 cm of the nipple or were larger than 2.0 cm in diameter. As clinical signs are absent in 50 per cent of cases with nipple involvement, the former practice of removing the apparently normal nipple before mastectomy and "banking" it for reconstructive purposes has been abandoned. From the clinical standpoint, two nipple changes are notable—retraction and Paget's disease. Inversion of the nipple is often a normal condition, but when cancer is responsible the nipple is fixed and cannot be everted as is otherwise usually possible. On closer examination, an underlying mass may be felt (Fig. 6–12).

The gross changes known as Paget's disease were first accurately described and associated with carcinoma of the breast by Sir James Paget in 1874. This lesion represents intraepithelial progression of carcinoma from a primary tumor within the breast through proximal ducts to the surface of the nipple (Jacobacus, 1904). Resembling a benign dermatitis of the nipple, and not always associated with a mass, it is sometimes treated by the unwary for prolonged periods with topical medications. The lesion can take on a variety of appearances, from moist and eczematoid to dry and psoriatic, or it may appear as a red granular erosion (Fig. 6–13). Symptoms include itching, burning, and a sensation of sticking in the involved area.

As spread of Paget's disease is centrifugal from ductal orifices on the nipple, it is evident that lesions confined to the nipple or to the nipple, areola, and even the surrounding skin can be Paget's disease. Extramammary Paget's disease can appear on the skin in wide distribution wherever aprocine glands are found, primarily in the anogenital and axillary areas but also in the ear canals and on the eyelids (Helwig and Graham, 1963; Kawatsu and Miki, 1971). It has also involved the epidermis superficial to cutaneous metastases of breast cancer (Greenwood and Minkowitz, 1971).

The microscopic features of Paget's disease

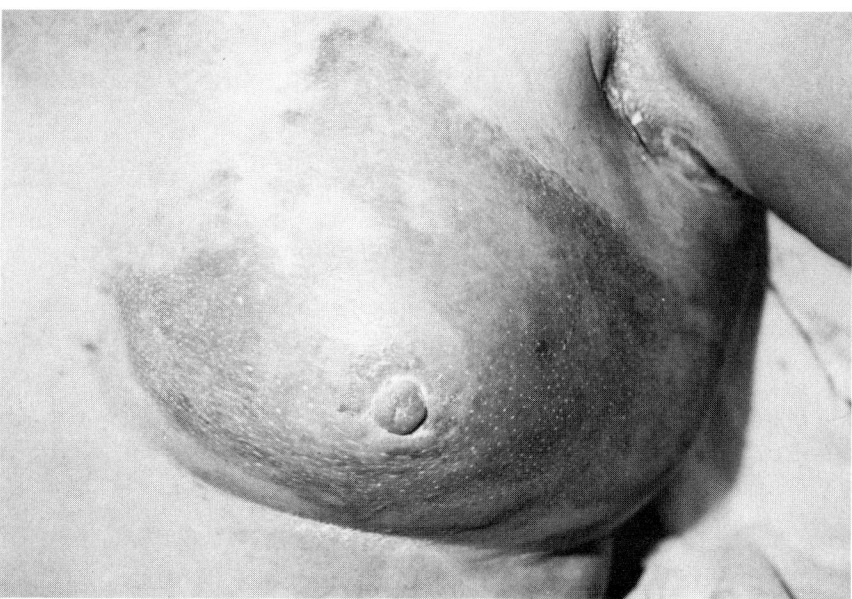

Figure 6–11. An inflammatory carcinoma of the breast demonstrating erythema and edema of the dermis with a peau d'orange appearance. Invasion of dermal lymphatics is a histologic hallmark of this lesion and the prognosis is poor.

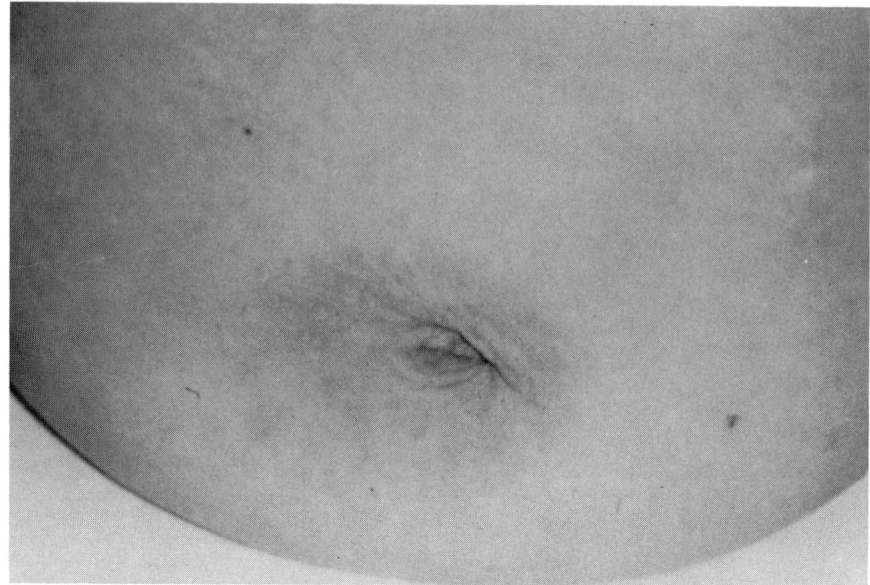

Figure 6–12. Nipple retraction is the only outward sign of this large carcinoma in the adjacent portion of the breast.

can be present with or without a detectable skin change. In only one of seven mastectomies with histologic Paget's disease examined by Lagios and colleagues (1979) was a clinical change recognized on the nipple. The histologic picture consists of large cells with pale cytoplasm and large nuclei (Paget's cells) within the epidermis (Fig. 6–14). These migrating cancer cells were described not by Paget but by Darrier in 1889. They almost always signal the presence of additional invasive or in situ carcinoma within the breast.

The characteristic lesion may exist with or without a palpable tumor mass in the breast. The prognosis of a patient without a mass is better than that of a patient who has a mass (Salvadori et al., 1976). At EFSCH, six patients without a mass had a 5-year survival rate of 83 per cent after radical mastectomy, as opposed to a 5-year survival of 33 per cent for 12 patients with a mass. The superior survival rate was attributable to a low incidence of involved axillary nodes and a high proportion of nonaggressive histologic types.

In summary, a biopsy of the involved nipple is indicated when Paget's disease is suspected or when any benign appearing lesion of the nipple, persistent itching, or discomfort does not resolve after a brief trial of local therapy. A biopsy diagnosis of Paget's disease is proof of mammary cancer and an indication for effective cancer therapy.

The Physical Examination

Careful physical examination has a time-honored role in evaluation of breast disease, and it remains indispensable for the detection and clinical staging of mammary carcinoma. The majority of breast cancers are still discovered in this way by physicians or patients themselves. A survey of 12,315 breast cancers by the American College of Surgeons showed that 73 per cent were found by the patient, 23 per cent by physician examination, and 4 per cent by mammography (Nemoto et al., 1982).

Approximately 70 per cent of all breast cancers are palpable and almost 50 per cent of tumors measuring 0.6 to 1.0 cm in diameter are detectable on clinical examination (Wolfe, 1974). Detectability increases with mass size and with time spent in the examination (Fletcher et al., 1985). Technologic advances have produced no substitutes for the information that is gained through palpation. The technique is not a self-evident one; both careful training and experience contribute to a skilled examination (Hall et al., 1977). The knowledge that the prognosis for cure correlates inversely with tumor size is an incentive for a careful examination. For routine examination of premenopausal women, 1 week after onset of the last menstrual period is best;

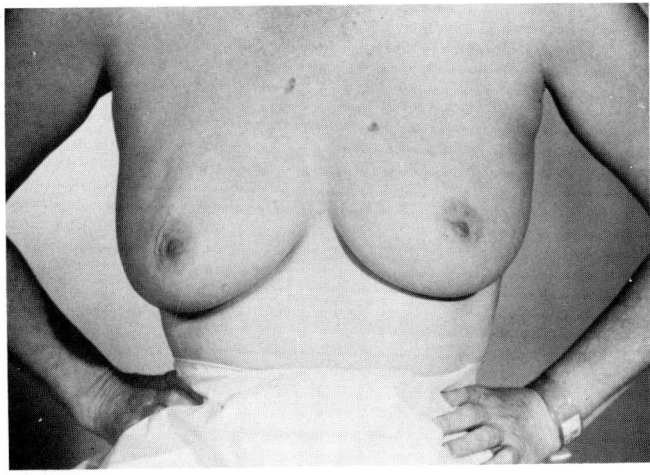

Figure 6–18. Inspection with the patient's hands pressed against her hips fixes the pectoralis major muscle and its fascia. Attachment to the skin and fascia produces skin retraction or deviation of the breast during this maneuver. Slight skin retraction evident on the right breast of this patient was due to cancer.

more, particular attention can be paid to this area during the examination.

Examination of the regional lymph nodes is performed most advantageously with the patient seated and precedes palpation of the breast. Regional nodes that lend themselves to examination are the axillary, infraclavicular, and supraclavicular groups. The axillary group is a primary site for regional metastases from carcinoma, whereas the supraclavicular nodes are involved secondarily. The infraclavicular nodes are actually apical axillary nodes that can be felt deep to the muscle in the deltopectoral triangle when they are enlarged. The coracoid process can be felt in this area and should not be mistaken for adenopathy. The internal mammary nodes are also primary recipients of lymphatic drainage, but normally they cannot be felt, as they are located within the bony thorax along the sternal margin between the pleura and the intercostal muscles.

After examination of the supraclavicular and infraclavicular nodes, which may be done from in front of or behind the patient (Figs. 6–19 and 6–20), the patient is positioned for examination of the axilla with her arms at her side, a position that relaxes the axillary fascia. To examine the left axilla, the physician's left hand steadies the shoulder to keep it from rising while the right hand examines (Fig. 6–21). Slight inward pressure with the heel of the left hand tends to keep nodes centralized in the axilla. The fingers of the right hand are cupped slightly and inserted high into the axilla before approximating them to the chest wall. By this means, nodes are trapped rather than pushed away. As the fingers then move inferiorly along the chest wall, nodes can be felt to escape, characteristically "popping" from under the fingers. The right axilla is examined in similar fashion, reversing the position of the hands. The size, number, consistency, and

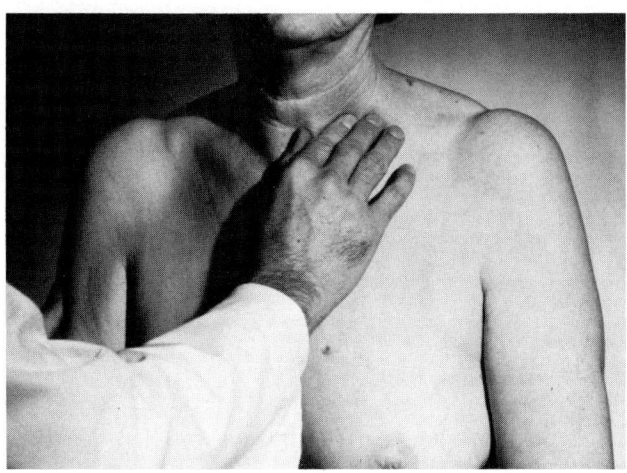

Figure 6–19. Palpation of supraclavicular nodes while the patient is seated. Attention is also given to the prescalene nodes located behind the lower end of the sternocleidomastoid muscle.

quiries are made concerning the presence of discomfort or pain in the breasts, masses, swelling, heaviness, skin changes, or nipple discharge. Of additional importance are the nature and results of previous operations, mammograms, or aspirations, the use of oral contraceptives or estrogens for replacement therapy, and the date of the last menstrual period (onset). Inquiries should be made about the patient's practice of breast self-examination and the presence of mammary cancers in members of the patient's family. Of epidemiologic significance are inquiries about the patient's age at menarche, the number of pregnancies, parity, and age at first childbirth. It is important to have information regarding the patient's menopausal status. If she is postmenopausal, whether artificially or naturally, the age at menopause should be recorded. Sometimes it cannot be determined from the patient's history whether a previous pelvic operation or hysterectomy included complete castration or not; proper treatment may require further pursuit of this information.

INSPECTION

The breasts are inspected in a good light with the patient seated facing the examiner (Fig. 6–16). They should have smooth outlines and be generally symmetric and of approximately the same size, although it is not unusual for

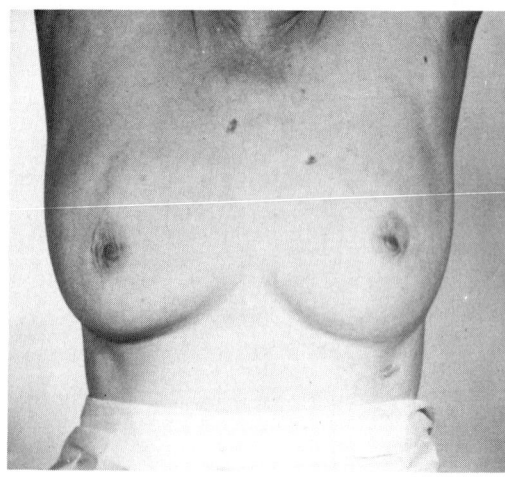

Figure 6–17. The breasts are inspected with the patient's arms extended above her head. This maneuver will sometimes elicit retraction of the skin when it is not otherwise evident.

one breast to be noticeably larger. A particularly small breast can be a sign of Poland's syndrome, in which the sternal head of the pectoralis major muscle is also missing; in severe cases the arm and hand are deformed. Accessory breasts or nipples should be noted. The presence of erythema, ulceration, edema, or skin nodules is noteworthy. The nipples should have similar directionality (normally slightly outward) and should be inspected for inversion or signs of Paget's disease. An increased venous pattern may be associated with mammary cancer, and dimpling, retraction, or localized flattening of the skin can be a sign of trouble. The presence and location of scars are noted.

Inspection should be performed first with the patient's arms at her side and then with them extended above her head (Fig. 6–17). The patient is directed next to place her hands on her hips and press inward on them. These positions serve to elicit retraction of the skin in the vicinity of a carcinoma as the position of the breast changes between the skin and the pectoral muscles (Fig. 6–18).

PALPATION

If the patient seeks consultation because of a lump, it is helpful at the outset to have her locate and demonstrate it. Feeling the site, the physician can often appreciate immediately whether her concern is well founded; further-

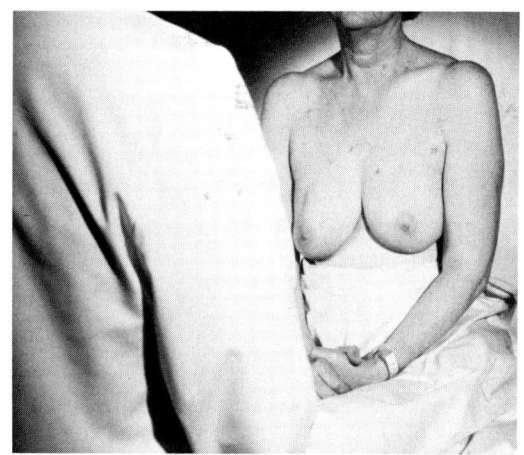

Figure 6–16. The breasts are inspected with the patient seated and facing the examiner. In this particular case the right breast is lower than the left and a carcinoma in the upper outer quadrant dimples the overlying skin. Asymmetry, changes in the nipple or skin, and prominent veins are other signs that may be due to cancer.

conducted a study in which four experienced surgeons examined 100 patients, 41 of whom were admitted to a hospital for biopsy of breast lesions, and 59 other inpatients, none of whom had known breast disease. Fifteen of the former (37 per cent) proved to have cancer on subsequent biopsy. Based on physical examinations, the opinion that an abnormality was present varied from 37 to 74 per cent; that a mass was present varied from 32 to 42 per cent; and that a malignancy was present varied from 13 to 19 per cent. A biopsy was recommended for 28 to 39 per cent of patients. The examiners correctly recommended biopsies for 80 to 93 per cent of the 15 cancers but also for 50 to 77 per cent of the benign lesions. (In only 16 per cent of cases did all four surgeons agree about the presence of a mass.) The surgeons' judgments that a mass was malignant varied in accuracy from 53 to 69 per cent. Most observer variation arose from difference in opinion about patients who did not have cancer. In this study no recommendation for bi-

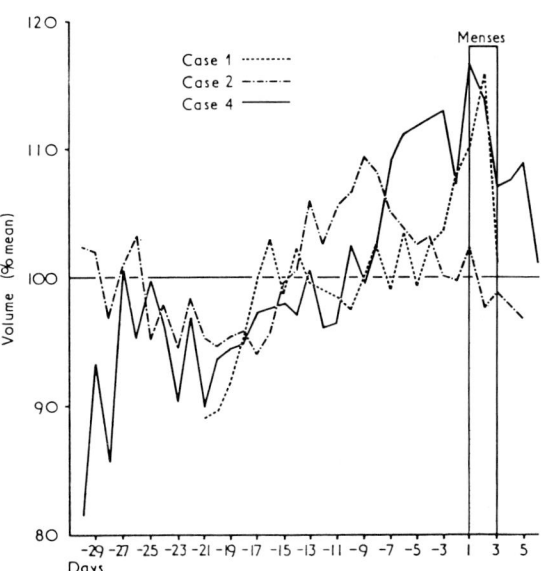

Figure 6–15. Volumetric measurements of the breasts of three premenopausal women during a complete menstrual cycle show that breast volume is least approximately 21 days before onset of the next menses, and therefore approximately 7 days after onset of the menstrual flow. Volume changes in all normal cycles were expressed as percentages of mean volume for each cycle and plotted backward from the first day of menses. (From Milligan, D., et al.: Changes in breast volume during normal menstrual cycle and after oral contraceptives. Br. Med. J., 29:494, 1975. Reprinted with permission.)

opsy would have been made for 7 to 20 per cent of cancers that presented as physical abnormalities. It is because of this hazard, as well as the limitations of other complementary examinations, such as mammography, that biopsy should be considered for any persistent mass or other unexplained abnormality of the breast.

The addition of mammography to the physical examination increases the accuracy of evaluation to over 90 per cent, as does the combination of palpation with fine needle aspiration and cytologic examination (Rimsten et al., 1975; Lewis et al., 1976). At present 40 per cent of cancers found in screening clinics are not detectable at all on physical examination (Baker, 1982).

A proper examination includes a medical history followed by inspection and palpation of the breast and regional lymph nodes.

MEDICAL HISTORY

The medical history is directed toward eliciting suggestive symptoms and evaluating risk. In-

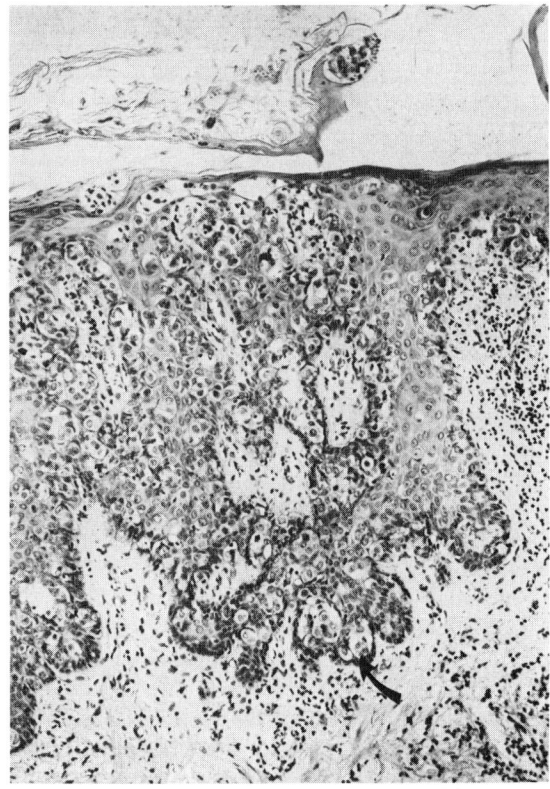

Figure 6–14. Paget's disease of the breast in a histologic section. Characteristic large cells with clear cytoplasm (Paget cells) representing intraepithelial carcinoma replace and distort the epidermis of the nipple.

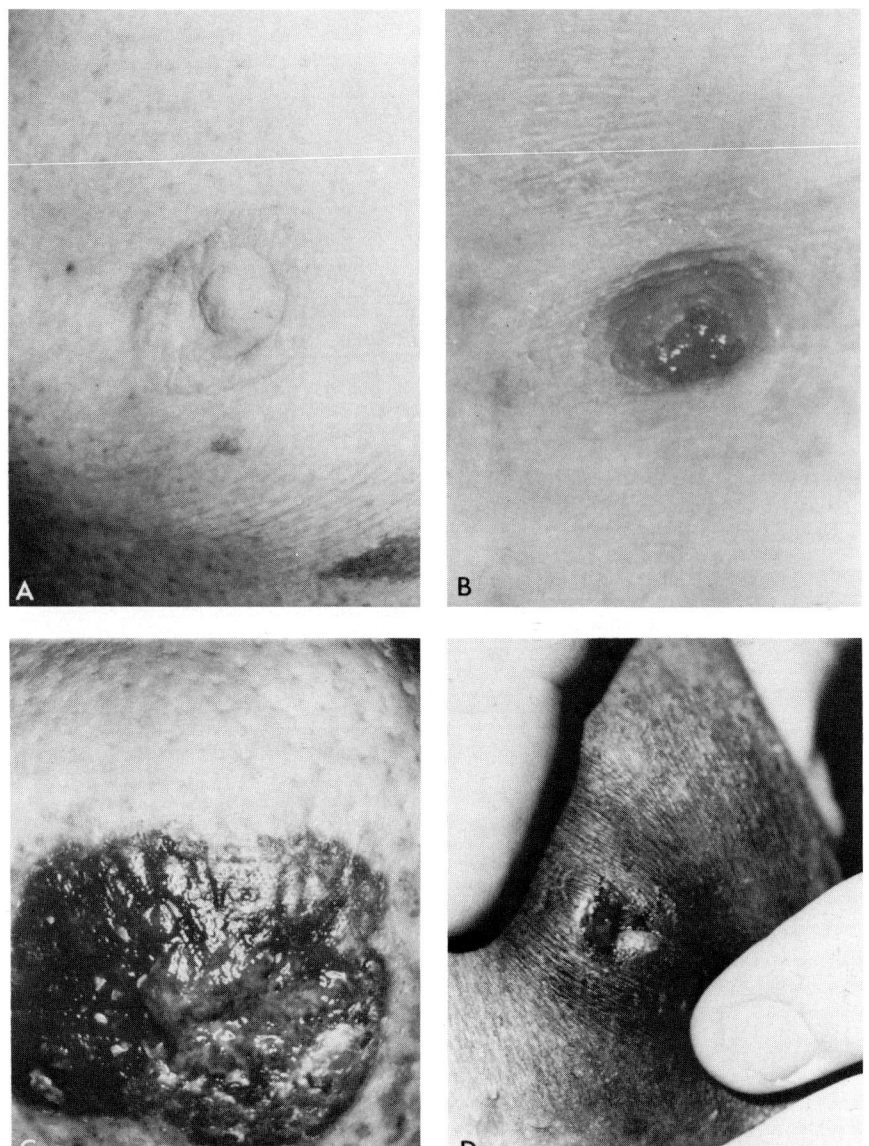

Figure 6–13. Four cases of Paget's disease illustrate its clinical variations. *A*, The nipple is thickened, but the epithelium is intact and the appearance mimics a chronic eczema. *B*, A small moist area of granulation is confined to the papilla of the nipple. *C*, Paget's disease destroys the entire nipple-areolar complex and is associated with edema of the surrounding skin. *D*, Minimal changes produced only a spot of moisture and were largely hidden within an inverted nipple.

engorgement of the breast is then minimal and masses will be most evident (Fig. 6–15).

Attention to the breasts should be a part of every physical examination. A conscientious effort in this regard, accompanied by monthly self-examinations by an enlightened female population, will help to optimize the yield of early cancers.

The opinion of an experienced examiner that a mass does or does not represent cancer is usually correct (Rimsten et al., 1975). The opinion that it definitely represents cancer is correct in 70 to 90 per cent of cases, and that it is benign is correct in 90 per cent of cases. The accuracy is not always this high, however, and variation is considerable. The initial experience in our own screening clinic was that only 37 per cent of breast abnormalities judged "suspicious" enough to biopsy were cancer (see Fig. 6–27). Boyd and coworkers (1981)

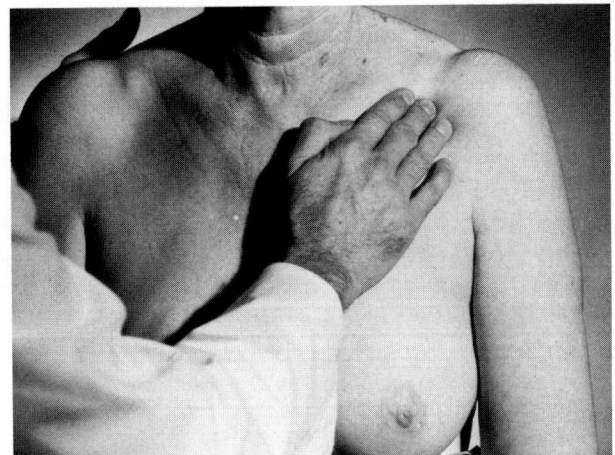

Figure 6–20. An attempt is made to detect enlargement of infraclavicular nodes located in the deltopectoral groove. These are, in fact, apical axillary nodes. A prominent coracoid process should not be mistaken for adenopathy.

fixation of nodes to the skin or deep fascia are noted, as is tenderness or lack of it. The axillae of obese patients as well as the supraclavicular areas may contain a soft fat pad that obscures lymph nodes. The former should not be mistaken for adenopathy, but sometimes nodes can be felt within it.

It is least informative and can be misleading to palpate the breast in the upright position when it is pendulous and folded on itself. More accurate information is obtained with the patient in a supine position and the side to be examined elevated slightly with a pad or pillow. In this position, the breast is flattened and thinned on the chest wall. The entire breast should be gently and thoroughly examined with the flats of the fingertips, remembering to include the tail of Spence, which extends toward the axilla. The upper outer quadrant demands particular attention because it is here that most carcinomas arise. This is facilitated by examining each breast while standing at the opposite side of the table. As an aid to thoroughness the examiner may conceptualize the breast as a wheel and palpate each spoke in turn from the hub to the periphery; others visualize a pinwheel and, beginning at the center, palpate in circles of increasing size. Breast tissue can extend to the clavicle, to the midline of the sternum, into the epigastrium, laterally into the axilla, and to the posterior axillary line (Hicken, 1940). These are the boundaries of the examination.

During the examination, it is advantageous to have the patient's arm abducted with her hand comfortably behind her head (Fig. 6–22). The subareolar area is frequently softer and more compressible than the remainder of the breast, occasionally causing the ridge of normal breast tissue at its rim to be mistaken for a mass. The same is true for the ridge of firm breast tissue near the inframammary fold, which is often evident to a greater or lesser extent in both breasts. A true mass, however,

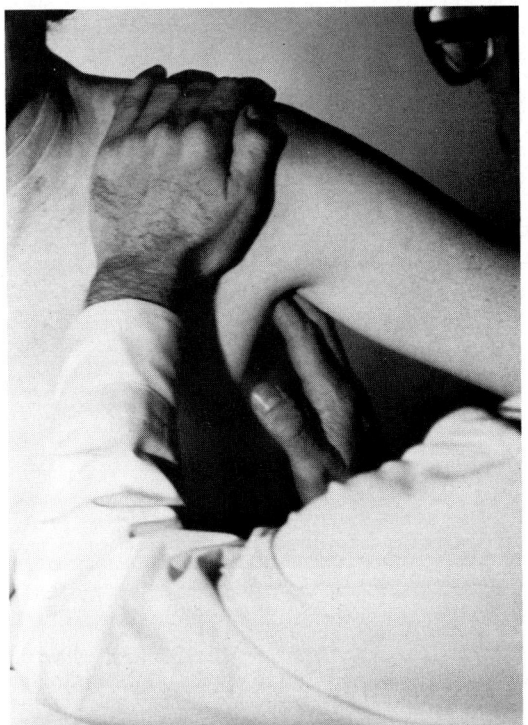

Figure 6–21. The technique is shown for palpating axillary lymph nodes. The fingers of the examining hand are cupped and inserted high into the axilla before being drawn down to trap nodes against the chest wall. Pressure with the other hand keeps the shoulder from moving upwards and moves anterior nodes into the center of the axilla, where they are more easily felt. Less abduction than is shown here improves the examination.

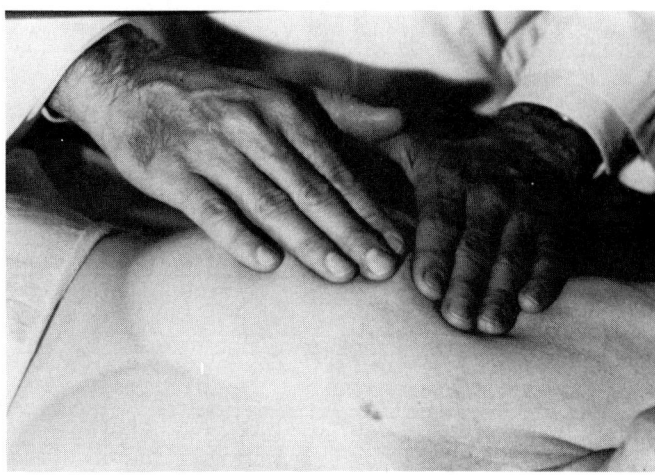

Figure 6-22. Palpation of the breast is performed with the flats of the fingertips. The patient is in a supine position with the side that is being examined slightly elevated and the arm abducted.

ordinarily has margins on all sides and is asymmetric with the other breast. Women with chronic cystic disease can have diffusely granular breasts or breasts with irregular firmness. In these circumstances it must be determined whether a "dominant mass" is present. Any density that is different in quality or quantity from the general consistency must be considered a dominant mass. In equivocal cases, simultaneous palpation of both breasts (Fig. 6–23) can help determine if pathologic asymmetry exists. If the presence of a density is truly equivocal, an acceptable practice in premenopausal women is to repeat the examination 1 week after onset of the next menstrual cycle. If the finding is due to hormonal stimulation, it may have resolved. Interruption of oral contraceptives, or of estrogens in postmenopausal women, may also help to resolve the issue.

The importance of deciding whether a mass or a dominant nodule is present cannot be overemphasized, for an affirmative decision demands that its nature be ascertained. Masses are carefully described with respect to size (centimeters), shape, mobility, attachment to skin or deep fascia, tenderness, consistency and location (Fig. 6–24). A useful mnemonic is to describe each *MASS* with *T*ender, *L*oving *C*are (M = Mobility, A = Attachments, S = Shape, S = Size, T = Tenderness, L = Location [i.e., quadrant], and C = Consistency). Failure of the skin to move independently of the mass establishes attachment. Fixation of a mobile mass when the patient presses with her hand firmly against her hip establishes attachment to the pectoral fascia. Immobility with the arm relaxed indicates that the mass is fixed to the chest wall, that is, the ribs and intercostal muscles.

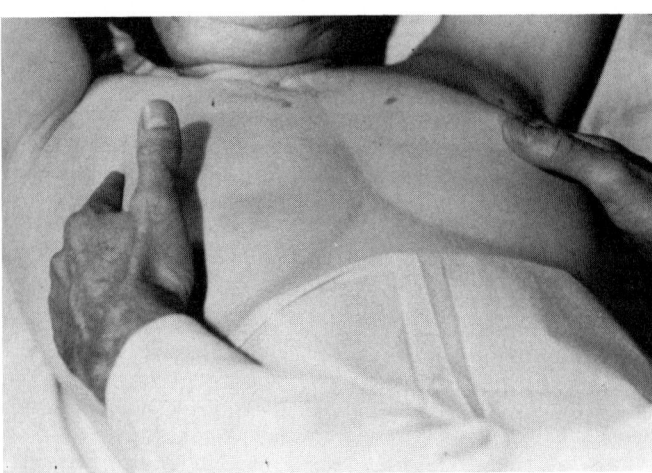

Figure 6-23. Bilateral simultaneous palpation of the breasts is sometimes useful to determine if asymmetry is present.

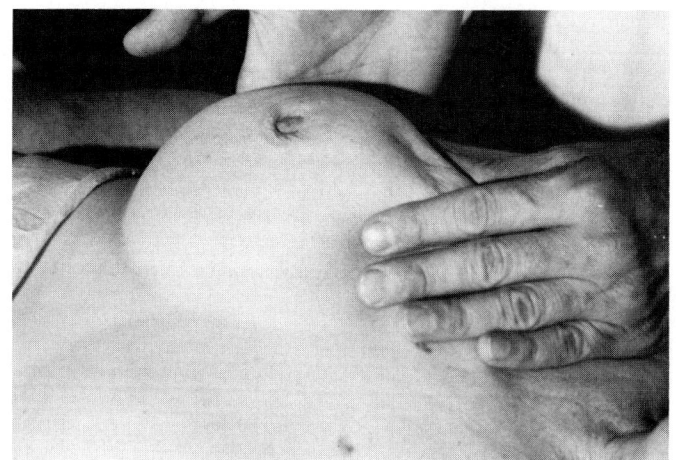

Figure 6–24. Attachment of a mass to the overlying skin can be demonstrated by squeezing the skin as shown. The skin remains fixed and creates a furrow over the mass, the "plateau" sign.

Finally, the nipple is gently squeezed with the thumb and index finger to elicit discharge. Success is favored by beginning low around the areola and stripping the ducts upwards. This is done gently to avoid discomfort and a second time after repositioning the fingers to exert pressure at 90 degrees. Discharge is tested for occult blood. The number and location of discharging ducts are recorded as well as the color and amount of the discharge.

BREAST SELF-EXAMINATION (BSE)

Women should begin monthly self-examinations of the breast at age 21 years according to the American Cancer Society. Beginning this early may be particularly wise for those with a strong family history of breast cancer. The potential advantages that can accrue from establishing a routine justify the small amount of time that is required. One week after menstruation begins, when there is least sensitivity and congestion, is best for premenopausal women (see Fig. 6–15). The beginning of each month serves as an easily remembered routine for postmenopausal women.

A convenient time for the examination is during bathing; wet, soapy skin and fingers optimize the ability to feel masses. The examination includes two parts, in whatever order is convenient: (1) View the breasts in a mirror with the arms at the side, then extended over the head, and finally with the hands pressed firmly against the hips, which serves to exaggerate dimpling and retraction. (2) Each quadrant of the breast and the nipple is palpated systematically with the fingers of the opposite hand while the ipsilateral arm is extended above the head. The examination includes palpation of the axilla and squeezing the nipples for discharge.

Women most likely to practice BSE are those who have been shown how to perform it, who are confident with it, and whose mother has had breast cancer (Bennett et al., 1983). A number of studies have demonstrated that breast cancers found in women who regularly practice breast self-examination are smaller and less often have produced axillary metastases than those in women who do not, and survival after treatment is superior (Foster et al., 1978; Feldman et al., 1981; Foster and Costanza, 1984).

TRANSILLUMINATION

Cutler popularized transillumination of the breast with his initial report in 1929. Transillumination with a bright light sometimes permits the differentiation of cystic from solid masses; in a darkened room, the former transmit light whereas the latter produce a darkened area in the translucent breast. Lipomas also transmit light. Areas of inflammation have diffuse opacity; traumatic hematomas are densely opaque, uneven, and characteristically disappear slowly; ductal papillomas have an intense opacity with a sharp outline. Small masses are difficult to evaluate, however, and a dark shadow does not distinguish a benign from a malignant mass.

Diaphanoscopy is a more recent method of transillumination introduced in 1977. It uses a quartz halogen light source in the red portion of the spectrum, and images can be recorded and photographed for permanent record (Girolamo and Leis, 1982). Some advantages are better tissue penetration and less diffusion than with earlier techniques. The procedure is harmless, but it is time consuming, dense breasts do not transilluminate well, and the method does not replace either physical examination or mammography. In one evaluation, diaphanoscopy produced excessive false positive results, found no cancers not already suspected on clinical examination, and failed to identify some that were suspected (Angquist et al., 1981).

FINE NEEDLE ASPIRATION

Fine needle aspiration of masses is a convenient and expeditious method of differentiating cysts from solid tumors and can be used at the time of the initial examination. Unless a hematoma is produced, it will not interfere with the accuracy of a subsequent mammogram.

The risk of missing an intracystic carcinoma is small. Intracystic carcinomas of the breast are rare (Table 6–5). According to Goode and associates (1955), only two were found among 281 carcinomas of the breast at Baylor University over 4 years. Rosemond and colleagues (1969) found only three among 3000 cyst aspirations. These unusual tumors ordinarily yield bloody fluid on aspiration and leave a residual mass. They will not be missed if prompt excision of the lesion is practiced when needle aspiration: (1) produces no fluid, (2) produces fluid that is bloody, (3) does not result in complete disappearance of the mass, or (4) is followed by rapid accumulation of the fluid (<2 weeks) and more than two aspirations are required. Following these guidelines, Goode and associates aspirated the breast masses of 267 consecutive women. In 210 cases an average of 8.1 ml of turbid green or amber fluid was obtained, and the masses disappeared completely. Fifty-seven women from whom no fluid was obtained had excisions of their lesions, and five carcinomas were found. The routine cytologic examination of fluid from cysts is advocated by some (Abramson, 1974; McSwain et al., 1978), but the yield of unsuspected carcinoma is negligible if the guidelines just cited are followed (Table 6–6).

It is difficult to defend the routine excision of masses that can be identified by needle aspiration or ultrasound as simple cysts. Occasionally occult cancers are found adjacent to simple cysts when the latter are removed. This discovery is fortuitous, however, and no evidence is at hand that occult cancers favor the vicinity of a simple cyst.

Fine needle aspiration of masses to identify simple cysts is a safe and effective method of reducing the number of unproductive biopsies and is an early step in evaluation of a mass. It can be performed with a 21 gauge needle and a 10 ml syringe without local anesthesia with no more, and usually less, discomfort than a routine venipuncture. The skin is wiped with alcohol or another antiseptic, and sterile precautions are observed. The mass is steadied with the fingers of one hand and the needle is directed into the mass with a single thrust at an angle to the chest wall (Fig. 6–25). If fluid is obtained, the cyst is emptied. If a mammogram is also reassuring, repeat physical examination in 2 weeks is all that is necessary.

A unique glycoprotein isolated from cyst fluid, termed gross cystic disease fluid protein (CDP), has been identified in the serum of women with metastatic breast cancer and is under evaluation as a marker for disease progression and regression during therapy (Haagensen et al., 1982).

Resistance to the passage of a needle usually identifies a solid mass even before aspiration is attempted. If a mass is solid, the opportunity is present to obtain a fine needle aspiration cytology (FNAC), sometimes erroneously termed a fine needle aspiration biopsy, or FNAB. This is accomplished as follows: After engaging the mass, the needle is passed repeatedly through the tumor at different angles while maintaining suction on the syringe (Fig. 6–26). Suction is released before withdrawing

Table 6–5. INTRACYSTIC BREAST CARCINOMA

	Number	Cystic Carcinomas	Per Cent
Abramson (1974)	3000 cysts	3	0.1
Gatchell et al. (1958)	9000 carcinomas	48	0.5
Czernobilsky (1967)	2500 carcinomas	14	0.5
Rosemond et al. (1969)	1275 cysts	1	0.1

Table 6–6. CYTOLOGY OF BREAST CYST FLUID

	Number of Cysts	False Positive*	False Negative	Carcinoma Without Clinical Sign
McSwain et al. (1978)	595	36%	(1) 0.2%	1†
Abramson (1974)	1275	0%	(1) 0.07%	0

*Classes 4 and 5.
†Prompt excision precluded determining whether the cyst would have refilled promptly.

the needle from the breast (Wanebo et al., 1984). The needle is removed from the syringe, air is drawn into the syringe, the two are reconnected, and then the cellular contents of the needle are blown out onto a glass slide, which is smeared using another slide. The two slides are immediately dropped into 95 per cent alcohol. Air drying must be avoided. The advantages of this technique are that it is quick, easy, and inexpensive. When the cytologic preparation is read as definitely cancer by an experienced cytopathologist, the opinion is seldom incorrect (Kher et al., 1981; Malberger et al., 1981), obviating the need for biopsy for histologic diagnosis in the opinion of some (Rimsten et al., 1975; Kaufman et al., 1983; Vorherr, 1984; Wanebo et al., 1984). In the opinion of most, however, FNAC is a useful adjunct to patient evaluation rather than diagnostic (Russ et al., 1978; Kline et al., 1979; Shabot et al., 1982; Bell et al., 1983). As shown in Table 6–7, false negative results are frequent and false positives are rare but do occur. Cellular papillomas and fat necrosis are most likely to produce false positive results. Diverse opinions on FNAC are given in Table 6–8. Despite its accuracy, a positive cytologic examination cannot distinguish preinvasive from invasive cancer. This author requires a

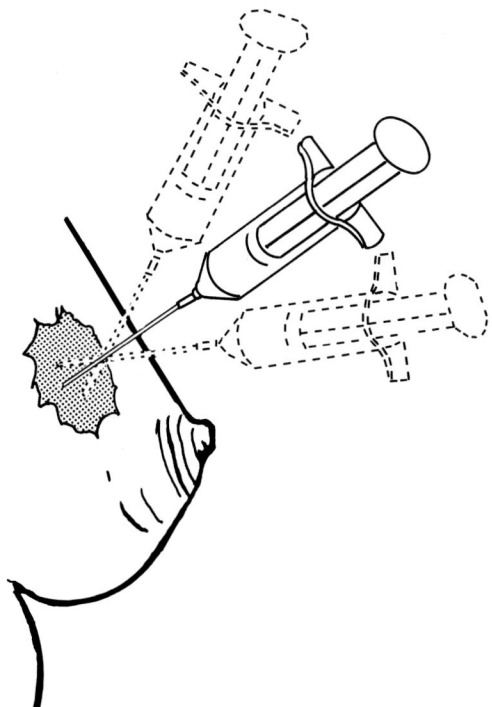

Figure 6–26. The technique for fine needle aspiration cytology of solid breast tumors is shown. A 21 gauge needle and a small syringe are used. After engaging the mass, suction is applied to the syringe while the needle is passed back and forth through the tumor at several angles. Suction is released before the needle is withdrawn to avoid aspirating normal tissues. The entire specimen will be within the needle and it is expelled onto a glass slide by first disconnecting the needle from the syringe, drawing air into the syringe, reconnecting the needle, and blowing the specimen out onto a glass slide. To avoid air drying, the specimen is smeared immediately with another glass slide and both are dropped into 95 per cent alcohol.

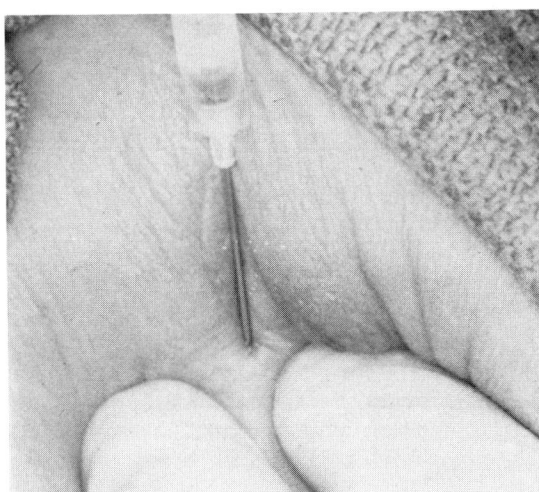

Figure 6–25. Aspiration of palpable masses can be performed as an office procedure to rapidly distinguish cystic from solid lesions. The patient can be assured that there is minimal discomfort and the skin is prepared with an alcohol wipe. Drapes and gloves are not necessary, although they are shown here; a small needle (21 gauge) and syringe are suitable equipment. One pass generally is sufficient to determine the nature of the lesion; if fluid is encountered, it is aspirated entirely.

Table 6–7. FINE NEEDLE ASPIRATION CYTOLOGY (FNAC) OF SOLID BREAST MASSES*

	Total FNACs	Sensitivity +/CAs	Specificity −/Benign	False Positive†	False Negative	Accuracy
Abele et al. (1983)	92	88%	97%	0	13%	93%
Bell et al. (1983)	583	69%	67%	0	17%	68%
Kaufman et al. (1983)	163	90%	97%	2%	12%	93%
Frable and Frable (1982)	588	91%	98%	2%	9%	95%
Malberger et al. (1981)	206	92%	95%	0	8%	94%
Kher et al. (1981)	80	94%	93%	0	6%	94%
Kline et al. (1979)	3545	66%	98%	0	10%	95%
Zajdela et al. (1975)	2772	88%	89%	0.3%	12%	89%
Rosen et al. (1972)	206	82%	100%	0	18%	84%
Franzen and Stenkvist (1968)	1713	76%	93%	0.1%	24%	92%
Total	9948	82%	94%	0.2%	18%	89%

*Confirmed histologically.
†Total = 13.
This table shows the correlation of 9948 fine needle aspiration cytologies of breast masses with biopsies that were read as either positive or negative for malignancy. The procedure is highly accurate in practiced hands, and false positives are unusual.

histologic diagnosis prior to treatment, but positive cytologic findings can serve to prepare the patient for the probable diagnosis, to justify a staging evaluation, and to justify a one-stage biopsy and treatment as suggested by Lannin et al. (1986).

Mammography

Mammography has a unique role in the detection of mammary cancer. Cancers can be detected earlier by mammography than by any other noninvasive means. It is indispensable for complete evaluation of symptomatic adults and is invaluable for the screening of asymptomatic women.

Table 6–8. FINE NEEDLE ASPIRATION CYTOLOGY

"Although histologic confirmation is always recommended before proceeding with mastectomy, a positive cytologic diagnosis can suffice when clinically advanced carcinoma is present or when there are medical contraindications to surgical treatment."
                                              Russ et al. (1978)

"With close cooperation between the surgeons and the cytopathologist, an almost completely accurate preoperative diagnosis of palpable mammary masses can be achieved."
                                              Malberger et al. (1981)

"When FNAC is unequivocally positive for malignancy, routine frozen section examination preceding mastectomy becomes, in our opinion, unnecessary."
                                              Kaufman et al. (1983)

The development of mammography began in 1913, when Salomon correlated the clinical, pathologic, and roentgenologic characteristics of 3000 amputated breasts, noting many of the roentgenographic features of breast tumors. By the late 1920s, several workers were investigating modifications of this technique and its applications to breast disease (Egan, 1972). In 1929, Warren (1930) was able to show an 85 to 95 per cent diagnostic accuracy of this method in 119 cases of breast disease, but the results remained inconsistent, and only a few investigators continued to evaluate the method (Leborgne, 1953; Gershon-Cohen et al., 1962). New impetus was provided in 1960 by Egan, who developed improved images using a high milliamperage, low kilovoltage technique, and standardized positional views. The method and interpretations proved reproducible and resulted in widespread adoption of mammography as an adjunct to physical examination. Further notable advances included the development of xeromammography by Wolfe (1976), which provided reduced radiation exposure and improved resolution, and more recently, low dose film mammography. Tissue patterns on xeromammograms have been correlated with personal risk for breast cancer by Wolfe (1976).

At present, two forms of mammography are in use, low dose film mammography and xeromammography. Two views of each breast, the mediolateral and the cephalocaudad views, taken at right angles to each other, constitute a standard examination, although other special views can be taken (oblique views and spot

Table 6–9. MAMMOGRAMS FOR 241 PALPABLE BREAST MASSES*

Mammogram	Biopsy	
	Cancer	Benign
No lesion	13 (16%)†	101 (64%)
Focal lesion	32 (39%)	47 (30%)
Cancer	37 (45%)	11 (7%)

*Mammography must be used in conjunction with physical examination, as 16 per cent of palpable cancers were missed by mammography. A small number of benign lesions (7 per cent) were also misdiagnosed as cancer on mammography.
†29 to 66 years old.
Consecutive cases at the Medical College of Wisconsin.

enlargements). Radiation exposure to the midbreast is less than 40 millirads per view for low dose film mammography and approximately 400 millirads for xeromammography.

Mammography is able to visualize nonpalpable and often unsuspected lesions; tumors smaller than 0.5 cm in diameter are often discovered. However, as visualization depends on a radiodensity that is different from that of surrounding tissues, easily palpable masses may remain undetected by mammography. Twelve to 16 per cent of clinically demonstrable cancers are not visualized on mammograms. This figure has reached 41 per cent in women less than 50 years old (Niloff and Sheiner, 1981) (Tables 6–9 and 6–10). Thus, although mammography is an invaluable complement to the physical examination, it is not a substitute for it and should always be used in conjunction with a physical examination.

The clinician must recognize the need for biopsy despite a negative mammogram should the presence of cancer be suspected on the basis of physical findings. The probability of a breast biopsy resulting in a diagnosis of cancer on the basis of the physical examination and a mammogram was explored by Lewis and colleagues (1976) and is shown graphically in Figure 6–27.

Mammography is indicated as a part of the diagnostic evaluation of all symptomatic women over the age of 30 years. The breasts of women younger than 30 are more sensitive to the mutagenic effects of irradiation, and the incidence of occult cancer is negligible in this age group, so that the irradiation exposure involved is unjustified (Stone et al., 1977). Furthermore, the tissues are sufficiently dense to make the examination of little usefulness. Mammography is of less value for evaluating the nature of a mass than for detecting a lesion that may have gone unnoticed. If a mass or other lesion is not felt, a mammogram provides additional assurance that a clinically occult lesion is not present. Mammography is also indicated before any surgical procedure on the breast of an adult woman and for evaluating the breast as the likely site of an occult primary tumor when metastatic carcinoma is found in an axillary lymph node.

Guidelines for screening asymptomatic populations with mammography are now well established (Cancer Letter, 1977). The American Cancer Society recommends the guidelines shown in Table 6–11. In addition, an annual mammogram is indicated for women of any age who have previously been treated for cancer of one breast.

In the only randomized trial of screening conducted in the United States (the HIP study)

Table 6–10. SENSITIVITY OF MAMMOGRAPHY FOR PALPABLE CANCERS

References	Number of Cancers	Positive Mammograms	Sensitivity	False Negatives
Strax (1976)	246	164	67%	33%
Baker (1982)	1205	1019	85%	15%
<50 years old	481	381	79%	21%
≥50 years old	724	638	88%	12%
McClow (1973)	156	135	87%	13%
Lesnick (1977)				
<45 years old	50	21	42%	58%
Egeli and Urban (1979)	520	412	79%	21%
<50 years old	154	108	70%	30%
≥50 years old	366	304	83%	17%
Medical College of Wisconsin	82	69	84%	16%

Several sources document that mammograms fail to detect many cancers that are palpable on physical examination (false negatives) and are more likely to be inaccurate in young women than in older women. Dense breasts, geographic misses, and poor technique contribute to the problem. For this reason mammograms must be supplemented with a physical examination.

	MAMMOGRAM		
PHYSICAL EXAMINATION	Normal	Benign	Suspicious
Normal		0/32 (0%)	50/155 (32%)
Benign	6/112 (5%)		
Suspicious	31/152 (20%)	3/52 (6%)	72/83 (87%)

Figure 6–27. The probability of finding cancer with a biopsy is correlated with the results of physical examination and mammography. Each aids detection of cancer independently. (From Lewis J. D., et al.: Which breast to biopsy: An expanding dilemma. Am. Surg., *184*:253, 1976. Reprinted with permission.)

annual physical examinations and mammography resulted in a 24 per cent reduction in 10 year mortality rate from breast cancer (Shapiro et al., 1982). No reduced mortality rate was demonstrated by this landmark study for women under 50 years old, although a recent review of the HIP data suggests a delayed benefit in these younger patients (Habbema et al., 1986). A trial of screening with mammography in Sweden (Tabar et al., 1986) and one in the Netherlands (Verbeek et al., 1984) have both found survival benefit in women older than 50 years of age.

Ultrasonography

Ultrasonic examination of the breast has established a useful place in detection. In special situations it can be a valuable complement to physical examination and mammography. It is noninvasive and does not involve radiation exposure.

Kobayashi (1982) reviewed the development of ultrasonic detection. Early development by Wild and associates in 1952 began with a unidimensional A-mode display, which rapidly developed into a two dimensional imaging technique described as an "echograph." Howry and coworkers reported the first echographic demonstration of a scirrhous carcinoma using a two dimensional B-mode radioscanner in 1954. At present, two techniques for breast ultrasonography are in use. The first is hand-held real time ultrasonography that can be used to explore various regions of the breast. Direct contact with the skin of the breast is made with a lubricant used to eliminate the gas-tissue interface, and a two dimensional gray scale image is produced. The second technique is dedicated whole breast computed ultrasonography with multiple step sections. The air-surface interface is eliminated either by placing a polyvinyl water bag containing degassed water on the skin with the patient in the supine position, or alternatively, by placing the patient prone with the breast immersed in a tank of water.

On an echogram, echogenic structures appear bright and nonechogenic structures dark. In differentiating benign from malignant lesions, three features are worthy of note: (1) the boundary echo and shape, (2) the internal echos, and (3) posterior shadowing. Characteristically, benign lesions have a regular, smooth, and round or oval boundary. They are free of internal echos (cysts) or have homogeneous, uniform-sized internal echos (fibroadenomas). The lateral shadow sign may be present (anechoic distal projections from the borders of the lesion). The deep margin is characteristically bright and echogenic, projecting posteriorly as a "tadpole sign." By contrast, boundary echoes of malignant lesions are irregular and jagged. The internal echoes are nonhomogeneous, and the posterior margin is obscure, with a dark, anechoic shadow projecting posteriorly, the middle shadow sign (Kobayashi, 1982). Cancers may have variable features, as described by Maturo and colleagues (1982) in four categories: (1) a hypoechoic mass with uneven discontinuous boundaries, nonuniform internal echos, and a poorly defined back wall with variable posterior sonic attenuation; (b) a hyperechoic focus appearing as a bright mass with a discrete posterior shadow; (c) a disrupted mammary parenchyma

Table 6–11. AMERICAN CANCER SOCIETY GUIDELINES FOR ASYMPTOMATIC WOMEN, 1983

Age (Yr)	
≥20	Breast self-examination monthly
20–40	Physical examination every 3 years
>40	Physical examination yearly
35–40	Baseline mammogram
40–49	Mammogram every 1–2 years*
>50	Mammogram yearly

*On physician's recommendation based on assessment

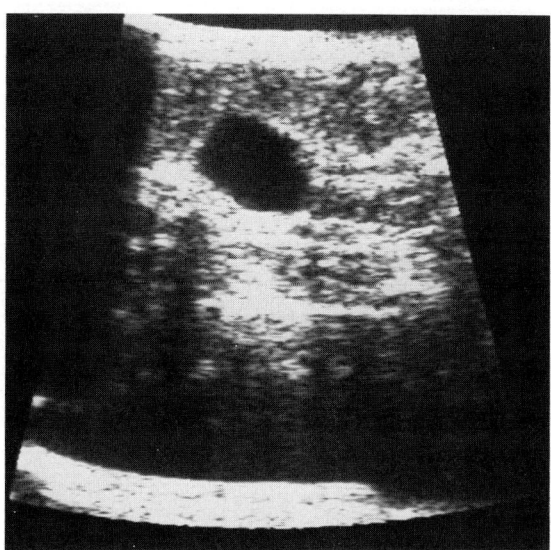

Figure 6–28. Real time hand-held ultrasonic image of a simple cyst demonstrating well-defined margins, an interior free of echoes, border shadows projecting posteriorly, and a bright echogenic posterior margin.

cent of minimal breast cancers are detected (Rosner and Blaird, 1985).

Ultrasonography excels, however, in identifying lesions in radiologically dense premenopausal breasts and in identifying cysts. Thus, it is an excellent complement to mammography, particularly in the young adult, and can readily distinguish the cystic or solid nature of a palpable mass or a nonpalpable density detected on mammography. Furthermore, a normal ultrasonic examination can be valuable when physical examination and mammography are inconclusive.

The indications for breast ultrasonography suggested by Brascho are given in Table 6–12. Rubin and colleagues (1985) found ultrasonography a useful adjunct to the x-ray mammogram in three groups of patients: (1) those with dense breasts and localized symptoms or a suspicious area on x-ray mammogram; (2) patients with nonpalpable abnormalities discovered on x-ray mammogram; and (3) those with palpable masses considered indeterminant on an x-ray mammogram. It is also useful for guiding needle aspiration of nonpalpable cystic structures. Ultrasonography is most accurate in cyst detection, but it should not be used as the sole imaging method because of its inability to detect microcalcifications and its difficulty in demonstrating small solid lesions, particularly in the fatty breast (McSweeney and Murphy, 1985).

In a premenopausal woman with a palpable breast mass, fine needle aspiration can distinguish a cyst from a solid tumor more quickly and less expensively than ultrasonography, so its value in this situation is less than it is in evaluating the deep-lying, nonpalpable mass detected mammographically.

with an irregular echogenic zone and a discrete distal acoustic shadow; (d) an atypical cystic mass with an anechoic center, poorly defined edges, and posterior bright sonic enhancement (Figs. 6–28 to 6–30).

Ultrasonic examinations are least accurate in detecting cancers in the fatty postmenopausal breast and poor in detecting microcalcifications, which are present in approximately 35 per cent of early breast cancers. In addition, small breast cancers will often escape detection. The accuracy of ultrasonography in detecting cancers less than 2 cm in diameter is no more than 57 per cent, and only 23 per

Figure 6–29. Ultrasonic image of a fibroadenoma, which appears dark, with a smooth outline. Echoes from its homogeneous interior are relatively few but appear as bright spots; variable shadowing projects posteriorly. Boundaries are marked by X for measuring purposes. (Courtesy of John R. Milbrath, M.D.)

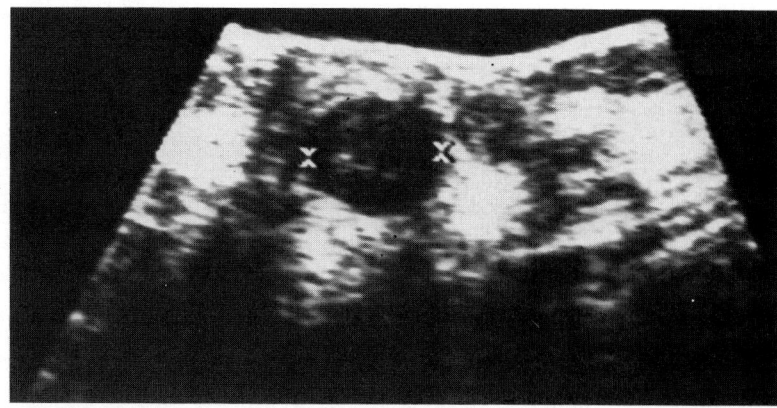

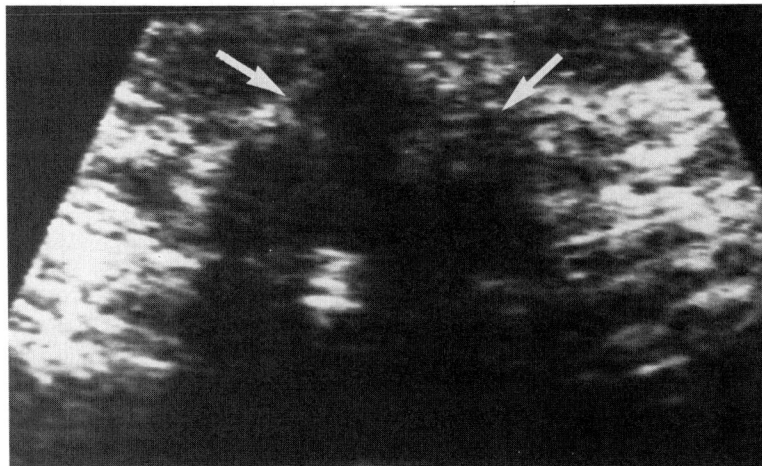

Figure 6–30. Ultrasonic image of a carcinoma, which appears as a dark area with irregular borders and internal echoes; a large, dark shadow projects posteriorly. (Courtesy of John R. Milbrath, M.D.)

Computed Tomographic Scanning of the Breast

Computed tomography (CT) of the breast is of relatively recent origin and is still under evaluation. Of interest is that the results of breast scanning with CT body scanners are equal to those of dedicated CT mammographic units. It is also evident that the limitations of CT prevent it from replacing conventional mammography in the evaluation of breast disease. CT mammography does have the capacity to detect some breast cancers that are occult by other methods. It permits visualization of both the axillary and the internal mammary lymph nodes and provides excellent visualization of the deep mammary and retromammary tissues. Detection is facilitated by asymmetry in the architecture of the breast tissue and the fact that breast cancers concentrate intravenously injected iodinated contrast dyes to a much greater degree than do benign lesions, resulting in marked contrast enhancement of cancers on postinjection scans. Tumors as small as 2 mm have been detected, and there is no definite relationship between size and contrast medium enhancement. Chang and associates (1982) suggested several situations in which CT scanning of the breast may be of value. These include the detection of cancers in dense breasts when mammography is of limited value owing to lack of tissue contrast, the detection of mammographically and physically unsuspected very small breast cancers, and the detection of breast cancer when axillary lymph node biopsy is positive and mammograms fail to demonstrate a primary lesion. The detection of unsuspected primary tumors in the contralateral breast is also possible.

On the other hand, CT has important liabilities. One is a high dose of irradiation per examination, which may vary between 3.2 and 1.2 rad skin dose per examination, depending upon the number of tomographic slices (Doust et al., 1981). This is approximately 15 times the dosage received with low dose film mammography and is high enough to exclude CT as a screening method. Other disadvantages include the unnecessary radiation to other parts of the thorax during the examination, the need for intravenous contrast medium injection to optimize the results, the high cost of the examination, and the lengthiness of the procedure.

Another disadvantage of CT scanning is that malignant microcalcifications without an associated mass cannot be identified owing to the averaging effect within the CT computer matrix. This is a serious limitation, as not only

Table 6–12. INDICATIONS FOR BREAST ULTRASONOGRAPHY

Young patients
Pregnant women
Dense breasts
Fibrocystic disease
Palpable mass
Adjunct to x-ray
Women with prostheses
Women who refuse x-ray
Previous breast neoplasm

From Brascho, D. J.: Ultrasound of the female breast; f the art. Ala. J. Med. Sci., 19:83, 1982. rmission.

the presence of calcium but also its pattern is important in deciding for or against the need for biopsy.

Thermography

Thermography refers to the measurement and imaging of surface heat patterns. Two methods of breast thermography exist: telethermography and cholesteric plate thermography. All objects absorb and emit heat as infrared radiation. By definition, black bodies absorb all infrared radiation that falls on them and emit it as a function of their absolute temperature. The breast is an excellent black body, and the heat emitted can be detected by remote infrared-sensitive scanning devices. The second method involves placing in contact with the skin a flexible Mylar film plate impregnated with cholesteric esters, which change colors at various temperature ranges, thereby producing a visible pattern.

Cancers ordinarily produce more heat than surrounding tissues owing to their high metabolism, and if this is transmitted to the skin directly or through veins draining the cancer, it can produce abnormal surface heat. Lawson (1956) was the first to use thermography for detection of breast disease, finding an average temperature increase of 1.2°C (2.27°F) over two mammary carcinomas. Increased sensitivity and resolution have resulted from improved technology, but fundamental problems remain with specificity and interpretation. The heat patterns of breasts are not entirely symmetric, preventing either from functioning as a control for the other. Patterns change during pregnancy and the menstrual cycle. Subcutaneous fat is an effective insulator, shielding the skin from the heat of small, deep-seated tumors. Although veins absorb heat from deep-lying carcinomas and transmit it to the surface, their warm pattern may be evident only at a site remote from the cancer. Unfortunately, increased heat is not specific for cancer. Benign lesions, such as plasma cell mastitis, adenosis, epithelial hyperplasia, and islands of functioning breast tissue surrounding cysts can produce elevated skin temperatures. As a detection method, the worth of thermography remains unproved, and it has not established a place in routine evaluation of the breast. Up to one third of asymptomatic women have abnormal thermograms (Isard et al., 1972). A similar proportion of women with benign lesions have abnormal thermograms (King and King, 1982). Furthermore, a substantial number of cancers are missed. False positive results exceed those of clinical examination, and one quarter to two thirds of all proved cancers are not detected by thermograms (Table 6–13). At present two points seem clear: (1) An abnormal thermogram alone is not an indication for biopsy except in unusual circumstances; and (2) a normal thermogram is not sufficiently reliable to exclude women from further examination.

Biopsy

Histologic examination provides the definitive diagnosis of mammary carcinoma. Only by removing a sample of tissue sufficient for histologic preparation can a diagnosis be made with ultimate confidence. The accuracy of the information obtained is limited only by the accuracy of sampling and morphologic interpretation. As a negative biopsy can be due to sampling error, cancer cannot be excluded unless all pathologic tissue is removed and examined thoroughly. Therapy for cancer should be predicated on histologic verification of its presence. Pertinent issues are the indications for biopsy, the techniques, and the timing.

INDICATIONS FOR BIOPSY

The indications for biopsy include a persistent mass or dominant nodule, a persistently dis-

Table 6–13. THERMOGRAPHY IN 502 PATIENTS*

	Number of Examinations	Sensitivity	False Positives
Infrared thermography†	792	33.3%	6.4%
Plate thermography†	718	36.4%	11.7%
Clinical examination		69.0%	1.4%

*This study illustrates continuing problems with thermography as a cancer detection method. Thermography detected only one third of proven cancers and false positives totaled more than 11%.
†Neither type of thermogram detected 5 of 11 carcinomas.
Based on data from Sterns, E. E., et al.: Thermography in breast diagnosis. Cancer, 50:323, 1982.

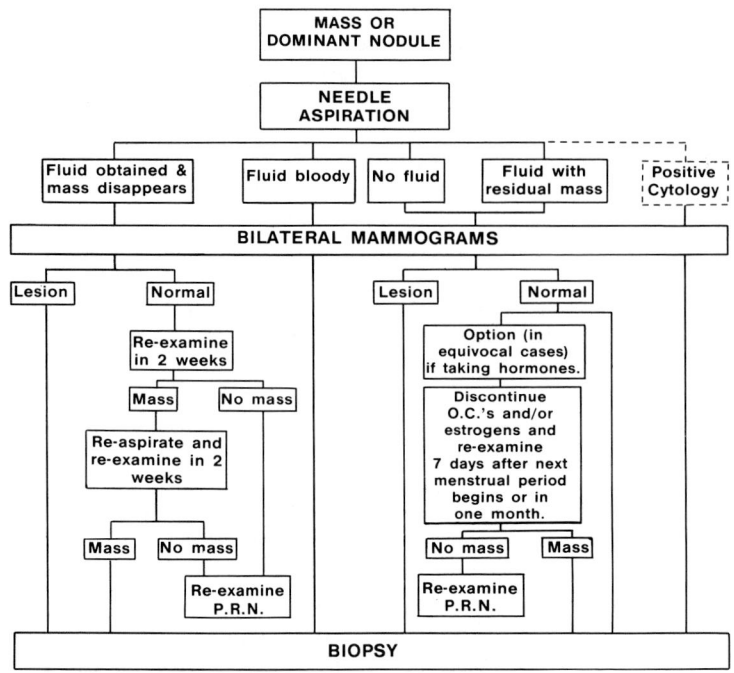

Figure 6–31. This algorithm pertains only to the management of palpable breast masses and demonstrates the integration of needle aspiration, mammograms, and biopsy in diagnosis. Although a cytologic examination of cyst fluid is not routine or essential to successful diagnosis, if positive cytologic findings are obtained on cyst fluid or tissue aspirate, a biopsy is indicated. A more comprehensive algorithm is presented in the chapter on surgical management pertaining to palpable and non-palpable lesions (Fig. 13–1).

charging duct, an abscess or unexplained inflammatory signs, unexplained nipple changes, and suspicious mammographic signs. Elective biopsy of the normal breast may be indicated, as discussed in Chapter 22 under *Cancer of the Second Breast*. A decision for biopsy of a palpable mass may be made using the scheme shown in Figure 6–31.

PERMANENT VERSUS FROZEN SECTIONS

The most accurate method for histologic examination of tissues is with stained paraffin sections, the only disadvantage being the 24 to 48 hours required to process the tissues. The convenience and theoretical advantage of an immediate diagnosis and treatment spurred the development of "frozen sections" by Welch (Sparkman, 1962) and by Wilson (1905) at the turn of the century. The technique of frozen section has reached a level of sophistication that permits the diagnosis with at least 98 per cent accuracy within 15 to 20 minutes after tissue is obtained. Thus, diagnosis and therapy can be completed during one period of general anesthesia in "one step." In a review of 556 consecutive breast biopsy specimens examined with frozen sections, no false positive reports ...osis of cancer in 145 cases ...e of doubt regarding the interpretation, a diagnosis was deferred for paraffin sections in 5.4 per cent of biopsies, and 8 (2.1 per cent) of 381 biopsies initially interpreted as benign proved to contain carcinoma on further examination with permanent sections. Lesions that can cause problems with interpretation on frozen section are papillary lesions, sclerosing adenosis, florid adenosis, atypical ductal hyperplasia, fat necrosis, and in situ lobular carcinoma (Kagali, 1983). These are best diagnosed on permanent paraffin sections. In general, frozen section is a highly reliable technique except for occasional instances of initial sampling error or in which small foci of carcinoma require confirmation on permanent preparations. The majority of initial false negative results prove to be non-invasive cancers with a good prognosis. Even when immediate treatment is not anticipated, frozen section may still be desirable so that cancers can be identified and submitted for hormone receptor determination while the tissue is still viable, and patients can receive expeditious answers.

Immediate Versus Delayed Mastectomy

The theoretical basis for "one step" diagnosis and treatment arose early in the twentieth

Table 6–14. BIOPSY VERSUS PROGNOSIS AFTER RADICAL MASTECTOMY FOR CARCINOMA AT THE ELLIS FISCHEL STATE CANCER HOSPITAL

Biopsy	Number of Cases	Local Recurrence (%)*	Distant Metastasis (%)*
None	190	18.4	37.3
With immediate mastectomy	307	16.9	35.1
With delayed mastectomy (1–630 days)	205	19.0	33.6

*Within 5 years.

Note: No significant influence on local recurrence or distant metastasis of mammary carcinoma can be attributed to a biopsy prior to mastectomy or to a delay between a diagnostic biopsy and mastectomy.

century when it was believed that trauma to a cancer, such as a biopsy for diagnosis, could cause its immediate and extensive spread through lymphatics. Halsted (1907) taught, "The excision of a specimen for macroscopic or microscopic examination is never resorted to except just before operation." He also stated, "If then, on incision, the tumor proved to be malignant, the complete operation should be performed immediately" (Halsted, 1898). Tyzzer appeared to confirm this hazard by demonstrating increased metastases in animals after repeated massage of primary cancers (Tyzzer, 1913). Later Cole and associates showed large numbers of tumor cells released into regional veins during surgical manipulation of cancers (Cole, 1973). This anxiety about biopsy established for many decades the one step procedure as a principle of management.

Despite the theoretical possibility of spreading cancer with the trauma of a biopsy, it has proved to have no detectable influence on prognosis. At EFSCH, patients who had biopsies prior to treatment fared as well as those in an earlier series in which no biopsies were performed (Table 6–14). A delay of several days or even longer between biopsy and treatment appears to have no adverse effect upon prognosis, an observation confirmed with personal data (Table 6–15) and by others (Table 6–16). For the most part, these studies can be faulted for small numbers and inadequate controls. Fisher and colleagues (1985) found no adverse effect of delay on survival of 1640 patients whether or not residual cancer was found at the site of biopsy and regardless of intervals of up to 14 days between biopsy and mastectomy, compared with 510 concomitant but nonrandomized controls who had one step diagnosis and treatment. It would appear that any risk inherent in the trauma of biopsy and a modest delay of treatment is too small to measure easily or is inconsequential to the prospects for cure. Long delays (> 3 months) permit greater opportunity for obvious clinical tumor progression, and the results of treatment tend to deteriorate (Charlson, 1985). Thus, a decision to delay mastectomy can safely be made, and should be made, whenever the histologic diagnosis is in doubt.

With the safety of a "two step" approach to diagnosis and treatment reasonably established, it has been appreciated that there are a number of important advantages, with the result that outpatient biopsy under local anes-

Table 6–15. SURVIVAL VERSUS DURATION OF DELAY BETWEEN BIOPSY AND RADICAL MASTECTOMY IN CLINICALLY LOCALIZED CASES, EFSCH, 1940 TO 1958*

Delay (Days)	Total Number of Cases	Number	5 Year Survival (Per Cent)	Median Tumor Diameter (cm)
No biopsy	49	28	57.1	3.0
Biopsy at surgery	133	94	70.7	2.0
1–7	51	33	64.7	3.0
8–14	36	23	63.9	2.8
15–21	17	8	47.1	3.3
22–28	13	8	61.5	2.3
29–35	11	10	90.9	1.5
36–42	7	6	85.7	1.8
More than 42	15	9	60.0	1.5

*The duration of delay between biopsy and radical surgery is not correlated with the per cent 5 year postoperative survival. Patients with a prolonged delay, however, had smaller tumors and a disproportionate number of less aggressive histologic types. No deleterious effect of biopsy or of a delay before mastectomy of up to 42 days can be shown on prognosis.

Table 6–16. BIOPSY WITH DELAYED MASTECTOMY*

	Number of Cases	Duration of Delay	5 Year Survival	Controls and 5 Year Survival	Conclusion
Nohrman (1949)	91	0–3 days 4–14 days 15+ days	81% 74% 71%	Own, historical (78%)	3 days' delay OK
Pierce et al. (1956)	96	6 mo	61.1% 44% Ax+ 75% Ax–	Own, historical (60%), 554 cases	No harm
Jackson and Pitts (1959)	51	2–145 days	62.7%	Others, historical	No harm
Sayago and Sirebrenik (1959)	40		14% Ax+	Own, historical (82%), Ax+	30 days' delay OK
Prechtel and Hallbauer (1979)	64	7 days		Own, historical Worse if > 3 cm diameter and Ax+ 15 cases	7 days' delay OK
Knapp and Mullen (1976)	58	0–46 days	72.4%	Own, historical, 48% (31 cases)	No harm
Abramson (1976)	41	1–30 days	79.5% 44.5% Ax+ 90% Ax–	Others, historical	No harm
Fisher (1985)	164	27 days	Stages I & II 59%	Own, concomitant (52%), 510 cases	14 days' delay OK; no information on longer delay

*A number of studies have failed to demonstrate an adverse effect of delay between biopsy and mastectomy. Almost all, however, have included inadequate numbers of cases or lacked randomized concomitant controls, permitting small differences to be missed. In general, no adverse effect on survival has been demonstrated by modest delays in treatment.

thesia, followed when necessary by cancer treatment after an interval, has become common practice (Charlson, 1985; Stein, 1982; Bertario et al., 1985). The benefits include less investment of time for the patient, reduced hospital expenses, and the psychologic advantages of a prompt diagnosis (Saltzstein et al., 1974). If the lesion is benign, which most will be, the issue is brought to a speedy and cost-effective conclusion; if malignant, a short interval before treatment permits time for staging procedures, for further pathologic or surgical consultation if desirable, and for discussion of treatment options based on a secure diagnosis. A hazard is the occasional wound infection or hematoma, which may require that treatment be further delayed or modified.

TECHNIQUES OF BIOPSY

There are essentiallly two techniques for obtaining a histologic diagnosis, core needle biopsy and "open" or "surgical" biopsy.

Core Needle Biopsy. Core needle biopsies can be performed under local anesthesia as an office procedure. With little discomfort it is possible to remove a small core of tissue from virtually any site within the breast. As accurate sampling is paramount, superficial masses and those measuring 2 cm or greater in diameter are the most suitable targets. Sterile precautions and a 2 to 3 mm incision in the skin through which to insert the needle are required. Care must be taken not to penetrate the chest wall or incise tissues that would not ordinarily be removed with a subsequent mastectomy should it be required. Instruments for this purpose include rotating drills (Meyerowitz, 1976) and various needles designed for the purpose. The Travenol disposable Tru-Cut needle is the author's preference (Roberts et al., 1975). This is a swift and expedient method for confirming the presence of cancer. False positive results are virtually nonexistent; because of potential sampling error, negative findings are inconclusive (Table 6–17). A negative result requires surgical biopsy. The tumor sample obtained with a Tru-Cut needle is ordinarily not sufficient to permit a biochemical determination of estrogen and progesterone receptors.

Surgical Biopsy. Surgical biopsy refers to removal of tissue through a surgical incision. It is best performed in a surgical suite, but it may be accomplished with local or general anesthesia, depending on circumstances and

Table 6–17. CORE NEEDLE BIOPSY

	Number	Sensitivity	Accuracy	False Negatives	False Positives
Tru-Cut					
Foster (1982)	30 carcinomas	90%		10%	0
Roberts et al. (1975)	87 carcinomas	67%			0
Blamey (1982)	932 carcinomas	76%		19%	
Drill					
Meyerowitz (1976)	135 carcinomas		99%	1.6%	0
Sieninski and Dabska (1976)	600 carcinomas	87%	94%		0

preferences. As two of every three biopsies reveal benign disease, it is important that scars be reasonably cosmetic. The lines of tension in the skin of the breast are generally concentric with the nipple, and incisions that follow these lines result in thin scars. Incisions for biopsy should follow them insofar as possible, although allowance must be made for keeping biopsy incisions within the bounds of a future mastectomy or local wide tumor removal (lumpectomy) should it be planned for treatment (Fig. 6–32). The most cosmetically ac-

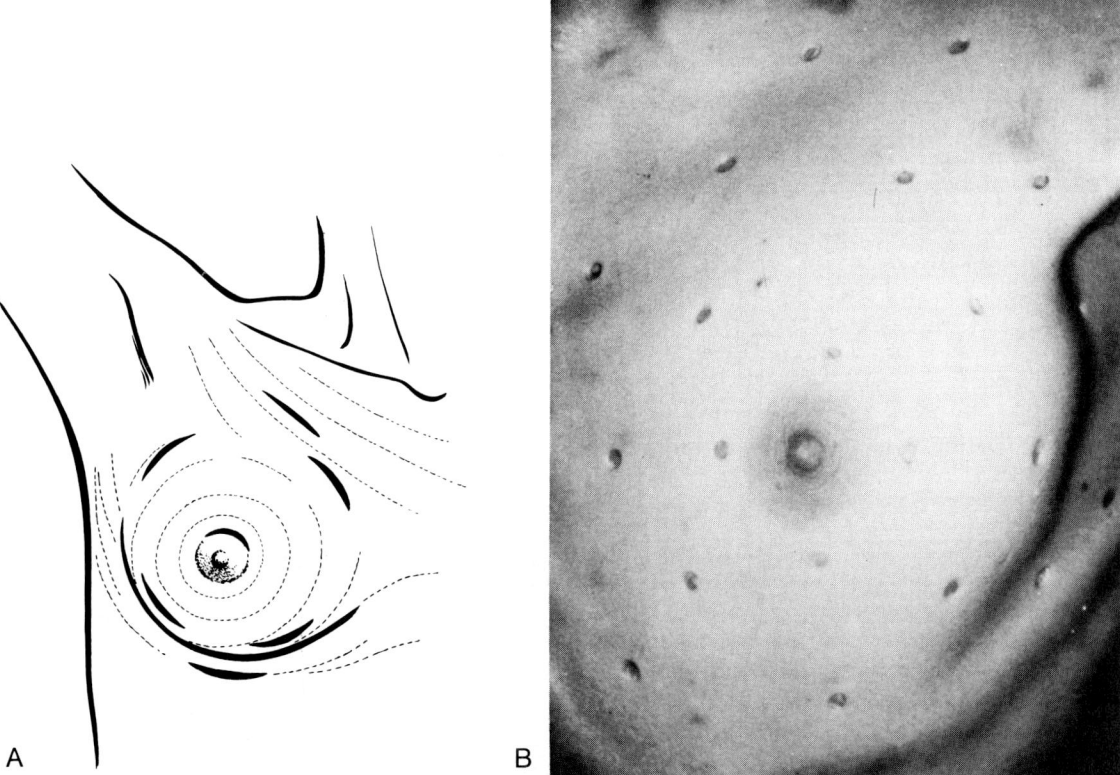

Figure 6–32. *A,* Lines of skin tension on the female breast based on studies done at the EFSCH using the technique of Langer are illustrated in this figure. The stress of gravitational pull described by Kraissl may be superimposed on large pendulous breasts (Kraissl, 1951). In general, dermal tension is concentric with the nipple, becoming transverse over the sternum and diagonal on the extreme upper lateral anterior chest. Periareolar or concentric incisions follow these lines of tension; they are, therefore, optimally cosmetic and generally provide adequate exposure for biopsies. Periareolar incisions should not extend more than half the circumference of the areola. A discharging ductal system, though radial to the nipple, can be adequately excised through a periareolar incision. If a substantial amount of breast tissue is to be removed, radial incisions are preferable for the lower hemisphere of the breast to preserve the distance between the nipple and the inframammary fold. *B,* An example of Langer's technique used to study lines of skin tension on the female breast (autopsy case). The distortion of circular skin defects makes a pattern concentric with the nipple.

ceptable scar results from an incision that lies just within the color margin of the areola. Most centrally located lesions can be approached in this manner, a modest amount of flap development sometimes being necessary. Injecting a tiny amount of Evans blue (<0.1 ml) into smaller or less discrete masses as a marker when this approach is used ensures accurate removal; masses easily palpable before an incision is made can often become elusive after the operation begins.

Surgical biopsies may be either "incisional" (removal of only a part of a tumor) or "excisional" (removal of the entire gross tumor or lesion). Small lesions, that is, those 1 cm or less in diameter, are best excised completely with minimal disturbance to the mass. This provides optimal tissues for the pathologist, and, if the tumor is benign, serves as adequate treatment. If the surgical margins are normal, it can also serve as a satisfactory lumpectomy for cancer in preparation for treatment with primary irradiation. Removal of a small sample of large masses usually provides a diagnosis and is preferable to a wide dissection. If a diagnosis of cancer is not forthcoming on frozen section, the remaining abnormal tissue or mass is removed for examination.

Whenever an entire tumor is removed for diagnosis, the specimen should be transported to the laboratory in ice and kept frozen so that estrogen and progesterone receptor determinations may be performed should it prove to be carcinoma.

Biopsies should be performed with a scalpel, not with electrodissection, as the latter can devitalize tissue and reduce detectable estrogen receptors (Rosenthal, 1979). It is probably preferable to obtain receptors on tissue removed at biopsy rather than on residual tumor in the mastectomy specimen; the residual tumor may be insufficient for analysis, and the warm ischemic time during mastectomy theoretically can reduce receptor content. Although Leight and colleagues (1984) found no clinically significant changes in estrogen receptors (ER) before and after mastectomy in 21 cases, the progesterone receptors (PgR) did decrease (Table 6–18). Biopsy incisions should be closed only after meticulous hemostasis and without drains. It is also important not to attempt suture closure of the breast tissue, as it will reconstitute itself in a more natural way than the surgeon can contrive (Fisher, 1985). It is sufficient to close only the subcutaneous fat and the skin. Wearing a brassière for support the first few days improves healing and comfort, and the incision should be kept dry until it is healed.

SKIN BIOPSY

In two instances, biopsy of the skin of the breast is important for diagnosis (i.e., when Paget's disease or inflammatory carcinoma is suspected). Excision of a small full-thickness ellipse from the involved areola or a punch biopsy of it can establish the presence of Paget's disease, and in the absence of a mass this is sufficiently definitive for treatment. Only local anesthesia is necessary, and the biopsy can be performed on an outpatient basis.

It is desirable to demonstrate invasion of dermal lymphatics to confirm a diagnosis of inflammatory carcinoma of the breast pathologically, and a full-thickness ellipse of skin is more likely to do this than is the small sample obtained with a punch biopsy tool. The specimen should be from edematous skin, and a biopsy sample should also be taken of the subjacent mass, or if a mass is not present, of the underlying breast tissue at the same time for corroboration and for estrogen receptor analysis.

In many instances locally advanced ulcerated carcinomas can be diagnosed with a small wedge of skin excised from the infiltrated cutaneous margin. As this area may already be anesthetic, the brief procedure can often be done without anesthesia.

Table 6–18. STEROID RECEPTORS FROM MASTECTOMY SPECIMENS*

fmol/mg Protein	ER Biopsy	ER Mastectomy	PR Biopsy	PR Mastectomy
<3	3	3	8	10
3–20	8	5	3	2
>10	10	13	6	5

*This represents a series of cases in which estrogen receptors (ER) and progesterone receptors (PR) were measured on cancers both before and after mastectomy. Estrogen receptor concentrations did not decline after the period of warm ischemia during mastectomy and were, therefore, valid for clinical purposes. However, two of nine tumors that were positive for progesterone receptors prior to mastectomy became negative afterward, and this determination may be less satisfactory if obtained from a mastectomy specimen.

Data from Leight et al. (1984).

BIOPSY OF NONPALPABLE LESIONS

With current emphasis on early diagnosis using screening mammography, the surgeon is increasingly confronted with the problem of biopsying nonpalpable lesions, usually suspicious small densities, architectural distortions, or clustered microcalcifications. These cases represent the optimum in early diagnosis, but without a mass to guide the surgeon, accurately locating and removing the site of suspected pathology without undue morbidity may be a problem. Quadrant excisions are not necessary (Schwartz and Siegelman, 1966). A number of useful techniques are now available for precise localizations (Hall and Frank, 1979; Hoehn et al., 1982; Feig, 1983). The two most widely used are the spot method and the fine hooked wire. Both require teamwork between the radiologist, the surgeon, and the pathologist. The simplest is the spot method (Simon et al., 1972), which this author uses as follows: The

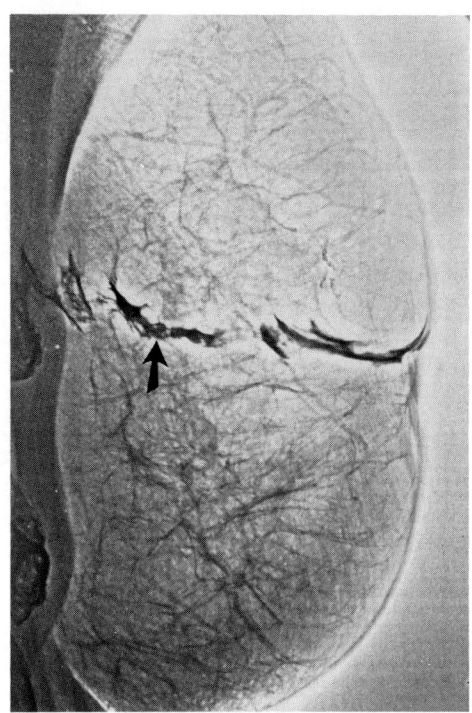

Figure 6–34. Localization of microcalcifications using the spot technique. In this case the streak of radiopaque marking fluid overlies and obscures the suspicious cluster of microcalcifications (arrow).

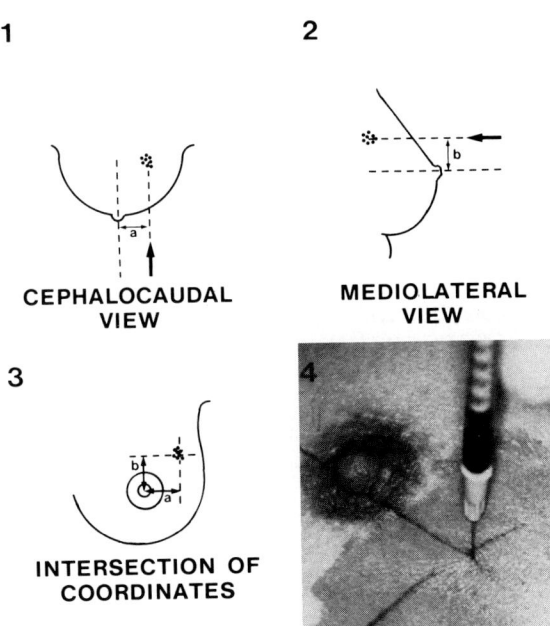

Figure 6–33. The spot technique described in the text is a useful method for localizing nonpalpable lesions; a mixture of ethiodol and a vital blue dye is injected at the junction of coordinates taken from mediolateral and cephalocaudal mammographic views. A mammogram then establishes the relation of the spot of contrast to the lesion, and the visible dye subsequently provides a reference point. (After Feig, S. A.: Localization of clinically occult breast lesions. Radiol. Clin. North Am., 21:155, 1983. Used with permission.)

lateral distance from the midnipple to the site of suspicion is measured and recorded in both the mediolateral and cephalocaudal mammograms. Shortly prior to biopsy the patient is taken to the mammography suite, and with the breast positioned in turn as it was for each of the two views, the vertical and horizontal axes are marked on the skin. Their intersection marks the approximate site of the lesion. The patient is then placed in the supine position as she would be for biopsy, and at the intersection of the coordinates 0.2 to 0.5 ml of a half-and-half solution of concentrated (37 per cent) radiopaque contrast solution (Ethiodol) and Evans blue dye is injected vertically into the breast using a tuberculin syringe and a 1.5 inch, 25 gauge needle (Fig. 6–33). The injection is continuous as the needle is withdrawn, and at its point of exit a small blue spot is left on the skin for reference. The mammogram is repeated immediately, and the position of the streak of radiopaque Ethiodol is noted with respect to the target site (Fig. 6–34). At the time of biopsy, the incision is made directly over the probable site of the lesion, and the Evans blue dye provides a visible reference for the location of the target. This permits accurate removal with sacrifice of only a modest amount of tissue. Generally no more than a 2.0 to 2.5 cm diameter divot of breast tissue is removed. The procedure can be performed under local anesthesia.

The hooked wire technique introduced by Funderburk and Flax (1976) is somewhat more complicated. In the mammography suite, similar measurements are made from the previous mammograms, and a needle is inserted into the breast at the approximate site of the lesion. By alternately repeating the mammogram and adjusting the needle, its tip is brought to lie in, or within 1 cm of, the target. A fine hooked wire is then inserted through the needle so that its barbed point is lodged at the site of interest, and the needle is removed. The wire remains as a guide for the surgeon, and the tissues at its point are removed (Fig. 6–35). It is a wise precaution to inject a drop of Evans blue dye through the guide needle prior to inserting the wire so that if the wire is dislodged prematurely during biopsy the target is still stained for identification. A more recent technique is to image the breast in the craniocaudal view under a special transparent grid.

The lesion will be visualized under one of the perforations, and the needle is inserted through the perforation, accurately impaling the lesion. The needle tip can be adjusted in the medial-lateral view to more closely approximate the target. This technique avoids accidentally penetrating the pleural space.

When clustered calcifications constitute the target tissues, an immediate specimen radiograph is obtained to ascertain that they were removed before closing the incision (Rosen et al., 1974; Bauermeister, 1975). If they are not in the initial specimen, more tissue is removed and radiographed. The specimen radiograph is an essential part of this technique, as it not only confirms that an accurate biopsy was performed but also enables the radiographer to pinpoint the suspicious calcifications for the pathologist's examination. As the lesions are small and the important diagnostic material is scant, frozen sections are generally not performed for fear of losing or damaging it. Saving all of the material for paraffin sections is customary. If the target is a density or small mass, a specimen radiograph is not helpful, and the surgeon's only recourse is to slice the specimen at the operating table to determine grossly whether it contains a lesion corresponding to that seen on mammography. In all instances in which no cancer is found, a mammogram is repeated in 3 to 4 months to ascertain that the tissue in question was in fact removed and to provide a new baseline for future reference.

BIOPSY OF THE DISCHARGING DUCT

Cytologic examination of fluid from a discharging duct is usually accurate when positive, but it does not replace a tissue diagnosis; false negative results are frequent and false positive findings occasionally occur. The former totaled 16.4 per cent and the latter 2 per cent in Leis' 560 cases of nipple discharge (Leis et al., 1985). As a consequence, diagnosis cannot be based on the cytology of nipple discharge, but when positive results are found, the cause must be pursued.

When a mass is associated with a discharging duct, the probability of finding cancer is increased and the mass is removed for diagnosis. In the absence of a mass, removal of the lesion causing the discharge requires a microductectomy. Its accuracy can be improved by using vital dye and a lacrimal probe. Local anes-

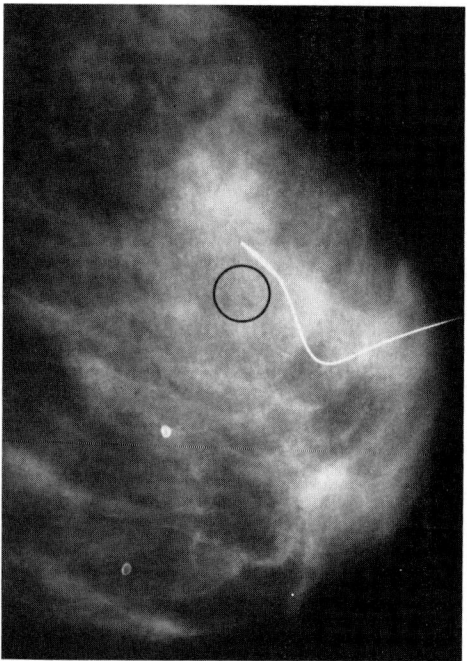

Figure 6–35. Hooked wire in place adjacent to clustered microcalcifications (circle) to guide biopsy. The wire and guide needle is available commercially from Frank Breast Biopsy Guide, Ransack Corporation, Avon, Massachusetts.

Table 6–19. NIPPLE DISCHARGE WITHOUT MASS OR ABNORMAL MAMMOGRAM—PERSONAL SERIES

Number of cases	12
Ages	25–66 (median, 50)
Gross blood	10 (83%)
Spontaneous	9 (75%)
Atypical cytology	1/4
Diagnoses	
Ductal carcinoma in situ	1 (8%)
Chronic cystic mastopathy	1
Duct ectasia	2
Epithelial hyperplasia	2
Ductal papilloma	6 (50%)

thesia is adequate, and the operation is performed through a periareolar incision. Prior to the incision, the discharging duct is cannulated with a plastic catheter (a 22 gauge angiocatheter serves well), and Evans blue dye is injected. This will fill the ductal system and stain the abnormal tissues. The removal of all stained tissues ensures removal of the lesion. The second aid is a lacrimal probe in the discharging duct, which serves to identify it. A flap of areola is elevated until the discharging duct is identified, and the entire ductal system from the base of the nipple to its periphery is removed. Unless cancer is obvious, diagnosis with permanent paraffin sections is preferred, as determining the benign or malignant nature of papillary lesions on frozen section can be difficult. In the absence of a mass, Chaudary and colleagues (1982) found cancer in 5.9 per cent of 254 explorations. In most instances, the lesion was a duct papilloma (45 per cent), ductal ectasia (31 per cent), or fibrocystic disease (9.6 per cent). In 22 cases in which no lesion was found, two patients later developed carcinoma in the breast, a figure similar to 2 to 7 per cent in other series. Thus, when a lesion is not found it may have been missed, and these patients should remain under continuing surveillance. Cancer was found in 8 per cent of a small personal series in which discharge was unassociated with a mass or an abnormality on mammograms (Table 6–19).

RESULTS OF BREAST BIOPSIES

The indications for and results of a personal series of 448 consecutive breast biopsies are shown in Table 6–20. A palpable mass was the most frequent indication (72 per cent), but nonpalpable lesions accounted for one quarter of the total. Among the latter, clustered microcalcifications predominated (29 per cent). Miscellaneous indications included nipple changes and breast edema.

Overall, almost one third (29 per cent) of the biopsies resulted in a diagnosis of cancer, as did slightly more than one third of biopsies for masses. Purely mammographic lesions were cancers in 18 per cent of cases, comparable with the 11 to 29 per cent reported in the literature (Cheek and Sears, 1978; Blichert-Toft et al., 1982; Lefor et al., 1984; Nehme and Macksood, 1984). The most ominous finding was a density that contained fine microcalcifications. Microcalcifications without a mass proved to be cancer in 21 per cent of the cases; other reports give percentages that range from 17 to 33 per cent in this circumstance (Egan et al., 1980; Roses et al., 1980; Powell et al., 1983). Ordinarily five or more fine calcium specks within a 0.5 cm × 0.5 cm area were

Table 6–20. CONSECUTIVE BREAST BIOPSIES*

Indication	Total	Cancer
Palpable mass	322 (72%)	108 (34%)
Mammogram only	110 (25%)	20† (18%)
Microcalcifications	57	12 (21%)
Density	40	2 (5%)
Microcalcifications + Density	13	6 (46%)
Nipple discharge only	12 (3%)	1 (8%)
Miscellaneous	4 (<1%)	3 (75%)
Total	448	132 (29%)

*This table shows the results of a personal series of 448 consecutive breast biopsies for various indications. Subclinical lesions found only on mammography accounted for 25 per cent of the cases. Overall, 29 per cent of the biopsies were diagnostic of cancer. Palpable masses proved to be cancer in 34 per cent and mammographic lesions in 18 per cent. Nipple discharge unaccompanied by mass or abnormal mammogram was caused by cancer in 8 per cent. Miscellaneous indications included nipple lesions and signs of inflammatory cancer.
†15% in situ

160 6 • Diagnosis

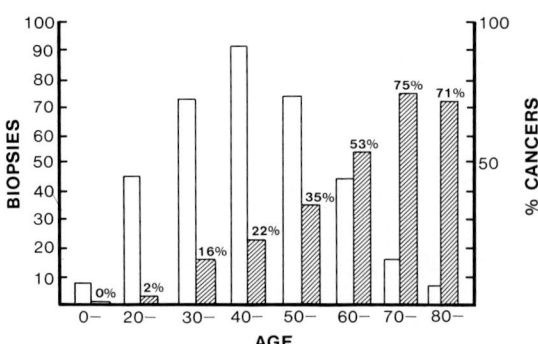

Figure 6–36. Although most breast biopsies involve patients between the ages of 30 and 60 years, the proportion of biopsies that yield cancer increase progressively with age. Open columns indicate the number of biopsies; the shaded columns indicate the percentages of cancers.

considered suspicious, but as few as three specks were biopsied, and one such case proved to be cancer. Clinically occult masses or densities without calcifications often proved to be fibroadenomas or intramammary lymph nodes and had a low rate of malignancy (5 per cent). Mammographically discovered cancers have a good prognosis; 15 per cent in this series were in situ cancers, three times higher than with breast cancers overall. In the experience of others, this frequency ranges widely, from 9 per cent to 40 per cent, and only 10 per cent of nonpalpable cancers are associated

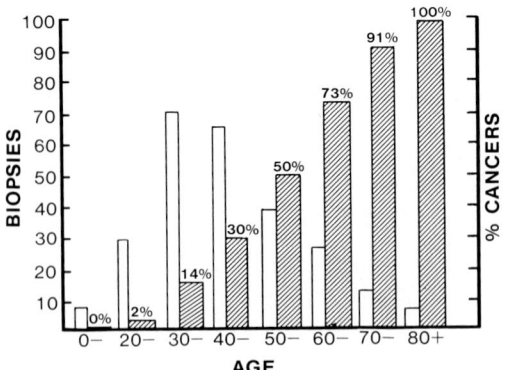

Figure 6–37. The results of a personal series of breast biopsies for palpable masses show a direct correlation between age and the probability of cancer. Open columns indicate the number of biopsies; the shaded columns indicate the percentage of cancers.

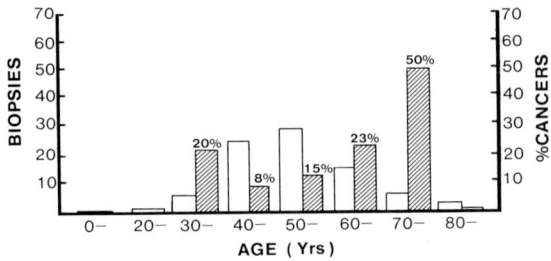

Figure 6–38. Eighty-one consecutive breast biopsies for subclinical mammographic lesions demonstrate a direct relationship between age and the probability of cancer, although one that is not as strong as for palpable masses.

with axillary nodal metastases at the time of treatment. As seen in Figure 6–36, the probability of a biopsy diagnosis of cancer increases with age. Under age 30 years, the frequency was less than 2 per cent; for women over 70 years old, three fourths of biopsies revealed cancer. The relationship of risk with age is even more impressive for palpable masses (Fig. 6-37), of which more than 90 per cent were cancer in women over 70 years of age. For purely mammographic lesions (Fig. 6–38), advancing age was still related to increasing probability of cancer, but not as strongly as with palpable masses. Noteworthy is that 23 per cent of the cancers were in women less than 50 years old.

Early Diagnosis

The short-term surveys on Trends in Cancer Management in the United States by the Commission on Cancer of the American College of Surgeons provide a perspective of the current status of breast cancer discovery (Nemoto et al., 1982). The survey of 12,315 breast cancer patients nationwide showed that, as stated earlier, 73 per cent of all cancers were found by the patient, 23 per cent by physicians, and 4 per cent by mammography. Younger women were more likely to discover their cancers than were older women. Mammography made its greatest impact on patients between the ages of 50 and 74 years, although it almost equaled other methods of discovery for women of ages 45 to 49 years. In this survey, mammography was considered underutilized for black patients. When the diagnosis after first symptoms was delayed more than 3 months, cancers tended to be larger and more aggressive. Cancers discovered by mammography were less likely to have metastases in the axillary lymph nodes. Unfortunately, this survey did not contain end result data or controls, and conclusions can only be inferred by interpretation of the descriptive data in the survey. The cases were inadequately stratified by known prognostic determinants for this to be meaningful. Trends in patterns of practice do not establish that accumulative disease morbidity and mortality rates are being altered by these trends, and caution has to be exercised in interpreting their public health significance. An update of this survey (Wilson et al., 1984) showed a continuation of the trends.

Mammary carcinomas do progress with time. The primary tumor enlarges; adjacent tissues such as the skin, pectoral muscles, and ultimately the chest wall are invaded; and at some point distant metastases appear, converting what was a local process into a disseminated and incurable disease. Spontaneous regression of mammary carcinoma is rare and temporary (Lewison, 1976).

The duration of symptoms might reasonably be expected to correlate with the signs of progression, and patients who bring themselves to medical attention promptly might be expected to have earlier signs and to have better case rates than those who delay. Yet it is not possible to demonstrate a strong relationship between the duration of symptoms and curability (Table 6–21). This may reflect the varied biologic behavior of cancers and the human reaction to them. That is to say, cancers that grow rapidly, produce alarming symptoms, and swiftly become incurable cause patients to seek early consultation, whereas more indolent cancers are less alarming to the patient and remain curable even when consultation is delayed for many months. Indeed, some reviews have shown an improved prognosis with increasing delay, probably a function of selection (Bloom, 1950).

Nevertheless, large tumor size, the presence of metastases in axillary lymph nodes, and advanced clinical stage are all associated with a poor prognosis, and each becomes more prevalent with increasing duration of the symptomatic period before treatment. Bloom (1965) demonstrated a correlation between advancement of disease and duration of symptoms, with higher grade tumors progressing most quickly. The EFSCH data demonstrated a small increase in tumor diameter and an increase in the percentage of patients with histologically involved axillary lymph nodes as

Table 6–21. DURATION OF SYMPTOMS CORRELATED WITH 5 YEAR SURVIVAL AFTER RADICAL MASTECTOMY (700 CASES AT EFSCH, 1940 TO JUNE 1958)

Duration of Symptoms (mo)	Total Number of Cases	5 Year Survivors	
		Number	Per Cent of Total*
1	58	38	65.0
2	65	35	53.8
3	68	38	55.9
4	49	30	61.2
5	33	13	39.4
6	67	38	56.7
7	21	8	38.1
8	30	16	53.3
9	14	8	57.1
10–12	92	40	43.5
13–24	102	58	56.9
25–36	33	15	45.5
37–48	23	16	69.6
49 and up	45	24	53.3

*A chi square test fails to show a significant difference in 5 year survival for the 14 categories. Chi square = 17.2763, df = 13, p > 0.20.

Note: The duration of symptoms before mastectomy is correlated with the proportion of 5 year survivors afterwards. No distinct association can be shown between a brief duration of symptoms and favorable 5 year survival.

the duration of symptoms lengthened (Table 6–22). The same was observed at Memorial Hospital (New York City) by Pilipshen and colleagues (1984), who found, however, that delay had no influence on nodal involvement if tumor size was constant.

Despite the evidence to support prompt consultation, delay is too often the rule. Contributing to delay are ignorance of the signs of breast cancer, lack of money for treatment, the absence of pain, hope that the mass would "go away," and fear that the mass might be cancer (Gold, 1964; Lynch and Krush, 1969). Unfortunately, physicians sometimes contribute to further delay by "watching" breast masses, by unjustified confidence in their ability to distinguish clinically between benign and malignant masses, or by too much confidence in a "negative" mammogram.

This situation can be improved through educational programs. Women need to be instructed on self-examination of the breast and perform it at least once a month. Too often they neglect this practice or are ignorant of the proper technique. Women have demonstrated ability to find masses 1 cm in diameter and sometimes smaller in their breasts. At this size, only 28.5 per cent of carcinomas have

Table 6–22. DURATION OF SYMPTOMS VERSUS SIGNS OF MAMMARY CARCINOMA (700 CASES OF MAMMARY CARCINOMA TREATED WITH RADICAL MASTECTOMY AT EFSCH, 1940 TO 1958)*

Duration of Symptoms (mo)	Total Number of Cases	Median Tumor Diameter (cm)	With Positive Axillary Nodes		With Ulceration		With Edema		With Erythema	
			Number	Per Cent†	Number	Per Cent	Number	Per Cent	Number	Per Cent
1–2	123	3.0	56	46	4		9		8	
3–4	117	3.0	51	44	4		9		13	
5–6	100	3.5	57	57	3	6	12	10	8	9
7–8	51	3.5	31	61	8		10		9	
9–10	26	3.5	15	58	0		1		3	
11–12	80	3.5	54	68	9	—	10	—	6	—
13–18	29	3.1	17	59	5		2		3	
19–24	73	4.0	45	62	22		12		14	16
25–36	33	4.5	26	79	7	23	4	14	4	
37–48	23	4.1	16	70	4		5		5	
49 and up	45	3.5	29	64	8		5		7	

*The percentage of patients with metastases to axillary nodes and with grave skin signs increases with increasing duration of symptoms.

†A chi square test indicates that the percentage of patients with axillary node metastases increases significantly with lengthening duration of symptoms. Chi square = > 47.9, $p < 0.001$.

Note: The duration of symptoms is correlated with signs of tumor progression. As the duration of symptoms increases, median tumor diameter enlarges and the frequency of nodal metastasis increases, as does the frequency of ulceration, edema, and erythema.

developed axillary metastases (see Fig. 12–11). Second, the public should know that the majority of breast cancers can be cured if detected early and treated properly. At least 95 per cent of preinvasive and minimally invasive breast cancers are cured (Peters et al., 1977). This knowledge can eliminate unjustified despair associated with the diagnosis of cancer and promote early consultation. Physicians must appreciate that any sign of disease in the breast is potentially attributable to cancer until proved otherwise, and they must act accordingly.

Substantial progress against mammary cancer can be made by ceasing to wait for symptoms to appear. The capacity to detect breast cancers while still asymptomatic through regular physical and mammographic examinations has been amply demonstrated by the Breast Cancer Detection Demonstration Projects (BCDDP) screening experience, in which 42 per cent of cancers were found by mammography alone; 32.4 per cent of the 3557 cancers were in situ or less than 1 cm in diameter, and only 20 per cent were associated with nodal metastases (Baker, 1982). The high frequency of preinvasiveness and the low frequency of nodal metastases characteristic of these occult cancers promise an excellent prognosis.

REFERENCES

Abele, J. S., Miller, T. R., Goodson, W. H., III, et al.: Fine-needle aspiration of palpable breast masses. A program for staged implementation. Arch. Surg., 118:859, 1983.

Abramson, D. J.: A clinical evaluation of aspiration of cysts of the breast. Surg. Gynecol. Obstet., 139:531, 1974.

Abramson, D. J.: Delayed mastectomy after outpatient breast biopsy. Long-term survival study. Am. J. Surg., 132:596, 1976.

Adashi, E. Y.: Diagnostic evaluation of hyperprolactinemia. Resident & Staff Physician, 31:15PC, 1985.

Anguist, K. A., Holmlund, D., Liliequist, B., et al.: Diaphanoscopy and diaphanography for breast cancer detection in clinical practice. Acta Chir. Scand., 147:231, 1981.

Ashikari, R., Rosen, P. P., Urban, J. A., et al.: Breast cancer presenting as an axillary mass. Ann. Surg., 183:415, 1976.

Baker, L. H.: Breast cancer detection demonstration project: Five-year summary report. CA 32:194, 1982.

Barber, K. W., Jr., Dockerty, M. B., and Clagett, O. T.: Inflammatory carcinoma of the breast. Surg. Gynecol. Obstet., 112:406, 1961.

Bauermeister, D. E.: The pros and cons of routine specimen radiography. *In* Gallager, H. S. (Ed.), Early Breast Cancer Detection and Treatment. New York, John Wiley & Sons, 1975, p. 159.

Bell, C. A.: A system of operative surgery, 1814, ii, p. 136; cited in Lee and Tannenbaum (1924).

Bell, D. A., Hajdu, S. I., Urban, J. A., et al.: Role of aspiration cytology in the diagnosis and management of mammary lesions in office practice. Cancer, 51:1182, 1983.

Bennett, S. E., Lawrence, R. S., Fleischmann, K. H., et al.: Profile of women practicing breast self-examination. J.A.M.A., 249:488, 1983.

Bertario, L., Reduzzi, D., Piromalli, D., et al.: Outpatient biopsy of breast cancer. Influence on survival. Ann. Surg., 201:64, 1985.

Blamey, R. W.: The diagnosis and prognosis of breast cancer. Practitioner, 226:1385, 1982.

Blichert-Toft, M., Dyreborg, U., Bogh, L., et al.: Nonpalpable breast lesions: Mammographic wire-guided biopsy and radiologic-histologic correlation. World J. Surg., 6:119, 1982.

Bloom, H. J.: Further studies on prognosis of breast carcinoma. Br. J. Cancer, 4:347, 1950.

Bloom, H. J.: The influence of delay on the natural history and prognosis of breast cancer: A study of cases followed for five to twenty years. Br. J. Cancer, 19:228, 1965.

Boyd, N. F., Sutherland, H. J., Fish, E. B., et al.: Prospective evaluation of physical examination of the breast. Am. J. Surg., 142:331, 1981.

Brascho, D. J.: Ultrasound of the female breast; current state of the art. Ala. J. Med. Sci., 19:83, 1982.

Bryant, T.: Diseases of the Breast. Woods Medical and Surgical Monographs, Vol. 4. 1889, pp. 35–322.

Busk, T., and Clemmesen, J.: The frequencies of left-sided and right-sided breast cancer. Br. J. Cancer, 1:345, 1947.

Byrd, B. F., Jr., and Stephenson, S. E., Jr.: Inflamed or inflammatory carcinoma of the breast. Am. Surg., 28:303, 1962.

Cancer Letter, Vol. 3 (43), October 28, 1977. J. D. Boyd (Ed.).

Chang, C. H. J., Nesbit, D. E., Fisher, D. R., et al.: Computed tomographic mammography using a conventional body scanner. Am. J. Radiol., 38:553, 1982.

Charlson, M. E.: Delay in the treatment of carcinoma of the breast. Surg. Gynecol. Obstet., 160:393, 1985.

Chaudary, M. A., Millis, R. R., Davies, G. C., et al.: Nipple discharge. The diagnostic value of testing for occult blood. Ann. Surg., 196:651, 1982.

Cheek, J. H., and Sears, A. D.: Results of breast biopsies for mammographic findings. Am. J. Surg., 136:726, 1978.

Cole, W. H.: The mechanisms of spread of cancer. Surg. Gynecol. Obstet., 137:853, 1973.

Copeland, E. M., and McBride, C. M.: Axillary metastases from unknown primary sites. Ann. Surg., 178:25, 1973.

Copeland, M. M., and Higgins, T. G.: Significance of discharge from the nipple in nonpuerperal mammary conditions. Ann. Surg., 151:638, 1960.

Cutler, M.: Transillumination as an aid in the diagnosis of breast lesions, with special reference to its value in cases of bleeding nipple. Surg. Gynecol. Obstet., 48:721, 1929.

Czernobilsky, B.: Intracystic carcinoma of the female breast. Surg. Gynecol. Obstet., 124:1, 1967.

Darrier, M. J.: La maladie de Paget, du mamelon. Soc. de Biol Ser., 9, 1:294, 1889.

Devitt, J. E.: Management of nipple discharge by clinical findings. Am. J. Surg., 149:789, 1985.

Donnelly, B. A.: Primary "inflammatory" carcinoma of the breast. A report of five cases and a review of the literature. Ann. Surg., 128:918, 1948.

Doust, B. D., Milbrath, J. R., and Doust, V. L.: CT scanning of the breast using a conventional CT scanner. J. Comput. Tomog., 5:296, 1981.

Egan, R. L.: Mammography. 2nd Ed. Springfield, Ill., Charles C Thomas, 1972, p. 5.

Egan, R. L., McSweeney, M. B., and Sewell, C. W.: Intramammary calcifications without an associated mass in benign and malignant diseases. Radiology, 137:1, 1980.

Egeli, R. A., and Urban, J. A.: Mammography in symptomatic women 50 years of age and under, and those over 50. Cancer, 43:878, 1979.

Ellis, D. L., and Teitelbaum, S. L.: Inflammatory carcinoma of the breast. A pathologic definition. Cancer, 33:1045, 1974.

Ewing, J.: Biopsy in mammary cacner. Mil. Surgeon, 72:322, 1933.

Feig, S. A.: Localization of clinically occult breast lesions. Radiol. Clin. North Am., 21:155, 1983.

Feldman, J. G., Carter, A. C., Nicastri, A. D., et al.: Breast self-examination, relationship to stage of breast cancer at diagnosis. Cancer, 47:2740, 1981.

Feuerman, L., Attie, J. N., and Rosenberg, B.: Carcinoma in axillary lymph nodes as an indicator of breast cancer. Surg. Gynecol. Obstet., 114:5, 1962.

Fiessinger, N., and Mathieu, P.: Thrombo-phlébites des veines de la paroi thoracoabdominale. Bull. Mem. Soc. Med. Hop. Paris, 46:352, 1922.

Fisher, B.: Reappraisal of breast biopsy prompted by the use of lumpectomy. Surgical strategy. J.A.M.A., 253:3585, 1985.

Fisher, E. R., Sass, R., and Fisher, B.: Biologic considerations regarding the one and two step procedures in the management of patients with invasive carcinoma of the breast. Surg. Gynecol. Obstet., 161:245, 1985.

Fletcher, S. W., O'Malley, M. S., and Bunce, L. A.: Physicians' abilities to detect lumps in silicone breast models. J.A.M.A., 253:2224, 1985.

Foster, R. S., Jr.: Core-cutting needle biopsy for the diagnosis of breast cancer. Am. J. Surg., 143:622, 1982.

Foster, R. S., Jr., and Costanza, M. C.: Breast self-examination practices and breast cancer survival. Cancer, 53:999, 1984.

Foster, R. S., Jr., Lang, S. P., Costanza, M. C., et al.: Breast self-examination practices and breast-cancer stage. N. Engl. J. Med., 299:265, 1978.

Frable, M. A., and Frable, W. J.: Fine-needle aspiration biopsy revisited. Laryngoscope, 92:1414, 1982.

Franzen, S., and Stenkvist, B.: Diagnosis of granular cell myoblastoma by fine-needle aspiration biopsy. Acta Pathol. Microbiol. Scand., 72:391, 1968.

Funderburk, W. S., and Flax, R. L.: Localization of nonpalpable carcinoma of the breast utilizing xeromammography: Technique A. Breast, 2:28, 1976.

Gatchell, F. G., Dockerty, M. B., and Clagett, O. T.: Intracystic carcinoma of the breast. Surg. Gynecol. Obstet., 106:347, 1958.

Gershon-Cohen, J., Yiu, L. S., and Berger S.M.: The diagnostic importance of calcareous patterns in roentgenography of breast cancer. AJR, 88:1117, 1962.

Girolamo, R. F., and Leis, H. P., Jr.: Diaphanography: A fourth dimension in the diagnosis of breast disease? Breast, 8:16, 1982.

Gold, M. A.: Causes of patients' delay in diseases of the breast. Cancer, 17:564, 1964.

Goode, J. V., McNeill, J. P., and Gordon, C. E.: Routine aspiration of discrete breast cysts. Report of 267 breast aspirations. Arch. Surg., 70:686, 1955.

Grant, C. S., Goeliner, J. R., Welch, J. S., et al.: Fine-needle aspiration of the breast. Mayo Clin. Proc., 61:377, 1986.

Greenwood, S. M., and Minkowitz, S.: Paget's disease in metastatic breast carcinoma. Arch. Dermatol., *104*:312, 1971.

Haagensen, C. D.: Diseases of the Breast. Philadelphia, W.B. Saunders, 1971, p. 74.

Haagensen, C. D.: Diseases of the Breast. Philadelphia, W.B. Saunders, 1971, p. 501.

Haagensen, C. D., Bodian, C., and Haagensen, D. E., Jr.: Breast Carcinoma. Risk and Detection. Philadelphia, W.B. Saunders, 1981, p. 63.

Haagensen, D. E., Jr.: Tumor markers for breast carcinoma. Clin. Lab. Med., *2*:543, 1982.

Habbema, J. D. F., Van Oortarssem, G. J., Van Putten, D. J., et al.: Age-specific reduction in breast cancer mortality by screening: An analysis of the results of the Health Insurance Plan of Greater New York study. JNCI, *77*:317, 1986.

Hall, D. C., Goldstein, M. K., and Stein, G. H.: Progress in manual breast examination. Cancer, *40*:364, 1977.

Hall, F. M., and Frank, H. A.: Preoperative localization of nonpalpable breast lesions. Am. J. Roentgenol., *132*:101, 1979.

Halsted, W. S.: A clinical and histological study of certain adenocarcinomata of the breast. Ann. Surg., *28*:557, 1898.

Halsted, W. S.: The results of radical operations for the cure of carcinoma of the breast. Ann. Surg., *46*:1, 1907.

Hatteland, K., and Kluge, T.: Mondor's disease, a subcutaneous form of periarteritis nodosa? Acta Chir. Scand., *129*:67, 1965.

Helwig, E. B., and Graham, J. H.: Anogenital (extramammary) Paget's disease. Cancer, *16*:387, 1963.

Hicken, N. F.: Mastectomy: A clinical pathologic study demonstrating why most mastectomies result in incomplete removal of the mammary gland. Arch. Surg., *40*:6, 1940.

High, R. M., and Watne, A. L.: The axillary mass in occult breast carcinoma. Case reports and overview. Am. Surg., *50*:630, 1985.

Hoehn, J. L., Hardacre, J. M., Swanson, M. K., et al.: Localization of occult breast lesions. Cancer, *49*:1142, 1982.

Isard, H. J., Becker, W., Shilo, R., et al.: Breast thermography after four years and 10,000 studies. AJR, *115(4)*:811, 1972.

Jackson, P. P., and Pitts, H. H.: Biopsy with delayed radical mastectomy for carcinoma of the breast. Am. J. Surg., *98*:184, 1959.

Jacobacus, H. C.: Paget's disease und sein Verhaltnis zum Milchdrusenkarzinom. Virchows Arch. Anat., *178*:124, 1904.

Kagali, V. A.: The role and limitations of frozen section diagnosis of a palpable mass in the breast. Surg. Gynecol. Obstet., *156*:168, 1983.

Kaplan, I. W., and Reinstine, H.: Occult carcinoma of the breast. Am. Surg., *20*:575, 1954.

Kaufman, M., Bider, D., and Weissberg, D.: Diagnosis of breast lesions by needle aspiration biopsy. Am. Surg., *49*:558, 1983.

Kawatsu, T., and Miki, T.: Triple extramammary Paget's disease. Arch. Dermatol., *104*:316, 1971.

Kemeny, M. M., Rivera, D. E., Terz, J. J., and Benfield, J. R.: Occult primary adenocarcinoma with axillary metastases. Am. J. Surg., *152*:43, 1986.

Kher, A. V., Marwar, A. W., and Raichur, B. S.: Evaluation of fine needle aspiration biopsy in the diagnosis of breast lesions. Indian J. Pathol. Microbiol., *24*:100, 1981.

King, B. J., and King, J. R. N.: Cholesteric plate thermography in breast disease: Correlation with biopsy data. Breast, *8*:13, 1982.

Kline, T. S., Joshi, L. P., and Neal, H. S.: Fine-needle aspiration of the breast: Diagnoses and pitfalls. A review of 3545 cases. Cancer, *44*:1458, 1979.

Knapp, R. W., and Mullen, J. T.: Triage for the breast biopsy. Am. J. Surg., *131*:626, 1976.

Kobayashi, T.: Ultrasonic detection of breast cancer. Clin. Obstet. Gynecol., *25*:409, 1982.

Kraissl, C. J.: The selection of appropriate lines for elective surgical incisions. Plastic Reconstr. Surg., *8*:1, 1951.

Lagios, M. D., Gates, E. A., Westdahl, P. R., et al.: A guide to the frequency of nipple involvement in breast cancer. A study of 149 consecutive mastectomies using a serial subgross and correlated radiographic technique. Am. J. Surg., *138*:135, 1979.

Lannin, D. R., Silverman, J. F., Pores, W. J., et al.: Cost-effectiveness of fine needle biopsy of the breast. Ann. Surg., *203*:474, 1986.

Lawson, R. N.: Implications of surface temperatures in the diagnosis of breast cancer. Can. Med. Assoc. J., *75*:309, 1956.

Leborgne, R. A.: The Breast in Roentgen Diagnosis. Montevideo, Uruguay, Impresora Uruguaya S.A. Juncal 1511, 1953.

Lee, B. J., and Tannenbaum, N. E.: Inflammatory carcinoma of the breast. Surg. Gynecol. Obstet., *39*:580, 1924.

Lefor, A. T., Numann, P. J., and Levinsohn, E. M.: Needle localization of occult breast lesions. Am. J. Surg., *148*:270, 1984.

Leight, G. S., Jr., Wells, S. A., Jr., and McCarty, K. S., Jr.: Sex steroid receptor concentration in breast carcinoma tissue: Effect of devascularization during mastectomy. Surgery, *95*:256, 1984.

Leis, H. P., Jr., Cammarata, A., and LaRaja, R. D.: Nipple discharge: Significance and treatment. Breast, *11*:6, 1985.

Lesnick, G. J.: Detection of breast cancer in young women. JAMA, *237*:967, 1977.

Lewis, J. D., Milbrath, J. R., Shaffer, K. A., et al.: Which breast to biopsy: An expanding dilemma. Ann. Surg., *184*:253, 1976.

Lewison, E. F.: Spontaneous regression of breast cancer. *In* Conference on Spontaneous Regression of Cancer. National Cancer Institute Monograph 44, November 1976.

Lucas, F. V., and Perez-Mesa, C.: Inflammatory carcinoma of the breast. Cancer, *41*:1595, 1978.

Lynch, H. T., and Krush, A. J.: Breast carcinoma and delay in treatment. Surg. Gynecol. Obstet., *128*:1027, 1969.

Malberger, E., Toledano, C., Barzilai A., et al.: The decisive role of fine needle aspiration cytology in the preoperative work-up of breast cancer. Isr. J. Med. Sci., *17*:899, 1981.

Manual for Staging of Cancer 1983. American Joint Committee for Cancer Staging and End-Results Reporting, 1983, pp. 127–133.

Maturo, V. G., Zusmer, N. R., Gilso, A. J., et al.: Ultrasonic appearance of mammary carcinoma with a dedicated whole-breast scanner. Radiology, *142*:713, 1982.

McClow, M. V., and Williams, A. C.: Mammographic examinations (4030): Ten-year clinical experience in a community medical center. Ann. Surg., *177*:616, 1973.

McSwain, G. R., Valicenti, J. F., Jr., and O'Brien, P. H.: Surg. Gynecol. Obstet., 146:921, 1978.

McSweeney, M. B., and Murphy, C. H.: Whole-breast sonography. Radiol. Clin. North Am., 23:157, 1985.

Meyerowitz, B. R.: Drill biopsy confirmation of breast cancer. Arch. Surg., 111:826, 1976.

Milligan, D., Drife, J. O., and Short, R. V.: Changes in breast volume during normal menstrual cycle and after oral contraceptives. Br. Med. J., 29:494, 1975.

Mondor, H.: Tronculite sous-cutanée subaigue de la paroi thoracique anterolateral. Mam. Acad. Chir. Paris, 65:1271, 1939.

Murad, T. M., Contesso, G., and Mouriesse, H.: Nipple discharge from the breast. Ann. Surg., 195:259, 1982.

Nehme, A. E., and Macksood, M. J.: Nonpalpable breast lesions: Diagnosis and management. Breast, 16:19, 1984.

Nemoto, T., Natarajan, N., Smart, C. R., et al.: Patterns of breast cancer detection in the United States. J. Surg. Oncol., 21:183, 1982.

Nicolesco, S., and Velciu, V.: Tumors arising from heterotopic mammary rudiments. Gynec. Obstet., 67:241, 1968.

Niloff, P. H., and Sheiner, N. M.: False-negative mammograms in patients with breast cancer. Can. J. Surg., 24:50, 1981.

Nohrman, B. A.: Cancer of the breast. Clinical study of 1,042 cases treated at Radiumhemmet 1936-41. Acta Radiol., 77(Suppl):1, 1949.

Paget, J.: On disease of the mammary areola preceding cancer of the mammary gland. St. Barth. Hosp. Rep., 10:86, 1874.

Parikh, K. J., and Singer, J. A.: Pathologic ectopic breast tissue. Breast, 9:16, 1983.

Patel, J., Nemoto, T., Rosner, D., et al.: Axillary lymph node metastasis from an occult breast cancer. Cancer, 47:2923, 1981.

Peters, T. G., Donegan, W. L., and Burg, E. A.: Minimal breast cancer. A clinical appraisal. Ann. Surg., 186:704, 1977.

Pierce, E. H., Gray, H. K., and Dockerty, M. B.: Surgical significance of isolated axillary adenopathy. Ann. Surg., 145:104, 1957.

Pierce, E. H., Clagett, O. T., McDonald, J. R., et al.: Biopsy of the breast followed by delayed radical mastectomy. Surg. Gynecol. Obstet., 103:559, 1956.

Pilipshen, S. J., Gerardi, J., Bretsky, S., et al.: The significance of delay in treating patients with potentially curable breast cancer. Breast, 10:16, 1984.

Powell, R. W., McSweeney, M. B., and Wilson, C. E.: X-ray calcifications as the only basis for breast biopsy. Ann. Surg., 197:555, 1983.

Prechtel, K., and Hallbauer, M.: Ein beitrag zur Prognose des Mammakarzinoma nach zweizeitigem Operationsverfahren. Geburtshilfe. Frauenheilkd., 39:187, 1979.

Richards, G. J., Jr., and Lewison, E. F.: Inflammatory carcinoma of the breast. Surg. Gynecol. Obstet, 113:729, 1961.

Rimsten, A., Stenkvist, B., Johanson, H., et al.: The diagnostic accuracy of palpation and fine-needle biopsy and an evaluation of their combined use in the diagnosis of breast lesions. Report on a prospective study in 1244 women with symptoms. Ann. Surg., 182:1, 1975.

Roberts, J. G., Preece, P. E., Bolton, P. M., et al.: The "tru-cut" biopsy in breast cancer. Clin. Oncol. 1:297, 1975.

Rosemond, G. P., Maier, W. P., and Brobyn, T. J.: Needle aspiration of breast cysts. Surg. Gynecol. Obstet., 128:351, 1969.

Rosen, P. P.: Frozen section diagnosis of breast lesions. Recent experience with 556 consecutive biopsies. Ann. Surg., 187:17, 1978.

Rosen, P. P., Snyder, R. E., and Robbins, G.: Specimen radiography for nonpalpable breast lesions found by mammography: Procedures and results. Cancer, 34:2028, 1974.

Rosen, P., Hajda, S. I., Robbins, G., et al.: Diagnosis of carcinoma of the breast by aspiration biopsy. Surg. Gynecol. Obstet., 134:837, 1972.

Rosenthal, L. J.: Discrepant estrogen receptor protein levels according to surgical technique. Am. J. Surg., 138:680, 1979.

Roses, D. F., Harris, M. N., Gorstein, F., et al.: Biopsy for microcalcification detected by mammography. Surgery, 87:248, 1980.

Rosner, D., and Blaird, D.: What ultrasonography can tell in breast masses that mammography and physical examination cannot. J. Surg. Oncol., 28:308, 1985.

Rubin, E., Miller, V. E., Berland, L. L., et al.: Hand-held real-time breast sonography. AJR, 144:623, 1985.

Russ, J. E., Winchester, D. P., Scanlon, E. F., et al.: Cytolic findings of aspiration of tumors of the breast. Surg. Gynecol. Obstet., 146:407, 1978.

Salomon, A.: Beitrage zur Patholgie und Klinik der Mammacarcinoma. Arch. Klin. Chir., 101:573, 1913.

Saltzstein, E. C., Mann, R. W., Chua, T. Y., et al.: Outpatient breast biopsy. Arch. Surg., 109:287, 1974.

Saltzstein, S. L.: Clinically occult inflammatory carcinoma of the breast. Cancer, 34:382, 1974.

Salvadori, B., Fariselli, G., and Saccozzi, R.: Analysis of 100 cases of Paget's disease of the breast. Tumori, 62:529, 1976.

Sayago, C., and Sirebrenik, D.: Surgical biopsy as a disseminating factor in breast cancer. Acta Un. Int. Canc., 15:1161, 1959.

Schwartz, A. M., and Siegelman, S. S.: A technique for biopsy of nonpalpable breast tumors. Surg. Gynecol. Obstet., 123:1320, 1966.

Seidman, H.: Cancer of the Breast. American Cancer Society Professional Education Publication, New York, 1972, p. 28.

Seltzer, M. H., Perloff, L. J., Kelley, R. I., et al.: The significance of age in patients with nipple discharge. Surg. Gynecol. Obstet., 131:519, 1970.

Shabot, M. M., Goldberg, I. M., Schick, P., et al.: Aspiration cytology is superior to Tru-Cut needle biopsy in establishing the diagnosis of clinically suspicious breast masses. Ann. Surg., 196:122 1982.

Shapiro, S., Venet, W., Strax, P., et al.: Ten- to fourteen-year effect of screening on breast cancer mortality. JNCI, 69:349, 1982.

Sieninski, W., and Dabska, M.: Usefulness of drill biopsy in the diagnosis of breast tumors. Cancer, 38:2567, 1976.

Simon, N., Lesnick, G. J., Lerer, W. N., et al.: Roentgenographic localization of small lesions of the breast by the spot method. Surg. Gynecol. Obstet., 134:572, 1972.

Smith, D. J., Palin, W. E., Katch, V. L., and Bennett, J. E.: Breast volume and anthropomorphic measurements: Normal values. Plast. Reconstr. Surg., 78:331, 1986.

Smith, J., Payne, W. S., and Carney, J. A.: Involvement of the nipple and areola in carcinoma of the breast. Surg. Gynecol. Obstet., 143:546, 1976.

Sparkman, R. S.: Reliability of frozen sections in the diagnosis of breast lesions. Ann. Surg., 155:924, 1962.

Stein, H. D.: Ambulatory breast biopsies. The patient's choice. Am. Surg., 48:221, 1982.
Sterns, E. E., Curtis, A. C., Miller, S., et al.: Thermography in breast diagnosis. Cancer, 50:323, 1982.
Stone, A. M., Shenker, I. R., and McCarthy, K.: Adolescent breast masses. Am. J. Surg., 134:275, 1977.
Strax, P.: Results of mass screening for breast cancer in 50,000 examinations. Cancer, 37:30, 1976.
Tabar, L., Fagerberg, C. J. G., Gad, A., et al.: Reduction in mortality from breast cancer after mass screening with mammography. Lancet, 1:829, 1985.
Taylor, G. W., and Meltzer, A.: "Inflammatory carcinoma" of the breast. Am. J. Cancer, 33:33, 1938.
Tyzzer, E. E.: Factors in the production and growth of tumor metastases. J. Med. Res., 28:309, 1913.
Verbeek, A. L. M., Hendriks, J. H. C. L., Holland, R., et al.: Reduction of breast cancer mortality through mass screening with modern mammography: First results of the Nijmegan Project—1975–1981. Lancet 1:1222, 1984.
Vilcoq, J. R., Caloe, R., Ferme, F., et al.: Conservative treatment of axillary adenopathy due to probable subclinical breast cancer. Arch. Surg., 117:1136, 1982.
Vorherr, H.: Breast aspiration biopsy. Am. J. Obstet. Gynecol., 148:127, 1984.
Wanebo, H. J., Feldman, P. S., Wilhelm, M. C., et al.: Fine needle aspiration cytology in lieu of open biopsy in management of primary breast cancer. Ann. Surg., 199:569, 1984.
Wang, C. C., and Griscom, N. T.: Inflammatory carcinoma of the breast. Results following orthovoltage and supervoltage radiation therapy. Clin. Radiol., 15:167, 1964.
Warren, S. L.: Roentgenologic study of breast. AJR, 24:113, 1930.
Westbrook, K. C., and Gallager, H. S.: Breast carcinoma presenting as an axillary mass. Am. J. Surg., 122:607, 1971.
Wilson, L. B.: A method for the rapid preparation of fresh tissues for the microscope. J.A.M.A., 45:1737, 1905.
Wilson, R. E., Donegan, W. L., Mettlin, C., et al.: The 1982 national survey of carcinoma of the breast in the United States by the American College of Surgeons. Surg. Gynecol. Obstet., 159:309, 1984.
Wolfe, J. N.: Breast patterns as an index of risk for developing breast cancer. AJR, 126:1130, 1976.
Wolfe, J. N.: Analysis of 462 breast carcinomas. AJR, 121:846, 1974.
Yorkshire Breast Cancer Group: Symptoms and signs of operable breast cancer, 1976–1981. Br. J. Surg., 70:350, 1983.
Zajdela, A., Ghossein, N. A., Pillerow, J. P., et al.: The value of aspiration cytology in the diagnosis of breast cancer: Experience at the Foundation Curie. Cancer, 35:499, 1975.

CHAPTER 7

MYRON MOSKOWITZ

Breast Imaging

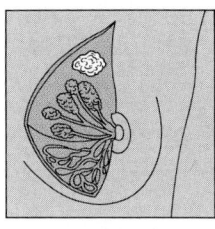

In the relatively recent past the role of breast imaging, specifically mammography, has been poorly understood and little appreciated by at least some members of the surgical community (Lesnick, 1977; Devitt, 1979; Mahoney et al., 1979). This has been provoked in part by failure of imaging specialists to acknowledge the limitations as well as the benefits of these ancillary clinical aids.

There is a clear-cut separation between using imaging techniques for diagnosis and using them for detection or screening (Moskowitz, 1979; Kopans et al., 1984a). In the former circumstance the clinician needs to answer a specific, clinical question. On the other hand, for screening the objective is to detect the suspected disease in an asymptomatic population when the cancer is small and most amenable to therapy. In this circumstance the test needs to "cull out" abnormals from the large number of normals. To impose the experience gained from one of these situations onto the other results in confusion.

Regarding breast disease, the problem is compounded by the fact that over the millenia breast cancers have been classically discovered either by the patient or by clinical palpation. Out of this experience has arisen a great body of expertise. Generally, this expertise is such that the predictive value, or positive biopsy rate, ranges from 20 to 33 per cent. Advocates for a new technique may claim a 97 per cent "accuracy" (often undefined) rate, a 98 per cent sensitivity rate, and a 99 per cent specificity rate. Unfortunately, these unrealistic claims may be derived from studies that are poorly controlled, based on series of cases selected because of clinically suspicious, large cancers, and interpreted after the results of palpation, and occasionally biopsy, are known.

It is doubtful that there is, or ever will be, a breast imaging method that, by itself, can be expected to be 97 to 100 per cent sensitive. It would appear that the sensitivity of mammography is on the order of 80 to 90 per cent (Baker, 1982). If a surgeon requests imaging consultations for palpable masses and receives reports that miss these palpable cancers 20 per cent of the time, his or her natural reaction is to reject the method as useless (Lesnick, 1977; Devitt, 1979; Mahoney et al., 1979; Mahoney and Csima, 1983).

For example, in Mahoney and coworkers' study (1979), a classic example of tautology in action, a population of women were screened with clinical examination, reserving mammography for those women in whom clinical examination was abnormal or questionable. You will recall that mammography will not find about 20 per cent of palpable cancers. When palpable lesions were missed by mammography, the impression was gained that screening mammography was unnecessary, as all the cancers in this series were picked up clinically. Because preclinical detection virtually could not exist in this circumstance, the tautology was fulfilled.

On the basis of data from the Breast Cancer Detection Demonstration Projects (BCDDP) (Baker, 1982), if this same experiment were performed with mammography being the primary examination and clinical examination reserved for abnormal or suspicious cases, only 30 to 60 per cent of cases could be expected to be detected by clinical methods. The impression would then follow that clinical examination is worthless as a screening tool.

These extremes are both fallacious and totally disregard the fact that each method contributes independently to detection of cancer (Baker, 1982; Moskowitz, 1983c; Strax, 1984). Failure to appreciate this point can contribute to delay in diagnosis and may be associated with clinically significant upstaging of the disease. The diagnosis of breast cancer should be based on histologic evaluation.

If biopsy is necessary to make the diagnosis of cancer, of what value are imaging studies? In this chapter the answers to this question are explored for the imaging modalities currently available.

Sensitivity, specificity, accuracy, and predictive values are measures used to evaluate diagnostic tests. To avoid semantic confusion, the following definitions are used for each of these parameters in this chapter:

1. Sensitivity (True Positive Rate [TP]): The ratio of the number of cancers correctly identified versus all cancers present.

2. Specificity (True Negative Rate): The portion of normal examinations correctly called negative.

3. False Positive Rate (FP): The fraction of normal patients incorrectly called positive, expressed as a percentage. In this chapter the term false positive rate (FP) will often be used in lieu of specificity.

4. Predictive Value (PV): The ratio of correct positive diagnoses to all tests called positive. In the case of breast cancer, if correctly calculated, this should equal the percentage yield of cancers among cases biopsied.

5. Accuracy: This term is perhaps misused more than any of the others. It represents the ratio of all correct diagnoses (positive and negative) to all outcomes. This category is of little relevance, particularly in screening situations in which the frequency of disease is expressed as a few cases per 1000. For example, if an investigator were to screen a population of 10,000 asymptomatic volunteers in which there resided as many as 100 with cancers and arbitrarily, without reference to the test itself, diagnose all tested women as normal or free of cancer, the "accuracy" of the test would be 0.99 and yet every cancer would have been misdiagnosed!

It is also possible to have an acceptable positive predictive value and yet be operating close to, or even at, random chance levels.

For example, let us assume a population of 400 patients were referred for imaging. Further assume that the subsequent course of clinical events demonstrated 100 cancer cases in that population. Let us say that the test identified 50 of the cancers correctly. In addition, 200 normal patients were incorrectly called positive. The predictive value, or expected biopsy yield, would be 20 per cent, an acceptable clinical level. However, a moment's reflection reveals that 50 per cent of normal persons were called abnormal (FP), and 50 per cent of persons with cancer were called abnormal (TP). In point of fact, this test was operating on a random chance level.

In a representative sample of the literature, sensitivity rates for mammography (TP) ranging from 65 to 97 per cent have been reported (Moskowitz, 1983b). The mean TP rate in these series was 84 per cent. The false positive rate was reported to range from 1 per cent to a high of 48 per cent with a mean of 9 per cent. Even in the worst case situation (48 per cent FP), the TP-FP ratio was better than chance alone. Generally speaking, the articles reporting higher sensitivities resulted from diagnostic situations in which masses tended to be larger. In the BCDDP the TP rate for mammography was a little better than 80 per cent if cases occurring within 12 months of a negative screen are considered.

In the author's center, about 7 to 9 per cent of cases were missed by both clinical examination and mammography. Forty-six per cent of all cases were identified by mammography alone. Physical examination alone was responsible for detecting 16 per cent of cases not detected by mammography, and the remainder were found by both.

Recent data reported by Sickles (1984b) show that in his referred practice, 64 per cent of cases were detected by clinical examination and the remainder by mammography alone.

Taken as a whole, these data would indicate that it is most reasonable to expect that the TP rate for mammography will be in the range of 80 to 85 per cent; its false positive rate may be as high as 13 per cent in diagnostic situations, and about 5 per cent in screening situations. Clearly, mammography and clinical examination contribute different cases to detection or screening. It is painfully clear that no test that will miss, or misdiagnose, up to 20 per cent of cancers can be used to exclude cancer when there is a dominant palpable mass. However, given a suspicious mammographic finding and a negative clinical examination, the surgeon who ignores the mammographic report does so at his or her, and the patient's, peril.

X-Ray Mammography

It is tempting to suggest that x-ray mammography is the oldest of imaging techniques for the breast. However, it was probably long preceded by simple light transillumination. Nevertheless, radiographic mammography has been in clinical use for over 30 years. The radiographic parameters for differentiating benign and malignant masses are well known. A relationship between microcalcifications and breast cancer is recognized. Although it is apparent that the calcifications are not so specific as originally thought, the presence of calcifications remains an invaluable clue to the diagnosis and, perhaps, prognosis of tiny carcinomas (Galkin et al., 1977; Snyder, 1980; Hajek et al., 1983; Moskowitz, 1983c; Paterok et al., 1983; Prorok et al., 1983; Anastassiades et al., 1984; LeGal et al., 1984; Meyer et al., 1984; Kopans et al., 1985b).

Strax and coworkers (Shapiro, et al., 1982; Strax, 1984) demonstrated that the combination of mammography and clinical examination, applied to an asymptomatic population, could help lower mortality rates from this disease. The recently reported results of the Swedish trial (Tabar et al., 1985) and Dutch studies (deWaard et al., 1984; Verbeek et al., 1984; Verbeek, 1985) not only demonstrate that mammographic screening alone can contribute to the detection of cancers 5 mm and smaller in screened women of all ages, but also reproduce the earlier findings of the Health Insurance Plan (HIP) study regarding mortality reduction almost exactly.

The HIP of New York study was a prospective, matched cohort study; the Swedish trial (Tabar et al., 1985) a population based, controlled trial; the Nijmegen study (Verbeek et al., 1984; Verbeek, 1985) a case-control study; and the Breast Cancer Detection Demonstration Projects (Baker, 1982) were simply what their names implied.

The results from the first three controlled studies have surprisingly similar results, namely screening for breast cancer can reduce breast cancer mortality by one third in the intermediate term (i.e., 4 to 6 years postscreening), and this benefit appears to be limited to women over the age of 50 years at entry. In HIP (Shapiro et al., 1982), long-term follow-up shows a later (7 to 15 year) mortality reduction for both older and younger women. In the HIP study, this was accomplished with annual mammography and clinical examination, whereas in the Swedish and Dutch studies, only single mediolateral oblique view mammography was used.

As indicated earlier, for women 40 to 49 years old, an early mortality reduction was not shown in HIP, perhaps related to a high detection threshold in this age group. For example, in the HIP study, mammography alone was responsible for detecting about 42 per cent of cancers in women 50 years and older. In the BCDDP studies (performed about 12 years later), it was also noted that in this age group mammography alone detected 42 per cent of cancers. However, in women age 40 to 49 years old in HIP, only 19 per cent of cases were detected by mammography alone, whereas in the BCDDP about 35 per cent were detected only by mammography. This is important because in HIP survival was best for those cases detected by mammography alone. Furthermore, about 40 per cent of cancers in the BCDDP were less than 1 cm in size, whereas very few of such cancers were detected in HIP. Thus, it appears that for younger women the threshold size of detection of cancer was relatively high in the HIP screen.

Despite this threshold, however, 7 years after beginning to screen, a reduction in mortality rate seems to have developed.

Is there an explanation for failure to observe a mortality reduction in the Swedish study in this age group? Let us see. Whereas HIP women of all ages were screened annually, in both the Swedish and Dutch studies women over age 50 were examined at 3 year intervals. Screening for women aged 40 to 49 was performed at 2 year intervals. If these intervals were beyond the lead time gained by screening, even though threshold sensitivity was lowered meaningfully, the following might have occurred: an excess number of cancers would be expected to occur between screens; the proportion of Stage II or higher disease would be excessive, and a large portion of the cases detected at the second screen would already have passed beyond the threshold of curability, despite being screen detected.

In an earlier model, Fox and coworkers (1978) (Table 7–1) predicted that for a randomly selected, asymptomatic population, the mean detection lead time gained by screening of women age 35 to 49 years old would be about 2 ± 0.5 years. For older women the estimations were 3.5 ± 0.5 years. Key to that model was the ability to project the detectable prevalence of cancer by age. The model correctly predicted the age-specific, detectable prevalence subsequently found in both the Swedish and Dutch trials. Therefore, there is reason to believe that the lead time predictions are reasonably close to correct.

Now after 10 complete years of follow up of the author's own cohort of 6000 younger

Table 7–1. AGE-SPECIFIC LEAD TIME GAINED BY SCREENING*

	(1) Fox et al (1978)	(2) BCDDP Calculated	(3) BCDDP Observed	(4) BCDDP Calculated
35–49	2 ± 0.5 yr	2 yr	<2 yr	1.6 yr
>50	3.5 ± 0.5 yr	2.9 yr	≅ 4 yr	2.5 yr

*This table shows the age-specific projected lead time gained by screening over the nonscreened setting for the Cincinnati BCDDP and all other BCDDPs. The actual, or observed, lead time for Cincinnati is shown in column 3.

women and 4500 older women (Figure 7–1, Table 7–1), the actual observed lead time for younger women is less than 2 years, and for older women it appears to be about 4.0 years.

If correct, these figures would suggest that the lead times chosen for the Dutch and Swedish screens are inappropriate for maximal effect, particularly in younger women. This is further attested to in the Dutch data (deWaard et al., 1984; Verbeek et al., 1984; Verbeek, 1985) (Table 7–2), which show that, in younger women, 56 per cent of cases occurred in the 2 year interval between screens, whereas in older women screened at 3 year intervals, only 28 per cent occurred between screens. Thus, even within the Dutch data the interval cancer rate for older women is less than for younger women despite the longer time between screens in older women.

Within the data from the BCDDP it can be seen (Table 7–3) that for women screened annually the interval rate is inversely related to lead time gained.

Another bit of supporting evidence for the effect of lengthening screen intervals is the increasing percentage of Stage II cancers by age in the Nijmegen cohorts (Verbeek et al., 1984; Verbeek, 1985) (Table 7–2). In older women, excluding noninvasive cancers, 36 per cent of cancers were Stage II or higher. This includes interval cases, cases detected at screening, and cases detected in women who did not return for their second appointment. In younger women, on the other hand, 49 per cent of cases were Stage II. Unfortunately, the numbers are too small for statistical significance, but the age-specific parallelism is striking.

Both of these effects (enhanced interval rate and more advanced staging), however, may well be the result of iatrogenic enhancement of length bias sampling effect.

Length bias sampling can be enhanced in several ways. Some number of rapidly growing tumors will always occur between screens. If the size threshold of detection is changed, more cases will be seen as interval cancers (Moskowitz, 1983c). If a low threshold is maintained, but the interval between screens is extended to the end of lead time or beyond, not only the number of cases of intermediate growth rate that occur between screens, but also the number of advanced cases that will be detected at the screen but whose course will not be altered by it, will be increased.

This clearly happened in the Nijmegen studies, in which a long screen interval was selected. Although the best survival was, as expected, in prevalence cases, screened detected cases experienced the poorest outlook, probably because a larger pool of more advanced disease was being created artificially. Interval cases survived at a better rate than expected, even better than incidence cases. This is probably because a greater number of more slowly growing tumors were allowed to reach clinical threshold at the end of lead time, but before the next screen.

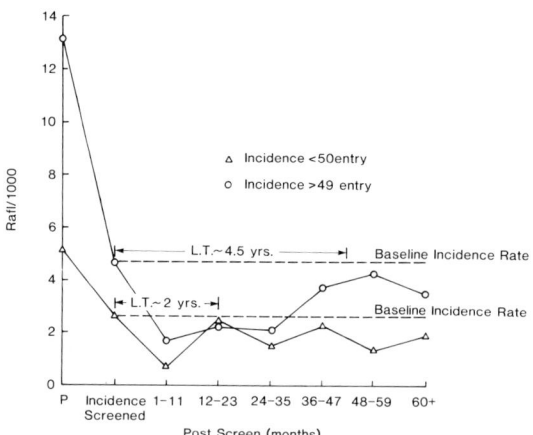

Figure 7–1. Lead time effect of screening observed in 10,500 volunteers. As expected, there is a high prevalence rate of breast cancer in the initial pass. During the 5 year period that screening was offered, the incidence screened rate per 1000 person-years is about 4.5 for women over age 49 at entry and about 2.5 for women 35 to 49 years old. When screening is discontinued, a sharp drop in incidence occurs in both age groups. The effect lasts for about 2 years in younger women and over 4 years in older women.

Table 7-2. SCREEN SENSITIVITY BY AGE IN NIJMEGEN, NETHERLANDS*

	Number of TP	TP Rate	FP Rate	Per Cent of Stage II+
Birth cohort 1925–1939	42/96	44%	56%	49%
Birth cohort 1910–1924	100/138	72%	28%	36%

*Note that in younger women, 56 per cent of cases occurred between screens (interval cancers), whereas in older women this rate was halved.

The data suggest that inappropriate screening intervals may prove to be a more fatal flaw than a less sensitive screen. If intervals are unduly lengthened, only the most slowly growing tumors will be detected by the screen. Therefore, short-term and intermediate-term mortality rates will not be reduced. The number of years required to observe any long-term effect may be exceedingly long. A less sensitive screen performed yearly may also not affect short-term mortality because it did not catch the rapidly growing tumors while they were small enough and most amenable to treatment. However, it may detect sufficient numbers of more slowly to intermediately growing tumors, perhaps not in a completely curable stage, but at a time when the course is still alterable, so that an intermediate and long-term effect can be achieved.

For younger women the screening sensitivity for all cancers, even the smallest, is improved by the combined use of aggressive clinical screening and mammography. In the author's series, 17 per cent of the minimal cancers found were detected by clinical examination alone (Moskowitz, 1983c). In the Swedish and Dutch trials, clinical examination was omitted. This omission may be an important contributing factor in failure to find a mortality decrease in the younger women.

If cancers in young women are not found when they are minimal, they will be detected later, when they are more advanced. For example, in the author's program in the post-screening period, failure to detect a significant portion of minimal cancers (5 mm or smaller) was accompanied by an excess rate of Stage II cancers (Table 7-4).

In the author's study of older women (Table 7-5) the 10 year cumulative survival for all invasive cancers occurring during screening (incidence, interval, and prevalent) is 71 per cent. In the case of invasive cancers, this represents an improvement of 29 percentage points in 10 year survival over breast cancer survival in the United States (Axtell et al., 1976). These data would lead us to believe that benefit the author obtained for older women is at least comparable to the results obtained in Falun (Sweden), Nijmegen (Netherlands), and New York. Because it may be argued that in older women small noninvasive cancers may never present as clinical tumors, they are not considered here in this analysis. If they were included, survival at 10 years would be 81 per cent.

It is only the results with younger women that appear anomalous. For young women, after 10 years of follow-up (Table 7-5), the survival rate (including prevalence, incidence, and interval cases) is 95 per cent. If noninvasive cancer is excluded, the overall survival is 88 per cent. Correcting for a 3.0 year lead time gained over clinical detection, the 10 year survival is projected to be 79 per cent. Thus, a 30 percentage point gain is seen by screening in this age group. (If a 2 year lead time was used, the gain would be more striking.) However, these women were screened annually, and a particularly vigorous and successful effort was made to detect noninvasive and minimal cancers. Given these considerations, there is every reason to believe that the survival rate noted represents a true alteration in the natural history of this disease in younger women.

Table 7-3. AGE-SPECIFIC LEAD TIME VERSUS INTERVAL RATES*

	All BCDDPs	Interval Cancers, Per Cent
35–39	1	33%
40–44	1.5	23%
45–49	1.8	18%
50–54	2.4	17%
55–59	2.25	13%
60–64	2.6	14%
65–69	2.6	12%
70–74	2.6	8%

*The relation of lead time (in years) gained by annual screening and interval cancer rates. As the lead time increases, the interval rates decrease.

RISKS OF SCREENING MAMMOGRAPHY

Ionizing radiation is carcinogenic. At high levels the breast carcinogenic effect, over time, is

Table 7-4. INCIDENCE OF CANCERS BY YEAR (AGE <50 YEARS AT ENTRY)*

	Prevalence	Screened	Months After Last Screen					Total Number Stage II Cancers	
			1-11	12-23	24-35	36-47	48-59	Screened	Postscreen
Number of persons	6000	12,600	6000	6000	6000	6000	6000	24,600	24,00
Number of cancers	31	32	5	16	9	13	8	18	28
Rate per 1000	5.2	2.5	0.83	2.77	1.5	2.2	1.3	0.73/1000	1.15/1000
Invasive cancer only	15	18	4	12	7	13	7	N.A.	N.A.
Rate per 1000	2.5	1.43	0.6	2.0	1.16	2.2	1.16		

*Note that in younger women the lead time is short, although there is a rebound shortly after cessation of screening. The average incidence for 4 years after screening is about 2 per 1000, or 22 per cent less than screened incidence. This may be the long-term effect of removing minimal cancers, or the result of excess "nonkilling cancers" found at screening. N.A., not applicable.

linearly related to dose. The effect of each dose of radiation is assumed to be cumulative to every preceding dose. This effect can be demonstrated in the women exposed to the atomic detonation in Japan (Committee on the Biological Effect of Ionizing Radiation, 1980), as well as Canadian women irradiated during pneumothorax therapy for tuberculosis (Myrden and Hiltz, 1969; Howe et al., 1982), for postpartum mastitis in the United States (Committee on the Biological Effect of Ionizing Radiation, 1980), and for treatment of benign conditions in Sweden (Baral et al., 1977).

All of these studies also demonstrate that the carcinogenic effect is clearly related to age at time of initial exposure to radiation. The greatest effect is seen in childhood, adolescence, and early adult life (ages 10 to 19 years). However, there is *no* important detectable effect on breast cancer incidence for exposure beginning at about the age of 40 years (Feig, 1983, 1984a, 1984b; Miller, 1985).

At levels of radiation in the diagnostic range it is doubtful that the effect is linear. Theoretically it could be linear, sublinear, or even supralinear. However, Miller (1985) and Howe and colleagues (1982), in a reanalysis of the Canadian fluoroscopy series, find strong evidence that the dose response seems to be quadratic-linear at the low levels. This is extremely important in that it means there is effectively a threshold effect. Miller and Howe and coworkers have estimated this to be at the 50 to 75 rad level. Modern mammography can deliver as little as 0.060 to 0.500 rad for a two-view examination. Digital mammography is on the horizon, and doses as low as 0.003 to 0.004 rad per examination may be possible.

The native cumulative risk for development of breast cancer is about 8 per cent, assuming no threshold. If a population of women were assumed to receive 1 rad per year to the breasts beginning at age 35 years, this lifetime cumulative risk would be increased to about 8.3 per cent. If the annual dose is only 0.1 rad, the cumulative effect would be 8.03 per cent.

At 1 rad per year, if there is a threshold effect at 50 rad, the population would have to reach age 90 years before the linear phase would be entered. At 0.1 rad per examination, the population would have to reach age 900 years. In either case, no effect could be seen for another 10 to 35 years. In this phase, note that the maximum risk is estimated to be 6

Table 7-5. CINCINNATI SURVIVAL RATES*

Months	1-11	12-23	24-35	36-47	48-59	60-71	72-83	84-95	96-107	108+
				Age >50 Years at Entry						
All	100%	100%	99%	99%	98%	98%	95%	95%	95%	95%
Invasive	100%	100%	97%	97%	94%	94%	88%	88%	88%	88%
				Age <49 Years at Entry						
All	100%	96%	94%	93%	93%	90%	87%	85%	83%	81%
Invasive	100%	94%	91%	90%	90%	85%	81%	78%	74%	71%

*Survival of breast cancer cases, younger and older women. This includes all cases found at initial (prevalence) screening, incidence (1 year intervals) screening, and cases occurring between screens (1-11 months). Includes cases found by mammography, clinical examination, by both methods, and those detected between screens by the patient herself.

cases per rad per 10^6 women, and that this is for women aged 10 to 19 years.

Because the target population is 40 years and older, the risk associated with modern mammography is essentially negligible (Feig, 1983, 1984a, 1984b; Miller, 1985).

It would appear to this observer that, at this time and for at least the next 5 years, good high quality mammography will be the mainstay of early breast cancer detection.

SCREENING RECOMMENDATIONS

As a result of the data generated from the HIP study and the BCDDP, the following guidelines for screening asymptomatic women have been suggested:

1. For women over the age of 50 years, annual mammographic and clinical examination should be performed.
2. For women aged 40 to 49 years, a baseline screening mammogram should be done with annual or biennial examinations thereafter, as indicated by risk factors or other considerations.

The author would suggest that, in view of the results of the Swedish and Dutch studies already cited and the lead time estimates and effects noted in this chapter, it would be rational to change these guidelines as follows:

1. Women over the age of 50 years can be screened at least every 2 years, and mammography alone seems to be sufficient.
2. Because no mortality reduction was shown in the controlled trials, it might be argued that no screening is required in the 40 to 49 year age group. However, for three reasons—the serious flaws in the design of those studies for younger women (already pointed out), the high yield of small cancers and low yield of large cancers in the BCDDP studies in younger women, and the fact that at this time there is no viable alternative—the author believes it is neither wise nor prudent to deny these women the potential benefit of early detection.
3. It is necessary to shorten the interval to 12 months between screens for this age group.
4. For these younger women, clinical examination should be offered.

TECHNICAL FEATURES

Xeroradiography uses the photoconductive principle, wherein a precharged selenium-coated plate is exposed to incoming x-ray. A residual charge proportional to the photon bombardment remains on the plate. Bipolar-charged particulate dust is sprayed onto the plate, and it adheres to the charged surface and, in turn, is printed onto an opaque paper.

Gas electron radiography is a variant of the photostatic principle using a sealed chamber of xenon gas as the ionizable material and a thin Mylar sheet on which the charge and powder are collected. This process is said to preserve the edge enhancing effect of xerography and the visual effect of film at a significantly lower dose.

Film screen, on the other hand, simply represents the classic light photon interaction with film, the light being generated by bombardment of x-ray photons of the screen within the cassette.

The xeroradiographic process produces a low contrast, flat image. Because of the edge enhancement effect, anatomic changes with relatively sharp borders stand out boldly. It is generally accepted that microcalcifications will readily be demonstrated owing to this edge enhancement effect.

The film screen image, on the other hand, is a high contrast one with a wide array of densities from white to black. It tends to favor the display of small, subtle areas of asymmetric density. In dense fibrous breasts, the image may be difficult to evaluate. Otherwise, in high quality film images, microcalcifications can usually be demonstrated, but a careful search pattern is important, backlighting must be reduced to diminished, and coning of extraneous light is very helpful. Although dense breasts render microcalcifications difficult to detect, use of a moving grid reduces scatter and greatly improves image quality.

Xeroradiography, because of its inherently low contrast, may lead the examiner to believe that dense breasts may be better visualized than with film. However, in my experience it is very doubtful that lesions are routinely seen better than they are on film.

An advantage that film offers that is not available with xeromammography is that the examiner can cone to an area of suspicious density for better detail. Owing to the toner-robbing effect with xeroradiography, severe coning is difficult. Magnification, however, can be performed with both. Magnification may be used as an alternative to coning, but it requires a somewhat greater exposure dose.

For the average 6 cm thick breast, the generally accepted range for midbreast absorbed dose by xerography systems is about 0.27 to 0.34 rad per exposure. Newer developments may reduce this level further. For film screen systems, doses as low as 0.03 rad have been noted, but generally, the midbreast dose ranges from 0.09 to 0.15 rad per exposure.

Xeroradiography is more forgiving of exposure error than is film mammography. In film mammography systems, exposure latitude is not as wide. This can be overcome to a great degree by phototiming devices. In both systems, positioning and adequate compression are important.

FILM SCREEN MAMMOGRAPHY VERSUS XEROMAMMOGRAPHY

Studies directly comparing xeromammography and film mammography are surprisingly few. Those that are available are often biased in design, and the results are almost predictable.

However, the range for true positive rates, as reported from representative papers in the literature for either film or xeroradiography, are generally close (Moskowitz, 1983b). The sensitivity for either form of imaging mammography varies from a low of 0.53 to a high of 0.98, and the specificity is generally similar as well. Overall, the trend suggests that film screen has the slighter edge.

Huppe and Schneider (1977) have reported that xeromammography and film mammography can reach the same diagnostic accuracy under optimal conditions. However, they note that with xeroradiography they had difficulty in detecting tiny microcalcifications that can be seen by high quality films. As noted earlier, supposedly one of the major advantages of xeroradiography is its ability to demonstrate calcifications better than film. Our experience with both, however, supports Huppe and Schneider's observations. On the other hand, Romanini and Bock (1982) believe that xeromammography and film mammography are alternative, rather than complementary, procedures.

The problem with most of the studies evaluating breast imaging is that they are often not blinded, the case material is sorely biased to large lesions, and the "gold standard" is often the method being evaluated. In terms of detection, it often is not possible to not sort out the added value of the imaging method to clinical examination alone.

Pagani and colleagues (1980) have suggested that the use of both Xerox and film technique will increase the pick up rate. Whether this is due to the different sensitivities of the two techniques or simply reflects the additive effect of more images is not known.

Insofar as mammography in general is concerned, the BCDDP studies have shown that mammography alone can detect from 30 to 50 per cent more cancers than clinical examination (Baker, 1982; Moskowitz, 1983a,c). The Swedish and Dutch trials (Andersson et al., 1979; Andersson, 1980; deWaard et al., 1984; Lundgren, 1979a, 1979b; Lundgren and Jakobsson, 1981; Lundgren and Helleberg, 1982; Tabar et al., 1985; Verbeek et al., 1984; Verbeek, 1985) demonstrated that the use of single view film mammography alone significantly increased the yield of early cancers over nonscreening, and this was clearly associated with a reduction in mortality in women over age 50 years (deWaard et al., 1984; Tabar et al., 1985).

In the BCDDP studies, to the author's knowledge, no glaring difference in early cancer detection was noted between centers using xeroradiography and those using film screen. However, the author does not believe that this particular question has yet been specifically addressed in the data analyzed to date.

Because it is not possible to state definitively that either film or xeroradiography is clearly superior to the other, decisions for use must be based on other considerations.

Whatever radiographic method is selected, it must be borne in mind that soft tissue imaging of the breast is very demanding. To paraphrase John Price: Mammography is best performed with dedicated equipment, in dedicated rooms, and by dedicated personnel and interpreted by dedicated radiologists (Price, 1985).

CLINICAL UTILITY OF MAMMOGRAPHIC SIGNS IN SCREENING

Generally speaking, the mammographic signs of breast cancer can be divided into the *direct* signs and the *indirect* signs. The direct signs can be further subdivided into primary signs and secondary signs.

The direct signs are those that reflect the radiographic shadow of the cancerous mass itself. This shadow has certain features that

Table 7-6. THE UNIQUE VALUE OF CERTAIN MAMMOGRAPHIC SIGNS IN THE PRESENCE OF A *POSITIVE CLINICAL EXAMINATION** OF THE BREASTS

Mammographic Sign	Number of Cancers Found by This Sign Alone		Percentage of Minimal Cancers			False-positive Rate of This Sign	Percentage of All Cancers Detected†	Predictive Value for Cancer Given This Sign	
	n	SE	Per Cent	n	SE			P	SE
Punctate calcification	8	(±2.8)	38.0%	3	(±1.7)	0.38%	3.90%	5.16	(±1.8)
Mass, possibly malignant	13	(±3.6)	15.4%	2	(±1.4)	0.30%	6.30%	10.65	(±2.8)
Mass, definitely malignant	7	(±0.0)	14.0%	1		0.01%	3.40%	100.00	(±0)
Mass, benign	6	(±2.4)	33.0%	2	(±1.4)	0.79%	2.90%	1.86	(±0.8)
Mass, questionable	4	(±2.0)	0.0%	0		0.25%	1.90%	3.88	(±1.9)
Vein dilation	1		100.0%	1		0.02%	0.48%	9.00	
Skin thickening	0		0.0%	0		0.00%	0.00%	0	
Nipple retraction	2	(±1.4)	50.0%	1		0.05%	0.90%	9.09	(±8.6)
Duct dilation	1		0.0%	0		0.22%	0.45%	1.08	(±1.0)

*Any localized abnormality.
†Percentage of 205 potentially detectable cancers identified by this sign alone.
SE, Standard error; n, number.
From Moskowitz, M.: The predictive value of certain mammographic signs in screening for breast cancer. Cancer, 51:1007, 1983. Reprinted with permission.

can be used to quantitate the probability of malignancy being present. These are the *primary* direct signs. *Secondary* direct signs are those that result directly from the presence of the cancer itself but that usually produce changes at some distance. In this latter category, for example, are skin thickening as a result of lymphatic permeation, skin or nipple retraction, or even cicatricial contraction of the whole breast.

When direct signs of breast cancer are present (primary or secondary) the lesion is usually well established, and the predictive value for mammography is usually reasonably high (see Tables 7–6 and 7–7).

The indirect signs of breast cancer are those that reflect changes within the breast that often occur in benign processes and, occasionally, in cancerous ones. As a result (when cancer is detected by these signs), the tumor is more often minimal (5 mm or less, or wholly noninvasive by light microscopy) than when direct signs are present. The predictive value of the secondary signs is, however, distinctly less than the predictive value of the primary signs (Moskowitz, 1979, 1983a,b,c; Sickles, 1984b). Even in these cases, however, the predictive value is greater than chance alone.

To bring some degree of quantification to mammographic interpretation, the author and colleagues have evaluated certain radiographic signs and diagnoses as they used them over a 5 year period of screening from 1973 to 1979 (Tables 7–6 and 7–7) in asymptomatic, self-selected women over age 35 years (average age at entry was 42.5 years). These signs will

Table 7-7. THE UNIQUE VALUE OF CERTAIN MAMMOGRAPHIC SIGNS IN THE PRESENCE OF A *NEGATIVE CLINICAL EXAMINATION* OF THE BREASTS

Mammographic Sign	Number of Cancers Found by This Sign Alone		Percentage of Minimal Cancers			False-positive Rate of This Sign	Percentage of All Cancers Detected*	Predictive Value for Cancer Given This Sign	
	n	SE	Per Cent	n	SE			P	SE
Punctate calcification	41	(±6.4)	71%	29	(±5.4)	0.88%	20.5%	11.50	(±1.7)
Mass, possibly malignant	15	(±3.9)	33%	5	(±2.2)	0.68%	7.3%	5.43	(±1.3)
Mass, definitely malignant	14	(±3.7)	14%	2	(±1.4)	0.04%	6.8%	73.68	(±10.7)
Mass, benign	6	(±2.4)	67%	4	(±2.0)	0.67%	2.9%	2.20	(±0.8)
Mass, questionable	0		0%			0.10%	0%	0	
Vein dilation	0		0%			0.00%	0%	0	
Skin thickening	0		0%			0.00%	0%	0	
Nipple retraction	0		0%			0.03%†	0%	0	
Duct dilation	0		0%			0.06%‡	0%	0	

*Percentage of 205 potentially detectable cancers identified by this sign alone.
†N = 13.
‡N = 26.
SE, Standard error; n, number.
From Moskowitz, M.: The predictive value of certain mammographic signs in screening for breast cancer. Cancer, 51:1007, 1983. Reprinted with permission.

be discussed in some detail because they impinge heavily on clinical decisions.

Smoothly Contoured, Solitary, Round Mass Larger than 1 cm. When such a mass was present with margins visible in their entirety, whether clinically palpable or not, the predictive value for cancer was about 2 per cent (± 0.8). Of the 12 cancers detected by pursuing this sign, half were minimal. These were either small cancers intimately attached to or within fibroadenomas or intracystic papillary carcinomas.

Spiculated, Stellate, or Knobby Mass. When this finding was present and clinical examination was negative, the predictive value for cancer was 74 per cent (± 10.7). If clinical examination revealed *any* positive finding, ranging from minimal thickening to fixed mass, the predictive value of these signs was 100 per cent. Only 14 per cent of the cancers detected by these findings were minimal; these minimal cancers constitute about 4 per cent of all the minimal cancers found during screening. Most cancers with this finding were present in the *first* year, and they accounted for 6 per cent of all the cancers of the author's group. Therefore, this sign is highly specific but very insensitive to minimal cancers and, when present, unequivocally requires biopsy. Fat necrosis and sclerosing duct proliferation (indurative mastopathy) may mimic this kind of cancer very closely. Occasionally certain features may be present that allow reasonably reliable differentiation from cancer.

Relatively Well Circumscribed Mass with Partial Loss of Border, or Too Dense for Size. When clinical examination was negative, the predictive value for this constellation of findings was about 5 per cent (± 1.3) (Fig. 7–2). When clinical examination was positive, the predictive value was about 11 per cent (± 2.8). Combined, the predictive value of this sign was about 7 per cent. However, about 25 per cent of cancers detected as a result of this finding represented minimal cancers. The FP rate for this sign approached 1 per cent. Twenty per cent of cancers with these findings were minimal, and they represent 13 per cent of all minimal cancers that occurred in this population. Today biopsy may be avoided in many of these cases if ultrasonography is available. However, for ultrasonography to be as reliable as aspiration in the diagnosis of cysts, strict criteria must be followed, and a number of cysts will still be explored (Boon and deGraaf Guillond, 1981; Sickles, 1984a; Sickles et al., 1984). If the lesion is solid on ultrasonography (in the cancer age group), excisional biopsy or aspiration cytology is needed. It is estimated that if ultrasonography is used to exclude cystic lesions, the probability of cancer in the remaining solid masses may be as high as 10 per cent.

MICROCALCIFICATIONS

The reported predictive value of microcalcifications varies widely in the literature (Paterok et al., 1983; Prorok et al., 1983; Anastassiades et al., 1984; Kopans, 1984; Kopans et al., 1984a; LeGal et al., 1984; Rasmussen, 1984;

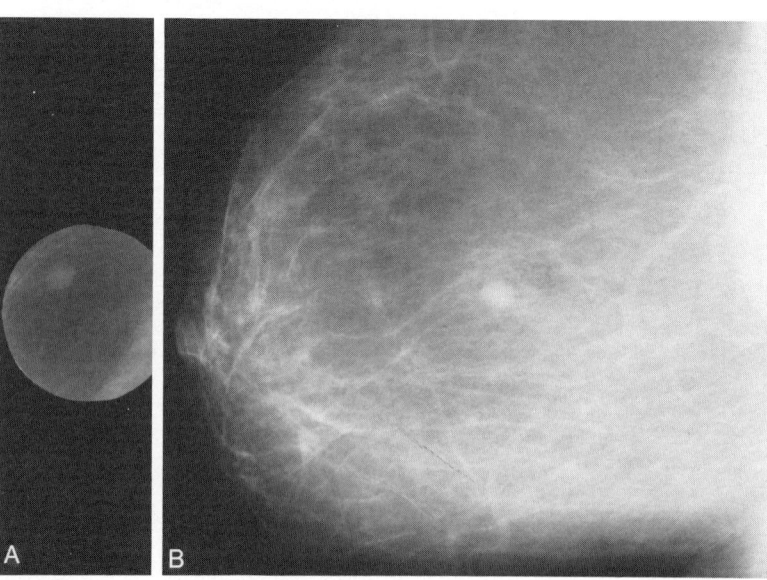

Figure 7–2. Note the small, relatively well-circumscribed mass. It is of relatively low density, but the coned view *(A)* demonstrates an undulating border betraying its solid nature. The partial loss of border and faint fibrillary retractions strongly suggest cancer. Pathologic diagnosis: 8 mm colloid carcinoma of the breast.

Dupont and Page, 1985). It has long been empirically recognized that certain kinds of microcalcifications are associated with a high probability of the presence of cancer (Snyder, 1980; Stamp et al., 1983; Boisselier et al., 1983; Anastassiades et al., 1984; Dupont and Page, 1985). Most early workers in mammography described these calcifications in association with soft tissue densities that often had radiographic features of malignancy.

As the use of mammography matured it became apparent that breast microcalcifications were not so specific as initially hoped. Often cancer-associated calcifications do not reside within the malignancy, but may be regional to it in as many as 60 per cent of the cases.

It is reasonable to divide microcalcifications into five categories, namely (1) clearly benign, (2) probably benign, (3) possibly cancer, (4) probably cancer, and (5) cancer. Categories 3, 4, and 5 will encompass most such cancers and keep a reasonably low, manageable, false positive rate and satisfactory predictive value.

It must be recognized that all calcifications within the breast are not equally predictive. Some calcifications do not enter into the differential diagnosis of malignancy and can be confidently excluded from biopsy. These are usually larger than 200 to 250 mm, often coarse calcifications, not usually clustered or lined up in a duct; or, if smaller, they are round and smooth, often hollow. On occasion a calcified blood vessel wall may mimic microcalcifications, but close inspection usually permits a firm diagnosis. The large coarse, linear ductal calcifications of secretory disease are not usually a differential diagnostic problem.

Skin calcifications may be mistaken for intramammary calcium. If the characteristic lobulated, hollow appearance of cutaneous calcium is not present or the calcifications do not project on the skin surface tangential to the x-ray beam, they may be difficult to distinguish from significant microcalcifications. Also, the soft tissue detail is such with modern mammography that care must be taken not to confuse the shadows of deodorant or talcum powder with breast microcalcifications.

Although microcalcifications have long been recognized to have an association with cancer and benign disease, it is only recently that an interest in the biochemical makeup of these radiographic shadows has been appearing in the literature (Galkin et al., 1977; Anastassiades et al., 1984). Galkin and associates' work suggests that there is indeed a biochemical difference in the tiny microcalcifications associated with cancer and those microcalcifications associated with bland, benign pathologic findings. It is intriguing that, on the basis of electron microscope spectroscopy, Galkin and colleagues suggest that some of these tiny particles are not calcium at all. They have reported the appearance of such metals as gold, lithium, zinc, and tin in the small dense spots seen in biopsy specimens.

The chief value of microcalcifications is that they are markers that permit the earlier detection of some breast cancers in asymptomatic women when the cancer is still wholly intraductal or, if invasive, less than 5 mm in size.

For example, in the author's own series, 42 per cent of all minimal cancers were detected by this radiographic sign.

In the author's screening program, when the only sign of suspicion was microcalcification, the predictive value was about 12 per cent; 71 per cent of these cancers were minimal. Given that, in nonscreened women in the United States about 20 to 25 per cent of all biopsies are cancerous, and 45 to 50 per cent are Stage II and higher disease, this appears to be an acceptable trade off. Although this approach has been unpopular in the past among radiologists as well as surgeons, there is a growing awareness that mass screening and detection of minimal cancer by indirect signs almost mandates a lower predictive value (Moskowitz, 1979, 1983a,c, 1984; Sickles, 1984b). This is only justifiable if the yield of minimal cancer can be increased and the absolute incidence of far advanced disease can be decreased. That it can do so is now clear (deWaard et al., 1984; Tabar et al., 1985).

The author's group tends to be more aggressive concerning biopsy in younger women when it is known that the yield per biopsy will be less, but the potential gain is greatest. As has been shown by postmortem studies of coroner's cases (Sandison, 1962; Pollei et al., 1986), no intraductal or minimal cancers are present in asymptomatic women below age 40 years, and few are present at ages 40 to 70 years. Therefore, those that are present should be sought out vigorously.

For older women with microcalcifications the author's group tends to be less aggressive, because as the population ages, many more subclinical, and probably indolent, cancers may be present (Sandison, 1962; Pollei, 1986). Therefore, the examination often is repeated in 3 months, and if there is no change, the assumption is made that the disease, if present, is not rapidly growing. Another examination is performed in 6 to 9 months, with monthly breast self-examination and appropriately timed interval clinical examinations. If all remains stable, annual mammography is again advised. If the calcium has developed as an interval finding and the screenee is in otherwise good general health, a biopsy is usually the most prudent course.

SIGN OF ASYMMETRY

The breasts are said to be "optical isomers," and any asymmetry is highly suspicious. It is self-evident that a cancer casting an image on one side is an asymmetric density. Martin and colleagues (1979), in reviewing interval cases occurring in several BCDDP studies, determined that an asymmetric density was the most frequently overlooked sign of cancer. However, nonspecific asymmetric areas of fibrosis occur frequently in the general population, and these, too, are "asymmetric densities."

In the author's experience, if obvious carcinomas or masses and areas of architectural distortion are excluded, asymmetry alone has been a very low yield sign. In the absence of a palpable abnormality in the author's screened population, no cancer was found by this sign alone. When accompanied by an area of clinical thickening or mass, the predictive value for cancer was 3 to 4 per cent. Currently, given asymmetric shadowing and no clinical finding, the author may ask the patient to return for a recheck mammogram examination in 6 months. Monthly breast self-examination is encouraged, and a clinical examination at 3 to 6 months is suggested. If there is any change, clinically or mammographically, biopsy is urged.

COST EFFECTIVENESS OF MAMMOGRAPHIC SCREENING

Whether mammographic screening is cost effective depends on the viewpoint of the observer and the context in which the question is being posed (Moskowitz, 1979; Turnball et al., 1979; Eddy, 1981, 1983; Mooney, 1981, 1982; Friedlander and Tattersall, 1982; Kays, 1983; Evans, 1984; O'Conner et al., 1985; Ward, 1985). The actual costs, and some associated comparisons, however, are measurable.

Screening mammography (not diagnostic imaging) can be performed at $35 to $45 per case, including interpretation fee, if (1) the volume of cases is sufficiently high, (2) highly skilled technologists are available, (3) images are developed in batches, (4) current images and old images are mounted on a multiviewer by a clerk, and (5) they are batch read by a skilled, experienced mammographer. This cost level for screening mammography is achievable (Ward, 1985) and is currently being done in Cincinnati in eight cooperating institutions.

If 20,000 self-selected women aged 40 to 49 years were screened annually at a cost of $40 per screen, with an average annual incidence rate of 2.5 per 1000, 50 cases would probably be found (Table 7–4), and the cost per case detected would be $16,000. If 10 biopsies were performed for every cancer detected, at $800 per outpatient biopsy, another $400,000 is added to the cost. Therefore, including biopsy, the total cost per cancer found, excluding prevalence cases, is $24,000. If prevalence cases were included, the cost per case detected would drop (Moskowitz, 1979).

If 35 per cent of the cancers found were less than 5 mm in diameter, there would be 16 more cases found at this stage than in the nonscreened situation. The cost of each added case found at this stage would be $75,000. Instead of 25 of the 50 women dying by the tenth year, only 3 to 10 would die (Table 7–5). Therefore, the cost per death averted at 10 years would be from $54,000 to $80,000.

These costs can be compared with reported costs (Turnbull et al., 1979; Boon and deGraaf Guillond, 1981; Schroeder et al., 1981; Friedlander and Tattersall, 1982; Lansky et al., 1983; Blommers, 1984; Long et al., 1984; Kelly et al., 1985) for other medical procedures, as follows: (1) cost per cervical cancer detected, $17,000; (2) cost for 10 years of renal dialysis, $230,000 to $320,000; (3) cost for first year of coronary bypass surgery, $13,500; and (4) $1200 to $1500 per day for the last month of life of terminal cancer patients. The costs for cardiac and hepatic transplant and use of artificial hearts are not considered here.

If prices are contained to reasonable levels, if high quality mammography can be assured, and if the limitations of screening are recognized, a significant impact on breast cancer can be achieved.

NEEDLE LOCALIZATION

It is self-evident that some means of assisting the surgeon in localizing nonpalpable lesions is necessary. To attempt blind resection or unaided quadrantectomy results not only in unnecessary deformity but also in an unacceptably high level of unresected lesions.

The technique for needle localization is limited only by the imagination of the equipment available (Chang et al., 1980; Snyder, 1980; Kopans et al., 1984b; El Yousef et al., 1985). It may vary from a simple method of estimating skin entry points from mammograms to highly sophisticated computerized equipment costing many thousands of dollars. Either a simple grid system or a coordinate system is highly satisfactory, and one of these is usually available with modern mammography units (Figs. 7–3 and 7–4). A satisfactory level of skill is achievable in a very short time.

Is it necessary to use special needles and wires? There are certainly a wide variety of localizing trocars, ranging from variants of miniharpoons to crimped wires passed into the breast through a needle trocar (Meyer et al., 1984; Rasmussen and Seerup, 1984; Homer, 1985; Kopans et al., 1985b). Generally speaking, the author has not found these to be necessary if the lesion is within 5 cm (2 inches) of the breast surface. Special instruments are of most help when the breast is very large and the lesion is deeply seated (i.e., central). Generally speaking, if a 22 to 25 gauge needle of

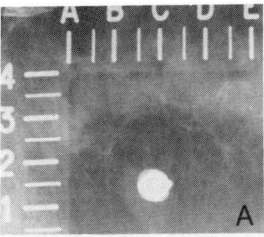
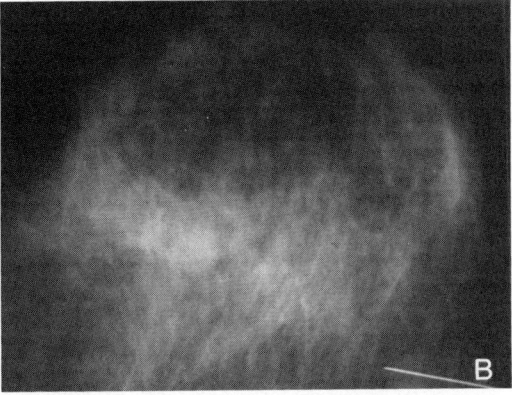

Figure 7–4. Coordinate system localization from the inferior approach. In this case the lesion was close to the chest wall and near the inframammary fold. This image was achieved with the x-ray apparatus inverted for the caudal view. This can also be done with a BB placed on the skin and multiple film localization.

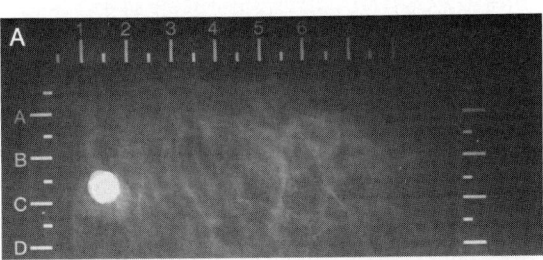
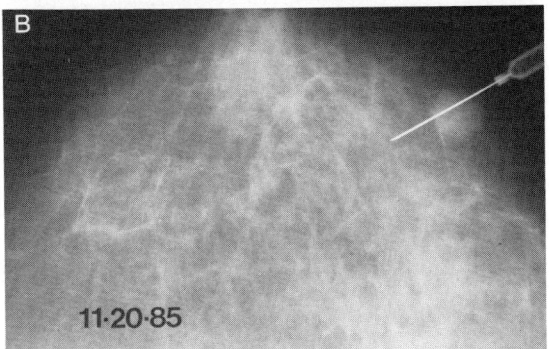

Figure 7–3. Needle localization coordinate system. A needle has been placed into a soft, circumscribed mass. Note that right angle films are used to verify that the lesion has been transfixed.

the appropriate length is selected for the estimated depth of the suspicious area (when the breast is noncompressed) and the full length of the needle is inserted up to the hub, the needles will usually stay in place for several hours or until removed by operating room personnel. The author has occasionally used collodion to hold the needles in place, and this seems to offer some measure of added protection.

It may be useful to insert more than one needle into the area of the abnormality (Fig. 7–5). This seems to be of more help when the calcifications are strung out in a fairly long linear array or cover a slightly larger area. The author tries to encompass the area of interest or the central area and an outer margin.

Methylene blue or radiopaque contrast agent, or both, may be injected. The author, however, rarely does this any longer.

Surgeons who review the position of the needles with the radiologist just prior to surgery are more successful in removing the suspected area at the first pass. Those who depend on the localization films alone, or on a map, seem to have more difficulty.

No matter how the procedure is performed, certain principles are straightforward and important:

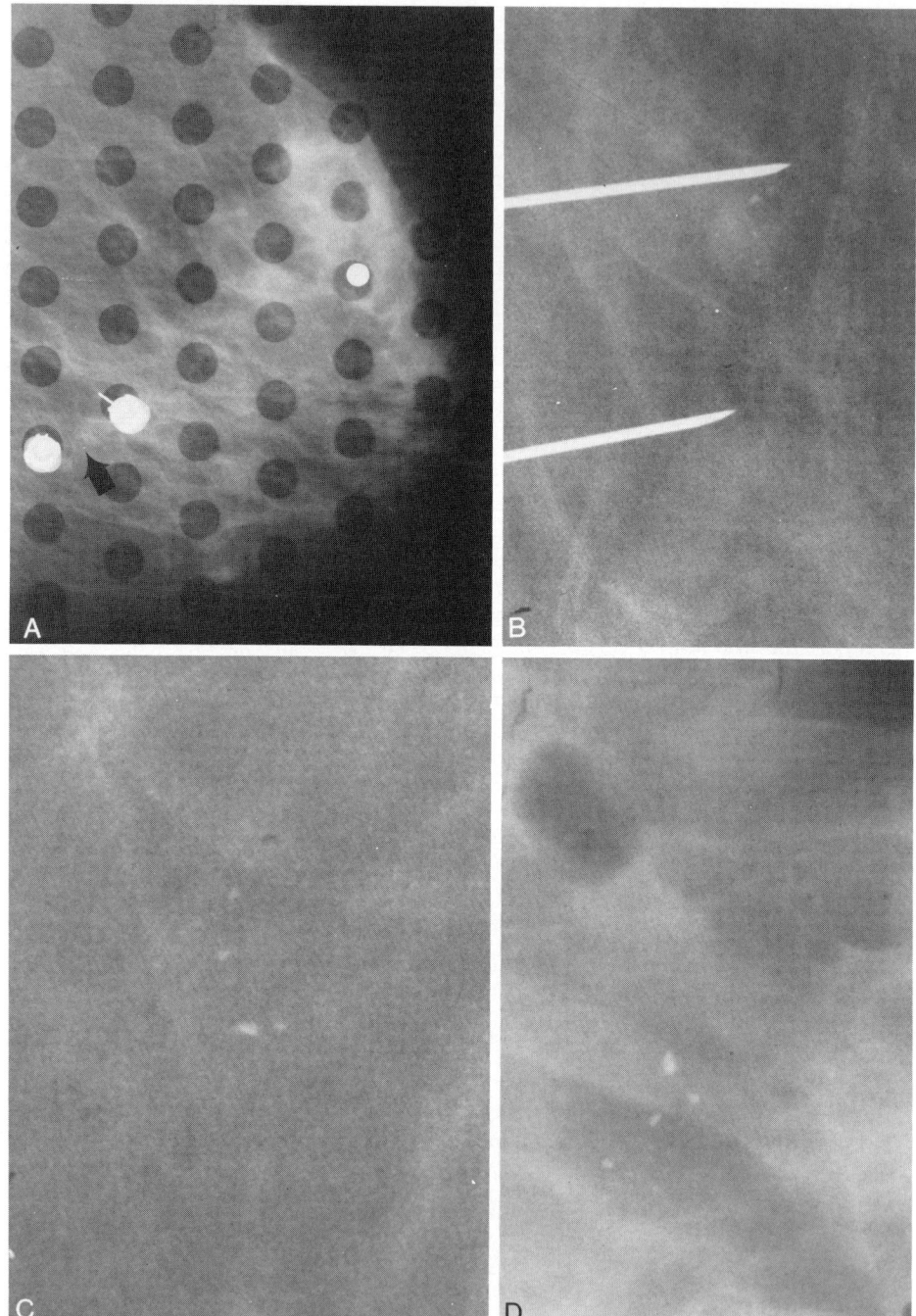

Figure 7–5. *A*, Needle localization from lateral aspect of breast using the perforated compression grid and multiple needles. *B*, Caudal view demonstrating the needle tips relative to the calcifications. *C*, Close-up view of calcifications as seen on the mammogram. *D*, Close-up of calcifications seen on the specimen radiograph. Pathologic diagnosis was intraductal carcinoma.

1. After preliminary localizing films are obtained, a needle of the appropriate length is inserted at the site of the shortest distance from skin to lesion. The length of the needle is based on the estimated depth of the lesion is the noncompressed breast.

2. Confirmatory films, at right angles to one another, must be obtained (Fig. 7–6). Any necessary adjustment to positioning requires a new set of films at right angles.

3. The localization is discussed and, ideally, reviewed directly with the operating surgeon in the physical presence of the patient. As experience is gained by the biopsy team, this becomes less necessary. However, until a good three dimensional reconstruction is established in the mind of the operating surgeon, this step is very useful. A map localizing the needle placement in reference to the lesion may be of help in the operating room.

4. If the biopsy is performed for microcalcifications, the specimen should be radiographed (Fig. 7–7). This only adds a few minutes to the biopsy procedure. If, in the course of evaluating the biopsy specimen, an obvious cancer is encountered, specimen radiography may be less important. Sectioning the specimen and tagging and radiographing it is helpful to the pathologist in narrowing the search for calcifications. It is obvious, however, that the pathologist needs to evaluate the total specimen provided.

If the biopsy was done not for calcifications but for some other radiographic sign, specimen radiography, in the author's experience, has been of less help. In this circumstance it is valuable for the radiologist to be present in the pathology laboratory when the biopsy specimen is macrosectioned. He or she can recognize if the gross lesion for which biopsy was recommended has been removed.

Failure to follow this course of action will increase the probability of leaving cancers in place, some of considerable size. On occasion, even following this course, the area of abnormality may be left behind (Fig. 7–8).

MAMMOGRAPHIC PATTERNS AND BREAST CANCER RISK

Since Wolfe (1976a,b) first described a possible relationship between certain mammographic patterns and the risk of developing breast cancer, many reports have appeared, some supporting and some rejecting his thesis (Egan and Mostellar, 1977; Mendell et al., 1977;

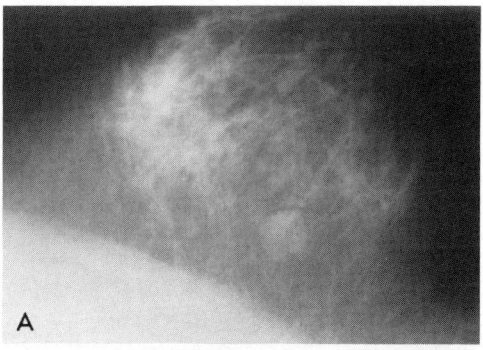
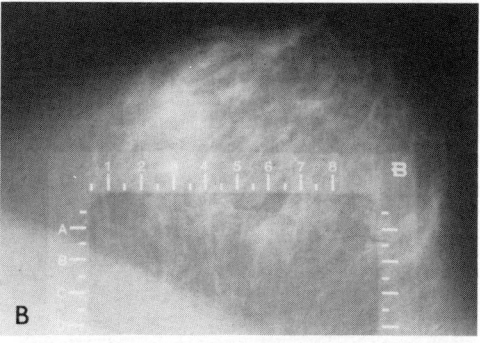
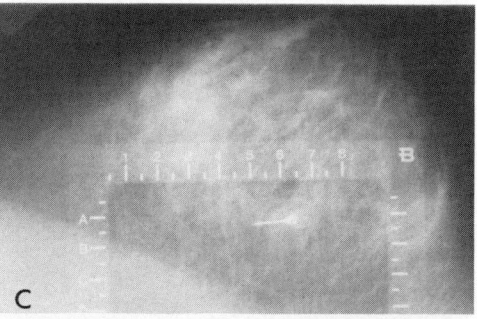
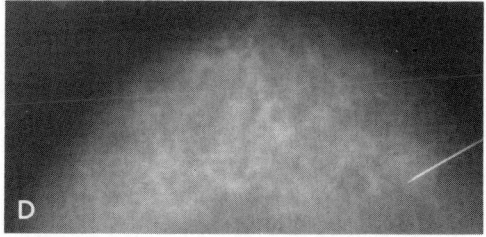

Figure 7–6. Another well-circumscribed lesion localized by coordinates. In the caudal view *(D)* the lesion looks transfixed. In the lateral view *(C)* it is obvious that the needle is about 3 mm superior to the lesion.

Moskowitz et al., 1980a; Moskowitz, 1982; Tabar and Dean, 1982; Chaudary et al., 1983; Danes, 1983; Witt et al., 1983; Boyd et al., 1984; Brisson et al., 1984; Verbeek et al., 1984; Witt et al., 1984; Horwitz et al., 1984; Kojima et al., 1984; Carlile et al., 1985; Spratt et al., 1985; Whitehead et al., 1985). Wolfe

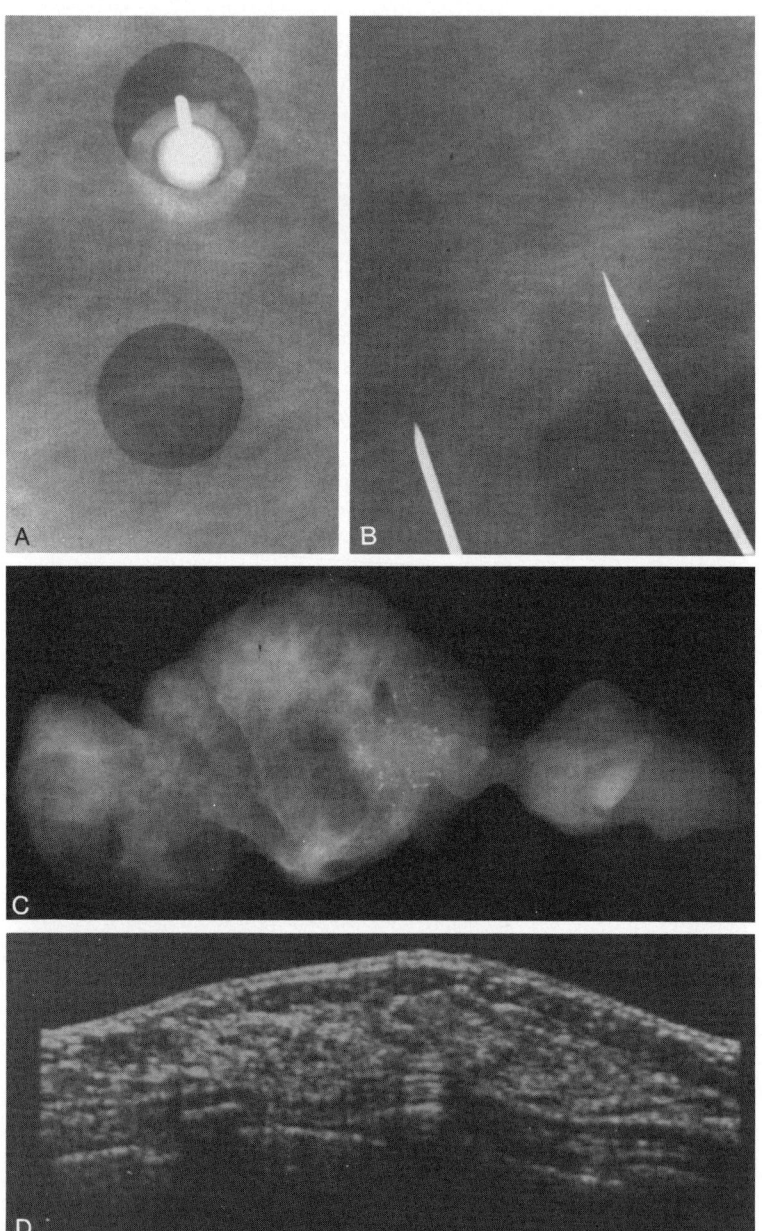

Figure 7–7. *A, B,* Needle localization in an area of clustered calcification surrounded by a poorly defined mass. No lesion was palpable. *C,* Specimen radiograph of same lesion. *D,* Negative ultrasonographic examination.

(1976a,b) originally estimated the highest risk pattern to be on the order of 30:1. Subsequently his estimates have been reduced considerably, although in a recent presentation (Wolfe et al., 1985) his group estimated a relative risk of 10:1.

In a blinded prospective study testing Wolfe's patterns, Moskowitz and coworkers (1980a) found a statistically significant correlation between Wolfe's high risk patterns and severe hyperplastic breast disease demonstrated by histology, but this could only be demonstrated if the two high risk groups were consolidated. Although the risk was statistically significant, it was only about 1.67 times the risk of the lower risk patterns. However, when the authors tested their interpretation of patterns against Wolfe's interpretation of the same cases, only a 50 per cent agreement rate was achieved.

Wellings and Wolf (1978) and Wilkinson and colleagues (1977) have presented data supporting Wolfe's observations. In that same time period, Egan and Mostellar (1977), Mendell and colleagues (1977), Rideout and Poor (1977), and Peyster and coworkers (1977) found only weak support or no support for a mammographic pattern and risk relationship.

More recently, Horwitz and colleagues (1984) reported the results of a case-control study wherein women were classified into high risk and low risk categories according to Wolfe's criteria. This study failed to show any significant difference in the proportion of high risk parenchymal patterns among patients who either were clinically normal or had clinical "fibrocystic disease" versus those with histologically confirmed breast cancer. It was believed that Wolfe's patterns could not be used to select women for breast screening.

Spratt and coworkers (1985) report no significant difference in the distribution of incidence cancers according to Wolfe's parenchymal pattern. However, only four patients with cancer were observed in 355 patients followed. The numbers are too small to draw a meaningful conclusion, as these authors point out. Similarly, they found no relation between various types of pathologic proliferative disorders and the distribution among Wolfe's parenchymal patterns. It must be noted, however, that these same authors did not find any significant excess risk of breast cancer among *any* of the various forms of "chronic cystic mastopathy." This is in somewhat stark contradistinction to the prospective long-term study recently reported by Dupont and Page (1985), who found a significant excess of cancers appearing in patients with atypical hyperplasia. Others (Black et al., 1972; Ashikari et al., 1974; Page et al., 1978; Moskowitz et al., 1980b; Boisselier et al., 1983) have also found consistent relationship between subsequent breast cancer risk and hyperplastic epithelial breast disease. As Spratt and colleagues point out, the failure to establish an association with patterns or subsequent risk may be a function of the small sample size.

Witt and associates (Witt et al., 1984; Ward, 1985) report that they reviewed the mammograms of 597 women whose images were obtained during the years 1971 to 1975. This was done prospectively and blindly, and 18 patients were excluded because of technically inadequate imaging. Subsequently, during the period of follow-up, ranging from 5 to 9 years, 12 cases of breast cancer developed, and they occurred with equal frequency in the low risk and high risk patterns. Again, however, the sample size is very small. Chaudary and colleagues (1983), in a matched study of about 1000 women over the age of 30 years, failed to demonstrate an association between the P2 mammographic pattern and breast cancer. Verbeek and coworkers 1984 reported the results of a prospective study based on the Nijmegen screening program. Patients were followed for 6 years, and they demonstrated a relative risk for women with P2 and DY* breasts of 0.7, with 95 per cent confidence limits of 0.2 and 2.4.

On the other hand, a prospective case-control study involving several of the BCDDP investigations has resulted in several supportive reports (Carlile et al., 1985; Whitehead et al., 1985). In these studies intensive training in patterns was given to the radiologists, and it was required that a satisfactory interobserver agreement rate with Wolfe's readings be achieved. Rates of agreement of 95 per cent were reported. To keep agreement high, atlas material was prepared and kept available at each institution. An excess risk on the order of 3.5:1 was noted, and mammographic patterns were found to be risk factors independent

---

*Wolfe (1976) introduced a classification system of four groups with increasing risk for breast cancer: N1 and P1 breasts are composed chiefly of fat; P2 consists of severe involvement with a prominent duct pattern; DY consists of severe involvement with dysplasia that often obscures the prominent duct pattern.

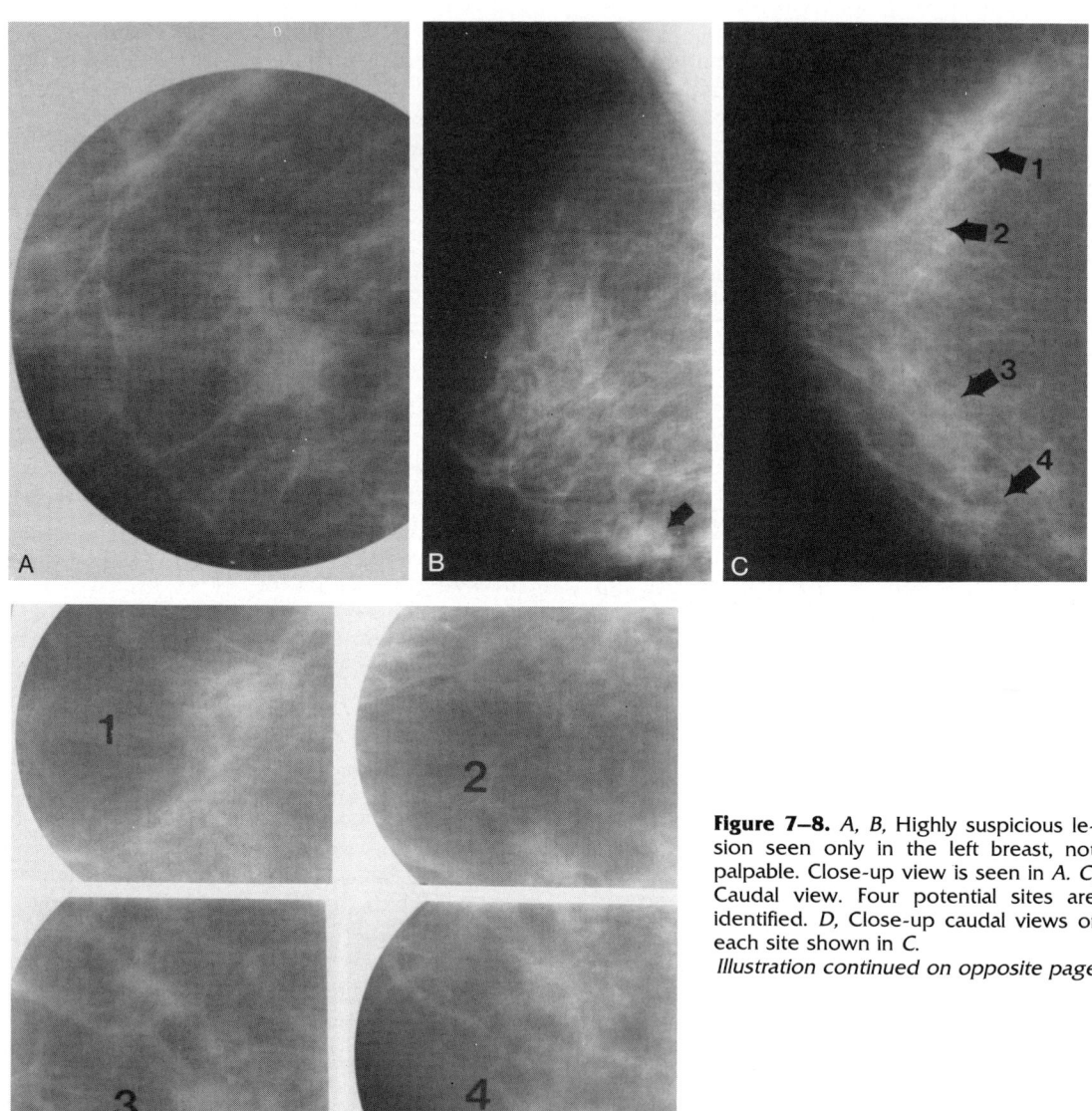

Figure 7–8. *A, B,* Highly suspicious lesion seen only in the left breast, not palpable. Close-up view is seen in *A. C,* Caudal view. Four potential sites are identified. *D,* Close-up caudal views of each site shown in *C.*
Illustration continued on opposite page

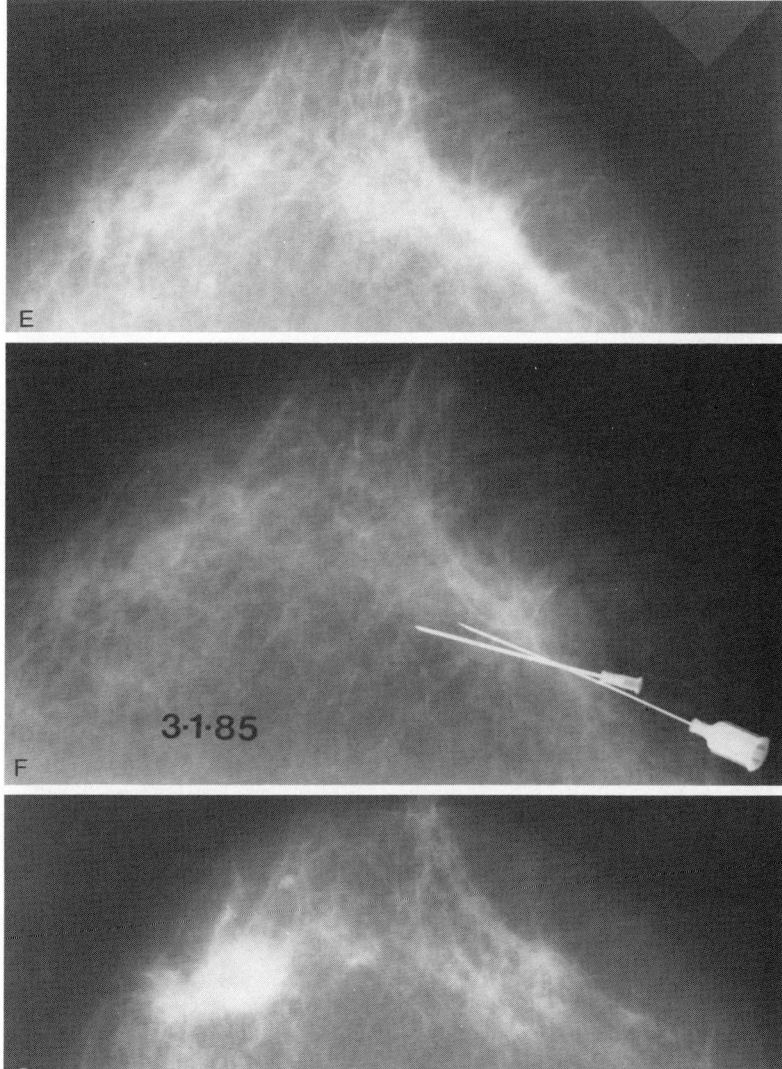

Figure 7–8 *Continued E,* One month later (2–18–85), the lateral site (4 in *D*) seems to have increased in density. *F,* Two weeks after *E* (3–1–85) needle localization at the lateral site revealed marked atypical hyperplasia. *G,* Seven months after *F,* an obvious cancer is present at the medial site.

of other common epidemiologic risk factors. These authors conclude that whereas risk estimates are statistically demonstrable, they are not of sufficient order of magnitude to use for management decisions for the individual woman, nor for selecting populations for screening.

In a subanalysis of this study, Whitehead and colleagues (1985) evaluated the possibility that dense breasts simply "mask" the presence of cancers, and that subsequent appearance of "new" lesions is not a risk marker but an artifact of density. Their analysis shows some masking effect, but Whitehead and coworkers believe there is an excess risk that is not accounted for by so-called masking.

Brisson and colleagues (1984) report the results of a case-control study of 362 women with newly diagnosed breast cancers identified in 1978–1979 and controls selected from 686 women referred for a "routine" mammogram. In this study, breast cancer was first confirmed histologically in the month preceding or in the 12 months following their examination, and, thus, the study essentially represents the results of a prevalence trial rather than a long-term incidence or prospective study. They found that an increase in body weight was associated with a marked reduction of the P2 or DY pattern so that 94 per cent of tall and thin women had a P2 or DY pattern, whereas only 19 per cent of short, stocky, and heavy women had a P2 or DY pattern. They also found that the concentration of nodular densities was inversely related to body weight but varied little with body height. When these authors did not adjust for body weight and height, they found that the P2 pattern had an excess relative risk compared to the N1 pattern of 2.0. When adjustments were made, a relative risk of 2.6 was found, with a range of 1.7 to 4.1 at the 95 per cent confidence level.

These authors also estimated the relative risk to be 4.4 (2.5–7.9) with correction for body weight and height based on the percentage of the breast affected by nodular densities and involvement of over 60 per cent of the breast. When the densities were homogeneous, the maximum relative risk was 2.0. It should be noted here that Myers and coworkers (1983) have reported that volumetric estimates of the percentage of breast involved by a given pattern are *not* highly reliable and reproducible.

Nevertheless, Brisson and colleagues conclude that the data show strong inverse association between mammographic features of breast tissue and body weight. They believe that the strength of the associations of mammographic features of breast cancer risk is underestimated in other studies as body size was not taken into account. It should be pointed out, however, that their study is essentially a study of prevalence cases, and prevalence studies have almost uniformly shown an excess risk as compared with incidence studies (Moskowitz, 1982). Furthermore, although a twofold to threefold excess relative risk may be large in epidemiologic terms, in practical terms for patient management or planning for screening it has little value. More specifically, selections of populations of women for screening based on all known risk factors will exclude 75 per cent of women who will subsequently develop breast cancer (Seidman, 1977).

Although these authors are able to increase the relative risk by adjusting for body height and weight, the differences observed between the uncorrected and corrected ranges fall well within the 95 per cent confidence interval for either. In addition, the ranges given for the confidence intervals of relative risk include the risk ranges presented by Moskowitz and colleagues (1980*a*), even though the latter group did not take into account body size.

Boyd and coworkers (1984) have reported the results of a literature review of 17 selected studies. They critically analyzed the methodologic standards that each of the studies reported. They concluded that "a large part of the controversy on this subject arises from the methodologic differences among the studies." Boyd and colleagues calculated the relative risks from the reported data and tabulated it in relation to the number of acceptable scientific methodologic criteria they judged to be present.

Of seven *prevalence* surveys analyzed, only a maximum of four criteria of a possible nine were met by any study, and the relative risk ranged from 0.24 to 1.60. Of five evaluatable *cohort* studies, two met seven of the criteria; one met five (although the authors credited it with only four); one met four; and one met three. In the two studies scoring seven criteria (both reported by the same author on the same data base), a relative risk of 7 to 8 was reported. The highest risk of 8 was reported by a study meeting only four of the standards set by Boyd and colleagues. Of the eight cohort studies, a relative risk exceeding 2 was found in two studies with a score of four, and in one study with a score of six.

These authors have concluded that studies that follow the usual scientific methods employed in the epidemiologic evaluation of risk generally have confirmed an association between mammographic pattern and breast cancer risk.

The data overall suggest that there is some slight excess risk of breast cancer in patients with P2 or DY pattern as compared to a parenchymal pattern composed mostly of fat, and that this is somehow related to body habitus. At present, the magnitude of the excess risk does not seem to be strong, and the uncertainty associated with its level precludes it from being clinically useful.

An interesting application of the use of parenchymal patterns has been suggested by Hinton and colleagues (Hinton et al., 1985), who reported that parenchymal patterns correlate relatively well with estrogen receptor (ER) content of tumors and prognosis. On the other hand, Nielsen and Poulsen (1985) have found no correlation between parenchymal pattern and ER content of tumors. They did find that high ER levels were present in spiculated masses. Well-defined masses or cancers found by calcification alone, or mammographically negative cancers, had a low ER level. The numbers are small but tend to follow the pattern previously reported by Broberg and colleagues (1983).

MAMMOGRAPHY FOR PURPOSES OTHER THAN SCREENING

For patients with symptoms, mammography may provide support for a clinical impression of malignant disease. However, if the clinical impression is strong and mammography is negative, delay in biopsy should not be allowed to occur.

Used preoperatively, mammography may help to stage and evaluate the extent of the disease. Magnification views, in particular, may show unsuspected foci of microcalcifications in addition to the major primary lesion. This is of great help in selecting patients for conservation surgery or radiation treatment.

Mammography is important as a clinical adjunct in following the residual breast in patients with unilateral mastectomy (Schalldach and Schumann, 1982) and is helpful in following the breasts of patients who have had breast preserving procedures (Dodd, 1984; Paulus, 1984).

Mammography can also occasionally be useful in defining early recurrences in the site of mastectomy or in the ipsilateral axilla if the patient has sufficient tissue remaining on the chest wall to make radiography possible.

When axillary nodes can be seen to be larger, and dense, or on rare occasions to contain spiculated microcalcifications in the presence of a known breast neoplasm, the positive predictive value for metastatic cancer is on the order of 90 to 95 per cent. However, these findings will identify only about 40 per cent of the patients who subsequently are proved to have lymph node involvement by axillary dissection (Kalisher et al., 1976; Coopmans de Yoldi et al., 1983).

In patients with breast prostheses, mammography and ultrasonography have limitations insofar as preclinical detection is concerned. Jensen and Mackey (1985) reported, however, that xeromammography is very useful in clarifying the nature of palpable masses under this circumstance. In their series, the mammogram proved that about 50 per cent of such palpable masses were prosthesis related.

In the author's opinion, the most important function of mammography lies in earlier detection (Shapiro et al., 1974; Fox et al., 1978; Andersson et al., 1979; Andersson, 1980; Baker, 1982; Shapiro et al., 1982; Council on Scientific Affairs, 1984; DeWaard et al., 1984; Gad et al., 1984; Hebert et al., 1984; Kambouris et al., 1984; Kopans et al., 1984a; Moskowitz, 1984; Rasanen et al., 1984; Verbeek et al., 1984; Watanabe, 1984; Editorial, 1985; Fox et al., 1985; Tabar et al., 1985; Verbeek, 1985). To date, there is no other method, including breast self-examination or clinical examination, that has been proved to be capable of reducing mortality in screened populations.

GALACTOGRAPHY

Galactography is simply retrograde injection of a radiographic contrast medium into a lactiferous duct, followed by appropriate radiographic imaging. The injection usually is accompanied by minimal discomfort unless the duct is ruptured. If there has been a duct discharge of long duration, the duct usually is relatively ectatic and cannulation is accomplished easily. If it is difficult to express a discharge, the procedure becomes, pari passu, similarly difficult to perform.

The author employs iothalamate meglumine (Conray 60) for this purpose and, generally, no more than 2 ml is necessary.

Galactography should not be done in the absence of a demonstrable discharge on the day of the examination, not only because of the difficulty involved in cannulating a nondischarging duct, but also because, if the duct is cannulated, it might be the wrong one. Indeed, the author has had the experience of initially cannulating a duct from which a small amount of serous fluid was expressed, and finding the underlying system to be perfectly normal. Further milking of the breast demonstrated a small bloody effluent from another site nearby; and galactography of this duct demonstrated an intraductal papillary lesion.

Some authors have gone so far as to call galactography the most important examination in the diagnosis of the secreting breast, and that it is indicated in all patients with spontaneous bloody or serous discharge (Kindermann et al., 1979; Peyster et al., 1979; Alberti and Troiso, 1982; Tabar et al., 1983). However, what can realistically be expected of this study is an excellent retrograde delineation of the anatomy of the duct injected. Ectasias, strictures, intraluminal filling defects, cut-offs, and duct displacement can be discerned. Multiple papillomas can be diagnosed confidently, but the cause of a larger, solitary mass (Fig. 7–9) cannot be determined short of biopsy. Unfortunately, as with most imaging procedures, a firm diagnosis of cancer can be rendered only occasionally. As DiPietro and coworkers (1979) point out, "in practice it should be the type of discharge that indicates surgery rather than the galactographic data."

In the author's experience the major value of this procedure has been to locate the site of the abnormality (ies), often reducing the magnitude of the surgical procedure necessary to assure resection of the papillary growth. If performed just prior to surgery, 0.1 ml of methylene blue may be mixed with the radiographic contrast medium. After injection for this purpose, the author puts a drop or two of collodion on the surface of the nipple to temporarily occlude the duct. If the duct has not been ruptured by the pressure of the injection, the contrast material will remain confined to the duct system.

In the presence of a spontaneous bloody or serous discharge, galactography may be helpful for further evaluation. In the author's opinion, other types of nipple discharge are even weaker relative indications for the study. The only absolute contraindication is known hypersensitivity to the contrast medium.

Although this author does not believe that galactography is the most useful test in the imaging armamentarium, and certainly it is not

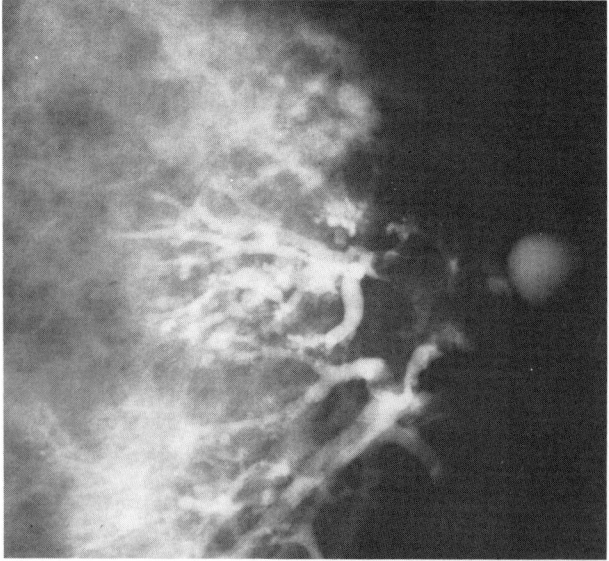
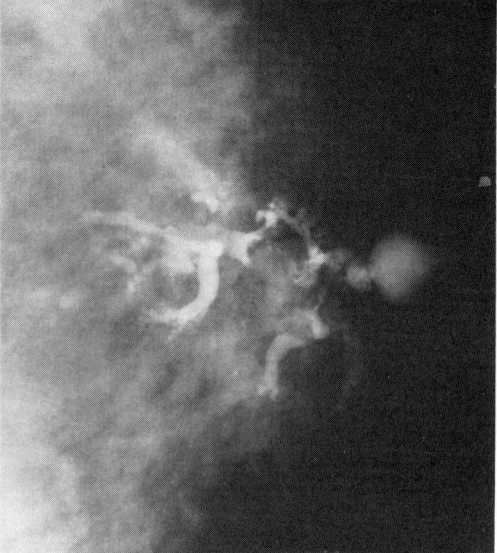

Figure 7–9. Ductogram. This is a large drop of contrast medium hanging from the nipple. About 1.5 cm deep to the nipple is a large filling defect. Pathologic examination proved this to be an intraductal papilloma. Note also the diffuse duct ectasia and an incidental stricture of a side duct just distal to the papilloma, about halfway between it and the nipple.

absolutely necessary in all cases of discharge, bloody or otherwise, it does appear that the method is probably being relatively underutilized considering the information that might be gained from it.

ULTRASONOGRAPHY

Ultrasonography is an important complementary breast imaging tool. It can do what no other imaging test can do: differentiate between cystic and solid masses (Jellins et al., 1977; Kobayashi, 1977; Harper and Kelly-Fry, 1980; Fleischer et al., 1983; Dempsey and Wilson, 1984; Egan and Egan, 1984; Rubin et al., 1985). In fact, Sickles and coworkers (Sickles, 1984a; Sickles et al., 1984) have clearly shown that when the ultrasonographic criteria for a cyst have been scrupulously observed, the predictive value for cysts is equal to that of needle aspiration. This is of extreme importance in evaluating certain mammographic findings that may be nonpalpable.

On the other hand, in the presence of an easily palpable mass, the diagnosis of cyst can be quickly established by needle aspiration. If the cyst is benign, this procedure has the added advantage of often being curative. In older women, however, intracystic papillary neoplasms are not uncommon, and ultrasonography, or pneumocytography at the time of aspiration, should be strongly considered. In cases of cysts that tend to recur, pneumocystography not only is useful for diagnosis but has also been reported to prevent benign cysts from refilling (Tabar et al., 1981).

Although it was initially thought that ultrasonography could ultimately substitute for screening mammography, the technique currently possesses neither the threshold sensitivity nor the specificity to make it a viable screening option. Put another way, minimal cancer cannot yet be detected with sufficient frequency to justify its screening use in asymptomatic women (Sickles et al., 1983; Dempsey and Moskowitz, 1984; Egan and Egan, 1984a; Kopans et al., 1984a, 1985a; Sickles, 1984a; Sickles et al., 1984b).

Wagai (1983) has used ultrasonography as part of a screening program in the Tokyo Prefecture from 1975 to 1981. It is worth critiqueing this study in some detail as it repeats some classic errors of study design.

Primary screening was performed with physical examination, reserving mammography and ultrasonography to evaluate suspicious areas. Thus, the most sensitive detection tool (mammography) was relegated to diagnostic status, and ultrasonography was used for its diagnostic capabilities. In this study, 30,000 women were screened, and only 20 cancers were found. As expected, all 20 cancers were detected by ultrasonography and clinical examination. The stage distribution of cancers found was: T0 = 0, T1 = 20 per cent and T2+ = 80 per cent. Considering that in the BCDDP, the Swedish trial, and the Dutch study, only 20 to 30 per cent of cases were Stage II, and 30 to 40 per cent were less than 5 mm in size, this distribution, reported by Wagai, represents a major step backward.

Recently Kopans and associates (1985a) have reported the results of a prospective study involving xeromammography, whole breast waterpath ultrasonography and clinical examination. The images were interpreted independently, and the population was a referred one. There were 125 cancers, of which 91 per cent were detected by clinical examination and 94 per cent by mammography. Eight clinical lesions were missed by mammography and 12 mammographic lesions were missed by clinical examination. Ultrasonography detected 64 per cent of the cancers, and all of these were palpable. To determine if there were cancers present in the group of "false" positives noted by ultrasonography but possibly missed by the other methods, long-term follow-up (4 years) was carried out. No case of cancer has yet occurred in 255 women who had lesions called suspicious by ultrasonography.

Therefore, in general, ultrasonography should not be used as a primary breast imaging tool, but should probably best be reserved to answer specific clinical questions or problems (Harper and Kelly-Fry, 1980; Fleischer et al., 1983; Harper et al., 1983; Kopans et al., 1984a, 1984b). In this way it can be clinically useful and reasonably cost effective.

For example, in the presence of a palpable abnormality not clearly diagnosable on x-ray mammography, ultrasonography may be particularly helpful (Harper and Kelly-Fry, 1980; Fleischer et al., 1983) (Fig. 7–10). In 186 malignancies demonstrated on sonography (Dempsey and Moskowitz, 1987), 14 were not noted on mammography.

The author has found that when a small, nonpalpable malignancy is seen only on one mammographic projection, an ultrasonographic examination may be a useful adjunct

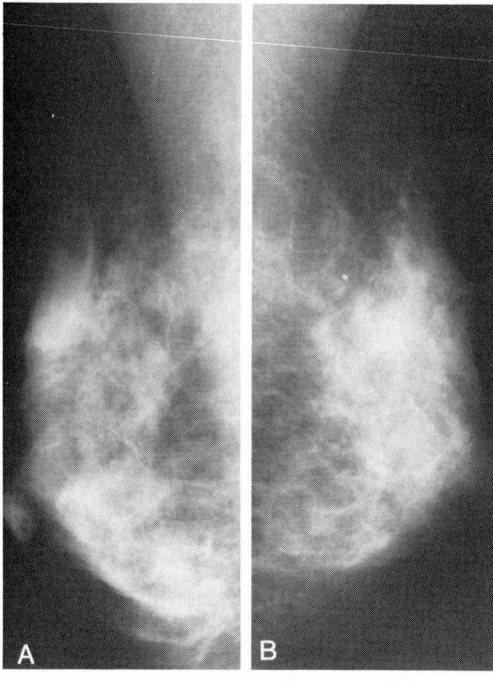
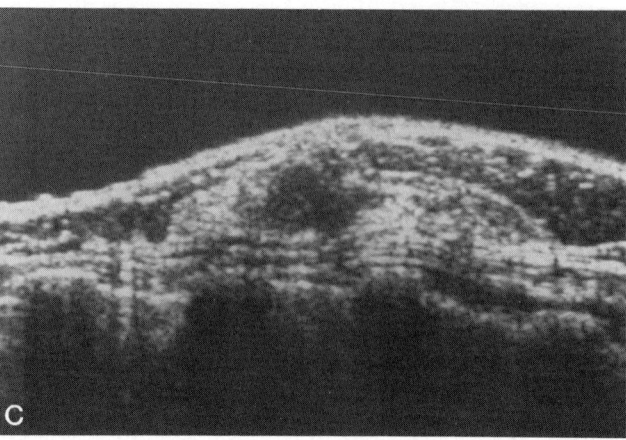

Figure 7–10. *A, B,* Dense breast pattern with a mass superior to the nipple on the left side. Owing to the surrounding density, a firm diagnosis cannot be made, but the findings favor benignity. *C,* Ultrasonography of the mass clearly reveals malignant characteristics.

for three dimensional spatial localization (Fig. 7–11).

Although most carcinomas are hypoechoic and some may cause acoustic shadowing (Kobayshi, 1977, 1979; Harper and Kelly-Fry, 1980; Harper et al., 1983), about 2 per cent will mimic a cyst. Close inspection may reveal some wall irregularity. Increasing the gain will usually demonstrate some increase in irregular central echoes, indicating its solid nature.

Fibroadenomas may present as ovoid, solid masses with well-circumscribed borders, regular internal echoes, and, perhaps, some increased through-transmission. Such a sonographic abnormality in a woman aged 14 to 25 years has a very high probability of being a fibroadenoma (Harper et al., 1983). Cystosarcoma phyllodes, benign or malignant, may have an identical sonographic picture. With the patient's increasing age, given these sonographic criteria, cancer can not be excluded.

Twenty-five per cent of 130 cancers reported by Kopans and associates (1982, 1985a) were solid and sharply defined (i.e., benign), solid masses by ultrasonographic criteria, and 12 per cent of cancers had retrotumoral enhancement rather than shadowing. Kasumi and coworkers (1982) report that about 20 per cent of 743 cancers they examined were circumscribed lesions. In the author's experience, malignant lesions with these characteristics will often be medullary carcinomas, occasionally lymphomas, and less frequently invasive necrotic ductal carcinomas.

As in other areas of the body, masses with mixed cystic and solid features could be the result of abscess, cyst with hemorrhagic debris, resolving hematoma, necrotic ductal cancer, or medullary cancer or lymphoma.

Decreased through-transmission (shadowing) seems to be related to fibrosis (Kobayashi, 1979; Harper et al., 1983) or dense calcifications (Fig. 7–12). Shadowing in the breast can be seen in the absence of malignancy or frank mass, and this may result from beam attenuation owing to intramammary fibrosis, fat necrosis, or normal breast structure. The nipple-areola complex regularly produces shadowing.

A problem with breast sonographic imaging, not to be taken lightly, is the fact that fat lobules may present as hypoechoic demarcated lesions and lead to false positive diagnoses. Although with experience this problem tends to diminish (Fig. 7–13), it does not completely disappear.

In patients with the clinical features of diffuse nodularity, mammography may show a dense breast with multiple nodular shadows or, surprisingly, a fatty, "clear" breast. On the other hand, it has been somewhat surprising to the author to find that sonography of the mammographically dense, nodular breast in

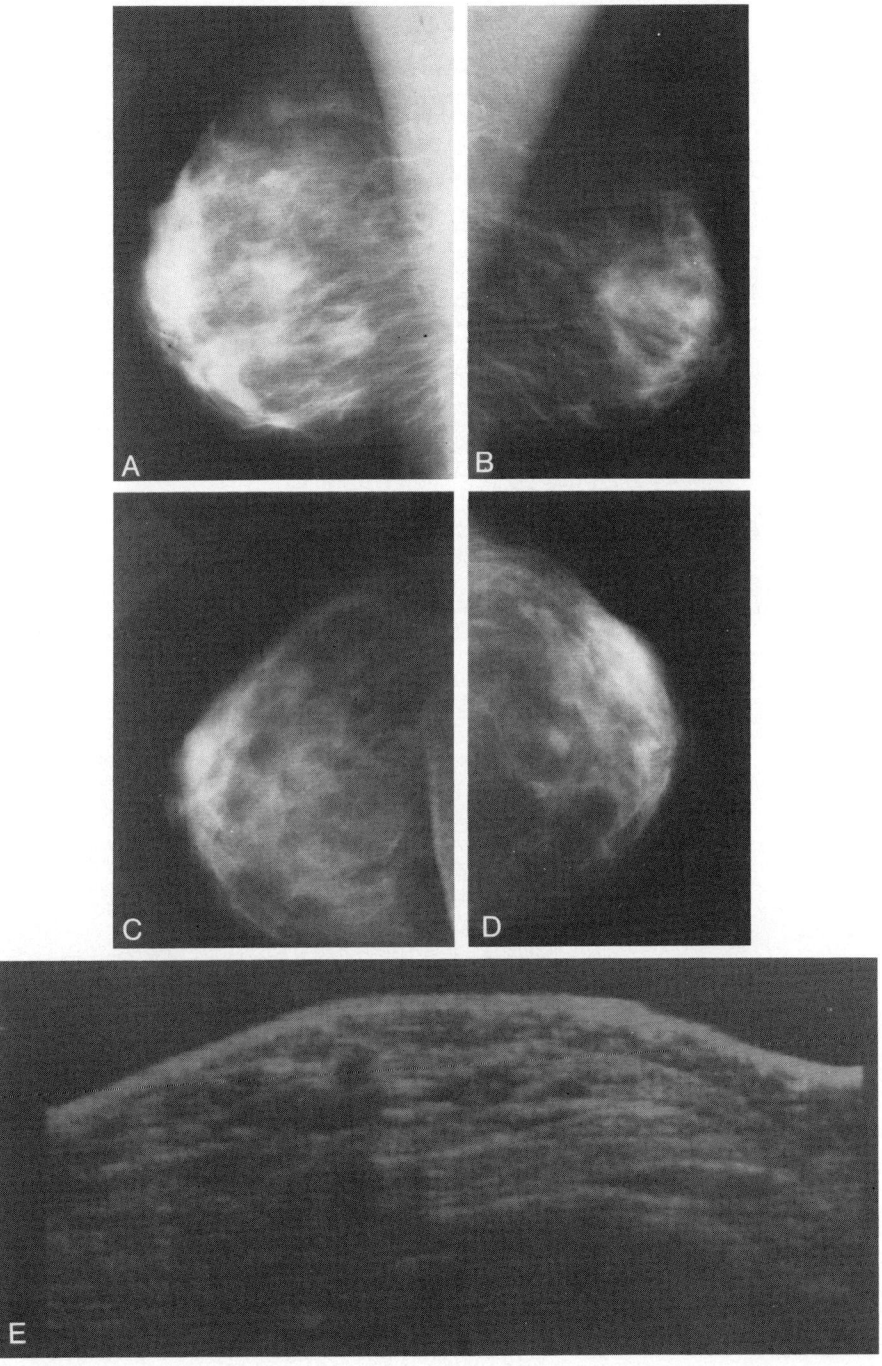

Figure 7–11. *A–D*, Obvious cancer is present in the upper aspect of the left breast in mediolateral oblique view, but is not seen in the caudal view. *E*, Transverse ultrasonography showing the location to be slightly medial.

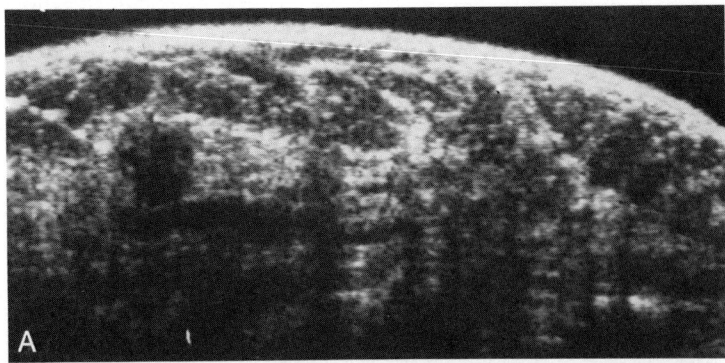
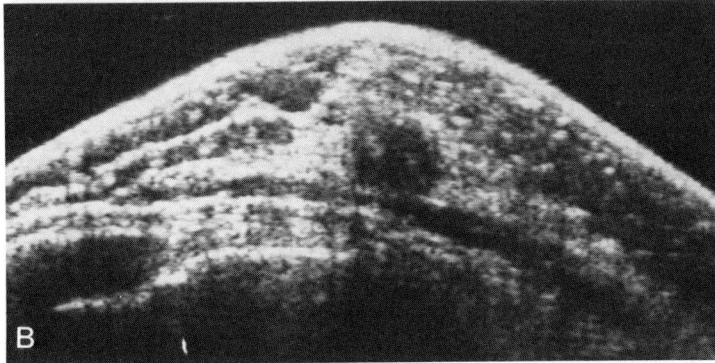

Figure 7–12. Note the irregular, hypoechoic mass without shadowing. The patient was a 31-year-old, pregnant woman with a palpable mass. The histologic diagnosis was medullary carcinoma.

Figure 7–13. This patient is a young woman with a palpable lump. Mammograms were not performed. Ultrasonographic examination was interpreted as lipoma. Pathologic diagnosis was "fatty tissue consistent with lipoma."

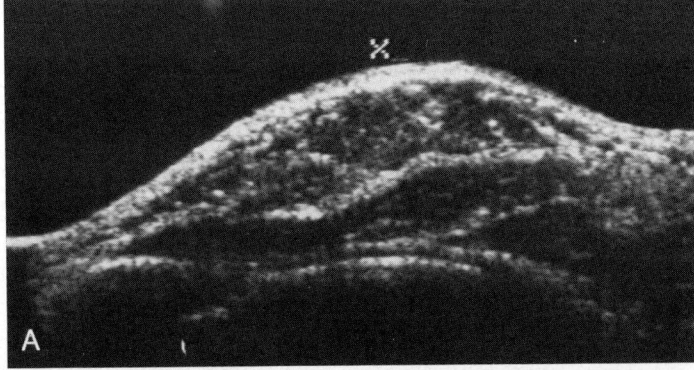
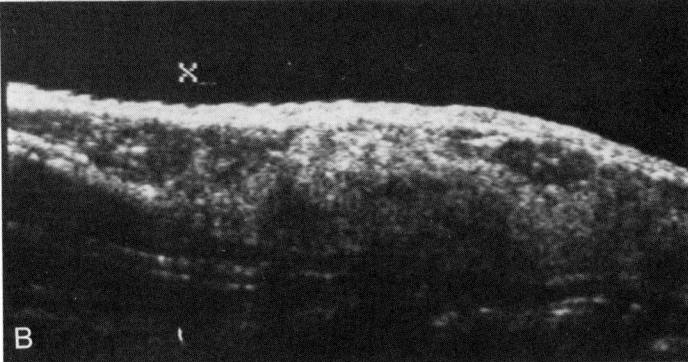

some women demonstrates that many of these "nodules" are not cysts but cannot be differentiated from normal glandular tissue. In other women, multiple cysts of varying size may be seen. Routine whole breast, or large segment, ultrasonographic evaluation of these women in the author's experience has produced many solid or shadowing foci, resulting in a high false positive rate and a very low true positive yield. If there is an area of clinical suspicion in such breasts, restricting the examination to that area may prove diagnostically rewarding. Therefore, the author currently does not recommend routine whole breast, or large segment breast, ultrasonography for dense or nodular breasts in the absence of a local area of clinical or mammographic suspicion.

In women with breast prostheses, the prone whole breast scanners may offer some help in evaluation of the "rind" of residual breast tissue (Cole-Beuglet et al., 1983), but the specificity, sensitivity, and predictive value relative to tumor size still remain to be established.

In Egan and coworkers' study (Egan et al., 1984) ultrasonography alone identified 15 of 31 (48 per cent) of cancers and mammography identified 24 (77 per cent). When positive for cancer, however, the predictive value of ultrasonography was 83 per cent. Generally it is the smallest lesions that can be detected by mammography that are missed by ultrasonography.

It is abundantly clear that ultrasonography can distinguish cysts from solid lesions, and in many cases has performed as well as mammography in symptomatic women with local findings (Texidor and Kazam, 1977; Kasumi et al., 1982; Harper et al., 1983), but it is not yet a screening tool. Perhaps improvements in technology will change this in the future.

DIAPHANOGRAPHY

In years gone by, when a physician desired to distinguish between a solid or cystic mass, he or she might have retired into a dark closet with the patient and a flashlight. After an appropriate period of dark adaptation, the flashlight was lit and applied to the suspect area. Some cysts would transilluminate, and solid lesions often would not, depending on size and proximity to the skin. The total cost of equipment involved was about 50¢. Today the light-tight closet is larger, a technologist often performs the examination, and the equipment consists of a light source, a TV receptor, a computer and floppy disk recorder, and color TV display. Soon to be added is a laser disk recorder. In addition, the procedure has acquired a new name. Instead of transillumination, it has acquired the title of diaphanography. The cost of the equipment alone is many thousands of dollars. It must be asked if this marvelous technologic wonder adds more information than a good flashlight and an attentive doctor.

Diaphanography is thought to depend in great part on the proclivity of some tissues to differentially absorb energy in the visible and near infrared portions of the electromagnetic spectrum. The TV recording device usually is sensitive to the shorter, near infrared range. In at least one currently popular instrument, the light source output varies rapidly between visible red and near infrared. The intensity of the source can be varied. The relative absorption of these two spectra is digitized, expressed as a ratio of absorption, and a color display corresponding to the absorption ratios is demonstrated on a TV screen.

As of this writing, active research programs are under way to determine rationales for differential absorption. It is clear that hemoglobin can absorb strongly in the near infrared range, but it is unclear if this is the sole cause of the image or abnormalities which may be seen.

The role of diaphanography has not yet been clearly elucidated. It still is in a state of Phase I clinical experimental evaluation.

Wallberg (1984) has reported the results of a retrospective review of 116 patients with breast cancer and 167 patients with benign disease. Eighty-four per cent of the cancer cases were examined because of palpable mass, axillary node involvement, or retraction of the skin or nipple. Wallberg reports that mammography sensitivity was 88 per cent, diaphanography was 85 per cent, and together a true positive rate of 95 per cent was achieved. In nine cases in which calcifications were the sole sign of suspicion, diaphanography was positive in seven. A disturbing note, however, is that in 12 per cent of patients with benign disease who had mammographically suspicious calcifications, biopsy was not done because the diaphanography was negative. Given mammography's proven track record, this seems a rather bold move and may alter the sensitivity significantly after a longer period of observation.

Muirhead and Seright (1984) missed only 2 of 11 cancers with diaphanography, one being a 5 mm lesion detected by mammography.

Sickles (1984a) has reported a stepwise increase in detection with increasing size. Twenty per cent of cancers less than 1 cm were detected and 76 per cent of cancers 2 cm and over were found.

Marshall and colleagues (1984) reported results in a population of 1000 women in whom 33 cancers were present. (The prevalence indicates quite clearly that the population is heavily skewed to symptomatic women.) There was one in situ cancer in this group and it went undetected, but 79 per cent of the invasive lesions were found. The sensitivity achieved by Marshall and colleagues was essentially the same for mammography as for diaphanography.

Geslien and coworkers (1985) in a nonblinded, Phase I study, found that 6 of 11 nonpalpable cases were detected by light scanning. Only 3 of 10 tumors less than 1 cm in size were found by this technique, however. These investigators did find one case that presented only as mammographic microcalcifications. The larger the tumor, the more likely it was to be found. These authors were unable to determine a definitive adjunctive role for light scanning at this time, and they also did not note a role for screening.

Anqvist and coworkers (1981) and Thomas (1981) report sensitivities of 38 per cent and 20 per cent, respectively, whereas Bartrum and Crow (1984) and Merritt and colleagues (Merritt et al., 1984; Merritt and Dempsey, 1985) report sensitivity on the order of 75 per cent.

Drexler and colleagues (1985) in a prospective, nonblinded study found that diaphanography detected only 58 per cent of the 26 cancers present in their series, did not pick up the two noninvasive ductal cancers, did identify two in three of the 5 mm cancers, and missed eight cancers less than 2 cm in size. From testing a physical model that they developed, they determined that diaphanography detection is a function of both size of lesion and depth in the breast. They also point out that the false positive rate was three times higher than that of mammography.

To date, these data can not justify the widespread use of diaphanography as a primary screening device. It is unclear to this observer that the data, overall, indicate it is a useful diagnostic device. The Phase I studies cited suggest some potential advantages, several major pitfalls, and areas in which technical development may be needed.

In the author's opinion, this device has not yet matured sufficiently to deserve widespread, general use in a nonexperimental setting. Certainly, in its current state of development, it should not be used to deter biopsy of suspicious areas identified by standard tests.

THERMOGRAPHY*

At this point it is tempting to state that thermography has no proved role in breast cancer detection and to let the matter go at that. However, so that the reader might better appreciate the problems with thermography and perhaps more specifically with the means by which the technique is evaluated, a more detailed review is undertaken here.

As pointed out earlier, the HIP study demonstrated a decreased mortality rate for a population screened for breast cancer compared with nonscreened controls. In that study, about 40 per cent of the cancers in the control population were Stage I or smaller, compared with 56 per cent for the study group.

Today in the United States in the absence of widespread screening, about 55 per cent of cancers are Stage I or less. If mortality rates are to be decreased by screening, the stage of detection must be lowered below 55 per cent Stage I. There is simply no evidence in the literature reviewed that thermography can contribute to lowering the stage at detection in any meaningful way. In fact, a body of data suggests that the converse is the case.

Wenth and Stein (1983) recently reviewed data presented by 26 investigators from the early 1960s into the mid-1970s; most were obtained prior to 1970. Their review showed that the combined data for 32,972 women (including 1998 breast cancer cases) yielded a sensitivity for thermography of 83.4 per cent, a specificity of 85.9 per cent, and a receiver operating characteristic (ROC) detectability index of 2.04. From these data, the authors concluded that thermography is a viable screening tool for breast cancer that should be restored to its "rightful" place. On the basis of these very data, rediscovered by Wenth and

---

*Much of this section is reproduced with permission from Moskowitz, M.: Journal of Reproductive Medicine, 30:451, 1985.

Stein, thermography was introduced into the Breast Cancer Detection Demonstration Projects (BCDDP).

The major problem with these data is that the studies that generated them failed to take into account the size and stage of tumors detected versus the size and stage of tumors that would become detectable by current mass screening methods.

A related, and not necessarily separate, problem is that many of the reported data were derived from symptomatic patients, and the results were extrapolated to the screening situation. This is simply not acceptable. Also, few if any of the studies were blinded, and, as a result, the independent value of a nonlocalizing screening test (particularly one which alone cannot generate a biopsy) is almost impossible to resolve.

That large tumors can be detected by thermography, clinical examination, breast self-examination, and simple inspection is not in question. That these methods can lower the stage of detection significantly is, indeed, in question. No statistical manipulation of data, despite its elegance and sophistication, can overcome the elementary failure of experimental design, beginning with the failure to ask the right question.

As indicated earlier, thermography was introduced into the BCDDP studies. Contrary to some recent reports (Haberman et al., 1980; Nyirjesy, 1982), most of the investigators in the BCDDP did undergo a period of training, and the equipment used was the state-of-the-art for the time. The method was not considered a diagnostic tool but was used as a risk indicator requiring short-term (6 months) follow-up of all cases positive on thermography and negative on all other techniques. It soon became apparent that the false positive rate was so high that short-term recall was not a viable, practical option. Worse yet was the fact that the sensitivity of thermography for the cancers being found in the BCDDP was very low. Because of its low true positive rate, thermography was dropped from the screening program.

Prior to this, a blinded, prospective study to evaluate the efficacy of thermography in detecting minimal and Stage I breast cancers was performed by Moskowitz and coworkers (1976a). It was found that these small cancers could not be identified at any rate greater than that of chance alone by expert observers. In fact, totally naive observers did as well as the experts. This observation caused a furor in the thermographic community, but only Threatt and colleagues (1980) repeated the study. Their investigation was not limited to minimal cancers, however. For in situ carcinomas, the same results were obtained. For all cancers, the overall detection rate could be pushed relatively little above the random chance line.

Haberman and coworkers (1979) have reported on the development of a computer-based interpretation of thermograms that were obtained under highly controlled environmental conditions. Although advanced cancers were found at a rate greater than that of chance, this was not found to be the case for cancers less than 5 mm, intraductal cancers, or in situ lobular cancers.

Reader Agreement

Even among expert thermographers, there is extreme interobserver disagreement in the interpretation of thermograms (Moskowitz et al., 1976a; Threatt et al., 1980; Stern et al., 1982). In all three series just cited, it is quite apparent that agreement on what constitutes a positive thermogram simply did not exist. In the study of Stern and coworkers the readers had been especially trained and tested, and still agreement was elusive.

Gautherie (1982a) has developed a computer-assisted interpretation schema that is said to eliminate this problem. Although computer-assisted interpretation should ensure greater consistency among observers, it is not obvious yet that it will affect risk prediction, cancer detection, or other variables. That will await the results of blinded prospective trials.

Thermography as a Screening Tool

An earlier critical review of the thermographic literature (Moskowitz, 1982) indicated that thermography offered little benefit as a screening device even in the hands of its advocates. At that time the data suggested that thermography simply could not detect the smaller cancers.

The data from Jones and colleagues (1975), for example, showed that thermography correctly identified 77 per cent of *clinical* lesions. However, only 10 per cent of 300 cancers in this study were undetectable clinically. Today, in mass screening centers, 40 to 60 per cent of cancers are undetectable clinically.

In Feig and coworkers' study (1977) only 31 per cent of cancers less than 1 cm were found by thermography, and 32 per cent of those between 1 cm and 2 cm were found. Sixty-two per cent of cancers larger than 2 cm were identified correctly. The thermograms were interpreted by thermographers with a long history of experience and interest in clinical thermography.

Clark and associates (1978) had a true positive rate of 84 per cent for thermography but only 5 per cent of 170 cancers were in situ at the time of detection. This represents no increase in yield of small cancers over that for nonscreening.

Rodes and colleagues (1977) state that "30 per cent of the early cancers found with mass screening will not be detected by infrared scanning, and the bulk of false negatives occur in those patients most amenable to therapy." Significantly this indictment of thermography as a screening device comes from proponents, not opponents, of the art.

The data obtained by Stark and coworkers (Stark et al., 1974; Stark, 1976) suggest that reliance on thermography may be responsible for a significant delay in detection of cancers that could be found earlier by a different approach to screening (Moskowitz, 1982).

Revesz (1978), in a model suggesting strategies for screening, simply fails to take into account stage at detection.

Haberman and colleagues (1980) published results of a large-scale screening effort. They examined 31,322 screenees, who received a total of 47,155 examinations. Ten per cent of these women were under the age of 40 years, and 14 per cent were at high risk. Mammography was not part of the screening examination. Seventy-one cancers were found: 56 screen detected; 10 within 12 months of a negative screen; and 5 more than 12 months later. The prevalence rate, therefore, was 2.1 per 1000 (66 in 31,322). This prevalence rate for this age population is, quite simply, low (vide infra).

Prevalence rates should reflect cancers that would normally "surface" during the initial year, some slowly growing cancers that might never surface, and some "dip" into future incidence, depending on the threshold sensitivity of the screen. For this age population it may be estimated that detectable breast cancer prevalence should be about three to four times the annual incidence. Prevalence of morphologically recognizable, but not detectable, cancers seems to be about 20 to 22 per 1000 (Moskowitz et al., 1976b; Pollei et al., 1986). Indeed, the population-based trials in Sweden and Holland are yielding prevalence rates of 6 to 7 per 1000 (Moskowitz, 1983a). The BCDDP, a nonrandomized nonpopulation-based screen, also yielded rates of this order (Baker, 1982). Although the HIP screen (Shapiro et al., 1973) in the 1960s found a prevalence rate of 2.73 per 1000, it is probable that the lead time gained was only 6 months to 9 months over the nonscreened population, contrasted with an estimated 2.0 to 3.5 years (depending on age) gained today.

It is difficult to determine stage distribution of the detected cancers from the data provided by Haberman and colleagues (1980), but approximately 60 per cent of the patients were free of axillary lymph node involvement. Although the 56 per cent Stage I disease in the HIP screen represented an improvement over the 40 per cent Stage I found in their control group, neither the HIP 56 per cent nor the 60 per cent Stage I found by Haberman and colleagues represents a clinically significant improvement over the 55 per cent Stage I distribution found in nonscreened populations in the United States today (Moskowitz et al., 1975; Third National Cancer Survey, 1975; Axtell et al., 1976). Furthermore, on the basis of the BCDDP data (Baker, 1982) and data presented by Andersson and colleagues (1979), Tabar and Gad (1981), and Rombach (1980), an adequate screen today can find up to 40 per cent of the cases while still less than 5 mm in size or wholly in situ, and up to 80 per cent of cancers while they are Stage I or less.

These data would suggest that Haberman and colleagues' reported screen was not sensitive to the detection of small tumors and, in fact, was not doing any more than could be achieved by physical examination alone.

Rosselli del Turco and coworkers (1983) stated that their own results "confirm that thermography can not play a primary role in breast cancer diagnosis, because of its high proportion of false negatives and false positives; its sensibility is significantly affected by the tumor size and its specificity by age."

Siu and colleagues (1982) examined 300 women referred for evaluation of symptoms of breast disease, aged 19 to 79 years; 22 cases of cancer were found. Clinical examination *guided by thermography* had a reported sensitivity of 71 per cent and specificity of 98 per cent. A statistical equation for "screening" was then derived from the information generated by these patients. Data derived from a high risk, symptomatic population in whom relatively large cancers exist in profusion simply cannot be extrapolated to a low risk, large population of asymptomatic women in whom just the opposite is the case.

Gohegan and coworkers (1980) report that in their BCDDP study, 16.5 per cent of the cancers they detected were less than 5 mm in size, and 27.8 per cent were 5 mm to 1 cm in size; 44 per cent were less than 1 cm in diameter. Of all cases in which lymph nodes were *not* involved, 42 per cent were detected by thermography. When lymph nodes were positive, thermography correctly identified 41.7 per cent of the cases. The false positive rates for thermography were estimated to range from 6 to 21 per cent.

Nyirjesy (1982) states, "We are aware of the fact that minimal or subclinical carcinomas can only be detected by mammograms and that thermograms are normal in many of these early tumors." Despite the statement, he believes that in his hands thermography is an important tool and goes on to buttress his argument with the following data:
1. 6459 thermograms were obtained in 2799 patients.
2. In this population were 34 cancers, 8 of which were less than 1 cm in size and 10 of which were between 1 cm and 2 cm.
3. The 6459 thermograms were read as:
   a. Th1 or Th2 (normal) = 63.5 per cent
   b. Th3 (atypical or doubtful) = 21.5 per cent
   c. Th4, Th5 (abnormal) = 15 per cent
4. True positive rate = 79 per cent. (It is not stated what fraction of the small cancers were detected.)

From these data, if it is assumed that all of the detected cancers occurred only in the Th4 and Th5 groups, the positive predictive value of thermography would be 2.7 per cent. If, as seems more likely, some cancers occurred in the Th3 group, the predictive value for cancer would be 1.1 per cent. From these data, it is not clear to this observer how thermography was helpful.

Graphic stress thermography (GST) has been proposed as an effective modification of thermography applicable to screening. Snyder and colleagues (1979) have shown in a group of patients already scheduled for biopsy at Memorial Hospital that GST had a sensitivity for cancer of approximately 90 per cent. In that same series, about 89 per cent of the patients with benign lesions were also considered positive.

Brooks and coworkers (1983) reported on 1030 patients who received 2012 thermographic studies using computerized evaluation after stress (GST). Of these, 289 patients were selected for mammography; from this group were distilled 61 patients for surgical consultation, and 31 of these were selected for biopsy. It is unclear from the report how the initial selection was made and even less clear how subsequent dichotomies were determined. In this group six cancers were detected, five of which were detected by GST. The average size of the lesions was 1.1 cm. Sufficient information is not presented to allow determination of the actual predictive value. It can only be estimated from the presented data. Assuming that all five detected cancers occurred in those patients with only a Class 3 examination, the predictive value of a positive test would be 1.3 per cent. Assuming that some cancers occurred in Class 2 as well as Class 3 GST scores, the predictive value of a positive test would equal 0.3 per cent.

Gautherie and colleagues (Gautherie and Gros, 1980; Gautherie, 1982a,c, 1983; Gautherie et al., 1982, 1983; personal communication) have presented extensive clinical and laboratory data to support all of the various claimed uses of thermography.

It would appear that neoplasms of some bulk and relatively advanced state can produce sufficient heat under laboratory conditions so that the heat can be measured and quantified. It is unclear, however, that in situ and 5 mm carcinomas can produce sufficient heat to be detected clinically at a significant rate. As fat is a very efficient thermal insulator and minimal amounts of heat at a depth would not reach the surface unless "piped" there by blood vessels, frequent detection of these lesions seems unlikely. It is tempting to postulate that capillary angiogenesis factor or elaboration of local tumoral effects induces sufficient blood flow when the cancers are tiny to allow measurable surface shunting to occur, but this is only speculation at this point.

However, at a meeting in Liege, Gautherie and coworkers (1985) presented preliminary data that suggest, for the first time, that thermography might be able to detect minimal cancers. They attribute this to improvements in thermographic technology and the development of specific and objective interpretation criteria. As they point out, however (1985), the small amount of heat produced by a minimal cancer "would exclude all possibility of detecting the tumor, whatever its depth may be." Gautherie and coworkers believe rather that the thermal abnormalities at the surface reflect local vascular changes accompanying the development of early cancer. The bulk of Gautherie and colleagues' reported work would suggest that such is not the case (Gautherie et al., 1982). For example, of 637 cancers occurring in a referral symptomatic population (1970–1980) only 13 per cent were in situ or nonpalpable or both. Only 27 per cent were less than 2 cm in size, including the 13 per cent already noted.

In Cincinnati, study of symptomatic women from 1950 to 1982 (Moskowitz et al., 1975), revealed that 55 per cent of the cases detected were Stage I or less. This rate is significantly greater than the 27 per cent reported by Gautherie and colleagues.

It might be argued that as the patients evaluated were symptomatic women, the prevalence of advanced cancers would be higher than if screened. Gautherie and colleagues (Gautherie, 1983; Gautherie et al., 1983) provided us with information to test this hypothesis.

In a group of 106 patients selected for screening by thermography, 69.5 per cent of the clinically palpable cancers were Stage II at detection, and by histologic criteria, 97.5 per cent were State II or higher.

Of the total 106 cancers, only 27 per cent were Stage I or less, including 13.2 per cent minimal breast cancer (as defined by Gautherie) and 4 per cent in situ disease. In the author's screened situation, approximately 20 per cent of cases are Stage II or higher; 80 per cent are Stage I or less, including 50 per cent less than 1 cm; 40 per cent are less than 5 mm; and 20 per cent are noninvasive. The author's figures generally are reflected in the BCDDP as a whole (Baker, 1982).

Thus, in the hands of Gautherie and coworkers there was no difference in stage at detection whether patients were referred for evaluation of a mass or were screened. Needless to say, at this junction of knowledge, this is not the goal of a screening process.

Overall, the data strongly suggest that small, deep-seated cancers do not emit sufficient thermal signals to be detected at the surface of the breast. Larger cancers, more peripherally located and usually palpable, may be detected.

Thermography as Risk Indicator

It has been postulated that thermography is a risk indicator for subsequent development of breast cancer (Gautherie and Gros, 1980; Almaric et al., 1983; Hobbins, 1983). It is probably most difficult to design an adequate, nonbiased, prospective trial to measure this parameter among all the aspects discussed. Unless the study is performed in a blinded fashion on an asymptomatic population with adequate controls, a sufficient number of screenees, and long-term follow-up, and unless it is associated with an independent, highly sensitive screening process, a self-fulfilling tautology will ensue; each observation will feed and flow into the other.

Moskowitz and colleagues (1981) have performed a blinded prospective study comparing liquid crystal thermography to generally accepted histopathologic parameters of high risk prediction. An international expert in thermography taught the technical performance, critiqued and rejected technical failures, and interpreted the study images without knowledge of the clinical, historical, or mammographic information. Cases with high risk histopathologic findings were not detected at a rate greater than that of chance alone.

Gautherie and Gros (1980) report on 740 patients who met their criteria for isolated, suspicious thermographic findings. Within 10 years, approximately 40 per cent of these patients have developed a breast cancer. Compared with thermographically negative women in the study, this represents a tenfold increase in risk. However, most of the subsequently detected carcinomas that occurred within the group with suspected lesions occurred within *18 months* of a previously negative clinical and mammographic examination.

Rather than thermography representing an excess risk indicator, perhaps in light of the data reviewed earlier concerning size and threshold of Gautherie and coworkers' primary detecting method, an alternative explanation might prevail:

1. On the basis of the data of Gautherie and colleagues, the threshold sensitivity of the clinical and mammographic evaluation at their institution is between Stage I and Stage II or higher (predominantly Stage II).

2. There are undoubtedly cancers that are Stage I or borderline Stage II that are currently not being detected by the relatively insensitive physical examination and mammography performed at Gautherie's center. (Such a high threshold level of detection for their clinical and mammographic tests suggests that early detection is being sacrificed for a high positive predictive value.)

3. The missed lesions subsequently reach the unusually high threshold of detectability achieved by their clinicians and radiologists in 12 to 18 months.

4. By this time, the lesions are mostly Stage II or higher.

5. As a result of being found at an advanced state, the cancers generally have a poor prognosis.

Gautherie and coworkers (1982) published an interesting descriptive chapter of their methodology. To a major degree this can explain some of the apparent discrepancies in their data (Gautherie and Gros, 1980; Gautherie, 1982b, 1983) and those generated by other prospective studies (Moskowitz et al., 1976a; Threatt et al., 1980; Moskowitz et al., 1981; Baker, 1982; Stern et al., 1982; Moskowitz, 1983b).

To begin, their case material is derived from evaluation of symptomatic, referred patients. For reasons discussed earlier, extrapolation of these data to an asymptomatic, self-selected population is, to say the least, dangerous.

The thermograms were analyzed by a preliminary "blind" reading. This preliminary blind study was then followed by "a careful comparison of the distinct thermal signs with regard to the physical findings in order to eliminate those signs that become less significant than would have appeared to be the case if the thermograms were considered by themselves" (Gautherie et al., 1982). Already a potentially major bias has been introduced.

As noted earlier, 73 per cent of the 637 cancers found in this population were clinical Stage II or higher. Of the tumors that were staged as "smaller" tumors, 43 were in situ, 38 ranged in size from 1.5 cm to 4 cm, and 92 were between 1 cm and 2 cm and were palpable. Therefore, only 43 (7 per cent) could be considered minimal by either of the generally accepted criteria for minimal cancer that are currently in use. The remainder represent, by today's standards, large cancers.

Gautherie and coworkers state that it is acceptable to miss 24 per cent of cancers smaller than 2 cm because some of the missed tumors were as small as 4 mm and probably had a slow growth rate. Perhaps that is so. It appears, however, that far more than 24 per cent of cancers less than 2 cm in size were missed.

That 28 per cent of 130 cancers larger than 1.5 cm in size were nonpalpable in their series is a remarkable observation. Given this perspective, it is easy to understand why 87 per cent of these nonpalpable cases were thermographically positive. Sixty per cent of the few in situ carcinomas that they found were also regarded as positive. Given the low detection rate of these cancers, by Gautherie and coworkers, it is safe to assume that for the most part they were reasonably large, probably multifocal, comedo carcinomas, many of which were probably palpable. In fact, in a blinded prospective study, Moskowitz and colleagues (1981) found some evidence to support this speculation.

Given the data by Threatt and coworkers (1980), Moskowitz and colleagues (1976a), Nyirjesy (1982), Feig and colleagues (1977), Haberman and coworkers (1980), Jones and colleagues (1975), Clark and associates (1978), and Stern and coworkers (1982) that expert thermographers do not find minimal breast cancers, and the fact that most of the cancers in the series reported by Gautherie and colleagues developed within 18 months of an otherwise negative screen, it is far more likely that the apparent risk prediction of thermography is more an artifact of procedure than it is an indicator of risk.

In the author's hands thermography does not appear to be a significant predictor of subsequent breast cancer risk. Although this alone does not indict thermography, the fact that so many authors can not replicate the data found by Gautherie and associates or by Amalric and coworkers would indicate at least that this method is not ready for general use. From the data reviewed, the value of thermography in evaluation of the human breast has not been proved.

Thermography is an experimental tool for breast evaluation. Gautherie and coworkers' approach to standardizing interpretation represents at least a positive step. Perhaps prospective trials adequately designed, asking appropriate questions and based on an adequately screened population, can determine in an objective way, once and for all, what thermography can or cannot contribute to the diagnosis of diseases of the human breast.

OTHER BREAST IMAGING MODALITIES

Magnetic resonance imaging (MRI) is still very new on the scene. It appears to be quite specific for cysts, may be able to detect cancer in fatty breast, is limited in detection of cancer in dense breasts, and is not yet able to find cancer detected only by microcalcifications on mammography (Egan and Mostellar, 1977; Mansfield et al., 1980; Alcorn et al., 1985; Wolfman et al., 1985). At this time, MRI seems to be an expensive way to achieve a result equal to ultrasonography. With the development of newer approaches and newer technology, and perhaps less emphasis on imaging and more on biology, MRI can prove useful in clarifying the natural history of precancerous lesions and cancer (El Yousef et al., 1984, 1985; McSweeney et al., 1984a).

Computed tomography (CT) of the breast seems to require intravenous contrast media (Chang et al, 1980; Kopans et al., 1984a). This requirement, the cost, and number of patients per hour sorely limit the use of CT as a screening tool. In certain highly selected cases, it may prove useful as a diagnostic test, or occasionally to localize in three dimensional space a lesion that can be seen only on one mammographic view.

Digital mammography is on the horizon (McSweeney et al., 1984b; Kopans, personal communication). Early work (Ackerman et al., 1985; Watt et al., 1985) suggests it may have an adjunctive diagnostic role when used with contrast media. It has the added potential advantages of (1) image enhancement; (2) expert system development; (3) perhaps automated prescreening; and (4) extremely low dose. Its ultimate role at this time is still conjectural.

Summary

Breast imaging seems finally to have come of age. If it is used appropriately, fewer and fewer deaths from breast cancer should occur. Less bickering among the professionals (Baum, 1985; Skrabanek, 1985) and a greater cooperative effort are needed if the full benefit of the scientific advances in this area are to be realized.

REFERENCES

Ackerman, L. V., Watt, A. C., Shetty, P., et al.: Breast lesions examined by digital angiography. Work in progress. Radiology, 155:65, 1985.

Alberti, G. P., and Troiso, A.: Secreting breast: The role of galactography. Eur. J. Gynaecol. Oncol, 3:96, 1982.

Alcorn, F. S., Turner, D. A., Clark, J. W., et al.: Magnetic resonance imaging in the study of the breast. RadioGraphics, 5:631, 1985.

Almaric, C., Geraud, D., Thomassin, L., et al.: The persistently abnormal isolated infrared thermogram: The highest known risk for breast cancer. Acta Thermograph., 7:91, 1983.

Anastassiades, O. T., Bouropoulou, V., Kontogeorgos, G., et al.: Microcalcifications in benign breast disease. A histological and histochemical study. Pathol. Res. Pract., 178:237, 1984.

Andersson, I.: Mammographic screening for breast carcinoma: A cross sectional, randomized study of 45-69 year old women. University of Lund, Malmo General Hospital, S-214 01 Malmo, Sweden, 1980.

Andersson, I., Andren, L., Hildell, J., et al.: Breast cancer screening with mammography: A population based, randomized trial with mammography as the only screening mode. Radiology, 132:273, 1979.

Anguist, K. A., Holmlund, D., and Liliequist, B.: Diaphanoscopy and diaphanography for breast cancer detection in clinical practice. Acta Chir. Scand., 147:231, 1981.

Ashikari, R., Huvos, A. G., Snyder, R. E., et al.: A clinico-pathologic study of atypical lesions of the breast. Cancer, 33:310, 1974.

Axtell, L., Asire, A., and Myers, M. (Eds.): Cancer patient survival. Report No. 5. Washington, D. C., U. S. Department of Health, Education and Welfare, Publ. No. (NIH) 77–992, 1976.

Baker, L. H.: Breast Cancer Detection Demonstration Project: Five year summary report. CA, 42:194, 1982.

Baral, E., Larsson, L. E., and Mattson, B.: Breast cancer following irradiation of the breast. Cancer, 40:2905, 1977.

Bartrum, R. J., and Crow, H. C.: Transillumination light scanning to diagnose breast cancer: A feasibility study. AJR, 142:409, 1984.

Baum, M.: Breast cancer controversies (letter to the editor). Lancet 2:564, 1985.

Black, M. M., Barclay, T. H. C., Cutler, S. J., et al.: Association of atypical characteristics of benign breast lesions with subsequent risk of breast cancer. Cancer 29:338, 1972.

Blommers, T. J.: Transplant and dialysis: The cost/benefit question. Iowa Med., 74:15, 1984.

Boisselier, P., Durand, J. C., Veith, F., et al.: Prognosis of breast epithelioma detected by microcalcifications in the absence of a palpable tumor. Presse Med., 12:1411, 1983.

Boon, M. E., and deGraaff Guilloud, J. C.: Cost effectiveness of population screening and rescreening for cervical cancer in the Netherlands. Acta Cytol., 25:539, 1981.

Boyd, N. F., O'Sullivan, B., Fishell, E., et al.: Mammographic patterns and breast cancer risk: Methodologic

standards and contradictory results. JNCI, 72:1253, 1984.
Brisson, J., Morrison, A. S., Kopans, D. B., et al.: Height and weight, mammographic features of breast tissue, and breast cancer risk. Am. J. Epidemiol., 119:371, 1984.
Broberg, A., Glas, U., Gustafsson, S. A., et al.: Relationship between mammographic pattern and estrogen receptor content in breast cancer. Breast Cancer Res. Treat., 3:201, 1983.
Brooks, P. G., Gart, S., Heldfond, A. J., et al.: Breast screening in the primary care office: A plea for early detection. J. Reprod. Med., 27:685, 1983.
Carlile, T., Kopecky, K. J., Thompson, D. J., et al.: Breast cancer prediction and the Wolfe classification of mammograms. J.A.M.A., 254:1050, 1985.
Chang, C. H. J., Sibala, J. L., Fritz, S. L., et al.: Computed tomography in detection and diagnosis of breast cancer. Cancer, 46:939, 1980.
Chaudary, M. A., Gravelle, I. H., Bulstrode, J. C., et al.: Breast parenchymal patterns in women with bilateral primary breast cancer. Br. J. Radiol., 56:703, 1983.
Clark, R. M., Rideout, D. F., and Chart, P. L.: Thermography of the breast: Experiences in diagnosis and follow up in a cancer treatment centre. Acta Thermograph., 3:155, 1978.
Cole-Beauglet, C., Schwartz, G., Kurtz, A. B., et al.: Ultrasound mammography for the augmented breast. Radiology, 146:737, 1983.
Committee on the Biological Effect of Ionizing Radiation: The effects on populations of exposure to low levels of ionizing radiation. Washington, D. C., National Academy of Sciences, National Research Council, 1980.
Coopmans de Yoldi, G. F., Andreoli, C., Costa, A., et al.: Lack of efficacy of xeroradiography to preoperatively detect axillary lymph node metastases in breast cancer. Breast Cancer Res. Treat. 3:373, 1983.
Council on Scientific Affairs: Early detection of breast cancer. J.A.M.A., 252:3008, 1984.
Danes, J.: Wolfe's risk groups and the incidence of breast carcinoma. Sb. Lek., 85:24, 1983.
Dempsey, P. J., and Moskowitz, M.: Is there a role for breast sonography? In McGraham, J. P. (ed.): Clinics in Diagnostic Ultrasound, Vol. 20. New York, Churchill Livingstone, 1987, pp. 17–36.
Dempsey, P. J., and Wilson, P. C.: The use of automated sonography in total clinical breast evaluation. Clin Diagn. Ultrasound, 12:57, 1984.
deWaard, F., Collette, H. J. A., Rombach, J. J., et al.: The DOM Project for the early detection of breast cancer, Utrecht, The Netherlands. J. Chron. Dis., 37:1, 1984.
Devitt, J. E.: Mammography: A surgeon's experience. Can. Med. Assoc. J., 120:1370, 1979.
DiPietro, S., Coopmans de Yoldi, G., Bergonzi, S., et al.: Nipple discharge as a sign of preneoplastic lesions and occult carcinoma of the breast: Clinical and galactographic study in 103 consecutive patients. Tumori, 65:317, 1979.
Dodd, G. D.: Mammography. State of the art. Cancer, 53(Suppl. 3):652, 1984.
Drexler, B., Davis, J. L., and Schofield, G.: Diaphanography in the diagnosis of breast cancer. Radiology, 157:41, 1985.
Dupont, W. D., and Page, D. L.: Risk factors for breast cancer in women with proliferative breast disease. N. Engl. J. Med., 312:146, 1985.
Eddy, D. M.: Screening for breast cancer. Proceedings of the Nineteenth Annual National Conference on the Diagnosis, Detection and Treatment of Breast Cancer, San Diego, Calif., March 1981.
Eddy, D. M.: Finding cancer in asymptomatic people. Estimating the benefits, costs and risks. Cancer, 51(Suppl. 12):2440, 1983.
Editorial: Lancet, 1:851, 1985.
Egan, R. L., and Egan, K. L.: Detection of breast carcinoma: Comparison of automated water-path whole-breast sonography, mammography, and physical examination. AJR, 143:493, 1984.
Egan, R. L., and Mosteller, R. C.: Breast cancer mammography patterns. Cancer, 40:2087, 1977.
Egan, R. L., McSweeney, M. B., and Murphy, F. B.: Breast sonography and the detection of cancer. Recent Results Cancer Res., 90:90, 1984.
El Yousef, S. J., Duchesneau, R. H., and Alfidi, R.: Nuclear magnetic resonance imaging of the human breast. RadioGraphics, 4:113, 1984.
El Yousef, S. J., O'Connell, D. M., Duchesneau, R. H., et al.: Benign and malignant breast disease: Magnetic resonance and radiofrequency pulse sequences. AJR, 145:1, 1985.
Evans, J.: Radiologic seminar CCXXXVIII: Mammography—benefit and risk. J. Miss. State Med. Assoc., 25:151, 1984.
Feig, S. A.: Hypothetical breast cancer risk from mammography. Recent Results Cancer Res., 90:1, 1984a.
Feig, S.: Radiation risk from mammography: Is it clinically significant? AJR, 143:469, 1984b.
Feig, S.: Assessment of the hypothetical risk from mammography and evaluation of the potential benefit. Radiol. Clin. North Am., 21:173, 1983.
Feig, S. A., Shaber G. S., Schwartz, G. F., et al.: Thermography, mammography and clinical examination in breast cancer screening: Review of 16,000 studies. Radiology, 122:123, 1977.
Fleischer, A. C., Muhletaler, C. A., Reynolds, V. A., et al.: Palpable breast masses: Evaluation by high frequency, hand-held real-time sonography and xeromammography. Radiology, 148:813, 1983.
Fox, S., Baum, J. K., Klos, D. S., et al.: Breast cancer screening: The underuse of mammography. Radiology, 156:607, 1985.
Fox, S. H., Moskowitz, M., Saenger, E. L., et al.: Benefit/risk analysis of aggressive mammographic screening. Radiology, 128:350, 1978.
Friedlander, M. L., and Tattersall, M. H.: Counting the costs of cancer therapy. Eur. J. Cancer Clin. Oncol., 18:1237, 1982.
Gad, A., Thomas, B. A., and Moskowitz, M.: Screening for breast cancer in Europe: Achievements, problems, and future. Recent Results Cancer Res., 90:179, 1984.
Galkin, B. M., Feig, S. A., Patchefsky, A. S., et al.: Ultrastructure and microanalysis of "benign" and "malignant" breast calcifications. Radiology, 124:245, 1977.
Gauthrie, M.: Improved system for the objective evaluation of breast thermograms. Prog. Clin. Biol. Res., 107:897, 1982a.
Gauthrie, M.: Temperature and blood flow patterns in breast cancer during natural evolution and following radiotherapy. Biomed. Thermol., 107:21, 1982b.
Gauthrie, M.: Thermobiological assessment of benign and malignant breast diseases. Chicago Gynecological Society, Holmes Lecture, April 1983.
Gauthrie, M., and Gros, C. M.: Breast thermography and cancer risk prediction. Cancer, 45:51, 1980.
Gauthrie, M., Haehnel, P., Walter, J. P. et al.: Long term assessment of breast cancer risk by liquid crystal thermal imaging. Prog. Clin. Biol. Res., 107:279, 1982.

Gautherie, M., Haehnel, P., and Walter, J. P.: Thermovascular disorders in in situ and minimal breast cancer. In Evaluation du Risque de Cancer Mammaire, Chimotherapie Primiere. Proceedings of the International Symposium of Senology, Liege, Belgium, November 1985.

Gautherie, M., Kotewicz, A., and Gueblez, P.: Accurate and objective evaluation of breast thermograms: Basic principles and new advances with special reference to an improved computer assisted scoring system. International Conference on Thermal Assessment of Breast Health, Washington, D. C., July 1983.

Geslien, G. E., Fisher, J. R., and Delaney, C.: Transillumination in breast cancer detection: Screening failures and potential. AJR, 144:619, 1985.

Gohegan, J. K., Rodes, N. D., Blackwell, S. W., et al.: Individual and combined effectiveness of palpation, thermography, and mammography in breast cancer screening. Prev. Med. 9:713, 1980.

Haberman, J. D.: Mass screening for breast cancer by electronic infrared pattern recognition. Final report, phase II (October 1976–June 1979). Oklahoma City, University of Oklahoma Health Sciences Center, Department of Radiological Sciences, 1979.

Haberman, J. D., Love, T. J., and Fracis, J. E.: Screening a rural population for breast cancer using thermography and physical examination techniques: Methods and results—a preliminary report. Ann. N.Y. Acad. Sci., 335:492, 1980.

Hajek, P., Binder, W., Kumpan, W., et al.: Lokalisationsgerät zur Feinnadelpunktion nicht papabler Veränderungen in der Mamma. Röntgenalatter, 36:285, 1983.

Harper, A. P., and Kelly-Fry, E.: Ultrasound visualization of the breast in symptomatic patients. Radiology, 137:465, 1980.

Harper, A. P., Kelly-Fry, E., Noe, J. S., et al.: Ultrasound in the evaluation of solid breast masses. Radiology, 146:731, 1983.

Hebert, G., Carrier, R., McFarlane, D. V., et al.: Guidelines for detection of breast cancer: An update on investigative methods. A report to the Ad Hoc Committee on Mammography of The Canadian Association of Radiologists. J. Can. Assoc. Radiol., 35:6, 1984.

Hinton, C. P., Roebuck, E. J., Williams, M. R., et al.: Mammographic parenchymal patterns: Value as a predictor of hormone dependency and survival in breast cancer. AJR, 144:1103, 1985.

Hobbins, W.: INITIAL (quarterly newsletter for Thermal Image Analysis), 4:1, 1983. Produced by Wisconsin Breast Cancer Detection Foundation, Madison.

Homer, M. J.: Nonpalpable breast lesion localization using a curved-end retractable wire. Radiology, 157:259, 1985.

Horwitz, R. I., Lamas, A. M., and Peck, D.: Mammographic parenchymal patterns and risk of breast cancer in postmenopausal women. Am. J. Med., 77:621, 1984.

Howe, G. R., Miller, A. B., and Sherman, G. J.: Breast cancer mortality following fluoroscopic irradiation in a cohort of tuberculosis patients. Cancer Detect. Prev., 5:175, 1982.

Huppe, J. R., and Schneider, H. J.: Comparative film mammography and xeromammography (German). ROFO, 126:361, 1977.

Jellins, J., Kossoff, G., and Reeve, T. S.: Detection and classification of liquid-filled masses in the breast by gray-scale echography. Radiology, 125:205, 1977.

Jensen, S. R., and Mackey, J. K.: Xeromammography after augmentation mammoplasty. AJR, 144:629, 1985.

Jones, C. H., Greening, W. P., Davey, J. B., et al.: Thermography of the female breast: A five year study in relation to the detection and prognosis of cancer. Br. J. Radiol., 48:532, 1975.

Kalisher, L., Chu, A. M., and Peyster, R. G.: Clinicopathological correlations of xeroradiography in determining involvement of metastatic axillary nodes in female breast cancer. Radiology, 121:333, 1976.

Kambouris, T., Kotoulas, K., and Pontifex, G.: The diagnostic value of xeromammography in clinically occult breast cancer. Radiologe, 24:L230, 1984.

Kasumi, F., Fukami, A., Kuno, K., et al.: Characteristic echographic features of circumscribed cancer. Ultrasound Med. Biol., 8:369, 1982.

Kays, H. W.: Cost effective cancer screening. J. Indiana State Med. Assoc., 76:324, 1983.

Kelly, M. E., Taylor, G. J., Moses, H. W., et al.: Comparative cost of myocardial revascularization: Percutaneous transluminal angioplasty and coronary artery bypass surgery. J. Am. Coll. Cardiol., 5:16, 1985.

Kindermann, G., Paterok, E., Weishaar, J., et al.: Early detection of ductal breast cancer: The diagnostic procedure for pathological discharge from the nipple. Tumori, 65:555, 1979.

Kobayashi, T.: Gray-scale echography for breast cancer. Radiology, 122:207, 1977.

Kobayashi, T.: Diagnostic ultrasound in breast cancer: Analysis of retrotumorous echo patterns correlated with sonic attunuation by cancerous connective tissue. JCU, 7:471, 1979.

Kojima, O., Majima, T., Uehara, Y., et al.: Radiographic parenchymal patterns in Japanese females as a risk factor for breast carcinoma. World J. Surg., 8:414, 1984.

Kopans, D. B.: "Early" breast cancer detection using techniques other than mammography. AJR, 143:465, 1984.

Kopans, D. B., Meyer, J. E., and Sadowsky, N.: Breast imaging. N. Engl. J. Med., 310:960, 1984a.

Kopans, D. B., Meyer, J. E., Lindfors, K. K., et al.: Breast sonography to guide cyst aspiration and wire localization of occult solid lesions. AJR, 143:489, 1984b.

Kopans, D. B., Meyer, J. E., and Lindfors, K. K.: Whole breast US imaging: Four year follow up. Radiology, 157:505, 1985a.

Kopans, D. B., Lindfors, K. K., McCarthy, K. A., et al.: Spring hookwire breast lesion localizer: Use with rigid-compression mammographic systems. Radiology, 157:537, 1985b.

Kopans, D. B., Meyer, J. E., and Steimbock, R. T.: Breast cancer: The appearance as delineated by whole breast water-path ultrasound scanning. J. Clin. Ultrasound, 10:313, 1982.

Lansky, S. B., Black, J. L., and Cairns, N. U.: Childhood cancer. Medical costs. Cancer, 52:762, 1983.

LeGal, M., Chavanne, G., and Pellier, D.: Diagnostic value of clustered microcalcifications discovered by mammography (apropos of 227 cases with histological verification and without a palpable breast tumor). Bull. Cancer (Paris), 71:57, 1984.

Lesnick, G. J.: Detection of breast cancer in young women. J.A.M.A., 237:967, 1977.

Long, S. H., Gibbs, J. O., Crozier, J. P., et al.: Medical expenditures of terminal cancer patients during the last year of life. Inquiry, 21:315, 1984.

Lundgren, B.: Population screening for breast cancer by single view mammography in a geographic region in Sweden. JNCI, 62:1373, 1379, 1979a.

Lundgren, B.: Positioning for oblique projection in mammography (letter to the editor). AJR, 132:858, 1979b.

Lundgren, B., and Helleberg, A.: Single oblique view mammography for periodic screening for breast cancer in women. JNCI, *68*:351, 1982.

Lundgren, B., and Jakobsson, S.: Repeat screening by single oblique view mammography. Breast Cancer Res. Treat., *1*:273, 1981.

Mahoney, L., and Csima, A.: Use and abuse of mammography in the early diagnosis of breast cancer. Can. J. Surg., *26*:262, 1983.

Mahoney, L. J., Bird, B. L., and Cooke, G. M.: Annual clinical examination. The best available screening test for breast cancer. N. Engl. J. Med., *301*:315, 1979.

Mansfield, P., Moris, P. G., Ordidge, R. J., et al.: Human whole body imaging and detection of breast tumors by NMR. Phil. Trans. R. Soc. Lond. (Biol.), *289*:503, 1980.

Marshall, V., Williams, D. C., and Smith, K. D.: Diaphanography as a means of detecting breast cancer. Radiology, *150*:339, 1984.

Martin, J., Moskowitz, M., and Milbrath, J. R.: Breast cancer missed by mammography. AJR, *132*:737, 1979.

McSweeney, M. B., Small, W. C., Cerney, V., et al.: Magnetic resonance imaging in the diagnosis of breast disease: Use of transverse relaxation times. Radiology, *153*:741, 1984*a*.

McSweeney, M. B., Sprawls, P., and Egan, R. L.: Enhanced-image mammography. Recent Results Cancer Res., *90*:79, 1984*b*.

Mendell, L., Rosenbloom, M., and Maimark, A.: Are breast patterns a risk index for breast cancer? A reappraisal. AJR, *128*:547, 1977.

Merritt, C. R., and Dempsey, P.: Presentation refresher course. Radiological Society of North America meeting, Chicago, November 1985.

Merritt, C. R., Sullivan, M. A., Segaloff, A., et al.: Real time transillumination: Light scanning of the breast. RadioGraphics *4*:989, 1984.

Meyer, J. E., Kopans, D. B., Stomper, P. C., et al.: Occult breast abnormalities: Percutaneous preoperative needle localization. Radiology, *150*:335 1984.

Miller, A. B.: Presentation at World Health Organization Committee meeting, Moscow, USSR, October, 1985.

Mooney, G. H.: Radiology and risk: An economist's perspective. Br. J. Radiol., *54*:861, 1981.

Mooney, G.: Breast cancer screening. A study in cost effectiveness analysis. Soc. Sci. Med., *16*:1277, 1982.

Moskowitz, M.: Screening is not diagnosis. Radiology, *133*:265, 1979.

Moskowitz, M.: Mammographic parenchymal patterns: More controversy. J.A.M.A., *247*:210, 1982.

Moskowitz, M.: Minimal breast cancer redux. Radiol. Clin. North Am., *21*:93, 1983*a*.

Moskowitz, M.: Screening for breast cancer: How effective are our tests? CA, *33*:26, 1983*b*.

Moskowitz, M.: The predictive value of certain mammographic signs in screening for breast cancer. Cancer, *51*:1007, 1983*c*.

Moskowitz, M.: Mammography to screen asymptomatic women for breast cancer. AJR, *413*:457, 1984.

Moskowitz, M., and Fox, S. H.: Cost analysis of aggressive breast cancer screening. Radiology, *130*:254, 1979.

Moskowitz, M., Fox, S. H., Brun del Re, R., et al.: The potential of liquid crystal thermography in detecting significant mastopathy. Radiology, *140*:659, 1981.

Moskowitz, M., Gartside, P., Gardella, L., et al.: The breast cancer screening controversy: A perspective. AJR, *129*:537, 1977.

Moskowitz, M., Gartside, P., and McLaughlin, C.: Mammographic patterns as markers for high risk benign breast disease and incident cancers. Radiology, *134*:293, 1980*a*.

Moskowitz, M., Gartside, P., Wirman, J. A., et al.: Proliferative disorders of the breast as risk factors for breast cancer in a self selected population: Pathologic markers. Radiology, *134*:289, 1980*b*.

Moskowitz, M., Milbrath, J., Gartside, P., et al.: Lack of efficacy of thermography as a screening tool for minimal and stage 1 breast cancer. N. Engl. J. Med., *295*:249, 1976*a*.

Moskowitz, M., Saenger, E. L., Gartside, P. S., et al.: Benefit versus risk in mammographic screening: One approach. Proceedings of the Eighth Annual National Conference of Radiation Control, Springfield, Ill., May 1976*b*.

Moskowitz, M., Russel, P., Fidler, J., et al.: Breast cancer screening: Preliminary report of 207 biopsies performed in 4128 volunteer screenees. Cancer, *36*:2245, 1975.

Muirhead, A., and Seright, W.: Clinical experience with the diaphanograph machine. Ann. R. Coll. Surg. Engl., *66*:123, 1984.

Myers, L. E., McLelland, R., Stricker, C. S., et al.: Reproducibility of mammographic classifications. AJR, *141*:445, 1983.

Myrden, J. A., and Hiltz, J. E.: Breast cancer following multiple fluoroscopies during artificial pneumothorax treatment of pulmonary tuberculosis. Can. Med. Assoc. J., *100*:1032, 1969.

Nielsen, N. S. M., and Poulsen, H. S.: Relation between mammographic findings and hormone receptor content in breast cancer. AJR, *145*:501, 1985.

Nyirjesy, I.: Breast thermography. Clin. Obstet. Gynecol., *25*:401, 1982.

O'Connor, G. T., Schneider-Jones, G. M., Leshen, M., et al.: The potential effects of mammographic screening as recommended by the American Cancer Society: A modeling study. Meeting abstract. Society of Medical Decision Making, 1985.

Pagani, J. J., Bassett, L. W., Gold, R. H., et al.: Efficacy of combined film screen/xeromammography. AJR, *135*:141, 1980.

Page, D. L., Vander Zwaag, R., Rogers, L. W., et al.: Relation between component parts of fibrocystic disease complex and breast cancer. JNCI, *61*:1055, 1978.

Paterok, E. M., Egger, H., and Willgeroth, F.: More than 1500 radiologically indicated breast biopsies. Microcalcifications and the pathologic galactogram, 1964–1982. Geburtshilfe. Fraunheilkd., *43*:721, 1983.

Paulus, D. D.: Conservative treatment of breast cancer: Mammography in patient selection and follow up. AJR, *143*:483, 1984.

Peyster, R. G., Kalisher, L., and Cole, R.: Mammographic parenchymal patterns and the prevalence of breast cancer. Radiology, *125*:387, 1977.

Peyster, R. G., and Kalisher, L.: Galactography. Rev. Interam. Radiol., *4*:57, 1979.

Pollei, S. R., Mettler, F. A., Bartow, S., et al.: Occult breast cancer: Prevalence and radiographic detectability. Radiology, *163*:459, 1987.

Price, J.: Personal communication, 1985.

Prorok, J. J., Trostle, D. R., Scarlato, M., et al.: Excisional breast biopsy and roentgenographic examination for mammographically detected microcalcification. Am. J. Surg., *145*:684, 1983.

Rasanen, O., Auranen, A., and Gronross, M.: Screening for breast cancer in Finland. Presented at Third Meeting of the European Group for Breast Cancer Screening, Dusseldorf, Germany, August 1984.

Rasmussen, O. S., and Serrup, A.: Preoperative radiographically guided wire marking of nonpalpable breast lesions. Acta Radiol. Diagn., 25:13, 1984.

Revesz, G.: Breast cancer screening: Predictive values and strategies. Acta Thermograph., 3:150, 1978.

Rideout, D. F., and Poor, P. Y.: Patterns of breast parenchyma on mammography. J. Can. Assoc. Radiol., 28:257, 1977.

Rodes, N. D., Farrell, C., and Blackwell, C. W.: Missouri's role in breast cancer detection. Missouri Med., 74:689, 1977.

Romanini, A., and Bock E.: Mammography and xeromammography. Min. Ginecol., 34:851, 1982.

Rombach, J. J.: Breast cancer screening: Results and implications for diagnostic decision making. Brussels, Alphen Aan Den Rijn, Stafleu's Scientific Publishing Co., 1980.

Rosselli del Turco, M., Santoni, R., Ciatto, S., et al.: The role of infrared thermography, mammography, and physical examination in the diagnosis of breast cancer. Acta Thermograph., 8:86, 1983.

Rubin, E., Miller, V. E., Berland, L. L., et al.: Hand held real-time breast sonography. AJR, 144:623, 1985.

Sandison, A. T.: An autopsy study of the adult human breast. National Cancer Institute Monograph. Washington, D. C., U. S. Department of Health, Education and Welfare, No. 8, June, 1962.

Schalldach, U., and Schumann, E.: The significance of mammography in follow up care of mammary carcinoma patients for detection of bilateral carcinoma. Zentralbl. Chir., 107:462, 1982.

Schroeder, S. A., Showstack, J. A., and Schwartz, J.: Survival of adult high-cost patients. Report of a follow up study from 9 acute care hospitals. J.A.M.A., 245:1446, 1981.

Seidman, H.: Screening for breast cancer in younger women: Life expectancy gains and losses. An analysis according to risk indicator groups. Cancer, 27:66, 1977.

Shapiro, S., Goldberg, J. D., and Hutchison, G. B.: Lead time in breast cancer detection and implications for periodicity of screening. Am. J. Epidemiol., 100:357, 1974.

Shapiro S., Strax, P., Venet, L., et al.: Changes in 5 year breast cancer mortality in a breast cancer screening program. Seventh National Cancer Conference Proceedings. Philadelphia, J. B. Lippincott, 1973.

Shapiro, S., Venet, W., Strax, P., et al.: Ten to fourteen year effects of breast cancer screening on mortality. JNCI, 69:349, 1982.

Sickles, E. A.: Breast cancer detection with transillumination and mammography. AJR, 142:841, 1984a.

Sickles, E. A.: Mammographic features of "early" breast cancer. AJR, 143:461, 1984b.

Sickles, E. A., Filly, R. A., and Callen, P. W.: Breast cancer detection with sonomammography and mammography: Comparison using state-of-the-art equipment. AJR, 140:843, 1983.

Sickles, E. A., Filly, R. A., and Callen, P. W.: Benign breast lesions: Ultrasound detection and diagnosis. Radiology, 151:467, 1984.

Siu, O., Ghent, W. R., Colwell, B. T., et al.: Thermogram aided clinical examination of the breast-an alternative to mammography for women 50 or younger. Can. J. Publ. Health, 73:232, 1982.

Skrabanek, P.: Screening for disease: False premises and false promises of breast cancer screening. Lancet, 2:316, 1985.

Snyder, R. E.: Specimen radiography and preoperative localization of nonpalpable breast cancer. Cancer, 46:950, 1980.

Snyder, R. E., Watson, R. C., and Crux, N.: Graphic stress telethermography (GST): A possible supplement to physical examination in screening for abnormalities of the female breast. Am. J. Diagn. Gynecol. Obstet., 1:197, 1979.

Spratt, J. S., Alagia, D. P., Greenberg, R. A., et al.: Association of chronic cystic mastopathy, xeromammographic patterns, and cancer. Cancer, 55:1372, 1985.

Stamp, G. W., Whitehouse, G. H., McDicken, I. W., et al.: Mammographic and pathological correlations in a breast screening programme. Clin. Radiol., 34:529, 1983.

Stark, A. M.: The significance of an abnormal breast thermogram. Acta Thermograph., 1:33, 1976.

Stark, A. M., and Way, S.: The use of thermovision in the detection of early breast cancer. Cancer, 33:1664, 1974.

Stern, E. E., Curtis, A. C., Miller, S., et al.: Thermography in breast diagnosis. Cancer, 50:323, 1982.

Strax, P.: Mass screening for control of breast cancer. Cancer, 53(Suppl. 3): 665, 1984.

Tabar, L., and Dean, P. B.: Mammographic parenchymal patterns: risk indicators for breast cancer? J.A.MA., 247:185, 1982.

Tabar, L., Dean, P. B., and Pentek, Z.: Galactography: The diagnostic procedure of choice for nipple discharge. Radiology, 149:31, 1983.

Tabar, L., and Gad, A.: Screening for breast cancer: The Swedish trial. Radiology, 138:219, 1981.

Tabar, L., Pentek, Z., and Dean, P. B.: The diagnostic and therapeutic value of breast cyst puncture and pneumocystography. Radiology, 141:659, 1981.

Tabar, L., Fagerberg, C. J. G., Gad, A., et al.: Reduction in mortality from breast cancer after mass screening with mammography. Lancet, 1:829, 1985.

Texidor, H. S., and Kazam, E.: Combined mammographic-sonographic evaluation of breast masses. AJR, 128:409, 1977.

Third National Cancer Survey: Incidence Data. National Cancer Institute Monograph No. 41, March 1975. Washington, D. C., U. S. Department of Health, Education and Welfare, Publ. No. (NIH) 75–787.

Thomas, B. A.: Breast transillumination using the sinus diaphanograph. Br. Med. J., 283:1057, 1981.

Threatt, B., Norbeck, J. M., and Ullman, N. S.: Thermography and breast cancer: An analysis of a blind reading. Ann. N.Y. Acad. Sci., 335:501, 1980.

Turnbull, A. D., Carlon, G., Baron, R., et al.: The inverse relationship between cost and survival in the critically ill cancer patient. Crit. Care Med., 7:20, 1979.

Verbeek, A. L. M.: Population screening for breast cancer in Nijmegen: An evaluation of the period 1975–1982. Nijmegen, Netherlands: Katholieke Universiteit Nijmegen, 1985.

Verbeek, A. L. M., Henriks, J. H. C.L., Peeters, P. H. M., et al.: Mammographic breast pattern and the risk of breast cancer. Lancet, 1:591, 1984.

Wagai, T.: Results of screening trials in Japan. In Jellins, J., and Kobayashi, T. (Eds.): Ultrasonic Examination of the breast. New York, John Wiley & Sons, 1983, p. 275.

Wallberg, H.: Diaphanography: A clinical and experimental study of benign and malignant mammary diseases. Huddinge, Sweden: Doctoral thesis, Department of Surgery, Karolinska Institute, 1984.

Ward, S. M.: Wall Street Journal, New York, N. Y., July 30, 1985.

Watanabe, H.: Current issues and future prospects of mass screening for breast cancer. Gan. No. Rinsho. *30*(Suppl. 6):598, 1984.

Watt, A. C., Ackerman, L. V., Shetty, P. C., et al.: Differentiation between benign and malignant disease of the breast using digital subtraction angiography of the breast. Cancer, *56*:1287, 1985.

Wellings, S. R., and Wolf, J. N.: Correlative studies of the histological and radiographic appearance of the breast parenchyma. Radiology, *129*:299, 1978.

Wenth, J., and Stein, M. A.: Efficacy of breast cancer screening by thermography. Acta Thermograph., *8*:76, 1983.

Whitehead, J., Carlile, T., Kopecky, K. J., et al.: Wolfe mammographic parenchymal patterns. A study of the masking hypothesis of Egan and Mosteller. Cancer, *56*:1280, 1985.

Wilkinson, E., Clapton, C., Gordonson, J., et al.: Mammographic parenchymal patterns and the risk of breast cancer. JNCI, *59*:1397, 1977.

Witt, I., Hansen, S., and Brunner, S.: Risk of developing breast cancer in relation to the mammographic findings. Ugeskr. Laeger., *145*:237, 1983.

Witt, I., Hansen, H. S., and Brunner, S.: The risk of developing breast cancer in relation to mammography findings. Eur. J. Radiol., *4*:65, 1984.

Wolfe, J. N.: Breast patterns as an index of risk for developing breast cancer. AJR, *126*:1130, 1976a.

Wolfe, J. N.: Risk for cancer development determined by mammographic parenchymal pattern. Cancer, *37*:2486, 1976b.

Wolfe, J. N., Saftlas, A. F., and Salane, M.: Association of radiographic dysplasia and breast carcinoma: A case control study. *In* Evaluation due Risque de Cancer Mammaire, Chimothérapie Première. Proceedings of the International Symposium of Senology, Liege, Belgium, November 1985.

Wolfman, N. T., Moran, R., Moran, P. R., et al.: Simultaneous MR imaging of both breasts using a dedicated receiver coil. Radiology, *155*:241, 1985.

CHAPTER 8

CARLOS M. PEREZ-MESA

Gross and Microscopic Pathology

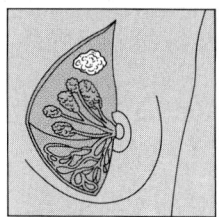

Everything is the same, everything is always different.
GERTRUDE STEIN

The heterogeneity of carcinoma of the breast is manifested in a myriad of overt or subtle differences in tumor behavior. Some of these differences can have recognizable histopathologic changes, whereas others escape the most astute and experienced observer. The dynamics of the processes of neoplasia are largely unknown and obviously cannot be contained in rigid concepts. New formulations based on other than the conventional histopathologic criteria are being added continuously, offering new vistas. In this chapter an attempt is made to delineate the clinical relevance of what is most commonly recognized in the morphologic appearance of breast carcinoma without covering in scope or in depth the information available in monographs.

Classification

All classifications, to avoid being sterile philosophic abstractions, by their own nature are imperfect and incomplete. The difficulties of devising from the pathologist's point of view a classification of tumors of the breast are well known.[60, 207, 215] The continuous additions, subtractions, and modifications of concepts and methods of study reflect both the complexity and lack of complete understanding of the pathobiology of breast disease and the tenacity of the student. Classifications based on only one parameter are flawed by failing to take into account the heterogeneity of breast tumors in their gross appearance, pattern of growth, and microscopic composition and the difficulty in determining their histogenetic and cytogenetic topography. When only one parameter is used, tumors of different morphology and diverse clinical behavior can be placed inappropriately under similar categories. With the application of newer and more advanced technology, it has become possible to measure properties of tumors and biochemical markers not previously measurable. Refinement of the present classification of breast tumors will come by discovering new parameters of prognostic significance, which, it is hoped, will provide bases for new classifications.[134] However, until the data obtained are critically analyzed and supported by careful clinical observation it is preferable to maintain the histopathologic classification that has been in use.

Carcinoma of the breast takes origin from the epithelium of mammary ducts and acini.[74] It has become increasingly accepted, however, on the basis of studies by Wellings and colleagues,[224] that ductal carcinoma originates from the terminal duct lobular units rather than from larger ducts. Morphologic characteristics along with possible topographic histogenesis allow the recognition of various tumor types. Foote and Stewart[71] in 1946 devised a classification that subsequent studies have corroborated. With minor modifications their schema is followed here.

Invasive Carcinoma
Invasive ductal carcinoma, not otherwise specified (NOS)
Medullary carcinoma
Mucinous (colloid) carcinoma
Papillary carcinoma
Invasive lobular carcinoma
Tubular (orderly) carcinoma

Noninvasive Carcinoma
Intraductal carcinoma
Lobular carcinoma, in situ (lobular neoplasia)

Rare Types of Invasive Carcinoma
Adenocystic carcinoma
Squamous cell carcinoma
Carcinoma with pseudosarcomatous metaplasia
Secretory carcinoma, juvenile type
Signet ring cell carcinoma
Lipid-rich carcinoma
Sudoriferous carcinoma
Glycogen-rich clear cell carcinoma
Carcinoid tumors
Mucoepidermoid carcinoma
Oat cell carcinoma

Special Manifestations of Breast Carcinoma
Paget's disease of the nipple
Inflammatory carcinoma

Invasive Carcinoma

INVASIVE DUCTAL CARCINOMA

Invasive ductal carcinoma in its pure form is estimated to represent between 50 and 75 per cent of all invasive types. In this category are included all tumors without an identifiable type; these are labeled ductal carcinoma not otherwise specified (NOS).

The gross features are well known; generally, the tumor is a poorly marginated mass of varied consistency. The fibrous tissue content, when abundant, imparts the characteristic hardness (scirrhous) (Fig. 8–1); when the cut surface is retracted, the tumor is found to be grayish-yellow with radiating streaks running centrifugally. Chalky streaks, which occur frequently, although not exclusively, in this type of tumor represent elastic tissue condensation along large mammary ducts (elastosis). Their dimensions vary; they can be so small that they escape clinical detection, necessitating special radiographic techniques and careful gross and microscopic inspection, or so large as to occupy the entire mammary gland, the covering skin, and subjacent musculature (Fig. 8–2). Infrequently, more than one dominant mass is recognizable; the frequency increases in proportion to the dimensions of the largest tumor. The tumor margins can be circumscribed, indicating an expansile type of growth; serrated, with an infiltrative type of growth; or of mixed type. The microscopic appearance depends on differentiation based on nuclear anaplasia, the presence of necrosis, inflammatory cell infiltrate, and the quality or quantity of the stroma. The stroma can be so pronounced that it occupies most of the tumor. Because of variations in the proportion of cells and stroma, this type of tumor has also been designated infiltrating ductal carcinoma with productive fibrosis, scirrhous carcinoma and carcinoma simplex. Among the invasive carcinomas, ductal carcinomas, NOS, are associated with the highest percentage of treatment failure. This tumor lends itself more than any other type to study of parameters of predictive value, including the nature of margins, whether circumscribed or serrated, and the presence of inflammatory infiltration. The histologic grade is generally accepted as most closely reflecting its aggressiveness or lack of it (see later discussion).

MEDULLARY CARCINOMA

Medullary carcinoma, a clinically and morphologically distinct type of breast carcinoma, was originally described by Geschickter[83] and further characterized by Moore and Foote.[141] It has been also designated as encephaloid carcinoma, bulky carcinoma, circumscribed and solid carcinoma, and medullary carcinoma with lymphoid stroma. It represents between 5 and 7 per cent of all invasive carcinomas. At gross inspection it appears as a globoid soft mass, with well-circumscribed margins. It possesses a fleshy, homogeneous, generally spongy cut surface. A pinkish-gray discoloration is present, or when hemorrhage or necrosis occurs, dark red or yellowish areas may be seen. Grossly, the tumor can be confused with a fibroadenoma. Its pattern of growth is of the expansile, pushing type (Fig. 8–3). Microscopically medullary carcinoma is typified by anastomosing solid sheets of medium to large anaplastic cells with syncytial growth, indistinct

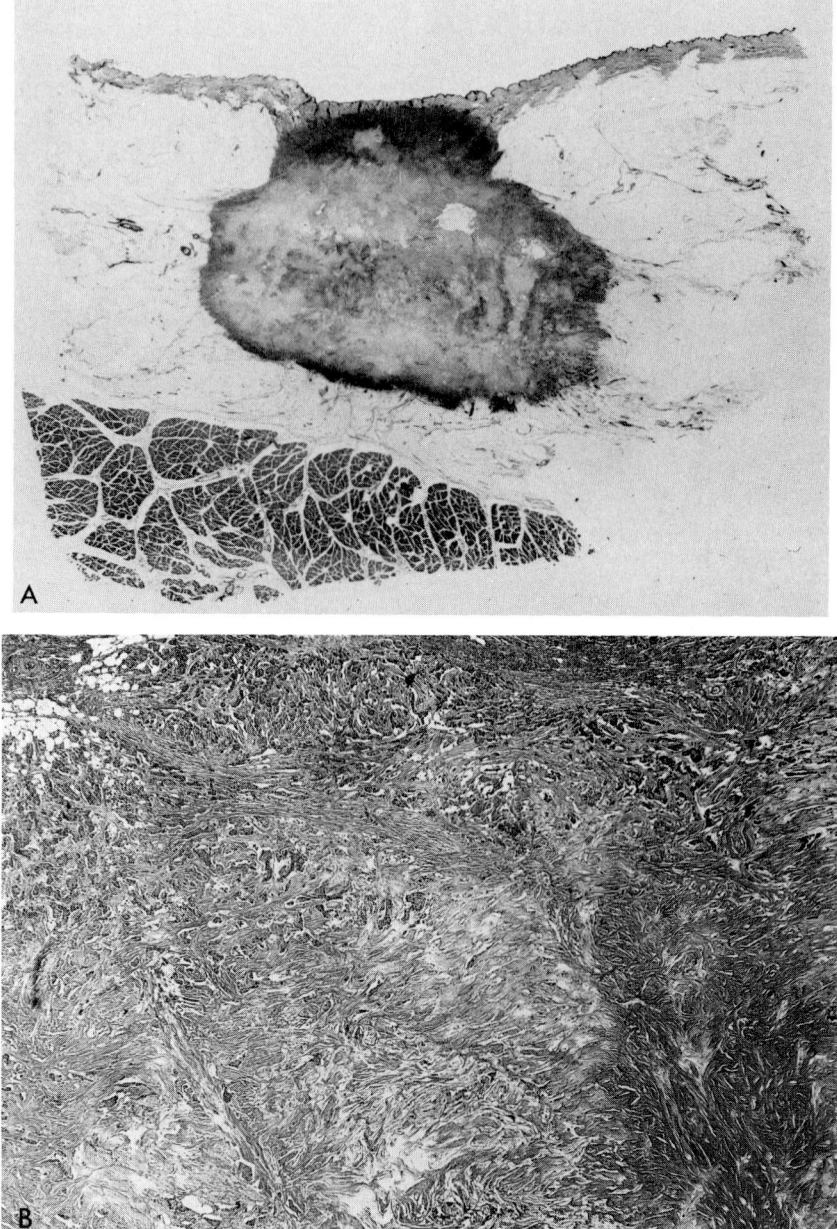

Figure 8–1. *A*, Whole section of the breast depicting invasive ductal carcinoma not otherwise specified (NOS) with pronounced fibrosis in most of the tumor. Darker area, mostly toward the periphery, represents the epithelial component of tumor. *B*, Center of tumor, with intense fibrosis.

borders, and frequently vesicular nuclei and prominent nucleoli. Mitoses are abundant. Characteristically, lymphoid cells are abundant in the stroma, although intratumoral fibrosis is negligible and generally absent. The lack of or presence of minimal intraductal components or glandular arrangements round out the microscopic features of these tumors. Despite the ominous appearance of the tumor cells, the prognosis is generally excellent.[25, 69, 141, 173] Tumors of 3 cm or less tend to have a very favorable prognosis. Even when metastases occur, the 10-year survival for this type of tumor is 84 per cent, versus 63 per cent for infiltrating ductal carcinoma. Distinction from atypical medullary carcinoma should be made as the behavior of the atypical type is similar to that of infiltrating ductal carcinoma,

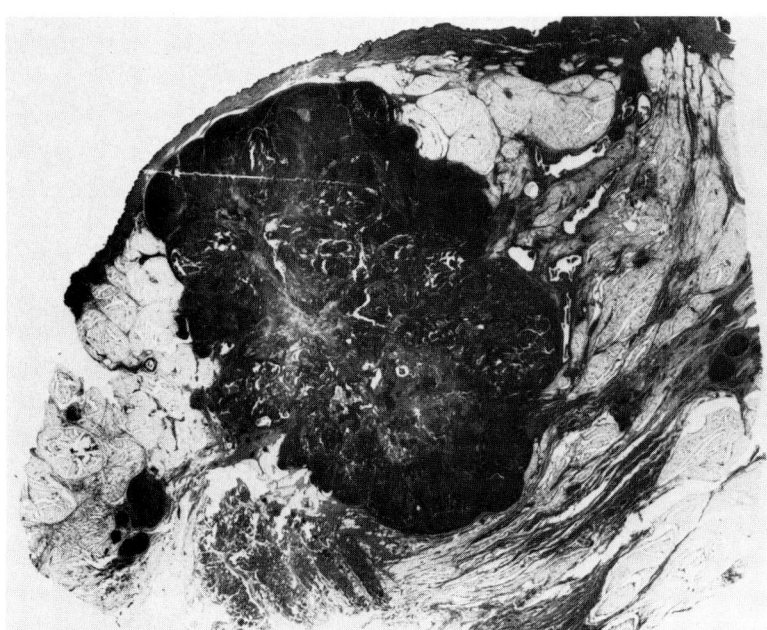

Figure 8–2. Large section of entire breast, showing tumor with extensive involvement, including pectoralis muscle and skin. Notice sharply circumscribed margins and the presence of other, smaller tumors.

NOS.[60, 175] The designation of medullary carcinoma must be restricted to tumors showing the morphologic criteria just described, as the term has been loosely applied to cellular tumors without any other distinguishing feature.

Hsu and colleagues[103a] found a qualitative difference in the type of plasma cells associated with medullary carcinoma and those associated with ductal carcinoma. The former were predominantly IgA plasma cells, and the tumor cells contained both IgA and secretory component (SC). Plasma cells associated with ductal carcinoma were IgG type. These differences reflect a degree of functional differentiation and may account for the favorable prognosis associated with medullary carcinoma.

MUCINOUS CARCINOMA

Since the early 19th century, the distinct morphologic and biologic properties of mucinous carcinoma have been recognized[84, 193]; colloid, gelatinous, myxomatous, and mucoid are other terms used in its designation. The frequency of this type varies between 1.5 and 5 per cent of all breast cancers. It tends to occur in older women, and its growth is slower than the conventional invasive ductal carcinoma. Protrusion of the nipple (see Fig. 6–3 in Chapter 6) and a sensation of "swish" on firm palpation are clinical signs ascribed to it.[95a] However, these signs are rarely observed (Fig. 8–4). In its pure form, the tumor is well circumscribed, without a capsule, soft, gray-yellow, and with a syrupy or gelatinous appearance. The size varies from less than 1 cm to masses occupying the entire breast thickness.

Microscopically, the mucinous carcinoma is composed of pools of mucin, which are pale and homogeneous, with slender bands of fibrovascular tissue dividing the tumor into incomplete compartments where small cells form nests, solid sheets, tubules, papillae, or sieve-like patterns. The tumor cells are uniform, with a well-defined membrane, and are hyperchromatic, with regular nuclei and infrequent nucleoli. The cytoplasm is abundant, foamy, and vacuolated and can contain mucin. The interface of the extracellular mucin with the surrounding tissue is sharp and without inflammatory reaction. Not infrequently, infiltrating ductal carcinomas, NOS, coexist with mucinous carcinoma, and this category is labeled "mixed." The differences in behavior between the pure and mixed tumors are well demonstrated.[200] In a recent report,[170] 3 of 95 patients with pure mucinous carcinoma had axillary lymph node metastases, contrasting with 37 of 112 with mixed mucinous carcinoma. The evolution of the mixed category runs parallel to that of infiltrating ductal carcinoma, NOS. Although it has long been identified as a special tumor type, there is a dearth of studies of mucinous carcinoma and specifically a lack of uniformity in defining its diagnostic criteria. In

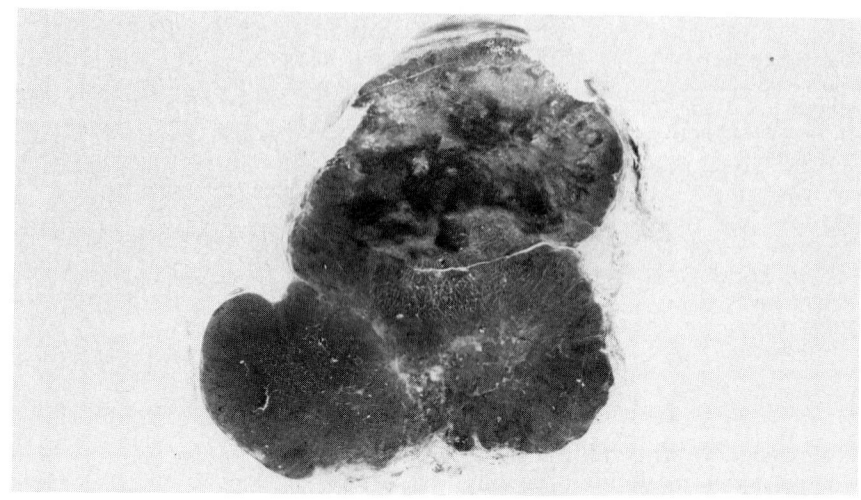

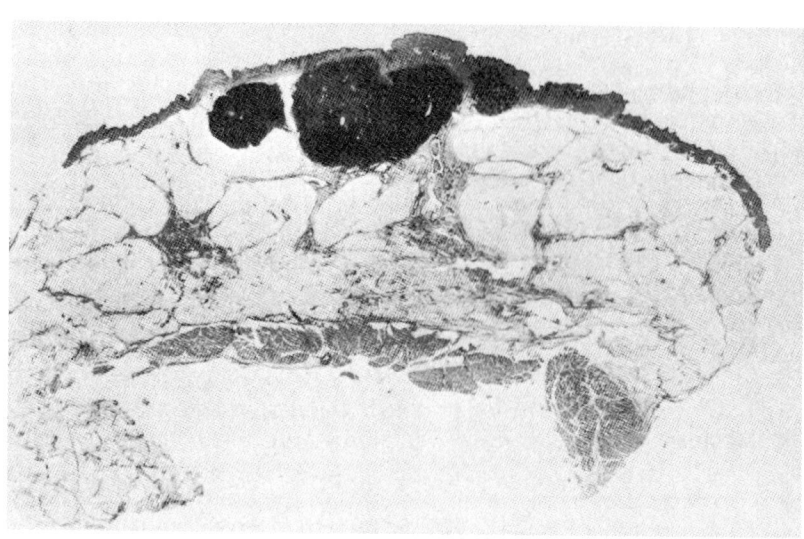

Figure 8–3. *A,* Sharply delineated, lobulated margins of medullary carcinoma. Paler and darker areas represent necrosis and hemorrhage. *B,* Whole mount of breast showing two adjacent but separate masses.

Illustration continued on opposite page

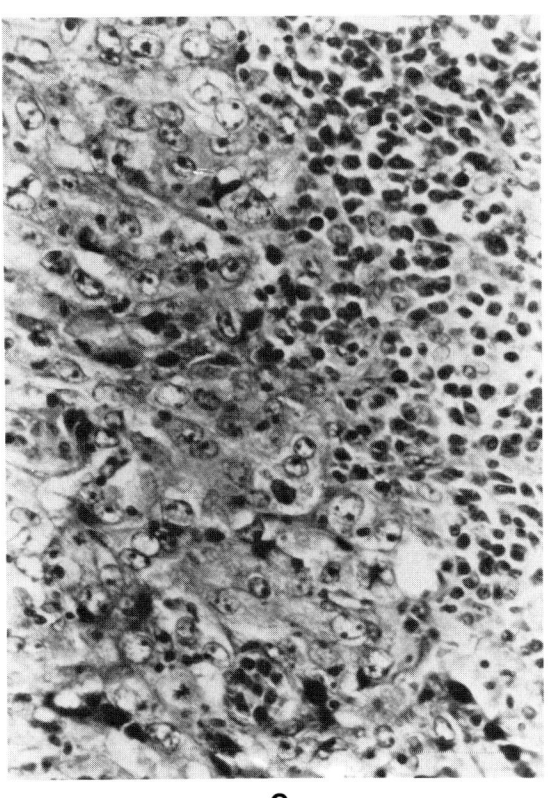

Figure 8–3 Continued C, Microscopic appearance, showing undifferentiated cells and the lymphoid stroma.

most of these studies, the definition varies from a precise and restricting one ("pure mucinous carcinoma, in which no infiltrating ductal carcinoma is present"[137, 153]) to a more vague characterization ("containing large amounts of extracellular epithelial mucus, sufficient to be visible grossly and recognizable microscopically surrounding and within tumor cells"[207]). It is important for pathologists to state in their reports the relative proportion of infiltrating ductal carcinoma and mucinous carcinoma because of their differing behaviors.

Despite the generally accepted view of the benign course of mucinous carcinoma, Rosen and Wang[188] cautioned that more than 10 years are necessary in the follow-up to appreciate the full potential lethality of this tumor. Forty-one patients with pure mucinous carcinoma were followed and nearly half of them died owing to tumor spread 12 years or more after diagnosis. In the author's files are six patients of a group of 15 who died of metastasis from pure mucinous carcinoma 10 to 22 years after mastectomy.

Argyrophilic granules have been found in mucinous tumors.[25, 38, 64] In a recent study of 202 mucinous tumors, Rasmussen and colleagues[171] found 25 per cent containing argyrophilic granules; however, no demonstrable differences existed morphologically or in clinical behavior between tumors with and without granules.

A variant of intracellular mucin-producing carcinoma has been recognized,[193] consisting of infiltrating malignant cells containing mucin in their cytoplasm displacing the nucleus toward the periphery (signet ring cells). The variant is more aggressive than extracellular mucinous carcinoma. Controversy has surrounded the histogenesis of this form, as some consider it a variant of invasive lobular carcinoma of ductal origin or colloid carcinoma; others contend that it is a well-defined pathologic entity. These tumors are described separately within the group of rare tumors.

INVASIVE PAPILLARY CARCINOMA

Invasive papillary carcinoma is an uncommon neoplasm representing between 0.3 to 3 per cent of all breast carcinomas.[13, 63] There is a dearth of published studies about this type of tumor, and, as others have commented, its separation from other benign papillary lesions is controversial and difficult.[68, 145, 146] No clear distinction is established from its noninvasive counterpart. The number of cases available to study is small, and the clinical behavior is so favorable that it increases the difficulty of morphologic and clinical delineation. The tumor affects most frequently postmenopausal, nonwhite women and is associated with nipple discharge in 25 per cent of cases.

The growth of invasive papillary carcinomas is slow and expansile in type; size, which is not given in some studies, varies. In Murad and coworkers' study,[146] the size ranged from microscopic to 4.5 cm in greatest dimension. In the author's cases, the mean size was 2.5 cm. The tumor is well circumscribed, and the gross appearance has been described as gray, tan, friable, and hemorrhagic. Occasionally, its filiform character can be recognized on the cut surface (Fig. 8–5A).

Microscopically (Fig. 8–5B–D), a papillary arrangement is the sine qua non. Several patterns can be recognized: papilliform, characterized by long or short blunt stalks, with or without a fibrovascular core; adenomatoid, in

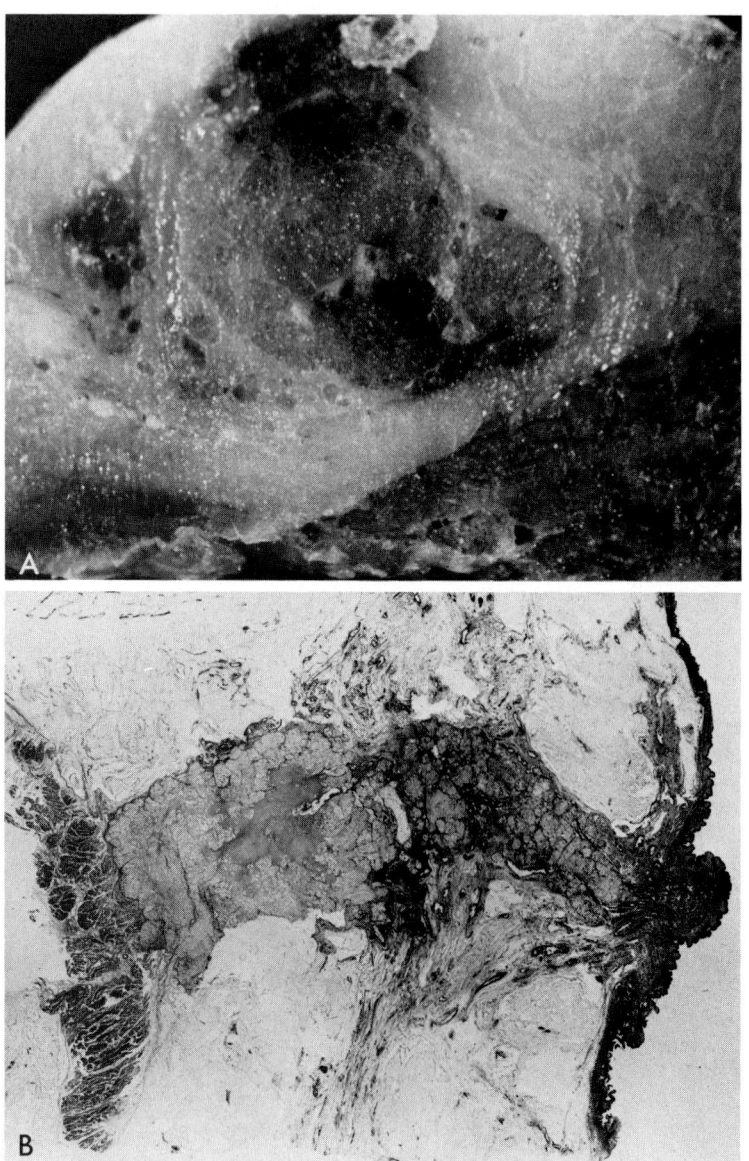

Figure 8–4. *A*, Close view of the cut surface, with the characteristic gelatinous appearance. *B*, Whole section of a breast depicting mucinous carcinoma infiltrating the skin and subjacent musculature. Darker areas toward center represent hemorrhage. Note the prominent nipple.

Illustration continued on opposite page

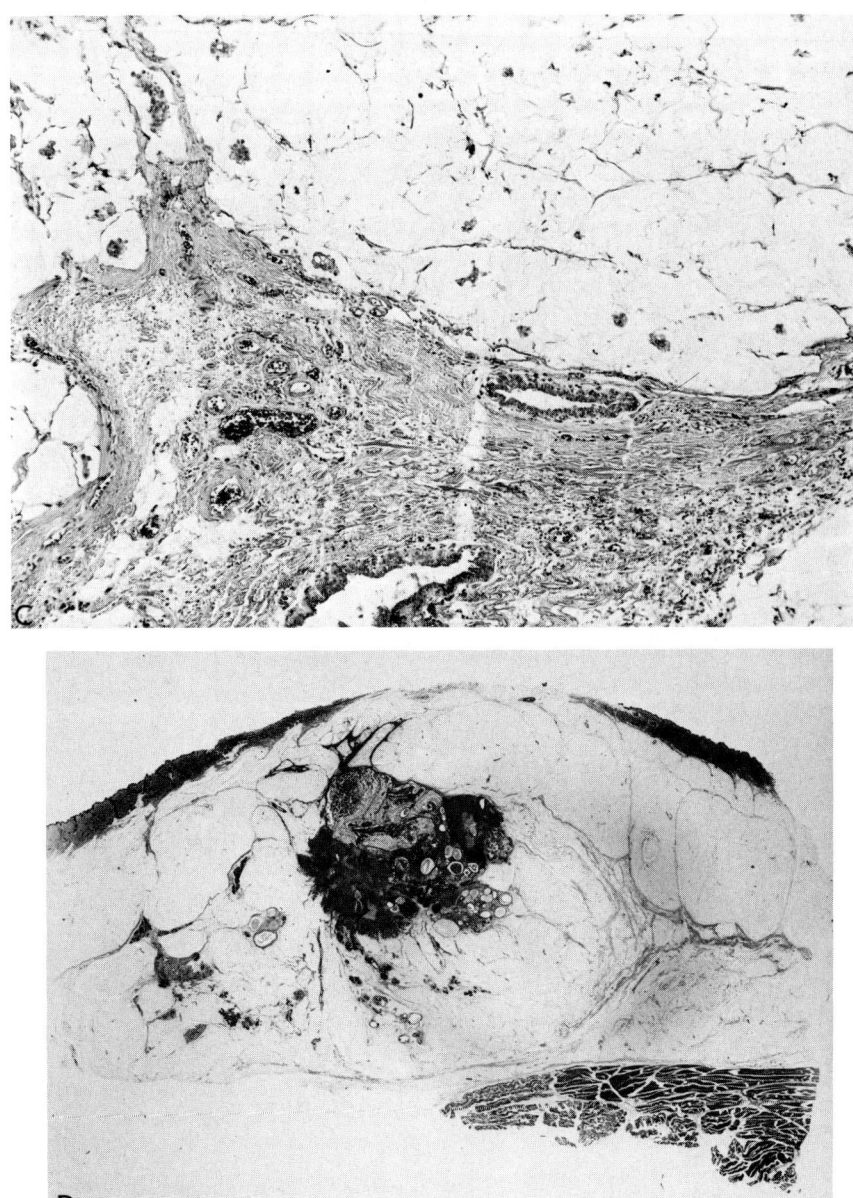

Figure 8–4 *Continued C,* Tumor margin is sharp and characteristically without inflammatory reaction. *D,* Whole mount of breast showing "mixed" mucinous carcinoma (lighter area).

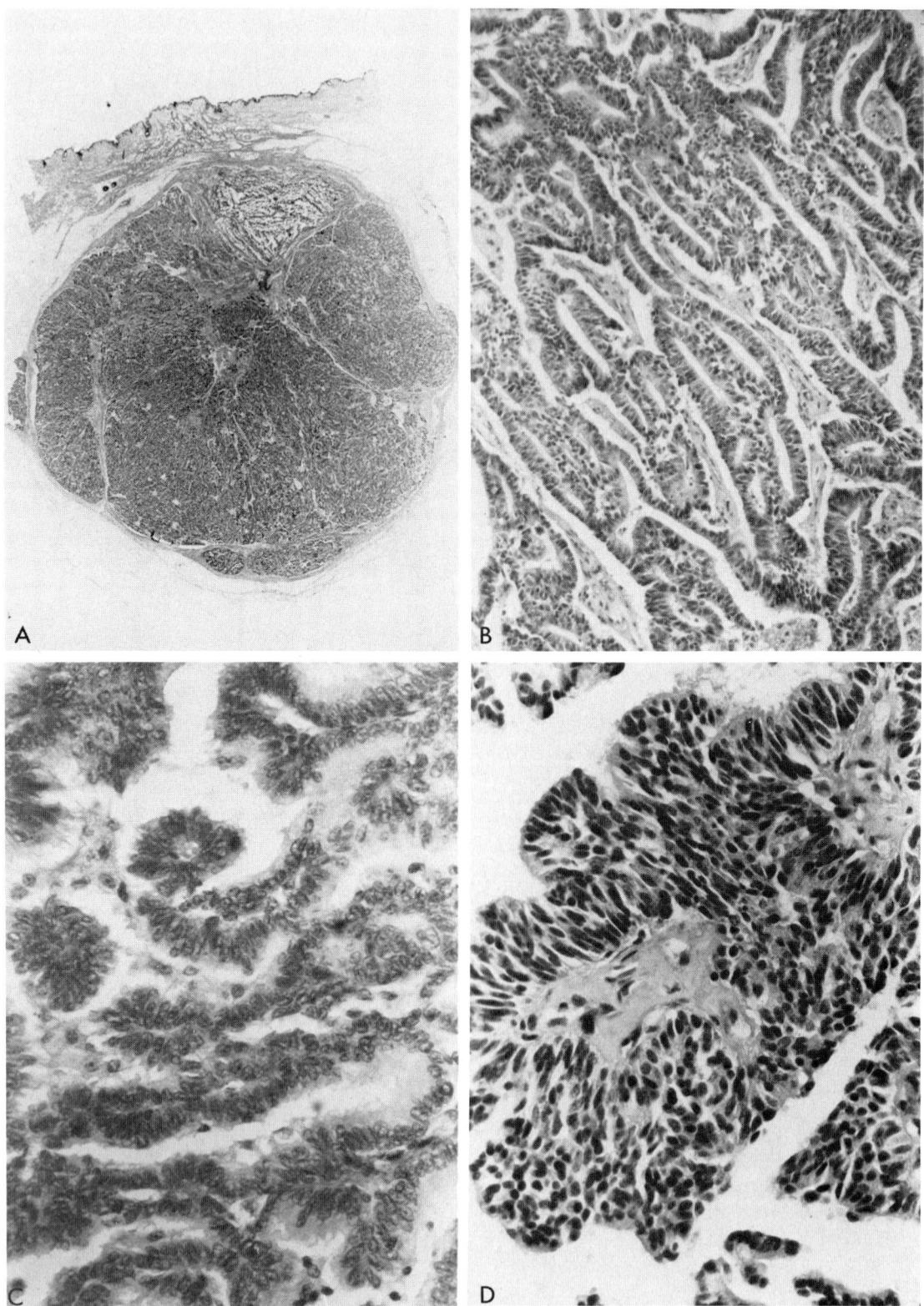

Figure 8–5. *A*, Cross section of papillary tumor, circumscribed with foci of invasion. Recognizable filiform structure is present. *B–D*, Various patterns (adenomatoid, papilliform). Note recognizable fibrous core and anaplasia in *D*.

which there is fusion of the papilla with the formation of glands; and microcystic, in which the lesion involves smaller ducts and the papillae are short. Combinations of these patterns can occur. The covering epithelial cells are distributed in single or multiple rows of a single cell type, predominantly well differentiated and of moderate nuclear grade. Variations can occur, and the differentiation of invasive papillary carcinoma from benign papillary lesions can be difficult. However, the presence or absence of a single cell type, not the existing number of cell layers, is pivotal in the distinction between papillary carcinoma and papilloma. Kraus and Neubecker[117] tabulated the most predominant characteristics of each lesion, and the data can be helpful in the diagnosis. However, numerous exceptions can occur, and careful observations and experience are required for correct interpretation. Azzopardi[12, 13] emphasized practical caveats in helping to establish a diagnosis.

The prognosis of this type of tumor is excellent, and although in a minority of cases metastases to the axillary lymph nodes can occur, this cancer does not usually threaten the life of the patient.

There is a rare variant of papillary carcinoma termed intracystic papillary carcinoma, which, despite its infrequency, has generated more publications than its more common congener[32, 45, 81, 107, 136, 203] (Fig. 8–6). It is difficult to identify the degree of malignant potential of this variant, as in some studies it is not clear whether the investigators are describing invasive or noninvasive carcinoma. The reported incidence of intracystic carcinoma is 0.5 to 2 per cent of all breast tumors. The tumor usually appears as a papillary carcinoma arising from the wall of a large cyst. Carter and associates[32] reviewed 41 cases of intracystic papillary carcinoma of the breast and found a highly favorable prognosis. Twenty-nine patients who had mastectomy had no recurrence after an average follow-up of 5 years. Eleven axillary dissections revealed no metastases. Eight of 11 patients treated with local excision were free of recurrence after an average of 10 years, but three patients in whom the lesions were associated with ductal carcinoma in situ had reappearance of tumor. The average age of the patients was 63 years, and in 85 per cent the presenting sign was a mass. Twenty-two per cent had nipple discharge, and 15 per cent pain. Only 2 of 11 patients developed recurrence after local excision, and both of these

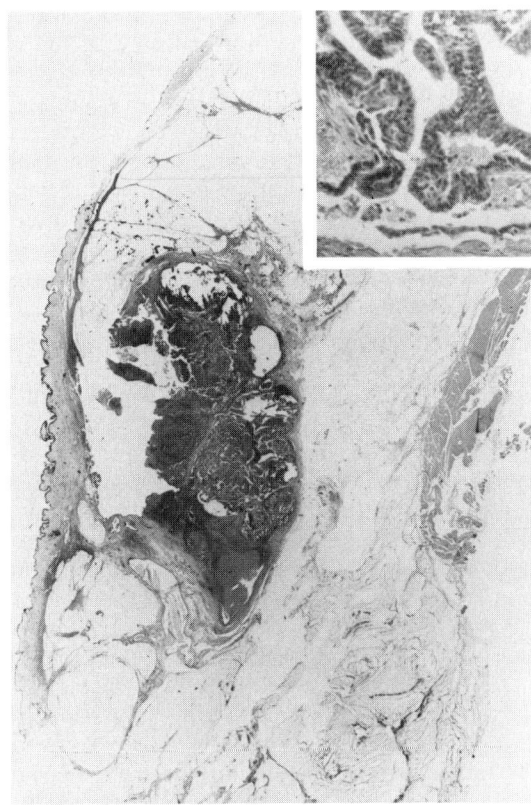

Figure 8–6. Whole section of breast showing a large cyst with a papillary tumor that protrudes into the cystic cavity. There is a "capsule" toward the periphery with foci of hemorrhage. Inset depicts the papillary pattern lined by a single type of cell with minimal anaplasia.

had concurrent ductal carcinoma in situ of the breast. Hunter and Sawyers[107] reported seven cases of intracystic papillary carcinoma of the breast. Six were treated with modified or radical mastectomy and one with simple mastectomy and postoperative irradiation. Only one patient had recurrence and died 2 years postoperatively with osseous metastases. Modified mastectomy was the recommended treatment. One of six patients (16 per cent) with axillary dissections was found to have metastases. Other authors have reported a 25 per cent and a 36 per cent incidence of nodal metastases.[45, 136]

INVASIVE LOBULAR CARCINOMA

Invasive lobular carcinoma is considered the invasive counterpart of lobular carcinoma in situ and similarly can be multicentric and bilateral. Both types frequently coexist. The invasive lobular carcinoma can occur independently or in combination with other tumor types. Its incidence varies from 0.7 per cent[13, 53] to 20 per cent of all invasive carcinomas, reflecting differences in diagnostic criteria rather than ethnic, geographic or environmental factors. The gross appearance is not different generally from invasive ductal carcinoma, NOS, especially those with abundant fibrous stroma. Occasionally, however, the tumors are palpable but not recognized by the naked eye or with imaging techniques. The "classic" histopathologic features as described in 1941[70, 144] consist of a homogeneous population of small, bland-appearing cells characteristically lacking cohesiveness, which may be distributed diffusely in the stroma, in a linear fashion (Indian file), or concentrically around mammary ducts (bull's-eye, targetoid) (Fig. 8–7A,B). Other histopathologic variants, however, have been described (Fig. 8–7C–F). Fechner[55] described a variant characterized by solid aggregates of tumor cells; Steinbrecher and Silverberg[204] noted the presence of mucus and intracytoplasmic vacuoles and signet ring formation in the tumor cells; Fisher and coworkers[62] noted a variety in which cells with features of invasive lobular carcinoma were also forming tubules (tubulolobular). Martinez and Azzopardi[126] described the alveolar variant, characterized by aggregates of monomorphic cells arranged in globules (alveoli) of 20 cells or more. The mixed category includes combinations with the classic type or with some of the variants. To explain the morphologic variants, it has been postulated that lobular carcinoma arises not from the lobules but rather from the "terminal secretory unit" composed of the lobules and the terminal ducts.[179a] The addition of new variants augments the complexity of the diagnosis of this type of tumor and obviously increases its incidence. Differences in the prognosis among the variants have been reported,[50] with the solid and mixed variants being associated with the poorest prognosis and the classic and the alveolar types with the best prognosis. Differences have been noted in the metastatic pattern between infiltrating lobular carcinoma and ductal carcinoma, NOS. The former occurs with greater frequency in the skeleton, retroperitoneum, and viscera.[97] A "histocytoid" appearance of some metastatic foci has been described.[5, 103] Conflicting opinions exist concerning treatment response between invasive lobular carcinoma and ductal invasive carcinoma. Although some studies suggest no differences, others reveal a better prognosis for the former.

TUBULAR CARCINOMA

Tubular carcinoma has also been referred to as an "orderly" and well-differentiated carcinoma because its microscopic hallmark is the presence of well-delineated tubules or glands in a fibrous stroma.[30, 31, 48, 129, 154, 161, 206, 209] These tumors were considered rare in the earliest publications, estimated at between 0.4 and 1 per cent of cancers in symptomatic populations using conventional methods of detection. In more recent studies their incidence has increased, now estimated to constitute as many as 9 per cent of all invasive carcinomas when discovered in asymptomatic populations during mass screening. A 5 per cent incidence of pure tubular carcinoma has been obtained in a Breast Cancer Screening Project in Columbia, Missouri.[164, 177] Further increase in the incidence is recorded, reaching 21.1 per cent, when tubular carcinomas associated with other tumor types are included (mixed category).[206, 214] The gross appearance is characterized by a poorly circumscribed mass that is grayish-tan, firm or hard on retracted cut surface, and with infiltrative margins. No distinguishing features from ductal carcinomas, NOS, with fibrous production can be noted on gross inspection. Their size varies from as small as 0.2 cm to as large as 12 cm in diameter. It is difficult to determine in some studies if the recorded size includes only pure types. The size of these tumors has been noted to increase in proportion to the degree of association with other tumor types, suggesting that many invasive ductal carcinomas are initially tubular carcinomas, becoming larger when they become less differentiated.[154] Microscopically (Fig. 8–8), they are characterized by glands or tubules distributed haphazardly or in an orderly fashion, often with angulated contours, lined by a single row of monomorphous cells with good nuclear grade and rare mitoses. Frequently apocrine snouts project into the lumina of the tubules. The intervening stroma is abundant, showing desmoplasia and frequently occupying the center of the lesion. In situ carcinoma (lobular, cribriform, or papillary) can be associated with these tumors. The presence of in situ carcinoma as well as the lack of basal membrane and of the lobular outline configuration helps distinguish tubular carcinoma

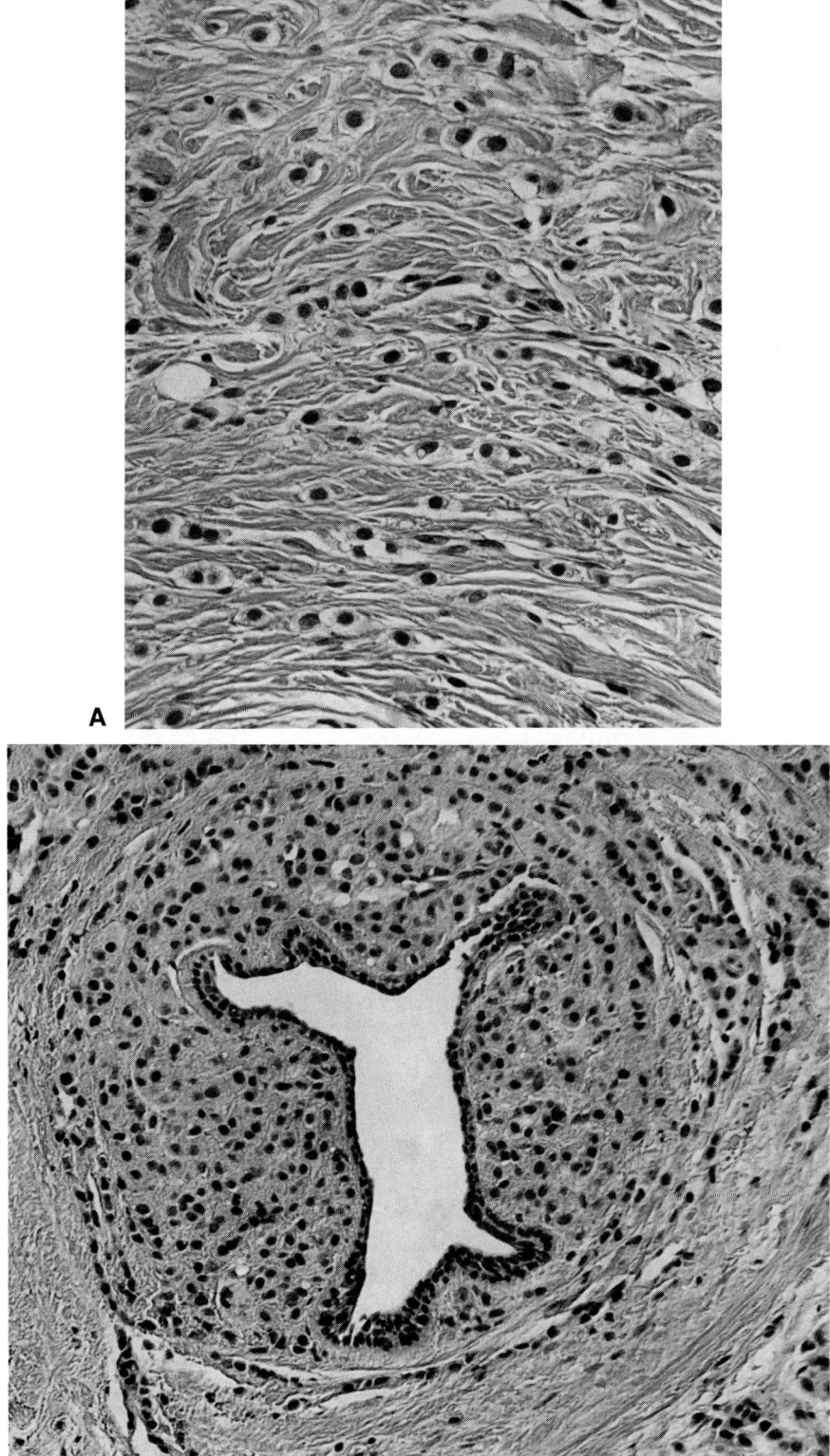

Figure 8–7. *A*, Invasive lobular carcinoma (small cell carcinoma) showing the "classic" type with linear distribution of tumor cells. *B*, A typical target board arrangement of lobular carcinoma cells around a nontumorous duct.

Illustration continued on following page

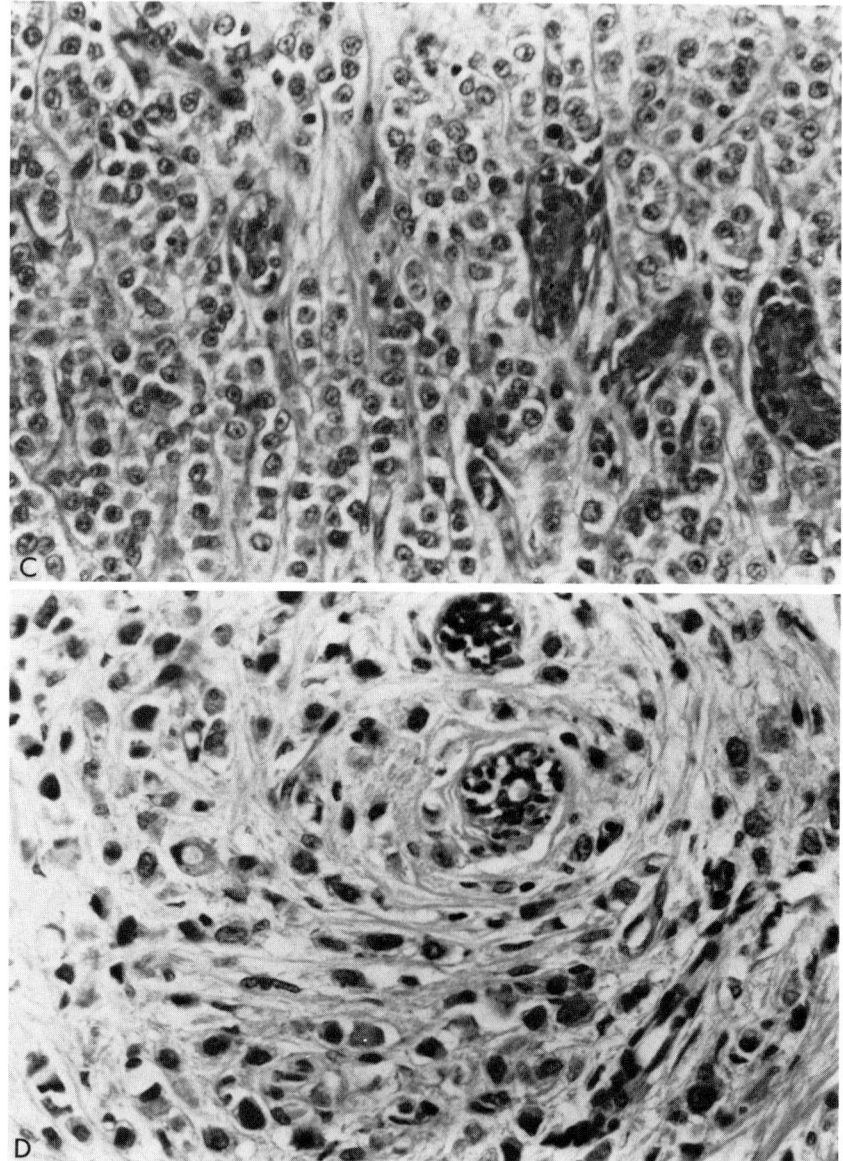

Figure 8-7 *Continued C,* Solid type of tumor distribution. In other areas the pattern was classic together with in situ component. *D,* Notice the targetoid distribution as well as signet-ring cells.

Illustration continued on opposite page

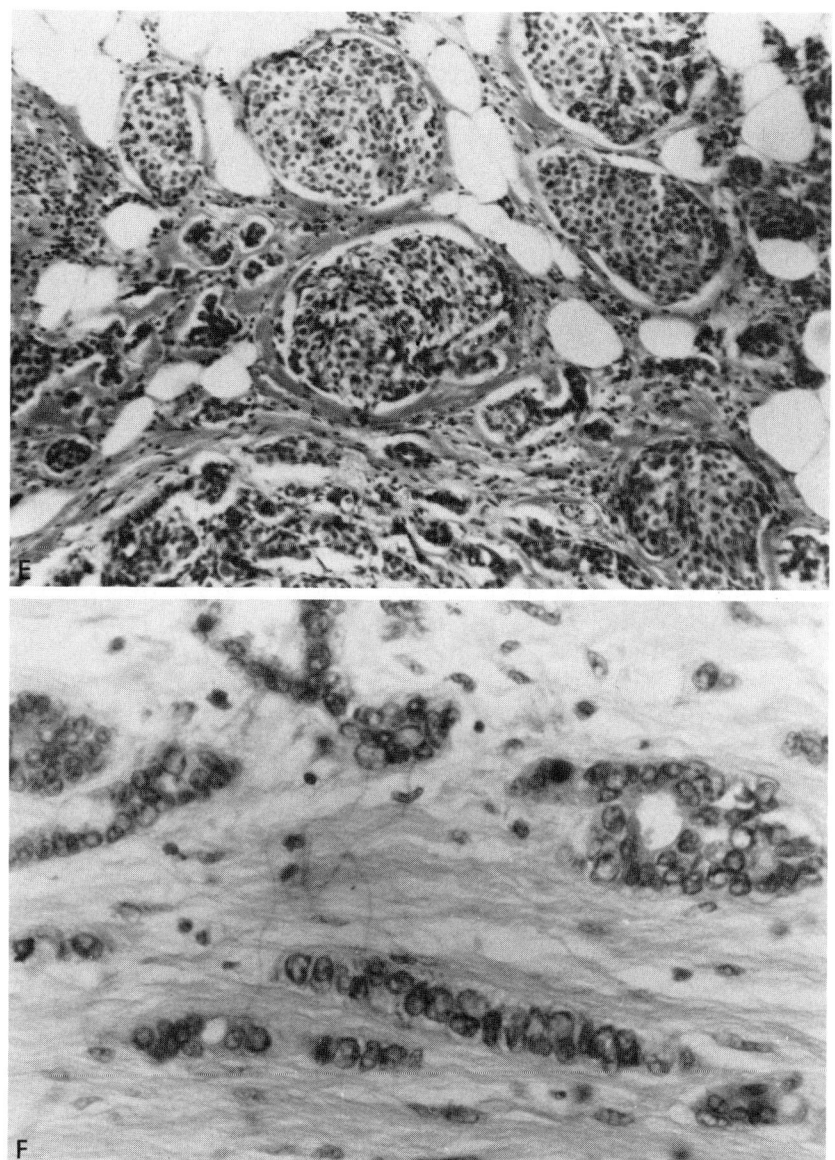

Figure 8–7 *Continued E,* Alveolar pattern of lobular carcinoma with tumor cells forming round aggregates. *F,* Tubulo-lobular pattern. Note the tubules merging with the linear arrangement of the tumor cells.

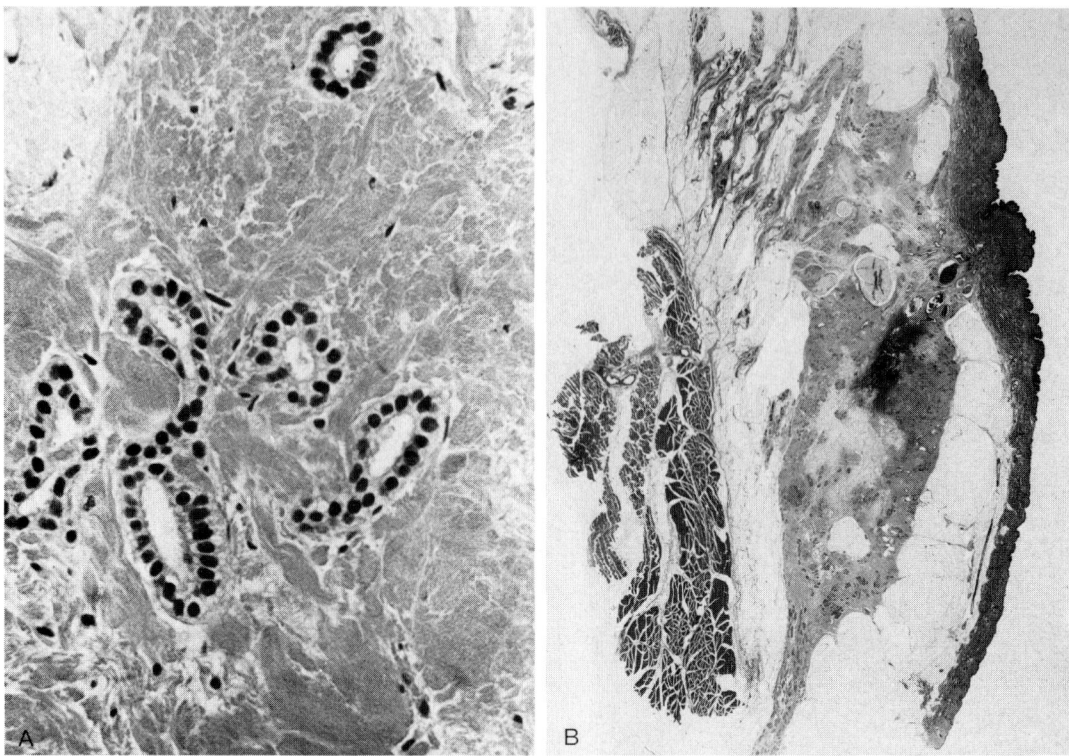

Figure 8–8. *A*, Tubular carcinoma; well-formed glands lined by a single row of cells, monomorphous, with bland nuclei. Apocrine snouts are visible. *B*, Whole breast section showing tubular carcinoma in the darkest area. In other segments of the specimen lobular carcinoma in situ is also present.

from sclerosing adenosis. The criteria for "pure" tubular carcinoma vary, but tumors are considered pure when 75 to 100 per cent of the tumor is tubular.[161, 206, 209, 214] Tumors are considered mixed when a minimum of 50 per cent of the bulk of the tumor is tubular carcinoma. It is important to underline that tubular carcinoma should be distinguished from well-differentiated, low grade, invasive ductal carcinoma, NOS. Axillary lymph node metastases occur in from 0 to 18.6 per cent, reflecting the composition of the tumor (pure or mixed) as well as its size. The prognosis for this tumor is excellent, but it depends on the proportion of the associated type of invasive tumor. In the study of Taylor and Norris,[206] including 33 cases, only one patient died from the tumor; in another study, no metastases occurred and no deaths were related to this tumor when more than 75 per cent of the lesion was composed of tubular carcinoma.[40a] The recommended treatment varies, but the most frequently employed method is modified radical mastectomy.

One hundred tubular carcinomas were reviewed by Peters and associates.[165a] In the pure form, tumor size was small and no metastases were found. Sixteen pure tubular carcinomas occurred predominantly in the right breast, generally in the upper outer quadrant. No recurrences and no deaths were noted from this tumor. As the tubular component in carcinomas diminished, the size and biologic aggressiveness increased. Nodal metastases were noted only when the tubular component constituted 75 per cent or less of the tumor. Peters and colleagues estimated the incidence of pure tubular carcinomas as 0.7 per cent and the total incidence of all carcinomas containing tubular elements as 2 per cent. Multicentric foci have been observed in 50 per cent of cases, and local excision is inappropriate as it has regularly been followed by recurrence.

Noninvasive Carcinoma

INTRADUCTAL CARCINOMA OF THE BREAST

The diagnosis of intraductal carcinoma, or ductal carcinoma in situ (DCIS), includes only tumors in which the carcinomatous growth is confined within the boundaries of preexisting mammary ducts. There are no discrete clinical characteristics because pure intraductal carcinomas are not often palpable, and their detection occurs because of their association with fibrocystic conditions.[111] In some instances, bloody nipple discharge or Paget's disease can lead to its diagnosis. A total of 23 intraductal carcinomas were diagnosed in one screening of 10,187 asymptomatic women.[177] In 20 instances, no palpable mass was noted during physical examination, performed by highly specialized, skilled personnel. In only three patients the mammographic study was considered within normal limits, whereas the remainder showed suspicious architectural distortions, of which 17 exhibited foci of calcification.[164] The gross appearance of this type of tumor is variable. It can exhibit features of unremarkable mammary tissue or fibrocystic changes, or it can show a comedo appearance, resulting from necrosis within the affected ducts. The tumors are multicentric and bilateral in up to 33 per cent and 10 per cent of cases, respectively. It is estimated that DCIS represents between 1 and 3 per cent of all breast cancers; however, in screening of asymptomatic populations, the incidence is higher, reaching 17 per cent of all cancers detected in the Columbia, Missouri, project.[177]

Microscopically (Fig. 8–9), these tumors are characterized by ducts filled with carcinomatous cells arranged in papillary, cribriform, or solid patterns, with or without central necrosis. The papillary form produces the well-known comedo appearance. Combinations of all patterns can coexist, however. An uncommon mucinous variant has been described.[66] The complexity and variety of the cellular proliferations within the ducts have received descriptive and colorful designations, such as serpentine, roman bridge, clinging, and cartwheel, patterns that are helpful in their identification. The differential diagnosis between atypical proliferation (borderline lesions) and intraductal carcinoma can be difficult; it is no less difficult to demonstrate the absence of stromal infiltration in intraductal carcinomas or to delineate the boundaries of the tubular wall or its basement membrane in every affected structure. The diagnostic spectrum at both ends of intraductal carcinoma lacks clear delineation.

The diagnosis of this type of tumor demands from the pathologist a careful and extensive sampling of the specimen. It is recommended that a minimum of six blocks per tumor and 4 to 10 sections per block be examined to establish the diagnosis.[176] The integrity of the affected tubular wall may be difficult to demonstrate in each affected ductal structure despite the use of special stains; even immunohistochemical methods can give inconsistent results.[68] The routine use of electron microscopy is not practical. Some studies tend to demonstrate that permeation of the ductal wall can occur before it is recognized by light microscopy, which can perhaps explain axillary metastasis in intraductal carcinoma.[157, 179] Despite careful studies using the most rigorous scrutiny, an element of subjectivity persists in the diagnosis. The natural history of the tumor is incompletely known, and the number of cases studied are insufficient to establish the ideal treatment.[18, 34, 158] The prognosis for this tumor is excellent and, as in other in situ carcinomas, a rate of 100 per cent cure is theoretically possible.[10, 86, 181] An estimated 5 per cent of tumors diagnosed as intraductal carcinoma metastasize to the axillary lymph nodes,[15, 190] which dramatizes the difficulty in ascertaining the in situ character of the tumor in all instances. Careful, continued observation of the small number of cases that have been treated with methods other than conventional mastectomy[68, 120, 140] may offer better understanding of the disease in the future.

LOBULAR CARCINOMA IN SITU

Nearly half a century after its initial description in 1941,[70, 144] lobular carcinoma in situ still remains a subject of controversy. There is agreement, however, that the lesion is multicentric (about 80 per cent) and bilateral (between 15 and 40 per cent).[70, 87] Lobular carcinoma in situ represents as little as 6 per cent to as many as 14 per cent of all breast cancers.[180, 222, 225]

This is a nonpalpable lesion that is clinically silent and is recognized only by microscopic examination, as it lacks any distinguishing gross characteristic features. Most of the time, lobular carcinoma in situ is an incidental microscopic finding, the breast biopsy having been done because of another benign or malignant lesion. Mammography may demonstrate linear or stippled calcifications, many of which are located in neighboring normal lobules. About 90 per cent occur in premenopausal women with a mean age of 44 years. Histologically (Fig. 8–10), the tumor is characterized by small cells with variable cytoplasm, homogeneous uniform nuclei, and rare

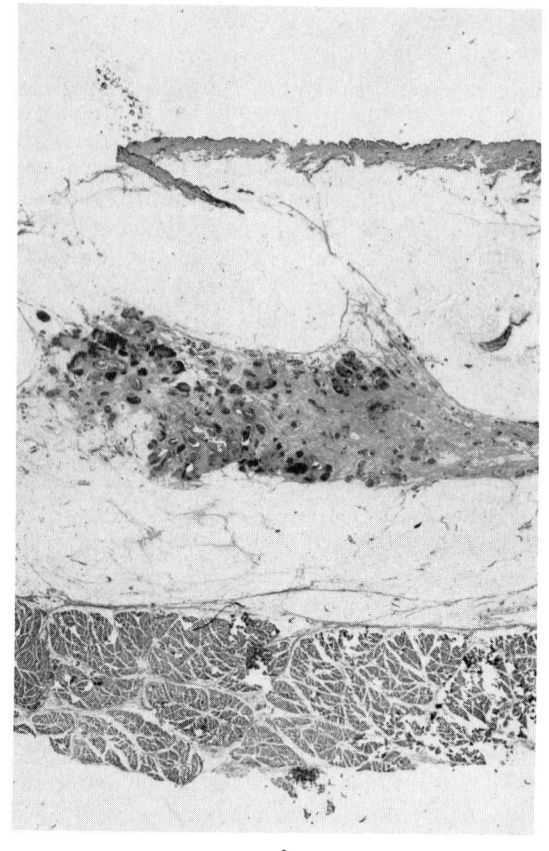

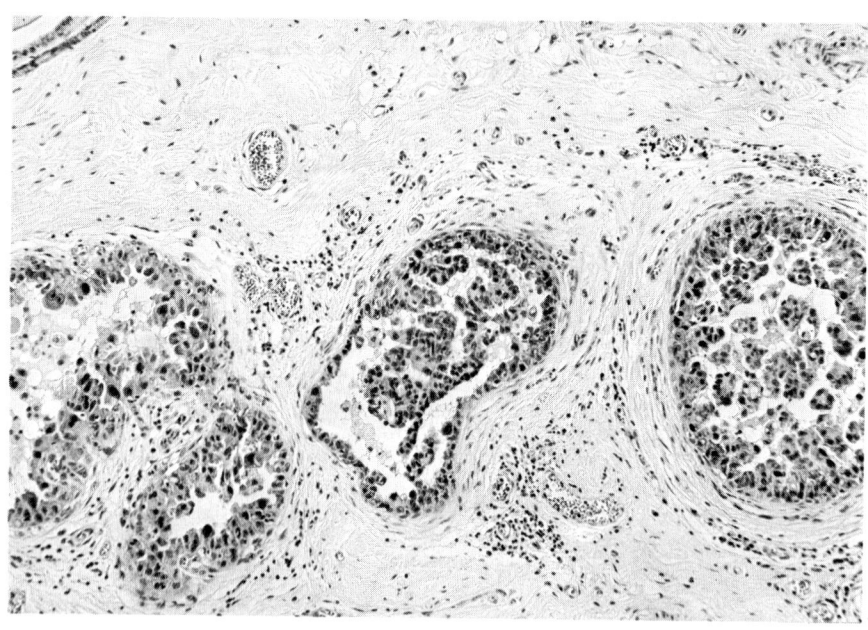

Figure 8–9. *A*, Whole breast mount showing foci of intraductal carcinoma. Tumor is represented by the darker areas. *B*, Papillary pattern with central necrosis and calcification.

Illustration continued on opposite page

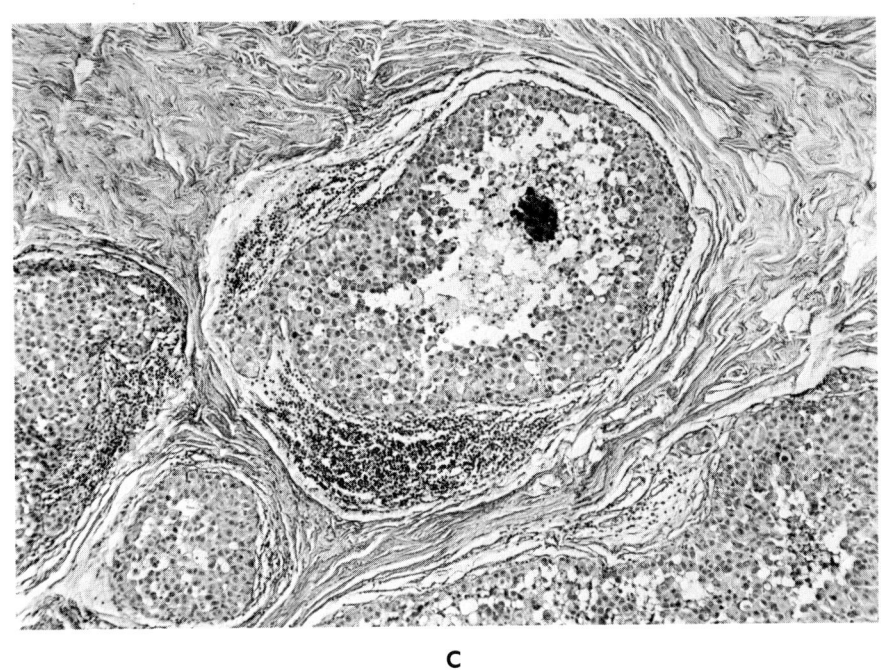

C

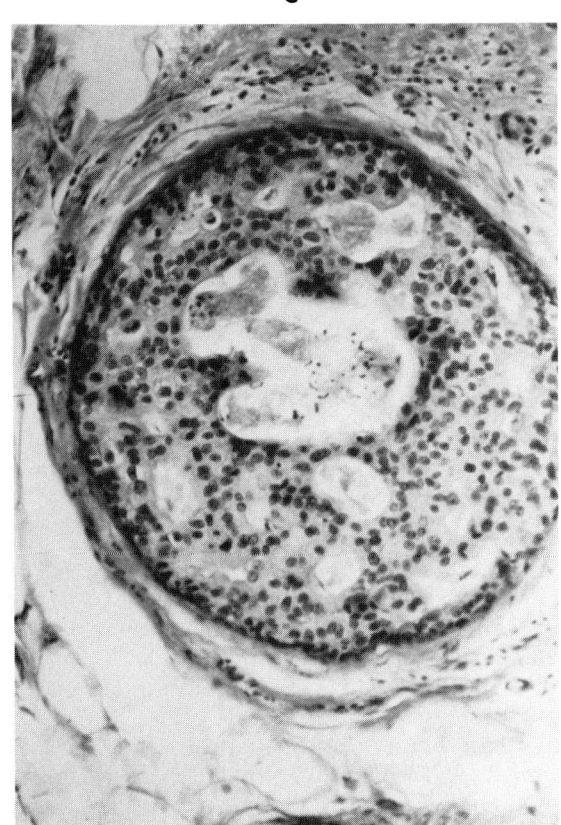

D

Figure 8–9 *Continued C*, Comedo pattern with central necrosis and calcification. *D*, Cribriform pattern with punch-out round spaces.

Illustration continued on following page

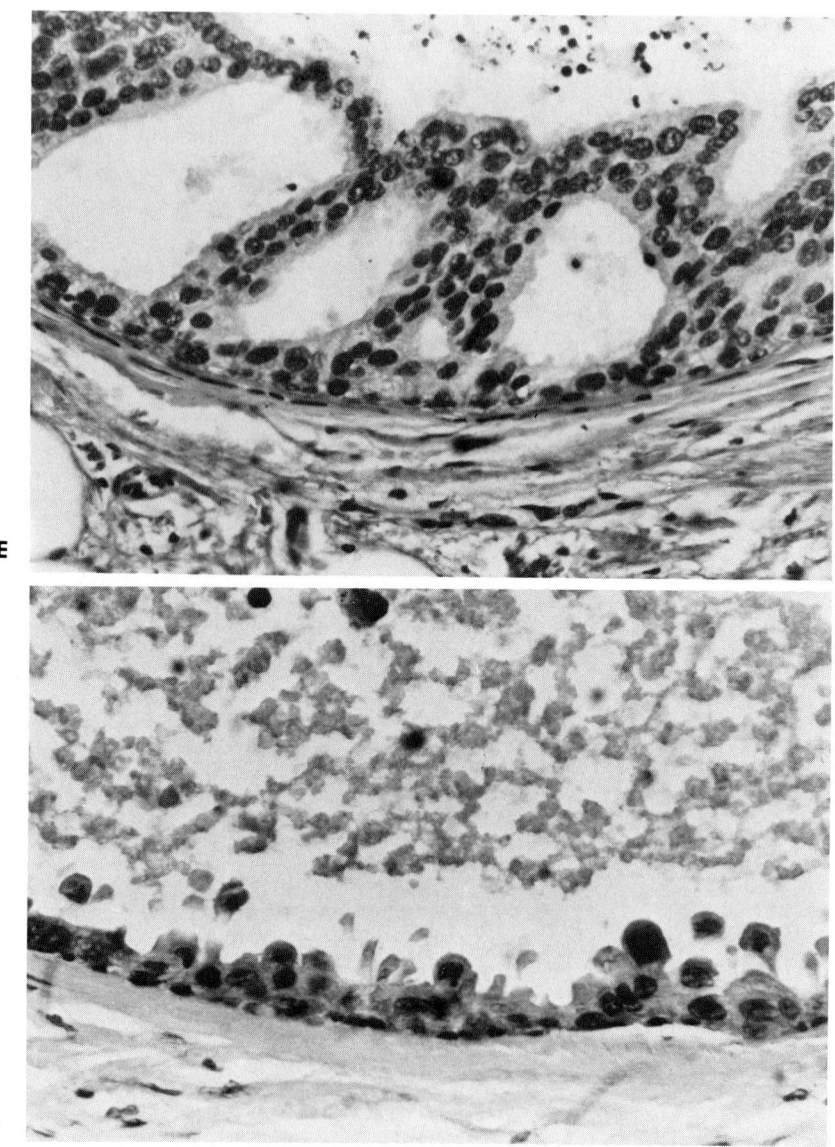

Figure 8–9 Continued *E,* "Roman bridges." Note the cellular anaplasia. *F,* Central necrosis leaving a few cells applied to the periphery ("clinging carcinoma").

mitotic figures; these cells fill the acini and distend the lobules. Larger ducts can also be involved by the proliferating cells.

Lobular carcinoma in situ can be associated with other invasive tumors (e.g., ductal carcinoma NOS, invasive lobular carcinoma, and others with special histology, e.g., tubular carcinoma and papillary carcinoma) and with benign tumors such as fibroadenoma.[89]

To some investigators, this lesion is only a marker of chronic cystic mastopathy, preneoplastic, with or without the potential to become malignant (lobular neoplasia)[94, 95]; to others, however, it is a true neoplasm, malignant, and a harbinger of invasion. Thus, correspondingly different ways of managing the lesion are advocated.[94, 183] The data obtained from untreated patients have not resolved all the uncertainties. The possible risk of developing an invasive carcinoma in the breast harboring lobular carcinoma in situ has been estimated at from 4 to 27 per cent for the ipsilateral breast and 10 per cent for the contralateral breast.[7, 94, 131, 183] The risk varies, depending on follow-up years. Noninterventionists have recommended close clinical surveillance, whereas

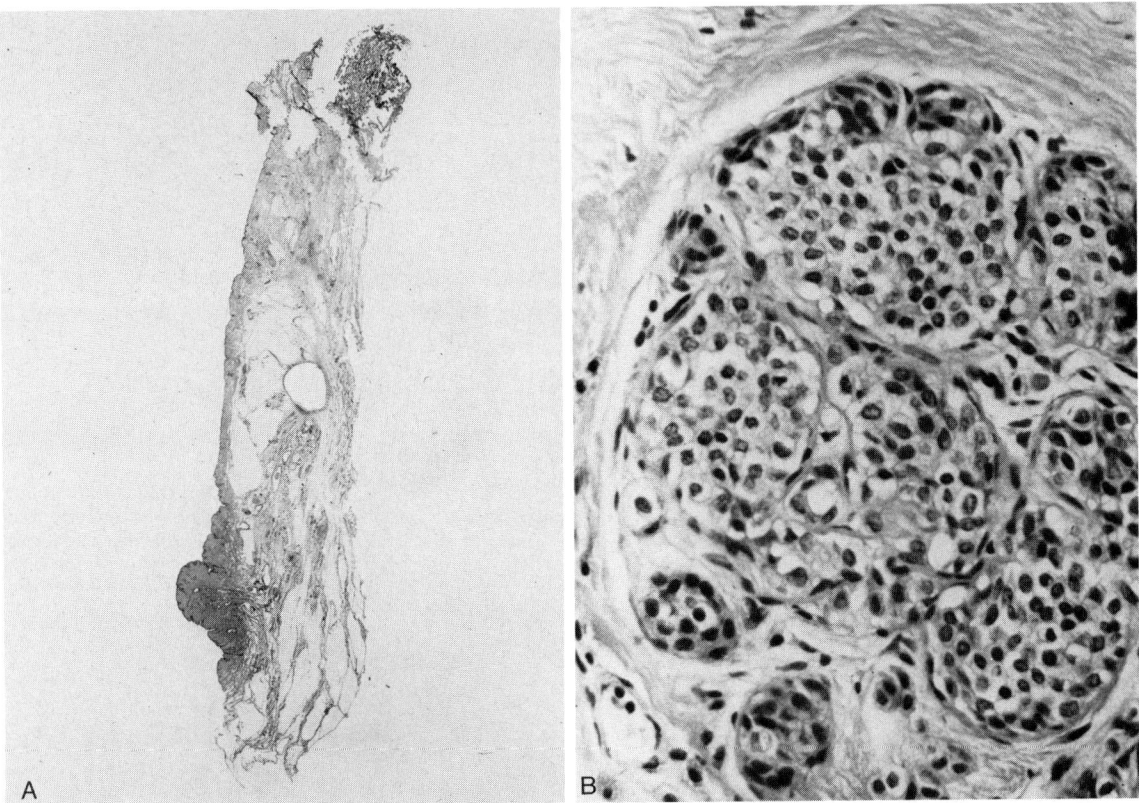

Figure 8–10. *A*, A focus of lobular carcinoma in situ is seen in the right side of the breast parenchyma in this whole breast section. Several cystic structures are present. *B*, Microscopic appearance of lobular carcinoma in situ.

others offer various kinds of mastectomy. The issue remains controversial.[6–8]

Rare Types of Invasive Carcinoma

ADENOID CYSTIC CARCINOMA

Adenoid cystic carcinoma of the breast is an uncommon type of breast adenocarcinoma, akin morphologically to other tumors more commonly observed in the major and minor salivary glands and in other locations, such as the tracheobronchial tree, lacrimal glands, tongue, nasopharynx, external ear canal, prostate, Bartholin's gland, and cervix.[35, 60, 116, 123, 165]

Although light microscopy and ultrastructural examination show no differences between tumors from different locations, biologically the behavior patterns of breast tumors and salivary gland tumors are strikingly different. In a recent study, only seven instances of 106 reported cases showed distant metastases, characteristically without axillary lymph node involvement. In only one case was axillary metastasis present at the time of diagnosis.[165]

These tumors appear as a small mass, usually near the nipple. They have been found to be positive for estrogen receptors. Grossly, the tumors are circumscribed, but not encapsulated, with a firm consistency and a variegated color without necrosis. They tend to grow slowly; in one of the author's cases, the slow growth of the tumor was observed during mammographic studies obtained over a period of 6 years.

Microscopically (Fig. 8–11), the characteristic cell is small, with scanty cytoplasm, hyperchromatic and uniform nuclei, infrequent mitoses, and unremarkable nucleoli, which are distributed in various patterns (cribriform, forming ducts, or in solid aggregates) in a pure form or in a combination of arrangements. The stroma is an integral part of the tumor and can be myxoid, hyaline, or various combinations of these, forming "cylinders" around

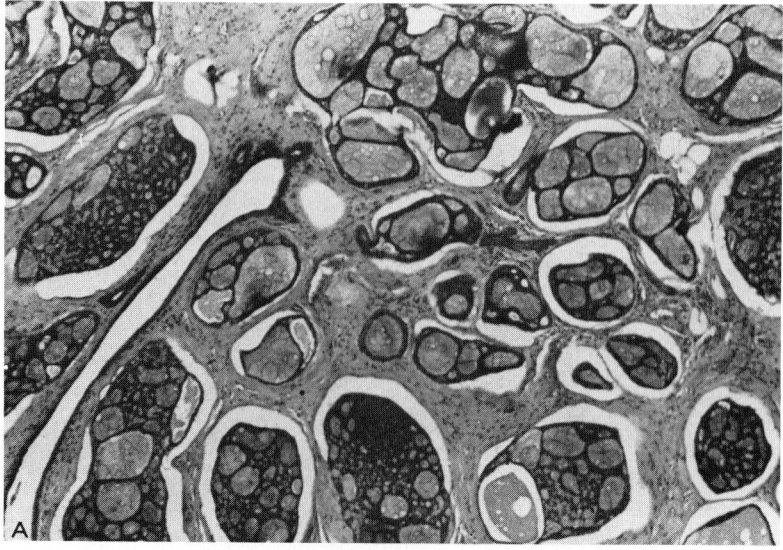
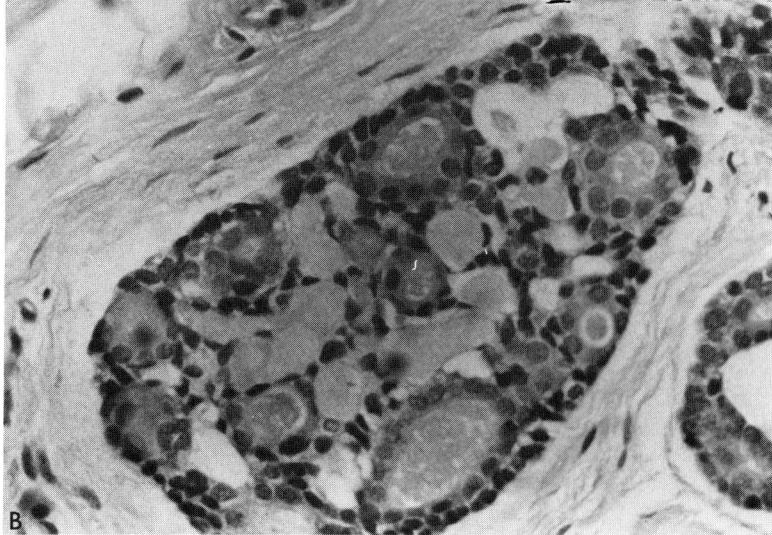

Figure 8–11. Low (A) and high (B) power views of adenocystic carcinoma. Notice the cribriform pattern and the stroma forming cylinders around and within the tumor.

and within the nests of tumor cells—justifying the name of cylindroma, as it is also known in other anatomic locations.

SQUAMOUS CELL CARCINOMA

Pure squamous cell carcinoma of the breast is rare. Frequency is difficult to estimate as cases of invasive carcinomas with focal squamous metaplasia have been included in some publications. Fisher and colleagues[61] reported an incidence of 3.6 per cent of squamous metaplasia in 1000 cases of invasive breast carcinoma. As Willis[227] noted, "Squamous cell carcinomas are rarer than is expected since breast developed from ectoderm." Figures fluctuate between 0.5 and 2 per cent of all breast cancers. Before a breast tumor is considered a pure squamous carcinoma, it is necessary to exclude tumors arising from the skin or its appendages,[28, 41] from the nipple, or from old mammary abscesses. Microscopically (Fig. 8–12A), the tumor shows conventional features of squamous cell carcinoma, including cellular stratification, presence of intercellular bridges, pearl formation, variable anaplasia, atypical mitoses and infiltration of the stroma. No mucin should be present in the cytoplasm. Obviously, no other type of tumor should coexist. Squamous metaplasia (Fig. 8–8B), which is benign, can occur rarely after breast

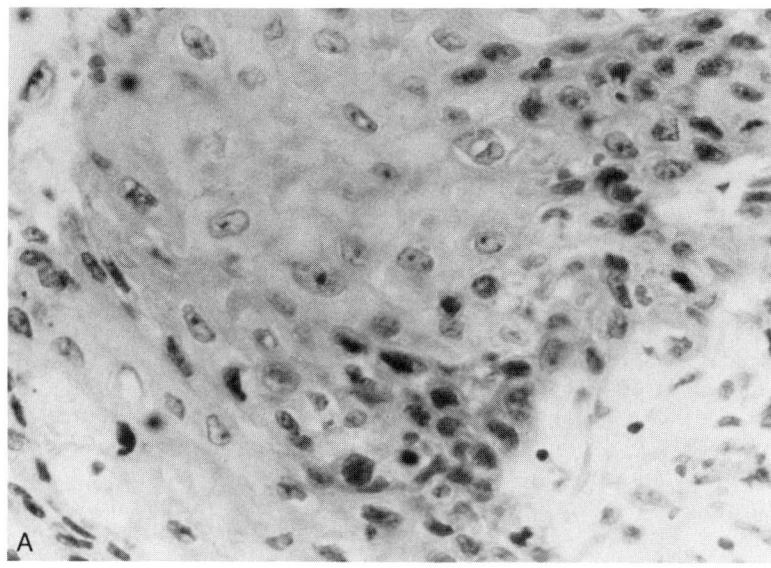
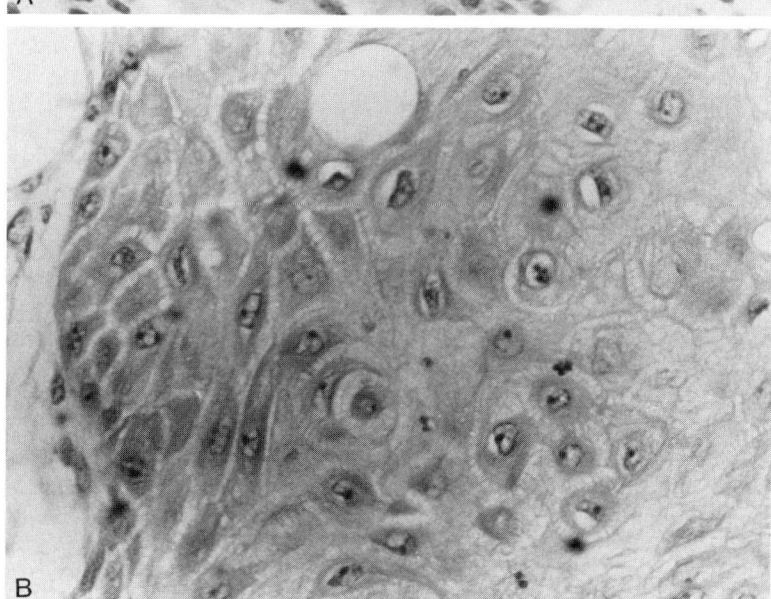

Figure 8–12. *A*, Squamous cell carcinoma. Note stratification, intercellular bridges, and atypical mitosis; metastatic foci in the axillary lymph nodes showed similar appearance. *B*, Squamous metaplasia after extensive infarction of the breast. Note well-oriented squamous epithelium without atypia. (Courtesy of Mitchell Rosenholtz, M.D.)

infarction and can be distinguished by lack of microscopic malignant features. In cases of cystosarcoma phyllodes or in spindle cell tumors, as well as in even rarer mucoepidermoid carcinomas,[162] areas of squamous cell carcinoma can be found. It is difficult to predict with confidence the natural history as the reported cases are few.

Only three pure primary squamous carcinomas of the breast were found among 4000 breast cancers by Toikkanen[209a] in Finland. They appeared to originate from the glandular tissue of the breast and followed an aggressive clinical course. All three patients died of dissemination after radical mastectomy. All the tumors were large and presented with necrosis and a cystic appearance. Lafreniere and coworkers[119a] reported on three cases of pure squamous cell carcinoma from the University of Miami School of Medicine, which brought the reported number of cases to a total of 21. Again, the cystic nature of these tumors was evident, with fluid varying from whitish to green, cloudy, straw-colored, bloody, or necrotic. The average age of patients was 53 years. The tumors measured from 2 to 12 cm in diameter. In one case the tumor was negative for estrogen receptors. Lafreniere and colleagues recommended an intensive work-up for other sites of primary squamous cell tumors known to metastasize to the breast (e.g., oral cavity, bronchus, esophagus, kidney, pelvis, bladder, ovary, and cervix). Only one of their three patients had nodal metastases, and all three were living free of recurrence for up to 24 months.

CARCINOMA WITH PSEUDOSARCOMATOUS METAPLASIA

This is an uncommon type, of which about 200 cases have been described, mostly in the form of case reports. Their distinctive feature is the mixture of malignant epithelial and mesenchymal components. The latter may include mature and immature bone, cartilage, and dense and loose stroma with sarcomatous appearance distributed in diverse combinations and proportions (Fig. 8–13). Transition between the epithelial and the pseudosarcomatous tumor cells has been demonstrated by light and electron microscopy. If no epithelial elements are identified, the tumor should be considered a sarcoma. This type of tumor appears to be more aggressive than nonmetaplastic carcinomas.

Kaufman and associates[112] described 26 cases of breast carcinoma demonstrating pseudosarcomatous metaplasia. Metaplastic elements included mature and immature bone, cartilage, myxoid stroma, fibromyxoid stroma, dense spindle cell stroma, and anaplastic stroma with giant cells, which resulted from dedifferentiation of epithelial cells. The tumors were more aggressive than pure epithelial carcinomas, with an overall survival rate of 44 per cent. The tumors tended to be large, averaging 4.7 cm in diameter. Lymph nodes were involved in 25 per cent. Although metastases to regional lymph nodes showed only the epithelial cancer, systemic metastases manifested the metaplastic elements seen in the primary tumor. TNM clinical stage and the relative preponderance of epithelial and pseudosarcomatous elements correlated with prognosis. Patients with tumors in which there was a pseudosarcomatous predominance had a poorer prognosis than those with predominantly epithelial components (28 per cent versus 62 per cent 5-year survival).

Carcinomas with metaplasia should be distinguished from the even less common spindle cell tumor, which has been diagnosed in other locations (oral cavity and larynx) and which is considered a variant of squamous cell carcinoma.[14, 82]

SECRETORY CARCINOMA

Described in 1966 by McDivitt and Stewart,[133] this tumor with distinct histologic features was initially thought to affect only children and adolescents[39, 156, 168]; however, it may occur occasionally in adults.[2, 155] Secretory carcinoma is a proper designation because of the distinct microscopic appearance. Secretory carcinoma is an indolent tumor without characteristic clinical features, the presence of a mass being the main complaint. At gross inspection, these are discrete, firm lesions generally with a sharply delineated margin, and can be confused with a fibroadenoma. Size varies from 1 to 12 cm or more in diameter. The tumor cells exhibit a granular cytoplasm. The microscopic appearance consists of acinar structures containing secretory material in the lumina and in the cytoplasm. The secretory material has been characterized as acid mucopolysaccharides, mostly in sulfated groups. The prognosis is excellent in children.

Tavassoli and Norris[204a] reported on 19 examples of secretory carcinoma of the breast and pointed out that not all patients are juveniles. Ages ranged from 9 to 69 years, with a median of 25 years. Six patients were 30 years of age or older, and one was a 9 year old boy. Four of the 19 patients (21 per cent) had axillary lymph node metastases and one of these (5 per cent of the total) died with disseminated tumor. These authors demonstrated Mucicarmine-positive material in the cells, separating them from lipid-rich carcinomas that stain with Oil Red O. They recommended wide excision as adequate treatment for children but advised modified mastectomy for patients more than 20 years old because of the capability of axillary nodal and distant metastases. Akhtar and colleagues[2] reported on three cases of secretory carcinoma of the breast in adults and stated that only 20 cases had been reported previously. The relatively favorable prognosis was noted. The tumors measured up to 5 cm in diameter. One patient had axillary nodal involvement but none had recurrence after less than 1 year of follow-up. A total mastectomy with axillary nodal dissection was recommended for adults.

SIGNET RING CELL CARCINOMA

Signet ring carcinomas are an aggressive subtype of breast cancer, distinct from extracel-

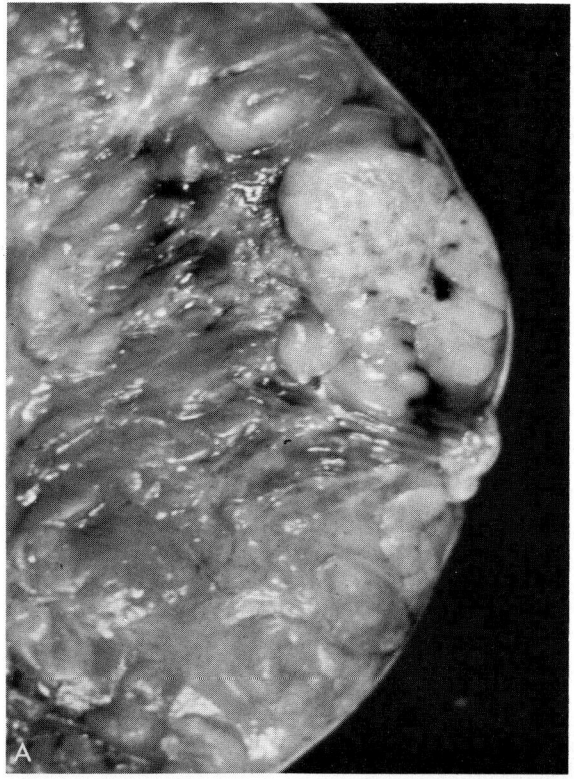
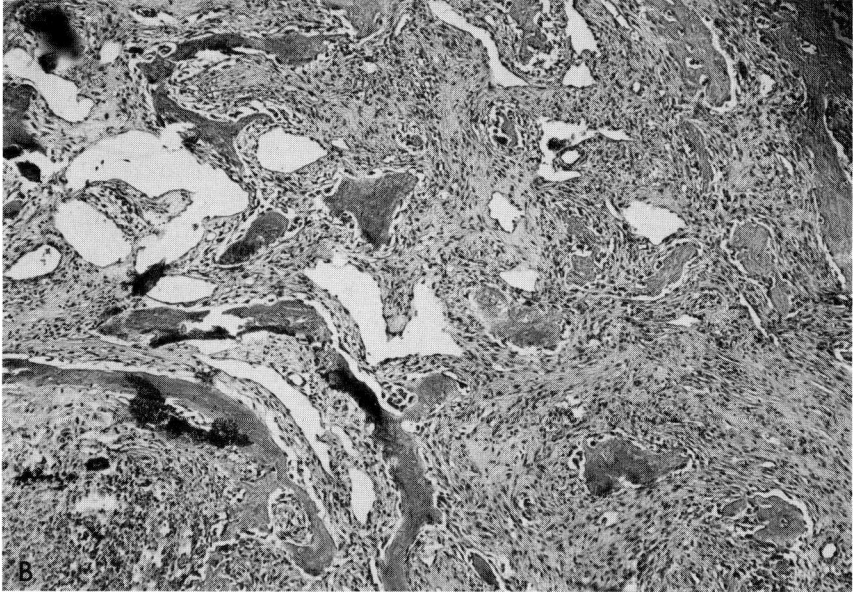

Figure 8–13. This carcinoma of the breast in a 67 year old woman displayed considerable osseous formation and produced extensive metastases to the gastrointestinal tract. A, The primary tumor appeared circumscribed. B, Many bone spicules are present in the tissues.

Illustration continued on following page

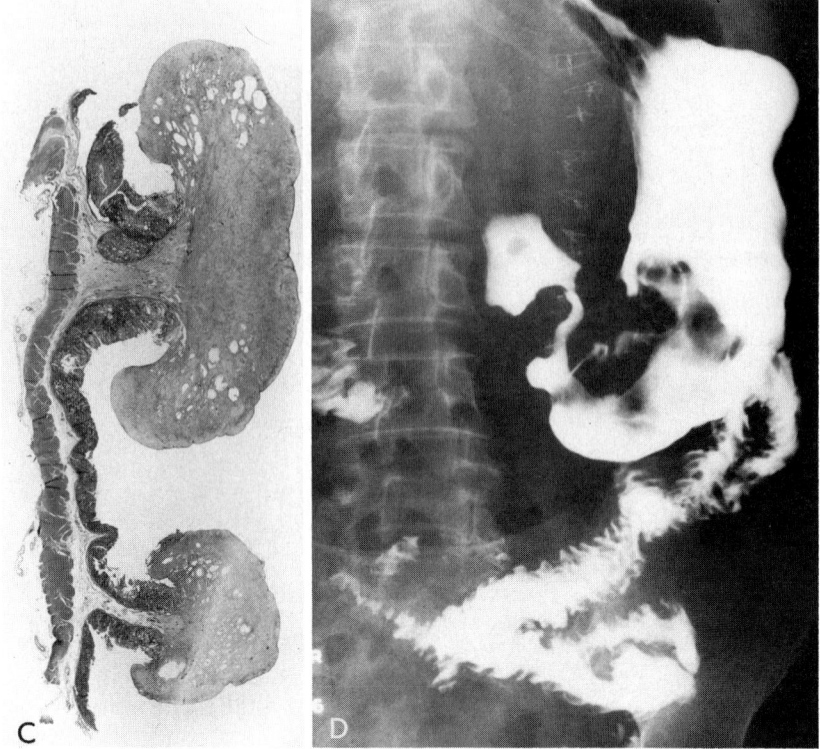

Figure 8–13 *Continued C,* Photomicrograph of the polypoid gastric metastases. *D,* Multiple polypoid metastases in the stomach demonstrated with a barium swallow. The patient developed dissemination 1 year after a radical mastectomy and died 2 years later.

lular mucinous carcinoma. They constitute about 2 per cent of all breast cancers and are derived from lobular rather than ductal carcinoma.[138] Signet ring cell carcinoma was first described by Saphir[193] in 1941 as a variety of mucinous carcinoma. Controversy exists concerning its histogenesis. To some authors this tumor represents a variant or part of the spectrum of invasive lobular carcinoma[76, 204] because of similarities in their patterns of growth (e.g., linear arrangement of the tumor cells, the coexistence of lobular carcinoma in situ, and the characteristic appearance of the metastatic deposits in the lymph nodes [sinus catarrh]). To other investigators it is a distinct pathologic entity.[98] It is the diffuse infiltration of signet ring cells that is the distinguishing feature (Fig. 8–14). These cells have peripherally located nuclei and the cytoplasm contains mucicarmine and periodic acid–Schiff (PAS)-positive material that is diastase resistant. The mixed forms show areas of infiltrating ductal or lobular carcinoma (or their in situ forms) as well as extracellular mucinous carcinoma. In its pure form it is more aggressive than both the extracellular mucinous carcinoma and other types of invasive lobular or ductal carcinoma.[105, 138] When this form is associated with lobular carcinoma there is an increased risk of bilaterality.

Signet ring cell carcinomas show an unusual metastatic pattern with a tendency to involve serosal surfaces or to produce retroperitoneal fibrosis, thereby mimicking gastrointestinal disease. They are associated with a poor prognosis. Sixty per cent of 24 patients studied by Merino and LiVolsi[138] had died of their cancers within 7 years. A rare type of intraductal signet ring cell carcinoma has been recently described.[59] There is morphologic evidence that at least some invasive signet ring cell carcinomas arise from intraductal signet ring cancer.[59] This lesion has been noted with medullary, tubular, ductal, and lobular invasive carcinomas.

LIPID-RICH CARCINOMA

Lipid-rich carcinoma is an aggressive tumor.[1] At the time of the biopsy many of the patients

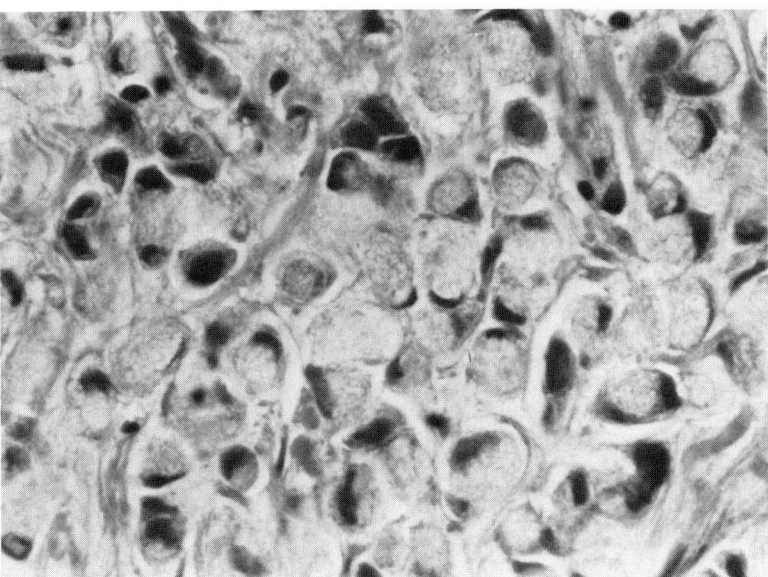

Figure 8–14. Intracellular mucinous carcinoma: Compact aggregate of signet-ring cells with peripheral nuclei and foamy cytoplasm, positive for mucus.

have metastases in the axillary nodes, and more than half die within 2 years after the diagnosis is established. The presenting clinical manifestation is a mass in the breast. The gross appearance is deceptive, lacking the conventional features of ductal carcinoma and sometimes mimicking a benign process. Microscopically, the tumor is characterized by large cells with clear, bubbly cytoplasm, irregular nuclei, and prominent nucleoli. The cytoplasmic content is positive for neutral lipids. Ultrastructural studies demonstrate that the lipid content is a result of secretory activities by the cell and is not a degenerative product. The tumor has infiltrating margins and invades the stroma without gland formation. In the series reported by Ramos and Taylor,[169] areas of intraductal and lobular carcinoma in situ were found in some tumors.

SUDORIFEROUS CARCINOMA

Sudoriferous carcinoma, a rare tumor, is also known as apocrine carcinoma, sweat gland carcinoma, oncocytic carcinoma, or carcinoma with apocrine metaplasia.[72, 93, 143] This tumor has no unique gross features distinguishing it from the ordinary infiltrating ductal carcinoma. Microscopically (Fig. 8–15), it is composed of large cells with an eosinophilic, pale, opaque cytoplasm resembling the cells of apocrine glands of the skin. Generally, it is well differentiated, with the cells arranged in tubular or glandular patterns. The origin and identity of the apocrine type of tumor cell exhibited by this neoplasm are in question. Some authors believe these tumors represent either embryonal inclusions of sweat gland structures within the breast, focally degenerative changes, or metaplasia. Many authorities consider the cancer a rare form of infiltrating ductal carcinoma with characteristic light microscopic appearance and distinct ultrastructural features. Others, however, do not consider it a pathologic entity.[178]

GLYCOGEN-RICH CLEAR CELL CARCINOMA

Few examples have been described of this rare neoplasm.[16, 104] The tumor is composed of clear cells containing glycogen in the cytoplasm and arranged in a papillary or solid pattern. Similarities have been noted to breast bud epithelial cells of the 13 week human embryo and to clear cell tumors of the female genital tract, salivary gland, and lung. Only two cases have been described and no lymph node metastases or distant dissemination occurred. Interestingly, both tumors were positive for estrogen receptors.

CARCINOID TUMORS

In 1979, Cubilla and Woodruff[43] reported a group of breast tumors with cytoplasmic argy-

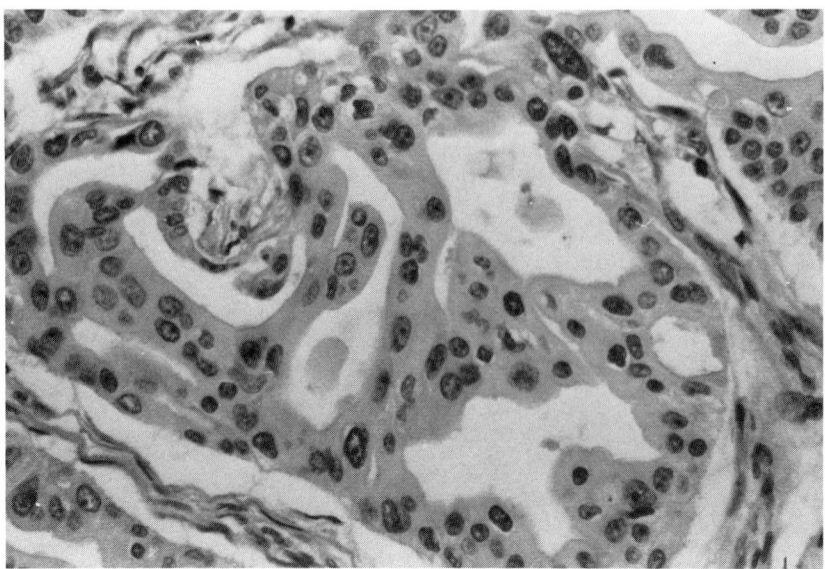

Figure 8–15. Sudoriferous carcinoma is a rare lesion that mimics sweat glands in its appearance. Tumor cells are large and possess eosinophilic cytoplasm.

rophilic granules, negative argentaffin reaction, and dense-cored granules of neurosecretory type ultrastructurally. None of the patients exhibited carcinoid syndrome or other endocrine symptoms. Subsequently, similar tumors have been reported in which hormonal substances were demonstrated using immunohistochemical localization or tissue extraction methods.[40, 113, 128, 197] Although some of these lesions resembled carcinoid tumors, the group is heterogeneous, with various patterns and types showing similar cytoplasmic argyrophilia, including ductal carcinomas, lobular carcinomas, carcinomas of uncertain origin, and mucinous (colloid) carcinomas. The histogenesis is uncertain.[163] To some authors it represents a carcinoid tumor arising from neuroendocrine cells present in normal breast tissue. To other investigators,[56] it is a variant of breast carcinoma that during the neoplastic transformation from primitive basal ductal cells differentiated into argyrophilic secretory cells. Interestingly, no relation has been established between the presence of cytoplasmic argyrophilia and clinical behavior of the tumors.[64, 171]

MUCOEPIDERMOID CARCINOMA

Mucoepidermoid carcinoma, a rare tumor described in 1979 by Patchefsky and colleagues,[162] exhibits microscopically a combination of mucus-forming glands and well-differentiated stratified squamous epithelium similar to low grade mucoepidermoid carcinomas of the salivary gland. Probably they originate in the ductal epithelium. The cases are few and the follow-up too short to establish prognosis.[61]

OAT CELL CARCINOMA

Small cell neuroendocrine (oat cell) carcinomas, histologically and ultrastructurally similar to those in the lung, have been described in a variety of extrapulmonary locations, including trachea, esophagus, salivary gland, stomach, bowel, pancreas, prostate, cervix, and skin. Their clinical evolution and therapeutic response run parallel to their pulmonary prototype. A similar type has been recently described in the breast,[219] characterized by small, anaplastic cells and containing neurosecretory granules on electron microscopy. The view advanced by the investigators is that it represents an anaplastic carcinoma with exclusively neuroendocrine differentiation.

Special Manifestations of Breast Carcinoma

PAGET'S DISEASE OF THE BREAST

The clinical description by James Paget in 1874 remains unsurpassed.[159] The eczematoid and erosive lesion of the nipple and areola are fairly constant as clinical signs, as is the presence of large, foamy cells in the epidermis, which constitute its histopathologic hallmark (Fig. 8–16). However, the underlying carcinomas vary in their clinical and pathologic characteristics.[11, 164] The lesions can be palpable or nonpalpable. They can infiltrate the breast parenchyma, or growth can be restricted to the confines of the ductal epithelium. The lesions can have "good" histology (intraductal carcinoma), or they can occur with tumors associated with a dismal prognosis, such as "inflammatory" carcinoma.[125] The carcinoma can even be limited to the most distal lactiferous ducts or to the epidermis of the nipple only.[121, 147, 160]

This vast array of the different underlying

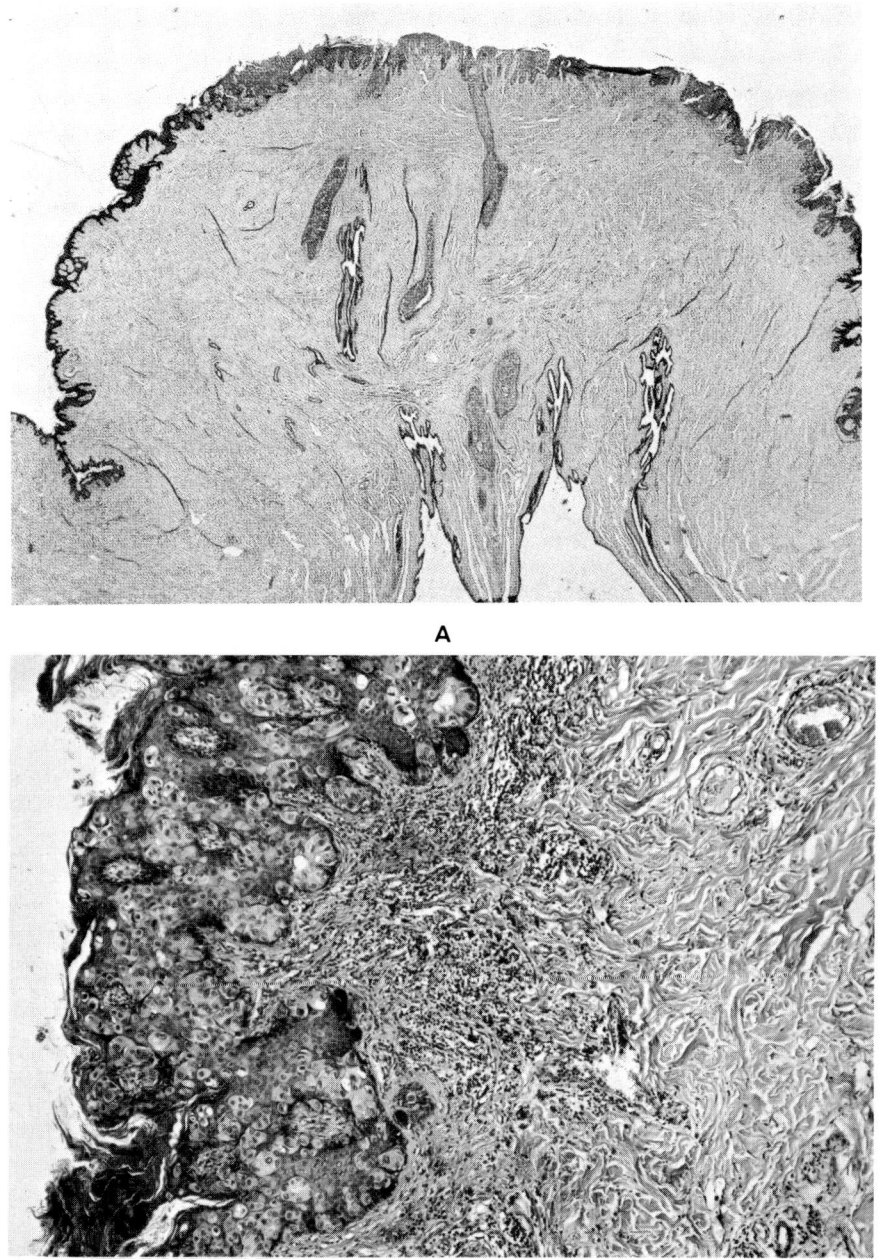

Figure 8–16. *A*, A low-power photomicrograph of the nipple shows lactiferous ducts engorged with ductal carcinoma and extensive changes characteristic of Paget's disease in the epidermis. *B*, High-power magnification of the epidermis of the nipple demonstrates extensive infiltration by the large cells with clear cytoplasm characteristic of Paget's disease.

malignancies justifies to some authors the exclusion of Paget's disease of the nipple as a special kind of breast carcinoma.[215]

Controversy still surrounds the nature and origin of the Paget's cells. Probably the prevalent view is that they represent an epidermotrophic upward migration to the nipple epithelium of malignant cells originating in the underlying tumor. Other views include the intraepidermal or in situ theory, which appears to be supported by the following evidence[121, 147, 178, 210]: (1) lack of continuity between the tumor and the nipple epithelium; (2) absence of underlying tumor in some cases, despite careful search in the specimen, as frequently occurs in extramammary Paget's disease; (3) occurrence of Paget's disease in ectopic nipples; (4) the existence of epithelial heterotopias within nipples; (5) demonstration by electron microscopy of intercellular bridges between Paget's cells and keratinocytes, as well as hemidesmosomes with the basal lamina of the epidermis.

The results of immunohistochemical studies showing common cell markers between Paget's cells, skin appendages, and breast carcinoma not shared by other cellular components of the skin, such as melanocytes and keratinocytes, are not entirely conclusive. It is still not clear if Paget's cells appear before or after the breast carcinoma.

As has been shown in various studies, the prognosis is related to the aggressiveness of the subjacent carcinoma, varying with the type of neoplasm and its clinical characteristics.[42] The existence of a palpable mass and the lymph node status are the main forces dictating the course of the disease.

INFLAMMATORY CARCINOMA

This manifestation of breast carcinoma is characterized clinically by skin erythema, "peau d'orange" edema, increased local temperature, pain and tenderness, with enlargement and induration of the affected breast.[205] Although it is possible to suspect the diagnosis on clinical grounds, a confirmatory biopsy should be obtained as benign inflammatory conditions and some infiltrative carcinomas with or without skin ulcerations can mimic this entity.[54]

Conversely, the clinical manifestations can be so subtle that they go undetected and their presence can be demonstrated only after the histopathologic study of the mastectomy specimen (occult inflammatory carcinoma).[191]

Inflammatory carcinoma represents a whole spectrum of clinical manifestations. Its low frequency (1 to 4 per cent of all breast carcinomas) contributes to the difficulties of precise clinical delineation. In an earlier study, 20 per cent of all patients with inflammatory carcinoma received topical anti-inflammatory treatment during the early phases of the disease.[125] The presence of diffuse thickening of the skin of the affected breast on mammography is usually present together with the clinical manifestations and may be the only mammographic sign.

The gross characteristics are variable and frequently no dominant mass is recognized, only diffuse induration of the parenchyma and the presence of satellite tumor deposits of variable size and location (Fig. 8–17).

Plugging of the dermal and intramammary lymphatics by tumor cells constitutes the histopathologic hallmark.[125, 205] In the dermis, cellular infiltrate may be absent or variable. Poorly differentiated or undifferentiated ductal carcinomas, NOS, are mostly responsible for this presentation. At the time of diagnosis, tumor has frequently spread into the axillary lymph nodes. This represents one of the most dreadful manifestations of breast cancer.

Rarely, local manifestations of "inflammatory" carcinoma can occur in the skin of the breast, resulting from metastasis from primary tumors in other sites,[100, 118, 213] including the ovaries, stomach, tonsils, lungs, and pancreas. This form has been designated, among other names, as carcinoma erysipelatoides.[100] Its inflammatory characteristics are the result of plugging of lymphatics by the metastatic tumor.

Clinicopathologic Correlation

Characteristics of tumors with prognostic significance can be tested and verified only if the data are collected uniformly and consistently.[130, 152] The use of a protocol will provide such information.[176] A printed form with blanks to be filled with the requested data should be available in the laboratory to record the gross and microscopic details of the specimen. Basic information to be obtained includes side, site, dimension of lesion, pertinent clinical details, and the exact identification of the procedure used to obtain the specimen. The need to maintain the broadest communication

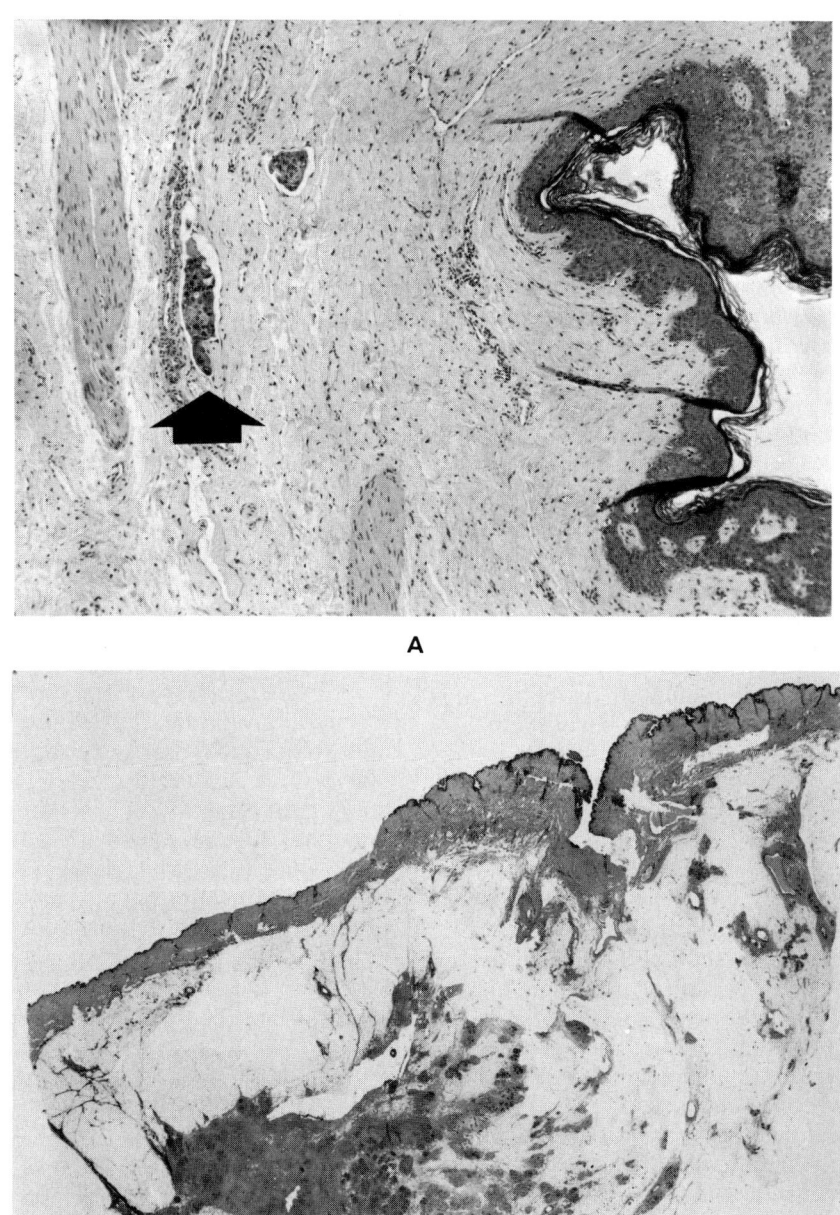

Figure 8–17. *A*, Section of skin from a breast with inflammatory carcinoma demonstrating tumor emboli in lymphatics of the lower dermis. *B*, Inflammatory carcinoma. Extensive infiltration of the breast by multiple tumor deposits is present with plugging of lymphatics. The dermis is thickened.

between surgeons and pathologists has been dramatized by the increasing number of specimens from asymptomatic patients containing nonpalpable lesions and also the growing frequency of excisional biopsies as the sole means of ablative therapy.[57] The proper handling of this type of specimen requires the utmost cooperation between professionals. Specimen mammograms are obviously mandatory for specimens from asymptomatic patients and are extremely helpful for excisional biopsies. Precise and clearly explained procedures should be followed to maintain uniformity and consistency in collecting the needed data. The frequent opportunity to correlate radiographs of lesions with gross and microscopic characteristics enables pathologists to increase their own usefulness.

The tumor size and the characteristics of its margins can be determined with precision. Comparing specimen mammograms with the patient's mammograms offers the additional advantage of verifying the exact location of the lesion, a useful datum for future reference. The separation of axillary lymph nodes into levels can be facilitated by identifying marks placed by the surgeon; in their absence, nodes from the middle and lower level can be grouped together.

Numerous methods to increase the harvest of lymph nodes have been developed.[115] An adequate number of lymph nodes can be dissected by a time-efficient procedure that consists of washing the axillary content in running water (for no more than 15 minutes, to avoid water artifacts) and immediately dissecting the specimen on a translucent surface (glass or plastic) with a light source underneath. The nodes will stand out as dark structures in a yellow background. When handling mastectomy specimens special attention should be given to the nipple, including its appearance and relation to tumor site, and tissue samples should be taken in both vertical and horizontal planes, including the subareolar fat. If specimen mammographic equipment is available, it is advantageous to utilize Egan's methods or modifications to identify and to sample parenchymal alterations, palpable or nonpalpable, for a more comprehensive histopathologic analysis.[53a] Use of this method may provide more precise delineation of the differences that exist between a multifocal and a multicentric lesion. This is a pivotal notion that pervades discussions between those who advocate and those who oppose segmental resection of breast tumors as a mode of therapy.

Tumors have measurable morphologic features, which in different degrees influence or reflect the clinical course of breast tumors. Lymph node status, tumor size, tumor differentiation, and tumor grade in addition to tumor type are among the pathologic parameters that closely correlate with patient survival; others include tumor margins, inflammatory infiltrates, and lymphatic and blood vessel invasion. Although a few parameters appear to exert an independent influence as prognostic discriminants, by and large their effect is strongest when considered in combination.[4]

LYMPH NODE STATUS

Metastasis to the axillary lymph nodes remains the most reliable index of aggressiveness of breast carcinoma.[67] Patient survival is reduced to nearly half when there are tumor deposits in the axillary nodes. However, there are qualifiers of prognosis other than the mere presence of metastasis. The number of positive lymph nodes appears to be more important than their level in the axilla[202] or than the total number of lymph nodes found in the dissection. The discovery of additional metastatic nodes by using multiple level sections of negative lymph nodes does not alter the prognosis significantly.[167] When metastases are confined within the limits of the nodes and are 2 mm or less in diameter (micrometastases), the prognosis is much less adverse than when the metastases are larger and the tumor extends to the perinodal fat.[109, 185] Even the number of metastatic nodes has differing prognostic significance; when metastasis occurs to a single node, the survival rate is only a little lower than that for patients with no metastases in the axilla.[142, 185, 186] A decrease in survival is observed in postmenopausal women with four or more metastatic lymph nodes, whereas the outcome in premenopausal patients is less favorable when only two or more lymph nodes are involved. A single nodal metastasis, when the affected node is larger than 2 cm in diameter (macrometastasis), has a prognosis equal to that for patients with two or more positive lymph nodes.[196] Evaluation of the subcategories of patients on the basis of the foregoing considerations is necessary to fully estimate the prognostic relevance of the axillary status.

HISTOLOGIC TUMOR TYPE

A gradient of aggressiveness is seen within carcinoma of the breast. In analyzing the characteristics of long-term survivors the prevalence of "special" histopathologic tumor types is noted, in contrast to the predominance of infiltrating ductal carcinomas, NOS, among short-term survivors.[51] The lesser biologic aggressiveness of the special histologic types can be identified by the pathologist as these tumor types possess recognizable gross and microscopic features.[79, 207] Ackerman and Rosai classified carcinomas of the breast into four categories after assessing certain tumor characteristics and their prognostic significance.[178]

Type I (Not Invasive)
Intraductal carcinoma (with or without Paget's disease)
Intraductal papillary carcinoma
Lobular carcinoma in situ (lobular neoplasia)

Type II (Invasive, Circumscribed Margins, Infrequent Metastasis)
Pure mucinous carcinoma
Tubular carcinoma
Invasive papillary carcinoma
Medullary carcinoma

Type III (Invasive, Moderately Metastasizing)*
Invasive ductal carcinoma, NOS
Intraductal carcinoma with invasion
Invasive lobular carcinoma

Type IV (Invasive Undifferentiated Carcinoma)
Tumors indisputably invading blood vessels, regardless of type

The relative proportions of each tumor type have been estimated in various studies[60, 150, 176]: ductal carcinoma, NOS, 52 to 67 per cent; medullary carcinoma, 3 to 6.2 per cent; lobular carcinoma in situ, 3 to 8.5 per cent; mucinous carcinoma, 2 to 2.4 per cent; papillary carcinoma, 0.3 to 3 per cent; tubular carcinoma, 1.2 to 1.5 per cent; Paget's disease, 0.5 to 2.2 per cent. These tumors exist in combination with ductal carcinomas, NOS; coexistence has been estimated to occur in between 17 per cent and 30 per cent of cases. Carcinomas occurring in combination with ductal carcinomas most frequently were invasive lobular, 6 per cent; tubular, 4.5 per cent; papillary, 2 per cent; colloid, 0.5 per cent. Fisher and colleagues[60] noted that in "pure" ductal carcinomas, NOS, lymphatic invasion, palpable lymph nodes, and greater histologic differentiation occur more frequently than in combined forms.

---

*All carcinomas not definitely classified as Type I, II, or IV constitute Type III.

TUMOR SIZE

One of the most reliable indicators of prognosis is the dimension of the tumor. The larger its size, the greater the possibility of axillary metastases and also of treatment failure. In tumors measuring less than 1 cm in diameter, axillary metastases occur in between 5 and 25 per cent of cases.[15, 194]; 90 per cent of the patients survive more than 5 years.[124] The 5-year survival is reduced to 65 per cent when tumors are 2 to 2.5 cm in diameter.[150] Further size increments produce further increases in metastasis to the axillary lymph nodes and reductions in survival. The study of Say and Donegan[194] demonstrates this direct correlation. The dimensions of the neoplasm, however, are not the only factor associated with survival as tumors with similar dimensions have different survival when lymph node metastases exist.[58, 143, 185, 186] Advances in technology have been responsible for the detection of small "early" carcinomas in asymptomatic women before they become clinically recognizable. The size distribution of the tumors detected in asymptomatic and symptomatic patients and the frequency of lymph node metastases[164, 177] are depicted in Figure 8–18.

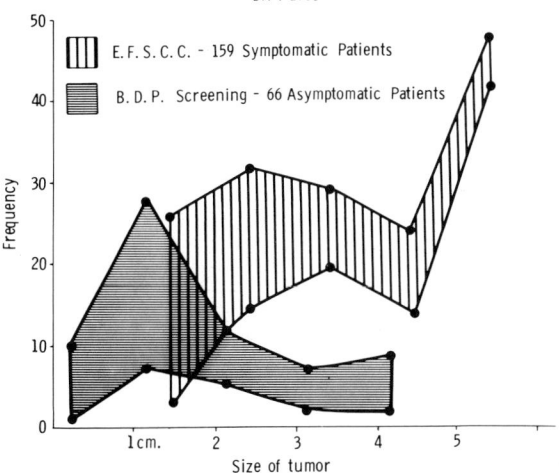

* Tumors included in this analysis represent invasive ductal carcinomas of no special type (N.O.S.) diagnosed and treated during same period of time.

Figure 8–18. Breast cancers detected by screening of asymptomatic women tend to be smaller and few have nodal metastases. Lower lines in each profile represent number of cases with metastases in each size category.

More than 15 years have elapsed since Gallagher and Martin[77] introduced the concept of minimal breast cancer; still a lack of agreement remains concerning its significance and value. Minimal breast cancer was initially defined to include all cases of in situ (noninvasive) mammary carcinoma of both lobular and ductal type and all invasive carcinomas of ductal and lobular types that measured 5 mm or less in greatest diameter.[166] Subsequently, this definition was amplified to include tumors with "good" histologic features (such as mucinous, papillary, and tubular carcinomas) and invasive carcinomas of 1 cm in diameter or less. The concept was developed to signify the existence of an "extremely early" phase of mammary carcinoma, "treatable with local measures alone."[78] Although different tumor entities were encompassed, they shared similarities and might be accordingly staged and treated.[99] The initial acceptance of the concept was facilitated by the lack of sufficient interest in breast carcinomas with good prognostic features.[221] It also coincided with the increased use of new technologic methods able to discover tumors in asymptomatic patients. Interestingly, tumors with the criteria of minimal breast cancer constituted 10 per cent of all breast tumors in tumor registries, and in breast cancer demonstration projects they represented more than 40 per cent of cancers discovered during initial screening.[172] However, some authors believe that the concept has outlived its purpose,[221] and that grouping together tumors of such complex and uncertain biology is inappropriate.

TUMOR DIFFERENTIATION AND NUCLEAR GRADE

The relationship between the microscopic characteristics of tumors and their clinical behavior has been recognized since the end of the 19th century. Although attributed to von Hansemann (1893),[218] it was Dennis (1891)[47] who first formulated the concept for tumors of the breast. Dennis noted that "the more typical the structure, the better the prognosis . . . the more embryonic the structure of the tumor the greater the liability of recurrence." In 1925, Greenough[91] for the first time systematically studied the correlation of histologic differentiation of breast tumors with patient survival. The criteria used were based on the degree of tubule formation and the characteristics of the tumor cells and their nuclei, including uniformity or variations in size, shape, tinctorial properties, and mitotic ratio. Greenough's study, based on 73 patients, demonstrated a close relation between cancer "cures" and well-differentiated tumors. Although his views were not endorsed by the majority of his contemporaries, Greenough's classification represents with some variations the basis for most current systems of grading breast tumors according to their differentiation.[24, 26, 27, 66, 195, 211] Rigorous application of the criteria permits the separation of tumors into categories of differentiation, particularly infiltrating ductal carcinomas, NOS. The use of these criteria in special types of tumors, such as medullary, papillary, or mucinous carcinomas, is not as fruitful as tumor type possesses its own prognostic characteristic independent of grade.[49, 51] The existence of more than one pattern of differentiation in the same tumor is not a deterrent for use of these criteria. It is still possible to score independently each pattern and determine the proportion from the total tumor bulk or record only the more anaplastic portion of the pattern. Likewise, if more than one tumor type is present (e.g., ductal carcinoma, NOS, with mucinous or tubular carcinoma), the estimated proportion of each type can be so stated. In a study by Andersen and coworkers,[9] 1048 patients with invasive ductal carcinomas, NOS, without lymphatic metastasis considered a favorable prognostic group were classified according to their histopathologic grade (WHO).[208] (The grades were as follows: Grade I: Well-marked glandular formation, occasional hyperchromasia or mitotic activity, and uniformity of nuclei, including size, shape, and tinctorial characteristics. Grade II: Tumors occupying a position intermediate between Grades I and III. Grade III: Negligible or absent glandular formation, more than three hyperchromatic or mitotic figures per high power field and marked nuclear pleomorphism.) Within the first year after mastectomy, the recurrence rates of tumors graded as I, II, and III were 4, 9, and 14 per cent respectively. The nuclear grade of tumors is determined by assessing the variations in size, mitotic ratio, chromatin pattern of the nuclei, and presence or absence of nucleoli. Nuclear grade is considered by Black and colleagues[21, 22] to be of greater prognostic significance than tubule formation. Grades are determined on a scale from 0 to 4, with 0 being the most undifferentiated and 4 the most differentiated.

Fisher and coworkers[66] inverted the order of the grading to a more conventional schema and reduced the grades of the scale; in their schema the grades ranged from 1 to 3, with 3 being the least differentiated. An attempt to integrate the prognostic value of both the degree of tubule formation and of the nuclear grade of tumors has been proposed by Fisher and associates.[66] In this system, both nuclear grade and histologic grade (tubule formation) are evaluated on a scale of 1 to 3. Their results, obtained in the analysis of 1500 invasive breast cancers, have been consistent with survival rates.

Criticism has been leveled at this method because of lack of consistency and reproducibility, as differences of about one third occurred when the grading of tumors by various observers was compared.[44, 92] However, the discrepancies can be reduced to acceptable levels with simplification of the system and strict observance of the criteria. Grading is a simple and relatively quick process that can provide useful prospective and retrospective information concerning prognosis independently or in combination with other tumor markers.[52]

TUMOR MARGINS

Greater aggressiveness has been noted in invasive breast carcinomas with irregular serrated margins than in tumors with well-circumscribed, knobby borders. Ingleby and Gershon-Cohen[110] in 1960 and Gold and coworkers[88] in 1972 observed such characteristics based on mammographic imaging. Lane and associates[122] in 1961, using histopathologic methods, made similar observations. Tumors exhibiting well-delineated, sharply defined contours with an expansile type of growth were associated less frequently with axillary lymph node metastasis than tumors whose margins were serrated and infiltrative (Fig. 8–19). The 10-year survival of patients with circumscribed tumor margins was 80 per cent, in contrast with only 38 per cent in patients with irregular tumor contours. No direct relation was found between lymph node metastasis, survival, and tumor size when the tumor had regular expansile borders. Patients having tumors smaller than 2.5 cm with irregular borders had a 10-year survival of 52 per cent. For those with larger tumors and irregular borders, survival was reduced to 25 per cent. Lane and coworkers also found a direct relationship between tumor profile and axillary lymph node metastasis. Fisher and colleagues[60] found tumor circumscription, both gross and microscopic, associated with negative axillary nodes. Kouchoukos and associates[119] found a significant difference in the incidence of metastasis to the axillary lymph nodes on comparing tumors with pushing borders and infiltrative borders; however, no difference was found in survival rate. Silverberg and colleagues,[199] however, noted lower survival rates in patients with circumscribed tumors despite less axillary involvement. More recently, Carter and associates,[33] studying invasive tumors in 330 patients, found significant differences in axillary lymph node metastasis and 10-year survival in patients with circumscribed versus infiltrative margins but no differences when the characteristics of the tumor border were used as the only discriminator; however, when the presence of tumor necrosis was included in the equation, tumors with necrosis and infiltrative margins behaved more aggressively than did tumors with no necrosis and expansile borders.

It appears that although the quality of the margins of tumors is a reflection of pattern of growth, it is not the dominant force in tumor behavior; however, when considered in association with other variables, it can provide useful prognostic information.

INFLAMMATORY INFILTRATE

The cellular inflammatory infiltrate with breast tumors has been considered an index of immune reaction in the host-tumor relationship. Its prognostic significance has been assessed both quantitatively and qualitatively in numerous studies with diverse conclusions. Black and colleagues indicated that there was a relationship between patient survival and the intensity of the lymphocytic infiltration of tumors. In a study including 222 patients, Hamlin[96] assessed the cellular response to tumors, both quantitatively and qualitatively, including size, location, type, grade of differentiation, in addition to the age of the patient and clinical status. This study demonstrated a relationship between cellular response, prognosis, and tumor differentiation. Berg[17] found a relationship between plasma cell infiltration and survival. Humphrey and coworkers[106] studied the immunologic responsiveness of breast cancer patients and concluded that lymphocytic infiltra-

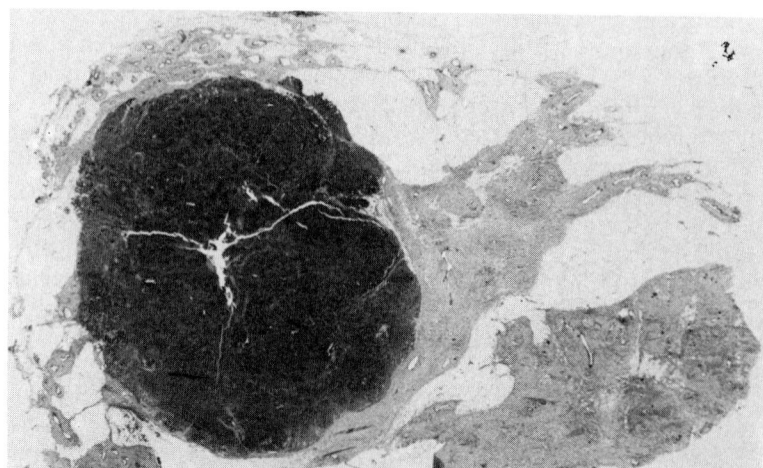

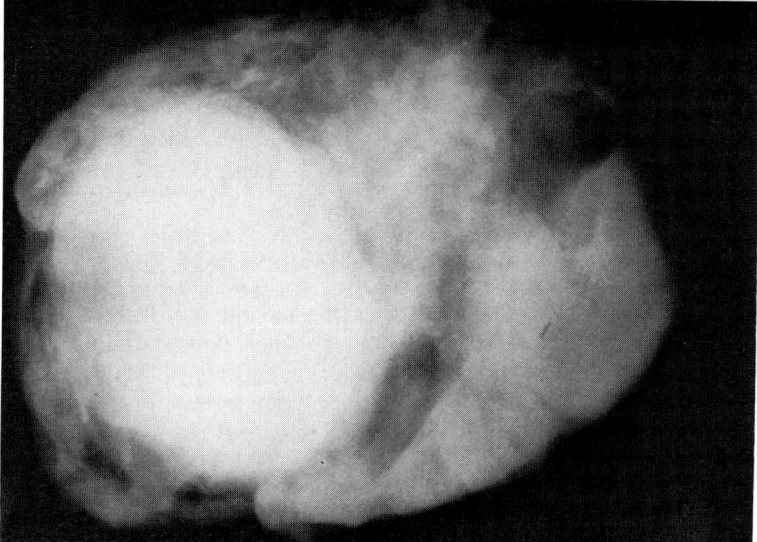

Figure 8–19. *A, B,* This specimen radiograph and photomicrograph illustrate a carcinoma (medullary) with a circumscribed margin.

Illustration continued on opposite page

tion of the primary tumor was an indicator of favorable prognosis. However, in several studies, when lymphocytic infiltration was considered in association with other variables, an opposite conclusion was reached.[37] Tumor anaplasia increases with the intensity of the inflammatory infiltrate, whereas an inverse relationship exists with estrogen receptor level.[36, 139, 184]

Using immunoperoxidase techniques, Shimokawara and colleagues[198] noted in tissue sections a correlation between the intensity of T cell infiltration and the clinical course of patients with breast carcinoma. As T cell infiltration was significantly high in those tumors without axillary lymph node metastasis, the possibility that T cell infiltration represents an index of host resistance against cancer is suggested.

LYMPHATIC INVASION

Lymphatic tumor emboli have been shown to be of prognostic significance; clusters of tumor cells within lymphatics at the periphery of tumors are associated with local or systemic recurrence. The emboli are more significant if tumors are larger than 1 cm in diameter. In seven studies encompassing 1602 patients with stage T1 N0 M0 cancers, lymphatic tumor permeation showed prognostic value in only one (Fig. 8–20).

In the estimation of Fisher and colleagues,[67] lymphatic invasion is related more closely to lymph node status than to treatment failure as 33 per cent of patients surviving 10 years showed such invasion. In a study of patients surviving 25 years,[46] lymphatic invasion occurred in 63 per cent.

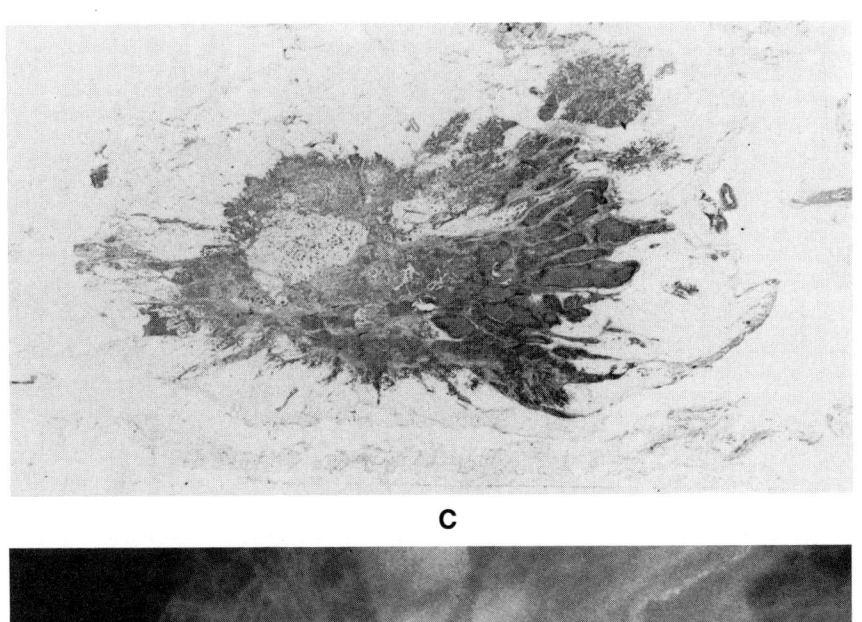

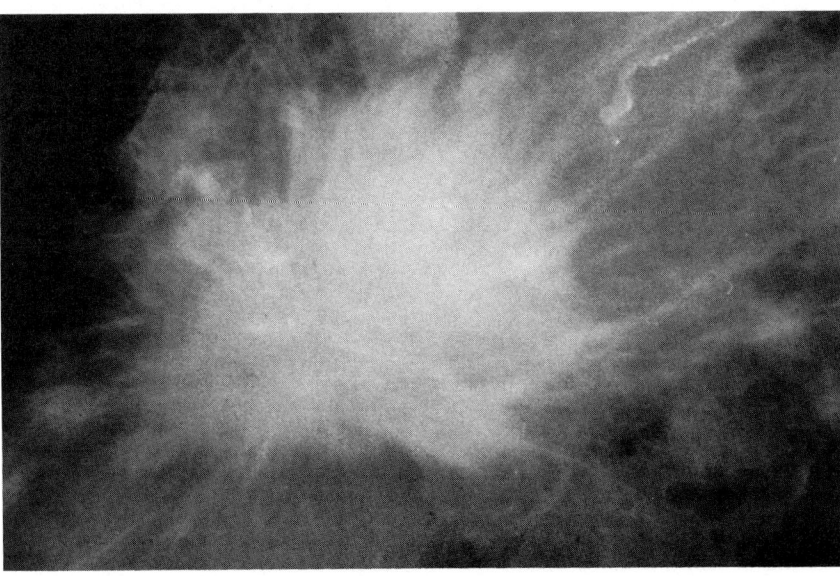

Figure 8–19 Continued C, D, Infiltrative tumor margins are illustrated in this case by both a photomicrograph (C) and a radiograph (D).

It is important, however, that strict criteria be used to identify lymphatic invasion as technical artifacts can mimic the phenomenon. Gilchrist and associates were unable in a double-blind study to find unanimity among experienced pathologists in detecting lymphatic invasion.[85]

BLOOD VESSEL INVASION

The frequency of blood vessel invasion varies according to published reports from 4 per cent to 51 per cent[19, 67, 192]; this fluctuation appears to be related to the broad spectrum of criteria used for such determination.[19, 67, 90, 223] It is possible that the true incidence may occupy an intermediate location between both extremes. When blood vessel invasion is assessed in combination with nodal status, its influence on prognosis has more predictive value. Early recurrence occurs in 70 per cent[223] of patients when both blood vessels and nodes are involved by tumor. Only 12 per cent[192] of patients survive for 5 years when both findings are present.

The prognostic significance of such findings has been disputed by Fisher and colleagues,[67] who found 3.6 per cent and 7.8 per cent of vascular invasion in patients without recurrence and in those with treatment failure, respectively.

HISTOPATHOLOGIC RISK FACTORS WITH PROGNOSTIC VALUE IN $T_1N_0M_0$ PATIENTS WITH BREAST CANCER								
Author	Number of Patients	Tumor Grade	Histologic Type	Tumor Margin	Tumor Lymphoid Infiltrate	Tumor Lymphatic Invasion	Tumor Vascular Invasion	Other
Thomas, et al ANN SURGERY 190:129, 1979	203	+		+		+	+	
Fracchia, et al SURG GYN OBST 151:375, 1980	520	0		⊕		+		Tumor size +
Nealon, et al SURGERY 89:279, 1981	228	+		+		+	+	
Roses, et al AM J CLIN PATH 78:817, 1982	122	0	+	0	0	+	0	Necrosis, Cellularity Fibrous response Neural Invasion
Ketterhagen, et al SURG GYN OBST 188:120, 1984	69	+		+		+	+	
Rosen, et al ANN SURGERY 193:15, 1981	382	+	+		0	+	+	
Bilik, et al AM J SURGERY 151:460, 1986	78	+			+		+	

+ Effect　　0 No Effect　　⊕ Inconclusive

Figure 8–20. Histopathologic parameters analyzed in seven separate studies encompassing 1602 patients.

Receptor Proteins

The determination of estrogen and progesterone receptors in breast carcinoma is a useful guide in selecting patients for hormonal manipulation.[3, 37, 65, 80, 220, 221, 228] Breast cancer patients whose tumors are rich in estrogen and progesterone receptors have a better prognosis and are more responsive to hormonal administration than those with no receptors or with low levels. The presence of receptor proteins indicates a retention of the regulatory controls of the mammary epithelium. However, the estrogen receptor value by itself is insufficient as a therapeutic and prognostic guide and should be evaluated in conjunction with other parameters, including age of the patient and tumor differentiation.[139] Some studies indicate that estrogen receptor content is related to tumor differentiation.[37, 228] Tumors with high labeling indices with rapid rates of cellular replication are less frequently positive for estrogen receptors. Well-differentiated carcinomas are more frequently receptor positive than are poorly differentiated tumors. In one study, 71 per cent of 45 Grade I carcinomas and 36 per cent of 127 Grade III tumors were estrogen receptor positive. This relation is not apparent in tumors of special type, such as mucoid, tubular, and intraductal carcinomas. An inverse relationship exists between lymphocytic infiltration of tumors and the level of estrogen receptors.[36] It has been suggested that the lymphocytic infiltration can interfere with the measurement of estrogen receptor.[184] Several other factors can interfere with accurate determination of estrogen receptors, including faulty assay methodology, impairment of receptor mechanisms, interference from indigenous estrogens, and estrogen receptor heterogeneity of the tumor.[228] Appropriate selection of the tissue sample and an estimate of the proportion of tumor present can avoid spurious results.[217] Direct tissue determination of estrogen receptor using immunoperoxidase techniques is a promising development. They can be applied to specimens too small for biochemical assay, to cytologic preparations, and to fixed tissues.[69a]

Multicentric and Multifocal Carcinoma

The designations "multicentric" and "multifocal" when applied to malignant tumors of the breast commonly are used interchangeably; however, not only semantic distinctions but also biologic differences and therapeutic implications occur between the two. According to Fisher and colleagues, multicentric carcinomas are "foci of cancer in quadrants remote from dominant mass," whereas multifocal carcinoma is "cancer in the vicinity of or within the same quadrant."[68] The increasing use of breast conserving surgery, lumpectomy, sector mastectomy, quadrantectomy, tylectomy, and other operations prompted the publication of studies trying to demonstrate the ineffectiveness of such therapy.[182, 196, 229] Up to 55 per cent of mastectomy specimens contained residual carcinoma after biopsy of the tumor. Although they were dependent on the dimensions of the tumor even in tumors less than 2 cm in diameter, malignant changes were identified in up to 40 per cent of the specimens.[230] The majority of these lesions (up to 90 per cent), however, are in situ tumors. One study found that, hypothetically, lumpectomy alone for operable tumors no larger than 2 cm in diameter, of peripheral location, and without palpable lymph nodes or Paget's disease would have left cancer in 48 per cent of the patients.[230] In many studies it is not clear if the residual carcinoma was in the area of the previous incisional or excisional biopsy or in a distant quadrant. Tumors of the breast that are undeniably multifocal and multicentric do exist, however, and their pattern of growth can be diffuse.

Holland and coworkers,[102] in a careful study using specimen radiography, correlated the expected rate of tumor recurrence with the amount of tissue removed around the neoplasm and its size. The issue of multifocality and multicentricity is not completely settled.

Miscellaneous Factors

The assessment of host response to tumor has also been used as a prognostic indicator. However, the data are inconclusive and controversy still exists. Black and colleagues[21] postulated that there is an interdependence between the host response to tumor manifested by local tumor lymphocytic infiltration, sinus histiocytosis of the axillary lymph nodes, and the aggressiveness of the tumor judged by nuclear grade. Tsakralides and associates,[212] in a retrospective study of 186 cases with an average survival of 58 per cent at 10 years, was able to distinguish four different types of morphologic reactions in the regional lymph nodes that demonstrated prognostic value. The surviving patients were in the following categories: lymphocytic predominance, 75 per cent; germinal center predominance, 54 per cent; lymphocyte depletion, 33 per cent; and unstimulated, 39 per cent. Fisher and colleagues,[67] in an analysis of influential prognostic factors operative 10 years after mastectomy, found germinal center predominance to exert an adverse influence on disease-free survival in patients with negative lymph nodes. Lymphocytic predominance is a T cell proliferation, whereas germinal center predominance pattern is a B cell humoral antibody response; the unstimulated pattern expressed absent or weak antigens.

The study of biologic markers using immunohistochemical methods in breast carcinoma has demonstrated heterogeneity. Walker[220] identified five antigens: alpha-lactalbumin, secretory immunoglobulin A, alpha-human chorionic gonadotropin, beta-specific pregnancy protein, and carcinoembryonic antigen. Some tumor cells contain more than one antigen. Carcinomas with three or more antigens were predominantly present in well or moderately differentiated tumors. Because of lack of uniform methods, variability of antibody specificity, and unpredictability of cellular differentiation in neoplasia, antigen tumor determination is not at the present a reliable histopathologic tool.[226] Still, it represents a promising area to explore.

Fibrosis or desmoplasia in tumors (e.g., scirrhous carcinoma) has been considered a sign of poor prognosis. However, this has not been proved.

Focal elastosis has been reputed to indicate slower growth of tumor and to be associated with a higher rate of survival, but evidence has so far been disappointing or inconclusive.[231]

Summary

The identification and clinical application of pathologic parameters of prognostic value is the desire of the surgical pathologist. Consequently, the validity of the information obtained from the study of specimens must include pathologic factors that truly reflect the biologic properties of the tumor. The pathologist, as well as the surgeon, radiotherapist, and clinical oncologist, must continuously collect, measure, and evaluate characteristics of tumors that may influence their behavior, and then select the most appropriate method of treatment. However, the heterogeneity of biologic characteristics, the diversity of morphologic composition, and the numerous operating variables do not permit simplification. Multiple factors influence the prognosis of invasive mammary carcinomas. Despite increased information on tumor behavior, collection of data about tumor properties not previously obtainable, and newer treatment techniques, a few time-tested factors remain of prognostic importance. The most influential are the status of the axillary nodes, including the number of metastases, their size, and pattern of growth; primary tumor size; the type of tumor; and the degree of differentiation. These have remained good prognostic indices in long-term follow-up. Many other factors are important, but the extent of their influence is uncertain when judged independently.

REFERENCES

1. Aboumrad, M. H., Horn, R. C., and Fine, G.: Lipid secreting mammary carcinoma. Cancer, 16:521, 1963.
2. Akhtar, M. A., Robinson, C., Ali, M. A., et al.: Secretory carcinoma of the breast in adults. Light and electron microscopic study of three cases with review of the literature. Cancer, 51:2245, 1983.
3. Alanko, A., Heinonen, E., Schenin, T., et al: Significance of estrogen and progesterone receptors, disease-free interval and site of first metastasis on survival of breast cancer patients. Cancer, 56:1696, 1985.
4. Alderson, M. R., Hamlin, I., and Staunton, M. D.: The relative significance of prognostic factors in breast cancer. Br. J. Cancer, 25:646, 1971.
5. Allenby, P. A., and Chowdhury, L. N.: Histiocytic appearance of metastatic lobular breast carcinoma. Arch. Pathol. Lab. Med., 110:759, 1986.
6. Andersen J. A.: Lobular carcinoma in situ. A long-term follow-up in 52 cases. Acta Pathol. Microbiol. Scand. (A), 82:519, 1974.
7. Andersen, J. A., Fechner, R. C., Lattes, R., et al.: Lobular carcinoma in situ (lobular neoplasia) of the breast (a Symposium). In Summers, S. G., and Rosen, P. P. (Eds.): Pathology Annual, Part I. New York, Appleton-Century-Crofts, 1980, p. 193.
8. Andersen, J. A.: Lobular carcinoma in situ of the breast. Cancer 39:2597, 1977.
9. Andersen, J. A., Fishermann, K., Hou-Jensen, K., et al.: Selection of high-risk groups among prognostically favorable patients with breast cancer: An analysis of the value of prospective grading of tumor anaplasia in 1,048 patients. Ann. Surg., 194:1, 1981.
10. Ashikari, R., Hajdu, S. I., and Robbins, G. F.: Intraductal carcinoma of the breast (1960–1969). Cancer, 28:1182, 1971.
11. Ashikari, R., Park, K., Huvos, A. G., et al.: Paget's disease of the breast. Cancer, 26:680, 1975.
12. Azzopardi, J. G.: Benign and malignant proliferative lesions of the breast: A review. Eur. J. Cancer Clin. Oncol., 19:1717, 1983.
13. Azzopardi, J. G.: Problems in breast pathology. In Bennington, T. L. (Ed.): Major Problems in Pathology. Vol. 2. Philadelphia, W. B. Saunders, 1979.
14. Bauer, T. W., Rostock, R. A., Eggleston, J. C., et al.: Spindle cell carcinoma of the breast: Four cases and review of the literature. Hum. Pathol., 15:147, 1984.
15. Bedwani, R., Vana, J., Rosner, D., et al.: Management and survival of female patients with minimal breast cancer: As observed in the long-term and short-term surveys of the American College of Surgeons. Cancer, 54:3002, 1984.
16. Benish, B., Peison, B., Newman, R., et al.: Solid glycogen-rich, clear cell carcinoma of the breast: A light and ultrastructural study. Am. J. Clin. Pathol., 79:243, 1983.
17. Berg, J.: Morphological evidence for immune response to breast cancer. A historical review. Cancer, 28:1453, 1971.
18. Betsill, W. L., Rosen, P. P., Lieberman, P. H., et al: Intraductal carcinoma: Long-term follow-up after treatment by biopsy alone. Cancer, 239:1863, 1978.
19. Bettelheim, R., Penman, H. G., Thornton-Jones, H., et al: Prognostic significance of peritumoral vascular invasion in breast cancer. Br. J. Cancer, 50:771, 1984.
20. Bilek, R., Moore, C., Wolloch, Y., et al: Histopathologic high risk factors influencing the prognosis of patients with early breast cancer (T1N0M0). Am. J. Surg., 151:460, 1986.
21. Black, M. M., Barclay, T. H. C., and Hankey, B. F.: Prognosis in breast cancer utilizing histological characteristics of the primary tumor. Cancer, 37:2048, 1975.
22. Black, M. M., Opler, S. R., and Speer, F. D.: Survival in breast cancer cases in relation to the structure of the primary tumor and regional lymph nodes. Surg. Gynecol. Obstet., 100:543, 1955.
23. Blamey, R. W., Davis, C. J., Elston, C. W., et al.: Prognostic factors in breast cancer: The formation of a prognostic index. Clin. Oncol., 5:227, 1979.
24. Bloom H. J. G.: Prognosis in cancer of the breast. Br. J. Cancer, 4:259, 1950.
25. Bloom, H. J. G., Richardson, W. W., and Field, J. R.: Host resistance and survival in carcinoma of the breast—a study of 104 cases of medullary carcinoma in a series of 1,411 cases of breast cancer followed for 20 years. Br. Med. J., 3:181, 1970.
26. Bloom, H. J. G., and Richardson, W. W.: Histological grading and prognosis in breast cancer. Br. J. Cancer, 11:359, 1957.
27. Bloom, H. J. G.: The role of histology in the treatment of breast cancer. Br. J. Radiol., 29:488, 1956.
28. Bogomoletz, W. V.: Pure squamous cell carcinoma. Arch. Pathol. Lab. Med., 106:57, 1982.
29. Capella, C., Eusebi, V., Mann, B., et al.: Endocrine differentiation and mucoid carcinoma of the breast. Histopathology, 4:613, 1980.

30. Carstens, P. H. B., Huvos, A. G., Foote, F. W., et al.: Tubular carcinoma of the breast. Am. J. Clin. Pathol., 58:231, 1972.
31. Carstens, P. H. B.: Tubular carcinoma of the breast. A study of frequency. Am. J. Clin. Pathol., 70:204, 1978.
32. Carter, D., Orr, S. L., and Merino, M. J.: Intracystic papillary carcinoma of the breast after mastectomy, radiotherapy or excisional biopsy alone. Cancer, 52:14, 1983.
33. Carter, D., Pipkin, R. B., Shepard, R. H., et al.: Relationship of necrosis and tumor border to lymph node metastasis and ten year survival in carcinoma of the breast. Am. J. Surg. Pathol., 2:39, 1978.
34. Carter, D., and Smith, R. R. L.: Carcinoma in situ of the breast. Cancer, 40:1189, 1977.
35. Cavanzo, F. J., and Taylor, H. B.: Adenocystic carcinoma of the breast. Cancer, 24:740, 1969.
36. Chabon, A. B., Goldberg, J. D., and Venet, L.: Carcinoma of the breast: Inter-relationships among histopathologic features estrogen receptor activities, and age of the patient. Hum. Pathol., 16:368, 1982.
37. Chua, D. Y. F., Pang, M. W. Y., Rauff, A., et al.: Correlation of esteroid receptors with histologic differentiation in mammary carcinoma: A Singapore experience. Cancer, 56:2228, 1985.
38. Clayton, F., Sibley, K. R., Ordonez, N. G., et al: Argyrophilic breast carcinomas: Evidence for lactational differentiation. Am. J. Surg. Pathol., 6:323, 1982.
39. Close, M. B., and Mazimow, N. G.: Carcinoma of the breast in young girls. Arch. Surg., 91:386, 1965.
40. Coombes, R. C., Estay, G. C., Detre, S. I., et al: Secretion of immuno reactive calcitonin by human breast carcinomas. Br. Med. J., 4:197, 1975.
40a. Cooper, H. S., Patchefsky, A. S., and Krall, R. A.: Tubular carcinoma of the breast. Cancer, 42:233, 1978.
41. Cornog, J. L., Mobini, J., Steiger, E., et al.: Squamous carcinoma of the breast. Am. J. Clin. Pathol., 55:410, 1971.
42. Crichlow, R. W., and Czernobilsky, B.: Paget's disease of the male breast. Cancer, 24:1033, 1969.
43. Cubilla, A. L., and Woodruff, J. M.: Primary carcinoid tumor of the breast: A report of eight patients. Am. J. Surg. Pathol., 1:283, 1977.
44. Cutler, S. J., Black, M. M., Friedell, G. H., et al.: Prognostic factors in carcinoma of the female breast. II. Reproducibility of histopathological classification. Cancer, 19:75, 1966.
45. Czernobilsky, B.: Intracystic carcinoma of the female breast. Surg. Gynecol. Obstet., 124:93, 1967.
46. Dawson, P. J., Ferguson, D. J., and Karrison, I.: The pathologic findings of breast cancer in patients surviving 25 years after radical mastectomy. Cancer, 50:2131, 1982.
47. Dennis, F. S.: Recurrence of carcinoma of the breast. Trans. Am. Surg. Assoc., 9:219, 1891.
48. Deos, P. H., and Norris, H. J.: Well-differentiated (tubular) carcinoma of the breast: A clinical pathological study of 145 pure and mixed cases. Am. J. Clin. Pathol., 78:1, 1982.
49. Dixon, J. M., Andersen, T. J., Elton, R. A., et al.: Prognosis in breast cancer. Br. J. Surg., 71:393, 1984.
50. Dixon, J. M., Andersen, T. J., Page, D. L., et al.: Infiltrating lobular carcinoma of the breast. Histopathology, 6:149, 1982.
51. Dixon, J. M., Page, D. L., Andersen, T. J., et al.: Long term survivors after breast cancer. Br. J. Surg., 72:445, 1985.
52. Dockerty, M. V.: The grading and typing of carcinoma of the breast. J. Iowa Med. Soc., 54:289, 1964.
53. Donegan, W. L., and Perez-Mesa, C. M.: Lobular carcinoma; an indicator for elective biopsy of the second breast. Am. Surg., 176:178, 1972.
53a. Egan, R. L., Ellis, J. T., and Powell, R. W.: Team approach to the study of diseases of the breast. Cancer, 23:847, 1969.
54. Ellis, D. L., and Teitelbaum, S. L.: Inflammatory carcinoma of the breast. A pathologic definition. Cancer, 33:1045, 1974.
55. Fechner, R. E.: Histologic variant of infiltrating lobular carcinoma of the breast. Hum. Pathol., 6:373, 1975.
56. Fetissof, F., DuBois, M. P., Arbelle-Brassart, B., et al: Argyrophilic cells in mammary carcinoma. Hum. Pathol., 14:127, 1983.
57. Fisher, B.: Reappraisal of breast biopsy prompted by the use of lumpectomy. JAMA, 253:3585, 1985.
58. Fisher, B., Slack, N. H., Bross, I. D. J., et al.: Carcinoma of the breast: Size of neoplasm and prognosis. Cancer, 24:1071, 1969.
59. Fisher, E. R., and Brown, R.: Intraductal signet ring cell carcinoma: hitherto undescribed form. Cancer, 55:2533, 1985.
60. Fisher, E. R., Gregorio, R. M., Fisher, B., et al.: The pathology of invasive breast cancer: A syllabus derived from findings of the National Surgical Adjuvant Breast Project (Protocol No. 4). Cancer, 36:1, 1975.
61. Fisher, E. R., Gregorio, R. M., Palekar, A. S., et al.: Mucoepidermoid and squamous cell carcinoma of breasts with reference to squamous metaplasia and giant cell tumor. Am. J. Surg. Pathol., 7:15, 1983.
62. Fisher, E. R., Gregorio, R. M., Redmond, C., et al.: Tubulolobular invasive breast carcinoma: A variant of lobular invasive carcinoma. Hum. Pathol., 8:679, 1977.
63. Fisher, E. R., Palekar, A. S., Edmon, C., et al.: Pathologic findings from the National Surgical Adjuvant Breast Project (Protocol No. 4). VI. Invasive papillary cancer. Am. J. Clin. Pathol., 73:313, 1980.
64. Fisher, E. R., Palekar, A. S., and NASBP collaborators: Solid and mucinous varieties of so-called mammary carcinoid tumors. Am. J. Clin. Pathol., 72:209, 1979.
65. Fisher, E. R., Redmond, C. K., Liu, H., et al.: Correlation of estrogen receptor and pathologic characteristics of invasive breast cancer. Cancer, 45:349, 1980.
66. Fisher, E. R., Redmond, C., and Fisher, B.: Histologic grading of breast cancer. In Summers, S. G., and Rosen, P. P. (Eds.): Pathology Annual, Part I. New York, Appleton-Century-Crofts, 1980, p. 239.
67. Fisher, E. R., Sass, R., Fisher, B., et al.: Pathologic findings from National Surgical Adjuvant Project for Breast Cancers (Protocol No. 4). X. Discriminants for tenth year treatment failure. Cancer, 53:712, 1984.
68. Fisher, E. R., Sass, R., Fisher, B., et al.: Pathologic findings from National Surgical Adjuvant Project for Breast Cancers (Protocol No. 6). I. Intraductal carcinoma (DCIS). Cancer, 57:197, 1986.
69. Flores, L., Arlen, M., Elguezabal, A., et al: Host-tumor relationships in medullary carcinoma of the breast. Surg. Gynecol. Obstet., 139:683, 1974.
69a. Flowers, J. L., Burton, G. V., Cos, E. B., et al.: Use of monoclonal antiestrogen receptor antibody to evaluate estrogen receptor content in fine needle

aspiration breast biopsies. Ann. Surg., *203*:250, 1986.
70. Foote, F. W., and Stewart, F. W.: Lobular carcinoma in situ. Am. J. Pathol., *17*:491, 1941.
71. Foote, F. W., and Stewart, F. W.: A histologic classification of carcinoma of the breast. Surgery, *19*:74, 1946.
72. Frable, W. J., and Kay, S.: Carcinoma of the breast: Histologic and clinical features of apocrine tumors. Cancer, *2*:756, 1968.
73. Fracchia, A. A., Rosen, P. P., and Ashikari, R.: Primary carcinoma of the breast without axillary lymph node metastasis. Surg. Gynecol. Obstet., *151*:375, 1980.
74. Fraser, J.: A study of malignant breast by whole section and key block section methods. Surg. Gynecol. Obstet., *45*:266, 1927.
75. Fridell, G. H., Goldenberg, I. S., Masnyk, R. J., et al.: Identification of breast cancer patients at high risk of early recurrence after radical mastectomy: Description of study. JNCI, *53*:603, 1974.
76. Gad, A., and Azzopardi, J. G.: Lobular carcinoma of the breast. A special variant of mucin-secreting carcinoma. J. Clin. Pathol., *28*:711, 1975.
77. Gallagher, H. S., and Martin, J. E.: Early phases in the development in breast cancer. Cancer, *24*:1170, 1969.
78. Gallagher, H. S.: Minimal breast cancer, concepts and results of treatment. Clin. Oncol., *1*:389, 1982.
79. Gallagher, H. S.: Pathologic types of breast cancer; their prognosis. Cancer, *53*:623, 1984.
80. Gapiniski, P. V., and Donegan, W. L.: Estrogen receptor and breast cancer. Prognostic and therapeutic implications. Surgery, *88*:386, 1980.
81. Gatchell, F. G., Dockerty, M. B., and Clagett, O. T.: Intracystic carcinoma of the breast. Surg. Gynecol. Obstet., *106*:347, 1958.
82. Gersell, D. J., and Katzenstein, A.-L.: Spindle cell carcinoma of the breast: A clinicopathologic and ultrastructural study. Hum. Pathol., *12*:550, 1980.
83. Geschickter, C. F.: Diseases of the Breast: Diagnosis, Pathology and Treatment. 2nd Ed. Philadelphia, J. B. Lippincott, 1945, p. 565.
84. Geschickter, C. F.: Gelatinous mammary carcinoma. Ann. Surg., *108*:321, 1938.
85. Gilchrist, K. W., Gould, V. E., Hirshl, S., et al.: Intraobserver variation in the identification of breast carcinoma and intra-mammary lymphatics. Hum. Pathol., *13*:170, 1982.
86. Gillis, D. A., Dockerty, M. B., and Clagett, O. T.: Preinvasive intraductal carcinoma of the breast. Surg. Gynecol. Obstet., *110*:555, 1960.
87. Giordano, J. M., and Klopp, C. T.: Lobular carcinoma in situ: Incidence and treatment. Cancer, *31*:105, 1973.
88. Gold, R. H., Main, G., Zippin, C., et al.: Infiltration of mammary carcinoma as an indicator of axillary metastasis: A preliminary report. Cancer, *29*:35, 1972.
89. Goldman, R. L., and Friedman, N. B.: Carcinoma of the breast arising in fibroadenomas with emphasis on lobular carcinoma. Cancer, *23*:544, 1969.
90. Golinger, R. C., Gregorio, R., and Fisher, E. R.: Tumor cells in venous blood draining mammary carcinoma. Arch. Surg., *112*:707, 1977.
91. Greenough, R. B.: Varying degrees of malignancy in carcinoma of the breast. J. Cancer Res., *9*:453, 1925.
92. Gresham, G. A.: Grading of mammary carcinoma. Clin. Oncol., *2*:351, 1976.
93. Haagensen, C. D.: Diseases of the Breast. 2nd Ed. Philadelphia, W. B. Saunders, 1971.
94. Haagensen, C. D., Lane, N., Lattes, R., et al.: Lobular neoplasia (so-called lobular carcinoma in situ) of the breast. Cancer, *42*:737, 1978.
95. Haagensen, C. D., Lane, N., and Lattes, R.: Neoplastic proliferation of the epithelium of the mammary lobules. Adenosis, lobular, neoplasia, and small cell carcinoma. Surg. Clin. North Am., *52*:497, 1972.
95a. Halsted, W. S.: A diagnostic sign of gelatinous carcinoma of the breast. J.A.M.A., *64*:1653, 1915.
96. Hamlin, I. M. E.: Possible host resistance in carcinoma of the breast. A histological study. Br. J. Cancer, *22*:383, 1968.
97. Harris, M., Howell, A., Chrisshou, M., et al: A comparison of the metastatic pattern of infiltrating lobular carcinoma and infiltrating duct carcinoma of the breast. Br. J. Cancer, *50*:23, 1984.
98. Harris, M., Wells, S., and Vasudev, K. S.: Primary signet ring cell carcinoma of the breast. Histopathology, *2*:171, 1978.
99. Hartmann, W. H.: Minimal breast cancer: an update. Cancer, *53*:681, 1984.
100. Hazelrigg, D. E., and Rudolph, A. H.: Inflammatory metastatic carcinoma, carcinoma Erysipelatoides. Arch. Dermatol., *11*:69, 1977.
101. Histological Typing of Breast Tumors: International Histologic Classification of Tumors II. Geneva, World Health Organization, 1968.
102. Holland, R., Veling, S. H. J., Mravunac, M., et al.: Histologic multifocality of Tis, T1–2 breast carcinomas. Implications for clinical trials of breast-conserving surgery. Cancer, *56*:979, 1985.
103. Hood, C. I., Font, R. L., and Zimmerman, L. E.: Metastatic mammary carcinoma in the eyelid with histiocytoid appearance. Cancer, *31*:793, 1973.
103a. Hsu, S. M., Raine, L., and Nayak, R. N.: Medullary carcinoma of breast: An immunohistochemical study of its lymphoid stroma. Cancer, *48*:1368, 1981.
104. Hull, M. T., Priest, J. B., Broadie, T. A., et al.: Glycogen-rich, clear cell carcinoma of the breast: A light and electron microscopic study. Cancer, *48*:2003, 1981.
105. Hull, M. T., Seo, I. S., Battersby, J. S., et al.: Signet ring cell carcinoma of the breast: A clinical pathological study of twenty-four cases. Am. J. Clin. Pathol., *73*:31, 1980.
106. Humphrey, L. J., Singla, O., and Volenec, F. J.: Immunologic responsiveness of the breast cancer patient. Cancer, *46*:893, 1980.
107. Hunter, C. E., Jr., and Sawyers, J. L.: Intracystic papillary carcinoma of the breast. South. Med. J., *73*:1484, 1980.
108. Hutter, R. V. P.: The influence of pathologic features on breast cancer management. Cancer, *46*:961, 1980.
109. Huvos, A. G., Hutter, R. V. P., and Berg, J. W.: Significance of axillary macrometastasis and micrometastasis in mammary carcinoma. Ann. Surg., *173*:44, 1971.
110. Ingleby, H., and Gershon-Cohen, J.: Comparative Anatomy, Pathology and Roentgenology of the Breast. Philadelphia, University of Pennsylvania Press, 1960, p. 359.
111. Editorial: Intraduct carcinoma of the breast. Lancet, *2*:24, 1984.
112. Kauffman, M. W., Marti, J. R., Gallagher, H. S., et al.: Carcinoma of the breast with pseudosarcomatous metaplasia. Cancer, *53*:1908, 1984.
113. Kenako, H., Hojo, H., Ashikawi, S., et al.: Norep-

inephrine producing tumors of bilateral breasts: A case report. Cancer, 41:2002, 1978.
114. Ketterhagen, J. P., Quackenbush, S. R., and Haushalter, R.: Tumor histology as a prognostic determinant in carcinoma of the breast. Surg. Gynecol. Obstet., 158:120, 1984.
115. Kingsley, W. B., Peters, G. N., and Cheek, J. H.: What constitutes adequate study of axillary lymph nodes in breast cancer? Ann. Surg., 201:311, 1985.
116. Koss, L. G., Brannan, C. D., and Ashikari, R.: Histologic and ultrastructural features of adenoid cystic carcinoma of the breast. Cancer, 26:1271, 1980.
117. Kraus, F. T., and Neubecker, R. V.: The differential diagnosis of papillary tumors of the breast. Cancer, 15:444, 1962.
118. Krishnan, E. U., Phillips, A. K., Randell, A., et al.: Bilateral metastatic inflammatory carcinoma in the breast from primary ovarian carcinoma. Obstet. Gynecol., 55(Suppl.):94S, 1980.
119. Kouchoukos, N. T., Ackerman, L. V., and Butcher, H. R., Jr.: Prediction of axillary nodal metastases from the morphology of primary mammary carcinomas. Guide to operative therapy. Cancer, 20:948, 1967.
119a. Lafreniere, R., Moskowitz, L. B., and Ketcham, A. S.: Pure squamous cell carcinoma of the breast. J. Surg. Oncol., 31:113, 1986.
120. Lagios, M. D., Westdahl, P. R., Margolin, F. R., et al.: Ductal carcinoma in situ; relationship of extent of noninvasive disease to the frequency of occult invasive multicentricity, lymph node metastasis and short-term treatment failures. Cancer, 50:1309, 1982.
121. Lagios, M. D., Westdahl, P. R., Rose, M. R., et al.: Paget's disease of the nipple. Alternative management in cases without or without minimal extent of underlying breast cancer. Cancer, 54:545, 1984.
122. Lane, N., Goksel, H., Salerno, R. A., et al.: Clinical pathologic analysis of surgical curability of breast cancers: A minimum ten year study of a personal series. Ann. Surg., 153:483, 1961.
123. Lawrence, J. V., and Mazur, M. T.: Adenoid cystic carcinoma. A comparative pathologic study of tumors in salivary gland, breast, lungs and cervix. Hum. Pathol., 13:916, 1982.
124. Leis, H. P., Cammarata, A., and LaRaja, R. D.: Update and potentially curable breast cancer therapy. Contemp. Surg., 36:1, 1985.
125. Lucas, F. B., and Perez-Mesa, C. M.: Inflammatory carcinoma of the breast. Cancer, 41:1595, 1978.
126. Martinez, V., and Azzopardi, J. G.: Invasive lobular carcinoma of the breast: Incidence and variance. Histopathology, 3:467, 1979.
127. Masse, S. R., Rioux, A., and Beauchesoe, C.: Juvenile carcinoma of the breast. Hum. Pathol., 12:1044, 1981.
128. Mavligit, G. M., Cohen, T. L., and Sherwood, L. M.: Ectopic production of parathyroid hormone by carcinoma of the breast. N. Engl. J. Med., 285:154, 1971.
129. McDivitt, R. W., Boyce, W., and Gersell, D.: Tubular carcinoma of the breast: Clinical and pathological observations concerning 135 cases. Am. J. Surg. Pathol., 6:401, 1982.
130. McDivitt, R. W.: Breast cancer. Hum. Pathol., 9:3, 1978.
131. McDivitt, R. W., Hutter, R. V. P., Foote, F. W., Jr., et al.: In situ and lobular carcinoma: A prospective followup study indicating correlative patient risk. J.A.M.A., 201:82, 1967.
132. McDivitt, R. W., Stewart, F. W., and Berg, J. W.: Tumors of the Breast: An Atlas of Tumor Pathology. Series 2. Fascicle 2. Washington, D.C., Armed Forces Institute of Pathology, 1968.
133. McDivitt, R. W., and Stewart, F. W.: Breast carcinoma in children. J.A.M.A., 195:388, 1966.
134. McDivitt, R. W., Stone, K. R., Craig, R. B., et al.: A proposed classification of breast cancer based on kinetic information. Cancer, 57:269, 1986.
135. McGuire, W. L., Carbone, P. P., Sears, M. E., et al.: Estrogen receptors in human breast cancer; an overview. In McGuire, W. L., Carbone, P. P., Vollmer, E. P. (Eds.): Estrogen Receptors in Human Breast Cancer. New York, Raven Press, 1975, p. 1.
136. McKittrick, J. E., Doane, W. A., and Failing, R. M.: Intracystic papillary carcinoma of the breast. Am. Surg., 55:195, 1969.
137. Melamed, M. R., Robbins, G. F., and Foote, F. W.: Prognostic significance of gelatinous mammary carcinoma. Cancer, 14:699, 1961.
138. Merino, M., and LiVolsi, V. A.: Signet ring carcinoma of the female breast: A clinicopathologic analysis of twenty-four cases. Cancer, 48:1830, 1981.
139. Mills, R. R.: Correlation of hormone receptors with pathological features in human breast cancer. Cancer, 46:2869, 1980.
140. Mills, R. R., and Thyne, G. S. J.: In situ intraduct carcinoma of the breast: A long-term follow-up study. Br. J. Surg., 62:957, 1975.
141. Moore, O. S., and Foote, F. W., Jr.: The relatively favorable prognosis of medullary carcinoma of the breast. Cancer, 2:635, 1949.
142. Morrow, M., and Foster, R. S.: Staging of breast carcinoma: A new rationale for internal mammary node biopsy. Arch. Surg., 116:748, 1981.
143. Mossler, J. A., Barton, T. K., Brinkhaus, K. S., et al.: Apocrine differentiation in human mammary carcinoma. Cancer, 46:2463, 1980.
144. Muir, R.: The evolution of carcinoma in the mamma. J. Pathol. Bacteriol., 52:155, 1941.
145. Murad, T. M., Contesso, G., and Mourisse, H.: Papillary tumors of large lactiferous ducts. Cancer, 48:122, 1981.
146. Murad, T. M., Swaid, S., and Pritchett, P.: Malignant and benign papillary lesions of the breast. Hum. Pathol., 8:379, 1977.
147. Nadji, M., Morales, A. R., Girtanner, R. E., et al.: Paget's disease of the skin. A unifying concept of histogenesis. Cancer, 50:2203, 1982.
148. Nealon, T. F., Nkongho, A., Grossi, C. E., et al.: Treatment of early carcinoma of the breast (T1N0M0) on the basis of histological characteristics. Surgery, 89:279, 1981.
149. Nehme, A. E.: Paget's disease of the male breast: A collective review and case report. Am. Surg., 42:289, 1976.
150. Nemoto, T., Vana, J., Bedwani, R. N., et al.: Management and survival of female breast cancer. Results of a National Survey by the American College of Surgeons. Cancer, 45:2917, 1980.
151. Nime, F. A., Rosen, P. P., Thaler, H. T., et al.: Prognostic significance of tumor emboli in intramammary lymphatics in patients with mammary carcinoma. Am. J. Surg. Pathol., 1:25, 1977.
152. Norris, H. J., and Austin, A. M.: Overview of prognostic factors in mammary carcinoma. Breast, 11:9, 1985.
153. Norris, H. J., and Taylor, H. B.: Prognosis of mucinous (gelatinous) carcinoma of the breast. Cancer, 18:879, 1965.

154. Oberman, H. A., and Fidler, W. J.: Tubular carcinoma of the breast. Am. J. Surg. Pathol., *3*:387, 1979.
155. Oberman, H. A.: Secretory carcinoma of the breast in adults. Am. J. Surg. Pathol., *4*:465, 1980.
156. Oberman, H. A., and Stephens, P. J.: Carcinoma of the breast in childhood. Cancer, *30*:470, 1972.
157. Ozello, L., and Sampitak, P.: The epithelial-stromal junction of intraductal carcinoma of the breast. Cancer, *26*:1186, 1970.
158. Page, D. L., DuPont, W. D., Rogers, L. W., et al.: Intraductal carcinoma of the breast; follow-up after biopsy only. Cancer, *49*:751, 1982.
159. Paget, J.: On diseases of the mammary aereola preceding carcinoma of mammary gland. St. Bart. Hosp. Rep., *10*:87, 1874.
160. Paone, J. F., and Baker, R. R.: Pathogenesis and treatment of Paget's disease of the breast. Cancer, *48*:825, 1981.
161. Parel, F. F., and Richardson, L. D.: The histologic and biologic spectrum of tubular carcinoma of the breast. Hum. Pathol., *14*:694, 1983.
162. Patchefsky, A. S., Frauenhoffer, C. M., Krall, R. A., et al.: Low-grade mucoepidermoid carcinoma of the breast. Arch. Pathol. Lab. Med., *103*:196, 1979.
163. Pearse, A. G. E.: Carcinoid of the breast—fact or figment. Am. J. Surg. Pathol. *1*:303, 1977.
164. Perez-Mesa, C. M., and Blackwell, C.: Unpublished data.
165. Peters, J. W., and Wolff, M.: Adenoid cyst carcinoma of the breast. A report of eleven new cases: A review of the literature and discussion of biologic behavior. Cancer, *52*:680, 1982.
165a. Peters, G. N., Wolff, M., and Haagensen, C. D.: Tubular carcinoma of the breast. Clinical pathologic correlations based on 100 cases. Ann. Surg., *193*:138, 1981.
166. Peters, T. G., Donegan, W. L., and Berg, E. A.: Minimal breast cancer: A clinical appraisal. Ann. Surg., *186*:704, 1977.
167. Pickren, J.: Significance of occult metastasis. Cancer, *14*:1266, 1961.
168. Ramirez, G., and Ansfield, F. J.: Carcinoma of the breast in children. Arch. Surg., *96*:222, 1968.
169. Ramos, C. V., and Taylor, H. B.: Lipid rich carcinoma of the breast: A clinicopathological analysis of thirteen examples. Cancer, *33*:812, 1974.
170. Rassmussen, B. B.: Human mucinous breast cancer and their lymph node metastasis:a histologic review of 247 cases. Pathol. Res. Pract., *180*:377, 1985.
171. Rassmussen, B. B., Rose, C., Thorpe, S. M., et al.: Argyrophilic cells in 202 human mucinous breast carcinomas. Relation to histopathologic and clinical factors. Am. J. Clin. Pathol., *84*:737, 1985.
172. Report of the Working Group to Review the National Cancer Institute–American Cancer Society Breast Cancer Detection Demonstration Project. JNCI, *62*:639, 1979.
173. Richardson, W. W.: Medullary carcinoma of the breast. A distinctive tumor type with a relatively good prognosis following radical mastectomy. Br. J. Cancer, *104*:415, 1956.
174. Ridenhour, C. E., Perez-Mesa, C. M., and Hori, J. M.: Paget's disease of the nipple. Cancer Bull., *21*:15, 1969.
175. Ridolfi, R. R., Rosen, P. P., Port, A., et al.: Medullary carcinoma of the breast: A clinicopathological study with 10 year follow-up. Cancer, *40*:1365, 1977.
176. Rilke, F., Andreola, S., Carbone, A., et al.: The importance of pathology in prognosis and management of breast cancer. Semin. Oncol., *5*:360, 1978.
177. Rodes, N. D., Lopez, M. J., Pearson, D. K., et al.: The impact of breast cancer screening on survival; a 5–10 year follow-up study. Cancer, *57*:581, 1986.
178. Rosai, J.: Ackerman's Surgical Pathology. 6th Ed. St. Louis, C. V. Mosby, 1981.
179. Rosen, P. P.: Axillary lymph node metastasis in patients with occult noninvasive breast cancer. Cancer, *46*:1298, 1980.
179a. Rosen, P. P.: Coexistent lobular carcinoma in situ and intraductal carcinoma in a single lobular duct unit. Am. J. Surg. Pathol., *4*:241, 1980.
180. Rosen, P. P., Braun, D. W., Lingholm, B., et al.: Lobular carcinoma in situ of the breast: preliminary results of treatment by ipsilateral mastectomy and contralateral breast biopsy. Cancer, *47*:813, 1981.
181. Rosen, P. P., Braun, D. W., and Kinne, D. E.: The clinical significance of preinvasive breast cancer. Cancer, *46*:918, 1980.
182. Rosen, P. P., Fracchia, A. A., Eurban, J. A., et al.: Residual mammary carcinoma following simulated partial mastectomy. Cancer, *35*:739, 1975.
183. Rosen, P. P., Liberman, P. H., Braun, D. W., et al.: Lobular carcinoma in situ of breast: detailed analysis of 99 patients with average follow-up of 24 years. Am. J. Surg. Pathol., *2*:225, 1978.
184. Rosen, P. P., Menendez-Botet, C. J., Nesselbaum, J. S., et al.: Pathological review of breast lesions analyzed for estrogen receptor protein. Cancer Res., *35*:3187, 1975.
185. Rosen, P. P., Saigo, P. E., Braun, D. W., et al.: Axillary micro- and macrometastasis in breast cancer. Ann. Surg., *194*:591, 1981.
186. Rosen, P. P., Saigo, P. E., Braun, D. W., et al.: Prognosis in Stage II (T1N0M0) breast cancer. Ann. Surg., *194*:576, 1981.
187. Rosen, P. P., Saigo, P. E., Braun, D. W., Jr., et al.: Predictors of recurrence in Stage I (T1N0M0) breast cancer. Ann. Surg., *193*:15, 1981.
188. Rosen, P. P., and Wang, T.-Y.: Colloid carcinoma of the breast: Analysis of 64 patients with long-term follow-up. (Abstract). Am. J. Clin. Pathol., *73*:304, 1980.
189. Roses, D. F., Bell, D. A., Flotte, T. J.,: Pathologic predictors of recurrence in stage I (T1N0M0) breast cancer. Am. Clin. Pathol., *78*:817, 1982.
190. Rosner, D., Bedwani, R. N., Vana, J., et al.: Noninvasive breast carcinoma. Results of a national survey by the American College of Surgeons. Ann. Surg., *192*:139, 1980.
191. Saltzstein, S. L.: Clinically occult inflammatory carcinoma of the breast. Cancer, *34*:382, 1974.
192. Sampat, M. B., Sirsat, M. V., and Gangaharan, P.: Prognostic significance of blood vessel invasion in carcinoma of the breast in women. J. Surg. Oncol., *9*:623, 1977.
193. Saphir, O.: Mucinous carcinoma of the breast. Surg. Gynecol. Obstet., *72*:908, 1941.
194. Say, C. C., and Donegan, W. L.: Invasive carcinoma of the breast. Prognostic significance of tumor size and involved axillary lymph nodes. Cancer, *34*:468, 1974.
195. Scarff, R. W., and Torloni, H.: Histological typing of breast tumors. Geneva, World Health Organization, 1968 (International Histological Classifications of Tumors).
196. Schwartz, G. F., Patchefsky, A. S., Feig, S. A., et

al.: Multicentricity of nonpalpable breast cancer. Cancer, 45:2913, 1980.
197. Sheth, N. A., Suraiva, T. N., Sheth, A. R., et al.: Ectopic production of human placental lactogen by human breast tumors. Cancer, 39:1693, 1977.
198. Shimokawara, I., Imamura, M., Yamanaka, N., et al.: Identification of lymphocyte subpopulations in human breast cancer and its significance: An immunoperoxidase study with anti-human T- and B-cell sera. Cancer, 49:1456, 1982.
199. Silverberg, S. G., Chitale, A. R., and Levitt, S. H.: Prognostic significance of tumor margins in mammary carcinoma. Arch. Surg., 102:450, 1971.
200. Silverberg, S. G., Kay, S., Chitale, A. R., et al.: Colloid carcinoma of the breast. Am. J. Clin. Pathol., 55:355, 1971.
201. Smart, C. R., Myers, M. H., and Gloeckler, L. A.: Implications from SEER data on breast cancer management. Cancer, 41:787, 1978.
202. Smith, J. A., III, Gomez-Araujo, J., Gallagher, H. S., et al.: Carcinoma of the breast. Analysis of total lymph node involvement vs. level of metastasis. Cancer, 39:527, 1977.
203. Squires, J. E., and Betsill, W. L., Jr.: Intracystic carcinoma of the breast. A correlation of cytomorphology, gross pathology and clinical data. Acta Cytol., 25:267, 1981.
204. Steinbrecher, J. S., and Silverberg, S. G.: Signet ring cell carcinoma of the breast: The mucinous variant of infiltrating lobular carcinoma? Cancer, 37:828, 1976.
204a. Tavassoli, F. A., and Norris, H. J.: Secretory carcinoma of the breast. Cancer, 45:2404, 1980.
205. Taylor, G., and Meltzer, A.: Inflammatory carcinoma of the breast. Am. J. Cancer, 33:33, 1938.
206. Taylor, H. B., and Norris, H. J.: Well-differentiated carcinoma of the breast. Cancer, 25:687, 1970.
207. The World Health Organization Histological Typing of Breast Tumors–second edition. Am. J. Clin. Pathol., 78:806, 1982.
208. Nealon, T. F., Jr., Nkonghu, A., Grassi, C., et al.: Pathological identification of poor prognosis stage I (T1N0M0) cancer of the breast. Ann. Surg., 190:129, 1979.
209. Tobon, H., and Salazar, H.: Tubular carcinoma of the breast: Clinical, histological and ultrastructural observations. Arch. Pathol. Lab. Med., 101:310, 1977.
209a. Toikkanen, S.: Primary squamous cell carcinoma of the breast. Cancer, 48:1629, 1981.
210. Toker, C.: Clear cells of the nipple epidermis. Cancer, 25:601, 1970.
211. Tough, I. C. K., Carter, D. Z., Fraser, J., et al.: Histological grading in breast cancer. Br. J. Cancer, 23:294, 1969.
212. Tsakralides, V., Olson, P., Kersey, J. H., et al.: Prognostic significance of the regional lymph node histology in cancer of the breast. Cancer, 34:1259, 1974.
213. Tschen, E. H., and Apisarnthanarax, P.: Inflammatory metastatic carcinoma of the breast. Arch. Dermatol., 117:120, 1981.
214. van Bogaert, L. J.: Clinicopathological hallmark of mammary tubular carcinoma. Hum. Pathol., 13:558, 1981.
215. van Bogaert, L. J., and Maldague, P.: Histological classification of pure primary epithelial breast cancer. Hum. Pathol., 9:175, 1978.
216. van Bogaert, L. J., and Maldague, P.: Infiltrating lobular carcinoma of the female breast: deviations from the usual appearance. Cancer, 45:979, 1980.
217. van Netten, H. P., Algard, F. T., Coy, P., et al.: Estrogen receptor assay on breast cancer microsamples: Implications of percent carcinoma estimation. Cancer, 49:2383, 1982.
218. von Hansemann, D. P.: Histologic grading of carcinoma of the breast. Cited in Haagensen, C. D.: Diseases of the Breast. 2nd Ed. Philadelphia, W. B. Saunders, 1971.
219. Wade, P. M., Mills, S. E., Read, M., et al.: Small cell neuroendocrine (oat cell) carcinoma of the breast. Cancer, 52:121, 1983.
220. Walker, R. A.: Biological markers in human breast carcinoma. J. Pathol., 137:109, 1982.
221. Walmark, N.: Minimal breast cancer, advance or anachronism. Can. J. Surg., 28:252, 1985.
222. Warner, N. E.: Lobular carcinoma of the breast. Cancer, 23:840, 1969.
223. Weigand, R. A., Isenberg, W. M., Russo, J., et al.: Blood vessel invasion and axillary lymph node involvement as prognostic indicators for human breast cancer. Cancer, 50:962, 1982.
224. Wellings, S. R., Jensen, H. M., and Marcum, R. G.: An atlas of subgross pathology of the human breast with reference to possible precancerous lesions. JNCI, 55:231, 1975.
225. Wheeler, J. E., Enterline, H. T., Roseman, J. M., et al.: Lobular carcinoma in situ of the breast. Cancer, 34:554, 1974.
226. Wick, M. R.: Immunochemical markers of benignancy and malignancy. Arch. Pathol. Lab. Med., 110:180, 1986.
227. Willis, R. A.: Pathology of Tumors. 4th Ed. London, Butterworths, 1967, p. 237.
228. Withliff, J.: Steroid-hormone receptors in breast cancer. Cancer, 53:630, 1983.
229. Morganstern, L., Kaufman, P. A., and Friedman, N. B.: The case against thylectomy for carcinoma of the breast. The factor of multicentricity. Am. J. Surg., 130:251, 1975.
230. Pickren, J. W., Satchidanand, Y. K., Lane, W. W., et al.: Lumpectomy for mammary carcinoma. A retrospective analysis of 40 presumptive candidates from a surgical series. Cancer, 54:1692, 1984.
231. Humeniuk, V., Forrest, A. P. M., Hawkins, R. A., et al.: Elastosis in primary breast cancer. Cancer, 52:1448, 1983.

CHAPTER 9

JOHN STRAUCH MEYER

Cell Kinetics of Breast and Breast Tumors

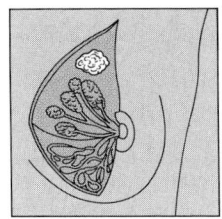

This chapter consists of three parts. The first part, *Overview of Cell Kinetics,* is intended for readers who are not conversant with the terminology and theory of cell kinetics and flow cytometry and for those who desire a review of these topics. The second section, *Cell Kinetics of Normal Breast and Benign Epithelial Hyperplasias,* provides a background against which the altered kinetics of cancers can be appreciated. The third section, *Cell Kinetic and DNA Flow Cytometric Measurements in Breast Carcinoma,* is a review of kinetic and DNA flow cytometric data with a discussion of their clinical applicability.

Overview of Cell Kinetics

MITOTIC COUNTS

Initially, the counting of mitotic cells was the only approach to cell kinetic analysis. Mitotic counts are well established for prognosis of mesenchymal tumors (Stout, 1948; Russell et al., 1977), including cytosarcomas of the breast (Norris and Taylor, 1967). Occasional reports have associated high mitotic indices with poor survival in breast carcinomas (Bloom and Richardson, 1957; Wallgren et al., 1976; Parl and Dumont, 1982). However, mitotic counts have not achieved widespread usage in epithelial tumors of the breast. The reasons are the relative scarcity of mitoses in breast carcinomas coupled with the variable admixture of stroma with epithelium in the carcinomas, which makes estimation by counts per high power field relatively meaningless. Furthermore, the discrimination of mitoses from pyknoses, karyorrhexis, and other nuclear artifacts in carcinomas with necrosis is difficult.

RADIOLABELING OF DNA AND THE CELL CYCLE

The advent of radioactive labeling of DNA provided a practical means for assessing cellular proliferation that is particularly useful in epithelial tumors (Figs. 9–1 and 9–2). The first attempts to label cells during DNA synthesis (S phase) employed radioactive phosphorus (Howard and Pelc, 1951) or carbon-14 labeled formate (Lajtha, 1957). Both of these labels were nonspecific but were preferentially incorporated into the DNA of S-phase cells (Lajtha, 1957). Thymidine labeled with tritium on the methyl group, introduced by Taylor and coworkers (1957), is a specific label for DNA because thymidine is incorporated only into DNA, and the methyl group evidently is not transferred to other pyrimidine bases. It soon was evident that all replicating cells engage in DNA synthesis during a discrete period of the interval between mitoses. The S phase is separated from mitosis by two intervals, G_1 and G_2. G_1 is relatively long and follows immediately after mitosis and ends at the beginning of the S phase. G_2 is relatively short (usually 2 to 4 hours) and separates the S phase from mitosis (M). (These two intervals in apparent activity were seen as gaps, hence the abbreviations G_1 and G_2.) The entire period between mitoses is termed the "cell cycle" (Fig. 9–3).

MEASUREMENT OF DURATION OF CELL CYCLE AND ITS SEGMENTS

Several methods for measuring cell cycle segment transit times (durations for G_1, S, G_2 and

250

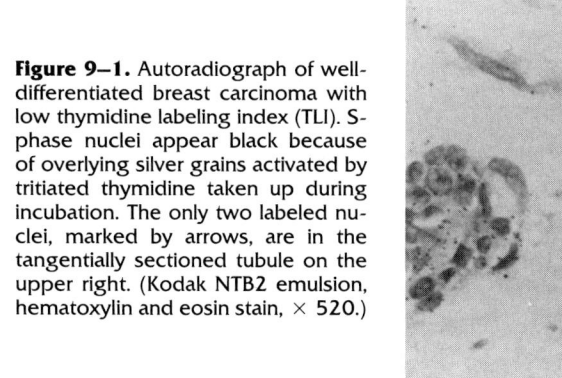

Figure 9–1. Autoradiograph of well-differentiated breast carcinoma with low thymidine labeling index (TLI). S-phase nuclei appear black because of overlying silver grains activated by tritiated thymidine taken up during incubation. The only two labeled nuclei, marked by arrows, are in the tangentially sectioned tubule on the upper right. (Kodak NTB2 emulsion, hematoxylin and eosin stain, × 520.)

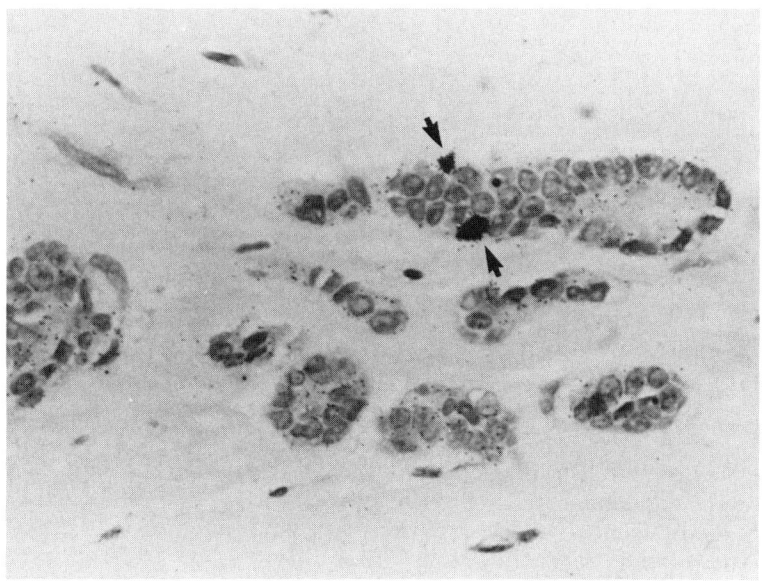

M) have been developed and are thoroughly reviewed by Steel (1977). In general, these methods are not practical for routine clinical application because they require administering radioactive DNA precursors or mitosis-arresting agents (colchicine, vinca alkaloids) to patients and performing serial biopsies. Quastler and Sherman (1959) developed the classic fraction of labeled mitoses (FLM) method. A single injection of tritiated thymidine is administered and biopsies are taken at regular intervals for several days to plot the percentage of labeled mitoses (Fig. 9–4). From these data the duration of the cell cycle and its segments can be deduced (Mendelsohn and Takahashi, 1971; Steel, 1977).

KINETIC AND MICROENVIRONMENTAL HETEROGENEITY

Populations of neoplastic cells invariably show a good deal of heterogeneity with regard to

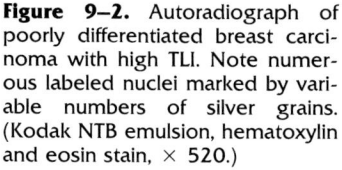

Figure 9–2. Autoradiograph of poorly differentiated breast carcinoma with high TLI. Note numerous labeled nuclei marked by variable numbers of silver grains. (Kodak NTB emulsion, hematoxylin and eosin stain, × 520.)

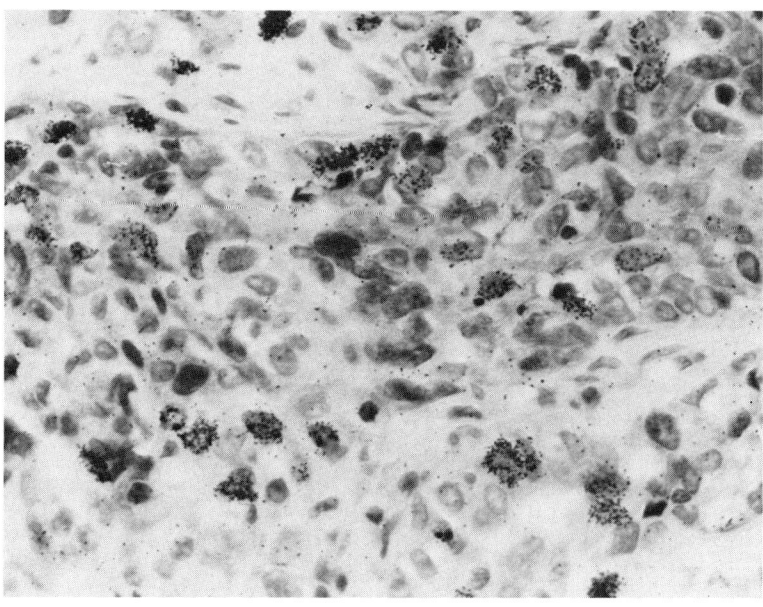

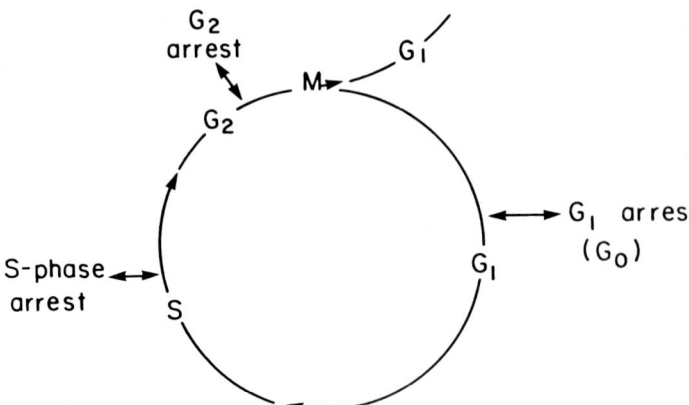

Figure 9–3. Cell cycle diagram. After mitosis (M), the daughter cells enter G_1, where they may become arrested (G_0). When conditions for growth improve, G_0 cells can reenter the mitotic cycle. G_1 cells progress to DNA synthesis (S), but, if conditions deteriorate, may become arrested in the S phase. On completion of DNA synthesis, a cell is in G_2 until the onset of the next mitosis.

cell cycle transit times. Prolongation of cell cycle segments for nutritional and respiratory reasons is now well established for both in vitro and in vivo conditions. Trowell (1952) calculated that the theoretical limiting radius of a cluster of nonvascularized cells with ordinary rates of oxygen consumption would be 0.32 mm (weight, 0.14 mg). Tissue culture conditions can be adjusted to produce cell death, noncycling cells, or cells that move through the cycle at much reduced rates (Dell'Orco, 1974). Similar conditions occur in vivo as a result of imbalance between growth of neoplastic cells and nutrient blood vessels. In this context of heterogeneity, the FLM method is strongly influenced by rapidly cycling cohorts, which rise above the background of more slowly cycling cells in the FLM curve.

For this reason, as Hamilton and Dobbin (1983) have shown, the FLM method may grossly underestimate the mean cell cycle time. Sufficient heterogeneity is usually present among even the rapidly cycling cells in human tumors so that a second FLM peak seldom is seen (Mendelsohn and Takahashi, 1971; Steel, 1977). Thus, the values for lengths of cell cycles and their segments derived from FLM curves are more representative of the healthier, more active cells than of the less well nourished cells.

ARREST OF PROGRESSION IN THE CELL CYCLE

Cells grown in culture as spheroidal aggregates show slowing of progression through the rep-

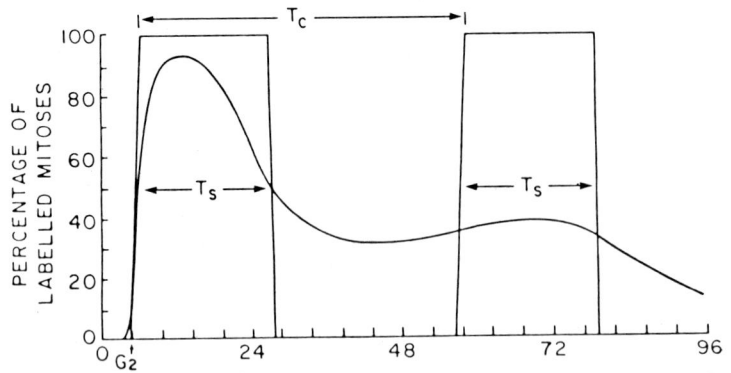

Figure 9–4. Idealized and representative fraction of labeled mitoses (FLM) curves for breast carcinoma. If the population of neoplastic cells all had the same invariable cell cycle transit times with total cycle time (T_c) of 43 hr, G_1 of 20 hr, T_s (DNA synthesis time) of 18 hr, G_2 of 4 hr, and mitosis of 1 hr, the result would be a series of parallelograms. After a single injection of tritiated thymidine (^{3}H-TdR), at time zero, the first labeled mitotic figures would appear at 4 hr, and the percentage of labeled mitoses would rise to 100 per cent as the last unlabeled mitoses reached completion 1 hr later. After 17 hr, unlabeled mitoses, representing cells in late G_1 at the time of injection of ^{3}H-TdR, would appear and within 1 hr the last of the labeled cells would have completed mitosis. All of the mitoses would then be unlabeled. As the daughter cells from the first mitosis enter mitosis again, the second wave of the FLM curve develops. Because tumors have wide dispersions of durations of cell cycle phases, the actual FLM curve varies markedly from the ideal, and synchrony of the labeled cohort is lost so quickly that a clear second wave may not be seen. Variation in the length of G_2 may prevent the FLM from reaching 100 per cent even in the first wave. Estimates for the cell cycle are derived from the FLM curve as follows: T_c from the distance between peaks, T_s from the width of the first peak as half height, G_2 from the time of first appearance of labeled mitoses, and G_1 by subtraction.

licative cycle with increasing distance from the surface, finally progressing to complete arrest in one segment or another and still more centrally becoming necrotic. Wibe and coworkers found that the thickness of viable cells in tumors grown as spheroids is about 80 μm (Wibe et al., 1981). Progressing inward from the surface, the relative number of cells in G_1 increased and the relative number in S decreased. Landry and coworkers (1982) and Allison and associates (1983) presented evidence for arrest also in the S and G_2 phases. Similar changes have been observed in thymidine labeling studies of experimental tumors with extensive necrosis and perivascular growth. In these so-called "corded" tumors (Tannock, 1968), Jones and Camplejohn (1983) found that the mean distance between zones of necrosis and blood vessels was 80 μm, similar to that of the zone of viability at the surface of spheroids. The mean number of layers of cells per cord was 10.3. Numbers of noncycling cells increased progressively with distance from blood vessels, and nonproliferative fractions were estimated as 64 per cent in the inner zones and 94 per cent in the outer zones. Cells with patterns of radioresistance typical of noncycling hypoxic cells exist in mouse mammary carcinomas as small as 1 mm in diameter (Suit and Shalek, 1963; Rockwell et al., 1972). Therefore, they should be expected to occur in micrometastases as well as in clinically evident tumors.

THE G_0 CONCEPT AND GROWTH FRACTION

The concept of a facultatively nonproliferative compartment in tumors was elaborated by Mendelsohn as a means of explaining the differential sensitivities of oxygenated and hypoxic cells to radiation therapy (Mendelsohn, 1960, 1962). Evidence that hypoxic cells are nonproliferative or have prolonged cell cycle durations and can survive higher doses of potentially lethal radiation than well oxygenated cells is well accepted among radiation biologists (Kennedy et al., 1980; Rockwell, 1983; Moulder and Rockwell, 1984). It has led to a number of clinical studies using either high oxygen tensions (to decrease numbers of hypoxic cells), low oxygen tensions (to protect host tissues by rendering them hypoxic also), or drugs such as misonidazole that sensitize hypoxic cells to radiation (Chapman, 1979). Mendelsohn defined G_0 cells as cells that do not traverse the replicative cell cycle but are capable of doing so at some time when conditions become more favorable. A neuron would not be considered a G_0 cell because it is not capable of reentering the cycle. However, a liver cell can be considered as G_0 (although not for reason of hypoxia). Given the proper stimulus (partial hepatectomy, for example), the hepatocyte is capable of DNA replication and division. Initially the G_0 compartment was considered to communicate with G_1. More recently, cells arrested in G_2 have been observed in both normal tissues (Sauerboern et al., 1978) and tumors (Coninx et al., 1983). S phase–arrested cells have also been identified in tumors (Darzynkiewicz et al., 1980; Allison et al., 1985). Whether these cells, arrested in cell cycle segments other than G_1, are capable of progression in the cell cycle and are therefore truly G_0 is not year clear. Abundant evidence shows that hypoxic cells in experimental tumors under both in vivo and in vitro conditions are capable of growth when conditions become favorable and can reestablish tumors when transplanted into new hosts (Kennedy et al., 1980).

DURATION OF CELL CYCLE AND ITS SEGMENTS

Summarized results from studies of human tumors both in vivo and in vitro show the following approximate durations: G_1, 58 hr; S, 19 hr; and G_2, 6 hr or less; total cell cycle, 85 hr (Meyer, 1981). These figures appear to apply to breast carcinoma in addition to a spectrum of other tumors, but they are only generalizations and approximations, and they probably are representative of only the better nourished cells.

From FLM studies of breast carcinomas, Post and coworkers (1977) reported a DNA synthesis time of 24 hr, Terz and coworkers (1977) reported 12.5 hr, and Straus and Moran (1977) reported 18 hr. Two in vitro studies by the double labeling technique yielded results between 18 and 22 hr (Sklarew et al., 1977; Schiffer et al., 1979). The FLM studies indicate a G_2 duration of approximately 4 or 5 hr (Post et al., 1977; Terz et al., 1977).

Time-lapse cinematographic studies of cell lines derived from human tumors show that the duration of mitoses (excluding prophase) is usually less than 30 min, with the greater portion of this time taken up by metaphase (Sisken et al., 1985). In three breast carcinoma lines, metaphases averaged 23, 40, and 60 min, anaphases lasted 4, 4, and 5 min, and cytokinesis lasted 3, 3, and 3 min, respectively. Total durations of histologically recognizable mitosis were 30, 47, and 68 min in the three cell lines (Sisken et al., 1985). As most measurements of the duration of the S phase for breast carcinoma are near 19 hr, the number of S phase cells is clearly approximately 20 times the number of M phase cells at any given time. S phase counts therefore have a great statistical advantage over M phase counts.

THE THYMIDINE LABELING INDEX: IN VIVO AND IN VITRO THYMIDINE LABELING

The earliest thymidine labeling indices (TLI) were achieved by injection of tritiated thymidine (^{3}H-TdR) into the patient shortly prior to biopsy or excision of the tumor (Baserga et al., 1962; Clarkson et al., 1965; Hoffman and Post, 1967; Shirakawa et al., 1970). Straus and coworkers (Straus and Moran, 1980; Straus et al., 1982) have published the only extensive studies of in vivo TLIs of breast carcinoma. They observed mean TLIs of 5.2 per cent in 13 patients with T1–3 carcinomas, 9.0 per cent in 10 patients with T4 carcinomas (local extension without distant spread), and 13.2 per cent in nine patients with metastatic breast carcinoma (Straus and Moran, 1980). They also noted decreased survival rates in all stages, including metastatic disease, with TLIs in excess of 8 per cent. Their frequency distribution of TLIs after in vivo labeling resembles the author's distribution from in vitro labeling (Meyer et al., 1986). Convincing evidence that in vitro and in vivo TLIs are essentially the same is furnished by several comparative studies with tumors in laboratory animals (Rajewsky, 1965; Steel and Bensted, 1965; Fabrikant et al., 1969; Meyer and Bauer, 1975; Meyer and Connor, 1977).

EFFECTS OF OXYGENATION AND INTRACELLULAR PRECURSOR POOLS ON DNA THYMIDINE LABELING

DNA synthesis in mammalian cells requires oxygenation. Incubation of small blocks or slices with ^{3}H-TdR at atmospheric oxygen tension may result in labeling only to a depth of five to 10 cells beneath the surface. Labeling tends to be less deep in poorly cellular tumors or in those with low TLIs than in tumors that are highly cellular and have high TLIs. When labeling is only superficial, the TLI is difficult to determine and may easily be underestimated. Fabrikant and coworkers (1969) demonstrated that the depth of labeling is increased by increasing the oxygen tension. Near maximum effects were achieved with 3 to 4 atmospheres (atm) of oxygen. Under these circumstances, well-labeled cells were found as much as 0.5 mm beneath the surface, but at atmospheric oxygen tension, labeling did not occur more than 0.1 mm beneath the surface. However, the author has observed in many highly cellular, high TLI breast carcinomas that even with hyperbaric oxygenation the depth of labeling is relatively poor. This presumably is because of rapid degradation of ^{3}H-TdR as it diffuses between the malignant cells (Rubini et al., 1966; Maurer, 1981).

Large intracellular pools of thymidine phosphates will dilute any ^{3}H-TdR transported into cells, and intensity of labeling of DNA will be decreased thereby. Furthermore, high levels of thymidine triphosphate may inhibit thymidine kinase, the enzyme responsible for phosphorylation of exogenous ^{3}H-TdR and its transport across the cell membrane (Fig. 9–5). A second factor that may influence the success of thymidine labeling is intracellular synthesis of thymidylate. The principal precursor of thymidine phosphate is deoxyuridine phosphate (Heidelberger, 1982). Synthesis of thymidine phosphate is effected by the enzyme thymidylate synthetase from deoxyuridine phosphate in the presence of the coenzyme tetrahydrofolate reductase. One practical way to decrease intracellular thymidine phosphate pools is to block thymidylate synthetase with 5-fluorouracil (5-FU) or its derivative, 5-fluoro-2′-deoxyuridine (FUdR), thereby preventing synthesis of thymidylate (Heidelberger, 1982). Several studies have demonstrated that blockade of cellular thymidylate synthesis increases the incorporation of exogenously supplied thymidine or thymidine analogues (Dormer et al., 1975; Meyer and Facher, 1977; Chavaudra and Malaise, 1979; Hamilton et al., 1984; Ellward and Dormer, 1985).

The data in Table 9–1 show that thymidylate synthetase blockade may enhance the detection of S-phase cells by thymidine labeling. Intracellular thymidylate synthesis may be particularly important in occasional tumors, as

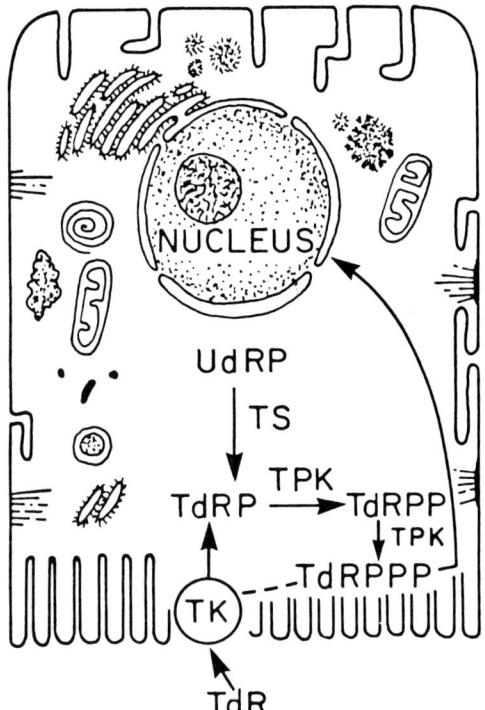

Figure 9–5. Simplified diagram of cell showing paths for uptake and phosphorylation of thymidine (TdR) to thymidine monophosphate (TdRP) by the enzyme thymidine kinase (TK) located in the cell membrane. TdRP can also be produced within the cell through methylation of deoxyuridine monophosphate (UdRP) by the enzyme thymidylate synthetase (TS). TdRP is phosphorylated by thymidine phosphokinase to the diphosphate TdRPP (TPK) and again to the triphosphate TdRPPP, which serves as a substrate for DNA polymerase. TdRPPP in high concentrations inhibits thymidine kinase, a mechanism through which the cell avoids accumulation of excess levels of thymidine phosphates.

reported by Hamilton and Dobbin (1982). These murine mammary carcinomas were labeled very well with titrated deoxyuridine through the thymidylate synthetase pathway. When ^{3}H-TdR was supplied, labeling was poor but was made equivalent to that achieved with tritiated deoxyuridine when thymidylate synthetase was blocked with FUdR (Hamilton et al., 1984). The author and colleagues have observed higher TLIs after in vitro labeling with use of hyperbaric oxygen and thymidylate synthetase inhibition than others have observed without these measures. Without blockade of thymidylate synthetase, DNA labeling with ^{3}H-TdR or 5-bromo-2'-deoxyuridine (BUdR) could give misleading results in certain carcinomas.

DNA MEASUREMENTS BY MICRODENSITOMETRY

The first DNA measurements of tumor cell nuclei were done by microdensitometry after Feulgen staining. This is a cumbersome technique, but it allows visual selection of the nuclei to be studied. Each nucleus must be positioned under the microscope for measurements of light absorption or fluorescence if a fluorescent DNA stain is used. Cytologic specimens rather than tissue sections must be used to ensure that the nuclei being measured are intact.

DNA MEASUREMENTS BY FLOW CYTOMETRY

The principle of DNA flow cytometry is analogous to that of the familiar Coulter counter of the hematology laboratory, but fluorescence emission rather than electrical conductance is measured. As cells flow through the instrument rapidly and in single file, they intercept a beam of light. After staining with a fluorescent dye that is stoichiometric for DNA, the cells will emit a pulse of light proportional to DNA content. The light is allowed to pass through a filter toward a photoelectric detector and amplifier. The resultant electrical pulse is

Table 9–1. THYMIDINE LABELING INDICES OF PRIMARY INVASIVE BREAST CARCINOMA

Author	Method*	Number	TLI		
			Median	*Mean*	*Range*
Straus and Moran (1980)	1	13		5.2	
Gentili et al. (1981)	2	541	2.8	4.8	0.09–40.7
Meyer and Hixon (1979)	3	128	2.1	3.7	0.05–18.6
Meyer et al. (1986)	4	757	5.2	7.1	0.05–35.6

*1, In vivo; 2, in vitro, atmospheric oxygen; 3, in vitro, hyperbaric oxygen; 4, in vitro, hyperbaric oxygen and thymidylate synthetase inhibition.

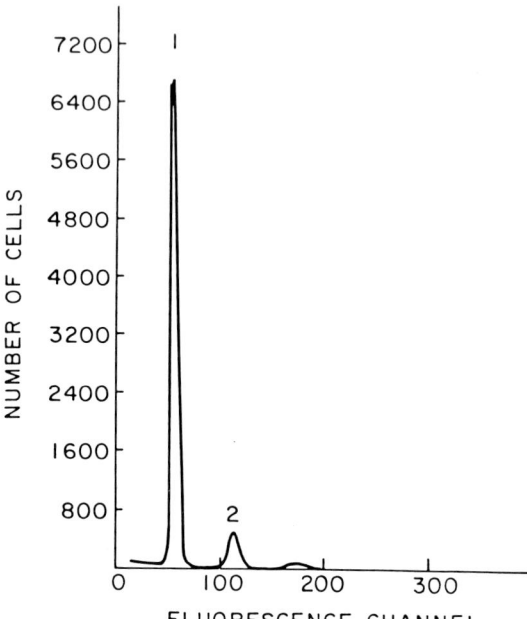

Figure 9–6. DNA histogram of breast carcinoma with diploid DNA content and a low percentage of S-phase cells (%S). Peak 1 represents G_1 and G_0 cells, peak 2 G_2 and M cells. Because few S-phase cells are present, the curve between the two peaks approaches the baseline. The low peak to the right of peak 2 represents doublets or triplets. As computed from the histogram, %S = 3 per cent; TLI = 3 per cent. This histogram and those in Figures 9–7 to 9–10 were obtained on cell suspensions stained with 4′,6-diamidino-2-phenylindole (DAPI) and run on a Partec PAS II flow cytometer.

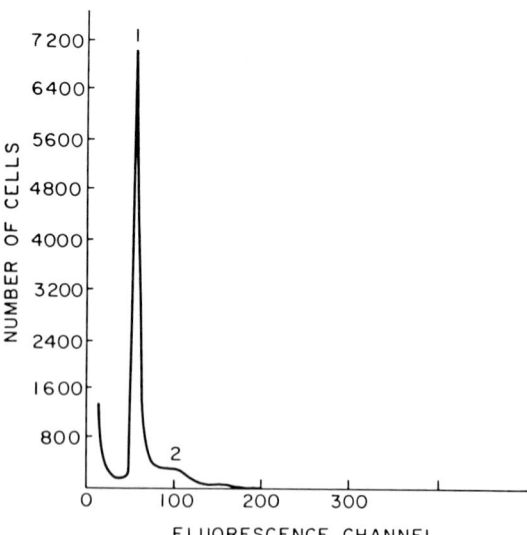

Figure 9–7. Diploid DNA content with a high %S in an adenocarcinoma of the lung. Such high S-phase fractions are unusual in diploid breast carcinomas. Peaks are identified as in Figure 9–6. Debris is seen to the left of peak. %S = 23 per cent; TLI = 24 per cent.

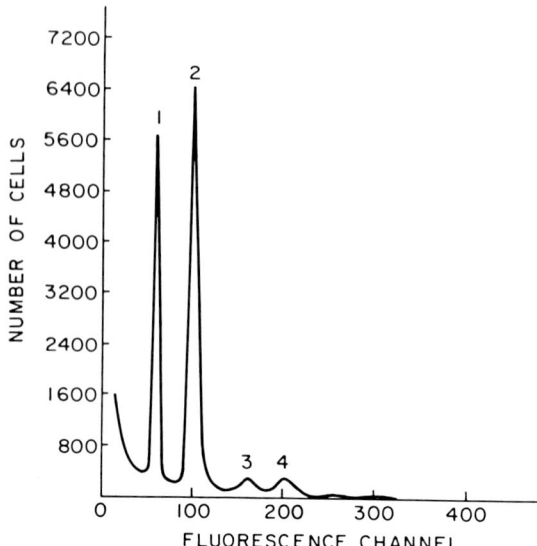

Figure 9–8. Breast carcinoma with an aneuploid (hyperdiploid) peak (peak 2). The diploid G_1-G_0 cells are to the right (peak 1). Peak 3 represents the G_2-M diploid cells and falls in the S region of the hyperdiploid portion of the histogram. Peak 4 represents the G_2-M hyperdiploid cells. %S = 13 per cent; TLI = 6.7 per cent; DNA index = 1.69.

transmitted to a computer, and a histogram is generated by plotting the number of cells with different DNA contents (Figs. 9–6 to 9–10). For detailed information, the reader is referred to reviews by Laerum and Farsund (1981), Braylan (1983), and Muirhead and colleagues (1985) and the detailed treatise of Shapiro (1985).

Flow cytometry offers the advantages of speed and automation but has the disadvantage of nonselectivity. The instrument records data from all cells, both the malignant cells of interest and associated benign cells. Development of markers selective for breast carcinoma cells eventually may permit exclusion of contaminating cells, but at present the DNA histogram represents a mixture of neoplastic cells and the associated benign cells (lymphocytes, histiocytes, granulocytes, fibroblasts, endothelial cells, and others) that contaminate all breast carcinomas.

PLOIDY ANALYSIS OF FLOW CYTOMETRIC DNA HISTOGRAMS

Flow cytometry resolves distinct peaks in the DNA histograms that correspond to G_1 and G_2 populations. Cell populations fall into two classes, diploid or aneuploid. Diploid as used

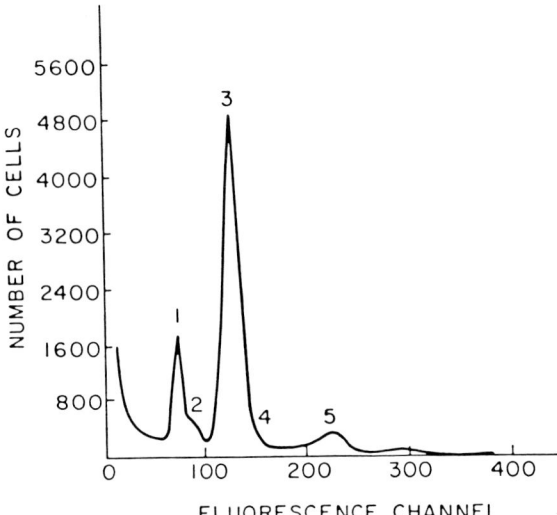

Figure 9–9. Breast carcinoma with two hyperdiploid populations. One (peak 3) has a DNA index of 1.74. The second is a small population with a DNA index of approximately 1.1 that appears as a shoulder on the G_1-G_0 diploid peak (peak 1). %S = 13 per cent for the major hyperdiploid population; TLI = 13 per cent.

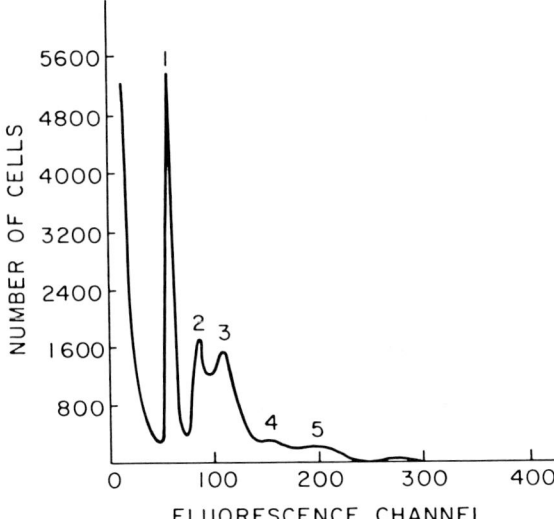

Figure 9–10. Breast carcinoma with two hyperdiploid peaks with DNA indices of 1.49 and 1.89 (peaks 2 and 3). The shoulder on peak 3 represents G_2-M diploid cells (peak 4), and peak 5 represents G_2-M cells of the hyperdiploid populations. %S = 35 per cent; TLI = 22 per cent.

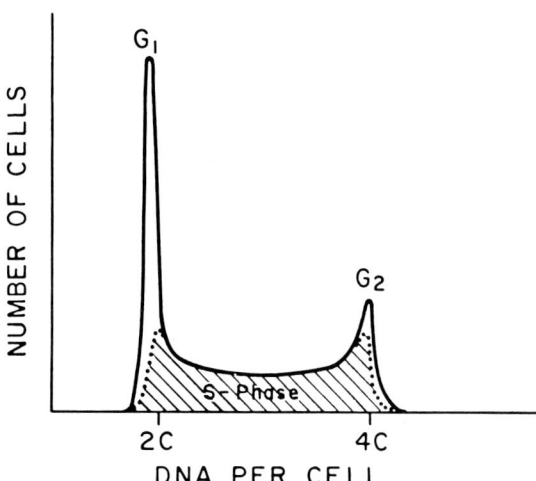

Figure 9–11. DNA histogram showing the U-shaped distribution of S-phase cells caused by the slow pace of DNA synthesis near the beginning and end of the S phase. This results in a disproportionate fraction of S-phase cells being near the extremes of S rather than in the middle. Presence of many S-phase cells under the G_1 and G_2 peaks complicates the estimation of %S from DNA histograms.

in the context of flow cytometry means DNA content indistinguishable from that of normal cells but does not imply a completely normal chromosomal pattern. Most of the aneuploid populations, which because of their tight DNA distributions are thought to be clonally derived, fall between G_1 diploid and G_2 diploid peaks or in the tetraploid (diploid G_2) position.

Roughly 20 to 40 per cent of breast carcinomas have no detectable aneuploid cells ("diploid carcinomas"), and 60 per cent have aneuploid cells detected ("aneuploid carcinomas"). Of the aneuploid carcinomas, only about 1 per cent are hypodiploid (less than normal DNA content), approximately 80 per cent are hyperdiploid or tetraploid, and 20 per cent are hypertetraploid (more than twice the normal DNA content) (Kute et al., 1981; Olszewski et al., 1981; Raber et al., 1982; McDivitt et al., 1985).

KINETIC INFORMATION FROM FLOW CYTOMETRIC DNA HISTOGRAMS

The S-phase cells have DNA contents intermediate between those of G_1 and G_2 cells. In DNA histograms, they are distributed between the beginning of the G_1-G_0 peak and the G_2-M peak. Because of the relatively slow pace of DNA synthesis early and late in the S phase, relatively more S-phase cells fall under the G_1-G_0 and G_2-M peaks than might be expected (Fig. 9–11) (Culpin and Morris, 1985). To account for the appearance of an S-phase cell in the extreme range of either peak, consider the multiple factors that can influence the size of the electronic pulse generated by a single fluorescent cell. These factors include the speed of flow through the light beam, variability in exciting beam intensity, course through the beam, orientation of the fluorescent nucleus and quenching within the cell and in its immediate environment, and output of the photomultiplier tube. Thus, a single G_1 cell that is repeatedly run through the instrument would produce a histogram with a normal distribution resembling the peaks generated by multiple cells. A very early S-phase cell with only a slight excess above the G_1 DNA content would produce a similar peak.

Various mathematical models have been proposed for analysis of DNA histograms, but for the most part they yield similar results (Baisch et al., 1982). Dean and associates (1982) observed inherent errors of 5 to 10 per cent (coefficient of variation) for measurements of G_1-G_0, S, and G_2-M on replicate runs. A single measurement could produce an error as large as 40 per cent for G_2-M and 15 to 20 per cent for G_1-G_0 and S (Dean et al., 1982). With a low percentage of S, the relative error of measurement could be still greater.

In exponentially growing cell cultures, the percentage of S determined by flow cytometry is closely similar to the TLI, and cells in the S region of the DNA histogram have been shown to be uniformly labeled after exposure to tritiated thymidine (Sheck et al., 1980). When conditions for growth are not ideal, as in many neoplasms where zones of vascular insufficiency occur, cells may become arrested in the S phase as discussed earlier. This may result in an excess of the percentage of S from flow cytometry over the TLI. Although in some studies of breast carcinomas the mean percentage of S has been as low as 3.7 to 7.5 per cent (Haag et al., 1984, 1987; McDivitt et al., 1984), which is close to the mean TLI in the author's laboratory, in other studies the mean percentage of S has been reported as 9 to 14 per cent (Kute et al., 1981; Olszewski et al., 1981b; Raber et al., 1982; Taylor et al., 1983; Meyer et al., 1984b). The lowest results reflect methods of computation of percentage of S from DNA histograms that attempt to correct for presence of debris and other artifacts. When debris is subtracted, the distributions of percentage of S and TLI become closely similar (Haag et al., 1987). Whether these corrections are appropriate is controversial. It appears unlikely that cells in early or late S, when the pace of DNA synthesis is slow, are being missed by thymidine labeling techniques that produce high grain counts over S-phase cells. Bose and coworkers combined computerized microfluorimetry for DNA analysis with autoradiography and showed that all mid-S cells of mouse bone marrow were labeled after 2 days of autoradiographic exposure and that all cells in early and late S were labeled after 8 days of exposure (Bose et al., 1984). Therefore the debris subtraction, which reduces the median percentage of S to the level of the median TLI, appears to be necessary for accurate evaluation of breast carcinomas by flow cytometry.

Cell Kinetics of Normal Breast and Benign Epithelial Hyperplasias

Breast epithelium has long been known to be responsive to ovarian hormones. Only recently has the proliferative activity been studied quantitatively. DNA synthesis takes place in epithelium of the lobule and the postlobular ducts ("breast ducts") at all stages of the menstrual cycle, but it is most intense during the progestational phase of the cycle (Masters et al., 1977; Meyer, 1977). In young women, the rate of cell production construed from the TLI is sufficient to renew all cells in the lobule in as little time as 1 month (Meyer, 1977). It is possible, however, that only a portion of the epithelium is renewed, in which case its turnover time would be even shorter. The rate of cell renewal decreases toward the menopause and is markedly diminished after the menopause. This helps explain the well known atrophy of the lobule that occurs at this time. The results of mitotic counting in the lobule are conflicting. Anderson and coworkers (1982) observed a peak in the mitotic index during the progestational phase, but Vogel and coworkers (1981) observed it late in the estrogenic phase.

The postlobular ducts show slower rates of cell renewal (lower TLIs) in premenopausal women than do the lobules (Table 9–2), but the TLIs of the postlobular ducts do not decrease appreciably after the menopause. Meyer and Connor (1985) observed a mean TLI for all phases of the menstrual cycle of 1.0 per cent of 59 premenopausal women, with a median of 0.44 per cent and a range of 0.00

Table 9–2. TLI OF NORMAL AND BENIGN PROLIFERATIVE EPITHELIUM

Type of Epithelium	Number	TLI		
		Mean ± SE*	Median	Range
Normal lobule	101	0.09 ± 0.13	0.41	0.00–8.9
Normal postlobular duct	87	0.71 ± 0.12	0.36	0.00–7.2
Lobular hyperplasia	19	0.82 ± 0.22	0.60	0.00–3.1
Intraductal hyperplasia, nonpapillary	27	0.79 ± 0.16	0.33	0.00–2.5
Intraductal hyperplasia, papillary	15	1.02 ± 0.36	0.38	0.00–4.8
Blunt duct adenosis	7	0.68 ± 0.28	0.60	0.00–2.2
Sclerosing adenosis	6	0.47 ± 0.12	0.53	0.10–0.75
Cyst	34	0.56 ± 0.33	0.20	0.00–5.8
Intraductal papilloma	14	1.22 ± 0.33	0.71	0.00–5.9

*SE, Standard error of mean.

to 8.8 per cent. Corresponding values for 16 postmenopausal women for the TLI of the lobular epithelium were a mean of 0.26 per cent, median of 0.18 per cent, and range 0.00 to 1.01 per cent. In 50 premenopausal women, the postlobular ducts had a mean TLI of 0.75 per cent, median of 0.29 per cent, and range of 0.00 to 6.0 per cent. In 16 postmenopausal women, the mean ductal TLI was 0.41 per cent, the median was 0.34 per cent, and the range was 0.00 to 0.93 per cent (Meyer and Connor, 1985). These findings suggest that the postlobular ducts are less responsive to ovarian hormones than is the epithelium of the lobule.

Benign epithelial proliferations of the breast generally have TLIs that resemble those of normal breast epithelium. The TLIs of breast carcinomas, as will be shown later, may be as low as those of the normal breast epithelium and its benign proliferations, but some breast carcinomas have much higher TLIs than have been observed in the benign epithelium.

Cell Kinetic and DNA Flow Cytometric Measurements in Breast Carcinoma

CLASSIC CELL KINETICS OF BREAST CARCINOMA

The three fundamental kinetic characteristics to be considered in this section are cell cycle phase durations, growth fraction, and cell loss. Available information about these variables comes from a few FLM studies in vivo and in vitro studies using double labeling techniques (Wimber and Quastler, 1963). Difficulties with giving radioactive precursors to patients and uncertainties about the reliability of in vitro results limit the scope and reliability of our knowledge (Table 9–3).

The duration of the S phase is of potential clinical importance because a number of cytotoxic drugs (for example, arabinosyl cytosine and 6-thioguanine, and to a large extent 5-fluorouracil, its derivative 5-fluoro-2'-deoxyuridine [FUdR], and methotrexate) specifically kill S-phase cells (Heidelberger, 1982). The proportion of S-phase cells in an exponentially growing population is related to the S phase duration, as described by Steel (1977) in the following:

$$(1) \qquad t_c = 0.75 \, (t_s/\text{TLI})$$

where t_c is the duration of the cell cycle, t_s is the duration of the S phase, the TLI is a measure of the proportion of S-phase cells, and 0.75 is a constant related to the position of the S phase in the cell cycle. This equation ignores the possibility of a G_0 population. Should such be present, the equation would overestimate the t_c for the cycling population.

The long duration of S phase relative to M gives S phase measurements a great advantage in speed and accuracy over M phase measurements. Mitotic cells can be confused with relatively common pyknotic and fragmenting nu-

Table 9–3. ESTIMATES OF CYCLE PHASE TRANSIT TIMES OF BREAST CARCINOMA CELLS

Phase	Transit Time
Complete cycle	One to many days
G_1	One to many days
S	Approximately 18 hr
G_2	Approximately 5 hr
M, metaphase + anaphase	15 min to 1 hr
M, complete	30 min to 1.5 hr

clei, and mitoses are so scarce in many breast carcinomas that many hours of work are required to measure mitotic indices.

GROWTH FRACTION

The growth fraction is theoretically important because noncycling cells are relatively insensitive to radiation therapy (Rockwell, 1983; Moulder and Rockwell, 1984) or cycle-active cytotoxic agents (Laster et al., 1969; Schabel, 1975; Skipper and Schabel, 1982). Measurements of growth fraction of breast carcinoma from different laboratories have yielded values of 0.01 to 0.65 (Lelle, 1987; McGurrin, 1987; Meyer, 1981).

CELL LOSS

Cell loss is as important in determining the growth rate of a neoplasm as is cell production. Cells may be lost by death or migration. Necrosis and apoptosis (death of single cells) are prominent features of approximately one third of infiltrating breast carcinomas (Meyer et al., 1986), but cell death may be inconspicuous and difficult to estimate by microscopic inspection. The only method whereby cell loss can be estimated in breast carcinoma at present is by comparing the proliferative rate of the neoplastic cells with the measured growth rate of the tumor (Steel, 1977). Steel (1967) wrote the following equation for calculation of cell-loss (ϕ):

$$(2) \qquad \phi = 1 - (t_c/t_d)$$

where ϕ is the fractional rate of cell loss, t_c is the cell cycle time, and t_d is the measured doubling time. If no loss of cells occurred, a breast carcinoma with extremely high proliferative activity would double in volume in 36 hrs. Because no clinically evident tumor even approaches this rate of growth, cell loss must be high in rapidly proliferating carcinomas. Mean volume-doubling times for breast carcinomas have ranged from 109 to 327 days, and measurements of cell cycle time range from less than 1 to 4 days (Meyer, 1981). Even allowing for a large G_0 fraction, the mean rate of cell loss must be well over 50 per cent. Measurements of cell loss in various human cancers have ranged from 15 per cent to 85 per cent (Meyer, 1981). The degree of histologically detectable cell loss (necrosis, apoptosis) increases in proportion to the TLI of breast carcinoma.

FREQUENCY DISTRIBUTION OF THE TLI IN BREAST CARCINOMA

Infiltrative and in situ breast carcinomas have a broad range of TLIs, which extend from 0.1 per cent or less to 35 per cent (Meyer et al., 1986) (Fig. 9–12). Repeated studies have shown that the frequency distribution of the TLI of infiltrating breast carcinoma is highly positively skewed (Tubiana et al., 1975; Sklarew et al., 1977; Meyer and Hixon, 1979; Schiffer et al., 1979; Silvestrini et al., 1979; Meyer et al., 1986). The author and colleagues have found the same to be true for in situ carcinoma, although their highest TLIs are lower than those for invasive carcinomas. Furthermore, the TLIs of in situ carcinomas have been found to be proportional to those of associated invasive carcinomas (Meyer, 1986).

SPECIAL HISTOLOGIC TYPES OF BREAST CARCINOMAS HAVE CHARACTERISTIC TLIs

Table 9–4 describes the strong relationship between histologic type of carcinoma and the TLI. Certain carcinomas of established low-grade malignancy have low TLIs (Meyer et al., 1978, 1986). These include adenocystic, mucinous, papillary, and tubular carcinomas. Medullary carcinomas and tumors with some features of medullary carcinomas (atypical medullary carcinoma) consistently have high TLIs. That medullary carcinomas have a relatively good prognosis despite rapid proliferative rates at first seems anomalous, but the good prognosis is explained by their low rates of metastasis, not by slow progression once metastases have occurred. Several authors have observed that death from medullary carcinoma is restricted almost entirely to the first 5 years after diagnosis (Berg and Robbins, 1966; Hartviet, 1974; Ridolfi et al., 1977). The author and coworkers have observed that circumscription of the tumor border is an important determinant of probability of relapse in carcinomas with high TLI (Meyer et al., 1983).

Infiltrating lobular carcinomas have low TLIs but nonetheless do not have a particularly good prognosis, no doubt because of their

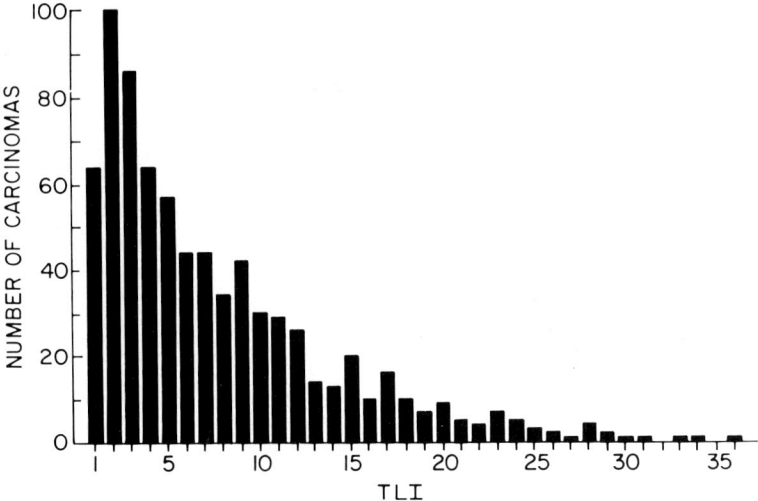

Figure 9-12. Frequency distribution of TLI in 757 primary, infiltrating breast carcinomas. (From Meyer, J. S., et al.: Breast carcinoma cell kinetics, morphology, stage, and host characteristics: A thymidine labeling study. Lab. Invest., 54:41, 1986. Reprinted with permission.)

highly infiltrative patterns and propensity to metastasize. However, their slow proliferative rates are reflected in long clinical courses. Ashikari and coworkers (1973) noted that in various clinical stages of infiltrating lobular carcinoma nearly as many deaths occurred between 5 and 10 years after primary treatment as in the first 5 years. Lobular carcinomas with moderately anaplastic nuclei (Grade II) have higher TLIs than those with minimal anaplasia (Grade I) (Meyer et al., 1986), but the prognostic implication of this difference is not yet known.

Only approximately 20 per cent of breast carcinomas belong to any of the well-defined special histologic types. The proliferative indices of the residual group, best designated "not otherwise specified" (NOS), as suggested by Fisher and coworkers (1975), reflect a broad range of TLIs that extends from approximately 0.1 to 35 per cent. Their behavior is as diverse as the spectrum of TLIs would suggest.

RELATIONSHIPS BETWEEN THE PROLIFERATIVE INDEX AND TUMOR GRADE

Just as the histologic type of breast carcinoma relates to the TLI, the grade of differentiation (histologic grade) and degree of nuclear anaplasia (nuclear grade) relate to TLI. The small group of NOS carcinomas with predominant gland and tubule formation have low TLIs, and the mean TLI increases with decreasing participation of cells in formation of lumens. However, some histologic Grade III carcinomas (lobular carcinomas and also carcinomas with solid growth patterns) have low TLIs. The mean TLI increases impressively with pro-

Table 9-4. TLI OF SPECIAL TYPES OF BREAST CARCINOMA

| | | TLI | | |
Type	Number	Mean	Median	Standard Deviation
Adenocystic	3	1.7	0.6	1.9
Linear large cell	4	9.9	11.2	6.3
Lobular	54	2.3	1.7	2.2
Medullary	24	16.6	16.2	5.6
Medullary, atypical	21	16.9	14.7	7.3
Metaplastic	2	10.1	10.1	2.1
Mucinous	20	2.0	1.5	1.4
Papillary	5	1.4	0.8	1.0
Tubular	10	1.3	1.0	1.0
Not otherwise specified (NOS)	581	7.1	5.5	5.9

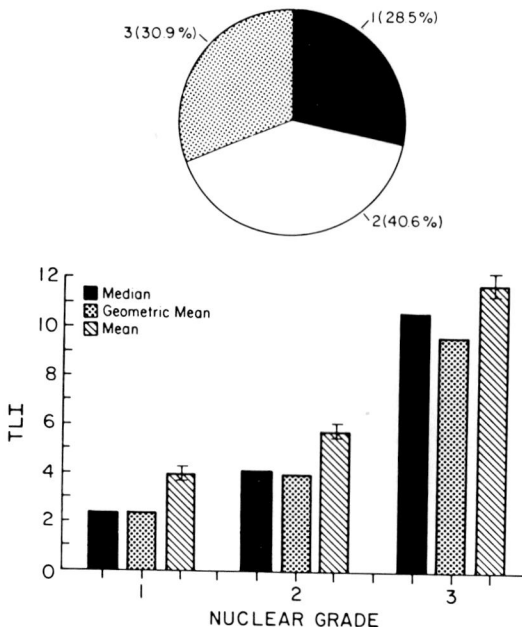

Figure 9–13. Relationship between the TLI of infiltrating breast carcinoma and the nuclear grade. The pie graph shows the relative proportions of patients with minimal (grade 1), intermediate (grade 2), and marked nuclear enlargement (grade 3). The bar graph demonstrates that enlargement of nuclei is associated with high TLI. (From Meyer, J. S., et al: Breast carcinoma cell kinetics, morphology, stage, and host characteristics: A thymidine labeling study. Lab. Invest., 54:41, 1986. Reprinted with permission.)

progesterone receptor (PgR) is well established (Meyer et al., 1977; Cooke et al., 1979; Silvestrini et al., 1979; Meyer et al., 1986). The relationship is true for both premenopausal and postmenopausal patients (Silvestrini et al., 1986). The correlation coefficients that the author's group has observed between ER and TLI or PgR and TLI, although significant, are not particularly high ($r = 0.2$ to 0.4), which reflects a good deal of variability in receptor assay results for all proliferative classes. Thus, a breast carcinoma with a high TLI is likely but not certain to be receptor negative, and carcinomas with low TLIs are sometimes not receptor positive. The relationship between PgR and TLI is not appreciably stronger than that between ER and TLI. Similar inverse relationships between ER content and percentage of S by flow cytometry also have been observed (Kute et al., 1981; Olszewski et al., 1981b; Raber et al., 1982; McDivitt et al., 1985).

gression of the nuclear grade from 1 to 3 (Meyer et al., 1986) (Fig. 9–13).

RELATIONSHIP BETWEEN AGE OF THE PATIENT AND THE PROLIFERATIVE INDEX

The TLI shows an impressive inverse relationship to age (Silvestrini et al., 1979; Meyer and Lee, 1980; Meyer et al., 1986) (Fig. 9–14). Young, premenopausal patients are likely to have high TLIs, and older, postmenopausal patients are likely to have low TLIs. Exceptions to this rule, however, are not rare.

RELATIONSHIPS BETWEEN THE PROLIFERATIVE INDEX AND STEROIDAL RECEPTOR CONTENT OF BREAST CARCINOMA

An inverse relationship between the TLI and content of either estrogen receptor (ER) or

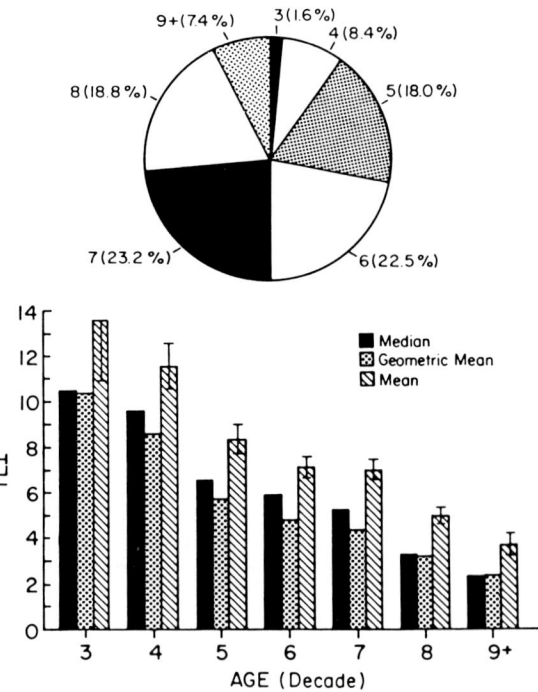

Figure 9–14. Relationship between TLI of infiltrating breast carcinoma and age at time of diagnosis. The pie graph shows the relative proportions of patients in each decade of age. The bar graph shows a steady decline in the median, geometric mean, and mean TLI with increasing age. (From Meyer, J. S., et al.: Breast carcinoma cell kinetics, morphology, stage, and host characteristics: A thymidine labeling study. Lab. Invest., 54:41, 1986. Reprinted with permission.)

Table 9–5. RELATIONSHIP OF TLI TO STAGE

Author	Method*	Number	Stage†	TLI Median	TLI Mean
Straus and Moran (1980)	1	13	T1–3		5.2
	1	10	T4		9.0
	1	9	Metastasis		13.2
Meyer et al. (1986)	3	325	A	4.5	6.7
	3	86	B	5.2	7.0
	3	22	C	8.5	8.0
	3	13	DL	12.2	12.7
	3	17	Metastasis	6.0	7.5

*1, In vivo; 3, in vitro, hyperbaric oxygen.
†Straus and Moran used the TMR system; T4 means local extension without distant spread. Meyer and Connor used the Columbia Clinical Staging system; DL means local extension without distant spread.

PROLIFERATIVE INDEX AND STAGE OF DISEASE

Tubiana and coworkers were the first to observe that locally aggressive breast carcinomas have high proliferative indices (Tubiana et al., 1975). This observation has been confirmed (Table 9–5). Nonetheless, only a weak relationship exists between the proliferative rate and number of axillary lymph node metastases (Tubiana et al., 1975; Schiffer et al., 1979; Bertuzzi et al., 1981; Raber et al., 1982; Meyer et al., 1986), showing that the metastatic potential in breast carcinoma is not closely tied to proliferative rate. This fact accounts for the broad clinical spectrum of behavior. The author's data suggest, however, that metastasis to the brain is associated with high TLI (Meyer et al., 1984a).

THE PROLIFERATIVE INDEX OF BREAST CARCINOMA AS A PROGNOSTIC FEATURE

Since the first report by Tubiana and associates (1975), evidence has been accumulated to establish the TLI as a powerful stage-independent indicator for the early course of breast carcinoma after primary treatment (Tubiana et al., 1975; Meyer and Lee, 1980; Straus and Moran, 1980; Gentili et al., 1981; Raber et al., 1982; Tubiana et al., 1984). Most reports have dealt with patients observed for only a few years, a report by Silvestrini and coworkers establishes that the TLI remains prognostic over a 6 year period (Silvestrini et al., 1985), and Tubiana and associates (1984) have demonstrated a relationship between TLI and relapse-free survival continuing over 10 years of observation. The predictive power of the TLI appears to be most striking in the low-stage patients (Fig. 9–15).

Limited association between the TLI and the stage of disease (Tubiana et al., 1975; Meyer and Hixon, 1979; Meyer and Lee, 1980; Silvestrini et al., 1986) indicates that proliferative indices will not be useful in predicting the status of the axillary lymph nodes. However, patients are less likely to relapse when their TLIs are low and are more likely to relapse when their TLIs are high, regardless of the nodal status. Any relationship between the TLI and the clinical stage of the disease is expressed primarily locally. Locally advanced carcinomas, and inflammatory carcinomas in particular, have high TLIs (Meyer et al., 1986).

Just as the TLI is prognostic independent of stage, it also is prognostic in both ER-positive and ER-negative tumor groups (Meyer et al., 1983; Silvestrini et al., 1985) (Fig. 9–16). Preliminary analysis of the author's data indicates that the same may be true for the PgR. Multivariate analysis showed no predictive power in the ER assay beyond its correlation with the TLI (Meyer et al., 1983).

DNA MEASUREMENTS IN BREAST CARCINOMA

By microdensitometric measurements of DNA in smears, breast carcinomas can be divided into four groups (Atkin, 1972; Auer et al., 1980b) (Table 9–6). Survival is distinctly higher for patients with predominantly diploid-tetraploid DNA contents in their breast carcinomas cells than for those with clearly aneuploid DNA content (Atkin, 1972; Auer et al., 1980b). In addition, aneuploid carcinomas

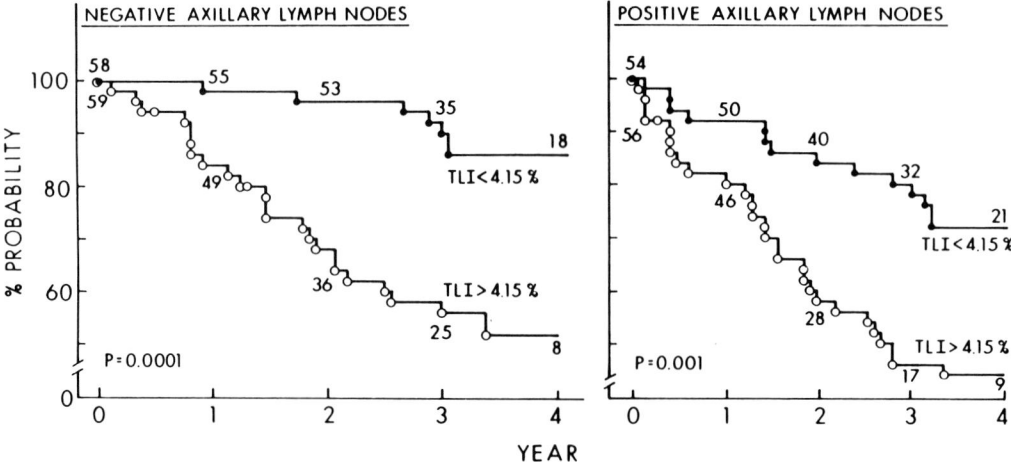

Figure 9–15. Prognostic value of the TLI in operable patients with invasive breast carcinoma in relationship to the axillary lymph nodal status. The TLI was predictive for relapse-free survival (vertical axis) in both groups. The number of patients at risk at a given time after total mastectomy and axillary lymph nodal dissection appears above the plot of relapse-free survival. (From Meyer, J. S., et al.: Prediction of early course of breast carcinoma by thymidine labeling. Cancer 51:1879, 1983. Reprinted with permission.)

(Types II and IV) are poor in estrogen receptor (ER), whereas diploid-tetraploid carcinomas (Types I and II) are often ER-rich (Auer et al., 1980a).

The DNA flow cytometric patterns of breast carcinomas express the presence or absence of aneuploid stem lines and the number of S-phase cells. Figures 9–6 to 9–10 illustrate different types of flow cytometric histograms.

From 44 to 92 per cent of breast carcinomas in various studies have contained aneuploid cell populations (Kute et al., 1981; Olszewski et al., 1981a; Bichel et al., 1982; Fosse et al., 1982; Raber et al., 1982; Barlogie et al., 1983; Taylor et al., 1983; Cornelisse et al., 1984; Coulson et al., 1984; Meyer et al., 1984b; McDivitt et al., 1986). The variability from one series to another may be caused by differences in stage distribution, adequacy of sampling, and flow cytometric resolution. The aneuploidy rate averaged from nine different laboratories is 70 per cent. Ewers and coworkers (1984) have demonstrated increasing rates of aneuploidy with increasing stage from T1 to

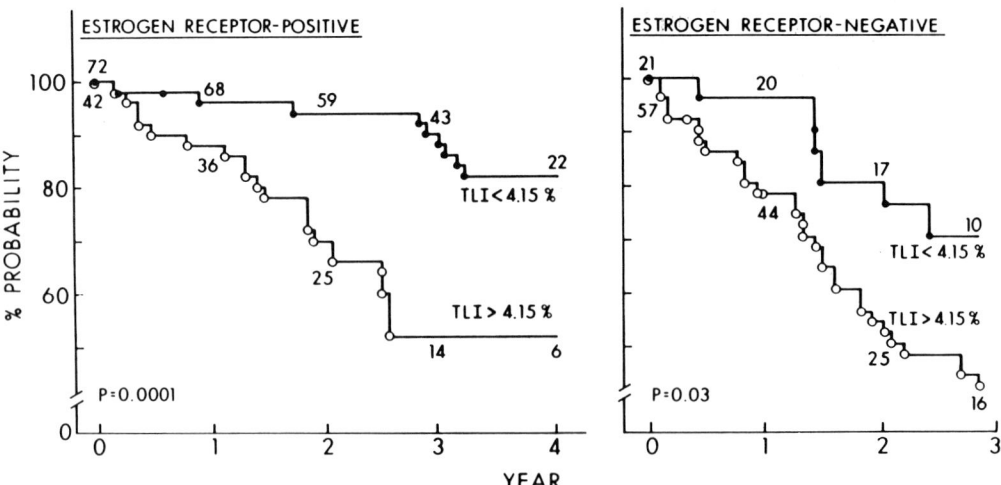

Figure 9–16. Prognostic value of the TLI in operable patients with invasive breast carcinoma subdivided according to estrogen receptor (ER) status. The TLI was predictive for relapse-free survival (vertical axis) in both groups. The number of patients at risk appears above each plot. (From Meyer, J. S. et al.: Prediction of early course of breast carcinoma by thymidine labeling. Cancer 51:1879, 1983. Reprinted with permission.)

Table 9-6. MICRODENSITOMETRIC CLASSIFICATION OF DNA CONTENT OF BREAST CARCINOMA CELLS*

DNA Type	Description	Frequency (%)	Estrogen Receptor	Long-Term Survival (%)
I	Single diploid modal DNA value	30%	Usually positive	50%
II	Both diploid and tetraploid DNA values	35%	Usually positive	50%
III	Modal DNA value between diploid and tetraploid	20%	Usually negative	25%
IV	Modal DNA value beyond tetraploid	15%	Usually negative	25%

*Based on data from Auer et al. (1980a,b); Atkin (1972); and Fossa et al. (1982).

T4. Various methods of preparation of the cell suspensions have yielded similar proportions of aneuploid carcinomas (Chassevent et al., 1984; Meyer et al., 1984b). Aneuploid breast carcinomas nearly always have excess DNA content; as noted earlier, only approximately 1 per cent are hypodiploid. Cytogenetic analysis has shown chromosomal abnormalities in diploid breast carcinomas (Barlogie et al., 1983; Tribukait, 1984). These chromosomal abnormalities are too minor to result in change in DNA content of a magnitude detectable by flow cytometry.

Aneuploidy and high percentage of S by flow cytometry are consistently associated with ER negativity, although the relationship has not been statistically significant in all studies (Kute et al., 1981; Olszewski et al., 1981a,b; Raber et al., 1982; Taylor et al., 1983; Cornelisse et al., 1984; Coulson et al., 1984). PgR and percentage of S are also negatively correlated, but to no greater degree than ER and percentage of S (Meyer et al., 1984a; McDivitt et al., 1986). Breast carcinomas with diploid DNA indices are more likely to be ER positive and PgR positive than are those with aneuploid DNA indices. Aneuploidy is also associated with high percentage of S (Kute et al., 1981; Olszewski et al., 1981b; Moran et al., 1984) and high TLI (Meyer et al., 1984b; McDivitt et al., 1985). Moran and coworkers (1984) have shown that the percentage of S, although consistently higher than the TLI, has the same relationships as the TLI to the age of the patient, histopathologic type of carcinoma, and nuclear grade.

A retrospective study in which nuclei were prepared from paraffin-embedded blocks demonstrated significantly increased relapse rates in patients with aneuploid tumors in comparison to diploid tumors (Wedley et al., 1984). Coulson and associates (1984) and Ewers and coworkers (1984) found the DNA index to be prognostic for short-term survival prospective studies. Their findings paralleled the microdensitometric observations of Auer and coworkers (1980b) and Atkins (1972) in that the higher the DNA index, the greater was the risk of early relapse. These studies indicate that the probabilities of relapse and death within 3 to 5 years of primary treatment are increased twofold or more if the carcinoma is aneuploid rather than diploid. No clear-cut data on relationships between flow cytometrically determined percentage of S and the course of breast carcinoma are available, but the good correlation between the TLI and the percentage of S by flow cytometry suggests that the percentage of S will be prognostic. However, overlapping peak prevent calculation of percentage of S in one third of carcinomas, even with the best flow cytometric resolution currently available (Taylor et al., 1983).

CYSTOSARCOMA PHYLLODES

Cytosarcoma phyllodes has the appearance of fibroadenoma with malignant-appearing stromal change. Actually the majority of these tumors have only locally malignant potential, and only a small minority have metastasized. Several authors have noted that the stromal mitotic index is predictive of the tumor's behavior (Norris and Taylor, 1967; Hart et al., 1978; Pietruszka and Barnes, 1978). The TLI of the stroma of fibroadenomas is uniformly low, but most cytosarcomas have higher stromal TLIs and also may have relatively high epithelial TLIs (Table 9-7). The author and colleagues have observed the highest proliferative indices in those cytosarcomas that exhibited malignant behavior.

Table 9–7. TLI OF FIBROADENOMA AND CYSTOSARCOMA

Tissue	Number	TLI		
		Mean	*Median*	*Range*
Fibroadenoma, epithelium	13	1.7	0.95	0.05– 4.2
Fibroadenoma, stroma	13	0.53	0.42	0.00– 1.30
Primary cystosarcoma, epithelium	5	2.0	2.7	0.35– 3.15
Primary cystosarcoma, stroma	5	3.7	1.3	0.10–13.11
Metastatic or recurrent cystosarcoma, stroma	3	8.4	5.0	3.00–15.63

Summary and Conclusions

The proliferative index by thymidine labeling is a relatively new and useful measurement with stage-independent, ER-independent prognostic power in breast cancer. It promises to be useful in selection of high risk patients both for stratification in controlled therapeutic trials and for selection of high risk patients for enrollment into therapeutic trials. Whether the proliferative index is best measured by DNA labeling or by flow cytometry is not yet established, but DNA labeling has the obvious advantage of specificity for the carcinoma and should be more reliable than derivation of percentage of S from DNA histograms. The DNA index is related to both the thymidine labeling index and the flow cytometric percentage of S and is a prognostic indicator, perhaps for that reason. It is not yet known whether the prognostic power of the DNA index is independent of its relationship to the proliferative rate. Further studies are indicated to establish the role of the proliferative index and the DNA index in selection of chemotherapeutic drugs or hormonal therapy. The association with high TLI with high chemotherapeutic remission rates in a survey of human cancers (Meyer, 1982) suggests that the proliferative index may be useful in selection of therapy for breast carcinomas.

REFERENCES

Allison, D. C., Ridolpho, P. F., Anderson, S., et al.: Variations in the (^{3}H) thymidine labeling of S-phase cells in solid mouse tumors. Cancer Res., *45*:6010, 1985.

Allison, D. C., Yuhas, J. M., Ridolpho, P. F., et al.: Cytophotometric measurement of the cellular DNA content of ^{3}H thymidine-labeled spheroids. Cell Tissue Kinet., *16*:237, 1983.

Anderson, T. J., Ferguson, D. J. P., and Raab, G. M.: Cell turnover in the "resting" human breast: Influence of parity, contraceptive pill, age and laterality. Br. J. Cancer, *46*:376, 1982.

Ashikari, R., Huvos, A. G., Urban, J. A., et al.: Infiltrating lobular carcinoma of the breast. Cancer, *31*:110, 1973.

Atkin, N. B.: Modal deoxyribonucleic acid value and survival in carcinoma of the breast. Br. Med. J., *1*:271, 1972.

Auer, G. U., Caspersson, T. O., Gustafsson, S. A., et al.: Relationship between nuclear DNA distribution and estrogen receptors in human mammary carcinomas. Anal. Quant. Cytol., *2*:280, 1980*a*.

Auer, G. U., Caspersson, T. O., and Wallgren, A. S.: DNA content and survival in mammary carcinoma. Anal. Quant. Cytol., *2*:161, 1980*b*.

Baisch, H., Beck, H. P., Christensen, I. J., et al.: A comparison of mathematical methods for the analysis of DNA histograms obtained by flow cytometry. Cell Tissue Kinet., *15*:235, 1982.

Barlogie, B., Raber, M. N., Schumann, J., et al.: Flow cytometry in clinical cancer research. Cancer Res., *43*:3982, 1983.

Baserga, R., Hennegar, G. C., and Kisieleski, W. E.: Uptake of tritiated thymidine by human tumors in vivo. Lab. Invest., *11*:360, 1962.

Berg, J. W., and Robbins, G. F.: Factors influencing long and short term survival of breast cancer patients. Surg. Gynecol. Obstet., *122*:1311, 1966.

Bertuzzi, A., Diadone, M. G., Di Fronzo, G., et al.: Relationship among estrogen receptors, proliferative activity and menopausal status in breast cancer. Breast Cancer Res. Treat., *1*:253, 1981.

Bichel, P., Poulsen, H. S., and Andersen, J.: Estrogen receptor content and ploidy of human mammary carcinoma. Cancer, *50*:1771, 1982.

Bloom, H. J. G., and Richardson, W. W.: Histologic grading and prognosis in breast cancer. Br. J. Cancer, *11*:359, 1957.

Bose, A. D., Ridolpho, P., and Meyne, J.: Lightly [^{3}H] TdR-labeled bone marrow cells are in G_1-G_2 (Abstract). Cell Tissue Kinet., *17*:669, 1984.

Braylan, R. D.: Flow cytometry. Arch. Pathol. Lab. Med., *107*:1, 1983.

Chapman, J. D.: Hypoxic sensitizers. Implications for radiation therapy. N. Engl. J. Med., *301*:1429, 1979.

Chassevent, A., Daver, A., Bertrand, G., et al.: Comparative flow DNA analysis of different cell suspensions in breast carcinoma. Cytometry, *5*:263, 1984.

Chavaudra, N., and Malaise, E. P.: In vitro incorporation of [^{3}H]TdR in human and murine solid tumors. Influence of 5-fluorouracil and/or hyperbaric oxygen on special distribution of labelling. Cell Tissue Kinet., *12*:597, 1979.

Clarkson, B., Ota, K., Ohkita, T., et al.: Kinetics of proliferation of cancer cells in neoplastic effusions in man. Cancer, *18*:1189, 1965.

Coninx, P., Liataud-Roger, F., Bousseau, A., et al.: Accumulation of noncycling cells with a G_2-DNA content in ageing solid tumors. Cell Tissue Kinet., 16:505, 1983.

Cooke, T., George, D., Maynard, P., et al.: Hormone receptors and cell kinetics in breast cancer (Abstract). Cancer Treat. Rep., 63:1190, 1979.

Cornelisse, C. J., de Koning, C. T., Moolenaar, A. J., et al.: Image and flow cytometric analysis of DNA content in breast cancer. Relation to estrogen receptor content and lymph node involvement. Anal. Quant. Cytol., 6:9, 1984.

Coulson, P. B., Thornthwaite, J. T., Wooley, T. W., et al.: Prognostic indicators including DNA histogram type, receptor content and staging related to human breast cancer patient survival. Cancer Res., 44:4187, 1984.

Culpin, D., and Morris, V. B.: Pattern of DNA synthesis and its effect on the classification of cells by flow cytometry. Cell Tissue Kinet., 18:1, 1985.

Darzynkiewicz, Z., Traganos, F., and Melamed, M. R.: New cell cycle compartments identified by multiparameter flow cytometry. Cytometry, 1:98, 1980.

Dean, P. N., Gray, J. W., and Dolbeare, F. A.: The interpretation and misinterpretation of DNA distributions measured by flow cytometry. Cytometry, 3:188, 1982.

Dell 'Orco, R. T.: Maintenance of human diploid fibroblasts as arrested populations. Fed. Proc., 33:1969, 1974.

Denekamp, J., and Kallman, R. F.: In vitro and in vivo labeling of animal tumours with tritiated thymidine. Cell Tissue Kinet., 6:217, 1973.

Dormer, P., Brinkmann, W., Born, R., et al.: Rate and time of DNA synthesis of individual Chinese hamster cells. Cell Tissue Kinet., 8:399, 1975.

Ellward, J., and Dormer, P.: Effect of 5-fluoro-2'-deoxyuridine (FdUrd) on 5-bromo-2'-deoxyuridine (BrdUrd) incorporation into DNA measured with a monoclonal BrdUrd antibody and by the BrdUrd/Hoechst quenching effect. Cytometry, 6:513, 1985.

Ewers, S.-B., Langstrom, E., Baldetorp, B., et al.: Flow-cytometric DNA analysis in primary breast carcinomas and clinicopathological correlations. Cytometry, 5:408, 1984.

Fabrinkant, J. I., Wisseman, C. L., III, and Vitak, M. J.: The kinetics of cellular proliferation in normal and malignant tissues. II. An in vitro method for incorporation of tritiated thymidine in human tissues. Radiology, 92:1309, 1969.

Fisher, E. R., Gregorio, R. M., and Fisher, B.: The pathology of invasive breast cancer: A syllabus derived from the findings of the National Surgical Adjuvant Breast Project (Protocol No. 4). Cancer, 36:1, 1975.

Fossa, S. D., Marton, P. F., Knudsen, O. S., et al.: Nuclear Feulgen DNA-content and nuclear size in human breast carcinoma. Hum. Pathol., 13:626, 1982.

Gentili, C., Sanfilippo, O., and Silvestrini, R.: Cell proliferation in relation to clinical features and relapse in breast cancers. Cancer, 48:974, 1981.

Haag, D., Feichter, G., Goerttler, K., et al.: Influence of systematic errors on the evaluation of the S phase portions from DNA distributions of solid tumors as shown for 328 breast carcinomas. Cytometry, 8:377, 1987.

Haag, D., Goerttler, K., and Tschahargane, C.: The proliferative index (PI) of human breast cancer as obtained by flow cytometry. Pathol. Res. Pract., 178:315, 1984.

Hamilton, E., and Dobbin, J.: [^{3}H]thymidine labels less than half of the DNA-synthesizing cells in the mouse tumor, carcinoma NT. Cell Tissue Kinet., 15:405, 1982.

Hamilton, E., and Dobbin, J.: The percentage labelled mitoses technique shows the mean cell cycle time to be half its true value in carcinoma NT. I. [^{3}H]thymidine and vincristine studies. Cell Tissue Kinet., 16:473, 1983.

Hamilton, E., Dobbin, J., and Kummermehr, J.: The relationship between the flash labelling index and the per cent S-phase cells in mouse tumors (Abstract). Cell Tissue Kinet., 17:298, 1984.

Hart, W. R., Bauer, R. C., and Oberman, H. A.: Cystosarcoma phyllodes. A clinicopathologic study of twenty-six hypercellular periductal stromal tumors of the breast. Am. J. Clin. Pathol., 70:211, 1978.

Hartviet, F.: Medullary carcinoma of the breast. Type I and type III tumors. Acta Pathol. Microbiol. Scand. A., 82:319, 1974.

Hedley, D. W., Rugg, C. A., Alun, B. P., et al.: Influence of cellular DNA content on disease-free survival of stage II breast cancer patients. Cancer Res., 44:5395, 1984.

Heidelberger, C.: Pyrimidine and pyrimidine nucleoside antimetabolites. In Holland, J. F., and Frei, E., III (Eds.): Cancer Medicine. 2nd Ed. Philadelphia, Lea & Febiger, 1982, p 801.

Hoffman, J., and Post, J.: In vivo studies of DNA synthesis in human normal and tumor cells. Cancer Res., 27:898, 1967.

Howard, A., and Pelc, S. R.: Nuclear incorporation of ^{32}P as demonstrated by autoradiographs. Exp. Cell Res., 2:178, 1951.

Jones, B., and Camplejohn, R. S.: Stathmokinetic measurement of tumor cell proliferation in relation to vascular proximity. Cell Tissue Kinet., 16:351, 1983.

Kempson, R. L., and Bari, W.: Uterine sarcomas. Classification, diagnosis and prognosis. Hum. Pathol., 1:331, 1970.

Kennedy, K. A., Teicher, B. A., Rockwell, S., et al.: The hypoxic tumor cell: A target for selective cancer chemotherapy. Biochem. Pharmacol., 29:1, 1980.

Kute, T. E., Muss, H. B., Anderson, D., et al.: Relationship of steroid receptor, cell kinetics and clinical status in patients with breast cancer. Cancer Res., 41:3524, 1981.

Laerum, O. D., and Farsund, T.: Clinical application of flow cytometry: A review. Cytometry, 2:1, 1981.

Lajtha, L. G.: Bone marrow cell metabolism. Physiol. Rev., 37:50, 1957.

Landry, J., Freyer, J. K. P., and Sutherland, R. M.: A model for the growth of multicellular spheroids. Cell Tissue Kinet., 15:585, 1982.

Laster, W. R., Jr., Mayo, J. G., Simpson-Herren, L., et al.: Success and failure in the treatment of solid tumors. II. Kinetic parameters and "cell cure" of moderately advanced carcinoma 755. Cancer Chemother. Rep., 53:169, 1969.

Lelle, R. J., Heidenreich, W., Stauch, G., et al.: The correlation of growth fractions with histologic grading and lymph node status in human mammary carcinoma. Cancer, 59:83, 1987.

McDivitt, R. W., Stone, K. R., and Meyer, J. S.: A method for dissociation of viable human breast cancer cells that produces flow cytometric kinetic information similar to that obtained by thymidine labeling. Cancer Res., 44:2628, 1984.

McDivitt, R. W., Stone, K. R., Craig, R. B., et al.: A comparison of human breast cancer cell kinetics measured by flow cytometry and thymidine labeling. Lab. Invest., 52:287, 1985.

McDivitt, R. W., Stone, K. R., Craig, R. B., et al.: A

proposed classification of breast carcinoma based on kinetic information. Cancer, 57:269, 1986.

McGurrin, J. F., Doria, M. I., Dawson, P. J., et al.: Assessment of tumor cell kinetics by immunohistochemistry in carcinoma of breast. Cancer, 59:1744, 1987.

Masters, J. R. W., Drive, J. O., and Scarisbrick, J. J.: Cyclical variations in DNA synthesis in human breast epithelium. JNCI, 58:1263, 1977.

Maurer, H. R.: Potential pitfalls of [^{3}H] thymidine techniques to measure cell proliferation. Cell Tissue Kinet., 14:111, 1981.

Mendelsohn, M. L.: The growth fraction: A new concept applied to tumors. Science, 132:1496, 1960.

Mendelsohn, M. L.: Autoradiographic analysis of cell proliferation in spontaneous breast cancer of C3H mouse. III. The growth fraction. JNCI, 28:1015, 1962.

Mendelsohn, M. L., and Takahashi, M.: A critical evaluation of the fraction of labeled mitoses method as applied to the analysis of tumor and other cell cycles. In Baserga, R. (Ed.): The Cell Cycle and Cancer. New York, Dekker, 1971, p. 58.

Meyer, J. S.: Cell proliferation in normal human breast ducts, fibroadenomas, and other ductal hyperplasia measured by nuclear labeling with tritiated thymidine. Hum. Pathol., 8:67, 1977.

Meyer, J. S.: Growth and cell kinetic measurements in human tumors. Pathol. Annu., 16(Part 2):53, 1981.

Meyer, J. S.: Potential value of cell kinetics in management of cancers of unknown origin. Semin. Oncol., 9:513, 1982.

Meyer, J. S.: Cell kinetics of histologic variants of in situ breast carcinoma. Breast Cancer Res. Treat., 7:171, 1986.

Meyer, J. S., and Bauer, W. C.: In vitro determination of tritiated thymidine labeling index (LI). Cancer, 36:1374, 1975.

Meyer, J. S., Bauer, W. C., and Rao, B. R.: Subpopulations of breast carcinoma defined by S-phase fraction, morphology, and estrogen receptor content. Lab. Invest., 39:225, 1978.

Meyer, J. S., and Connor, R. E.: In vitro labeling of solid tissues with tritiated thymidine for autoradiographic detection of S-phase nuclei. Stain Technol., 52:185, 1977.

Meyer, J. S., and Connor, R. E.: Cell proliferation in fibrocystic disease and postmenopausal breast ducts measured by thymidine labeling. Cancer, 50:746, 1985.

Meyer, J. S., and Facher, R.: Thymidine labeling index of human breast carcinoma. Enhancement of in vitro labeling by 5-fluorouracil and 5-fluoro-2'-deoxyuridine. Cancer, 39:2524, 1977.

Meyer, J. S., Friedman, E., McCrate, M. M., et al.: Prediction of early course of breast carcinoma by thymidine labeling. Cancer, 51:1879, 1983.

Meyer, J. S., and Hixon, B.: Advanced stage and early relapse of breast carcinomas associated with high thymidine labeling indices. Cancer Res., 39:4042, 1979.

Meyer, J. S., and Lee, J. V.: S-phase fraction of breast carcinoma in relapse: Relationships of remission-duration, estrogen receptor content, therapeutic responsiveness, and duration of survival. Cancer Res., 40:1890, 1980.

Meyer, J. S., McDivitt, R. W., Stone, K. R., et al.: Practical breast carcinoma cell kinetics: Review and update. Breast Cancer Res. Treat., 4:79, 1984a.

Meyer, J. S., Micko, S., Craver, J. L., et al.: DNA flow cytometry of breast carcinoma after acetic-acid fixation. Cell Tissue Kinet., 17:185, 1984b.

Meyer, J. S., Prey, M. U., Babcock, D. S., et al.: Breast carcinoma cell kinetics, morphology, stage and host characteristics; a thymidine labeling study. Lab. Invest., 54:41, 1986.

Meyer, J. S., Rao, B. R., Stevens, S. C., et al.: Low incidence of estrogen receptor in breast carcinomas with rapid rates of cellular replication. Cancer, 40:2290, 1977.

Moulder, J. E., and Rockwell, S.: Hypoxic fractions of solid tumors: Experimental techniques, methods of analysis, and a survey of existing data. Int. J. Radiat. Oncol. Biol. Phys., 10:695, 1984.

Muirhead, K. A., Horan, P. K., and Poste, G.: Flow cytometry: Present and future. Bio/Technology, 3:337, 1985.

Moran, R., Black, M., Alpert, L., et al.: Correlation of cell-cycle kinetics, hormone receptors, histopathology and nodal status in human breast cancer. Cancer, 54:1586, 1984.

Norris, H. J., and Taylor, H. B.: Relationship of histological features to behavior of cystosarcoma phyllodes: Analysis of ninety-four cases. Cancer, 20:2090, 1967.

Olszewski, W., Darzynkiewicz, Z., Rosen, P. P., et al.: Flow cytometry of breast carcinoma. I. Relation of DNA ploidy level to histology and estrogen receptor. Cancer, 48:980, 1981a.

Olszewski, W., Darzynkiewicz, Z., Rosen, P. P., et al.: Flow cytometry of breast carcinoma. II. Relation of tumor cell cycle distribution in histology and estrogen receptor. Cancer, 48:985, 1981b.

Parl, F. F., and Dupont, W. D.: A retrospective cohort study of histologic risk factors in breast cancer patients. Cancer, 50:2410, 1982.

Pietruszka, M., and Barnes, L.: Cytosarcoma phyllodes. A clinicopathologic analysis of 42 cases. Cancer, 41:1974, 1978.

Post, J., Sklarew, R. H., and Hoffman, J.: The proliferative patterns of human breast cancer cells in vivo. Cancer, 39:1500, 1977.

Quastler, H., and Sherman, F. G.: Cell population kinetics in the intestinal epithelium of the mouse. Exp. Cell Res., 17:420, 1959.

Raber, M. N., Barlogie, B., Latreille, J., et al.: Ploidy, proliferative activity and estrogen receptor content in human breast cancer. Cytometry, 3:36, 1982.

Rajewsky, M. F.: In vitro studies of cell proliferation in tumors. II. Characteristics of a standardized in vitro system for measurement of ^{3}H-thymidine incorporation into tissue explants. Eur. J. Cancer, 1:281, 1965.

Ridolfi, R. L., Rosen, P. P., Port, A., et al: Medullary carcinoma of the breast. A clinicopathologic study with 10 year follow-up. Cancer, 40:1365, 1977.

Rockwell, S.: Hypoxic cells as targets for cancer chemotherapy. In Cheng, Y.-C., Goz, B., and Minkoff, M. (Eds.). Development of Target-Oriented Anticancer Drugs. New York, Raven Press, 1983, p. 157.

Rockwell, S., Kallman, R. F., and Fajardo, L. F.: Characteristics of a serially transplanted mouse mammary tumor and its tissue culture-adapted derivative. JNCI, 49:735, 1972.

Rubini, J. R., Wescott, E., and Keller, S.: In vitro DNA labeling of bone marrow and leukemic blood leukocytes with tritiated thymidine. II. H^3 thymidine biochemistry in vitro. J. Lab. Clin. Med., 68:566, 1966.

Russell, W. O., Cohen, J., Enzinger, F., et al.: A clinical

and pathological staging system for soft tissue sarcomas. Cancer, 40:1562, 1977.

Sauerboern, R., Balmain, A., Goerttler, K., et al: On the existence of "arrested G_2 cells" in mouse epidermis. Cell Tissue Kinet., 11:291, 1978.

Schabel, F. M., Jr.: Concepts for systemic treatment of micrometastases. Cancer, 35:15, 1975.

Schiffer, L. M., Braunschweiger, P. G., Stragand, J. J., et al.: The cell kinetics of human mammary cancers. Cancer, 43:1707, 1979.

Shapiro, H.: Practical Flow Cytometry. New York, Alan R. Liss, 1985.

Sheck, L. E., Muirhead, K. A., and Horan, P.: Evaluation of the S-phase distribution of flow cytometric DNA histograms by autoradiography and computer algorithms. Cytometry, 1:109, 1980.

Shirakawa, S., Luce, J. I., Tannock, I., et al.: Cell proliferation in human melanoma. J. Clin. Invest., 49:1188, 1970.

Silvestrini, R., Diadone, M. G., and Di Fronzo, G.: Relationship between proliferative activity and estrogen receptors in breast cancer. Cancer, 44:665, 1979.

Silvestrini, R., Daidone, M. G., Di Fronzo, G., et al.: Prognostic implication of labeling index versus estrogen receptors and tumor size in node-negative breast cancer. Breast Cancer Res. Treat., 7:161, 1986.

Silvestrini, R., Daidone, M. G., and Gasparini, G.: Cell kinetics as a prognostic marker in node-negative breast cancer. Cancer, 56:1982, 1985.

Sisken, J. E., Bonner, S. V., Grasch, B. D., et al.: Alterations in metaphase durations in cells derived from human tumours. Cell Tissue Kinet., 18:137, 1985.

Skipper, H. E., and Schabel, F. M., Jr.: Quantitative and cytokinetic studies in experimental tumor systems. In Holland, J. F., and Frei, E., III (Eds.): Cancer Medicine. Philadelphia, Lea & Febiger, 1982.

Sklarew, R. J., Hoffman, J., and Post, J.: A rapid in vitro method for measuring cell proliferation in human breast cancer. Cancer, 40:2299, 1977.

Steel, G. G.: Cell loss as a factor in the growth of human tumours. Eur. J. Cancer, 3:381, 1967.

Steel, G. G.: Growth kinetics of tumours. Oxford, England, Clarendon Press, 1977.

Steel, G. G., and Bensted, J. P. M.: *In vitro* studies of proliferation in tumors. I. Critical appraisal of methods and theoretical considerations. Eur. J. Cancer, 1:275, 1965.

Stout, A. P.: Fibrosarcoma. The malignant tumor of fibroblasts. Cancer, 1:30, 1948.

Straus, M. J., and Moran, R. E.: Cell cycle parameters in human solid tumors. Cancer, 40:1453, 1977.

Straus, M. J., and Moran, R. E.: The cell cycle kinetics of human breast cancer. Cancer, 46:2634, 1980.

Straus, M. J., Moran, R., Muller, R. E., et al.: Estrogen receptor heterogeneity and the relationship between estrogen receptor and the tritiated thymidine labeling index in human breast cancer. Oncology, 39:197, 1982.

Suit, H. D., and Shalek, R. J.: Response of anoxic C3H mouse mammary carcinoma isotransplants (1–35 mm^3) to X irradiation. JNCI, 31:479, 1963.

Tannock, I. F.: The relation between cell proliferation and the vascular system in a transplanted mouse mammary tumor. Br. J. Cancer, 22:258, 1968.

Taylor, I. W., Musgroove, E. A., Friedlander, M. L., et al.: The influence of age on the DNA ploidy levels of breast tumors. Eur. J. Cancer Clin. Oncol., 19:623, 1983.

Taylor, J. H., Woods, P. S., and Hughes, W. L.: The organization and duplication of chromosomes using tritium-labeled thymidine. Proc. Natl. Acad. Sci. USA, 43:122, 1957.

Terz, J. J., Curutchet, H. P., Lawrence, W., Jr.: Analysis of the cycling and noncycling cell population of human solid tumors. Cancer, 40:1462, 1977.

Tribukait, B.: Clinical DNA flow cytometry. Med. Oncol. Tumor Pharmacother., 1:211, 1984.

Trowell, D. A.: The culture of lymph nodes *in vitro*. Exp. Cell Res., 3:79, 1952.

Tubiana, M., Chauvel, P., Ranaud, A., et al.: Vitesse de croissance et histoire naturelle du cancer du sein. Bull. Cancer, 62:341, 1975.

Tubiana, M., Pejovic, M. H., Chavaudra, N., et al.: The long-term prognostic significance of the thymidine labelling index in breast cancer. Int. J. Cancer, 33:441, 1984.

Vogel, P. M., Georgiade, N. G. Fetter, B. F., et al.: The correlation of histologic changes in the human breast with the menstrual cycle. Am. J. Pathol., 104:23, 1981.

Wallgren, A., Silfversward, C., and Eklund, G.: Prognostic factors in breast cancer. Acta Radiol. (Ther.), 15:1, 1976.

Wibe, E., Lindmo, T., and Kaalhus, O.: Cell kinetic characteristics in different parts of multicellular spheroids of human origin. Cell Tissue Kinet., 14:639, 1981.

Wimber, D. E., and Quastler, H.: A ^{14}C- and ^{3}H-thymidine double labelling technique in the study of cell proliferation in *Tradescantia* root tips. Exp. Cell Res., 30:8, 1963.

CHAPTER 10

JOHN S. SPRATT
JOHN A. SPRATT

Growth Rates

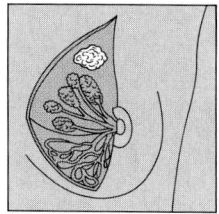

The purpose of this chapter is to review the growth kinetics of human mammary cancer. Growth is a characteristic of all true cancers, and the rate of growth is a fundamental determinant of the time required for any cancer to reach threshold size, size large enough to be detected or size large enough to produce symptoms, or to reach lethal proportions. Cancer development is at least a two-step process. First, the normal cell is "immortalized" and is capable of dividing indefinitely in tissue culture without ever becoming a fully differentiated or mature cell. Conversion to a cancer cell occurs through induction by chemical carcinogens or by certain oncogenes. The second change involves promotion of growth in the immortalized cell to the disorganized structure of cancer. Both suppression and enhancement occur at the molecular level. Suppression and cytodifferentiation of immortalized cells that are constantly replicating is an intense area of cytokinetic research, whose findings will have significant implications on future cancer prevention and treatment. However, this work has reached a level of only limited clinical application. Clinicians are encountering only the end results of these molecular processes on the actual growth of human breast cancers. This basic information is well advanced and essential for understanding the behavior of breast cancer in vivo. Before reviewing actual data, the principles and terminology of cytokinetics need to be summarized.

To appreciate the geometric perspective of cancer growth requires a perspective of the magnitude of changes that occur in size when a geometric or exponential variable changes. The double helix of DNA would fit in a box that was about 10^{-18} m^2; the nucleus of a cell, in a box 10^{-16} m^2; a blood cell in an arteriole, in a box 10^{-15} m^2. In comparison, a person could easily fit in a box that was 10^0 m^2, and the human hand, in a box that was 10^{-1} m^2.

An adult human is composed of 10^{13} cells. A cancer 1 cm^3 contains approximately 10^9 cells. Death from cancer can usually be expected with a tumor burden of 10^{12} cells (equivalent to 2^{40} cells or 40 net generations). Occasionally a cancer will exceed this, but there will always be a certain proportion of cancer cells to host cells which, if exceeded, will lead to death of the individual. The upper limit of this lethal proportion is on the order of 10^{12} to 10^{13} cells, or one tenth of the body cell composition. This would be less than 10 per cent of body weight when extracellular mass is considered. Critical or less critical locations for cancer cells allow for some variance in the lethal mass.

In many scientific discussions, powers of two rather than powers of ten are used. The following relationship permits conversion between the two powers:

$$(1) \qquad 10^x = 2^y,$$

$$(2) \qquad x \ln 10 = y \ln 2,$$

$$(3) \qquad y = \frac{x \ln 10}{\ln 2} \qquad x = \frac{y \ln 2}{\ln 10}$$

Most human cancer cells undergo binary division, then grow to a certain size or a certain age and repeat the process. In a variety of circumstances, subsets of cells may become nonproliferating. Growth is a multiplicative or geometric increase in proliferating cells; random errors in such a system are to be expected. Cell death is a prominent phenomenon in growing cancers. In the clinical arena, net accumulations of cells are observed.

The cell cycle can be divided into four phases: the presynthetic (G_1), the DNA synthesis (S), the postsynthetic (G_2), and the mitotic (M). M time, the shortest segment of the cycle, may be regarded as the fourth phase of the cell reproductive cycle or as the brief interval in the cycle when two daughter cells appear. The time a cell spends in each phase is subject to biologic variation that leads to a frequency distribution of cycle times that Steel (1967, 1972) considered normal, lognormal, gamma, or other.

The relationship between the mitotic index (MI) and tissue growth measurement was considered by Hoffman (1949). MI is defined as the ratio of the number of cells containing mitotic figures (m) to the total number of cells counted (N). The index m/N is proportional to the ratio of the time in mitosis (T) and the cell doubling time or cell cycle time (t_c). The duration of the intermitotic interval can be highly variable, affecting the value of t_c proportionately. T is also susceptible to considerable variation. These relative changes in relationships have limited the ability of MI to quantify growth rates accurately. However, correlations between the MI and the aggressiveness of breast cancer have been shown.

Parl and Dupont (1982) concluded that a high MI was the "*single* most important factor indicating high risk for death from cancer." Patients whose breast cancers had a high MI had a standardized mortality ratio (SMR) 2.7 times the mortality of the base population studied. Absence of tubule formation and nuclear anaplasia were associated with SMRs of 2.0 and 1.9 times the base rate. A combination of a high MI and an absence of tubule formation was associated with an SMR of 2.9, whereas a high MI and nuclear anaplasia had an SMR of 2.5. Well-defined tubules were associated with an SMR of 0.2; when combined with a low MI, the SMR was only 0.17. Thus, although the MI is only a crude parameter for measuring growth rates, it nevertheless has great prognostic significance alone or in conjunction with other histopathologic variables. In Chapter 9 Meyer discussed the various relationships between the tritiated thymidine labeling of mitoses with various aspects of breast cancer. Meyer's reviews in Chapter 9 reported correlations between in vitro thymidine labeling indices (TLI) of S-phase cells and patient age, various staging and histopathologic characteristics, estrogen and progesterone assay levels, and survivorship. The TLI frequency distributions were consistently lognormal. Cancers associated with high TLIs are larger, exhibit more inflammatory cell reaction, consist of more undifferentiated histologic patterns and show greater nuclear anaplasia, and contain more necrosis. The higher TLIs were also associated with cancers that tended to be well circumscribed. The TLIs were not associated significantly with race, axillary lymph node status, or the invasion of lymphatics and blood capillaries. TLIs were higher in younger women than in older women and tended to be reciprocally related to estrogen and progesterone receptor assay values.

TLI was directly related to the intensity of inflammatory cell response around the cancer and to cell death. For Meyer and coworkers, this suggested that inflammatory cell response was a secondary phenomenon, possibly relating to cell death. They concluded that the TLI values were an important, possibly causative determinant of morphologic patterns. TLI is definitely associated with the modulation of the disease's progress but is a weak determinant of the probability that metastasis will occur.

Post and colleagues (1977) studied the proliferative patterns of human breast cancer cells in vivo and used intravenously administered tritiated thymidine (^{3}H-TdR) as a pulse and as a continuous label. Tumor cells engaged in DNA synthesis ranged from 4 to 11 per cent. The periods ranged from G_2 + (½M) and for DNA synthesis were estimated to be about 4 hr each. They also observed a wide range of intermitotic intervals.

The three principal parameters that determine the net rates of growth of cancer are the cell cycle time of proliferating cells, the proportion of cells proliferating, and the extent of cell loss. This cell loss comes from exfoliation, metastasis, or cell death (Spratt and Ackerman, 1961; Pearlman, 1976). The shedding of cells into the circulation and development of metastasis formation are stochastic processes that can be defined by mathematical models (McGuire et al., 1974). A very small percentage of all cancer cells that metastasize actually survive. As these models are better tested with data from human cancer, they will become essential to the planning of optimum therapy.

Recent data reaffirm the developmental process for early metastases from human breast cancer. A longitudinal evaluation of the association of tumor volume, status of the axillary lymph nodes and remote metastases has been analyzed for 2663 women with breast cancer (Atkinson et al., 1986). The sample was drawn from 4609 women with mammographically measurable tumors at initial diagnosis, who had no evidence of lymph node metastasis (76 per cent of the total). Distant metastases were defined as any cancer outside the breast and its regional lymph nodes (axillary, internal mammary, and supraclavicular). Tumor volume was calculated from the measurements of length and width obtained from the mammograms. Data were accessed between 1955 and 1979. Certain categories of breast cancer in a total population of breast cancers have probably been excluded: those surfacing in intervals between mammograms and those not visible on mammograms. The authors' own data suggest that these are the more virulent cancers. The second critical omission is the failure to convey the histopathologic characteristics of small cancers. Meyer describes the critical importance of this in Chapter 9.

The study by Atkinson and coworkers (1986) shows the extremes of kinetic and metastatic behavior in the population. There was an "extraordinarily large contribution to metastasis of very small tumors." The metastatic potential per cancer cell actually *decreased* with increasing size. These investigators concluded that very small primary cancers exhibit a propensity for rapid diversity with cloning of cell lines with high metastatic potential, as do tumors that are subject to strong selection pressure (Fidler and Hart, 1982). At the opposite extreme, over 20 per cent of the very largest cancers had not produced diagnosable metastases within 300 months of follow-up. "Large" is defined as a chordal dimension of 7.5 to 8 cm and a volume of 200 ml. The volume effect differed according to nodal status.

The simple relationship of a small, predetectable cancer to its source of nutrition has an unequivocal but incompletely measured impact on the rates of growth and the rapid appearance of deceleratory growth. When tumors grow as cords of cells, the cords generally appear around the capillaries. However, necrosis of the cord cells occurs whenever the distance from cells to capillary exceeds 200 μm. Tissue oxygen approaches zero at that distance (Tannock and Steel, 1969). Whenever V_2 carcinoma is implanted into the avascular vitreous, a neoplastic node evolves that develops a necrotic center when a nodal diameter of 0.5 mm is reached (Brem, 1976).

The mean distance of cells from their nearest blood vessel is greater for larger tumors. Cells in mitosis are closer to blood vessels, but even with higher vascular density, necrosis is common. Intact blood vessels are often seen in areas of necrosis. When red cells were labeled with chromium (^{51}Cr), few appeared in the blood vessels in necrotic regions, suggesting that necrosis and intravascular stasis were commonly associated. The cell's average distance from its nearest capillary was 100 μm for the smaller tumors and 170 μm for the larger ones.

The diffusion length for any nutrient is the distance from an isolated blood vessel at which the nutrient's concentration falls to zero (Breur et al., 1976). Gullino (personal communication, 1985) estimated that a spherical conglomerate of cells with a diameter of 300 to 400 μm would have trouble maintaining uniform cell survivorship if it were totally dependent on diffusion of oxygen and nutrients. Angiogenesis, therefore, becomes essential for the sustained growth of a cancer. With angiogenesis comes the avenue for metastasis.

Thus, cell loss accelerates as the tumor enlarges. The loss seems predetermined by the distance oxygen and other nutrients can diffuse through tissues. If the rate of diffusion cannot keep up with the demands of cell metabolism, central cell death occurs, producing a deceleratory influence on the net growth rate of the neoplasm (Gullino et al., 1967).

Geometric Relationships

The geometric relationships that occur as a cancer grows are defined as follows:

$$(4) \qquad N = 2^n$$

where N equals the number of cancer cells and n equals the number of net generations of cancer cells.

If the specific volume of a primary locus of cancer is known, the number of cells in the locus may be estimated crudely by dividing the volume by the approximate volume of a cell (10^{-6} mm^3). More concise estimates of N have been obtained in the laboratory.

Meyskens and colleagues (1984) provided an estimate of the cells of 38 diverse histologic types that grew in tissue culture. The colonies grew into shapes such as oblate spheroids. The relationship of cells to colony size fitted the following linear regression with a correlation coefficient of 0.92:

(5) ln (number of cells/colony) =
0.87 − 2.80 ln (colony cells axis) +
2.38 ln (colony axis)

This provided an accurate prediction of the total number of cells counted. Estimations of the total number of cells based on a spherical shape resulted in an overestimation of the number of cells.

Estimating the number of cells in a colony of cancer cells growing in vivo in humans cannot approach this accuracy. With the data available, we can only estimate orders of magnitude, and use equation 4. The method of Meyskens and coworkers lends itself to clonogenic assays of cells in tissue culture in humans, but it can be applied only to an excised cancer relatively free of noncancerous stroma.

Consistent with the foregoing observations, Heuser et al. (1979b) have shown that the xeromammographic dimensions of mammary cancer fit best those of a spheroid. In determining the volume, the geometric formula for calculating the volume of spheroids was used. For estimating the number of cells, the volume was divided by the volume of a single cell rounded off to 10^{-6} mm^3 (Heuser et al., 1979a). Cell numbers are discussed later in this chapter.

For various colonies of cancer cells, the spread in the cell cycle time has been measured. The geometric mean of this spread is the value usually quoted. Cell cycle time, measured by using tritiated thymidine to label DNA during its synthesis in mitosis, gives a wealth of information on the cytokinetics of both normal and neoplastic tissues (Steel, 1972). Additional and summarized cytokinetic terms and their relations are as follows:

t_c = cell cycle time.
t_s = duration of DNA synthesis of proliferating cells.
LI = the labeling index that defines the ratio of the number of cells that incorporate tritiated thymidine into DNA during mitosis over the total number of cells. The ratio is expressed as the percentage of cells in mitosis during the time period of thymidine incorporation. LI = $\mu\, t_s/t_c$ for proliferating cells, when DT is more than 19 days and μ, the constant for the equation, is in the range of 0.7 to 0.8.
DT_{pot} = potential doubling time or time required for the volume to double once in the absence of cell loss (i.e., when all dividing cells survive).
DT_{act} = actual doubling time or actual time required for a cancer to double its volume once.

The DT_{act} represents the net effect of all cytokinetic parameters. Cell loss is a major and variable factor and DT_{act} is of longer duration than DT_{pot}. DT_{act} frequently can be calculated from gross serial measurements of growing human cancer taken from radiographs or the direct measurement of tumor masses. A margin of error is always present in measuring growth rates, but if this margin stays relatively constant, its effect on calculated rates is minimal.

If cell loss is the major variable factor and DT_{act} is of longer duration than DT_{pot}, the relation between them can be defined for a parameter of the rate of cell loss, ρ (rho). Cell loss is defined as a fraction of the rate at which cells are entering mitosis. For a 100 per cent loss of new cells, DT_{act} would be static. The relation is indicated by the following equation:

(6) $$\rho = 1 - \frac{DT_{pot}}{DT_{act}}$$

The frequency distribution that best describes the frequency distribution of many cytokinetic parameters, as well as other characteristics of cancers and their hosts, is a normal frequency distribution of the logarithm of the variate. Such a distribution occurs whenever the random errors of the variate are geometric or logarithmic rather than arithmetic or linear (i.e., a product rather than a sum of random events).

All standard statistical tests applicable to the more commonly displayed arithmetic normal distribution can be applied (Spratt, 1969a). The probability that a frequency distribution is, in fact, lognormal can be calculated by the Kolmogovov-Smirnov test (Bradley, 1968).

Various growth equations express the pattern of growth within a cancer. The pattern is determined by the complex and changing interactions of variables that affect the division and accumulation of cancer cells. Descriptions of the more commonly observed growth equations follow.

Linear Growth Equation

A cancer growing linearly has its linear dimensions increased by a specific increment each day, regardless of its size. Examples include the Jensen's rat sarcoma (Mayneord, 1932) and some human lung cancers (Spratt and Spratt, 1976). This pattern is thought to occur when all cellular proliferation is restricted to the periphery of the cancer. The equation is as follows:

$$(7) \quad R = \frac{d_1 - d_0}{t}$$

where R = linear rate of change in the diameter, usually expressed as mm/day
d_0 = greatest chordal dimension; or, in the case of spherical tumors, the diameter at first observation
d_1 = greatest chordal dimension or diameter at second observation
t = time elapsing between measurement of d_0 and d_1.

If the rate of a single growth vector or radius is desired, R must be divided by 2.

Exponential Growth Equation

A cancer growing exponentially or geometrically has a randomly steady increase in volume, unit, or unit time. Any cell population increasing in number by the randomly steady binary division of cells with negligible or at least steady state cell loss would follow this equation. For an exponential increase in volume, the equations are as follows:

$$(8) \quad V_1 = V_0 e^{bt} \text{ or } d_1^3 = d_0^3 e^{bt}$$

$$(9) \quad b = \frac{\ln V_1 - \ln V_0}{t} \text{ or } b = \frac{3(\ln d_1 - \ln d_0)}{t}$$

$$(10) \quad DT_{act} = \frac{\ln 2}{b}$$

where $\ln 2 = 0.69315$
V_0 = volume at first measurement, expressed in mm^3
V_1 = volume at second measurement, expressed in mm^3
d_0 = diameter at first measurement, expressed in mm
d_1 = diameter at second measurement, expressed in mm

t = time in days elapsing between measurement of V_0 and V_1 or between d_0 and d_1
b = exponential growth constant with the dimension of mm^3/mm^3/day
$\ln$ = a prefix indicating the natural logarithm of the variate
e = base of the natural logarithm, 2.71828.

By moving the decimal point of b three places to the right, the constant becomes a measure of the number of new cells per 1000 existing cells per day. When b is divided into the natural logarithm of 2 (0.69315), the actual doubling time DT_{act} is obtained in days. When more than two measurements exist, the most suitable growth equation can be more accurately determined by the use of regression analysis.

Deceleratory and Gompertzian Growth Equations

The Gompertz equation provides one of many options for considering deceleratory growth (Gompertz, 1825). Very few tissues can sustain exponential growth indefinitely, and deceleration of growth rate with increasing size becomes a necessity. Skehan (1984) concluded that deceleratory growth has to be a relatively universal phenomenon. This phenomenon expresses itself grossly by gradually lengthening actual tumor volume doubling time (DT_{act}) with increasing tumor size. Decelerating growth is the most frequent growth pattern exhibited by metazoa. All of the mechanisms that mediate or control it are not known, but patterns of communication between cells are essential, though incompletely understood. In addition to the Gompertz equation, deceleratory growth in cancer systems has also been modeled by the inverse cube root (ratio of volume to surface area) and by logistic and simple power functions. The various growth models are given in Table 10–1.

The relationship between the specific growth rate (SGR) and DT_{act} occurs in successive pairs of data points or size measurements, which are separated by an observation time, T_{obs}.

$$(11) \quad SGR = 100[-1 + 2^{Tu(\ln[S2/S1])/(0.69315)\, T_{obs}}]$$

$$(12) \quad DT_{act} = 16.636/\ln(1 + 0.01\, SGR)$$

where Tu is the unit of time, one day.

Table 10–1. MATHEMATICAL MODELS OF CANCER GROWTH

Family of Equation	Value of Root (N)	Equations
1. Nth root	$N = 1$	$SGR = R(1 - S^N/K^N)$
2.	$1/2$	
3.	$1/3$	
4.	$1/4$	
5. Inverse Nth root	$N = -1$	$SGR = \theta(1 - K^{-N}S^N)$
6.	$-1/2$	
7.	$-1/3$	
8.	$-1/4$	
9. Nth power	$N = 2$	$SGR = R(1 - S^N/K^N)$
10.	3	
11.	4	
12. Inverse Nth power	$N = -2$	$SGR = \theta(1 - K^{-N}S^N)$
13.	-3	
14.	-4	
15. Gompertz		$SGR = G(\ln K - \ln S)$
16. Exponential decay		$SGR = Re^{-GS}$
17. Hyperbolic		$SGR^{1/2} = G(1 - [\ln S/\ln K])$
18. Simple power		$\ln SGR = \ln G - (1/b) \ln S$

SGR, Specific (to size) growth rate; R, SGR at infinitesimal size (single cell level); S, tumor size; θ, SGR at infinite size; K, final size attained by tumor; G,b, arbitrary rate coefficients.
Adapted from Skehan, P.: *In* Skehan, P., and Friedman, S. J. (Eds.): Growth, Cancer, and the Cell Cycle. Clifton, N. J., Humana Press, 1984, p. 323.

The units for DT_{act} with this relationship are calculated in hours. Three growth phases were identified: acceleratory (increasing SGR), exponential (constant SGR), and deceleratory (decreasing SGR). Using data from the literature, analysis was applied to 58 data bases for normal tissue growth and 49 data bases of neoplastic tissue growth. Table 10–1 gives a comparison of these analyses.

Cancer growth rates have significant chronologic implications for cancer behavior. Skehan's model (1984) considers the implications of growth rates to the growth rates of the tissue of origin and provides an explanation for the survival of mutant cells when cancers develop in metazoa.

Skehan (1984) observed that exponential growth is rarely observed in vivo. The pattern for normal tissue and cancer is one of nonexponential kinetics in which growth decelerates continuously with time. This results in a progressive increase in the length of the actual tissue doubling time with the passage of time and an increase in tumor size. Growth-inhibitory negative feedback is predominantly responsible for this. Skehan used a variety of equations to describe the growth of normal and neoplastic tissue (Table 10–2). He consistently observed that cancers do not grow faster than their tissues of origin and that organized tissue growth is required for the maintenance of phenotypic homogeneity in the cells of metazoa. When feedback controls and contact inhibition are lost, progressive phenotypic heterogeneity is tolerated and becomes a characteristic of a true cancer.

There are insignificant qualitative and quantitative differences between the growth of normal and neoplastic tissues. In Chapter 9, Meyer showed the existence of nearly identical TLIs for normal and cancerous breast tissue by age. Because the rates are basically the same, Skehan hypothesized that the error in

Table 10–2. COMPARISON OF THE GROWTH OF NORMAL AND NEOPLASTIC TISSUES

	Tissue Growth	
Characteristic	Normal	Neoplastic
Exclusively or predominantly deceleratory	Yes	Yes
Deceleration related to mass inhibition	Yes	Yes
Most of growth inhibition or deceleration occurs while tissue or tumor mass still quite small	Yes	Yes
Inverse Nth root equations constitute the family of growth equations providing the best fit to observed data; Nth power equations provide the poorest fit	Yes	Yes

Adapted from Skehan, P.: *In* Skehan, P., and Friedman, S. J. (Eds.): Growth, Cancer, and the Cell Cycle. Clifton, N. J., Humana Press, 1984, p. 323.

cancer growth lies in the failure of cell recognition and mass inhibition, not in the actual rates. Cell replication rates in cancerous and normal tissue are too similar for cancerous growth to be attributed to them. Tumors behave like new types of tissue with normal growth regulation policies and control mechanisms but have an altered "recognitive determinant" (Skehan, 1984). Some cancers could even be a disorder of tissue neogenesis. Growth spurts come with the loss of deceleratory feedback. Proponents of this theory consider that contemporary use of antiproliferative drugs may be valueless as well as counterproductive. These drugs generally fail to improve the prognosis of most solid neoplasms.

By applying the various deceleratory growth equations to various cancer growth data sets, Skehan found the best fits to be with equations 1, 2, and 13 in Table 10-1 ($\rho = 0.560 - 0.669$). Equations 4 and 15 of Table 10-1 were second best. The authors selected Equation 15 of Table 10-1, the Gompertzian equation, to evaluate the implications of deceleratory growth on a breast cancer growth data base. This equation is a specific deceleratory growth rate formula. It is the exact solution to the following two differential equations:

(13) $$\frac{dV}{dt} = \lambda V$$

(14) $$\frac{d\lambda}{dt} = \alpha \lambda$$

Equation 13 states that tumor growth rate is the product of relative growth rate and volume. This is what is seen in exponential growth, where λ is constant. In the second equation, relative growth rate is time dependent. Alpha, the rate of decay of the relative growth rate, is a constant.

The Gompertzian growth equation derives thus:

(15) $$V = V_0 e^{(1 - e^{\alpha t})\beta/\alpha}$$

The independent variables that describe a given curve are α and β. Comparative plots of Gompertzian and exponential growth curves are shown in Figure 10–1. A cancer following Gompertzian growth grows rapidly while small and more slowly as its size increases. It approaches a horizontal asymptote determined by a size ($V = V_{max}$ as $t \to \infty$) that it never exceeds. The curve exhibits a steady decrease in its actual growth rate as it approaches the asymptote. A nomogram showing the interrelatedness of tumor volume and diameter, net number of cell generations, net or actual doubling time, and tumor duration is provided in Figure 10–2.

As the relative growth rate is constantly decreasing, the doubling time is continuously increasing. The doubling time equation can be solved as a function of time (equation 16) or as a function of tumor size (equation 17):

(16) $$DT_{act} = \frac{-1}{\alpha} \ln\left(1 - \frac{\alpha}{\beta} \ln 2e^{\alpha t}\right),$$

for $t < t_{1/2}$

(17) $$DT_{act} = \frac{-1}{\alpha} \ln\left(1 - \frac{\ln 2}{\ln(V_{max}/V)}\right),$$

for $V < \frac{1}{2} V_{max}$.

Doubling time has meaning only for a tumor that is less than half its maximal size ($V < \frac{1}{2} V_{max}$).

The time necessary for a tumor to grow to half maximal size ($\frac{1}{2} V_{max}$) is as follows:

(18) $$t_{(1/2)} = \frac{1}{\alpha} \ln\left(\frac{\beta}{\alpha \ln 2}\right)$$

Irregular Growth

Irregular growth has no specific rate formula. Different segments of the curve may have varying growth patterns and rates. This growth may occur with episodes of necrosis, slough, infection, spontaneous regression, regression under treatment, and unexplained accelerations and decelerations of growth. Random errors in measurement would contribute to some of the "irregularity."

Data Sources

Basic data on the rates of growth of human mammary cancer have been obtained indirectly by roentgenography and from labeling indices on human breast cancer in vivo or in vitro, using breast cancer tissue slices, by the

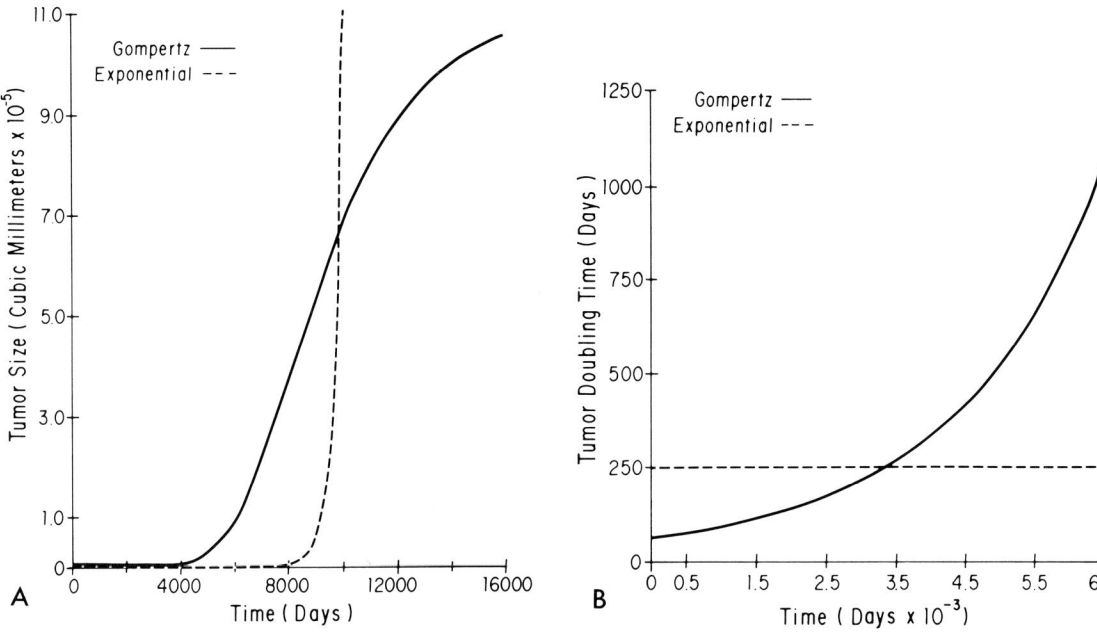
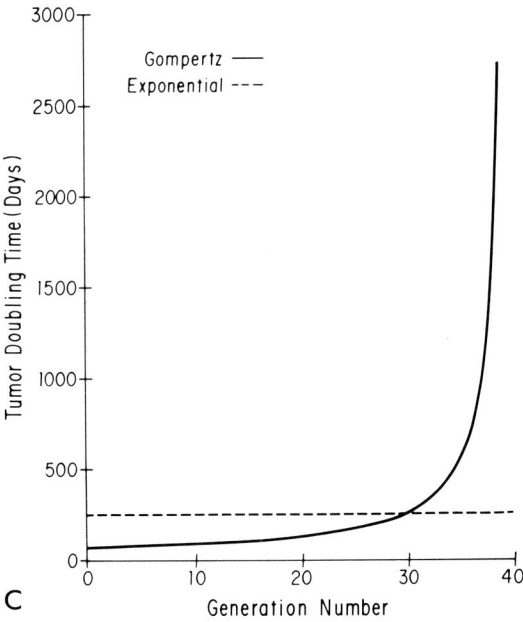

Figure 10–1. A–C, Graphic demonstration of the differences between exponential and Gompertzian growth with respect to tumor size and tumor duration (A), actual tumor volume doubling time and tumor duration (B), and actual tumor volume doubling time and the net number of tumor cell generation (C). (From Spratt, JA: Fitting deceleratory growth curves to human breast cancer data. Submitted for publication.)

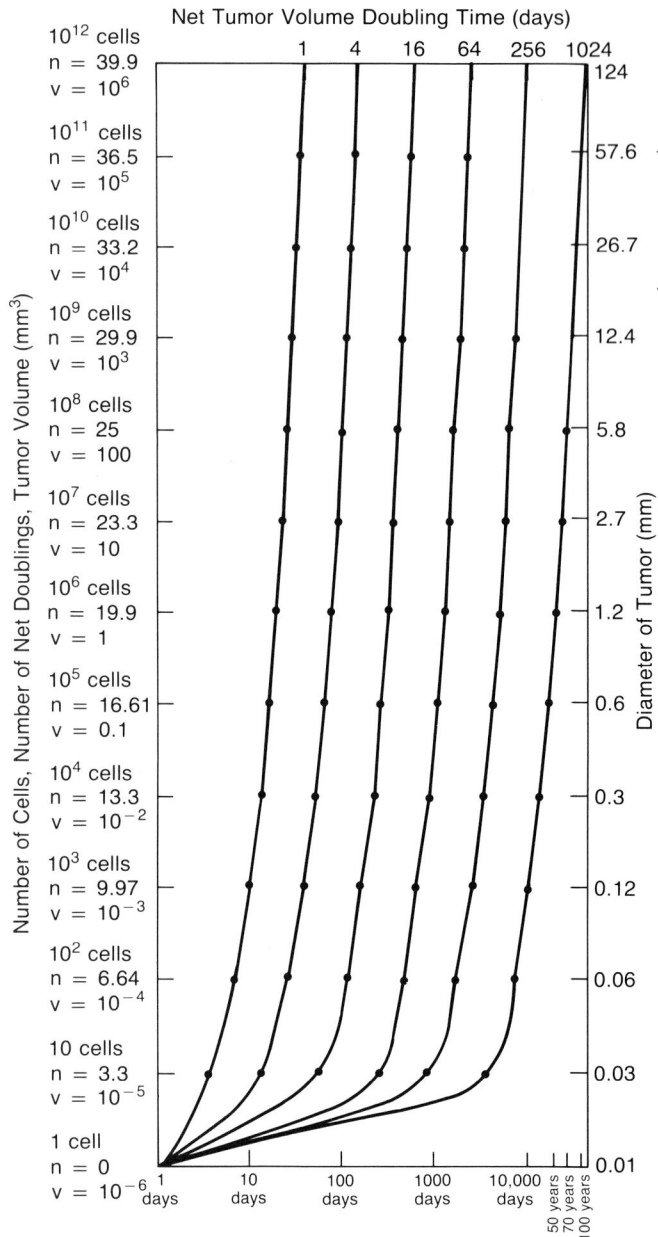

Figure 10-2. A nomogram showing the interrelations of number of cancer cells, net number of generations of cancer cells, tumor volume, tumor diameter, time elapsing from the inception of a cancer, and the net actual tumor volume doubling time (From Spratt, J. S., et al.: Geometry, growth rates, and duration of cancer and carcinoma *in situ* of the breast before detection by screening. Cancer Res., *46*:970, 1986. Reprinted by permission.)

incorporation of tritiated thymidine in the DNA of dividing cells. Direct measurements of skin and lymph node metastases have been made with calipers. A collection of growth curves derived from the measurement of pulmonary metastases from mammary cancer is given in Figure 10–3. These data were used to calculate the actual doubling times of the pulmonary metastases. The DT_{act} values are plotted in Figure 10–4. Mammograms have become a major source of data.

Data of this type generally form lognormal frequency distributions, but this cannot be shown unequivocally with the small sample sizes. The data and implications they might have on host survivorship, assuming both normal and lognormal frequency distributions, are given in Tables 10–3 through 10–7. These estimates also assume constant exponential growth based on doubling times measured after the cancer was large enough to measure grossly. Since this approach does not allow for

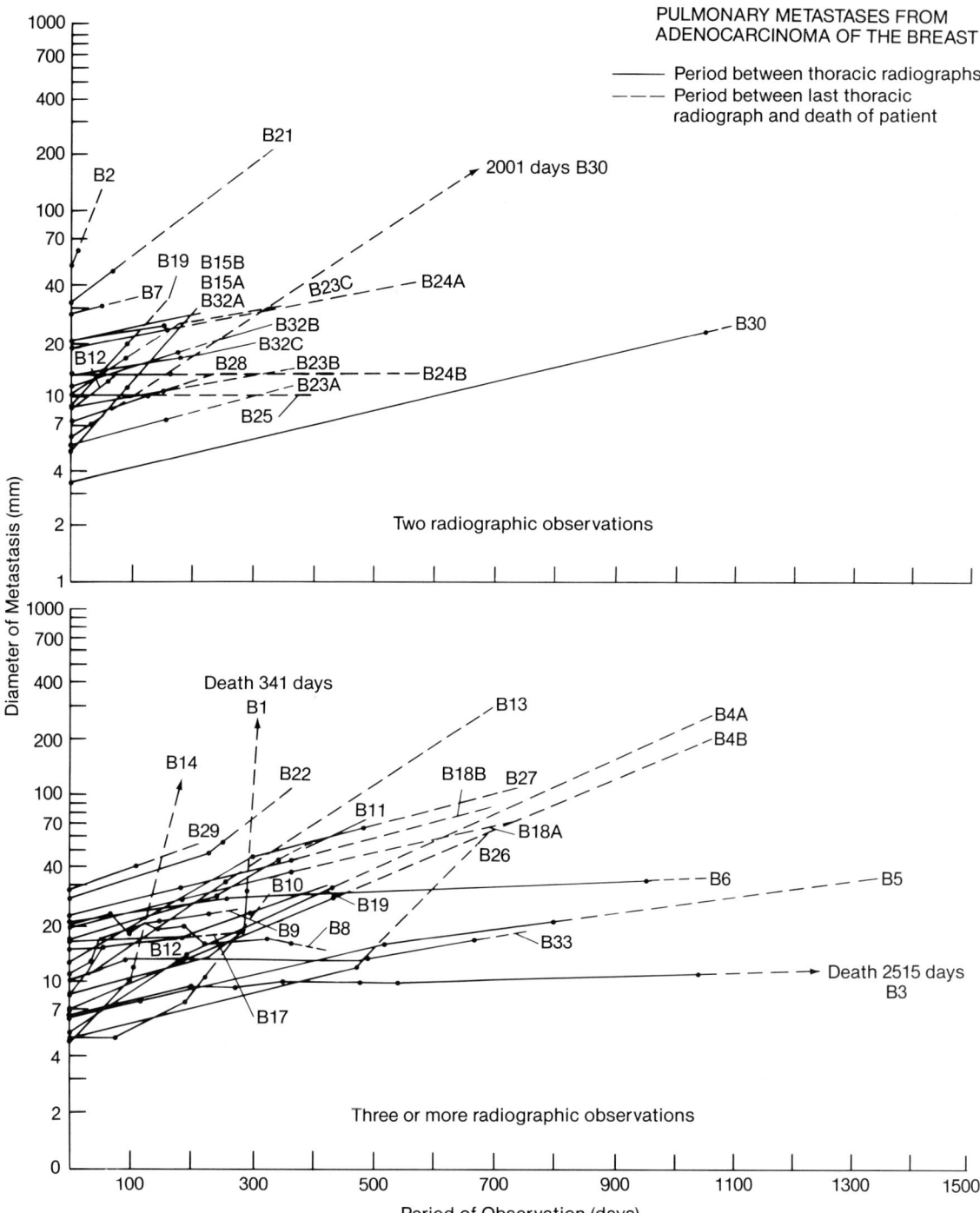

Figure 10–3. Each dot represents the measurement of the diameter of a special pulmonary metastasis from a breast cancer. The broken line beyond the last dot records the time between the last chest radiograph and the death of the host. These curves are for the fastest growing pulmonary metastasis in 29 different hosts. The frequency distribution of the growth rates was lognormal. The log mean (or linear median) doubling time (actual) was 82 days with a 99 per cent confidence range of 7 to 969 days. Equivalent exponential growth constant is 0.0085 with a 99 per cent confidence range from 0.0007 to 0.099. Moving the decimal point of these constants three places to the right gives the number of new breast cancer cells surviving each day per 1000 existing breast cancer cells, as varying from less than one to as many as 99 new cancer cells per 1000 existing cells per day. (From Spratt, J. S., and Spratt, T. L.: Rates of growth of pulmonary metastases and host survival. Ann. Surg., *159*:161, 1964. Reprinted with permission.)

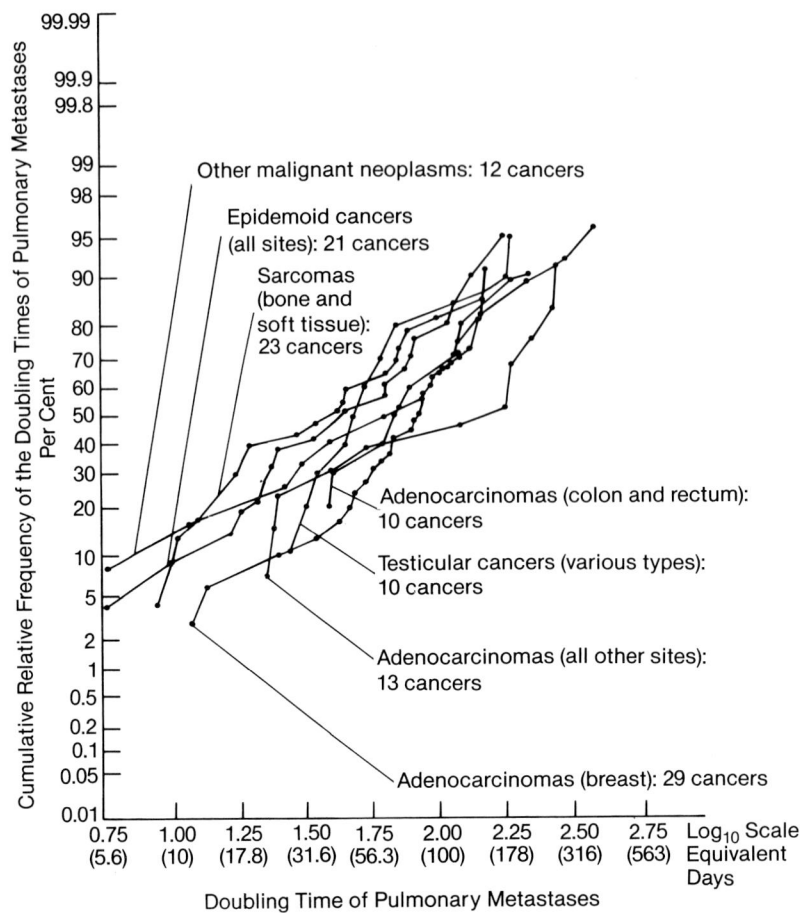

Figure 10–4. Accumulative relative frequency of the doubling times of pulmonary metastases from cancer of various sites, showing the comparative plot for metastatic adenocarcinoma of the breast. (From Spratt, J.S., and Spratt, T. L.: Rates of growth of pulmonary metastases and host survival. Ann. Surg., *159*:161, 1964. Reprinted with permission.)

Table 10–3. DOUBLING TIMES OF PRIMARY MAMMARY CANCERS OBSERVED BY MAMMOGRAPHY

Case Number	Observation Period (mo.)	Diameter at Operation (cm)	Doubling Time (days)	Natural Log of Doubling Time
1	6	2.0	23	3.1355
2	6	3.0	36	3.5835
3	12	3.0	37	3.6109
4	12	2.5	49	3.8918
5	23	2.0	57	4.0431
6	16	1.2	63	4.1431
7	20	3.2	75	4.3175
8	12	1.0	90	4.4998
9	20	0.4	120	4.7875
10	6	1.0	120	4.7875
11	30	0.8	130	4.8675
12	12	1.8	144	4.9698
13	12	2.0	144	4.9698
14	21	0.8	160	5.0752
15	30	0.6	180	5.1930
16	18	1.0	180	5.1930
17	54	2.0	200	5.2983
18	16	1.0	205	5.3230
19	6	0.7	209	5.3423

From Spratt, J. S., Kaltenbach, M. L., and Spratt, J. A.: Cytokinetic definition of acute and chronic cancer. Cancer Res., *37*:226, 1977. Reprinted with permission.

Table 10–4. CHARACTERISTICS OF THE FREQUENCY DISTRIBUTION OF THE ACTUAL DOUBLING TIMES (DT_{act}) OF PRIMARY MAMMARY CANCERS, ASSUMING LOGNORMALITY AND LINEAR NORMALITY

Deviation	Logarithmic		Linear (days)
	Logarithm	Days	
$+3\sigma$	6.6011	736	304
$+2\sigma$	5.9276	375	242
$+1\sigma$	5.2541	191	179
μ	4.5806	98	117
-1σ	3.9071	50	55
-2σ	3.2336	25	
-3σ	2.5601	13	

From Spratt, J. S., Kaltenbach, M. L., and Spratt, J. A.: Cytokinetic definition of acute and chronic breast cancer. Cancer Res., 37:226, 1977. Reprinted with permission.

rapid early growth and deceleration with time and size, the estimates are considered high.

Thermal properties of growing neoplasms have also been used as an indirect method of measuring tumor growth (Chato, 1980; Gautherie, 1980; Gullino, 1980; Eberhart et al., 1980). The theory and observations in the thermobiology of breast cancer and the differences between cancer and normal tissue formed the basis for promoting thermography as a diagnostic tool. These methods also confirm the greater sensitivity of breast cancer

Table 10–5. ACUTE AND CHRONIC SURVIVORSHIP IN DAYS AS CALCULATED FROM THE LOGNORMAL FREQUENCY DISTRIBUTION OF ACTUAL DOUBLING TIMES OF PRIMARY MAMMARY CANCERS

Probability of Surviving	Survivorship*
0.005 $(+3\sigma)$†	29,440
0.025 $(+2\sigma)$	15,000
0.158 $(+1\sigma)$	7640
0.500 (μ)	3920
0.842 (-1σ)	2000
0.975 (-2σ)	1000
0.995 (-3σ)	520

*These figures are calculated by multiplying the number of days in Table 10–4, column 3, by 40. Forty net doublings of a malignant clone of cells are estimated to produce a lethal mass of cancer cells. Thus, the time required to produce this lethal mass determines host survivorship.
†In parentheses μ = mean, σ = standard deviation about the mean.
From Spratt, J. S., Kaltenbach, M. L., and Spratt, J. A.: Cytokinetic definition of acute and chronic breast cancer. Cancer Res., 37:226, 1977. Reprinted with permission.

Table 10–6. ACUTE AND CHRONIC SURVIVORSHIP IN DAYS AS CALCULATED FROM THE LINEAR NORMAL FREQUENCY DISTRIBUTION OF ACTUAL DOUBLING TIMES OF PRIMARY MAMMARY CANCERS

Probability of Surviving	Survivorship*
0.005 $(+3\sigma)$†	12,160
0.025 $(+2\sigma)$	9680
0.158 $(+1\sigma)$	7160
0.500 (μ)	4680
0.842 (-1σ)	2200
0.975 (-2σ)	
0.995 (-3σ)	

*These figures are calculated by multiplying the number of days in Table 10–4, column 4, by 40.
†In parentheses μ = mean, σ = standard deviation about the mean.
From Spratt, J. S., Kaltenbach, M. L., and Spratt, J. A.: Cytokinetic definition of acute and chronic breast cancer. Cancer Res., 37:226, 1977. Reprinted with permission.

cells to heat compared with the thermal sensitivity of normal tissue. The combination of greater sensitivity of cancer cells to death from increased heat and the increase in temperature that occurs in a growing breast cancer provides one theoretical explanation for the high cell death rate in a growing cancer.

OBSERVATIONS OF ACTUAL DOUBLING TIMES

The first gross measurements of the rates of growth of primary breast cancers were provided by Gershon-Cohen and colleagues (1963). They studied 18 patients who had not

Table 10–7. ESTIMATED NUMBER OF DAYS ELAPSING BETWEEN THE INCEPTION OF A CLONE OF MAMMARY CANCER CELLS AND THE SMALLEST SIZE DISCERNIBLE BY MAMMOGRAPHY (ABOUT 22 DOUBLINGS)

Doubling Times from Table 10–4, Column 3	Table 10–4, Column 3 × 22
736	16,192
375	8250
191	4202
98	2156
50	1100
25	550
13	286

From Spratt, J. S., Kaltenbach, M. L., and Spratt, J. A.: Cytokinetic definition of acute and chronic breast cancer. Cancer Res., 37:226, 1977. Reprinted with permission.

had biopsies until two or more mammograms had been performed. Gross doubling times of primary mammary cancers were calculated. One case from the Cancer Research Center, Ellis Fischel State Cancer Hospital (EFSCH) was added (Tables 10–3 to 10–7). The median doubling time observed for 19 cases was 120 days, but it ranged from 23 to 209 days (Spratt et al., 1977).

Fournier and associates (1980) studied doubling times of 147 patients with primary breast cancers who were observed serially by mammography. Although unable to correlate the histologic characteristics of breast cancers with doubling times as measured by serial mammography, they did note that thermographic changes were more apt to be abnormal in faster growing breast cancers. Their measurements were based on multiple mammograms performed on 163 women; the longest period of observation of a single neoplasm was 11 years. The accuracy of their measurements varied ± 0.6 mm. The smallest cancer was 2 mm in diameter. They observed considerable variation with size, deceleration, regression, and nongrowth.

By 1982 Fournier and colleagues' data contained measurements and the dates for each case on tumor nucleus shadows observed on mammograms done on 202 patients. Data on 32 patients from the Breast Cancer Detection and Demonstration Project—Louisville (BCDDP-L) were added. These data were evaluated assuming both exponential and Gompertzian growth patterns.

Tumor size measurements were made in three dimensions. Volume was calculated as an ellipsoid. Exponential doubling times were calculated by performing a linear regression between ln V and the times between the various observations. The slope of this relationship is the relative growth rate.

Doubling time is the natural logarithm of 2 divided by the relative growth rate and is constant with exponential growth. The distribution of the doubling times was tested with the Kolmogorov-Smirnov test (Bradley, 1968). The distribution was lognormal with a log mean of 5.53 ± 0.81 days, which corresponds to 252 days.

To calculate Gompertzian growth curves, the following assumptions were made: (1) each cancer originated as one cell (2^0); and (2) the maximum size attainable was 2^{40} cells ($V_{max} = 2^{40}$). The usual lethal tumor mass is roughly 10^{12} cells or 40 net cellular generations (2^{40}).

Total body cell composition of an adult is about 10^{13} cells or $2^{40.8}$ cells. A lethal number of breast cancer cells would have a total body distribution equivalent to 10 per cent of all the cells in the host. Our measurements, unfortunately, are only of the tumor nucleus shadow seen on mammograms and predictably represent a decreasingly smaller percentage of the total body cell mass.

By specifying 2^{40} to equal V_{max} it can be shown that

(19) $\qquad \alpha = \beta/(40 \ln 2)$

so the Gompertz equation becomes:

(20) $\qquad V = V_0 e^{(1 - e^{-\alpha t}) 40 \ln 2}$

The doubling time formula in equations 16 and 17 can be simplified by substituting equation 19. In addition, doubling time could then be expressed as a function of generation number.

(21) $\qquad DT_{act} = \dfrac{-1}{\alpha} \ln \left(1 - \dfrac{1}{40 - n}\right)$

where n is the generation number.

The Gompertzian equation can be converted into linear form by taking the logarithm of each side of equation 15 twice. This equation is:

(22) $\qquad \ln \ln (V_{max}/V) = -\alpha t + \ln (\beta/\alpha)$

From our assumptions, β/α and V_{max} are known. The resulting equation is thus the relationship between tumor size and time where $-\alpha$ is the slope of this relationship. A standard regression analysis on $\ln \ln (V_{max}/V)$ versus time was calculated for each patient studied.

Using the Kolmogorov-Smirnov test, the distribution of alphas was examined. This distribution was not significantly different from a lognormal distribution with mean -7.813 ± 0.844 day^{-1}. The antilog of this number, the geometric mean of alpha, was $4.034 (10)^{-4}$ day^{-1}.

With Gompertzian growth, tumor doubling time is a function of tumor size. To compose sojourn time and doubling time data, assuming Gompertzian or exponential growth, the parameters must be specified. For example, doubling times could be compared to the size of a tumor when first detected. The mean diameter of the first mammographic tumor shadow in this study was 8.7 mm. That corresponds to a volume of 345 mm^3, which is the 28th net cellular generation of the tumor nucleus shadow on a mammogram. It should be emphasized that most tumors in this study were first detected at a larger size and only verified to be present at the 345 mm^3 size retrospectively.

A graph of the mean tumor growth for all patients, assuming both exponential and Gompertzian growth, is shown in Fig. 10–1A. The Gompertzian growth curve rises sooner but undergoes a progressively decreasing growth rate as tumor size increases. The exponential growth curve shows the tumor size to be very small until it reaches a sojourn time of approximately 8000 days. It then undergoes a rapid increase in size for the next 2000 days.

Doubling time is plotted as a function of sojourn time in Figure 10–1B. With exponential growth, mean doubling time was constant at 252 days. Assuming Gompertzian growth, however, the mean doubling time for the first cellular division was 62 days. Doubling time slowed to approximately 231 days at the time the tumors were discovered, then slowed even more to a mean of over 1000 days by the 6500th day of growth.

This same effect is illustrated in Figure 10–1C, where doubling time is plotted as a function of generation number. Exponential doubling time is constant, regardless of generation number. Gompertzian growth begins with a doubling time of 62 days for the first generation but approaches infinity at the 39th generation, the last generation for which doubling time has meaning.

Tissue culture and thymidine labeling studies have shown that the initial doubling time of mammary cancer cells runs from 12 to 48 hr (Tseng, 1986). Tumors approximately 1 cm^3 double with a mean of 261 days. Many large tumors have no demonstrable growth, indicating a further prolongation of the doubling time. Although exponential growth curves can be fitted accurately to some data in the range of clinical observation, they cannot allow for the rapid growth rates of smaller tumors. Gompertzian or other deceleratory growth curves may be fitted to available data to reflect more accurately tumor growth throughout its entire life span.

An important result of this type of analysis is estimating the sojourn time of a tumor from one cell through its clinically detectable size. Assuming Gompertzian growth for the data described, the mean sojourn time from one cell to 1 cm^3 of tumor was 3428 days with 95 per cent confidence intervals of 633 days to 18,569 days.

Other deceleratory growth rate formulas, suggested by Skehan (see Table 10–1), may allow more accurate mathematical modeling of breast cancer growth. Growth rates calculated from the measurement of tumor nucleus shadows on mammograms would be expected to be slower than the actual rate of increase in total body tumor burden if cells are being shed rapidly from cancers to take up metastatic growth elsewhere.

Fournier and coworkers (1980) reported a mean doubling time of 311 days. These data, composed of measurements of mammographically visible cancers, formed a lognormal frequency distribution of DT_{act} with a coefficient of correlation of 0.8899. The coefficient of correlation for a linear frequency distribution of Fournier and colleagues' data was 0.4763. Mammograms were repeated annually for the patients whose tumor growth was measured. This bias results in a significant truncation of the growth rate measurements by excluding very rapidly arising cancers, which can be assessed by considering the frequency with which cancers are diagnosed in the interval between annual mammograms. A population-based study is required to quantify this bias by identifying all cancers that surface in the intervals between annual mammograms.

INTERVAL SURFACING CANCERS

Panoussopoulas and associates (1977) reported the interval cancer discovery rates for a BCDDP study. The percentage of cancers diagnosed *between* annual mammograms was 29 per cent of all cancers diagnosed (24 of 89). Monitoring rates at which breast cancers were discovered between annual mammograms were essential for evaluating the worth of mammography and for estimating the potential truncation of the frequency distribution of mammographically measured growth rates by identifying the percentage of very rapidly appearing cancers (Spratt, J. S., in Panoussopoulas et al., 1977).

As an extension of this observation, data were later provided by Spratt and coworkers (1983) on "acute carcinoma of the breast." More acute cancers or "fast" carcinomas were associated with a more anaplastic nuclear grade in the cancer cells, absence of mammographic and microscopic calcifications in the cancer, age of patient less than 50 years old, mammographically dysplastic breasts, lack of a family history, and a prognosis poorer than with slower cancers. Significantly, slower cancers were associated with a circumscribed tumor margin and a papillary growth pattern. In this same population, the absence of calcifications and the presence of lymphatic invasion around the periphery of the primary cancer were associated with the early development of metastases in the axillary lymph nodes (Heuser et al., 1984).

The potential truncation of the DT_{act} data, which originates from the exclusion of the rates of acute, rapidly growing interval cancers, can be estimated in several ways. Dividing the lethal number of net doublings (about 40) into 365 days equals 9. Any breast cancer with a net actual doubling time of less than 9 days could arise de novo and kill the host between annual mammograms. If this estimate is recalculated from the threshold of mammographic detection (i.e., at a range of about 2 mm or 20 to 22 net doublings), 365 could be divided by 20 (40 minus 20), giving 18 days. Any breast cancer that could sustain a net actual doubling time of 18 days or less could grow from the threshold of mammographic detectability to the death of its host in less than 365 days. If the majority of breast cancers followed Gompertzian or decelerating growth in their predetectable period, the truncation problem would be even more serious. Not only can accurate reporting of breast cancer development rates *between* annual mammograms help evaluate the degree of truncation, but also careful follow-up of interval cancer cases can confirm whether faster growing cancers are also more rapidly lethal. Eventually, it will be possible to determine whether mammographic screening is having a real impact on the overall lethality of mammary cancer or whether it is simply dividing breast cancers into fast-growing and slow-growing subsets.

The BCDDP study provided an opportunity to define the entire frequency distribution of actual growth rates of primary mammary cancers. This distribution falls into three subsets. The first consists of cancers growing too rapidly to permit measurement by annual mammography. These are the interval surfacing cancers. The second is composed of cancers in which two or more mammographic observations annually permitted a measurement of growth and a calculation of growth rates. The third subset included very slow-growing cancers for which no measurement of growth occurred on mammographic observations at intervals of 1 year or longer.

During the BCDDP study at Louisville (Heuser et al., 1979a,b), there were 115 proved cancers in the 10,128 women receiving more than 30,000 mammograms over a 4-year period of annual screening. When the pathologic material was reviewed by a panel of national experts appointed for a quality control check on pathologic diagnoses, the University of Louisville had the lowest exception rate in the country among the 27 centers, giving the pathologic diagnoses a high degree of reliability. Serial measurements were possible with xeromammograms in 32 Louisville patients. Actual doubling times ranged from 109 to 944 days, with a median value of 324 days. The log mean doubling time was 327 days. The predominant geometric shape of small primary breast cancers was a spheroid, with the long axis following the direction of the ducts. The frequency distribution of the doubling times of these spheroids was lognormal.

Of these cases (49 of 115), 43 per cent were interval cancers. Nine of the 115 (7.8 per cent) or 9 of the 32 cancers measured serially (28 per cent) had cancers growing too slowly to permit measurement of growth. Incidence in interval cancers increased from 0.064 to 0.239 per cent over the first 3 years of the project and dropped to 0.144 per cent in the fourth year, when women who were less than 50 years old were excluded.

Galante (personal communication, 1986) summarized his continuing clinical characterization of breast cancers with different DT_{act} (Tables 10–8 and 10–9). He established some clear associations between DT_{act}, histopathologic cancer characteristics, nodal metastases, anatomic foci of metastases, and multicentricity. His data show that cancers with the shortest DT_{act} had more tumor necrosis, more frequent multicentricity, more frequent peritumoral lymphatic invasion, higher labeling indices, lower estrogen receptor assay values, more frequent nodal metastases, and more frequent soft tissue metastases. These data generally parallel many of Meyer's conclusions noted in Chapter 9.

Conclusions. A very large percentage of all breast cancers are exceedingly rapid in early or predetectable growth, and the annual mam-

Table 10–8. CHARACTERISTICS OF THE DIFFERENT GROUPS OF GROWTH FOR CANCER OF THE BREAST—EXPERIENCE WITH 193 CASES

Fast (16%): DT_{act} 1 to 30 days	
Highest percentage of necrosis (48.4%)	NS
Highest percentage of multicentricity (50%)	$p = 0.02$
Lowest percentage of estrogen receptor positivity (44.4%)	$p = 0.007$
Highest percentage of second tumor (16%)	$p = 0.03$
Intermediate (42%): DT_{act} 30.1 to 90 days	
High rate of ductal carcinomas (46%)	$p = 0.009$
Highest percentage of PLI (48.9%)	NS
Highest percentage of positive nodes (70%)	$p = 0.01$
Highest percentage of LI values	Mean, 7.6
High percentage of metastases to soft tissues (62.5%)	NS
Slow (17.6%): DT_{act} 90.1 days to $<\infty$	
Low percentage of necrosis (38.2%)	NS
High percentage of estrogen receptor positivity (77.8%)	$p = 0.007$
Very Slow (24.4%): DT_{act} ∞	
High percentage of mixed forms (43.2%)	$p = 0.09$
Lowest percentage of necrosis (36.2%)	NS
Lowest percentage of PLI (25%)	NS
Lowest percentage of multicentricity (8.7%)	$p = 0.02$
Highest percentage of estrogen receptor positivity (95%)	$p = 0.007$
Lowest LI values	Mean, 2.3
Lowest percentage of second tumor (2%)	$p = 0.03$

PLI, Peritumoral lymphatic infiltration; LI, labeling index; ∞ = infinity; NS, not significant.
Courtesy of E. Galante, Milan, Italy, 1986.

mogram has primarily subdivided breast cancers into fast and slow growing subsets. Faster growing cancers were much more likely to metastasize. These observations have numerous implications on the natural history of early breast cancer and on the development of mathematical models for the purpose of detection and evaluation of treatment. The Louisville BCDDP data provide the first report of a full spectrum of growth rates in a defined population of women who range in age from 35 to 70 years (Heuser et al., 1979a,b).

Intensified, effective training in breast self-examination (BSE) at monthly intervals may be the only available cost-effective method for the early detection of more breast cancers. However, as discussed in Chapter 19, the cancers discovered by BSE are relatively large. After correcting for lead time bias, the question that needs to be answered by controlled trial is "Will the earlier self-discovery of palpable cancers by BSE lead to a higher percentage of non-disseminated cancers that are curable by local-regional treatment?" Threshold size for discovery varies with the screening method and with the contrast between cancerous and noncancerous breasts.

Thoracic Radiographs

Coincident with the report by Gershon-Cohen and coworkers (1963) on mammographically measured DT_{act} were studies done at the Ellis Fischel State Cancer Hospital (Spratt et al., 1962; 1963a,b,c; Spratt and Spratt, 1964; Spratt, 1969). The data from these studies consisted of two or more thoracic radiographs on each of 21 patients who had 22 primary lung cancers and on 176 patients who had various types of cancer metastatic to the lung. The sizes of the metastases were lognormally distributed, and the limits on observed size were determined by the threshold of radiographic resolution and by lethal size. Initially no tumor was diagnosed by the radiologist if it was 3 mm in diameter or smaller. Generally, diagnosis was not established until tumors

Table 10–9. RELATIONSHIP BETWEEN HISTOLOGIC TYPE OF BREAST CANCER AND THE DOUBLING TIME

	Infiltrative Duct	Mixed Ductal	Lobular	Others	Mixed	Total
Fast	10	10	3	5	3	31
Intermediate	44	19	1	3	14	81
Slow	17	9	3	1	4	34
Very Slow	16	12	2	1	16	47
Total	87	50	9	10	37	193

$p = 0.009$
Courtesy of E. Galante, Milan, Italy, 1986.

achieved a diameter of 6 mm. This size is equivalent to 26.7 doublings of a 1000 μm^3 cell. A tumor 200 mm in diameter, equivalent to 40.8 doublings, was uniformly lethal. Thus, the segment of growth curve amenable to gross measurement was determined by the terminal 14 doublings in the life of the cancers (40.8 − 26.7 = 14.1).

In this sample were 29 patients with mammary cancer metastatic to the lung. The distribution of growth rates was lognormal, with a geometric mean of 83 days with 95 per cent confidence limits of 16 to 426 days. The number of cells dividing each day was quite small in comparison to the total cell mass. Growth curves for these 29 different breast cancers are shown in Figure 10–3.

Growth rates were compared for all types of tumors in this study. Sex, age, and tumor type did not affect the growth rate of primary pulmonary cancers or of metastases growing in the lung. Exceptions occurred with bone and soft tissue sarcomas, testicular and epidermoid carcinomas, and cancers in patients younger than 29 years. These grew significantly faster than cancers in other categories. A comparison of the frequency distribution of the DT_{act} of pulmonary metastases from breast cancer with metastases from other sites is shown in Figure 10–4.

Breur (1966a,b) reported the gross doubling times of six mammary cancers metastatic to the lung in patients who were from 52 to 71 years old. Doubling times ranged from 23 to 745 days. With sublethal doses of radiation, regrowth started right after the last fractional treatment. Breur used the rate of cancer regression that occurred with the fractionated treatments to estimate the dose needed to eradicate specific tumors. The same approach might be applied to an estimation of the tumoricidal dose of a chemotherapeutic agent that is needed to produce varying percentages of cell kill based on observed regression with fractional doses.

Cutaneous Metastases

Phillippe and Le Gal (1968), who reported on the growth rates of cutaneous nodules of mammary cancer recurrent after mastectomy, saw an order of magnitude similar to that calculated from radiographic measurements of pulmonary metastases. For 78 nodules, the average gross doubling time was 40 days, varying from 3 to 211 days.

Pearlman (1976) calculated the doubling time of breast cancers recurrent in mastectomy scars for 82 patients (Figs. 10–5 and 10–6). The scar recurrences observed by Pearlman and by Phillippe and Le Gal seemed to have faster growth rates than did primary cancers observed by mammography. Pearlman concluded, as these authors have, that the 5 year survival rate is not a meaningful parameter for such extreme variances in growth rate. The same can be said for any fixed end point survival rates.

Multiple Sites

Kusama and associates (1972) compared the median actual doubling times of metastatic breast cancers at various sites. They also considered the association between various characteristics in the population from which the data were derived and the doubling times. In each group, the frequency distribution of doubling times for a population of cancers was lognormal. The median gross doubling time, longest for primary cancers, was progressively shorter for pulmonary metastases, metastases in lymph nodes, and local metastases. The doubling times were shorter for patients under age 30 years and longer for those over age 60 years. Doubling times were no different for married and single women, for parous and nulliparous women, or for whites and blacks. No relationship could be established between doubling time and the presence or absence of axillary metastases. With the exception that tumors with doubling times of more than 8 months recurred infrequently, no relationship could be established between the probability of recurrence and doubling time. Cancers with 8 month doubling times might take more than 15 years to produce a grossly visible mass of neoplasm. Survival time was more favorable in patients with these cancers.

In a study of EFSCH data, the gross growth rates of 171 soft tissue metastases have been reported (Lee, 1970, 1972; Lee and Spratt, 1972). The frequency distributions of observed growth rates were lognormal. Sixty-six metastases were measured in patients who were not treated by systemic therapy; the gross doubling time was 17.1 days (geometric mean), with a 95 per cent confidence range of 3.4 to 86.1.

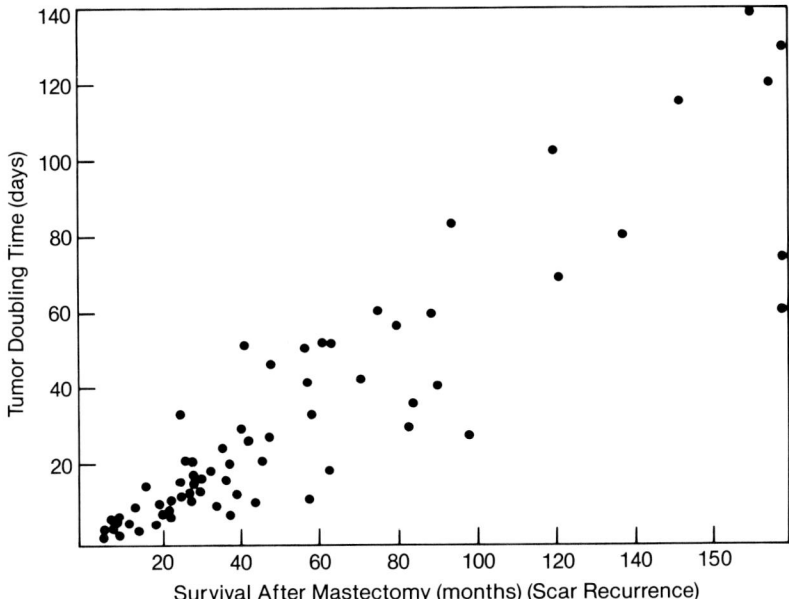

Figure 10–5. In this scattergram, survival in months after mastectomy has been correlated with the tumor growth rate in 67 patients with a mastectomy scar recurrence. There is an approximately linear relationship betwen doubling time and longevity. The distribution becomes scattered especially in the range of the longer doubling times. (From Pearlman, A. W.: Breast cancer—influence of growth rate on prognosis and treatment evaluation. Cancer, 38:1826, 1976. Reprinted with permission.)

For cancers treated subsequently, the ratios of the shrinkage rates after therapy to the growth rates before therapy had means of approximately 1 but varied from 0.2 to 4.2 with 95 per cent confidence.

Indirectly Measured Doubling Times

The doubling times estimated indirectly are related in an expected order of magnitude to the actual doubling times. Malaise and coworkers (1973) described the application of DNA labeling to human solid tumors, including available data from the literature. In most cases, cell division was measured by considering the need for thymidine in the production of DNA and the fact that DNA is manufactured by the cell only during the active synthesis phase of a mitotic cycle. By tagging thymidine with tritium, cell nuclei that have incorporated thymidine during DNA synthesis can be recognized by the effect of the radioactive emission from the tritium on a photographic emulsion. Thus, tritiated thymidine, which is given to a patient with cancer or included in the nutrient media into which viable cancer tissue specimens are placed, permits the measurement of the percentage of cells in an active mitotic cycle. This measurement is referred to as the tritiated thymidine labeling index (TLI).

The distribution of labeling indices for cancers with histologic characteristics in common tends to be lognormal or to follow other skewed frequency distributions. The labeling indices of groups of proliferative cells are proportional to the duration of DNA synthesis and to the cell cycle time. The data can be used to calculate the *potential* doubling time of the tumor cell population. This is not the actual doubling time of the cell population because of cell loss. With 100 per cent loss of new cells, actual growth might even be static.

Applying such considerations to laboratory data, Steel (1967) concluded that the duration of DNA synthesis in human tumors is not much greater than 15 hr, and that cell loss from many human cancers may exceed 50 per cent.

Among the 121 patients with adenocarcinoma reported by Malaise and coworkers (1973) 75 breast cancers were found. The DT_{act} time was 83 days, but the DT_{act} time based on labeling data was about 23.8 days.

Meyer and Bauer (1976) reported the TLI

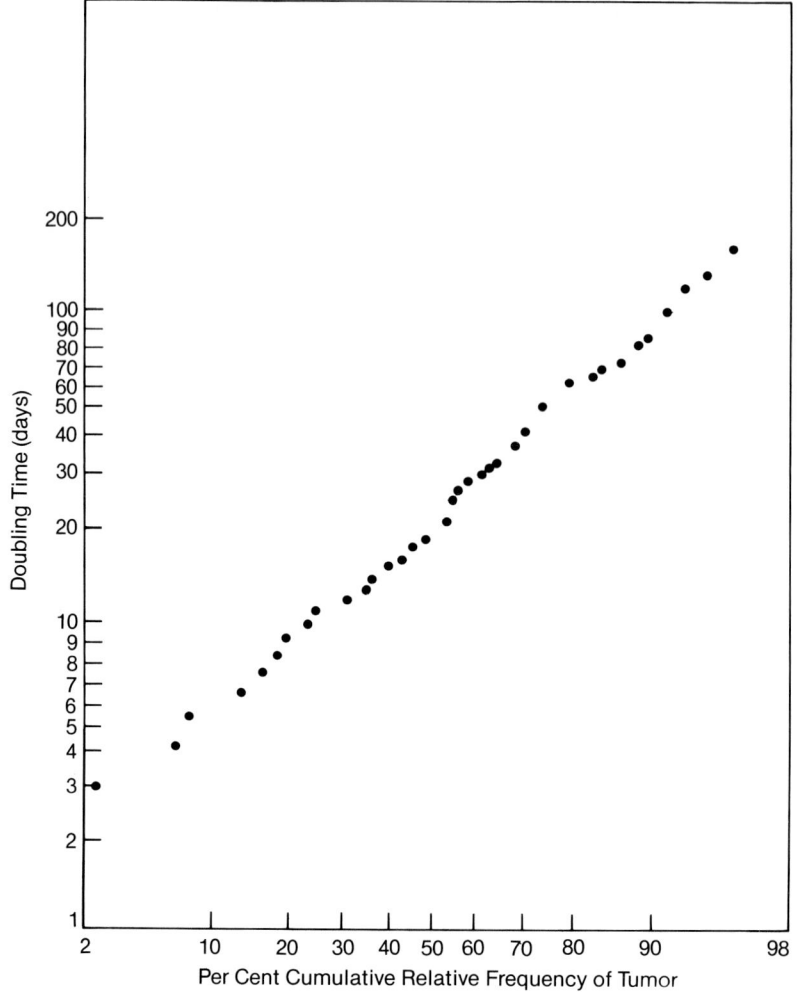

Figure 10–6. The growth curves of pulmonary metastases from adenocarcinoma of the breast. The dotted projection records survival after last chest x-ray. (From Pearlman, A. W.: Breast cancer—influence of growth rate on prognosis and treatment evaluation. Cancer, 38:1826, 1976. Reprinted with permission.)

by in vitro pulse labeling. TLI on nonneoplastic terminal breast ducts was significantly higher during the second half of the menstrual cycle, with a geometric mean of 1.5. This is equivalent to a 47 per cent turnover of duct cells during a menstrual cycle. Fibroadenomas showed a similar menstrual variation of TLI. The TLI range for cancers was from 0.04 to 18.6. The arithmetic mean was 3.7 and the geometric mean was 2.1. TLI tended to be higher in women less than 50 years old ($p > 0.05$) and when two or more axillary lymph nodes contained metastases. Updated results of these studies are given in Chapter 9.

CLINICAL DATA AND THE INDIRECT ASSESSMENT OF GROWTH RATES

An indirect method of assessing breast cancer growth rates by using the clinical history was emphasized by Charlson and Feinstein (1984). These investigators reconstructed entire chronologies of cancers, including history, physical examination, initial treatment, tumor histology, nodal involvement, and follow-up events, including additional treatments. The cancers were classified according to the TNM system. The index of cancer progression was developed for 219 women and validated for 465 additional women. By using the Cox proportional hazard model (Cox, 1972), they created prognostic distinctions within staging groups by relying on anatomic size and extent and on the presence or absence of nodal metastases. Using a qualitative method for comparing rates of cancer progression before treatment, they showed that the indices had a prognostic validity "independent of anatomic stage, nodal status, type of treatment, and other variables." Boyd and coworkers (1981) confirmed the validity of their indices. They divided cancers into "slow," "intermediate," and "rapid." These divisions must be regarded as arbitrary because extant data consistently exhibit a continual spectrum of growth rates distributed lognormally (Spratt, 1969a). This spectral phenomenon results in an overlap of the characteristics of arbitrary subdivisions. However, even with overlap, the concepts are useful in appreciating the importance of growth rate to prognosis. A cancer of long pretreatment duration may have a better prognosis than a cancer with a short pretreatment duration. Even in screening, this phenomenon appears with the more acute cancers that surface and are self-detected in the intervals between annual screens (Spratt et al., 1983).

Indirectly, growth rates may be expressed as rate of progression in evaluating survival, as noted by Pearlman and Jochimsen (1979). These authors studied 464 patients with recurrent breast cancer and used a convention of the R_1-R_2 intervals to compare different subsets of cases. The R_1-R_2 interval is defined as the period of time elapsing between the diagnosis and treatment of the first recurrence (R_1) and the appearance of a second recurrence (R_2).

The most important determinants were the anatomic site of the first recurrence and the tumor progression rate as quantified by the R_1-R_2 interval. Type of treatment had less influence on survival. The median survival from R_1 was 22 to 26 months for bone or soft tissue recurrences, 10 to 12 months for involvement of the pleura or lung, or both, and 4 to 6 months for liver or brain metastases, or both. Patients with longer R_1-R_2 intervals had better survival times than patients with shorter intervals at each anatomic site. Long R_1-R_2 intervals were present in about 50 per cent of patients with bone or soft tissue metastases. For patients with long R_1-R_2 intervals, survival was independent of the treatment method. Long R_1-R_2 intervals were present in only 16 to 20 per cent of the patients with visceral metastases who had undergone only local-regional treatment and in 37 to 38 per cent of those receiving systemic therapy. Survivorship was similar for local and systemic treatment. With visceral metastases, systemic treatment gave superior results. Pearlman and Jochimsen concluded that the combination of the anatomic site of first recurrence coupled with the R_1-R_2 interval provided a way of relating prognosis to the rate of metastatic tumor progression for metastases at different loci.

Potential Relation Between the Size and Duration of Primary Mammary Cancers and the Development of Metastases

Several approaches have been used to estimate how small a breast cancer is when it begins to metastasize. Through clearing studies of axillary contents removed at mastectomy, Pickren (1961; personal communication, 1977) identified all nodes in the axilla and step-sectioned each. Of the 200 patients in his series, 19 had a primary breast cancer that was 10 mm or smaller. The smallest cancer with associated axillary metastases was 8 mm. Of the two patients whose cancers were 8 mm in diameter and who had metastases, one had 11 positive lymph nodes (Table 10-10). The selection of these cases would introduce length biased sampling as a result of truncation by the exclusion of the most rapidly growing cancers.

There is also a biologic variant of breast cancer that never seems to metastasize, no matter how large the primary (Donegan, personal communication, 1977). In reviewing the EFSCH data, Donegan identified a subset of women who had mammary cancers larger than 9 cm in greatest chordal dimension with no lymph node metastases; their 5 year survival after radical mastectomy was 70 per cent.

Campbell and associates (1976) noted positive bone scans in 30 per cent of the women with Stage I breast cancer and in 35 per cent of the women whose cancers were less than 2 cm in greatest chordal dimension.

In both Pickren's and Campbell and coworkers' studies, the first metastasis must have occurred early, when the primary cancers were relatively small. From the EFSCH data, only seven patients who had radical mastectomies had primary cancers of less than 1 cm in diameter. Distant dissemination developed in three of these seven patients during follow-up. Rosen and colleagues (1980) documented the early expression of adverse cellular characteristics for T1N0M0 cancers that recur and cause death. Tumor emboli in lymphatics was most strongly linked with recurrence. Other factors were poor differentiation, marked lymphoid reaction to the cancer, and menarche beginning before age 12 years or after age 14 years. There was a very low risk of recurrence for tumors 1.0 cm or smaller and for tubular, medullary, or colloid cancers up to 2.0 cm. These cases were diagnosed and treated by at least a modified mastectomy. This selection pattern would be characterized by length biased sampling because more indolent cancers would be extant longer at a detectable size of under 2.0 cm. A population-based assessment of all cancers under 2.0 cm might be expected to present a higher proportion of adverse characteristics.

Table 10–10. ASSOCIATION OF LYMPH NODE METASTASES WITH PRIMARY CANCERS 10 MM IN DIAMETER OR LESS AS CONFIRMED BY CLEARING STUDIES AND STEP SECTIONS

Greatest Chordal Dimension of Primary Cancer (mm)	Number of Cancers	Number with Metastasis
10	5	1
9	1	1
8	7	2‡
7	1	0
5	2	0
4	1	0
0†	2	0
Total	19	4

†The cancers listed as "0" mm were microscopic in size and not recognized as gross nodules.
‡The two cancers 8 mm in diameter with metastases had respectively 1 and 11 axillary nodes containing metastatic cancer.
From Pickren, J. W.: Significance of occult metastases. A study of breast cancer. Cancer, 14:1266, 1961. Reprinted with permission.

Cell Shedding and Cell Death as Deceleratory Growth Rate Factors

In the kinetics of mammary cancer, the rate of cell shedding from the primary neoplasm into the vasal circulation and its relation to growth rates is a significant datum. A significant number of breast cancers disseminate before detection (Spratt et al., 1983). Breast cancer cells circulating in the blood have been reported on a number of occasions, but, in humans, the rate of shedding is difficult to quantify. Butler and Gullino (1975) provided insight into cell death and vasal shedding. Their model was an isolated hormone-dependent MTW9 rat mammary cancer from which all efferent blood could be collected. Regression could be induced by reduction of the mammotropin level in the rat. Tumor cells were identifiable by immunofluorescence. The growing tumors shed 3.2×10^6 cells/g of cancer/24 hr. The cell shedding rate, which compared growing and regressing tumors, was not significantly different. The number of cells in arterial blood was one twelfth of that in efferent tumor blood.

Butler and Gullino made the following conclusions: cell shedding via the bloodstream played only a minor role in the total cell loss from growing cancers; the hormone-produced regression was not associated with increased cell shedding; the shed tumor cells were rapidly cleared from circulating blood; and a 2 g carcinoma shed enough cells into the circulation to transplant itself every 24 hr. Cell loss during growth and regression was primarily attributable to cell death within the primary neoplasm in spite of this rate of shedding. The estimated cell destruction and necrosis within the tumor were consistent with measured amino acid nitrogen loss during regression. This loss accounted for 60 to 90 per cent of the tumor protein loss during regression. Furthermore, the rate of cell loss by shedding into the efferent venous blood remained constant whether tumor was growing or regressing. Although data do not exist for human mammary cancer, the same processes are at work and must start very early in the evolution of a breast cancer. Cancer cells are present in the venous blood draining human mammary cancers in 26 per cent of the patients with Stage I and II disease (Golinger et al., 1977). With sampling errors and intermittent shedding, it can be assumed that the true accumulative presence of venous shedding from early human cancers is much greater than 26 per cent.

Growth Rates of Predetectable Cancers Using Composite BCDDP Data

The accumulation of program data in BCDDP studies provided an opportunity to assess the duration and biologic behavior of preclinical breast cancer. The National Cancer Institute contracted for 27 separate BCDDP groups to screen 5000 asymptomatic self-referred women the first year and 5000 more the second year. These women had no prior history of breast cancer and were between 35 and 70 years old. This sample was not population-based and was nonrandomly selected, introducing sources of bias. As other demonstration projects that evaluated the feasibility of mass screening existed, there were no controls. It was, therefore, not possible to test hypotheses as to the benefit of this program.

Screening consisted of a standard history and physical examination, followed by mammographic and thermographic examinations of the breasts on admission into the project. At the first screen, women were taught the technique of breast self-examination (BSE). The first screen resulted in the discovery of the accumulated cancers in the study population. When this number was divided by the total number of women screened, the prevalence rate for the population was obtained at the entry point, the very first screening examination.

In each of the next 4 years of identical screening, additional cancers were discovered. These cancers fell into two subsets that were combined to obtain the total number of cancers that occurred in a single year. These subsets included cancers that were self-discovered in the intervals between annual screens and cancers discovered at annual screens. When the number of cancers discovered yearly was divided by the number of women screened that year, the annual incidence of cancers was obtained. When these rates were divided into the prevalence rates measured at the entry year, an estimate of disease duration before discovery was obtained (Spratt, 1982). This period, defined as the sojourn time from threshold (ST_t), approximates the time elapsing between threshold size and actual detection. Gould and coworkers (1978) reaffirmed that extant knowledge on breast cancer supported origin from a single cell but that the time between origin from that single cell and the attainment of threshold size could not be estimated with these data.

Two separate sets of data were available for this study. The first set of data is from BCDDP-L (Louisville) and is a subset of the second set of composite data from all the BCDDP studies. The characteristics of the first subset have been reported (Heuser et al., 1979a,b, 1984; Spratt et al., 1983). There were too few cases for significant stratification of many factors that might significantly associate with growth rates. The accumulated data for all 27 centers (Baker, 1984) gave meaningful stratification for patient age (Table 10–11). In all instances, time between the attainment of threshold size that might permit detection and the actual size at the time of detection (ST_t) was estimated by dividing the prevalence rate in the first year of screening by the annual incidence rates in the same population. This calculation was done under the assumption that the incidence rate remained constant during that period. Incidence does increase with age and probably with other factors, but in a short-term study there was little reason to assume a major change in incidence in a population of otherwise constant characteristics. There was some random variation in incidence.

A previous report on BCDDP-L data identified the significance of the association of younger age at mastectomy and the absence of microcalcifications with the more acute cancers that appeared in the interval between annual screening examinations (Spratt et al., 1983). Other factors associated with interval-surfacing acute cancers were anaplastic nuclear grade, mammographically classified dysplastic breasts, and the absence of a family history for breast cancer. Survivorship was also poor for the faster growing cancers (Buchanan et al., 1983; Heuser et al., 1979a,b, 1984; Spratt et al., 1983). The threshold size, below which mammary cancers were diagnosable on mammograms, ranged from 2.1 to 2.6 mm (Heuser et al., 1979a).

In the BCDDP-L data, the prevalence of breast cancers discovered at first screen was 0.40 per cent (41 cancers ÷ 10,128 women × 100). At screens 2 to 5, the incident cancers (discovered at annual screen plus those that surfaced and were diagnosed in the 12 months preceding the annual screen) exhibited an incidence rate from 0.18 to 0.37 per cent. The data from BCDDP-L are provided in Tables 10–12 and 10–23.

The times elapsing between the attainment

Table 10–11. ESTIMATION OF THE DURATION OF BREAST CANCERS BEFORE DETECTION IN BCDDP PROGRAMS OBTAINED BY DIVIDING FIRST YEAR (PREVALENCE) RATES BY ANNUAL INCIDENCE RATES IN YEARS 2 TO 5 ACCORDING TO AGE RANGES

Age (yr)	Year 1 Prevalent*	Years 2–5 Incident* (Range)	Prevalence Over Incidence (Year 1/ Incidence in Years 2–5)	Previous Column Converted to Days and Inverted†
35–39	1.0	0.8–1.0	1.25–1.00	365–456
40–44	2.4	1.6–2.1	1.50–1.14	416–548
45–49	5.1	2.1–2.8	2.43–1.82	664–887
50–54	6.6	2.4–3.0	2.75–2.20	803–1004
55–59	7.9	3.2–3.6	2.47–2.00	750–902
60–64	9.4	3.6–3.8	2.61–2.47	902–953
65–69	9.6	3.7–4.1	2.59–2.34	854–945
70–74	12.9	3.4–5.0	3.79–2.58	942–1383

*See definitions of "prevalent" and "incident" in the text.

†Ranges in this column provide an age-specific estimate of the sojourn time elapsing between mammographic threshold size and size at detection of breast cancers discovered in the BCDDP program. For an unknown increment of this estimated duration, cancers would have been below the threshold size permitting detection. Considerable variation around these values would be expected. The entire duration of the cancer from inception as a single cell to detection cannot be estimated with these data.

Data from Baker (1982). From Spratt, J. S., et al.: Geometry, growth rates, and duration of cancer and carcinoma *in situ* of the breast before detection by screening. Cancer Res., 46:970, 1986. Reprinted with permission.

of threshold size and detection (ST_t) from BCDDP-L are provided in Tables 10–13 and 10–14. The authors have separated invasive cancers (CA) and carcinoma in situ (CIS) to calculate the prevalence and incidence rates for each separately and to estimate the ST_t of each category. The estimated time lapsing between CIS and invasive cancer (CA) was determined and designated $ST_{CA\text{-}CIS}$. The estimated ST_t for CA detected in BCDDP-L is given in Table 10–14. The difference between the ST_t for CA and the ST_t for CIS estimates the span of time elapsing after CA transgresses the CIS stage but before detection (Table 10–15). This estimation is predicated on the assumption that CIS progresses to CA and that CAs go through a CIS phase. If a significant number of cancers bypass a detectable CIS period, the effect would simply negate the value of these estimates.

Table 10–12. ACCUMULATIVE SCREENING EXPERIENCE FOR INVASIVE CANCER AND CIS AT BCDDP-L

Screen	Cancers at Screen	Cancers Surfacing in 12 mo Preceding Screen	Total Cancers	CIS at Screen	CIS in 12 mo Preceding Next Screen	Total CIS
1 prevalent (10,128)*	41	—	41	6	—	6
2 (9497)	15	6	21	6	1	7
3 (8878)	23	10	33	4	2	6
4 (8483)	10	7	17	2	2	4
5 (7725)	20	4	24	3	0	3
No sixth screen	—	6†	—	—	—	—
Totals	109	27	136‡	21‡	5	26

*Numbers in parentheses represent number screened.

†Cancers known to have occurred in 12 months following fifth screen, but there was no sixth screen; thus true incidence is indeterminable for this period.

‡In three cases with cancer and one case with CIS, bilateral simultaneous lesions were present. These cases are tabulated singly rather than as two separate cancers.

CIS, carcinoma in situ.

From Spratt, J. S., et al.: Geometry, growth rates, and duration of cancer and carcinoma *in situ* of the breast before detection by screening. Cancer Res., 46:970, 1986. Reprinted with permission.

Table 10–13. ESTIMATION OF SOJOURN TIME OF CIS FROM THRESHOLD SIZE TO SIZE AT DETECTION IN BCDDP-L

Mathematical Step	Data from Table 10–11*	Prevalence Rate / Incidence Rate	ST_t Years	ST_t Days
Prevalence rate at first screen	6 / 10,128			
Composite incidence rate in years 2–5	20 / 34,583	0.0005924 / 0.0005783	1.0243818	373
Prevalence rate at first screen	6 / 10,128			
Annual incidence rate for next 4 years				
Year 1	7 / 9497	0.0005924 / 0.0007371	0.80363901	293
Year 2	6 / 8878	0.0005924 / 0.0006758	0.8765907	320
Year 3	4 / 8483	0.0005924 / 0.0004715	1.2564157	459
Year 4	3 / 7725	0.0005924 / 0.0003883	1.5256245	557

*Number of cases with carcinoma in situ (CIS) divided by number of women screened.
From Spratt, J. S., et al.: Geometry, growth rates, and duration of cancer and carcinoma *in situ* of the breast before detection by screening. Cancer Res., 46:970, 1986. Reprinted with permission.

The estimates in Table 10–11 are based on the accumulated data from all BCDDP studies. Previous studies on cancer data are affected by size at first observation. Growth rates confirmed a tendency of both to form lognormal frequency distributions (Spratt, 1969a). If this general tendency were applicable to the estimates of duration, the existence of a highly skewed distribution of ST_t and DT_{act} before detection could be assumed around the estimates in Table 10–11. The estimates approximate averages. Table 10–11 data provide the 95 per cent confidence limits of a lognormal distribution. Age, the only stratification performed on the composite data from all centers, makes a difference. The authors estimated that

Table 10–14. ESTIMATION OF THE SOJOURN TIME OF INVASIVE CA FROM THRESHOLD SIZE TO SIZE AT DETECTION IN BCDDP-L

Mathematical Step	Data from Table 10–11	Prevalence Rate / Incidence Rate	ST_t* Years	ST_t* Days
Prevalence rate at first screen	41 ÷ 10,128	0.0040482		
Composite incidence	95 ÷ 34,583	0.002747	1.473804	538
Prevalence rate at first screen / Annual incidence rate for next 4 years				
Year 1	41 ÷ 10,128 / 21 ÷ 9497	0.0040482 / 0.0022112	1.8307706	668
Year 2	41 ÷ 10,128 / 33 ÷ 8878	0.0040482 / 0.0037171	1.0890748	398
Year 3	41 ÷ 10,128 / 17 ÷ 9483	0.0040482 / 0.0017927	2.2581581	824
Year 4	41 ÷ 10,228 / 24 ÷ 7725	0.0040482 / 0.0031068	1.3030127	475

*Sojourn time (ST_t) equals time elapsing between the moment the cancer reaches threshold size and the actual time of detection. CA, Invasive cancer.
From Spratt, J. S., et al.: Geometry, growth rates, and duration of cancer and carcinoma *in situ* of the breast before detection by screening. Cancer Res., 46:970, 1986. Reprinted with permission.

Table 10–15. ESTIMATION OF SOJOURN TIME (ST$_{CA-CIS}$) ELAPSING BETWEEN DETECTION OF CIS IN BCDDP-L AND INVASIVE CANCER (DAYS)

Year of Screen	ST$_t$ in Days		Difference (ST$_{CA-CIS}$ in days)
	Invasive Cancer	CIS	
1	668	293	375
2	398	320	78
3	824	459	365
4	475	557	(Negative)
Composite	538	373	165

CA, Cancer; CIS, carcinoma in situ.
From Spratt, J. S., et al.: Geometry, growth rates, and duration of cancer and carcinoma *in situ* of the breast before detection by screening. Cancer Res., 46:970, 1986. Reprinted with permission.

Table 10–17. RELATION OF VOLUME, NUMBER OF CANCER CELLS, AND NUMBER OF NET CELL GENERATIONS AT FIRST OBSERVATION FOR CA WITH AXILLARY LYMPH NODE METASTASES (AX+) DETECTED BY XEROMAMMOGRAPHY

Case Code	Volume (mm^3)	Number of Cells (N)*	Number of Net Cell Generations (n)†
2147 (1)	335	3.35 × 10^8	28.32
8807 (2)	681	6.8 × 10^8	29.34
6129 (3)	824	8.24 × 10^8	29.62
6580 (4)	3535	3.54 × 10^9	31.72
2147 (5)	14,509	1.45 × 10^{10}	33.76
7069 (6)	179,646	1.80 × 10^{11}	37.39

*Mean (log) = 3.4514 ± 0.0426; 95 per cent limit = 3.3413 to 3.5615.
†$\bar{n}$ = 31.55 (28.26 to 35.22).
From Spratt, J. S., et al.: Geometry, growth rates, and duration of cancer and carcinoma *in situ* of the breast before detection by screening. Cancer Res., 46:970, 1986. Reprinted with permission.

over 50 per cent of the invasive CAs occurring in women under 40 years, and probably under age 45 years, were present for less than 1 year before detection.

With much longer durations of breast cancers occurring in women 45 years old and older, we must assume that both length and lead time bias would be highly significant factors in assessing any reduced mortality value attending screening in this age group. The duration of the cancer control window might be longer, permitting less frequent screenings.

The next step taken with BCDDP-L data used the previously reported volumes of cancers at the time of discovery on screening mammograms (Heuser et al., 1979a). The volume was calculated in cubic millimeters on the basis of radiographic dimensions and shape (Tables 10–16 to 10–18). The cancers assumed the shape of spheroids, and the volumes were calculated using the formula for a spheroid (Heuser et al., 1979a). The volume of a single cell was then assumed to be 10^{-6} mm^3. The number of cells was estimated by dividing the volume of the cancer by 10^{-6}. Tumor volume for the threshold size below which breast cancers were not discoverable by mammogram (2.1 mm) was calculated and is provided in Table 10–19. The number of significant figures for all data depends on the methods of measuring tumor size on mammograms. The calculation of tumor volume probably does not exceed two digits. More digits were carried through by computation; final figures may be rounded off. The dimensions of the tumor nucleus shadow on the mammograms were measured in two dimensions to the nearest millimeter with a millimeter scale.

The next step uses the formula fundamental to exponential growth, equation 4 ($N = 2^n$), where n is the net number of doublings of the original cancer cell and N is the estimated number of cells, as calculated from the previous paragraph. To solve for n, convert to the Naperian logarithmic form:

$$(23) \quad n \ln 2 = \ln N \text{ or } n = \frac{\ln N}{\ln 2}$$

Table 10–16. RELATION OF VOLUME, NUMBER OF CANCER CELLS, AND NUMBER OF NET CELL GENERATIONS AT FIRST OBSERVATION FOR CARCINOMA IN SITU OF THE BREAST DETECTED BY XEROMAMMOGRAPHY

Case Code	Volume (mm^3)	Number of Cells (N)*	Number of Cell Generations (n)†
6352 (1)	24	2.4 × 10^7	24.52
0050 (2)	28	2.8 × 10^7	24.74
5318 (3)	42	4.2 × 10^7	25.32
7014 (4)	113	1.13 × 10^8	26.75

*Mean (ln) = 3.2571 ± 0.0298; 95 per cent limits = 3.1735 to 3.3408.
†$\bar{n}$ = 25.98 (23.89 to 28.24).
From Spratt, J. S., et al.: Geometry, growth rates, and duration of cancer and carcinoma *in situ* of the breast before detection by screening. Cancer Res., 46:970, 1986. Reprinted with permission.

Table 10-18. RELATION OF VOLUME, NUMBER OF CANCER CELLS, AND NUMBER OF NET CELL GENERATIONS AT FIRST OBSERVATION FOR CA WITHOUT AXILLARY LYMPH NODE METASTASES (AX−) DETECTED BY XEROMAMMOGRAPHY

Case Code	Volume (mm³)	Number of Cells (N)*	Number of Net Cell Generations (n)†
9601 (1)	79	7.9×10^7	26.24
2074 (2)	79	7.9×6^7	26.24
5264 (3)	92	9.2×10^7	26.46
2684 (4)	151	1.51×10^8	27.17
7320 (5)	151	1.51×10^8	27.17
7059 (6)	189	1.89×10^8	27.49
4833 (7)	335	3.35×10^8	28.32
5607 (8)	448	4.48×10^8	28.74
1165 (9)	513	5.13×10^8	28.93
1818 (10)	760	7.6×10^8	29.50
3210 (11)	760	7.6×10^8	19.50
7324 (12)	943	9.43×10^8	29.81
4981 (13)	1,508	1.508×10^9	30.49
8748 (14)	1,593	1.59×10^9	30.57
0071 (15)	1,659	1.66×10^9	30.63
4489 (16)	1,767	1.77×10^9	30.72
2015 (17)	2,121	2.121×10^9	30.98
0266 (18)	3,394	3.39×10^9	31.66
3116 (19)	3,784	32.78×10^9	31.82
7673 (20)	6,285	6.29×10^9	32.55

*Mean (ln) = 3.3737 ± 0.0151; 95 per cent limits = 3.3421 to 3.4053.
†n̄ = 29.19 (28.28 to 30.12).

From Spratt, J. S., et al.: Geometry, growth rates, and duration of cancer and carcinoma *in situ* of the breast before detection by screening. Cancer Res., 46:970, 1986. Reprinted with permission.

The n value for breast cancers of threshold size, n_t (22 from Table 10-19) can be subtracted from the n values at actual discovery n_d (Tables 10-20 to 10-22), and the differences may be divided into the ST_t to estimate the average DT_{act} in this period (Tables 10-21 and 10-22). These estimates are shorter than those obtained from the direct mensuration of larger neoplasms reported previously.

As uniform quality control was exercised over mammography in the 27 BCDDP programs, the assumption was made that estimates of n in BCDDP-L would be approximately the same as n for the composite data for all BCDDP studies. The net difference for the n value at threshold size (n_t) and the n value of the detection size (n_d), or ($n_d - n_t$), can be divided into the ranges of ST_t for the national data from all the centers. Table 10-23 shows the potential variations in net DT_{act} for the predetectable growth of breast cancers among women of different ages. Greater reliability

Table 10-19. NUMBER OF NET GENERATIONS OF CANCER CELLS AT THRESHOLD SIZE (n_t)

Range of Diameters at Earliest Detection (mm)*	Tumor Volume (mm³)	N	n
2.1	4.85	4.85×10^6	22

*No breast cancer was diagnosed by mammographic exam at a size smaller than this in all categories ($p < 0.005$).

From Spratt, J. S., et al.: Geometry, growth rates, and duration of cancer and carcinoma *in situ* of the breast before detection by screening. Cancer Res., 46:970, 1986. Reprinted with permission.

exists for these composite data, as greater numbers exist. The variations are an expression of the randomness in incidence rates.

That estimated values of DT_{act} are shorter in the ST_t period is expected. Many breast cancers develop so rapidly in their early growth that they surface in the intervals between annual examinations. These observations provide additional justification for accepting that cancers follow Gompertzian or decelerating growth with growth undergoing time-dependent retardation of growth rate. The net effect is that growth becomes progressively slower as the cancers approach a maximum size asymptomatically. Early or predetectable growth rates would be the fastest rates attained.

The measurement of the DT_{act} of breast cancers observed serially by mammograms after they are larger and observable in the BCDDP-L data resulted in a mean DT_{act} of 325 days, ranging from 109 to 944 days for 23 cases. For nine additional cancers, there was no measurable growth in mammographic tumor nucleus shadows for as long as 4 years (Heuser et al., 1984). These data were truncated; and data that were necessary to deter-

Table 10-20. DIFFERENCE BETWEEN NUMBER OF NET CELLULAR GENERATIONS (n_d) AT DETECTION AND AT THRESHOLD SIZE (n_t = 22 or 23)

	$n_t = 22$	$n_t = 23$
CIS	4.022 ± 1.769808	3.022 ± 1.769808
Ax(−)	7.2495 ± 1.9596172	6.2495 ± 1.9596172
Ax(+)	9.70033 ± 3.4042704	8.70033 ± 3.4042704

From Spratt, J. S., et al.: Geometry, growth rates, and duration of cancer and carcinoma *in situ* of the breast before detection by screening. Cancer Res., 46:970, 1986. Reprinted with permission.

Table 10–21. ESTIMATIONS OF THE DT_{act} WITH 95 PER CENT RANGE FOR A LOGNORMAL DISTRIBUTION FOR CANCERS GROWING FROM THRESHOLD SIZE TO DETECTABLE SIZE BY XEROMAMMOGRAPHY

Age (yr)	ST_t (days)*	CIS $n_d - n_t$†	CIS DT_{act}‡	Cancer Ax− $n_d - n_t$†	Cancer Ax− DT_{act}‡	Cancer Ax+ $n_d - n_t$	Cancer Ax+ DT_{act}
35–39	365–465	3.98	92–117	7.19	51–65	9.55	38–49
40–44	416–547	1.89–6.24	105–137	6.28–8.12	58–76	6.26	44–57
45–49	664–887	(95%)	167–223	(95%)	92–123	13.22	70–93
50–54	803–1004		201–252		112–140	(95%)	84–105
55–59	750–902		188–227		104–125		79–94
60–64	902–953		227–239		125–133		94–100
65–69	854–945		215–237		119–131		89–99
70–74	942–1383		237–347		131–192		99–145
Extremes (95%)			59–732		50–220		28–221

*ST_t, Sojourn time, or time elapsing from the time a cancer reaches threshold size to time it is detected.
†n_d, Number of doublings or net cell generations required to attain the volume of a cancer at the threshold of detection by xeromammography; n_t, Number of doublings or net cell generations required to attain the volume of a cancer at the time actually detected by xeromammography.
‡DT_{act}, Mean time (days) for a cancer to double its volume.
From Spratt, J. S., et al.: Geometry, growth rates, and duration of cancer and carcinoma *in situ* of the breast before detection by screening. Cancer Res., 46:970, 1986. Reprinted with permission.

Table 10–22. ESTIMATION OF DT_{act} FOR CANCERS GROWING BETWEEN THRESHOLD SIZE (n_t) AND SIZE OF DETECTION (n_d) IN BCDDP-L

	ln (mean) $n_d = e$	95 Per Cent Limits	d.f.	n_t	$n_d - n_t$	$n_d - n_t$ (95 Per Cent)	ST_t	DT_{act}	DT_{act} (95 Per Cent)
CIS	25.98	23.89–28.24	45	22	3.98	1.89–6.29	373	94	197–60
Ca AX (−)	29.19	28.28–30.12	19	22	7.19	6.28–8.12	538	75	86–66
Ca Ax (+)	31.55	28.26–35.22	5	22	9.55	6.26–13.22	538	56	86–41

From Spratt, J. S., et al.: Geometry, growth rates, and duration of cancer and carcinoma *in situ* of the breast before detection by screening. Cancer Res., 46:970, 1986. Reprinted with permission.

Table 10–23. ESTIMATES OF THE DT_{act} FOR MAMMARY CANCERS DURING ST_t ACCORDING TO THE AGE OF WOMEN, CIS OR CANCER BY AXILLARY NODE STATUS

Age	ST_t days	CIS $n_d - n_t$	CIS DT_{act} (days)	Cancer AX− $n_d - n_t$	Cancer AX− DT_{act} (days)	Cancer AX+ $n_d - n_t$	Cancer AX+ DT_{act} (days)
35–39	365–465	4.02	90–116	7.25	50–64	9.7	38–48
40–44	416–547	4.02	103–136		56–75		43–56
45–49	664–887	4.02	105–221		91–122		68–91
50–54	803–1004	4.02	200–250		110–138		83–104
55–59	750–902	4.02	167–224		103–124		77–93
60–64	902–953	4.02	224–237		124–131		93–98
65–69	854–945	4.02	212–235		118–130		88–97
70–74	942–1383		234–344		130–191		97–143

From Spratt, J. S., et al.: Geometry, growth rates, and duration of cancer and carcinoma *in situ* of the breast before detection by screening. Cancer Res., 46:970, 1986. Reprinted with permission.

mine the DT_{act} of cancers that surfaced in the intervals between screens were missing. Previously reported data did not permit the determination of DT_{act} before tumor size became measurable on mammograms. The actual rate of cell division in the beginning of a cancer in the human breast is not known. According to Tseng (personal communication, 1984), human mammary cancer cells in tissue culture may exhibit cell doubling times of 24 to 36 hours and Gompertzian growth. Present data support the thesis that after the cancer is large enough to be seen on a mammogram, the DT_{act} is longer than in the predetectable period. With more data, it may be possible to correlate the decreasing growth rate that occurs with increasing size in human breast cancer to Skehan's predictions of decelerating growth (Skehan, 1984, and Tables 10–1 and 10–2).

Limitations on BSE Imposed by Rapid Early Growth and Spread

More rapid growth in predetectable breast cancer has immediate relevance on the relationship between breast self-examination (BSE) practices and breast cancer survival (Foster and Costanza, 1975). At 5 years, the survivorship of monthly BSE performers was 75 per cent (± 3 per cent), compared with 57 per cent (± 3 per cent) for the nonperformers. Death due to breast cancer was 14 per cent at 5 years for women performing BSE, in contrast to 26 per cent in nonperformers (p <0.001). Women performing BSE discovered, their cancers at an average size of 2.1 cm, compared with 3.2 cm for self-discovered cancers in those who did not perform BSE. In adjusting survivorship for lead time bias, Foster and Costanza concluded that survivorship remained significantly better in women performing BSE. However, they used a *uniform* cancer volume doubling time of 100 days to estimate lead time. This does not allow for the extreme variance in the doubling times and the change in DT_{act} with increasing tumor size. Their conclusions that BSE survivors had significantly better survivorship for lead times up to 3 years cannot be defended by this calculation.

Accumulating evidence supports the thesis that a significant number of new breast cancers grow more rapidly and metastasize in the predetectable period. As a consequence, many cancers that surface in the intervals between annual screening examinations will already have metastasized. This problem is more significant for women less than 45 years old. The enormous variations in average DT_{act} of grossly measurable cancers also complicate defining an optimum time interval between screening examinations. The clonogenic kinetic events that occur before a breast cancer is detectable undoubtedly have a major impact on prognosis, which may override the prognostic utility of anatomic staging. The prognostic differences with various anatomic stages may be an illusion that incompletely considers numerous sources of sampling bias and variations in kinetic and biologic behavior. Paralleling the early rapid increase in total cell mass is the variable tendency to metastasize that may be greater with the faster growing cancers. It is possible that many breast cancers have negative cancer control windows (i.e., metastasis occurs before the cancer reaches detectable size).

Using data from an older study (Table 10–3), the shortest gross doubling time measured for any primary breast cancer observed by mammography was 23 days; the longest, 209 days. Few persons survive after their tumor cells have undergone a net of 40 doublings; thus, 40 times this doubling time was used to speculate about the extreme duration of human breast cancer from inception to death. In the series of Gershon-Cohen and colleagues (1963), the shortest survival time was 23 × 40 = 920 days and the longest was 209 × 40 = 8320 days (22.8 years). Deceleratory growth rather than exponential growth would effect this variation.

Applying the DT_{act} of only 3 days reported by Phillippe and Le Gal (1968) for a cutaneous metastasis from breast cancer, breast cancers could be acutely lethal. Three days times 40 doublings could conceivably be associated with a mammary cancer growing from inception to lethal proportions in as little as 120 days. At the opposite extreme, Breur (1966a) reported a breast cancer with an actual doubling time of 745 days. This value times 40 equals 29,000 days, a period longer than the normal life span (27,375 days). A person with such a slowly growing cancer would be likely to die from old age before the cancer reached lethal proportions. In fact, long survivals are seen clinically without relying on the dormant cell theory to account for the very long symptom-free intervals.

Survival of patients at EFSCH from the time of first radiographic diagnosis of pulmonary metastases was also found to be lognormal with respect to time (Spratt and Spratt, 1964). Mean survival, corrected for measurement from a common point (a metastasis of 10 mm in diameter), was 310 days with 95 per cent confidence limits, ranging from 20 to 4780 days without treatment. This extreme variance in survival in mammary cancer must be considered before attributing benefit to newer therapeutic methods or combinations thereof. As length of survival and rates of growth both show extreme natural variance, the rate of growth and the time required to produce a lethal neoplastic mass may be the two most important characteristics of a mammary cancer (Spratt et al., 1977). Data on growth rate and survivorship are not yet of a quality and quantity necessary to describe the type of linear relation that probably exists between these two variables, but seeking this relationship is a useful area of research.

A simple relationship between doubling time and survivorship from first radiographic observation of pulmonary metastasis was determined for a small series of patients at EFSCH. A doubling time of 100 days was a critical point in the lethality of these cancers. With a doubling time of less than 100 days, 10 of the 14 (71 per cent) patients died within a year. With a doubling time of over 100 days, 5 of 5 patients, or 100 per cent, lived longer than 1 year.

Relation of Growth Rate to Differentiation

Differentiation, as classified by the anatomic pathologist, undoubtedly has a biophysical basis determined by such factors as cell size and cell membrane characteristics, which include cohesiveness, rate of cell loss, necrosis, and as yet incompletely defined differentiators. A poorly differentiated cancer might still be associated with a long survival of its host if the cancer had a long actual doubling time. Conversely, a well-differentiated cancer might have a short doubling time and short host survival. Meyer has made significant findings in this area (see Chapter 9).

Relation of Immune Factors to Growth Rate

Apart from the effect of tumor ablation by surgical resection, radiotherapy, or chemotherapy, the cytokinetics of mammary cancer and its growth and regression are influenced by immune factors (McGuire et al., 1974, 1975). No data exist for their influence on human mammary cancer growth rates. The potential for immunobiologic effect on growth rate is considered in Chapter 18.

Kinetics, Genetics, Heterogeneity, and Drug Resistance

Kinetics, genetics, cellular heterogeneity, and drug resistance are complexly interrelated. Each cellular generation has a mutation rate that through successive generations has greater phenotypic heterogeneity. The mutation rate, which seems to have an inevitable relationship to cancer cell division, cannot be reduced. Cancers whose cells are resistant to a single drug may have as few as 10^4 cells. By the time new cancers have reached a threshold of size that will permit discovery, the number of existing cells is very great and the cancer has progressed through many generations of cellular division. The probability of having no resistant cells reaches zero while the cancer is still quite small (Goldie and Coldman, 1979, 1984). Goldie and Coldman reviewed the importance of overall tumor growth kinetics to determine the response to chemotherapeutic agents. The theoretical relation between the chances of cure can be expressed as follows:

(24)   function ρ (rho) (cure) $= e^{-\alpha N}$

where α = the mutation rate per cell generation
N = the number of cells in the cancer
e = the base of the natural logarithms

Goldie and Coldman's model (1985) attempts to integrate the stem cell and somatic mutation hypotheses as an explanation for the emergence of drug resistance in cancer. The model recognizes the capacity of neoplasms to evolve a great range of phenotypic diversity compared with normal cell systems. Skehan's arguments (1984) address the inherent reasons for this phenotypic diversity and the survival of mutants. The phenomenon of resistance of a cancer to chemotherapy is similar to the development of antibiotic resistance by bacteria.

The probability that zero resistant cells are present is expressed with the following relationship:

$$(25) \quad P_o = \exp\left[-\alpha(N-1)\right],$$

where P_o is the probability, α is the mutation rate per cell generation, and N is the size of the cell population.

The model assumes no resistant cells at the onset of development of the neoplasm. If the original cell is not sensitive, drug resistance would be an initial phenotypic property of the neoplasm.

The plot of this function provides a sigmoid-shaped curve in which the probability of cure from drugs falls very quickly. Any treatment strategy that does not control the neoplasm increases the likelihood of double or even multiple levels of mutation, which in turn increases the probability of incurability.

The stem cell model of tumor growth may be applicable to neoplasms mimicking the normal cell removal system, in which the end cell is differentiated, nonrenewing, or dead, as with the hematopoietic system. Random stem cell loss magnifies the risk of drug resistance. A cancer characterized by a relatively high clonogenic cell mass, relatively low renewal probability, and high rates of mutation to resistance probably cannot be cured by current drug protocols.

The Goldie-Coldman model has been used to simulate many different treatment strategies. The disturbing constraint implied by this model is that it predicts a high probability of drug incurability whenever the number of cell generations is greater than 30. This produces a neoplasm of 10^9 (or 2^{30}) cells, for which the probability of zero drug resistance falls to zero. When all 10^9 cells are found together, this provides a neoplasm of less than 1 cm^3. Actually, with angiogenesis and the early propensity for vasal seeding, 10^9 cells diffused through breast and body could be associated with an exceedingly small primary neoplasm and still have a body tumor burden well in excess of 10^9 cells. From the standpoint of detection and screening strategy, the number of cell generations elapsing between the attainment of threshold size visible on mammograms (2^{22} cells) and 2^{30} cells is no more than eight net generations. The actual time lapsing between the attainment of threshold size and the discovery by screening varied from between 365 and 465 days at ages 35 to 40 years to between 942 and 1383 days at ages 70 to 74 years (Spratt et al., 1986). The authors suspect that the time period under the age of 35 years is much shorter. Clearly these cytokinetic factors near the threshold of detectability impose persistent limitations on the ability to control breast cancer by "early" detection (Spratt et al., 1986). As Goldie and Coldman (1984) observed, "the upper limit of curable size (by chemotherapy) of many solid tumors appears to be only at the lower range of *even microscopic tumor burden*." Because of the complex issue identified theoretically and in laboratory models, there are "still many unresolved questions in the area of drug resistance, especially as applied to the behavior of human cancer *in vivo*." In both the laboratory and clinical situation, drug resistance is a multifactorial problem on which incomplete knowledge has been gained. For example, Goldie and Coldman's model fails to explain the great variation in growth rates and the significance of biologic age. The models have become so complex that researchers in clinical trials for breast cancer will have to consider these implications in planning and evaluation.

Duration of Symptoms, Growth Rate, and Survival

The relationship between duration of symptoms before the treatment of breast cancer and survivorship also has implications for growth rate. Dennis and coworkers (1975) reported no significant correlation ($p > 0.05$) between delay attributable to either physician or patient and survivorship after treatment when survivorship is measured from the onset of symptoms to correct for lead time. They also reviewed the contradictory literature that antedated their report. Fisher and colleagues (1977) noted that both tissue necrosis within the cancer and the prevalence of highly malignant histologic grade decreased when the duration of symptoms antedating treatment exceeded 9 months. Though "ominous" prognostic findings increased with longer delay, the average monthly treatment failure rate was not altered. A trend was even noted toward a decline in monthly treatment failure rates when symptoms antedated treatment by more than 9 months. Thus, there is a documented trend for the rapidly appearing cancers to be more virulent and for the more chronic, more slowly growing cancers with longer duration of symptoms before treatment to progress more slowly after treatment.

Clinical Application of Growth Rates

Precise measurements of in vivo growth of most human breast cancers are at present insufficient to define an absolute relationship between gross rates of growth, tumor cell proliferation, cell loss, and survivorship in a specific host. Multiple events occur continuously in the life cycle of a cancer and its host, and the net effect reflects the interaction of these variables. The slope of the growth curves mirrors the net effect of many variables; these curves also reflect the changing relationship that may occur among these variables with the growth of cancer. Attempts made to extrapolate growth curves beyond the extent of observed data are subject to serious error.

The extreme variation in the prelethal duration of a breast cancer casts further doubt on the value of fixed end point (as 5 year) survival rate as a parameter for assaying the value of treatment. The slope of the survival curve or the interval rate of dying, measured at short intervals, is more compatible with the now well-documented extreme variation in cancer growth rates. For very acute breast cancers, even short periods of symptom-free survival may have great meaning for a patient. An extremely long treatment course, not providing a major lengthening of survival, might simply use up this short period. A more flexible model is needed for assaying the value of diagnosis and treatment in cohorts with varying survivorship, as is suggested in Chapter 30.

In summary, the cytokinetic properties of cancer cells, in relation to their host and their growth controlling and inhibiting factors, are significant determinants for understanding and controlling cancer in humans.

REFERENCES

Atkinson, E. N., Brown, B. W., and Montague, E. O.: Tumor volume, nodal status, and metastasis in breast cancer in women. JNCI, 76:171, 1986.

Baker, L. H.: Breast cancer detection demonstration project: Five year summary report. Cancer, 53:96, 1984.

Boyd, N. F., Meakin, J. W., Hayward, J. L., et al.: Clinical estimation of the growth rate of breast cancer. Cancer, 48:1037, 1981.

Bradley, J. V.: Distribution free statistical tests. Englewood Cliffs, N.J.: Prentice-Hall, 1968, p. 296.

Brem, S., Brem, H., Folkman, J., et al.: Prolonged tumor dormancy by prevention of neovascularization in the vitreous. Cancer Res., 36:2807, 1976.

Breur, K.: Growth rate and radiosensitivity of human tumours. I. Growth rate of human tumours. Eur. J. Cancer, 2:157, 1966a.

Breur, K.: Growth rate and radiosensitivity of human tumours. II. Radiosensitivity of human tumours. Eur. J. Cancer, 2:173, 1966b.

Buchanan, J. B., Spratt, J. S., and Heuser, L. S.: Tumor growth, doubling times and the inability of the radiologists to diagnose certain cancers. Radiol. Clin. North Am., 21:115, 1983.

Butler, T. P., and Gullino, P. M.: Quantitation of cell shedding into efferent blood of mammary adenocarcinoma. Cancer Res., 35:512, 1975.

Campbell, D. J., Banks, A. J., and Oates, G. D.: The value of preliminary bone scanning in staging and assessing prognosis of breast cancer. Br. J. Surg., 63:811, 1976.

Charlson, M. E., and Feinstein, A. R.: Rate of disease progression in breast cancer: a clinical estimate of prognosis within nodal and anatomical stages. JNCI, 72:225, 1984.

Chato, J. C.: Measurements of the thermal properties of growing neoplasms. Ann. N.Y. Acad. Sci., 335:67, 1980.

Cox, D. R.: Regression models and life tables. J. R. Statist. Soc., 34:187, 1972.

Dennis, C. R., Gardner, B., and Lim, B.: Analysis of survival and recurrence vs. patient and doctor delay in treatment of breast cancer. Cancer, 35:714, 1975.

Eberhart, R. C., Shitzer, A., and Hernandez, E. J.: Thermal dilution methods: Estimation of tissue blood flow and metabolism. Ann. N.Y. Acad. Sci. 335:107, 1980.

Fisher, E. R., Redmond, C., and Fisher, B.: A perspective concerning the relation of duration of symptoms to the treatment failure in patients with breast cancer. Cancer, 40:3160, 1977.

Foster, R. S., and Costanza, M. C.: Breast self-examination and breast cancer survival. Cancer, 53:999, 1975.

Fournier, D. von, Kubli, F., and Barth, V.: Growth rates of 147 mammary carcinomas. Cancer, 45:2198, 1980.

Gautherie, M.: Thermopathology of breast cancer: Measurement and analysis of in vivo temperature and blood flow. Ann. N.Y. Acad. Sci., 335:383, 1980.

Gershon-Cohen, J., Berger, S. M., and Klickstein, H. S.: Roentgenography of breast cancer moderating concepts of "biologic predeterminism." Cancer, 16:961, 1963.

Goldie, J. H., and Coldman, A. J.: A mathematical model for relating the drug sensitivity of tumors to their

spontaneous mutation rate. Cancer Treat. Rep., 63:1727, 1979.
Goldie, J. H., and Coldman, A. J.: The genetic origin of drug resistance in neoplasms: Implications for systemic therapy. Cancer Res., 44:3643, 1984.
Goldie, J. H., and Coldman, A. J.: A model for tumor response to chemotherapy: An integration of the stem cell and somatic mutation hypotheses. Cancer Invest., 3:553, 1985.
Golinger, R. C., Gregorio, R., and Fisher, E. R.: Tumor cell in venous blood draining mammary carcinoma. Arch. Surg., 112:707, 1977.
Gompertz, B.: On the nature of the function expressive of the law of human mortality, and on a new mode of determining the value of life contingencies. Phil. Trans. R. Soc. Lond., 115:513, 1825.
Gould, M. N., Jirtle, R., Crowley, J., et al.: Reevaluation of the number of cells involved in the neutron induction of mammary neoplasms. Cancer Res., 38:189, 1978.
Gullino, P. M.: Influence of blood supply on thermal properties and metabolism of mammary carcinoma. Ann. N.Y. Acad. Sci., 335:1, 1980.
Gullino, P. M., Grantham, F. H., and Courtney, A. H.: Utilization of oxygen by transplanted tumors *in vivo*. Cancer Res., 27:1028, 1967.
Heuser, L. S., Spratt, J. S., Kuhns, J. G., et al.: The association of pathologic and mammographic characteristics of primary human breast cancers with "slow" and "fast" growth rates and with axillary lymph node metastases. Cancer, 53:96, 1984.
Heuser, L. S., Spratt, J. S., and Polk, H. C., Jr.: Growth rates of primary breast cancers. Cancer, 43:1888, 1979a.
Heuser, L. S., Spratt, J. S., Polk, H. C., Jr., et al.: Relation between mammary cancer growth kinetics and the intervals between screenings. Cancer, 43:857, 1979b.
Hoffman, J. G.: Theory of mitotic index and its application to tissue growth measurement. Bull. Math. Biophys., 11:139, 1949.
Kusama, S., Spratt, J. S., Jr., Donegan, W. L., et al.: The gross rates of growth of human mammary carcinoma. Cancer, 30:594, 1972.
Lee, Y. T.: The lognormal distribution of growth and shrinkage rates of soft tissue metastases of breast cancer. Trans. Mo. Acad. Sci., 4:33, 1970.
Lee, Y. T.: The lognormal distribution of growth rates of soft tissue metastases of breast cancer. J. Surg. Oncol., 4:81, 1972.
Lee, Y. T., and Spratt, J. S., Jr.: Rate of growth of soft tissue metastases of breast cancer. Cancer, 29:344, 1972.
Liotta, L. A., Saidel, M. G., and Kleinerman, J.: Stochastic model of metastasis formation. Biometrics, 32:535, 1976.
Malaise, E. P., Chavaudra, N., and Tubiana, M.: The relationship between growth rate, labelling index and histological type of human solid tumors. Eur. J. Cancer, 9:305, 1973.
Mayneord, W. V.: On a law of growth of Jensen's rat sarcoma. Am. J. Cancer, 16:841, 1932.
McGuire, W. L., Chamness, G. C., Costlow, M. E., et al.: Hormone dependence in breast cancer. Metabolism, 23:75, 1974.
McGuire, W. L., Carbone, P. P., and Vollmer, E. P. (Eds.): Estrogen Receptors in Human Breast Cancer. New York, Raven Press, 1975.
Meyer, J. S., and Bauer, W. C.: Tritiated thymidine labelling index of benign and malignant human breast epithelium. J. Surg. Oncol., 8:165, 1976.
Meyskens, F. L., Jr., Thomson, S. P., and Moon, T. E.: Quantitation of the number of cells within tumor colonies in semisolid medium and their growth as oblate spheroids. Cancer Res., 44:271, 1984.
Morrison, P., and Morrison, P.: Powers of ten—a book about the relative size of things in the universe and the effects of adding another zero. San Francisco, Scientific American Library, W. H. Freeman, 1982.
Panoussopoulas, D., Chang, J., and Humphrey, L. J.: Screening for breast cancer. Ann. Surg., 186:356, 1977.
Parl, F. F., and Dupont, W. D.: A retrospective cohort study of histologic risk factors in breast cancer patients. Cancer, 50:2410, 1982.
Pearlman, A. W.: Breast cancer—influence of growth rate on prognosis and treatment evaluation. A study based on mastectomy scar recurrences. Cancer, 38:1826, 1976.
Pearlman, N. W., and Jochimsen, P. R.: Recurrent breast cancer: Factors influencing survival, including treatment. J. Surg. Oncol., 11:21, 1979.
Phillippe, E., and Le Gal, Y.: Growth of seventy-eight recurrent mammary cancers. Quantitative study. Cancer, 21:461, 1968.
Pickren, J. W.: Significance of occult metastases. A study of breast cancer. Cancer, 14:1266, 1961.
Post, J., Sklarew, R. J., and Hoffmann, J.: The proliferative patterns of human breast cancer cells in vivo. Cancer, 39:1500, 1977.
Rosen, P. P., Saigo, P. E., Braun, D. W., et al.: Predictors of recurrence in Stage I (T1N0M0) breast carcinoma. Ann. Surg., 193:15, 1980.
Skehan, P.: Cell growth tissue neogenesis and neoplastic transformation. *In* Skehan, P., and Friedman, S. J. (Eds.): Growth, Cancer and the Cell Cycle. Clifton, N.J., Humana Press, 1984, p. 323.
Spratt, J. A.: Fitting deceleratory growth curves to human breast cancer data. (Submitted for publication.)
Spratt, J. S.: The rates of growth of skeletal sarcomas. Cancer, 18:14, 1965.
Spratt, J. S.: The lognormal frequency distribution and human cancer. J. Surg. Res., 9:151, 1969a.
Spratt, J. S.: Locally recurrent cancer after radical mastectomy. Cancer, 20:1051, 1969b.
Spratt, J. S.: The relation of "human capital" preservation to health costs. Am. J. Econ. Sociol., 34:295, 1975a.
Spratt, J. S.: The physician's role in minimizing the economic morbidity of cancer. Sem. Oncol., 2:411, 1975b.
Spratt, J. S.: Epidemiology of screening for cancer. Curr. Probl. Cancer, 6:1, 1982.
Spratt, J. S., and Ackerman, L. V.: The growth of a colonic adenocarcinoma. Am. Surg., 27:23, 1961.
Spratt, J. S., and Spratt, J. A.: The prognostic value of measuring the gross linear radial growth of pulmonary metastases and primary pulmonary cancers. J. Thorac. Cardiovasc. Surg., 71:274, 1976.
Spratt, J. S., and Spratt, T. L.: Rates of growth of pulmonary metastases and host survival. Ann. Surg., 159:161, 1964.
Spratt, J. S., Chang, A. F-C., Heuser, L. S., et al.: Acute carcinoma of the breast. Surg. Gynecol. Obstet., 157:220, 1983.
Spratt, J. S., Greenberg, R. A., and Heuser, L. S.: Geometry, growth rates and duration of cancer and carcinoma *in situ* of the breast before detection by screening. Cancer Res., 46:970, 1986.
Spratt, J. S., Kaltenbach, M. L., and Spratt, J. A.: Cytokinetic definition of acute and chronic breast cancer. Cancer Res., 37:226, 1977.
Spratt, J. S., Spjut, H. J., and Roper, C. L.: The frequency distribution of the growth rates and the esti-

mated duration of primary pulmonary carcinomas. Acta Un. Int. Cancer, *19*:1270, 1963*a*.

Spratt, J. S., Spjut, H. J., and Roper, C. L.: The frequency distribution of the growth and the estimated duration of primary pulmonary carcinomas. Cancer, *16*:687, 1963*b*.

Spratt, J. S., Spjut, H. J., Ter-Pogossian, M., et al.: Correlation of primary pulmonary neoplastic growth curves with morphology, necrosis, survival and aetiology. Proceedings of the VIII International Cancer Congress, Moscow, U.S.S.R., 1962, p. 281.

Spratt, J. S., Ter-Pogossian, M., and Long, R. T. L.: The detection and growth of intrathoracic neoplasms. The lower limits of radiographic distribution, the antemortem size, the duration, and the pattern of growth as determined by direct mensuration of tumor diameters from random thoracic roentgenograms. Arch. Surg., *86*:283, 1963*c*.

Steel, G. G.: Cell loss as a factor in the growth rate of human tumours. Eur. J. Cancer, *3*:381, 1967.

Steel, G. G.: The cell cycle in tumours: An examination of data gained by technique of labelled mitosis. Cell Tissue Kinet., *5*:87, 1972.

CHAPTER 11

JAMES L. WITTLIFF

Steroid Receptor Analyses, Quality Control, and Clinical Significance

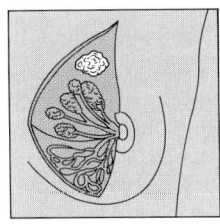

Since the original observations of Beatson (1896), the hormonal milieu of a patient has been known to influence significantly the growth rates of certain breast tumors. Clinical observations by Huggins and Bergenstal (1952), Luft and Olivecrona (1955), and others (Dao, 1972; Kennedy, 1974) since the turn of the century indicated that 25 to 40 per cent of breast cancers respond to the surgical removal of endocrine-producing glands, such as the ovaries in the premenopausal woman, or the adrenals or anterior pituitary in the postmenopausal patient. Administration of pharmacologic doses of estrogens, androgens, and so-called antihormones, such as tamoxifen (Nolvadex), also brought about breast tumor remissions (Hall, 1968; Fisher et al., 1983). Endocrine ablative surgery has been replaced largely by administration of antihormones, owing to increased knowledge of steroid hormone action and its relationship to hormonal response (Jensen et al., 1971; Wittliff, 1974, 1984; McGuire et al., 1975, 1977).

It is essential that the oncologist treating a breast cancer patient identify the individual most likely to respond to endocrine manipulation (Polk, 1986). Until recently, clinical factors such as previous response to hormone therapy, disease-free interval, age and menopausal status, and location of the dominant metastatic lesion were the principal criteria for selecting therapeutic regimens for women with breast cancer.

Investigations during the past 20 years have made significant progress toward elucidating the mechanism by which steroid hormones influence the differentiation and development of target organs (Buller and O'Malley, 1976; Clark and Peck, 1979; Wittliff and Dapunt, 1980; Moudgil, 1985). A prerequisite for responsiveness appears to be a cellular protein termed the steroid receptor or steroid binding protein. Receptor proteins are found in a variety of concentrations, ranging from 50 to 50,000 sites in target cells, but they are virtually absent in nontarget tissues. An important property is that the steroid hormones associate with their characteristic receptor protein in a manner exhibiting high affinity and ligand specificity.

Since the original report of Folca and co-workers (1961) indicating a greater uptake of labeled hexoestrol by breast tumors of patients showing a response to ablative therapy, numerous studies have shown that approximately one half of all biopsy specimens of malignant breast tumors contained estrogen receptors (Jensen et al., 1971; Wittliff, 1974, 1984; McGuire et al., 1975, 1977). Furthermore, 55 to 60 per cent of the patients exhibiting estrogen receptors were responsive to either administrative or ablative hormone therapies. The use of this single biochemical criterion (presence of estrogen receptors) by the oncologist

---

This chapter is dedicated to Dr. Thomas C. Hall, my first clinical mentor who shared his knowledge of and devotion to the application of basic science to problems of clinical medicine.

has increased by twofold or threefold the accuracy of selecting the patient with advanced breast cancer most likely to respond objectively to endocrine manipulation. Addition of the results from progestin receptor determinations further defines the endocrine responsive breast carcinomas (Proceedings of the NIH Consensus Development Conference, 1980; Clark et al., 1983; Fisher et al., 1983; Wittliff, 1984).

At present, both estrogen and progestin receptors are used routinely in the clinical management of breast cancer as predictive indices of a patient's response to endocrine therapy and as prognostic indicators of a patient's clinical course. Clearly, this is a decade of enormous progress in the field of hormone receptor studies of all types. Soon additional receptor tests will be added to the oncologist's armamentarium to combat breast cancer and other hormonally responsive neoplasms.

Steroid Hormone–Target Cell Interaction

The normal breast represents an organ in which hormonal interactions, both peptide and steroid, influence the molecular processes involved in proliferation, differentiation, and secretion. The major stages in the differentiation of the breast involve both parenchymatous and mesenchymal components. Although the specific role of each of the hormones is unknown, estrogens, progesterone, and certain glucocorticoids are known to influence these processes. Likewise, androgen is known to exert a negative control on the proliferation of breast epithelium during early development.

Several peptide hormones, such as insulin, prolactin, possibly growth hormone and certain growth factors, act in concert with the steroid hormones to bring about the orderly differentiation of the resting breast cell of the female to a structurally and functionally differentiated state. The functionally differentiated state is characterized histologically by an alveolar secretory appearance and by increased rates of synthesis of milk proteins, lipids, and lactose. Prior to the onset of lactation, the breast is composed predominantly of adipose cell surrounding a branched system of ducts of epithelial cells with connective tissue elements. As the gland differentiates during pregnancy and lactation, the tissue shifts its composition toward a higher concentration of lobuloalveolar cells, which are responsible principally for the synthesis of milk constituents. At the culmination of lactation, the mammary epithelium undergoes involution. These events appear to be regulated by a host of factors, of which hormone receptors are central to organized differentiation and development.

The concept underlying endocrine therapy is that certain tumor cells have retained the molecular mechanisms (receptors) to respond to the same hormonal perturbations as their normal progenitor cells. With specific hormone binding data, it is possible to derive information about the natural history of the lesion, such as transformation (dedifferentiation), which may result in the loss of receptors; it is also possible to exploit their presence by employing hormone therapy, as in the case of tamoxifen administration.

Current understanding of the sequence of events that follows the interaction of a steroid hormone with a target cell (Fig. 11–1) evolved from the original "two-step mechanism" suggested independently by Gorski and coworkers (1968) at the University of Illinois and by Jensen and colleagues (1968) at the University of Chicago. Uterine tissues from rodents were used for these early studies. Investigations from many laboratories with rodents and human tissues suggest that a similar cascade of events exists in normal and neoplastic mammary cells. Steroid hormones are transported in the plasma compartment by a number of proteins, including albumin, testosterone-estradiol-binding globulin (TeBG, formerly sex steroid binding globulin), and corticosteroid binding globulin (CBG), each with a characteristic affinity and capacity. Albumin binds estradiol-17β (Fig. 11–2), the native female sex hormone, reversibly with a dissociation constant (K_d) value of 10^{-5}M, whereas TeGB associates with the hormone exhibiting a K_d value of 10^{-7} to 10^{-8} M.

The unbound steroid enters the cell, apparently by passive diffusion, and combines with its specific receptor protein in a reaction termed uptake (Fig. 11–1). This step is characterized by a high degree of ligand affinity and specificity with the intracellular receptor. The exact location of the receptor in normal or neoplastic target cells is not clearly understood, although recent data suggest a nuclear location (King and Greene, 1984; Welshons et al., 1984). Prior to high affinity association with the nuclear matrix, the steroid-receptor

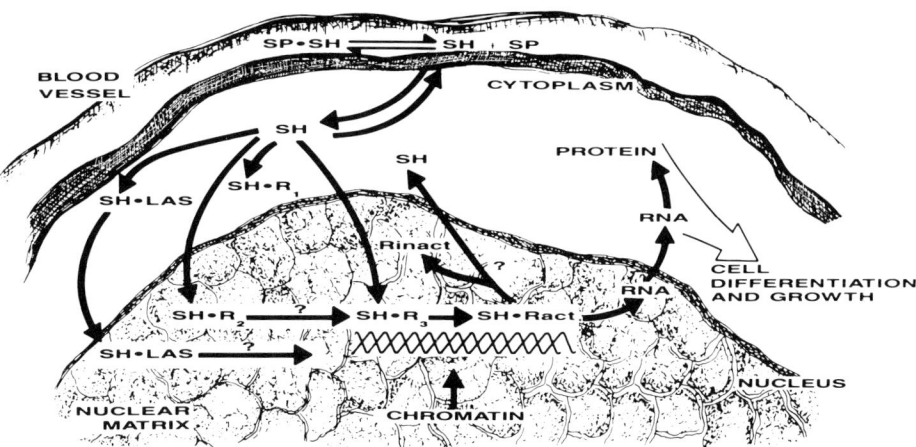

Figure 11–1. Proposed intracellular cascade of events following steroid receptor interaction with its receptor in a target cell. Steroid hormones (SH) normally circulate in the blood bound to albumin and certain specific serum proteins (SP) such as testosterone-estradiol-binding globulin TeBG and corticosteroid-binding globulin (CBG). Being lipids, steroids move across the cell membrane into the cytoplasm in a passive fashion and interact with their intracellular receptor proteins (R) in a reaction exhibiting high affinity and specificity. The exact location of the true receptor protein is unknown, but possibilities include sites associated with the nuclear membrane (R_1), nuclear matrix (R_2), and the chromatin (R_3). Following association with the steroid, an apparent activation takes place which may involve phosphorylation. The activated steroid-receptor complex (Sh•Ract) associates with acceptor sites in chromatin and stimulates the synthesis of nucleic acids and subsequently proteins characteristic of the biological response (differentiation and growth) to the specific steroid hormone. In addition, steroid hormones may associate with low affinity sites (LAS), whose subsequent pathway is uncertain. The details of these intranuclear events are unclear at present. However, the presence of a receptor protein in a cell appears to be a prerequisite for response to a steroid hormone stimulus.

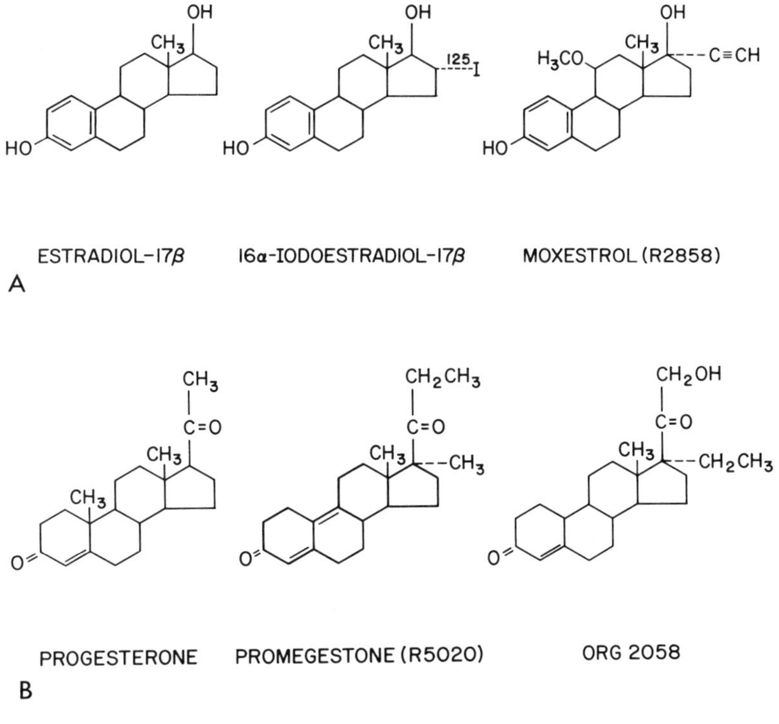

Figure 11–2. Ligands used in the determination of estrogen receptors (A) and progestin receptors (B).

complex must undergo an activation step, which may involve phosphorylation of the receptor (Moudgil, 1985). The activated steroid hormone–receptor complex then associates with the chromatin in an event called retention. This interaction stimulates RNA synthesis in a yet undisclosed manner, resulting in the formation of certain breast cell proteins. Thus, the steroid receptor appears to be a biologic prerequisite for responsiveness to hormonal perturbations; in its absence, alterations in macromolecular synthesis do not occur at physiologic hormone concentrations. Normal breast cells contain specific binding proteins for estrogen, progestins, glucocorticoids, and androgens in variable quantities, depending on the stage of mammary gland differentiation (Wittliff, 1975; Moudgil, 1985). Representative examples of radiochemically labeled ligands for estrogen and progestin receptors are shown in Figure 11–2.

Tissue Handling and Preparation

Breast biopsy specimens should be transported from surgery and pathology to the clinical chemistry laboratory either in the frozen state or chilled in a petri dish or plastic bag placed in ice. If possible, the specimen should be frozen immediately upon excision, at the time of frozen section diagnosis. However, an increasing number of specimens are transported directly to pathology for permanent section and may remain unfrozen for a considerable time. The specimen must be maintained on ice to retard receptor degradation. Recent studies indicate that the half-lives of estrogen and progestin receptors are highly variable in intact tumor biopsy specimens, ranging from as little as 30 minutes to no change in 6 hours at room temperature (Wittliff, 1987). A rule of thumb is that the tissue should be frozen within 30 to 45 minutes after surgery and, preferably, maintained on ice or in a refrigerator in the interim. If a specimen is to be shipped to a distant laboratory for analyses, the snap-cap vials used by electron microscopists for grid storage are superb for freezing in liquid nitrogen or on dry ice.

The pathologist plays an important role in preserving the biologic integrity of the tumor biopsy specimen prior to arrival in the laboratory. Important considerations are that the specimen sent for steroid receptor analyses is both representative of the tumor and large enough for receptor analysis. Usually no less than 200 mg and, preferably, 400 to 500 mg of tumor is required to determine both estrogen and progestin receptors. Intratumoral regional differences in steroid receptor status have been observed (Locher et al., 1984) emphasizing the need for submission of a representative sample. These results and others (Wittliff and Savlov, 1975; Meyer, 1986) suggest a clonal heterogeneity relative to receptor status.

Because human breast tumors are heterogeneous with regard to cell type, the author and colleagues examined the relationship between estrogen binding capacity and the proportion of tumor epithelium in a breast biopsy specimen (Wittliff et al., 1976). There did not appear to be a correlation between the quantity of estrogen receptors in a biopsy specimen and the proportion of tumor epithelium. It was noted, first, that numerous specimens containing less than 25 per cent tumor epithelium exhibited very high estrogen binding capacities. Second, the results indicated that the specific estrogen binding capacities of individual tumor specimens containing the same quantity of tumor epithelium were highly variable. The quantity of estrogen receptors in these tumors varied from undetectable levels to in excess of several hundred femtomoles (fmol) per milligram of cytosol protein. Although it may be expected that the estrogen binding capacity of normal mammary gland increases with increasing cellularity, this is not true of breast tumors. Thus, the quantitative differences in estrogen binding capacity are not due simply to the number of tumor cells in a biopsy specimen. Rather, this variation in activity reflects differences in the number of binding sites per breast tumor cell. This author has long recommended that, routinely, a small sample of the biopsy material sent for receptor analyses be fixed and stained to confirm the presence of tumor and its pathology (Wittliff et al., 1972, 1976).

After the biopsy specimen arrives in the laboratory, an extract is made of the tumor cells by homogenization in buffer. The thermostability of steroid receptors in tumor specimens has been difficult to assess, partially due to the heterogeneous nature of the tissue and the quantity of steroid receptors. However, it is clear from studies in vitro that steroid receptors are labile proteins that undergo degradation or ligand dissociation in a temperature dependent manner (Wittliff, 1975). Association of the ligand with the receptor clearly aids in stabilization, which leads to the suggestion that the time between cytosol preparation and introduction of the ligand should be as short as possible. Addition of sodium molybdate to homogenization buffer also aids in the stabilization of receptors released during cellular extraction (Raam and Teixeira, 1985).

Other aspects of tissue selection include a comparison of receptor levels in fresh mastectomy specimens and in biopsy specimens (Meyer et al., 1983). It appears only a small reduction occurs in the proportion of estrogen receptor positive mastectomy specimens compared with biopsy specimens, suggesting that either is clinically useful if maintained properly.

Determination of Steroid Hormone Receptors

CLINICAL PROCEDURES

The two methods currently accepted for the clinical determination of steroid receptors are the multipoint titration and sucrose gradient analyses (DeSombre et al., 1979; Wittliff, 1987). The titration procedure is the most commonly employed and uses dextran-coated charcoal to remove unbound steroid from that associated with intracellular receptors (Fig. 11–3).

As already stated, the exact location of steroid receptors in a cell is currently debated, but increasing evidence suggests a nuclear association (King and Greene, 1984; Welshons et al., 1984). Receptors are soluble proteins found in cytosolic extracts of target cells. Cytosol is accepted as an operational definition referring to the soluble portion of the cell, both nuclear and cytoplasmic. Most steroid receptors exist in the presence of other binding components, complicating measurements of their binding properties. Receptors associate with their particular steroid hormone in a reversible fashion and with high affinity and ligand specificity.

The rates of association and dissociation of steroid hormones with specific binding sites in cytosol from breast depend on incubation time and temperature according to the following reaction:

(1)
$$\text{Ligand} + \text{Receptor} \underset{k_{-1}}{\overset{k_1}{\rightleftharpoons}} [\text{Ligand-Receptor}]$$
$$\downarrow k_3 \qquad\qquad\qquad \downarrow k_2$$
$$\text{degradation} \qquad\qquad \text{degradation}$$

For example, the binding of ^{3}H-estradiol to its receptor is maximal at 4 hr at 0 to 3°C and remains virtually unchanged for 16 additional hours of incubation. At 25°C, apparent equilibrium is reached in 30 minutes and is maintained for 30 additional minutes before a gradual loss in binding activity is observed. Presumably, this loss is due to the degradation of the receptor protein itself, whether or not its binding sites are occupied by steroid. However, there is a possibility that irreversible dissociation of the steroid receptor complexes also occurs in some tumors. As a result of the temperature sensitivity of the estrogen-receptor and progestin-receptor complexes, the majority of binding reactions are performed at 0 to 3°C.

To demonstrate the affinity and concentration of steroid receptors in a cytosol preparation, aliquots are incubated with increasing concentrations of various labeled steroids for 5 to 18 hr at 0 to 3°C (Fig. 11–2). Routinely, 2,4,6,7-^{3}H-estradiol-17β and 17-methyl-^{3}H-promegestone (R5020) are used as labeled ligands to measure estrogen and progestin receptors, respectively (Fig. 11–3). An iodine-125 labeled estrogen (Fig. 11–2) has also been synthesized, which is also a satisfactory ligand for estrogen receptor determinations (Hochberg, 1979). Binding observed in the presence of an excess of unlabeled inhibitor is related to nonreceptor or nonspecific (low affinity, high capacity) association of the ligand. Specific binding is estimated as the difference between total and nonspecific binding (Fig. 11–3). Recently, a modified charcoal-gelatin assay has been described for estrogen receptors in very small biopsy specimens (Tandon et al., 1986). The use of a double-label procedure also increases sensitivity (Grill et al., 1984).

Using Scatchard analysis, the dissociation constant (K_d) or the association constant (K_a) may be determined from the slope of the plot according to the following equation:

$$\text{Slope} = -1/K_d, \text{ where } K_d = 1/K_a = k_{-1}/k_1$$

Here, k represents the rate constant for the association reaction, while k_{-1} represents the

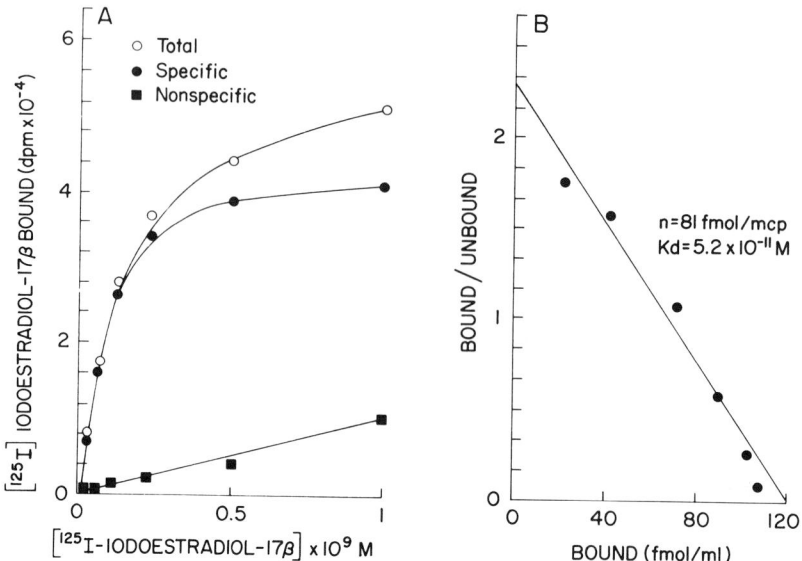

Figure 11–3. Titration analysis of estrogen receptors in human breast carcinoma. *A*, Aliquots (0.1 ml) of cytosol prepared from frozen human breast tumors were incubated in triplicate with 0.1 ml ^{125}I-iodoestradiol-17β solutions in homogenization buffer containing increasing amounts of radioactive ligand either in the absence (○) or presence (■) of a 200-fold excess of unlabeled diethylstilbestrol. Specific binding (●) was estimated as the difference between total binding (○) and binding in the presence of the competitor (■). *B*, The titration data from *A* were plotted according to the method of Scatchard. This dissociation constant (K_d) determined from the slope of the curve was 5.2×10^{-11} M for this preparation. The specific binding capacity (n) of the estrogen receptor complexes was estimated from the intercept on the x axis and gave a value of 81 fmol/mg of cytosol protein. (Reproduced by permission from Wittliff, J. L.: Steroid hormone receptors. *In* Pesce, A., and Kaplan, L. [Eds.]: Clinical Chemistry—Methods. St. Louis, The C. V. Mosby Co., 1987.)

rate constant for dissociation. The binding capacity is estimated from the intercept of the abscissa. By definition, the higher the affinity of the binding site, the lower the dissociation constant, which is a measure of the tendency of the steroid-receptor complex to dissociate. The rate of this first order process is highly dependent on both the type of ligand used in the assay and the kind of receptor being measured (Table 11–1). K_d values of 10^{-10} M to 10^{-11} M for the estrogen receptors and of 1 to 9×10^{-9} M to 1 to 9×10^{-10} M for progestin receptors when found on a patient's chart are good indicators that the biopsy specimen contains high affinity components.

Usually specific binding capacity is expressed in femtomoles (10^{-15} moles) of labeled steroid bound per milligram of cytosol protein. It is accepted, generally, that less than 3 fmol/mg cytosol protein represents a quantity of estrogen binding sites usually correlated with the lack of response of a breast cancer patient

Table 11–1. STEROID HORMONES AND ANALOGUES USED AS LIGANDS FOR STEROID HORMONE RECEPTORS

Estrogen Receptors	Progestin Receptors	Androgen Receptors	Glucocorticoid Receptors
^{3}H-estradiol-17β*	^{3}H-progesterone	^{3}H-testosterone	^{3}H-hydrocortisone
^{3}H-estrone	^{3}H-R5020	^{3}H-5α-dihydrotestosterone	^{3}H-corticosterone
^{3}H-estriol	(promegestone)*	^{3}H-R1881	^{3}H-dexamethasone*
^{125}I-iodoestradiol-17β*	^{3}H-R27987	(methyltrienolone)*	^{3}H-dexamethasone mesylate
^{3}H-R2858 (moxestrol)	^{3}H-Org 2058	^{3}H-cyproterone acetate	^{3}H-triamcinolone acetonide*
^{3}H-tamoxifen	^{3}H-medroxyprogesterone	^{3}H-mibolerone*	
^{3}H-tamoxifen-4OH	acetate		
^{3}H-tamoxifen aziridine			

*Most often employed in clinical assays.
Reproduced by permission from Wittliff, J. L.: Clinical analysis of steroid hormone receptors. *In* Pesce, A., and Kaplan, L. (Eds.): Clinical Chemistry—Methods. St. Louis, The C. V. Mosby Co., 1987.

Table 11–2. SPECIFIC BINDING CAPACITIES OF STEROID RECEPTORS IN BREAST TUMOR BIOPSY SPECIMENS ACCORDING TO PATIENT ENDOCRINE STATUS

Steroid Binding Capacity (fmol/mg cytosol protein)*		Endocrine Status of Patient	Receptor Status of Tumor
Estrogen	*Progestin*		
90 ± 9 (10–1335)	237 ± 22 (10–3038)	Premenopausal	ER$^+$, PR$^+$
83 ± 16 (10–568)	—	Premenopausal	ER$^+$, PR$^-$
—	84 ± 18 (10–1151)	Premenopausal	ER$^-$, PR$^+$
286 ± 18 (10–5693)	337 ± 28 (10–5922)	Postmenopausal	ER$^+$, PR$^+$
176 ± 29 (10–2807)	—	Postmenopausal	ER$^+$, PR$^-$
—	75 ± 26 (10–977)	Postmenopausal	ER$^-$, PR$^+$

*Measured by multipoint titration analyses using Scatchard plots. Mean ± standard error of the mean of number of determinations shown in Table 11–6. Range shown in parentheses. A level of > 10 fmol/mg cytosol protein was taken as an arbitrary cut-off point for the presence of receptors as utilized by the NSABP (Fisher et al., 1983).

From Wittliff, J. L.: Steroid hormone receptors in breast cancer. Cancer, *53*:630, 1984. Reprinted with permission.

given endocrine therapy of either the ablative or additive type (Proceedings of the NIH Consensus Development Conference, 1980; Wittliff, 1984). Although there is a "borderline" range of values from 3 to 10 or 20 fmol/mg cytosol protein, estrogen binding capacities of >10 fmol of estrogen appear to represent a clinically significant level (Fisher et al., 1983). The author's group has observed values of more than 5000 fmol/mg cytosol protein for the estrogen receptor and 6000 fmol/mg cytosol protein for progestin receptors in certain tumors (Table 11–2). The levels of estrogen receptors in breast tumor biopsy specimens from premenopausal patients appear considerably lower than those of postmenopausal women with breast carcinoma. In general, a higher progestin binding capacity was observed in tumor specimens from both premenopausal and postmenopausal women when the estrogen receptor was present in the tumor. However, a lower progestin receptor level was measured in the absence of estrogen receptors, supporting the suggestion that the formation of the progestin receptors is dependent on estrogen action (Horwitz et al., 1975).

Sucrose gradient centrifugation, which separates the various forms of the steroid receptors, assesses certain molecular properties of these proteins in a tumor extract (Fig. 11–4). Using this method, it has been determined that the sedimentation profiles of both estrogen and progestin receptors in human breast carcinomas fall into general categories (Wittliff, 1974): tumors that contain specific steroid binding components migrating at either 8 S (Svedberg units) only, at 4 S only, or at both 8 S and 4 S (Fig. 11–4), and those in which receptors are

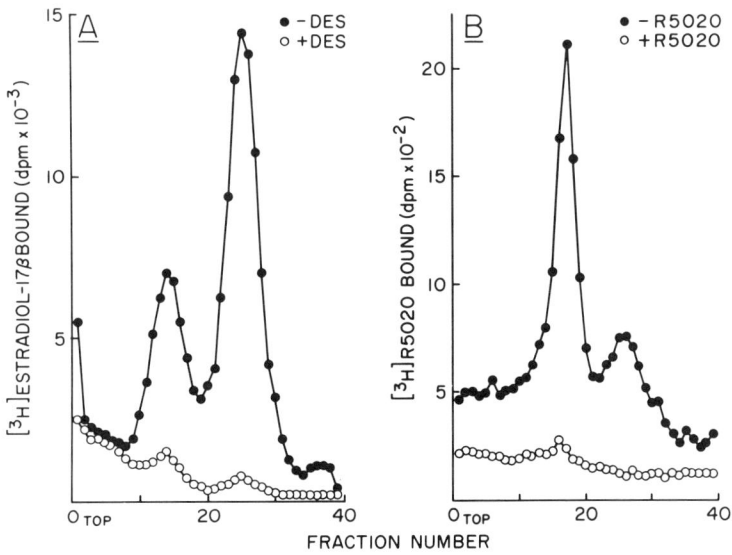

Figure 11–4. Sucrose density gradient separation of the isoforms of estrogen and progestin (R5020) receptors in human breast carcinoma. Tumor cytosol was reacted either with ^{3}H-estradiol-17β *(A)* or with ^{3}H-R5020 *(B)* for 4 hr at 3°C in the presence (○) or absence (●) of a 200-fold excess of unlabeled competitor. Note the presence of both 8 S and 4 S forms of these steroid receptors in the single breast carcinoma analyzed. (Reprinted with permission from *The Clinical Biochemistry of Cancer*, 1979. Copyright American Association for Clinical Chemistry, Inc.)

undetectable. The sedimentation coefficients of 8 S and 4 S are only approximate and are used operationally. The majority of breast tumors containing estrogen receptors exhibit both the 8 S and 4 S isoforms (Fig. 11–4). From 10 to 15 per cent of biopsy specimens contained only the 4 S specimens using sucrose gradient centrifugation with conditions of low ionic strength (Wittliff et al., 1978). As a result of the existence of two kinds of steroid receptors, each with four different types of profiles, there are at least 16 possible combinations. Clinical significance of this receptor polymorphism will be addressed later in this chapter.

A variety of software is available for performing the calculations required in the multipoint titration assay. Two commercially available programs have been developed independently by Beckman Instruments and by DuPont/NEN Products. A number of programs are also available from NIH sponsored efforts (Rodbard et al., 1980). The author's laboratory has developed a program from the multipoint titration assay and another that computes the specific binding capacities of the individual receptor isoforms, such as the 8 S and 4 S species separated by gradient centrifugation. These latter programs are available from the Hormone Receptor Laboratory, University of Louisville, Louisville, Kentucky.

EXPERIMENTAL METHODS

As a number of experimental methods were reviewed in detail in several recent reports (Wittliff, 1985, 1987; Wittliff and Wiehle, 1985), only brief mention of them will be made here. Table 11–3 outlines various methods of steroid receptor determination that may be used with the ligands listed in Table 11–1.

Steroid receptors are dynamic proteins whose properties of size, shape, surface charge, and hydrophobicity vary, depending on the conditions of their environments. Using various types of chromatography, these properties can be exploited so that the various species of the receptors can be separated. Early chromatographic methods used conventional gel filtration and ion-exchange chromatography (Wittliff, 1975). However, because of the extended times required for separation, many of the receptor species reported may have been products of reactions occurring with the packing matrices or as a result of the long incubation times.

To circumvent the problem of prolonged manipulation in receptor preparations, the use of high performance liquid chromatography (HPLC) in size exclusion, ion exchange, chromatofocusing, and hydrophobic interaction modes was developed for rapid, effective separation of receptor isoforms (Wittliff, 1985, 1986; Wittliff and Wiehle, 1985). HPLC separation has shown that receptors exhibit polymorphism. This is an indication that their composition is far more complicated than originally assumed. The author suggests the use of the term "fractionated receptors" to designate the pattern of the various steroid hormone–binding components (isoforms) displayed by a single receptor type (Wittliff, 1984) and predicts that sophisticated separation procedures, such as HPLC, will be used as a new generation of methods for the assay of steroid receptors in a tumor biopsy.

A representative profile of estrogen receptor isoforms separated on the basis of properties of size and shape using high performance size exclusion chromatography (HPSEC) is shown in Figure 11–5. Note the large variation in molecular weights of the receptor isoforms, similar to that seen with sucrose gradient centrifugation (Fig. 11–4).

Polymorphism of steroid hormone receptors also may be demonstrated by separating isoforms on the basis of surface charge properties using either ion exchange chromatography (HPIEC) (Wittliff and Wiehle, 1985) or chromatofocusing (HPCF) (Wittliff, 1986). Representative profiles of receptor isoforms are shown in Figures 11–6 and 11–7, which illustrate the two separation modes. The molecular heterogeneity of receptors in a tumor extract is easily detected within hours, and a small tissue sample (100 mg) is satisfactory for a complete assay. Table 11–4 summarizes some of the molecular properties of estrogen receptors in breast cells.

The clinical significance of isoform profiles is currently the subject of considerable research in the author's group. Various physiologic conditions appear to alter the relative amounts and distribution of isoforms of both estrogen and progestin receptors. Some of these parameters include patient age, endocrine status, and history of therapeutic manipulation. Application of "fractionated receptor" profiles to clinical management of breast cancer must await additional investigation.

Table 11-3. METHODS OF DETERMINING PRESENCE OF STEROID HORMONE RECEPTORS

Method	Principle	Usage	Comments
Titration	Sample incubated with increasing amounts of labeled steroid, with and without the presence of unlabeled inhibitor. Amount of specific binding plotted by Scatchard plot and the total number of binding sites and dissociation constant (K_d) are calculated.	Most frequently used	Requires largest sample size. Results dependent on ligand used.
Sucrose density gradient	Molecular forms of receptors of different sizes are separated on sucrose gradient following centrifugation. Location and number of sites present are determined by labeled ligand binding (with and without inhibitor).	Frequently used	Cannot calculate K_d by this method.
High performance liquid chromatography (HPLC) methods	Different receptor isoforms are separated by specific molecular property of receptors.	Research of molecular properties	Calculation of K_d values approximate by these methods.
a. Size exclusion	Following binding with labeled ligand, receptors are separated on basis of molecular size and shape.		
b. Ion exchange	Following binding with labeled ligand, receptors are separated on basis of their surface charge properties.		
c. Chromatofocusing	Following binding with labeled ligand, receptors are separated on basis of their isoelectric points.		
d. Hydrophobic interaction	Following binding with labeled ligand, receptors are separated on basis of different surface hydrophobicity.		
Immunofluorescence	Fluorescein-labeled steroid is bound to tissue steroid receptors. Amount of bound steroid is visualized by fluorescence microscopy.	Rare, experimental	Used for qualitative identification on small tissue biopsy specimens.
Immunohistochemical	Monoclonal antibody, specific for a steroid receptor, binds to tissue steroid receptor. Second antibody, labeled with peroxidase, is used to localize first antibody binding. Visualization of receptor in tissue with substrates for peroxidase stain.	Rare, experimental	Used for qualitative identification on small tissue samples.
Enzyme-linked immunoassay	Sandwich-assay with immobilized monoclonal antibody to receptor. Following binding of specific receptor, second monoclonal antibody labeled with horseradish peroxidase is bound. Quantitation using appropriate substrate is performed.	Research	Cannot be used to calculate K_d.

Reproduced by permission from Wittliff, J. L.: Clinical analyses of steroid hormone receptors. *In* Pesce, A., and Kaplan, L. (Eds.): Clinical Chemistry—Methods. St. Louis, The C. V. Mosby Co., 1987.

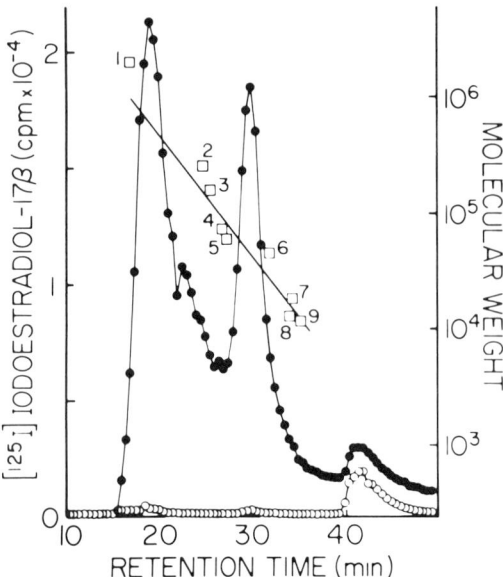

Figure 11–5. Identification and characterization of isoforms of the estrogen receptor from human breast cancer by high performance size exclusion chromatography (HPSEC). Cytosol was prepared from a sample of human breast cancer and incubated with 3 to 4 nM of ^{125}I-iodoestradiol-17β in the presence (○) and absence (●) of excess diethylstilbestrol (DES). A 200 μl aliquot of incubate was cleared of free steroid with dextran-coated charcoal and applied to a TSK 3000 SW chromatography column. Hemoglobin was added to all samples before analysis or reanalysis as an internal marker. In addition, the HPSEC system was calibrated using a series of pure proteins: (1) thyroglobulin, (2) catalase, (3) aldolase, (4) bovine serum albumin, (5) hemoglobin, (6) ovalbumin, (7) lysozyme, (8) myoglobin, and (9) cytochrome c. (From Wittliff, J. L., and Wiehle, R. D.: *In* Hollander, V. P. [Ed.]: Hormonally Responsive Tumors. New York, Academic Press, 1985, p. 383. Reprinted with permission.)

FLUORESCEIN-LINKED STEROID LIGANDS

Often breast carcinomas are discovered that contain an insufficient amount of tissue for titration analyses of estrogen and progestin receptors. Another approach to estimate the level of receptors in small biopsy specimens has been the use of fluorescein-linked steroid hormones (Chamness et al., 1980). This provides a nonradiochemical means of detecting receptors in histologic preparations of breast and endometrial cancer. The method involves the incubation of tissue slices with a fluorescein-linked estrogen and the visualization of the "receptor-bound" steroid under a fluorescence microscope.

Although the use of a fluorescein-linked steroid as a ligand for steroid hormone receptors would be desirable, especially for tissue biopsy sections of tumors, this procedure has been employed with very little success (Lonsdorfer et al., 1983). Thus far, the use of these compounds has two major disadvantages: (1) formation of estradiol as a derivative in the 17β position reduces the affinity of the ligand for the specific binding sites on the receptor, and (2) bonds between the fluorescent steroid ligand and the spacer are labile, so that assess-

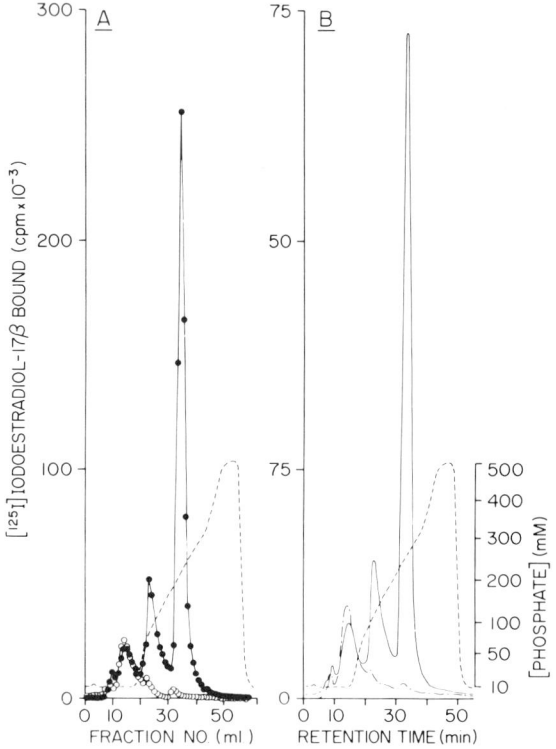

Figure 11–6. High performance ion exchange chromatography (HPIEC) separation of ionic isoforms of estrogen receptors from human breast cancer. Cytosol was prepared and incubated with 5 nM ^{125}I-iodoestradiol-17β as described earlier. Elution of the AX-1000 ion exchange column was performed on 200 μl of cytosol cleared of unbound ligand at 1.0 ml/min using a gradient of potassium phosphate at pH 7.4 (---). A, Fractions of 1 ml were collected and radioactivity measured manually with a gamma counter. B, Radioactivity was recorded continuously using the Beckman Model 170 Radioisotope Detector on-line with a conductivity flow cell. Total binding is indicated by • in A and by a solid line in B, and nonspecific binding is indicated by ○ in A and by —•—• in B. Recovery of radioactivity from the column was 97 per cent. Specific binding was 167 fmol receptor/mg cytosol protein determined by multipoint titration analysis. (From Boyle D. M., et al.: Rapid, high-resolution procedure for assessment of estrogen receptor heterogeneity in clinical samples. J. Chromatogr., *327*:369, 185. Reprinted with permission.)

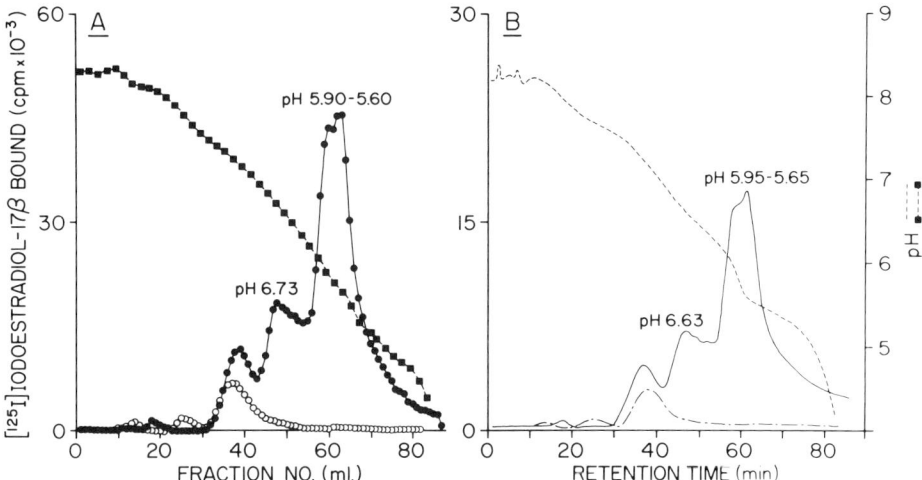

Figure 11–7. High performance chromatofocusing (HPCF) separation of ionic isoforms of estrogen receptors from human breast cancer. The sample of breast tissue and conditions used in this experiment were the same as described in the legend to Figure 11–6. The curves of bound ^{125}I-iodoestradiol-17β shown are the results of receptors separated in the presence (● in A; —•— in B) or absence (○ in A; — in B) of 200-fold excess of DES. Elution of the AX-500 column by a pH gradient was performed isocratically on 200 μl of cleared cytosol at 1.0 ml/min. The pH gradient is indicated as ■ in A and as ---- in B. A, Fractions of 1 ml were collected and radioactivity or pH was measured manually. B, Radioactivity and pH were recorded continuously using on-line Model 170 Radiosiotope Detector with flow-through electrode. Recovery of radioactivity from the column was 97 per cent. Specific binding was 167 fmol receptor/mg cytosol protein, determined by multipoint titration analysis. (From Boyle, D. M., et al.: Rapid, high-resolution procedure for assessment of estrogen receptor heterogeneity in clinical samples. J. Chromatogr., 327:369, 1985. Reprinted with permission.)

Table 11–4. COMPARISON OF PROPERTIES OF ESTROGEN RECEPTORS SEPARATED BY CONVENTIONAL METHODS AND VARIOUS MODES OF HPLC

Tissue	Sucrose Density Gradient Centrifugation	Sephacryl S-300	HPSEC (TSK 3000 SW Column)	DEAE-Cellulose	HPIEC (AX-1000 Column)	HPCF (AX-500 Column)
Human breast carcinoma	4–5 S and 8–9 S[a]		>61 A and 29–32 A[d]	0.03 M KCl 0.09 M KCl 0.22 M KCl[e]	52, 100, 190 mM phosphate[g]	pH 6.3, 5.3 4.8–3.5 shoulder[h]
MCF-7 cells	4–5 S and 8–9 S[b]	85 A and 65–70 A[b]	68 A[b]		55 and 180 mM phosphate[b]	pH 6.3 and 4.3[b]
Rat lactating mammary gland	4–5 S and 8–9 S[c]	>85 A, 70–72 A, and 28–30 A	>61 A[d]	0.02–0.05 M KCl 0.18–0.20 M KCl[f]	90 and 205 mM phosphate[g]	pH 6.8 and 6.5[i]

[a]Wittliff et al. (1972).
[b]Shahabi et al. (1984).
[c]Wittliff (1975).
[d]Wiehle et al. (1984).
[e]Kute et al. (1978).
[f]Wittliff et al. (1978).
[g]Wiehle and Wittliff (1984).
[h]Boyle et al. (1985).
[i]Hutchens et al. (1983).

HPSEC, High performance size exclusion chromatography; DEAE, Diethylaminoethylcellulose; HPIEC, high performance ion exchange chromatography; HPCF, high performance chromatofocusing; S, Svedberg units; A, Angstrom; KCl, potassium chloride.

ment of the affinity constant is made difficult because of the presence of contaminated free estradiol. The unequivocal determination of estrogen receptors in tissue preparations has not been possible because of these and other complicating factors, such as tissue autofluorescence and low affinity association (Berns et al., 1984).

IMMUNOCYTOCHEMICAL TECHNIQUES

The majority of the immunohistochemical techniques for localization of steroid hormone receptors use highly specific monoclonal antibodies directed against the partially purified receptor (Greene et al., 1980). Sections of freshly frozen tumor biopsy samples are prepared in a cryostat, and the slides are immersed immediately in 3.7 per cent formaldehyde-phosphate buffered saline at 25°C for 10 minutes. The tissue sections are then transferred to 100 per cent methanol for 4 minutes at −10°C followed by a 1 minute soak at −10°C in acetone. A peroxidase-antiperoxidase method for immunocytochemical staining has been employed. Normal goat serum serves as the blocking antibody, and the primary antibody is a monoclonal antibody to human estrogen receptor (Greene et al., 1984). The bridging antibody is goat anti-rat immunoglobulin; thus, the peroxidase-antiperoxidase complex must be of rat origin. Serial sections of breast should be prepared as control slides by incubation with rat immunoglobulin. Peroxidase activity is detected by use of the substrate diaminobenzidine. Evaluation of the immunohistochemical analysis is largely qualitative, although some workers (McCarty et al., 1985) divide the percentage of positively stained epithelial cells into various intensity categories using a system of 0, 1+, 2+, and so on.

Although this represents a nonradiochemical means of detecting these receptors in histologic preparations of cancer, the method is largely qualitative. At this point, the procedure is primarily for investigational use and is being correlated with conventional ligand-binding assays (King et al., 1985; McCarty et al., 1985). It is unclear whether these commercially prepared monoclonal antibodies (Abbott Laboratories, North Chicago, Ill.) react with the various isoforms of the steroid hormone receptors to the same extent (Sato et al., 1986). Furthermore, another disadvantage is that the immunohistochemical procedures are available only for the estrogen receptor. However, monoclonal antibodies to the progestin receptor are being developed in several laboratories and may become available for laboratory use in the late 1980s.

ENZYME-LINKED IMMUNOCHEMICAL ASSAY

This procedure is also based on a sandwich technique that involves two specific monoclonal antibodies prepared against the partially purified estrogen receptor (Greene et al., 1980, 1984). The first antibody (D-547) is immobilized on a polystyrene bead. Cytosol is prepared in either Tris or phosphate buffer containing 5 to 10 mM sodium molybdate and incubated with the polystyrene bead for 18 hr at 3°C. After incubation and complexing of the receptor with the monoclonal antibody (H-222), the bead is washed and a second monoclonal antibody that has previously been labeled with peroxidase is incubated with the bead. The horseradish peroxidase enzyme linked to the second antibody serves as a marker for the presence of the estrogen receptor. The intensity of the color produced as a result of the enzymatic action of the horseradish peroxidase on the substrate indicates the quantity of the receptor present in the cytosol. This procedure measures the mass of the receptor, in contrast to radioligand binding techniques, which measure the steroid binding capacity. However, most workers relate the enzyme immunoassay results to specific steroid binding capacity, expressed as femtomoles per milligram (fmol/mg) of cytosol protein. There appears to be considerable variation in the estrogen receptor levels measured by the multipoint titration assay compared to that observed with the enzyme immunoassay (EIA) (Mirecki and Jordan, 1985; Nakao et al., 1985; Raam and Vrabel, 1986; Symposium on Estrogen Receptor Determination with Monoclonal Antibodies, 1986) with a greater receptor level by the EIA method. Since the molecular basis of this difference is unclear, the assay is still under investigation.

Quality Control of Steroid Receptor Analyses

SOURCES OF VARIABILITY IN ASSAY PROCEDURES

An extensive problem has been the lack of uniformity in the methods of receptor analyses in the clinical laboratory and in the expression of specific steroid binding data (Wittliff et al., 1980, 1981; Sarfaty et al., 1981; Leclercq et al., 1984). Some of the common sources of variability in steroid receptor analyses by clinical laboratories which the author and colleagues have observed in the past 10 years are the following:

1. Type and range of steroid ligand concentrations
2. Concentration and type of competitive inhibitor
3. Incubation time and temperature
4. Concentration of cytosol protein and type of assay selected

In addition, there are a number of other parameters that may complicate steroid receptor analyses if not properly controlled. Among these are the following:

1. Metabolism of the ligand
2. Contribution of nonspecific (low affinity, high capacity) binding
3. Ligand-receptor dissociation
4. Ligand association with specific serum proteins, such as TeBG and CBG
5. Thermal lability in both the biopsy and cell-free preparations
6. Ionic strength lability
7. Occupancy of binding sites by endogenous hormone
8. Receptor "inhibiting" substances
9. Proteolysis

To ensure accurate quantification of the number of steroid binding sites in a biopsy specimen using a titration procedure and dextran-coated charcoal to remove unbound steroid, it is necessary to use a broad range of tritium-labeled ligand concentrations. These must include a sufficient number of points below the saturation level so that an interpretable Scatchard plot is generated (Fig. 11–3). From experience with laboratories participating in cooperative clinical trials, a considerable number used too many saturating concentrations of either ^{3}H-estradiol or ^{3}H-R5020 so that the points were "grouped" near the abscissa of the Scatchard plot, making it difficult to estimate the dissociation constant as well as number of specific binding sites accurately.

Another common source of variation is the concentration and type of competitive inhibitor used to estimate the contribution of nonspecific (low affinity, high capacity) binding. It appears this is largely due to contamination of tumor biopsy specimens by necrotic material and blood, which may contain albumin and other proteins, such as TeBG and CBG, known to associate specifically with steroid hormones. Diethylstilbestrol is a potent synthetic estrogen that does not bind to plasma proteins with high affinity. Thus, it is a useful inhibitor in estrogen receptor analyses (Fig. 11–3) as it associates only with intracellular binding components. The dissociation constant (K_d) of the diethylstilbestrol-receptor complexes in cytosol from breast tumors is approximately 10^{-9} M, which is higher than that of estradiol-receptor complexes (Wittliff et al., 1978). Routinely, the author uses a 200-fold excess of unlabeled diethylstilbestrol in a titration assay.

A similar quantity (200-fold excess) of unlabeled R5020, a synthetic progestin, is used with ^{3}H-R5020 to estimate low affinity, high capacity binding. Since R5020 and certain glucocorticoids may associate with similar binding sites (McGuire et al., 1977), it is advisable to use low nanomolar (nM) concentrations of ^{3}H-R5020 to avoid also measuring glucocorticoid receptors (Horwitz and McGuire, 1975). The principal advantage of using ^{3}H-R5020 as a ligand for the progestin receptor is that it does not associate to any great extent with CBG, known to bind progesterone, the natural progestin. Furthermore, it does not dissociate readily from the progestin receptor of mammary gland, as has been observed for progesterone, nor is it metabolized under the conditions of most clinical assays (Wittliff et al., 1981a).

If the sucrose gradient procedure (Fig. 11–4) is used to quantify steroid receptors, the investigator must be sure to use a saturating concentration of the tritium labeled ligand, usually 3 to 5 nM for either estradiol-17β or R5020, as suggested from titration analyses (Fig. 11–2). Furthermore, it is imperative to use a competitive inhibitor of ligand binding to estimate the receptor proteins clearly. Because albumin and other contaminating proteins sediment in the 4 S to 5 S region of the sucrose gradient, where certain receptor species migrate as well (Fig. 11–4), the ligand specificity should be evaluated. Using the newer techniques of HPLC for receptor isoform separation (Wittliff and Wiehle, 1985; Wittliff, 1986), unlabeled inhibitors are also employed to ensure specificity (Figs. 11–5 to 11–7).

QUALITY ASSURANCE PROGRAMS

Currently, both female sex steroid receptors are being analyzed annually in thousands of breast tumor biopsy specimens in the United States alone. As a means of examining the correlations of these data with responses to specific therapeutic techniques, certain clinical cooperative groups, particularly the National Surgical Adjuvant Breast Project (NSABP) and the Southeastern Cancer Study Group (SECSG) initiated experimental therapeutic protocols in the late 1970s requiring analyses of estrogen and progestin receptors of breast tumors (Wittliff et al., 1980, 1981a). Thus, the establishment of assay uniformity and quality control was imperative to ensure meaningful correlations between laboratory results and clinical response.

The following conclusions were drawn from the 1979 NIH Consensus Development Conference on Steroid Receptors in Breast Cancer (DeSombre et al., 1979; Proceedings of the NIH Consensus Development Conference, 1980) regarding assay procedures for steroid receptors:

1. Freeze tissue immediately in dry ice or in liquid nitrogen and transport frozen to the assay laboratory.

2. Retain an adjacent piece of tumor tissue for pathology evaluation to confirm that the assay sample consists of tumor.

3. If the assay is not performed on the same day, store the tumor at −70°C or colder. Prolonged storage is discouraged.

4. The most reliable methods of analyses for both estrogen and progestin receptors are (a) sucrose gradient sedimentation and (b) multipoint titration with Scatchard analysis.

5. Histochemical procedures that localize steroid receptors within tissue are not yet validated.

6. There is a need for quality control of steroid receptor assays.

Regarding the last point, the author's laboratory (Wittliff et al., 1980, 1981a) developed a national reference program in 1977 for establishing uniformity in steroid receptor analyses.

A variety of tissue reference powders were prepared composed of various quantities of frozen, pulverized organs such as uterus, breast, muscle and liver, as well as certain types of sera (of pregnancy), using tissue grinders and liquid nitrogen. Breast tumors also were added to certain powders. Each of these reference powders is formulated in such a manner as to contain different combinations of estrogen and progestin receptors (e.g., estrogen receptor positive, progestin receptor negative; estrogen receptor positive, progestin receptor positive, and so forth) at different test levels. The exact composition is based on the specific need of each clinical cooperative trial group. Thus far, this laboratory has cooperated with the NSABP, SECSG, Southwest Oncology Group (SWOG), Cancer and Leukemia Group B (CALGB), North Central Cancer Treatment Group (NCCTG), Eastern Cooperative Oncology Group (ECOG), and the College of American Pathologists to bring about greater uniformity in the analyses of steroid receptors and the expression of binding capacity data. Currently more than 400 laboratories in North America are participating in this quality assurance program. The author's group has also cooperated with laboratories on virtually every continent to bring about standardized methods (Wittliff, 1987) and quality assessed results for clinical management of breast cancer.

Briefly, a laboratory from an institution participating in a treatment trial of one of the cooperative groups is sent a set of two to four different tissue powders frozen in dry ice. Often three vials of each powder are included to evaluate the intra-assay variability of each receptor measurement. A vial of unknown protein concentration is included to assess the influence of variation in this important determination. The laboratory analyzes these using "in house" methods and returns the results to the headquarters of the cooperative group for comparison with data generated by other laboratories and by the Reference Laboratory at the University of Louisville. Criteria for evaluating agreement of the results are established by committees in each of the cooperative groups. Either the committee or the Reference Laboratory contacts each participating laboratory in writing regarding its performance relative to that of the other laboratories participating in the clinical trial. A representative survey report is shown in Table 11–5. This important information is available to the phy-

Table 11–5. INTERNATIONAL ONCOLOGY GROUP, STEROID RECEPTOR REFERENCE LABORATORY, UNIVERSITY OF LOUISVILLE, SUMMARY RESULTS FROM DECEMBER 15, 1986, SHIPMENT OF TISSUE REFERENCE POWDER

Laboratory	Specific Estrogen Binding Capacity (fmol/mg Cytosol Protein)		Specific Progestin Binding Capacity (fmol/mg Cytosol Protein)		Protein Unknown (mg/ml)
	Mean ± SD Ref. Powder I[a]	Mean ± SD Ref. Powder II[b]	Mean ± SD Ref. Powder I[a]	Mean ± SD Ref. Powder II[b]	
IN-AA	101 ± 6	0	145 ± 18	0	3.9
IN-AB	67 ± 24	4	137 ± 40	4	5.5
IN-AC	104 ± 32	18	46 ± 4	0	4.0
IN-AD	57 ± 6	0	220 ± 53	14	3.9
IN-AE	85 ± 29	0	133 ± 12	2	3.9
IN-AF	100 ± 4	0	72 ± 9	1	3.3
IN-AG	97 ± 4	2	121 ± 7	15	3.4
IN-AH	96 ± 6	2	162 ± 21	2	3.8
IN-AI	90 ± 17	0	147 ± 24	0	4.7
IN-AJ	44 ± 33	0	182 ± 31	0	6.2
U of L #1	95 ± 2	2	150 ± 8	2	3.1
Return Shipment #2	104 ± 4	3	164 ± 2	3	3.0
Target Values	98 ± 10	2	155 ± 5	2	3.6 ± 0.3
Kd values (× 10 −10M)	1.9 ± 0.4		2.4 ± 0.7		(Bradford)
Participating Labs	84 ± 28		137 ± 54		4.3 ± 0.9
range	44 − 104		46 − 220		3.3–6.2

[a] Reference Powder I designated as IN-225, IN-227, IN-228 (n=3)
[b] Reference Powder II designated as IN-226, IN-229 (n=2)
[c] Sucrose density gradient centrifugation method
Target and Kd values generated by multipoint titration analysis using dextran-coated charcoal.
Please note these were analyzed over a period of at least 10–12 weeks and may reflect some degradation.

Reference Powder Assays n = 15
Reference Powder Assays n = 15

Compliance Criteria					
Within	7 of 10	9 of 10	6 of 10	8 of 10	7 of 10
Above	0 of 10	1 of 10	1 of 10	2 of 10	3 of 10
Below	3 of 10		3 of 10		0 of 10

sician treating the patient by contacting the headquarters of the clinical trial group. It is essential that receptor assays on breast tumor biopsy tissue be conducted by laboratories meeting the compliance criteria of one or more of the quality assurance programs.

Factors Influencing the Level of Steroid Receptors

CLINICAL AND PHYSIOLOGIC FACTORS

A number of clinical and physiologic factors must be considered when assessing the significance of a steroid receptor level. These include (1) race, (2) sex, (3) age, (4) menopausal status, (5) day of cycle (premenopausal), (6) pregnancy and lactation, (7) organ site, (8) tumor cellularity and histologic differentiation, and (9) prior drug administration.

As discussed earlier (Table 11–2), the concentration of estrogen receptors in biopsy specimens of infiltrating ductal carcinoma show a broad spectrum of values ranging from zero to almost 6000 fmol/mg cytosol protein. Thus far, no single histologic feature has been found that might explain the variation in the levels of estrogen receptors in human breast tumors. However, Black and coworkers (1983) suggested that tumor cellularity and estrogen receptor levels were related to prognosis for operable breast cancer. Prognosis was actually better in patients with low cellularity.

Related to histopathology, Chua and associates (1985) reported a strong correlation between estrogen receptor level, age, and histologic grade of breast tumors from women in Singapore. Silfversward and coworkers (1980) reported a positive correlation between estrogen receptor content and degree of differentiation in ductal carcinoma. Cancer with lymphoid infiltration generally showed low estrogen receptor levels. Other studies (Rosen et al., 1975; Wittliff et al., 1976; Meyer et al., 1977; Mills, 1980; Chabon et al., 1982; Howat et al., 1983; Ponsky et al., 1984) have investigated the relationship of pathologic features and receptor status. At this time there is considerable variability in the results reported and a well-controlled interlaboratory study is recommended for assessing the relationship of parameters such as histologic classification, nuclear grade, DNA content, ploidy, and lymphocytic infiltration to receptor status. In general, it may be concluded that the presence of both sex steroid receptors implies retention of the regulatory mechanisms operating in the normal breast epithelium. Thus, a loss in receptor may be taken with other neoplastic features as a means of identifying patients at increased risk of tumor recurrence or mortality (Parl et al., 1984).

In the author's experience, the proportion of tumor cells to surrounding connective tissue and adipose cells does not appear to be correlated with a variation in estrogen binding capacity (Wittliff et al., 1976), although connective tissue appears to contribute to the quantity of progesterone receptors estimated in a biopsy specimen. This observation relates to the finding that fibroblasts may contain significant levels of specific progestin binding components. For this reason, it is imperative to use a biopsy specimen that contains as much of the malignant lesion as is possible. It is known that the adipose cells of normal breast do not contain specific estrogen receptors (Wittliff, 1975), although these cells have the ability to take up a considerable amount of the steroid hormones, presumably because of their lipid solubility. At present, it has not been determined if the level of a steroid receptor in a tumor biopsy specimen is a reflection of a heterogeneous cell population in which a variable number of tumor cells exhibit hormone sensitivity or a more homogeneous cell population in which individual cells contain variable numbers of estrogen receptor molecules. Analysis of this point is under investigation using the new immunocytochemical methods for detecting steroid receptors (King et al., 1985; McCarty et al., 1985).

Although several studies have investigated this aspect, there does not appear to be a correlation between steroid receptor status and either the size or location of the tumor in the breast, the axillary node status, or the clinical stage of the disease. It was initially reported (McGuire et al., 1975) that larger tumors contained lower quantities of estrogen receptors, presumably because of increased necrosis, but this has not been supported from later, more thorough investigations presented at the NIH Consensus Development Conference (Proceedings of the NIH Consensus Development Conference, 1980).

The endocrine status has influence on the endogenous concentration of estrogens in the plasma and in the tumor of the patient. Circulating estrogen and progesterone levels are known to influence the number of specific binding sites on receptor proteins occupied in vivo by the steroid hormones. For example, Maass and colleagues (Maass et al., 1972; Trams and Maass, 1976) and Pollow and associates (1980) have found that the estrogen binding capacity in target organs varies during the menstrual cycle; it is low in midcycle and is reduced further in the second phase. Trams and Maass and their colleagues (1976; Stegner et al., 1980) have also shown that there is insignificant binding of ^{3}H-estradiol to receptors in breast tumors from patients with plasma estradiol-17β levels exceeding 300 mg/ml.

Most studies indicate that both the incidence and the concentration of estrogen receptors in breast tumors are lower in premenopausal than in postmenopausal women (Tables 11–2 and 11–6). Clearly patient age has an influence on the level of receptors, with higher concentrations being exhibited by tumors from elderly patients (Wittliff, 1974; Alghanem and Hussain, 1985; McCarty et al., 1983). Apparently this is also due in part to the elevated levels of endogenous estrogen in plasma of premenopausal women, which may mask receptor binding sites. However, since estrogen is known to stimulate the formation of its own receptor as well as the progesterone receptor (Horwitz and McGuire, 1975; Horwitz et al., 1975), the level of circulating estrogen may not be the only factor. Elevated circulating progesterone levels in the premenopausal patient with breast cancer may reduce the formation of estrogen receptors in comparison with the level known to occur in the postmenopausal women, in whom progesterone levels are lower (Proceedings of the NIH Consensus Development Conference, 1980). Thus, it appears prudent to consider the menstrual status of a breast cancer patient when evaluating the significance of the specific steroid binding capacity in the selection of a therapeutic regimen.

In general, the levels of specific estrogen

receptors in biopsy specimens of metastatic breast carcinomas are similar to those observed in primary tumors (Proceedings of the NIH Consensus Development Conference, 1980; Wittliff and Dapunt, 1980; Hall et al., 1983). There is general agreement that the incidence of estrogen and progestin receptors is somewhat elevated in tumor biopsy specimens of postmenopausal patients compared with those of premenopausal women (Table 11–6). This may be due to the fact that metastatic lesions are often less differentiated than primary breast tumors. During malignant transformation, there may have been a loss of steroid hormone receptors, reflecting a more endocrine-independent growth pattern. A few studies reported at the Consensus Development Conference and later (Proceedings of the NIH Consensus Development Conference, 1980; Hull et al., 1983; Young et al., 1985) using multiple sequential biopsy specimens suggest that there may be a progressive loss of estrogen receptors in breast tumors with progression of the disease.

Hähnel and Twaddle (1985) have provided an excellent review of the relationship between estrogen receptors in primary and secondary breast carcinomas and in sequential primary breast cancers. No major discordance in estrogen receptor status was observed in 48 cases from their laboratory. In the majority (~80 per cent) of cases reviewed, estrogen receptor status of the asynchronous secondary tumor was the same as that of the primary tumor, even though variations in quantifiable receptor levels were observed in approximately half of the tumors. There was no consistent influence of site or time interval between primary and secondary tumor appearance on the variation in estrogen receptors. This author agrees with Hähnel and Twaddle's recommendation that whenever feasible steroid receptors should be reevaluated in the metastatic lesion.

Thus, the majority of investigations support the view that the presence of steroid receptors in a primary tumor correlates well (75 to 85 per cent) with the presence of receptors in metastatic lesions even though the time interval between these two events may be years. These data clearly indicate every primary breast tumor should be analyzed for steroid receptors even if the patient does not have metastatic disease. Later in the course of the breast carcinoma, receptor levels may become even more useful if the metastatic lesions have disseminated to organs such as bone and brain, which are not easily accessible for biopsy.

Table 11–6. DISTRIBUTION OF STEROID RECEPTORS IN TUMOR BIOPSIES ACCORDING TO PATIENT ENDOCRINE STATUS*

Receptor Status of Tumor Biopsy Specimen	Endocrine Status of Patient	
	Premenopausal	Postmenopausal
ER$^+$, PR$^+$	222 (45%)	520 (63%)
ER$^+$, PR$^-$	58 (12%)	128 (15%)
ER$^-$, PR$^-$	136 (28%)	137 (17%)
ER$^-$, PR$^+$	72 (15%)	41 (5%)
Total	488	826

*Fifty-five years of age was chosen as an age at which virtually every woman may be considered postmenopausal.

From Wittliff, J. L.: Steroid hormone receptors in breast cancer. Cancer, 53:630, 1984. Reprinted with permission.

The influence of interim therapies using cytotoxic drugs or antihormones must be taken into consideration. Studies by Allegra and coworkers (1978) suggested that intervening hormonal therapy selectively eliminates estrogen receptor containing cells, but chemotherapy apparently has little or no effect on the specific estrogen binding capacity of tumor biopsy specimens.

Wilking and colleagues (1984) observed that tamoxifen exhibited a small influence on estradiol-17β production in human breast tumors. Burke and coworkers (1978) reported that estrogen receptor levels were not altered by irradiation of human breast cancer cells and, furthermore, reappeared after removal of antiestrogen inhibition. Because of the half-life of tamoxifen-receptor complexes in vivo, it is recommended that Nolvadex administration be discontinued at least 3 weeks prior to biopsy for steroid receptor analyses. Literature from studies on cells in culture (Allegra and Lippman, 1980) and in patients (Carlson et al., 1984) clearly indicate that tamoxifen may work either as an estrogen agonist or as an estrogen antagonist, depending on its concentration. Furthermore, it may be used therapeutically to induce progestin receptors in human tumors (Mortel et al., 1981; Carlson et al., 1984).

Consideration of the organ sites of breast carcinoma metastases is one of the criteria used in the selection of therapy for the breast cancer patient. During the past decade this author and others (Proceedings of the NIH Consensus Development Conference, 1980; Wittliff, 1984) have demonstrated the presence of estrogen and progestin receptors in breast carcinoma metastases from the adrenal gland, bone, colon, contralateral breast, kidney, liver, lung, lymph nodes, muscle, omentum, ovary, skin, stomach, and thyroid gland. The incidence and specific steroid binding capacities of these metastatic lesions varied considerably; however, the ligand affinities and specificities of the sex hormone receptors were characteristic of those in normal tissues. At no time has a correlation been observed between the presence of steroid receptors and the organ site of these metastatic lesions in breast cancer patients.

The race of the patient apparently also has an influence on both clinical prognosis (Wynder et al., 1963; Morrison et al., 1973; Nemoto et al., 1980; Walker et al., 1984) and steroid receptor status (Nomura et al., 1977, 1984; Savage et al., 1981; Mohla et al., 1982; Pegoraro et al., 1986a,b). At this time relationship between receptor status and level with survival data considering white, black, and Asian patients is unclear. Important is the simultaneous development of reference ranges of sex steroid receptors in these racial groups and their clinical significance.

REFERENCE RANGES

As the multipoint titration assay described has been used in the author's laboratory for more than 15 years on literally thousands of biopsy specimens from breast cancer patients, well-defined reference ranges have been developed. As already noted, usually specific binding capacity is expressed as femtomoles (10^{-15} moles) of labeled steroid bound per milligram of cytosol protein. Because menopausal status is one of the factors influencing receptor level (Table 11–2), the reference ranges should be considered in terms of this factor (Bland et al., 1981; McCarty et al., 1983). Table 11–2 and Figure 11–8 provide examples of the ranges in steroid binding capacity in breast tumors from premenopausal patients (range, 10 to 3038 fmol/mg cytosol protein) and postmenopausal patients (range, 10 to 5922 fmol/mg cytosol protein). It is generally accepted (McGuire et al., 1975, 1977; Proceedings of the NIH Consensus Development Conference, 1980; Wittliff, 1984) that a level of greater than 10 fmol/mg cytosol protein of receptor is taken as a cut-off point for the presence of these receptors as utilized by the NSABP (Fisher et al., 1981, 1983). The sensitivity of the assay and the biologic data suggest that less than 3 fmol/mg cytosol protein is a clinically insignificant quantity in human breast tumors. K_d values of 1 to 9 × 10^{-10} M to 1 to 9 × 10^{-11} M are representative of the estrogen receptor, where 1 to 9 × 10^{-9} M to 1 to 9 × 10^{-10} M are indicative of the presence of high affinity progestin binding components.

Intra-assay variation by a single operator in the author's laboratory is indicated by a coefficient of variance of 5 to 11 per cent (Wittliff, 1987). Intralaboratory comparison of the performance of multipoint titration analyses by 3 or 4 operators in the author's laboratory gave coefficients of variance of 10 to 19 per cent. Comparison of interlaboratory performance by several of the survey programs conducted by the Reference Laboratory at the University of Louisville for clinical cooperative trial groups and the College of American Pathologists gave coefficients of variance of 40 to 65 per cent. These data are misleading in that the summaries contain the results from numerous laboratories that did not meet the compliance criteria required by the cooperative groups. The sample survey data presented in Table 11–5 provides an example of the manner in which the results are reported to the participants. Certainly, the reproducibility is significantly greater within an individual laboratory.

It should also be noted that some tumors exhibit the presence of both estrogen and progestin receptors whereas others exhibit only one of these receptors (Proceedings of the NIH Consensus Development Conference, 1980), as illustrated in Table 11–6. A fourth category does not exhibit either steroid hormone receptor. This distribution of receptor types is important to note, particularly that of the progestin receptor, for which the level is high in tumors from premenopausal patients in the presence of the estrogen receptor but considerably lower and rarely observed in patients who do not exhibit the estrogen receptor (Table 11–6). An example of the distribution of the two receptor types in premenopausal and postmenopausal patients with breast cancer is shown in Figure 11–8. In general, steroid hormone receptors are seen more often and at higher concentrations in breast tumors in postmenopausal patients than in those of premenopausal patients. In addition, the curious distribution in which the estrogen receptor is lacking and the progestin receptor is present is seen three times more often in biopsy specimens of premenopausal patients than in the postmenopausal patients (Bland et al., 1981). This appears to be due to the presence of

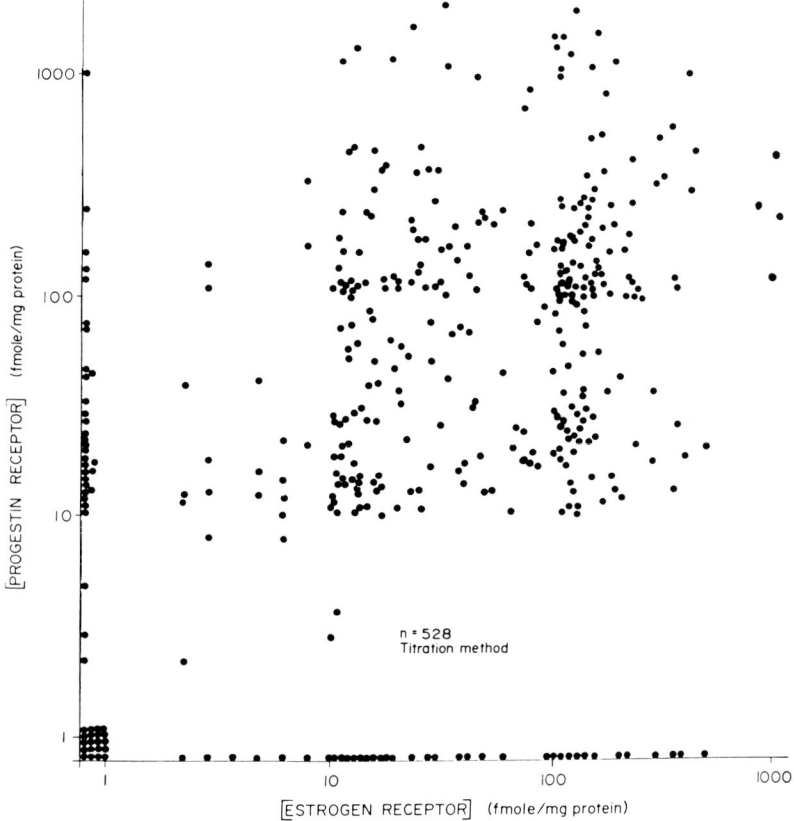

Figure 11–8. Distribution of estrogen and progesterone receptors in human breast tumors determined by multipoint titration analyses using dextran-coated charcoal to remove unbound steroids. Specific steroid binding capacities are expressed as fmol/mg cytosol protein. ^{3}H-Estradiol-17β and ^{3}H-R5020 were used to measure estrogen and progestin receptors, respectively. (From Wittliff, J. L.: Steroid hormone receptors in breast cancer. Cancer, 53:630, 1984. Reprinted with permission.)

circulating estrogens in the plasma in premenopausal patients, which thereby masks the steroid hormone receptors in a tumor biopsy specimen (Maass et al., 1972; McCarty et al., 1983).

As it appears that, in the presence of endogenous ligand or when associated with a hormonal type of drug, such as tamoxifen, the steroid hormone receptor associates more tightly with nuclear components (matrix and chromatin), radioligand binding procedures would be expected to provide in some biopsies an underestimation of the number of receptors. If the new enzyme immunoassay (EIA) monoclonal based antibody procedures (Greene et al., 1984; Raam and Vrabel, 1986) can be sufficiently validated both in the laboratory and with clinical response data, they will provide a logical avenue to estimate both ligand associated and nonassociated forms of the receptor in biopsy specimens. In this author's opinion, both enzyme immunoassays and immunocytochemical procedures for measuring these receptors require further investigation and standardization at this time (Wittliff, 1987).

It is known that the stage of differentiation of the normal mammary gland influences the level of receptor concentration in that target tissue (Wiehle and Wittliff, 1983). In this regard there are a few data defining the influence of stage of tumor differentiation on the level of estrogen and progestin receptors expected in a tumor biopsy (Proceedings of the NIH Consensus Development Conference, 1980). However, the relationship of stage of tumor differentiation and of patient age, menopausal status, day of cycle, and associated therapy complicates interpretations of the results. Therefore, it is essential that the relevant information be indicated on the assay request form prior to analysis.

HORMONE RECEPTOR LABORATORY
JAMES GRAHAM BROWN CANCER CENTER
SCHOOL OF MEDICINE
THE UNIVERSITY OF LOUISVILLE
LOUISVILLE, KY 40292

D86-075
11/20/86
law

Patient's Name: Smith, Mary Ann   Surgery Number: S86-4861

Hospital or Laboratory: Lamar Memorial   Hospital or Lab Number: W38-502

Physician's Name: Dr. N. Martin

Date of Surgery: November 11, 1986

Date of Tissue Acquisition: November 12, 1986

Date of Assay: November 12, 1986

Remarks: multipoint titration analyses

Technologist: C.H. Jones
C.H. Jones, MT (ASCP)

TYPE OF RECEPTOR

SPECIFIC STEROID BINDING CAPACITY (fmol/mg cytosol protein)	ESTROGEN	PROGESTIN	ANDROGEN	GLUCOCORTICOID
	62	153	136	--
DISSOCIATION CONSTANT (M)	1.4×10^{-10}	4.8×10^{-10}	2.5×10^{-10}	

INTERPRETATION:

Less than 3 fmol/mg cytosol protein (estrogen and progestin receptors) usually assumed to indicate a clinically insignificant level of steroid receptor (Cancer 46(12):2759–2963, 1980).

Greater than 10 fmol/mg cytosol protein usually correlated with an increased likelihood of an objective remission to endocrine therapy. Both the level of estrogen receptor and the presence of progestin receptor appear related to objective clinical response (New England J. Medicine, 301:1011–1012, 1979; Cancer 46(12):2759–2963, 1980; J. Clinical Oncology 1:227–241, 1983).

Clinical significance of androgen and glucocorticoid receptors under investigation.

Progestin receptors correlated with regression of endometrial carcinoma and progestin therapy (Obstet. Gynecol. 55:363, 1980; Am. J. Obstet. Gynecol. 141:539, 1981; Cancer 50:2157, 1982).

James L. Wittliff, Ph.D.
Director
(502) 588-5694/5216

Interstate License #16-1047
State License #200078

White: Physician's Copy — Yellow: Hospital Copy — Pink: Pathologist Copy — Gold: Laboratory Copy

Figure 11–9. Clinical report form for steroid receptor results on a hypothetical patient with breast carcinoma.

There are at least three studies indicating that ethnic origin has an influence on steroid binding capacity in the tumor biopsy (Savage et al., 1981; Mohla et al., 1982; Pegoraro et al., 1986a,b). A recent study (Crowe et al., 1986) reports a striking relationship between the interaction of estrogen receptor status and race in predicting prognosis for Stage I breast cancer patients. These preliminary data would suggest that reference ranges may vary in different areas of the world, depending on the population distribution. However, more studies will have to be performed before these reference ranges can be defined readily.

This author highly recommends that an individual laboratory develop its own distribution profiles of steroid hormone receptors, such as presented in Figure 11–8 and including the levels found in the various types of tumors, as presented in Tables 11–2 and 11–6. These should be compared with studies published in the literature to ensure that a laboratory is generating comparable information, thus indicating a valid procedure. A representative Clinical Report Form used in the author's laboratory is presented in Figure 11–9. Note that specific binding capacity, affinity constant (K_d value), and references related to interpretation are given. Also note that results from androgen and glucocorticoid receptors are often reported, which assist in establishing the degree of loss in hormone regulatory mechanisms in breast cancer cells (Wittliff, 1984, 1986). Allegra and colleagues (1979a,b) have evaluated the relationships between all of the steroid hormone receptors, revealing interesting correlations that the author's laboratory is currently pursuing.

Clinical Significance of Estrogen Receptors

During the past decade it was demonstrated conclusively that the presence of estrogen receptors provides a molecular basis for the distinction between human breast carcinomas that are responsive to hormonal therapy or to endocrine organ ablative surgery and those that are not. From studies of these steroid binding proteins in hormonally responsive tumors of rodents, Jensen and coworkers (1971) originally suggested that the ability of a breast carcinoma to bind estrogen may be predictive of a patient's response to endocrine therapy.

This was supported by their findings in which the presence of estrogen receptors in tumor biopsy specimens of patients was correlated with a favorable response to adrenalectomy. Since the original report of Folca and coworkers in 1961, numerous studies (Proceedings of the NIH Consensus Development Conference, 1980) have shown that approximately one half of all biopsy specimens of malignant breast tumors contain estrogen receptors.

The analyses of approximately 8000 breast tumor specimens over the past decade indicates that 60 to 65 per cent of primary lesions and 45 to 55 per cent of metastatic breast tumors exhibit more than 10 fmol/mg cytosol protein binding of estrogen receptors. Furthermore, 53 per cent of patients with breast tumors containing estrogen receptors were responsive to hormonal therapies of the additive or ablative type (Wittliff et al., 1978). The data given in Table 11–7 are the collective results from investigators participating in the NIH Consensus Development Conference in 1979. They represent the level of response (50 to 60 per cent) that may be expected of a breast cancer patient given hormonal manipulation when only estrogen receptor status is considered. These results are also in excellent agreement with the data presented in 1974 at the first International Workshop on Estrogen Receptors in Human Breast Cancer (Table 11–8). Unfortunately, the field has not progressed sufficiently to indicate the particular therapeutic method to be chosen.

Numerous investigations also support the thesis that the number of objective remissions in breast cancer patients given hormone therapy may be expected to increase with an elevation in specific estrogen binding capacity of the tumor. If the collective results of the reports from the NIH Consensus Development Conference are summarized, there appears to

Table 11–7. RELATIONSHIP BETWEEN ESTROGEN RECEPTOR (ER) STATUS OF BREAST TUMOR AND PATIENT'S OBJECTIVE RESPONSE TO ENDOCRINE THERAPY

Estrogen Receptor Status	
Responses/ER+ Tumors	**Responses/ER− Tumors**
522/977 (53%)	36/567 (6%)

Based on the collective papers presented at the NIH Consensus Development Conference on Steroid Receptors in Breast Cancer (DeSombre et al., 1979; Proceedings of NIH Consensus Development Conference, 1980).

Table 11–8. RELATIONSHIP BETWEEN ESTROGEN BINDING CAPACITY OF BREAST TUMOR BIOPSY SPECIMENS AND OBJECTIVE REMISSION AFTER AN ENDOCRINE MANIPULATION

Therapeutic Manipulation	Specific Estrogen Binding Capacity	
	Positive	**Negative**
Additive hormone treatment	59/105 (56%)	12/109 (11%)
Ablative endocrine therapy	59/107 (55%)	8/94 (8%)
Total	118/212 (56%)	20/203 (10%)

Based on the collective papers presented at the National Cancer Institute Workshop on Estrogen Receptors in Human Breast Cancer (McGuire et al, 1975).

be a spectrum of responses, ranging from less than 6 per cent at levels of estrogen receptors below 10 fmol/mg cytosol protein to more than 80 per cent objective remissions by patients with tumors containing several hundred or more femtomoles per milligram of cytosol protein. Recent results suggest that only methods of analyses providing quantification of the estrogen (and progestin) receptor should be used in the clinical laboratory. Likewise, the clinician should learn to discriminate the hormonal response potential of the breast cancer patient by evaluating both the specific binding capacity and the K_d (or K_a) values of estrogen and progestin receptors in a tumor (Fig. 11–9).

A new and exciting finding, which relates to the importance of analyses of estrogen receptors in primary lesions, evolved from the work of Knight and coworkers (1977). They found that patients with primary breast cancer containing estrogen receptors exhibited an increased disease-free survival when compared with women whose tumors did not contain estrogen receptors. The disease-free interval of Stage II patients appeared to be independent of the patient's menopausal status and the presence of metastases in the axillary lymph nodes. These data, which now have been supported by a number of studies (Bishop et al., 1979; Hähnel et al., 1979; Blamey et al., 1980; Gapinski and Donegan, 1980; Palshof et al., 1980; Stewart et al., 1983), indicate clearly that the estrogen receptor is useful not only as a predictive index of a patient's response to endocrine manipulation but also as a prognostic index of the course of the disease. Thus, quantitative results from estrogen receptor analyses should play a major role in the management of the patient with carcinoma of the breast, as is suggested by the adjuvant trial conducted by the National Surgical Adjuvant Breast Project (Fisher et al., 1981, 1983).

The relationship between estrogen receptor content of a tumor and ability to predict either disease-free survival or overall survival is at present unclear. However the important NSABP study (Fisher et al., 1987) showed the benefit of prolonging tamoxifen therapy for primary breast cancer in patients with greater than 10 fmol/mg cytosol protein of the steroid hormone receptors. Women 50 years of age or more receiving a third year of tamoxifen had a better disease-free survival rate and survival rate through their fifth postoperative year. Recent investigations suggest that these parameters also may be related to the stage of breast cancer and the race of the patient. Crowe and associates (1986) recently reported that estrogen receptor status and race, although both acting as important variables, interact when considering survival data. They conclude that black patients with estrogen receptor negative tumors, particularly if postmenopausal, are at very high risk of recurrence and death.

The reader is referred to Chapters 15 and 17 for a more detailed treatment of the clinical significance of these receptors.

Clinical Significance of Progestin Receptors

As already discussed, not all women with breast tumors containing estrogen receptors respond to hormone therapy. One possibility for this binding may be that there is a defect in the intracellular cascade of events that normally control biologic responsiveness to an endocrine stimulus. One of the approaches taken to assess the intactness of the estrogen response mechanism in breast tumors has been the determination of progestin receptors as suggested by Horwitz and coworkers (1975). The assumption is that progestin receptor formation in breast carcinomas is regulated by estrogen receptors in a fashion similar to the mechanism in rodent uterine tissues, as described by Rao and Meyer (1977). Thus, the simultaneous determination of the progestin receptor with the estrogen receptor (shown in Fig. 11–8) should increase the accuracy of selecting the breast cancer patient most likely to respond to hormone therapy.

Table 11–9. RELATIONSHIP BETWEEN STEROID RECEPTOR (ER, PR) STATUS OF BREAST TUMOR AND PATIENT'S OBJECTIVE RESPONSE TO ENDOCRINE THERAPY

Steroid Receptor Status*			
ER+, PR+	ER+, PR−	ER−, PR−	ER−, PR+
135/174 (78%)	55/164 (34%)	17/165 (10%)	5/11 (45%)

*Number of patients responding to treatment/number of women with receptor status designated.

Based on the collective papers presented at the NIH Consensus Development Conference on Steroid Receptors in Breast Cancer (Proceedings of the NIH Consensus Development Conference, 1980).

If the hypothesis is correct that the presence of a functional estrogen receptor is required for the formation of a progestin receptor, there should be a direct relationship between these two receptors in responsive cells. The majority of the breast tumors containing both receptors would be assumed to retain hormonal responsiveness (Degenshein et al., 1980).

A summary of results presented at the Consensus Development Conference (Proceedings of the NIH Consensus Development Conference, 1980) is given in Table 11–9. From studies of the steroid receptor status of the tumor biopsy specimen, it was found that 78 per cent of patients with breast tumors containing both receptors responded objectively to hormone therapy. If only the estrogen receptor was present, a 34 per cent response rate was observed, whereas only 10 per cent of patients responded to endocrine manipulation if neither receptor was present in the breast tumor. Surprisingly, 5 of 11 (45%) patients responded objectively to hormone therapy when only the progestin receptor was present. This appears puzzling if there is a relationship between estrogen and progestin receptors in responsive tumors and may be related to the endocrine status of the patient (McCarty et al., 1983; Alghanem and Hussain, 1985), as discussed earlier (Table 11–2). These latter data suggest that the progestin receptor may be particularly important in the selection of premenopausal patients for endocrine manipulation (Bland et al., 1981).

Results of an adjuvant trial that compared cytotoxic chemotherapy with and without tamoxifen also suggest that the progestin receptor may have particular significance (Fisher et al., 1983, 1987). Patients with increased levels of progestin receptors who received both cytotoxic chemotherapy and tamoxifen exhibited an increased disease-free survival. Clark and associates (1983) also concluded that progestin receptor level was of equal or greater value than that of the estrogen receptor for predicting the disease-free survival of patients with breast cancer.

Steroid Receptors in Male Breast Cancer

Breast cancer in men is often a hormone-dependent lesion in that approximately 65 per cent of patients with advanced disease respond to orchiectomy or adrenalectomy. Because of the physiologic and psychologic impact of orchiectomy and adrenalectomy, the problem of correlating endocrine manipulation with the presence of estrogen receptors in these tumors should be addressed. However, because these tumors are encountered infrequently, relatively few analyses have been reported. The collective study reported by Everson and colleagues (1980) found that estrogen receptors were present in the tumor biopsy specimens from 29 of 34 cases (85 per cent) of male breast cancer. There was a negative correlation of estrogen receptor concentration with patient age. Although the quantity of estrogen receptor appeared to be related to the level of progesterone receptor, the disease-free interval, and duration of response, these were not statistically significant. Clinical results from this report are not sufficient justification to base a therapeutic maneuver on the estrogen receptor status of a biopsy specimen in a manner analogous to that used for breast cancer of the female. More detailed analyses of both cytoplasmic and nuclear levels of these receptors may be useful, as suggested by Pegoraro and colleagues (1982).

Nine of 14 breast cancer biopsy specimens (64 per cent) from male patients had significant levels of progesterone receptors, and several exhibited androgen and glucocorticoid receptors (Everson et al., 1980). It has been the author's experience and that of others that few gynecomastia specimens exhibit estrogen receptors, and usually these are limited to the 4 S species as detected by sucrose gradient centrifugation.

The presence of estrogen receptors in the breast cancer of men suggests that some of these patients may be candidates for an endocrine manipulation other than orchiectomy or adrenalectomy. Because of the elevated concentrations of estrogen receptors in both primary and metastatic tumors, which the author has observed in a number of specimens during the past ten years, there is a possibility that inhibitors of estrogen binding, such as tamoxifen, may be useful therapeutically in the management of this disease. Only the participation of a large cooperative group in which numerous patients can be studied would warrant such a clinical trial.

Steroid Receptors in Chronic Cystic Mastopathy

During the past decade, a number of workers have investigated the presence of steroid receptors in nonmalignant lesions of the breast, such as chronic cystic mastopathy (fibrocystic disease) or fibroadenoma (Spratt et al., 1985). From determinations in more than 200 biopsies using either the titration method or sucrose gradient centrifugation, the author has rarely detected more than 10 fmol/mg cytosol protein (Wittliff et al., 1972, 1976). The majority of studies from other workers agree with these findings (Proceedings of the NIH Consensus Development Conference, 1980). However, significant binding of labeled estradiol has been reported for a few specimens of benign breast disease when measured by the tissue slice procedure. In general, it may be concluded that benign breast disease peripheral to the malignant lesion will not contribute significantly to the estrogen binding capacity. Thus, the possibility of a "false" estrogen receptor positive assay is excluded. However, fibroblasts may contain a significant level of progestin receptors complicating this measurement if excessive nontumorous tissue is present in the biopsy specimen (Wittliff, 1984, 1987).

Although normal breast tissue from women is known to concentrate ^{3}H-estradiol in vivo, the level of steroid retained is considerably lower than that found in tumor tissue. One explanation for this reduced binding is that normal breast tissue contains few epithelial cells during resting states other than pregnancy and lactation. Furthermore, it contains a predominance of adipose and connective tissue cells compared with most malignant breast tumors. To date, this author has detected specific estrogen receptors sedimenting at 8 S in normal breast tissue in only one patient. Results obtained in the author's laboratory suggest that the simple explanation of a lack of cellularity may not be the reason for the absence of estrogen receptors in normal tissue. Examination of the specific binding capacities of mammary glands from rats revealed that the levels of estrogen receptors were low in breast tissue from virgin and pregnant animals (Wiehle and Wittliff, 1983). These receptors increased throughout lactation, reaching a maximum just prior to weaning of the young, to levels comparable to that of infiltrating ductal carcinoma of the human breast. Normal breast tissue from pregnant or lactating women was not examined, however, for the obvious reason that it is rarely, if ever, available. The prediction is that these latter tissues would exhibit estrogen receptors with properties similar to those found in breast tumors. Since virtually all breast tumors are removed from women who are not pregnant or lactating, the inclusion of normal breast tissue in the biopsy specimen does not pose a problem so long as the sample is representative of the malignant lesion.

Absence of Estrogen Receptors in a Tumor Biopsy Specimen and Response to Cytotoxic Chemotherapy

The concept that the estrogen receptor may be useful in predicting a patient's response to chemotherapy is based on the assumption that the absence of one or more steroid hormone receptors reflects a loss of differentiated function (hormone control mechanisms), which might be correlated with a more rapid growth rate. Thus, these rapidly growing tumors may be more sensitive to chemotherapy than tumors that possess steroid hormone receptors. In support of this idea, Meyer and coworkers (1977, 1983) have shown that breast tumors without estrogen receptors exhibit a higher growth rate as measured by thymidine labeling and mitotic indices.

Knight and colleagues (1977) reported that patients whose primary breast cancer contained estrogen receptors have a prolonged disease-free survival compared with those women with receptor-negative tumors, independent of their menopausal status or the involvement of the axillary lymph nodes with tumor metastases. These workers also postulated that the lower incidence of estrogen receptors in breast tumor biopsy specimens of premenopausal women may account for their increased survival with adjuvant therapy as opposed to that of postmenopausal patients. This implies that the higher incidence of estrogen receptor–negative tumors in premenopausal patients may be associated with a greater sensitivity to cytotoxic chemotherapy. Several randomized trials of adjuvant chemotherapy in resectable breast cancer, conducted by the National Surgical Adjuvant Breast Project (Fisher et al., 1977) and by Bonadonna and coworkers (1977) in Europe, have shown that the major beneficiaries of this therapy were premenopausal patients with breast carcinoma. Although chemotherapy is known to cause ovarian suppression, it does not appear to be the reason for the increased survival of premenopausal women with breast cancer.

Allegra and coworkers (1978) were among the first to determine if a correlation existed between a higher growth rate of breast tumors and response to chemotherapy. Using a group of patients carefully matched with regard to age, menopausal status, Karnofsky performance index, disease-free interval, number of sites involved with metastases, and prior therapy, they suggested that premenopausal patients with tumors predominantly negative for the estrogen receptor may be more sensitive to chemotherapy than postmenopausal women with estrogen receptor positive tumors. The distribution of the treatments was similar for the two groups and consisted of doxorubicin hydrochloride (Adriamycin) and one or more additional chemotherapeutic agents. Thirty-four of 45 patients (75 per cent) with estrogen receptor negative tumors responded objectively, compared to only 3 of 25 women (12 per cent) with breast tumors containing estrogen receptors. Regardless of visceral involvement, patients with tumors lacking estrogen receptors had a higher response rate to chemotherapy. Furthermore, the presence of progestin receptors in a tumor does not appear to influence the response rate of patients given combination chemotherapy.

The relationship between specific estrogen binding capacity of a tumor biopsy and a patient's response to cytotoxic chemotherapy has been studied by a great number of investigators since the original suggestion by Allegra and coworkers (1978). Although a few groups reported results in agreement with this study during the 1979 Consensus Development Conference (Proceedings of the NIH Consensus Development Conference, 1980), others reached variable conclusions. The studies of Kiang and Kennedy (1977) and others (Proceedings of the NIH Consensus Development Conference, 1980) gave virtually opposite results, in that patients with breast tumors containing estrogen receptors exhibited an elevated response to chemotherapy. Other studies reported at this conference were unable to demonstrate any relationship between the estrogen receptor status of a breast tumor and a patient's response to cytotoxic chemotherapy, further complicating the picture. Examination of the reports of these studies suggests that there were considerable differences in the mode of patient selection, which may have considerable bearing on the outcome. It appears that a suitable means of evaluating this attractive hypothesis would be a well-controlled prospective study supervised by one of the cooperative groups and employing a quality assurance program for the analyses of steroid receptors. A more detailed discussion of this area is presented in Chapter 15.

Polymorphism of Estrogen Receptors as a Molecular Basis of Endocrine Responsiveness

In 1969, the author and coworkers began a long-term study to examine the original hypothesis expressed by Jensen and colleagues (1971) that the presence of specific estrogen binding components in breast carcinomas was predictive of a patient's response to endocrine therapy.

The distribution and levels of estrogen receptor isoforms in tumor biopsy specimens were examined and correlated with a breast cancer patient's response to endocrine therapy (Wittliff and Savlov, 1975; Wittliff et al., 1978; Wittliff, 1984). No objective remissions were observed in patients with advanced breast carcinoma whose tumor biopsy specimens were estrogen receptor negative regardless of the type of hormone therapy administered. Approximately 75 per cent of patients whose biopsy specimen revealed either 8 S species or both the 8 S and 4 S forms of the estrogen receptors exhibited objective remissions after receiving various types of hormone therapy. Of the 23 patients whose tumors contained exclusively or predominantly the 4 S species of estrogen receptors, only four responded objectively after receiving hormone therapy. These data suggested that the molecular forms of estrogen receptors in human breast cancer have clinical significance.

Steroid hormone receptors are proteins that show a great deal of size, shape, and charge heterogeneity (Table 11–4). To characterize further the estrogen binding components in the cytosol of breast tumors, DEAE-cellulose chromatography (Kute et al., 1978; Wittliff et al., 1981b) and more sophisticated procedures, such as high performance liquid chromatography (HPLC) (Wittliff, 1985, 1986), were employed to study the interrelationships of these elusive receptor proteins. The number of binding components, which the author has termed isoforms (Wittliff et al., 1981b), and their relative specific estrogen binding capacities were highly variable from tumor to tumor (Figs. 11–4 to 11–7). Whether these binding components represent distinct subunits or cleavage products owing to proteolytic digestion of the estrogen receptors is unknown. Similar molecular heterogeneity has been observed in progestin receptors (van der Walt and Wittliff, 1986). The findings using these procedures with partially purified forms of estrogen receptors from human breast carcinoma suggest that the molecular composition of the 8 S species from hormonally responsive tumors is different from that of unresponsive neoplasms containing these proteins. A major advance that aided in determining the nature of the interrelationships of various receptor isoforms is the availability of monoclonal antibodies to estrogen receptors (Greene et al., 1980, 1984).

Numerous workers in the field of estrogen receptors, particularly those working with uterine tissue (Puca et al., 1972; Notides et al., 1981), favor a model that contains a single type of subunit (Fig. 11–10A). The dimer is the species suggested to be most likely to occur at physiologic ionic strength. Regardless of the ionic strength of the environment in vitro, it is assumed that no more than four types of components are possible, as depicted. These include the mereceptor (3.5 S), which is presumed to arise as a result of proteolytic cleavage of higher molecular weight species (Sherman et al., 1978).

Employing a monoclonal antibody that Greene and coworkers (1980, 1984) produced against estrogen receptors from the MCF-7 human breast cancer cell line, the author and associates demonstrated that immunopurified isoforms of the estrogen receptors from extracts of these cells appeared to be associated with both protein kinase (Fig. 11–11) and phospholipid kinase activities (Baldi et al., 1986). Although unexpected, these enzyme activities were easily ascertained in vitro on femtomolar quantities of the receptors by virtue of the fact that the isoform–monoclonal antibody complexes were immobilized on a single polystyrene bead (Sato et al., 1986). A further novel use was that the receptor could be associated with ^{125}I-iodoestradiol-17β and could easily be measured in a gamma counter by placing the bead coated with labeled receptor into the counting well (Sato et al., 1986). The receptor directed a phosphorylation reaction requiring adenosine triphosphate (ATP) rather than guanosine triphosphate (GTP) as the phosphoryl donor (Fig. 11–11) and was highly dependent on the presence of Mg^{2+}. As seen in Figure 11–11, three phosphopeptides were eluted by detergent from the monoclonal antibody–coated bead associated with the purified estrogen receptor. Only estrogen receptor positive cell lines (MCF-7) exhibited the protein kinase activity; estrogen receptor negative breast cancer cell lines, such as the MDA and the T-47D, showed minimal or no activity (Baldi et al., 1986).

Recent observations from several groups implicate steroid receptor phosphorylation as a possible regulatory mechanism that alters the binding capacity of these molecules (Auricchio et al., 1981). Furthermore, an increasing number of protein hormone receptors, growth factors, and oncogenic transforming products have been shown to contain autophosphorylating activities and to exhibit the ability to phosphorylate exogenous substrates. The exciting observation that two oncogenic products, $p68^{v-ras}$ (Macara et al., 1984) and $pp60^{v-src}$ (Sugimoto et al., 1984), contain phospholipid kinase activity, has brought new insight in the phosphate transfer reaction related to tumor genesis.

The evidence that the immunopurified estrogen receptor directs autophosphorylating activity and phosphorylates phosphoinositides

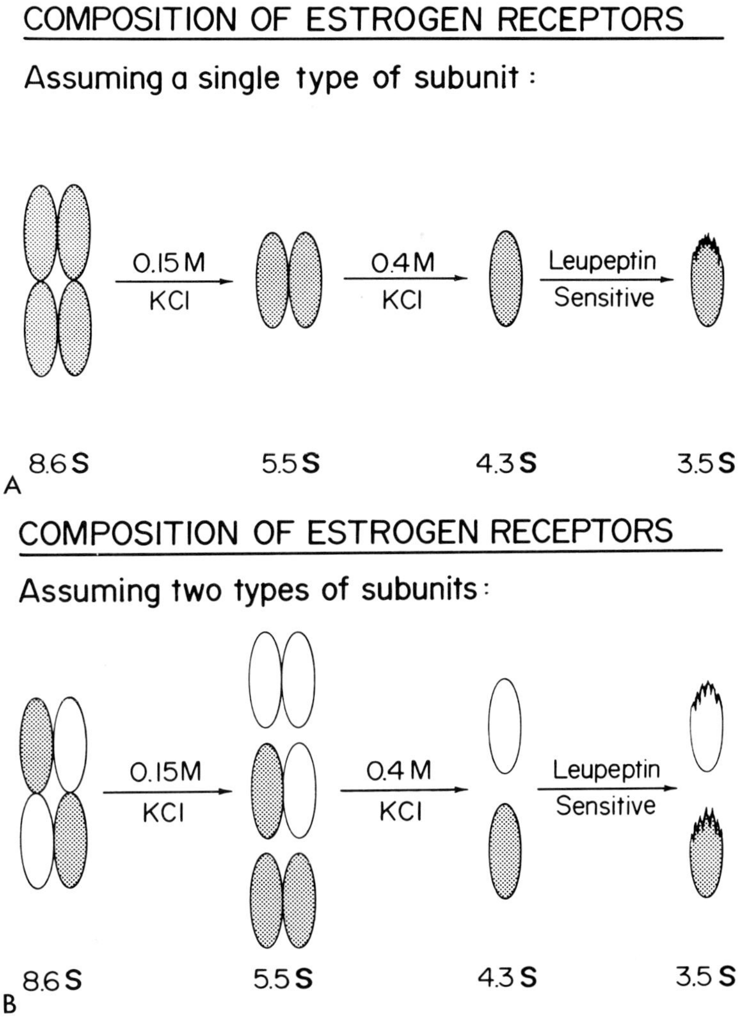

COMPOSITION OF ESTROGEN RECEPTORS

Assuming a single type of subunit:

Figure 11-10. Proposals regarding the composition of the estrogen receptor in hormone target organs of eukaryotes. (From Wittliff, J. L., et al.: In Soto, R., et al. [Eds.]: Physiopathology of Endocrine Diseases and Mechanisms of Hormone Action. New York, Alan R. Liss, 1981, p. 375. Reprinted with permission.)

A: 8.6 S → (0.15 M KCl) → 5.5 S → (0.4 M KCl) → 4.3 S → (Leupeptin Sensitive) → 3.5 S

COMPOSITION OF ESTROGEN RECEPTORS

Assuming two types of subunits:

B: 8.6 S → (0.15 M KCl) → 5.5 S → (0.4 M KCl) → 4.3 S → (Leupeptin Sensitive) → 3.5 S

(Baldi et al., 1986) led the authors to postulate a mechanism by which steroid hormone receptors may share similar properties with oncogene products, as recently discussed by Sluyser and Mester (1985). It should be mentioned, however, that the kinase activity exhibited by estrogen receptor molecules from MCF-7 breast cancer cells is a serine type kinase (Baldi et al., submitted for publication), in contrast to the tyrosine kinase mode exhibited by most of the oncogenic transforming products (Hunter and Cooper, 1985). Of course, considerable work is needed to establish a relationship between steroid hormone receptors and the synthesis of oncogenic products. However, these results suggest that the steroid binding site of the estrogen receptor represents *only* a portion of a more complex regulatory molecule.

The author's data from ion exchange chromatography, isoelectric focusing, and, more recently, HPLC, are more consistent with the model shown in Figure 11–10B (Wittliff et al., 1981b), illustrating protein polymorphism. In this model, the molecular heterogeneity of the estrogen receptor arises as a result of the various possible combinations of two unlike subunits. It is unclear, at present, which are the so-called native forms and which are proteolytic fragments retaining the ligand-binding domain in HPLC profiles of these receptors. These differences in separation characteristics may be due to a variety of physiologic reasons, including phosphorylation, protein-protein interaction, such as subunit association-dissociation, and possible protein–nucleic acid association. The authors have preliminary evidence that a high molecular weight component

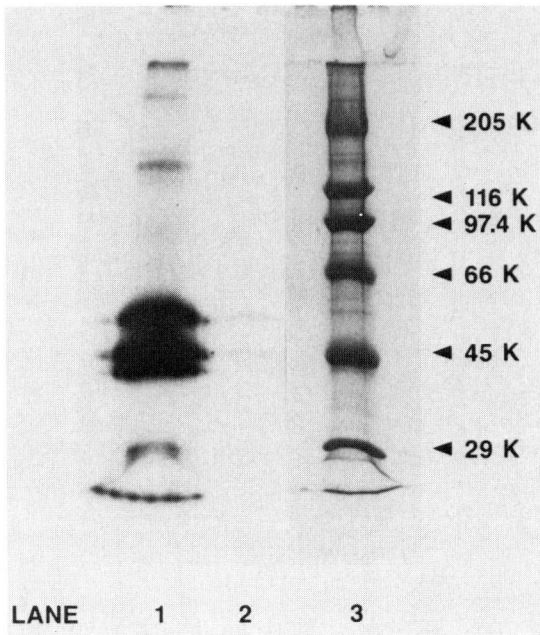

Figure 11–11. Nucleotide dependence of estrogen receptor (ER) autophosphorylation activity from MCF-7 cells. ER was purified from MCF-7 cytosol using immobilized monoclonal antibody. The immunocomplexes were washed extensively and incubated either with γ-^{32}P-ATP or γ-^{32}P-GTP. Reactions were terminated by removal of the reaction medium and the ^{32}P-labeled polypeptides were solubilized and separated by polyacrylamide-SDS gel electrophoresis. The slab gels used were dried and autoradiography was performed for 16 hr at 25°C. Lane 1, MCF-7 MAb-receptor complex incubated with γ-^{32}P-ATP as substrate, showing the presence of phosphorylated proteins with molecular weights of 57, 47, and 43 kilodaltons. Lane 2, Same as Lane 1, but γ-^{32}P-GTP was used as substrate. Note absence of phosphorylation activity. Lane 3 shows the corresponding molecular weight standards. Numbers on the right indicate the position of molecular weight standards in kilodaltons. (From Baldi, A., et al.: Estrogen receptor is associated with protein and phospholipid kinase activities. Biochem. Biophys. Res. Commun., *135*:597, 1986. Reprinted with permission.)

(>400,000 daltons) exists in cytosol from studies with molybdate using ^{125}I-iodoestradiol-17β and HPLC (Hofmann et al., unpublished data). This binding protein may be a precursor of the functional estrogen receptor. The author's current research is directed toward an understanding of the interrelationships of the various molecular species or isoforms of steroid hormone receptors and their role in target cell response. HPLC and ^{125}I-iodoestradiol-17β provide the means of exploring these receptor proteins at a molecular level that was not possible 5 years ago.

Conclusions and Future Considerations

Analyses of sex hormone receptors are important in the identification of the individual with breast cancer most likely to respond to additive or surgical ablative endocrine manipulation. These receptors are also indicators of uterine carcinomas with a high probability of progestin sensitivity, and, therefore, a good prognosis. Steroid hormone receptors are considered, along with clinical factors such as previous response to hormone therapy, disease-free interval, age, menopausal status, and location of the dominant metastatic lesion, as the principal criteria for selecting therapeutic regimens for these women.

The author had earlier suggested the use of the term *receptor fingerprint* or *isoform profile* to designate the pattern of specific steroid hormone binding components (isoforms) displayed by a single receptor type when separated according to properties of size, shape, surface charge, and hydrophobicity. For example, Figures 11–4 to 11–7 illustrate the isoform profiles of the estrogen receptors in several tissue specimens. The prediction is made that methods that separate receptor proteins on the basis of size and shape, such as sucrose gradient centrifugation and high performance size exclusion chromatography, or on the basis of surface ionic charge, such as isoelectricfocusing, ion exchange chromatography, and chromatofocusing, will play a greater role in the clinical laboratory in this decade. In contrast to a receptor fingerprint, the term *receptor profile* is suggested to indicate the presence of the different types (e.g., estrogen, progestin, androgen, glucocorticoid) of steroid hormone receptors in a single biopsy specimen. An example would be the patient whose breast tumor contained estrogen, progestin, and androgen receptors, as illustrated in Figure 11–9.

In general, when the estrogen receptor was present in the tumor, a higher progestin binding capacity was observed in tumor biopsies from both premenopausal and postmenopausal women. However, in the absence of estrogen receptors, a lower progestin receptor level was measured, supporting the suggestion that the formation of estrogen receptor is dependent on estrogen action. Similar values have been reported for biopsies of endometrial cancer.

Progress during the last 15 years has shown, with regard to breast cancer, the following results:
- The most reliable methods of determining estrogen and progestin receptors are (1) multipoint titration analysis with radio-labeled ligand using dextran-coated charcoal and (2) sucrose density gradient centrifugation.
- 55 to 65 per cent of primary breast tumors contain more than 10 fmol/mg cytosol protein of estrogen receptors.
- 45 to 55 per cent of metastatic breast tumors contain more than 10 fmol/mg cytosol protein of estrogen receptors.
- Estrogen receptors are present more often in breast tumors of postmenopausal women than in those of premenopausal women.
- Benign breast lesions, such as fibrocystic disease and fibroadenomas, usually contain less than 10 fmol/mg cytosol protein of estrogen receptor.
- 90 per cent of male breast carcinomas contain estrogen receptors and less than 50 per cent contain progestin receptors.
- Approximately 55 per cent of women with breast tumors containing estrogen receptors respond objectively to endocrine therapy, either additive or ablative.
- Less than 3 per cent of women with breast tumors lacking estrogen receptors respond objectively to hormone therapy.
- 45 to 60 per cent of primary or metastatic breast tumors contain progestin receptors.
- The presence of both types of female sex hormone receptors in a breast tumor indicates a 75 to 80 per cent likelihood that the patient will respond to endocrine manipulation, either additive or ablative.
- It has been suggested that the presence of the 8 S isoforms of the estrogen and progestin receptors in a breast tumor (as detected by sucrose gradient centrifugation) improves the accuracy of selecting the patient likely to respond to endocrine therapy. The clinical significance (or rather insignificance) of the 4 S isoform of these receptors is being debated at present.
- Both estrogen and progestin receptors exhibit polymorphism (presence of multiple isoforms) based on separation and characterization, using their properties of size, shape, surface ionic charge, and hydrophobicity and employing techniques such as HPLC. Molecular heterogeneity appears to be due to various types of receptor modification, such as phosphorylation, and to non-receptor-associated activities, such as protein kinase.
- There is a relationship between the quantity of both estrogen and progestin receptors in a breast tumor and a patient's response to endocrine therapy. The incidence of response to hormone therapy increases with increasing receptor levels.

It is recommended that both estrogen and progestin receptor analyses be performed on all tumor biopsies from patients with confirmed or suspected cases of breast and endometrial carcinoma prior to therapeutic manipulation. Laboratories that are in compliance with criteria assigned by quality assurance programs should be used to establish uniformity of methods and data expression of these receptors. Receptor profiles (i.e., the reporting of the presence of different types of receptors, including those of androgen, glucocorticoid, and other hormones) may be useful in the diagnosis of certain neoplasms. Receptor results may be used as (1) *predictive* indicators of an endocrine responsive tumor, and (2) *prognostic* indices of a patient's clinical course. Elevated levels of these receptors in a tumor biopsy specimen are associated with a greater probability of disease-free survival.

It is evident that both the quality (biologic integrity) and quantity (number of binding sites) of estrogen and progestin receptors in a biopsy specimen are useful biochemical parameters in the clinical management of the patient with carcinoma of the breast. These findings suggest that a new generation of laboratory tests will evolve in which the analyses will be performed directly on the tissue specimen. The tumor itself provides an enormous resource for the development of new markers of therapeutic response. Several of these currently under investigation are estrogen sulfotransferase, peroxidase, cytochrome P450–linked enzymes, and receptors for prolactin, insulin, epidermal growth factor, and prostaglandin. As a biochemist who chose with some apprehension to investigate human disease as his life's work, the author is reminded of the words of Alexander Pope in his *Essay on Man* (1734): "The proper study of mankind is man."

Acknowledgments

While at the University of Rochester, and presently at the University of Louisville, I have had the privilege of working with a multitude of talented graduate students and research fellows. Although their number precludes listing them individually, they are due special acknowledgment for their valued contributions and friendship. I wish to thank Dr. Thomas C. Hall, who introduced me to the study of human disease and shared his enthusiasm for discovery. Also, I am deeply appreciative of the encouragement and counsel given me by numerous clinical scientists, particularly Drs. Edwin D. Savlov, Robert A. Cooper, Jr., Arthur H. Keeney, Joseph C. Allegra, Thomas C. Day, Joseph Sanfilippo, Condict Moore, John S. Spratt, Hiram C. Polk, Jr., Bernard Fisher, John Durant, and Edwin R. Fisher. Ms. Linda Deuser is owed special acknowledgment for her careful efforts in the preparation of the typescript. I am especially grateful to my wife, Mitzie, who has been my right hand in the laboratory and at home.

Studies in the Hormone Receptor Laboratory during the past decade have been supported in part by grants from the American Cancer Society (BC-514B); Phi Beta Psi Sorority; USPHS grants CA-19657, CA-34211, CA-32102, CA-37429, CA-25224, CA-42154, and CA-31946 from the National Cancer Institute; and the College of American Pathologists.

REFERENCES

Alghanem, A. A., and Hussain, S.: The effect of age on estrogen and progesterone receptors in primary breast cancer. J. Surg. Oncol., 30:29, 1985.

Allegra, J. C., and Lippman, M. E.: The effects of 17β-estradiol to tamoxifen on the ZR-75-1 human breast cancer cell line in defined medium. Eur. J. Cancer, 16:1007, 1980.

Allegra, J. C., Lippman, M. E., and Thompson, E. B.: An association between steroid hormone receptors and response rate to cytotoxic chemotherapy in metastatic breast cancer. Cancer Treat. Rep., 62:1281, 1978.

Allegra, J. C., Lippman, M. E., Thompson, E. B., et al.: Distribution, frequency and quantitative analysis of estrogen, progesterone, androgen and glucocorticoid receptors in human breast cancer. Cancer Res., 39:1447, 1979a.

Allegra, J. C., Lippman, M. E., Thompson, E. B., et al.: Relationship between the progesterone, androgen, and glucocorticoid receptor and response rate to endocrine therapy in metastatic breast cancer. Cancer Res., 39:1973, 1979b.

Auricchio, F., Migliaccio, A., and Castoria, G.: Dephosphorylation of oestradiol nuclear receptor in vitro. Biochem. J., 198:699, 1981.

Baldi, A., Boyle, D. M., and Wittliff, J.L.: Estrogen receptor is associated with protein and phospholipid kinase activities. Biochem. Biophys. Res. Commun., 135:597, 1986.

Beatson, G. T.: On the treatment of inoperable cases of carcinoma of the mamma; suggestions for a new method of treatment with illustrative cases. Lancet, 2:104, 1986.

Berns, E. M. J. J., Mulder, E., Rommerts, F. F. G., et al.: Fluorescent ligands, used in histocytochemistry, do not discriminate between estrogen receptor-positive and receptor-negative human tumor cell lines. Breast Cancer Res. Treatm., 4:195, 1984.

Bishop, H. M., Blamey, R. W., Elston, C. W., et al.: Relationship of oestrogen-receptor status to survival in breast cancer. Lancet, 2:283, 1979.

Black, R., Prescott, R., Bers, K., et al.: Tumor cellularity, oestrogen receptors and prognosis in breast cancer. Clin. Oncol., 9:311, 1983.

Blamey, R. W., Bishop, H. M., Blake, J. R. S., et al.: Relationship between primary breast tumor receptor status and patient survival. Cancer, 46:2765, 1980.

Bland, K. L., Fuchs, A., and Wittliff, J. L.: Menopausal status as a factor in the distribution of estrogen and progestin receptors in breast cancer. Surg. Forum, 32:410, 1981.

Bonadonna, G., Rossi, A., Valagossa, P., et al.: The CMF program for operable breast cancer with positive axillary nodes: Updated analysis of the disease-free interval, site of relapse and drug tolerance. Cancer, 39:2904, 1977.

Boyle, D. M., Wiehle, R. D., Shahabi, N. A., et al.: Rapid, high-resolution procedure for assessment of estrogen receptor heterogeneity in clinical samples. J. Chromatogr., 327:369, 1985.

Buller, R. E., and O'Malley, B. W.: The biology and mechanism of steroid hormone receptor interaction with the eukaryotic nucleus. Biochem. Phar., 25:1, 1976.

Burke, R. E., Miva, J. G., Datta, R., et al.: Estrogen action following irradiation of human breast cancer cells. Cancer Res., 38:2813, 1978.

Carlson, J. A., Allegra, J. C., Day, T. G., Jr., et al.: Tamoxifen and endometrial carcinoma alterations in estrogen and progesterone receptors in untreated patients and combination hormonal therapy in advanced neoplasia. Am. J. Obstet. Gynecol., 149:149, 1984.

Chabon, A. B., Goldberg, J. D., and Venet, L.: Carcinoma of the breast: inter-relationship among histopathologic features, estrogen receptor activity and age of the patient. Hum. Pathol., 14:368, 1982.

Chamness, G. C., Mercer, W. D., and McGuire, W. L.: Are histochemical methods for estrogen receptor valid? J. Histochem. Cytochem., 28:792, 1980.

Chua, D. Y. F., Pang, M. W. Y., Rauff, A., et al.: Correlation of steroid receptors with histologic differentiation in mammary carcinoma. Cancer, 56:2228, 1985.

Clark, G. M., McGuire, W. L., Hubay, C. A., et al.: Progesterone receptors as a prognostic factor in Stage II breast cancer. N. Engl. J. Med., 309:1343, 1983.

Clark, J. H., and Peck, E. J., Jr.: Female Sex Steroids: Receptors and Functions. New York, Springer-Verlag, 1979.

Crowe, J. P., Jr., Gordon, N. H., Hubay, C. A., et al.: The interaction of estrogen receptor status and race in predicting prognosis for Stage I breast cancer patients. Surgery, 100:599, 1986.

Dao, T. L.: Ablation therapy for hormone-dependent tumors. Annu. Rev. Med., 23:1, 1972.

Degenshein, G. A., Bloom, N., and Tobin, E.: The value of progesterone receptor assays in the management of advanced breast cancer. Cancer, 46:2789, 1980.

DeSombre, E. R., Carbone, P. P., Jensen, E. V., et al.: Steroid receptors in breast cancer. N. Engl. J. Med., 301:1011, 1979.

Everson, R. B., Lippman, M. E., Thompson, E. B., et al.: Clinical correlations of steroid receptors and male breast cancer. Cancer Res., 40:991, 1980.

Fisher, B., Brown, A., Wolmark, N., et al.: Prolonging tamoxifen therapy for primary breast cancer. Ann. Intern. Med., 106:649, 1987.

Fisher, B., Redmond, C., Brown, A., et al.: Treatment of primary breast cancer with chemotherapy and tamoxifen. N. Engl. J. Med., 305:1, 1981.

Fisher, B., Redmond, C., Brown, A., et al.: Influence of tumor estrogen and progesterone receptor levels on the response to tamoxifen and chemotherapy in primary breast cancer. J. Clin. Oncol., 1:227, 1983.

Fisher, B., Sherman, B., Rockette, H., et al.: L-Phenylalanine mustard (L-PAM) in the management of premenopausal patients with primary breast cancer: Lack of association of disease-free survival with depression of ovarian function. Cancer, 44:847, 1977.

Folca, P. J., Glascock, R. F., and Irvine, W. T.: Studies with tritium-labeled hexoestrol in advanced breast cancer. Lancet, 2:796, 1961.

Gapinski, P. V., and Donegan, W. L.: Estrogen receptors and breast cancer: Prognostic and therapeutic implications. Surgery, 88:386, 1980.

Gorski, J., Toft, D., Shyamala, G., et al.: Hormone receptors: Studies in the interaction of estrogen with the uterus. Recent Progr. Hormone Res., 24:45, 1968.

Greene, G. L., Fitche, F. W., and Jensen, E. V.: Monoclonal antibodies to estrophilin: Probes for the study of estrogen receptors. Proc. Natl. Acad. Sci. USA, 77:157, 1980.

Greene, G. L., Sobel, N. B., King, W. J., et al.: Immunochemical studies of estrogen receptors. J. Steroid Biochem., 20:51, 1984.

Grill, H., Manz, B., Belozsky, O., et al.: Criteria for establishment of the double labeling assay for simultaneous determination of estrogen and progesterone receptors. Oncology, 41:25, 1984.

Hähnel, R., and Twaddle, E.: The relationship between estrogen receptors in primary and secondary breast carcinomas and in sequential primary breast carcinomas. Breast Cancer Res. Treat., 5:155, 1985.

Hähnel, R., Woodings, T., and Vivian, A. B.: Prognostic value of estrogen receptors in primary breast cancer. Cancer, 44:671, 1979.

Hall, T. C.: Chemotherapy of breast cancer. Clin. Obstet. Gynecol., 11:401, 1968.

Hochberg, R. B.: Iodine-125-labeled estradiol: A gamma-emitting analog of estradiol that binds to the estrogen receptor. Science, 205:1138, 1979.

Horwitz, K. B., and McGuire, W. L.: Specific progesterone receptors in human breast cancer. Steroids, 25:497, 1975.

Horwitz, K. B., McGuire, W. L., Pearson, O. H., et al.: Predicting response to endocrine therapy in human breast cancer: A hypothesis. Science, 189:726, 1975.

Howat, J. M. T., Barnes, D. M., Harris, M., et al.: The association of cytosol oestrogen and progesterone receptors with histological features of breast cancer and early detection of disease. Br. J. Cancer, 47:629, 1983.

Huggins, C., and Bergenstal, D. M.: Inhibition of human mammary and prostatic cancer by adrenalectomy. Cancer Res., 12:134, 1952.

Hull, D. F., III, Clark, G. M., Osborne, C. K., et al.: Multiple estrogen receptor assays in human breast cancer. Cancer Res., 43:413, 1983.

Hunter, T., and Cooper, J. A.: Protein-tyrosine kinases. Ann. Rev. Biochem., 54:897, 1985.

Hutchens, T. W., Wiehle, R. D., Shahabi, N. A., et al.: Rapid analysis of estrogen receptor heterogenity by chromatofocusing with high performance liquid chromatography. J. Chromatogr., 266:115, 1983.

Jensen, E. V., Suzuku, T., Kawashima, T., et al.: A two-step mechanism for the interaction of estradiol with rat uterus. Proc. Natl. Acad. Sci. (Wash.), 59:32, 1968.

Jensen, E. V., Block, G. E., Smith, S., et al.: Estrogen receptors and breast cancer response to adrenalectomy. Natl. Cancer Inst. Monogr., 34:55, 1971.

Kennedy, B. J.: Hormonal therapies in breast cancer. Sem. Oncol., 1:119, 1974.

Kiang, D. T., and Kennedy, B. J.: Factors affecting estrogen receptors in breast cancer. Cancer, 40:1571, 1977.

King, W. J., and Greene, G. L.: Monoclonal antibodies localize oestrogen receptor in the nuclei of target cells. Nature, 307:745, 1984.

King, W. J., DeSombre, E. R., and Jensen, E. V.: Comparison of immunocytochemical and steroid-binding assays for estrogen receptor in human breast tumors. Cancer Res., 45:293, 1985.

Knight, W. A., Livingston, R. B., Gregory, E. J.: Estrogen receptor as an independent prognostic factor for early recurrence in breast cancer. Cancer Res., 37:4669, 1977.

Kute, T. E., Heidemann, P., and Wittliff, J. L.: Molecular heterogeneity of cytosolic forms of estrogen receptors from human breast tumors. Cancer Res., 38:4307, 1978.

Leclercq, G., Toma, S., Paridaens, R., et al. (Eds.): Clinical Interest of Steroid Hormone Receptors in Breast Cancer. New York, Springer-Verlag, 1984.

Locher, G. W., Davis, B., Zava, D. T., et al.: Intratumoral regional differences in hormone receptor status of breast cancer. Geburtshilfe Frauenheilkd., 44:304, 1984.

Lonsdorfer, M., Clements, N. C., Jr., and Wittliff, J. L.: Use of high performance liquid chromatography in the elevation of the synthesis and binding of fluorescein-linked steroids to estrogen receptors. J. Chromatogr., 266:129, 1983.

Luft, R., and Olivecrona, H.: Hypophysectomy in man; experiences in metastatic cancer of the breast. Cancer, 8:261, 1955.

Maass, H., Engel, B., and Hohmeister, H.: Estrogen receptors in human breast tissue. Am. J. Obstet. Gynecol., 113:377, 1972.

Macara, I. G., Marinetti, G. V., and Balduzzi, P. C.: Transforming protein of avian sarcoma virus UR2 is associated with phosphatidylinositol kinase activity: Possible role in tumorigenesis. Proc. Natl. Acad. Sci. USA, 81:2728, 1984.

McCarty, K. S., Jr., Miller, L. S., Cox, E. B., et al.: Estrogen receptor analyses: correlation of biochemical and immunohistochemical methods using monoclonal antireceptor antibodies. Arch. Pathol. Lab. Med., 109:716, 1985.

McCarty, K. S., Jr., Silva, J. S., Cox, E. B., et al.: Relationship of age and menopausal status to estrogen receptor content in primary carcinoma of the breast. Ann. Surg., 197:123, 1983.

McGuire, W. L., Carbone, P. O., and Vollmer, E. P. (Eds.): Estrogen Receptors in Human Breast Cancer. New York, Raven Press, 1975.

McGuire, W. L., Raynaud, J. P., and Baulieu, E.-E., (Eds.): Progesterone Receptors in Normal and Neoplastic Tissues. New York, Raven Press, 1977.

Meyer, J. S.: Hormone receptors in human malignancy of unknown origin: Potential utility in clinical management. In Fer, M. F., Oldham, D., and Greco, A.

(Eds.): Tumors of Unknown Origin and Poorly Differentiated Neoplasms. Orlando, Florida, Grune & Stratton, 1986, p. 519.

Meyer, J. S., Rao, B. R., Stevens, S. C., et al.: Low incidence of estrogen receptor in breast carcinomas with rapid rates of cellular replication. Cancer, 40:2290, 1977.

Meyer, J. S., Schechtman, K., and Valdes, R., Jr.: Estrogen and progesterone receptor assays on breast carcinoma from mastectomy specimens. Cancer, 52:2139, 1983.

Mills, R. R.: Correlation of hormone receptors with pathological features in human breast cancer. Cancer, 46:2869, 1980.

Mirecki, D. M., and Jordan, V. C.: Steroid hormone receptors and human breast cancer. Lab. Med., 16:287, 1985.

Mohla, S., Sampson, C. C., Kahn, T., et al.: Estrogen and progesterone receptors in breast cancer in black Americans. Cancer (Phila.), 50:552, 1982.

Morrison, A. S., Black, M. M., Lowe, C. R., et al.: Some internation differences in histology and survival in breast cancer. Int. J. Cancer, 11:261, 1973.

Mortel, R., Levy, C., Wolff, J.-P., et al.: Female sex steroid receptors in postmenopausal endometrial carcinoma and biochemical response to an antiestrogen. Cancer Res., 41:1140, 1981.

Moudgil, V. K. (Ed.): Molecular Mechanisms of Steroid Hormone Action (German). Berlin, Walter de Gruyter, 1985.

Nakao, M., Sato, B., Koga, M., et al.: Identification of immunoassayable estrogen receptor lacing hormone binding ability in tamoxifen-treated rat uterus. Biochem. Biophys. Res. Commun., 132:336, 1985.

Nemoto, T., Vana, J., Bedwani, R. N., et al.: Management and survival of female breast cancer: Results of a national survey by the American College of Surgeons. Cancer, 45:2917, 1980.

Nomura, Y., Kobayashi, S., Takatani, O., et al.: Estrogen receptor and endocrine responsiveness in Japanese versus American breast cancer patients. Cancer Res., 37:106, 1977.

Nomura, Y., Yamagata, J., Takenaka, K., et al.: Steroid hormone receptors and clinical usefulness in human breast cancer. Cancer, 46:2880, 1980.

Nomura, Y., Tashiro, H., Hamada, Y., et al.: Relationship between estrogen receptors and risk factors in breast cancer in Japanese pre- and postmenopausal patients. Breast Cancer Res. Treat., 4:37, 1984.

Notides, A. C., Lerner, N., and Hamilton, D. E.: Positive cooperativity of the estrogen receptor. Proc. Natl. Acad. Sci. USA, 78:4926, 1981.

Palshof, T., Mouridsen, H. T., and Daehnfeldt, J. L.: Adjuvant endocrine therapy of primary operable breast cancer. Report on the Copenhagen breast cancer trials. Eur. J. Cancer, 16(Suppl. 1):183, 1980.

Parl, F. F., Schmidt, B. P., Dupont, W. D., et al.: Prognostic significance of estrogen receptor status in breast cancer in relation to tumor stage, axillary node metastasis, and histopathologic grading. Cancer, 54:2237, 1984.

Pegoraro, R. J., Nirmul, D., and Joubert, S. M.: Cytoplasmic and nuclear estrogen and progesterone receptors in male breast cancer. Cancer Res., 42:4812, 1982.

Pegoraro, R. J., Karnan, V., Nirmul, D., et al.: Estrogen and progesterone receptors in breast cancer among women of different racial groups. Cancer Res., 46:2117, 1986a.

Pegoraro, R. J., Nirmul, D., Reinach, S. G., et al.: Breast cancer prognosis in three different racial groups in relation to the steroid hormone receptor status. Breast Cancer Res. Treat., 7:111, 1986b.

Polk, H. C., Jr.: Improved understanding of mammary cancer and exemplar for surgical oncology. Cancer, 57:411, 1986.

Pollow, K., Schmidt-Gollwitzer, M., and Pollow, B.: Progesterone- and estradiol-binding proteins from normal human endometrium and endometrial carcinoma: A comparative study. In Wittliff, J. L., and Dapunt, O. (Eds.): Steroid Receptors and Hormone-Dependent Neoplasia. New York, Masson Publishing, 1980, p. 69.

Ponsky, J. L., Gliga, L., and Reynolds, S.: Medullary carcinoma of the breast: An association with negative hormonal receptors. J. Surg. Oncol., 26:76, 1984.

Proceedings of the NIH Consensus Development Conference on Steroid Receptors in Breast Cancer. Cancer, 46:2759, 1980.

Puca, G. A., Nola, E., Sica, V., et al.: Estrogen-binding proteins of calf uterus. Interrelationship between various forms and identification of a receptor-transforming factor. Biochemistry, 11:4157, 1972.

Raam, S., and Teixeira, T.: Effect of sodium molybdate on protein measurements: Quality control aspects of steroid hormone receptor assays. Eur. J. Cancer Clin. Oncol., 21:1219, 1985.

Raam, S., and Vrabel, D. M.: Evaluation of an enzyme immunoassay kit for estrogen receptor measurements. Clin. Chem., 32:1496, 1986.

Rao, B. R., and Meyer, J. S.: Estrogen and progestin receptors in normal and cancer tissue. In McGuire, W.L., Raynaud, J. P., and Baulieu, E. E. (Eds.): Progesterone Receptors in Normal and Neoplastic Tissues. New York, Raven Press, 1977, p. 155.

Rodbard, D., Munson, P. J., and Thakur, A. K.: Quantitative characterization of hormone receptors. Cancer, 46:2907, 1980.

Rosen, P. P., Menendez-Botet, C., Nisselbaum, J. S., et al.: Pathological review of breast lesions analyzed for estrogen receptor protein. Cancer Res., 35:3187, 1975.

Sarfaty, G. A., Nash, A. R., and Keightly, D. D. (Eds.): Estrogen Receptor Assays in Breast Cancer: Laboratory Discrepancies and Quality Assurance. New York, Masson Publishing, 1981.

Sato, N., Hyder, S. M., Chang, L., et al.: Interaction of estrogen receptor isoforms with immobilized monoclonal antibodies. J. Chromatogr., 359:475, 1986.

Savage, N., Levin, J., De Moor, N. G., et al.: Cytosolic oestrogen receptor content of breast cancer tissue in blacks and whites. S. Afr. Med. J., 59:623, 1981.

Schlick, E., Hewetson, P., and Ruffmann, R.: Adjuvant chemoimmunotherapy of cancer: Influence of tumor burden and role of functional immune effector cells in mice. Cancer Res., 46:3378, 1986.

Shahabi, N. A., He, Y. J., Wiehle, R. D., et al.: Characteristics of estrogen receptors in MCF-7 breast cancer cells. Amsterdam, Excerpta Medica, 1984, p. 1469.

Shahabi, N. A., Hyder, S. M., Wiehle, R. D., et al.: HPLC analysis of estrogen receptor by a multidimensional approach. J. Steroid Biochem., 24:1151, 1986.

Sherman, M. S., Pickering, L. A., Rollwagen, F. M., et al.: Meroreceptors: Proteolytic fragments of receptors containing the steroid-binding site. Fed. Proc., 37:167, 1978.

Silfversward, C., Gustafsson, J.-A., Gustafsson, S. A., et al.: Estrogen receptor concentrations in 269 cases of histologically classified human breast cancer. Cancer, 45:2001, 1980.

Sluyser, M., and Mester, J.: Oncogenes homologous to steroid receptor? (letter to the editor). Nature, *315*:546, 1985.

Spratt, J. S., Damian, P. A., Greenberg, R. A., et al.: Association of chronic cystic mastopathy, xerommammographic patterns, and cancer. Cancer, *55*:1372, 1985.

Stegner, H. E., Maass, H., Trams, G., et al.: Estrogen receptors and ultrastructural pathology of mammary carcinoma. *In* Dallenback-Hellweg, G. (Ed.): Functional Morphological Changes in Female Sex Organs Induced by Exogenous Hormones. Berlin, Springer-Verlag, 1980.

Stewart, J. F., Rubens, R. D., Millis, R. R., et al.: Steroid receptors and prognosis in operable (Stage I and II) breast cancer. Eur. J. Cancer Clin. Oncol., *19*:1381, 1983.

Sugimoto, Y., Whitman, M., Cantly, L. C., et al.: Evidence that the Rous sarcoma virus transforming gene product phosphorylates phosphatidylenositol and dracylglycerol. Proc. Natl. Acad. Sci. USA, *81*:2117, 1984.

Symposium on Estrogen Receptor Determination with Monoclonal Antibodies. Cancer Res., *46*(Suppl.): 4231S, 1986.

Tandon, A. K., Chamness, G. C., and McGuire, W. L.: Estrogen receptor in very small breast tumor specimens: a modified charcoal-gelatin assay. Cancer Res., *46*:3375, 1986.

Trams, G., and Maass, H.: Specific binding of estradiol and dihydrotestosterone receptors in human mammary cancers. Cancer Res., *37*:258, 1976.

van der Walt, L. A., and Wittliff, J. L.: Assessment of progestin receptor polymorphism by various synthetic ligands using HPLC. J. Steroid Biochem., *24*:377, 1986.

Walker, A. R. P., Walter, B. F., Tshyabalala, E. N., et al.: Low survival of South African urban black women with breast cancer. Br. J. Cancer, *49*:241, 1984.

Welshons, W. V., Lieberman, M. E., and Gorski, J.: Nuclear localization of unoccupied oestrogen receptors. Nature, *307*:747, 1984.

Wiehle, R. D., and Wittliff, J. L.: Alterations in sex-steroid hormone receptors during mammary gland differentiation in the rat. Comp. Biochem. Physiol., *768*:409, 1983.

Wiehle, R. D., and Wittliff, J. L.: Isoforms of estrogen receptors by high performance ion exchange chromatography. J. Chromatogr., *297*:313, 1984.

Wiehle, R. D., Hofmann, G. E., Fuchs, A., et al.: High performance size exclusion chromatography as a rapid method for the separation of steroid hormone receptors. J. Chromatogr., *307*:39, 1984.

Wilking, N., Carlström, H., Sköldefors, H., et al.: Estradiol formation and estrogen receptors in breast tumor tissue: Effect of tamoxifen on estrogen interconversions in breast tumor homogenate in vitro. Breast Cancer Res. Treat., *4*:149, 1984.

Wittliff, J. L.: Specific receptor of the steroid hormones in breast cancer. Semin. Oncol., *1*:109, 1974.

Wittliff, J. L.: Steroid-binding proteins in normal and neoplastic mammary cells. *In* Busch, H. (ed.): Methods in Cancer Research. Vol. II. New York, Academic Press, 1975, p. 293.

Wittliff, J. L.: Steroid hormone receptors in breast cancer. Cancer, *53*:630, 1984.

Wittliff, J. L.: Separation and characterization of isoforms of steroid hormone receptors using high-performance liquid chromatography. *In* Moudgil, V. K. (Ed.): Molecular Mechanisms of Steroid Hormone Action. Berlin, Walter de Gruyter, 1985, p. 791.

Wittliff, J. L.: HPLC of steroid-hormone receptors. LC-GC, Magazine of Liquid and Gas Chromatography, *4*:1092, 1986.

Wittliff, J. L.: Steroid hormone receptors. *In* Pesce, A., and Kaplan, L. (Eds.): Methods in Clinical Chemistry. St. Louis, C. V. Mosby, 1987, p. 767.

Wittliff, J. L., and DaPunt, O. (Eds.): Steroid Receptors and Hormone-dependent Neoplasia. New York, Masson Publishing, 1980.

Wittliff, J. L., and Savlov, E. D.: Estrogen-binding capacity of cytoplasmic forms of the estrogen receptor in human breast cancer. *In* McGuire, W. L., Carbone, P. O., and Vollmer, E. P. (Eds.): Estrogen Receptors in Human Breast Cancer. New York, Raven Press, 1975, p. 73.

Wittliff, J. L., and Wiehle, R. D.: Analytical methods for steroid hormone receptors and their quality assurance. *In* Hollander, V. P. (Ed.): Hormonally Responsive Tumors. New York, Academic Press, 1985, p. 383.

Wittliff, J. L., Hilf, R., Brooks, W. F., Jr., et al.: Specific estrogen-binding capacity of the cytoplasmic receptor in normal and neoplastic tissues of humans. Cancer Res., *32*:1983, 1972.

Wittliff, J. L., Beatty, B. W., Savlov, E. D., et al.: Estrogen receptors and hormone dependency in human breast cancer. Recent Results Cancer Res., *57*:59, 1976.

Wittliff, J. L., Lewko, W. M., Park, D. C., et al.: Steroid binding proteins of mammary tissues and their clinical significance in breast cancer. *In* McGuire, W. L. (Ed.): Hormones, Receptors, and Breast Cancer. New York, Raven Press, 1978, p. 325.

Wittliff, J. L., Heidemann, P. H., and Lewko, W. M.: Molecular basis of endocrine responsiveness in normal and neoplastic breast tissues. *In* Fleisher, M. F. (Ed.): The Clinical Biochemistry of Cancer. Washington, D. C., The American Association for Clinical Chemistry, 1979, p. 179.

Wittliff, J. L., Fisher, B., and Durant, J. F.: Establishment of uniformity in steroid receptor analyses used in co-operative clinical trials of breast cancer treatment. Recent Results Cancer Res., *71*:198, 1980.

Wittliff, J. L., Durant, J. R., and Fisher, B.: Methods of steroid receptor analyses and their quality control in the clinical laboratory. *In* Soto, R., DeNicola, A. F., and Blaquier, J. A. (Eds.): Physiopathology of Endocrine Diseases and Mechanisms of Hormone Action. New York, Alan R. Liss, 1981*a*, p. 397.

Wittliff, J. L., Feldhoff, P. A., Fuchs, A., et al.: Polymorphism of estrogen receptors in human breast cancer. *In* Soto, R., DeNicola, A. F., and Blaquier, J. A. (Eds.): Physiopathology of Endocrine Diseases and Mechanisms of Hormone Action. New York, Alan R. Liss, 1981*b*, p. 375.

Wynder, E. L., Kajitani, T., Kuno, J., et al: Comparison of survival rates between American and Japanese patients with breast cancer. Surg. Gynecol. Obstet., *117*:196, 1963.

Young, S. C., Burkett, R. J., and Stewart, C.: Discrepancy in ER levels of breast carcinoma in biopsy vs mastectomy specimens. J. Surg. Oncol., *29*:54, 1985.

CHAPTER 12

WILLIAM L. DONEGAN

Staging and Primary Treatment

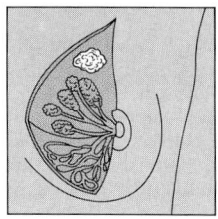

The objective of primary treatment is to provide initial management of the breast and regional lymph nodes that is appropriate for each individual patient. This decision is facilitated principally by histology, stage of the tumor, and the demonstrated effectiveness of various treatment alternatives. With respect to histology, epithelial cancers represent 99 per cent of all malignancies of the breast. They are the concern of this chapter; sarcomas are discussed in Chapter 27. The major influence of histology on treatment of carcinomas is whether they are noninvasive or invasive. These two types are considered separately, as is inflammatory carcinoma, which has distinguishing histologic and clinical features. As the disease advances beyond the noninvasive, or in situ, phase of growth its anatomic extent, or stage, assumes major importance.

This chapter is addressed largely to surgical treatment. Because the operations used in the past and present to treat breast cancer are numerous and their names are confusing, a diagram is provided for matching terminology with the anatomic features of the tissues removed (Table 12–1).

A permissive climate for evaluating therapeutic alternatives prevails at present that was unknown in the first half of this century, when allegiance to radical mastectomy was nearly uniform. This reevaluation, particularly as it pertains to breast conserving techniques, has attracted considerable attention from the public. Mastectomy has such social and emotional repercussions that concern has grown about the circumstances that make it necessary and the possible alternatives. The result has been that many states have passed laws regarding the management of breast cancer. These laws place a special legal obligation on the physician who manages breast cancer to be current and knowledgeable about all viable forms of treatment and to be fully informative to his patients about them. Examples are the following:

Massachusetts, 1979: Every patient "suffering from any form of breast cancer" has a right to "complete information on all alternative treatments which are medically viable."

California, 1980: "Failure . . . to inform a patient by means of a standardized written summary . . . of alternative efficacious methods of treatment . . . when the patient is being treated for any form of breast cancer" is unprofessional conduct.

Michigan, 1986: "A physician who is administering the primary treatment for breast cancer to a patient who has been diagnosed as having breast cancer shall inform the patient, orally and in writing, about alternative methods of treatment of the cancer, including surgical, radiological or chemotherapeutic treatments, or any other generally accepted medical treatment. The physician also shall inform the patient about the advantages, disadvantages and risks of each method of treatment."

Public interest is great enough that women seeking consultation are often well informed on the subject of breast cancer and aware of recent developments. They ask perceptive questions and are likely to seek second opinions before consenting to treatment. Furthermore, they are likely to have already had a biopsy elsewhere. If so, it is essential to review the slides to confirm the diagnosis, as well as to review mammograms and other laboratory and radiologic studies that may have been performed.

In the forefront of current developments are

Table 12–1. ANATOMIC STRUCTURES REMOVED IN VARIOUS OPERATIONS FOR CANCER OF THE BREAST

Type of Mastectomy	Tumor	Tumor with Part of Gland	Skin	Most of Gland	All of Gland	Areola	Pectoralis Minor Muscle	Pectoralis Major Muscle	Some of Low Ax. Nodes	Low Ax. Nodes (Level I)	Mid Ax. Nodes (Level II)	High Ax. Nodes (Level III)	Rotter's Nodes (Interpectoral)	Internal Mammary Nodes	Supraclavicular Nodes	Mediastinal Nodes
Lumpectomy or Tumorectomy	X															
Segmental or Quadrantectomy		X	X													
Subcutaneous				X												
Total (Simple)			X		X	X										
Total with Low Node Dissection (Modified Simple)			X		X	X				X						
Total with Axillary Dissection:																
Modified Radical (Auchincoloss)			X		X	X				X	X					
Modified Radical (Scanlon)			X		X	X				X	X	X				
Modified Radical (Patey)			X		X	X	X			X	X	X				
Radical Mastectomy (Halsted)			X		X	X	X	X		X	X	X	X			
Extended Radical (Urban)			X		X	X	X	X		X	X	X	X	X		
Extended Radical (Dahl-Iversen)			X		X	X	X	X		X	X	X	X	X	X	
Super-radical (Wangensteen)			X		X	X	X	X	X	X	X	X	X	X	X	X
Axillary Node Sample*									X							
Low Axillary Dissection*										X						
Low and Mid Axillary Dissection*										X	X					
"Complete" Axillary Dissection*										X	X	X				

*Performed in conjunction with lumpectomy or segmental mastectomy.

prospective randomized clinical trials of competing treatment techniques and sophisticated methods of data analysis. Although expensive, laborious and still imperfect, controlled clinical trials provide more satisfactory answers to clinical questions than formerly were available. They afford important insights about not only treatment but also about the malignant process, and they are given emphasis in the sections that follow.

Staging

Staging refers to the classification of breast cancer according to the anatomic extent of disease, each stage serving to aggregate cases having an approximately similar prognosis. Effective staging requires careful examination of clinical and pathologic information and accurate knowledge of end results. Ideally, it includes all presentations of the disease and results in a limited number of prognostically discrete categories, which are arranged in order of increasing gravity. It applies specifically to carcinoma, and only a histologic diagnosis gives it meaning.

Staging may be based solely on clinical evaluation (clinical stage) (e.g., physical examination, radiographs, and scans) or on information gained from surgical resections (pathologic stage). Although the latter is more accurate, the former is in some respects more useful. Clinical staging can be determined prior to therapeutic intervention and therefore provides a common baseline for comparing diverse methods of treatment, both resective and nonresective. Pathologic staging based on survey biopsies may also precede treatment, but detailed examination of resected tissues can be performed only after surgical treatment. Comparable pathologic information is not available after surgical and nonsurgical treatment, or after resections of unequal extent.

Some caveats are in order. It must be obvious that relegating the entire complex spectrum of breast cancer to a few categories is simplistic. Each stage must include considerable diversity, which results in loss of precision. It is also important to appreciate that although all presentations of the disease can be described and arranged stepwise with respect to prognosis, individual cases cannot be depended on to progress through all of the steps in an orderly fashion. Staging merely implies natural history. For example, a primary tumor may disseminate without involving regional lymph nodes as an intermediate step in the process. It is also apparent that staging based exclusively on anatomic features has important limitations. Growth rate, differentiation, and other biologic markers influence prognosis. Tumors with rapid growth rates characterized by high mitotic indices and striking aneuploidy can prove rapidly lethal despite small size and discovery at an "early" stage. Finally, staging is an evolving process, changing with new insights. As a consequence, it is not a substitute for accurate and complete factual information, which can be used for categorizing according to one or more systems. Staging is a useful abstraction, one that facilitates communication and provides some estimate of prognosis. It provides a basis for selection of treatment and for comparing results of alternative methods of treatment.

Staging has a long history. As a practical matter surgeons originally divided patients into two groups, "operable" or "inoperable," depending on whether they believed there was a chance of surgical cure or not. However, what was "operable" varied considerably in the perceptions of surgeons, encompassed a diverse mix of patients, and proved to be a poor basis on which to compare results. It was plain that, within this broad category, certain patients fared far better than others. Patients in whom the cancer was apparently confined to the breast were more likely to be cured than those who had axillary adenopathy. The latter in turn fared better than others with more widespread involvement. On the basis of these observations, Steinthal of Stuttgart (1905) suggested three groupings:

Steinthal's Groupings (Author's translation)
Group 1   Slowly growing tumors not larger than a plum confined to glandular tissue and not involving skin. Axillary lymph nodes are not clinically evident and are generally found only during an operation.
Group 2   Obvious tumors adherent to the overlying skin. Enlarged axillary lymph nodes are clearly evident.
Group 3   Most of the breast is diseased and the tumor has extended to the skin and deep tissues. Supraclavicular lymph nodes often are involved.

The majority of cases qualified for Group 2. Recurrences after resection were noted in 27.3 per cent of Group 1, 76 per cent of Group 2, and 100 per cent of Group 3 cases, and because of the discouraging results in Group 3, Steinthal recommended operation only when required for palliation. This classification was widely adopted in Germany and Scandinavia, but as it became plain that clinical evaluation of the axilla was inaccurate, Stages 1 and 2 were redefined in Scandinavia to mean the histologic absence or presence of metastases in axillary lymph nodes, in effect changing a clinical to a pathologic classification.

Later Lee and Stubenbord (1928) proposed a cumbersome classification called the clinical index of malignancy, based not only on the extent of the disease but also on the age of the patient and on the rate of tumor growth. This "biologic" system did not gain wide acceptance.

In 1940, the Manchester classification was developed at the Christie Hospital and Holt Radium Institute in Manchester, England. The Manchester system adhered strictly to clinical criteria for defining four stages, and therefore provided a common denominator for comparing diverse methods of management (Windeyer, 1949). The introduction of this four-stage system served to define two prognostically favorable categories and two poor ones. Stage III was characterized by contiguous advancement of the primary tumor into adjacent tissues and Stage IV by unremovable disease, either because of obvious dissemination or technical unresectability. The Manchester classification enjoyed wide acceptance in the British literature.

The Manchester System
Stage I   The growth is confined to the breast. Involvement of the skin directly over and in continuity with the tumor may be present provided the area is small in relation to the size of the breast.
Stage II   The growth is confined to the breast, but palpable mobile lymph nodes are present in the axilla.
Stage III   The growth extends beyond the

mammary parenchyma, as shown by
  (a) Skin invasion or fixation over an area large in relation to the size of the breast or skin ulceration.
  (b) Tumor fixation to the underlying muscle or fascia; axillary nodes, if present, are mobile.

Stage IV The growth extends beyond the breast area, as shown by fixation or matting of the axillary nodes, complete fixation of tumor to chest wall, deposits in supraclavicular nodes or in the opposite breast, satellite nodules, or distant metastases.

Three years later Portmann (1943) of the Cleveland Clinic introduced a four stage system based on both clinical and pathologic features, which took into consideration the extent of the primary tumor, skin involvement, and the extent of metastases. This mixed classification was symptomatic of continuing dissatisfaction with the inaccuracies of clinical staging.

Portmann Classification

Group or Stage I
  Skin: Not involved
  Tumor: Localized in breast and movable
  Metastases: None in axillary lymph nodes or elsewhere

Group or Stage II
  Skin: Not involved
  Tumor: Localized in breast and movable
  Metastases: Few axillary lymph nodes involved, no other metastases

Group or Stage III
  Skin: Edematous; brawny red induration and inflammation not obviously due to infection; extensive ulceration; multiple secondary nodules
  Tumor: Diffusely infiltrating breast; fixation of tumor or breast to chest wall; edema of breast; secondary tumors
  Metastases: Many axillary lymph nodes involved or fixed; no clinical or radiographic evidence of distant metastases

Group or Stage IV
  Skin: As in any other group or stage
  Tumor: As in any other group or stage
  Metastases: Axillary and supraclavicular lymph nodes extensively involved, and clinical or radiographic evidence of more distant metastases

Portmann found that 25 per cent of cases were Group I, 25 per cent were Group II, 30 per cent were Group III, and 20 per cent were Group IV, and survivals at 5 years after surgical treatment were 90 per cent, 50 per cent, 5 per cent, and 5 per cent, respectively. He recommended radical mastectomy alone for Group I, radical mastectomy and postoperative irradiation for Group II, and irradiation alone for Groups III and IV.

The Columbia Clinical Classification evolved from Haagensen and Stout's criteria for inoperability first published in 1943. These criteria were derived from careful study of 568 cases treated with radical mastectomy at Columbia–Presbyterian Medical Center in New York City from 1915 to 1935. At a time when radical mastectomy was being performed indiscriminately, this work served to define features of breast cancer that identified them as incurable with this operation. Breast cancer accompanied by pregnancy was removed from the original list, and it reached final form as follows:

Haagensen and Stout's Criteria of Inoperability
1. Extensive edema of the skin over the breast (involving more than one third of the skin of the breast)
2. Satellite nodules present in the skin
3. Carcinoma of the inflammatory type
4. Parasternal tumor nodules
5. Proved supraclavicular metastases
6. Edema of the arm
7. Distant metastases
8. Two or more of the following five grave signs of locally advanced carcinoma:
  a. Ulceration of the skin
  b. Edema of the skin of limited extent (less than one third of the skin of the breast)
  c. Fixation of the axillary lymph nodes to the skin or to the deep structures of the axilla
  d. Axillary lymph nodes measuring 2.5 cm or more in transverse diameter
  e. Solid fixation of the tumor to the chest wall

To these strictly clinical criteria of inoperability were added biopsy proof of metastases in parasternal lymph nodes or lymph nodes at the apex of the axilla, with such biopsies becoming a part of some patients' pretreatment evaluation. Haagensen and Stout's "triple biopsy" (biopsy of the primary tumor, apical axillary nodes, and internal mammary nodes), however, was not widely adopted.

The continuation of this work and the statistical assistance of Cooley ultimately resulted in the four stage Columbia Clinical Classification, in which the foregoing criteria of inoperability defined Stage D, and five "grave signs" of advancement identified Stage C.

The Columbia Clinical Classification

Stage A No skin edema, ulceration, or solid fixation of tumor to chest wall; axillary lymph nodes not clinically involved

Stage B No skin edema, ulceration, or solid fixation of tumor to chest wall; clinically involved axillary lymph nodes, but less than 2.5 cm in transverse diameter and not fixed to overlying skin or deeper structure of axilla

Stage C Any one of the five grave signs of comparatively advanced carcinoma:
1. Edema of skin of limited extent (less than one third of the skin over the breast)
2. Skin ulceration
3. Solid fixation of tumor to chest wall
4. Massive involvement of axillary lymph nodes (2.5 cm or more in transverse diameter)
5. Fixation of the axillary lymph nodes to overlying skin or deeper structures of the axilla

Stage D All other patients with more advanced carcinoma, including the following:
1. A combination of any two or more of the five grave signs listed in Stage C
2. Extensive edema of skin (involving more than one third of the skin over the breast)
3. Satellite skin nodules
4. The inflammatory type of carcinoma
5. Supraclavicular metastases, clinically apparent
6. Parasternal metastases, clinically apparent
7. Edema of the ipsilateral arm
8. Distant metastases

This classification was carefully conceived. It was widely accepted and in 1974 was used in an international cooperative study to compare results of various treatment methods in the United States and abroad (Haagensen et al., 1969). A long-term follow-up of personal experience with radical mastectomy and the Columbia Clinical Classification (CCC) was published by Haagensen and Bodian in 1984.

Stage-specific 10 year survival rates were as follows: A, 80 per cent (727 cases); B, 50 per cent (208 cases); C, 28.2 per cent (85 cases); D, 25 per cent (16 cases). Their ultimate assessment was that only Stages A and B were suitable for radical mastectomy; Stages C and D should be treated with irradiation. In this author's experience with the CCC, the four stages provide clear separation of survival with a continuum of deterioration from Stages A to D (Fig. 12–1). The subcategories of Stage C treated surgically are prognostically homogeneous, and the same can be said of Stage D (Fig. 12–2).

The CCC may be criticized for ignoring the prognostic importance of tumor size in early stages of the disease. The influence of this important variable is shown in Figure 12–3. The CCC likewise does not discriminate between objective findings in the axilla and the examiner's subjective opinion regarding involvement of the axillary lymph nodes. Furthermore, it does not distinguish between invasive and noninvasive cancers, having evolved during a period when in situ carcinomas were rare. These shortcomings are addressed in the more complex TNM system.

THE TNM CLASSIFICATION

In 1954 the International Union Against Cancer (UICC) initiated an effort to perfect a

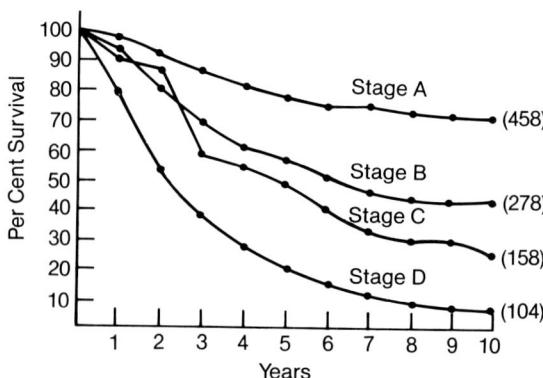

Figure 12–1. The relative survival of patients with invasive carcinoma at EFSCH, 1940–1965, treated with radical mastectomy according to the Columbia Clinical Classification (CCC). Relative survival deletes natural mortality and so when mortality from the disease ceases, the curve becomes flat. It is evident that this generally does not occur even after 10 years of observation. Stage D was composed of highly selected cases without obvious dissemination. The distinction between stages B and C is not as great as it is between others.

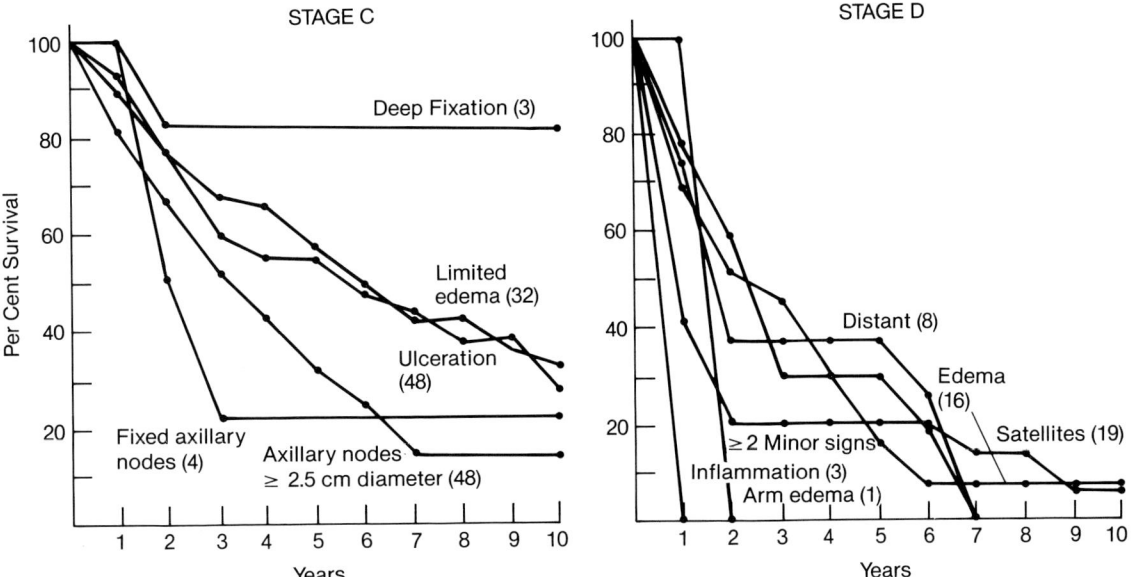

Figure 12–2. The relative survival of patients in subcategories of the CCC Stages C and D at EFSCH, 1940–1965, after radical mastectomy. Numbers in parentheses indicate number of cases. The patients are women with unilateral invasive carcinomas of the breast who have no previous mammary cancer, no pregnancies during symptoms or treatment, no simultaneous malignancies elsewhere, no previous therapy, and no adjuvant therapy with either irradiation or chemotherapy. Some overlap is evident (e.g., patients with large axillary nodes in Stage C have approximately the same survival as those with satellite nodules and edema in Stage D). Patients with limited edema of the breast or ulceration in Stage C, however, clearly have superior survival to all groups in Stage D. The few patients with either inflammatory carcinoma or edema of the arm in Stage D died rapidly, and none with distant metastases or two or more minor signs of local advancement survived for 10 years.

staging classification that would have worldwide acceptability (UICC Committee on Clinical Stage Classification, 1961). At the instigation of Denoix of France, a system based on meticulous description of the primary tumor (T), the regional lymph nodes (N), and distant metastases (M) was adopted. The subcategories of T, N, and M were then grouped in various combinations to describe four stages. The TNM concept was adopted by the American Joint Committee for Cancer Staging and End Results Reporting (AJC), but published in a somewhat different form in 1962, a year after the UICC version appeared. Efforts to evaluate the two systems and to reconcile differences generated several revisions. Using data collected from the California Tumor Registry, Zippin (1966) demonstrated that the AJC version failed to give sufficient consideration to tumor size, a feature it simply dicho-

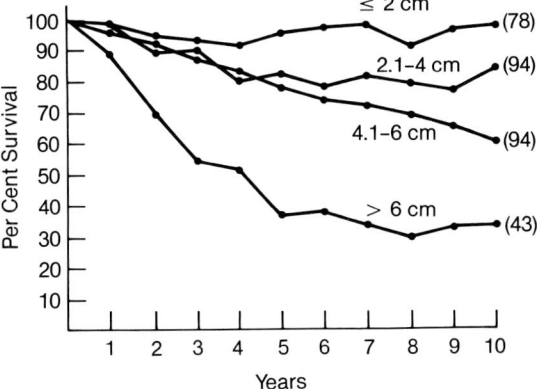

Figure 12–3. Relative survival of CCC Stage A carcinomas by tumor size after radical mastectomy for invasive carcinoma, EFSCH, 1940–1965. The prognosis of patients with Stage A carcinomas varies considerably depending on the maximum diameter of the primary tumor, a feature not considered in the staging system. Patients with carcinomas 2 cm or less in diameter fare well, and those with carcinomas greater than 6 cm in diameter fare poorly. Tumors with diameters of greater than 2 cm but not more than 6 cm appear to be a relatively homogeneous group prognostically.

Table 12–2. THE TNM CLASSIFICATION (1983) CURRENTLY IN USE FOR STAGING OF BREAST CANCER

I. Primary Tumor (T)

Clinical-diagnostic classification is the same as postsurgical resection–pathologic classification

- TX Minimum requirements to assess primary tumor cannot be met
- T0 No evidence of primary tumor
- TIS In situ cancer (in situ lobular, pure intraductal, and Paget's disease of the nipple without palpable tumor)

Note: Paget's disease with a demonstrable tumor is classified according to size of the tumor.
Inflammatory carcinoma is reported separately. (Cancers that lack microscopic dermal lymphatic permeation are not classified as inflammatory carcinoma.)

- T1 + Tumor 2 cm or less in greatest dimension
  - T1a No fixation to underlying pectoral fascia or muscle
  - T1b Fixation of underlying pectoral fascia or muscle
    - i. tumor ≤ 0.5 cm
    - ii. tumor $> 0.5 \leq 1.0$ cm
    - iii. tumor $> 1.0 \leq 2.0$ cm
- T2 + Tumor > 2 cm but not more than 5 cm in its greatest dimension
  - T2a No fixation to underlying pectoral fascia or muscle
  - T2b Fixation to underlying pectoral fascia or muscle
- T3 + Tumor > 5 cm in its greatest dimension
  - T3a No fixation to underlying pectoral fascia or muscle
  - T3b Fixation to underlying pectoral fascia or muscle
- T4 Tumor of any size with direct extension to chest wall or skin (chest wall includes ribs, intercostal muscles, and serratus anterior muscle, but not pectoral muscle).
  - T4a Fixation to chest wall
  - T4b Edema (including peau d'orange), ulceration of the skin of the breast, or satellite skin nodules confined to the same breast
  - T4c Both of the above

II. Nodal Involvement (N)

Definitions for Clinical-Diagnostic Stage

- NX Regional lymph nodes cannot be assessed clinically
- N0 Homolateral axillary lymph nodes not considered to contain growth
- N1 Movable homolateral axillary nodes considered to contain growth
- N2 Homolateral axillary nodes considered to contain growth and fixed to one another or to other structures
- N3 Homolateral supraclavicular or infraclavicular nodes considered to contain growth or edema of the arm (edema of the arm may be caused by lymphatic obstruction and lymph nodes may not then be palpable).

Definitions for Surgical Evaluative and Postsurgical Resection–Pathologic Stage

- NX Regional lymph nodes cannot be assessed (not removed for study or previously removed).
- N0 No evidence of homolateral axillary lymph node metastasis
- N1 Metastasis to movable homolateral axillary nodes not fixed to one another or to other structure
- N1a Micrometastasis ≤ 0.2 cm in lymph node(s)
- N1b Gross metastasis in lymph node(s)
  - I Metastasis > 0.2 cm but < 2.0 cm in one to three lymph nodes
  - II Metastasis > 0.2 cm but < 2.0 cm in four or more lymph nodes
  - III Extension of metastasis beyond the lymph node capsule (< 2.0 cm in dimension)
  - IV Metastasis in lymph node 2.0 cm or more in dimension
- N2 Metastases to homolateral axillary lymph nodes that are fixed to one another or to other structures
- N3 Metastasis to homolateral supraclavicular or infraclavicular lymph node(s)

Note: Homolateral internal mammary nodes considered to contain growth are included in N3.

III. Distant Metastasis (M)

- MX Minimum requirements to assess the presence of distant metastasis cannot be met.
- M0 No (known) distant metastasis
- M1 Distant metastasis present

Stage Grouping

Stage TIS	In situ
Stage X	Cannot stage
Stage I	T1ai, N0, M0
	T1aii, N0, M0
	T1aiii, N0, M0
	T1bi, N0, M0
	T1bii, N0, M0
	T1biii, N0, M0

Table 12–2. THE TNM CLASSIFICATION (1983) CURRENTLY IN USE FOR STAGING OF BREAST CANCER *Continued*

Stage Grouping *Continued*
- Stage II
  - T0, N1a or N1b, M0
  - T1a or T1b, N1a or N1b, M0
  - T2a or T2b, N0, M0
  - T2a or T2b, N1a or N1b, M0
- Stage IIIA
  - T0, N2, M0
  - T1a or T1b, N2, M0
  - T2a or T2b, N2, M0
  - T3a or T3b, N0, M0
  - T3a or T3b, N1, M0
  - T3a or T3b, N2, M0
- Stage IIIB
  - Any T, N3, M0
  - Any T4, any N, M0
- Stage IV
  - Any T, any N, M1

Measurements of 2 cm or less for T1a, T1b, and N1b do not necessarily need to be recorded.

---

tomized as 2.0 cm or less versus greater than 2.0 cm. A joint AJC-UICC TNM classification published in 1972 was encumbered by a large Stage III, which encompassed 50 per cent of all cases and was composed of many subgroups that overlapped prognostically with Stages II and IV. A further revision endorsed by both organizations appeared in 1977. Tumors with direct extension of the chest wall or skin were moved out of Stage III into Stage IV, as were those associated with edema of the arm and those with supraclavicular or infraclavicular adenopathy. Inflammatory carcinoma, requiring histologically proved dermal lymphatic invasion, remained in Stage IV.

The current version (Table 12–2 and Figure 12–4*A*) was agreed on in 1978 by the UICC and the renamed American Joint Committee on Cancer. It restricts Stage IV to cases with distant dissemination.

The system can be used as both a clinical classification (Clinical-Diagnostic Stage) or a pathologic one (Postsurgical Resection–Pathologic Stage), which involves pathologic examination of the whole breast and all axillary lymph nodes, as would be available from a total mastectomy and complete axillary lymph node dissection. A third category (Surgical Evaluative Stage), is derived from pathologic examination of the primary tumor and some of the axillary lymph nodes, as might be provided by a segmental mastectomy and axillary node sampling. The category is specified with a lower case prefix (e.g., cTNM, pTNM, or sTNM). Nodal involvement, local-regional recurrence, and survival after mastectomy according to TNM Clinical Diagnostic Stages are shown in Figure 12–4*B*.

Unfortunately, the complexity of the TNM classification makes it difficult to use. It is subject to periodic change and whether it will classify reliably the less frequent histologic types of cancers is not known. It will possibly undergo further change, underscoring the wisdom of recording clinical and pathologic data in all cases of breast cancer with the accuracy, objectivity, and completeness that permits them to be transported into any present or future staging system that may come into use. The clinician should consult the most recent publications of the American Joint Committee on Cancer to remain current on TNM staging.

The Yorkshire Breast Cancer group (1980) evaluated the 1974 version of the TNM system and found problems that probably persist. Surgeons and pathologists agreed on tumor size (T category) in only 54 per cent of cases, surgeons and radiologists in only 39 per cent, and radiologists and pathologists in 59 per cent. Assessment of the axilla was in error in 42 per cent of cases when judged clinically negative. The T0 category remains a problem. A physically occult primary tumor (manifested only by a palpable axillary metastasis) would be T0, but a physically occult mammographically measurable primary tumor could be T1 or higher, depending on size. It has been suggested that occult invasive tumors found on mammogram be included in the T0 category (Schwartz et al., 1984), rather than in the T1 category. Inflammatory cancer continues to be identified by dermal histologic examination only.

It is useful to appreciate that an unofficial and imprecise but generally understood staging terminology exists. Stage I without further

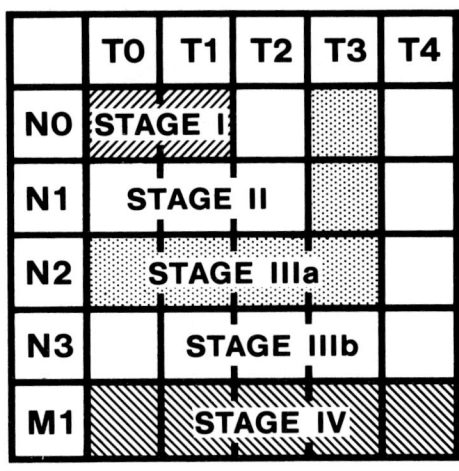

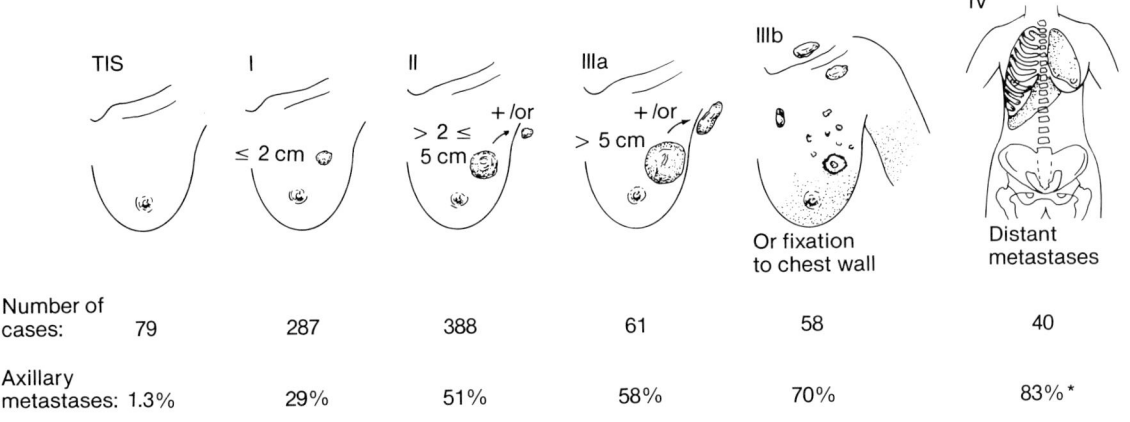

Figure 12–4. *A*, Grid showing the subsets of T, N, and M combined into clinical stages. *B*, cTNM stages are represented diagrammatically. The frequency of axillary metastases is shown for cases treated surgically at the Medical College of Wisconsin. *Surgical cases.

definition is understood to mean a tumor confined to the breast without involvement of adjacent tissues or regional nodes. Stage II means such a tumor associated with axillary metastases. Whether the former are clinically or pathologically identified is uncertain unless specified. Stage IV implies distant dissemination. Tumors with various local and regional advancement between Stages II and IV are Stage III.

Resources for Clinical Staging

A careful physical examination is the primary resource for clinical staging. Useful for identifying distant metastases are radiographs, serologic studies, computed tomography, and radioisotopic scans of the liver, bones, and brain. Appropriate use of scans depends on the reliability of the results and the probability of finding occult metastases. The most likely sites for initial dissemination are bones, lungs, and pleura; the liver and brain are considerably less frequent sites.

An extensive laboratory investigation is not appropriate before biopsy; a complete evaluation can be performed afterward if cancer is diagnosed. Before a biopsy of the breast is performed, adults should have bilateral mammograms. Mammograms are obtained despite the presence of a clinically obvious cancer to detect subclinical lesions in either breast that might require evaluation at the same time (Young et al., 1986).

HEMOGRAM AND CHEST RADIOGRAPHS

A hemogram and a radiograph of the chest are obtained in all cases before treatment. Anemia may indicate extensive bone marrow involvement, which may not be evident on a bone scan. Pulmonary metastases may be asymptomatic or betrayed by only a mild cough. Their presenting signs are pleural effusions or nodular pulmonary densities. Lymphangitic spread within the lungs is suggested by dyspnea and may provide few radiographic signs. Diffuse streaking from the hilar areas is characteristic of lymphangitic involvement; blood gas determinations and pulmonary function studies show compromise of ventilatory function. A solitary lesion of the lung in a woman with otherwise clinically localized cancer of the breast is more likely to be a primary carcinoma of the lung than a metastasis (Cahan and Castro, 1975). Among 42 women with breast cancer who had a solitary pulmonary nodule either initially or during follow-up, Casey and associates (1984) found that 52 per cent had primary lung cancer, 5 per cent had a benign lesion, and 43 per cent had metastatic breast cancer. This fact is of considerable significance for staging and treatment. It can be attributed to the rising frequency of lung cancer among women in the United States and the low frequency with which breast cancer produces a solitary metastasis. Histologic evaluation of solitary pulmonary lesions is in order, including a thoracotomy if necessary. A considerable number of women with asymptomatic lung cancers can be salvaged with resections. At the same time, the synchronous breast cancer can receive appropriate treatment.

BONE RADIOGRAPHS AND SCANS

A radiographic survey of the skeleton (ribs, skull, spine, pelvis, femora, and humeri) is unrewarding unless the patient has symptoms suggesting osseous metastases. Gibbons and associates (1961) examined 85 consecutive asymptomatic patients within 6 weeks after mastectomy. Eighteen per cent had benign abnormalities of bones and only one of the 85 had a possible asymptomatic metastasis. The latter was not histologically proved and had not progressed after 18 months.

Bone scans are considerably more sensitive than radiographs, being able to detect metastases before they become asymptomatic and up to 12 months before they can be demonstrated on radiographs. Unfortunately, they are nonspecific, and any osteoblastic activity produces abnormalities (e.g., that accompanying fractures, periosteal reaction to trauma, osteoarthritis, Paget's disease of bone, and primary bone tumors). Thus, radiographs of abnormalities are necessary for reliable interpretation. The combination of an abnormal bone scan and a normal radiograph is suggestive of early metastasis (Baker et al., 1977). The subsequent appearance of unexplained abnormalities in an initially normal bone scan is usually indicative of metastasis, although not always. According to a number of reports, patients with preoperative bone scans suspected of indicating cancer have a poor prognosis (Hoffman and Marty, 1972; Galasko, 1975; Citrin et al., 1976). In these cases, however, the bones are not always the first site of recurrence.

Recommendations for the use of bone scans have become conservative. Galasko (1975) found scans suggestive of metastases in 24 per cent of patients with clinically early breast cancers and advised that scans precede any decision about treatment. This opinion was shared by Charkes and associates (1975), who observed recurrence in 3 of 35 patients (9 per cent) who had positive preoperative scans. Opposing this view were Robbins and coworkers (1972), who observed that only 19 per cent of patients eventually developed osseous metastases after mastectomies, and often only after many years. Robbins and associates considered scans justified only with borderline operable cancers or in the presence of bone pain. Supporting these observations, Sklaroff and Sklaroff (1976) reported prolonged asymptomatic survival of 40 per cent of patients with abnormal preoperative bone scans. Baker and colleagues (1977) also advised selective use. These investigators found positive scans in only 1 of 64 patients (1.6 per cent) with TNM Stage I or II cancers and believed that the low yield failed to justify scans in these clinical stages. El-Domeiri and Shroff (1976) recommended scans for T2 cancers only if located centrally or medially, for patients with palpable axillary lymph nodes, and for those with some evidence of spread beyond the breast.

Komaki and associates (1979) found evidence of difficulty among radiologists in distinguishing between abnormalities due to benign and neoplastic processes. Scans initially read as suggestive of metastases were surprisingly frequent (32 per cent for TNM Stage I, 34 per cent for Stage II, 44 per cent for Stage III, and 75 per cent for Stage IV, respectively). After an average follow-up of 24 months, 21 per cent of the patients with Stages I, II and III collectively had developed disseminated cancer after initially normal bone scans, as had 41 per cent with abnormal (but not suspicious) bone scans and 38 per cent with suspicious bone scans. A suspicious scan was correlated with a poor prognosis in TNM Stages I and II but not with recurrence in bones.

Preoperative bone scans should be obtained in locally advanced cases and in those with signs or symptoms suggesting bony metastases. Abnormalities must be examined with radiographs before conclusions are drawn. Furthermore, an abnormality on scan in a radiologically normal bone should not preclude potentially curative treatment without histologic proof that it represents dissemination.

LIVER FUNCTION TESTS AND SCANS

Approximately 35 to 65 per cent of autopsied patients with cancer of the breast have hepatic metastases (Haagensen, 1971); the early detection of these metastases continues to present a challenge.

Isotopic scans are limited in sensitivity and plagued by false positive results, particularly in populations subject to nonneoplastic disease of the liver. Metastases less than 2 cm in diameter usually fail to be visualized (Castagna et al., 1972), and congenital cysts, pressure defects, and cirrhosis mimic metastasis. When metastases are present, scans are abnormal in up to 89 per cent of cases, but false positive findings range from 10 to 30 per cent (Sugarbaker et al., 1977). Focal defects are the most reliable indicators of metastases. If diffuse abnormalities are included, sensitivity is increased, but at the price of an increase in false positive rate.

Elevated serum alkaline phosphatase level remains one of the simplest and best methods of detecting hepatic metastases (Table 12–3). An abnormal value in a patient with breast cancer signals hepatic involvement with 85 per cent certainty. When the test is normal, it is accurate 88 per cent of the time. An elevated serum alkaline phosphatase level may be indicative of either hepatic or osseous metastases. Fractionating the alkaline phosphatase into its heat-stable and heat-labile portions may be helpful. A heat-stable fraction that is greater than 35 per cent of the elevated value generally indicates hepatic origins, whereas a lesser value suggests bony involvement.

In the nonjaundiced patient, multiple abnormal serologic tests of hepatic function (notably alkaline phosphatase, glutamic-oxaloacetic transaminase, and albumin) signal cancer in 92 per cent of cases. The addition of an abnormal liver scan increases this probability to near certainty. Castagna and associates (1972) found only one false positive diagnosis in 101 cases in which this combination was present. The evidence is that in the absence of hepatic enlargement or deranged hepatic functions, isotopic scans add little to detection. Felix and coworkers (1976) found only 13 per cent of hepatic scans positive in patients with metastases unassociated with an abnormal physical examination or abnormal serologic tests. Sugarbaker and associates (1977) found a combination of elevated carcinoembryonic antigen (CEA) and a positive liver scan highly correlated with hepatic metastases in patients with carcinoma of the breast and associated with a low false positive rate.

Computed tomography (CT) has largely replaced radioisotopic scans of the liver because of superior accuracy and definition. Cysts can be differentiated from solid lesions, and when combined with use of intravenous contrast material, which lingers in tumors, the size and number of metastases can be discerned with even greater accuracy. False negative results, which continue to occur, are attributable to nonfocal hepatic involvement, the lack of diferent radiodensity between normal liver and metastasis, and small lesions that fall between the planes that are imaged. In direct comparisons, CT scanning has proved superior to technetium-99 m sulfur colloid scintigraphy, ultrasonography, and magnetic resonance imaging for detecting metastases (Zeman et al., 1985).

Scans are best reserved for patients suspected of having metastases on the basis of hepatomegaly on physical examination or abnormal serologic tests (Sears et al., 1975; Felix et al., 1976; Wiener and Sachs, 1978). Focal defects in a liver scan, particularly when unaccompanied by clear evidence of disturbed hepatic function, require histologic confirma-

Table 12–3. ACCURACY OF SEROLOGIC TESTS OF HEPATIC FUNCTION AND LIVER SCINTISCANS IN DETECTING HEPATIC METASTASES OF MAMMARY CARCINOMA

Examination	Abnormal	Normal	Accuracy (%)	Per Cent Abnormal when Cancer Present (True Positives)	Per Cent Abnormal when Cancer Absent (False Positives)
Alkaline Phosphatase (AP)	X		85	58–71	12–40
		X	88		
SGOT**				60–74	31
SGPT†				21	
LDH‡				74	58
CEA§ (greater than 2.5 ng/ml)				76	25
AP + ALB‖ + SGOT	X		92		
AP + ALB + SGOT + BILI¶ + SGPT		X	70		
Liver Scan	X		20–78	89	14
		X	71		
Liver Scan + CEA (> 1.0 ng/ml)				89	0
Liver Scan + AP + SGOT + ALB	X		99		
		X	78		

Note: The accuracy, sensitivity, and specificity of serologic tests of hepatic function and radioisotopic scans in the detection of hepatic metastases from carcinoma of the breast are tabulated. The alkaline phosphatase and the liver scan are the single tests with greatest overall accuracy.
**Serum glutamic oxaloacetic transaminase.
†Serum glutamic pyruvic transaminase.
‡Lactic acid dehydrogenase.
§Carcinoembryonic antigen.
‖Albumin.
¶Bilirubin.
Based on data from Sugarbaker et al., 1977 (breast cancer only); Sears et al., 1975 (breast cancer only); and Castagna et al., 1972 (mixed cancers).

tion before concluding that they represent metastases.

BRAIN SCANS

Radionuclide brain scans are highly accurate, detecting 85 to 90 per cent of cerebral metastases. Intracranial metastases from cancer of the breast apparently are quick to make their presence known, however, and they are rarely detected in asymptomatic patients. Muss and coworkers (1976) reviewed the brain scans of 116 patients with metastatic cancer of the breast who had no symptoms of intracranial disease and found only one with an abnormality, the precise nature of which was never determined. Eleven of 37 patients with central nervous system symptoms (30 per cent) had abnormal scans initially and three (8 per cent) developed abnormalities later. The symptoms of the remaining 23 patients cleared spontaneously. Brain scans, therefore, are not indicated unless symptoms are suggestive of central nervous system metastases. Conversely, an abnormal brain scan in an asymptomatic patient is sufficiently rare to require further confirmation. As osteolytic metastasis in the skull will create abnormalities on brain scans, peripheral lesions should be further evaluated with roentgenograms of the skull or a bone scan to make this distinction. CT scans are similarly unproductive. Lewi and coworkers (1980) reported that CT scans of the brain in 61 asymptomatic patients detected no occult metastases.

BONE BIOPSIES

The results of routine bone marrow biopsies of the posterior iliac crest in 532 women with unilateral breast cancer were reported by Ridell and Landys (1979). When a radiologic examination of the skeleton was negative, positive biopsies were obtained with a prevalence of 1.6 per cent. Whenever there was any radiologic evidence of skeletal metastases, the prevalence of positive biopsies rose to 28 per cent. In the presence of a negative bone scan and normal radiograph, DiStefano and colleagues (1979) reported positive bone biopsies in only 2.8 per cent of 213 cases and Ingle and coworkers (1978) found positive bone biopsies in 4 per cent of 24 cases. In view of the low rate of detection in cases without some basis for suspicion, bone biopsies are not performed routinely.

SUMMARY

It might be observed that the more examinations performed, the greater is the chance of discovering asymptomatic metastases. Yet considering the time, expense, and morbidity involved and the frequency of false positive results, the value of exhaustive testing might be questioned.

For practical purposes after a tissue diagnosis of cancer is made, the following are recommended for clinical staging. The addition of other procedures depends on the presence of suggestive symptoms or signs.

1. A complete history and physical examination
2. A complete blood count
3. A radiograph of the chest (posteroanterior and lateral views);
4. Serologic tests of hepatic function, with a CT scan of the liver only if abnormalities are detected
5. A bone scan for TNM clinical Stage III and IV cases and those with bone pain. Radiographs are indicated if any abnormalities are evident on bone scan or if the patient has unexplained bone pain or anemia.
6. Bilateral mammograms.

Clinical Classification of Advanced Breast Cancer

Considerable variation is observed in the survival of patients with disseminated cancer of the breast. It is possible, by taking into consideration the body organs involved and their number, to achieve more accurate estimates of prognosis. This information can influence decisions relative to the urgency of palliative therapy. It also ensures that evaluating alternative methods of palliation is based on cases with a comparable prognosis.

Cutler and associates (1974) observed that patients with metastases in the liver, peritoneum, brain, or spinal cord had a rapid demise (median survival time of 6 months) and classified them as a "dire prognosis" group. The courses of others, including those with other visceral metastases, were influenced most notably by the number of organs involved. Patients with dissemination could be placed into three groups:

Group I   Metastases in only one organ system (median survival, 15 months)

Group II   Metastases in two or more organ systems (median survival, 12 months)

Group III   Metastases in the liver or central nervous system (median survival, 4 months)

Patients with postoperative recurrence were classified separately. Taking into consideration the fact that patients with the greatest interval between surgery and dissemination also had the longest survival after dissemination was discovered, Cutler and associates (1969) suggested four groups:

Classification of Cases with Postoperative Recurrence

Group I   All patients with a free interval of 5 years or longer or with a free interval of 2 to 5 years with only one organ system involved (Median survival within subcategories, 14 to 40 months).

Group II   Patients with a free interal of 2 to 5 years with two or three organ systems involved, those with a free interval of 1 to 2 years with one or two systems involved, and those with a free interval of less than 1 year with only one organ system involved (median survival in subcategories, 11 to 16 months).

Group III   Patients with a free interval of 2 to 5 years with four or more systems involved, 1 to 2 years with three or four systems involved, and less than 1 year with two or more systems involved (median survival in subcategories, 5 to 7 months).

Group IV   Patients with hepatic or central nervous system metastases (median survival in four subcategories, 5 to 11 months).

Evident in a review of patients with recurrence after mastectomy at the Medical College of Wisconsin (MCW) was the poor survival of those with metastases initially in the liver, peritoneum, or gastrointestinal tract (Tomin and Donegan, 1987). None lived beyond 3 years from the time metastases were discovered (median survival, 6 months). Patients with the most favorable outlook were those with initial local recurrence, followed by those with metastases to lymph nodes. An intermediate prognosis was shared by patients with initial metastases in bones (median survival, 30 months) and in lung or pleura (median survival, 21 months) (Fig. 12–5).

Pathologic Staging

The appeal of pathologic staging is the histologic certainty it provides. Most attention has been given in surgical cases to the pathologic staging of regional lymph nodes, particularly the axillary nodes. The inaccuracy of clinical determination is widely appreciated. Axillary lymph nodes contain metastases in approximately 40 per cent of cases without clinical adenopathy; the false positive error is 30 per cent when metastases are suspected (Fig. 12–6). The internal mammary nodes, hidden within the bony thorax, are not accessible for physical examination but often contain metastases.

INVASIVENESS

The single most important determinant of prognosis is whether the primary tumor is invasive or not. Noninvasive tumors are almost always cured by mastectomy.

NUMBER OF AXILLARY METASTASES

In cases of invasive carcinoma treated with mastectomy, the number of metastases in axillary lymph nodes is of paramount prognostic importance. The risk of treatment failure rises progressively and continuously with the absolute number of axillary metastases. The data in Table 12–4 demonstrate that survival, local

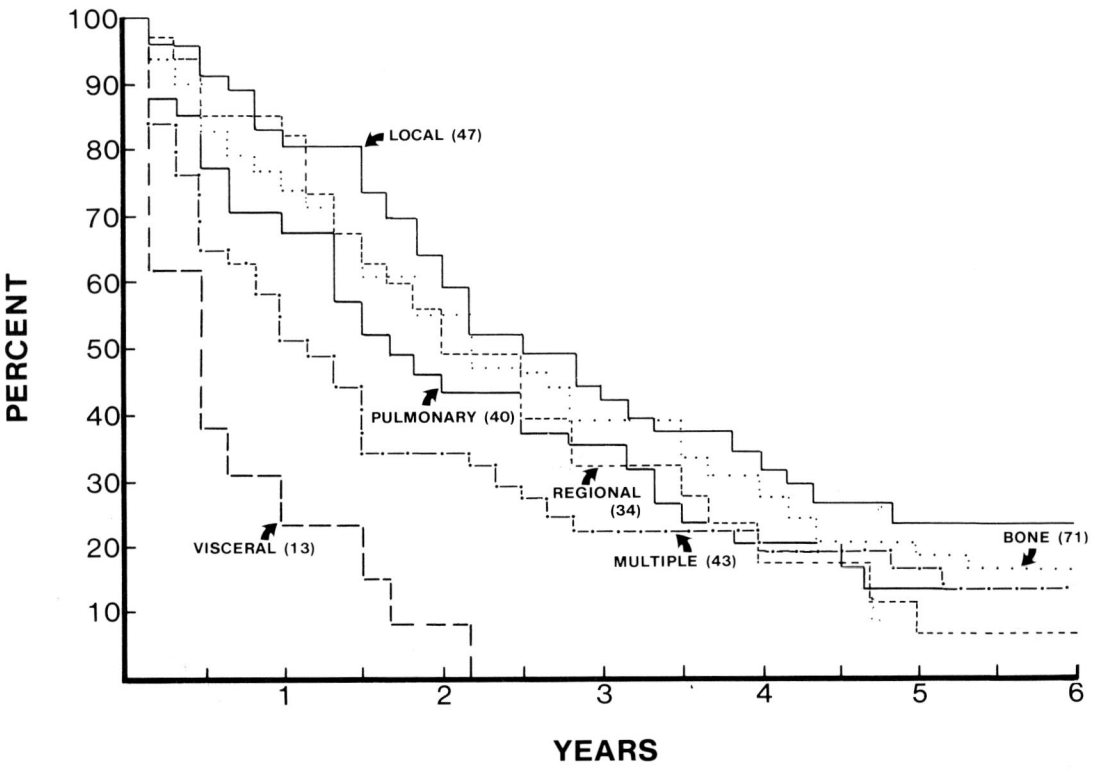

Figure 12–5. The survival of 248 cases of recurrent breast cancer at the Medical College of Wisconsin demonstrates that prognosis varies according to the site of initial recurrence. Recurrence in viscera (e.g., liver, brain, and intraperitoneal organs), the most unfavorable, and that associated with recurrence at multiple sites is also poor.

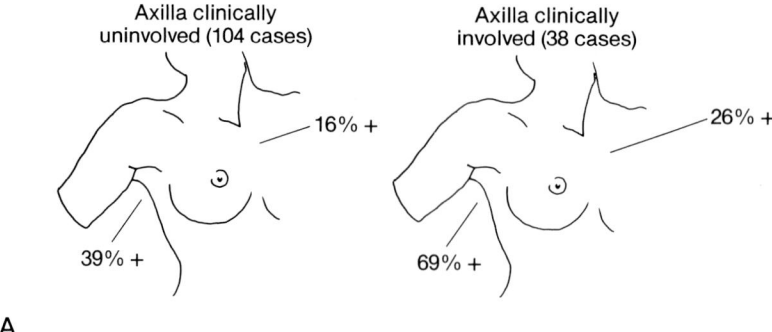

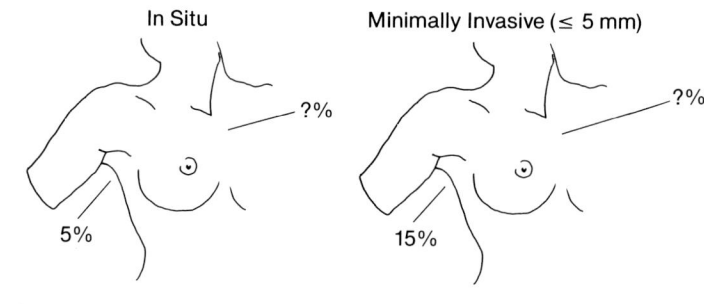

Figure 12–6. *A,* The frequency of metastatic cancer in axillary and internal mammary lymph nodes as determined from extended mastectomies by Sugarbaker. Clinical evaluation of the axilla is falsely negative in 39 per cent of cases and falsely positive in 31 per cent, respectively. The internal mammary nodes, which cannot be evaluated clinically, contain metastases in 16 per cent of localized cases and 26 per cent of cases with axillary adenopathy.

B, The frequency of axillary nodal metastases from minimal breast cancers is shown for 96 cancers in a review at the Medical College of Wisconsin. Five per cent of apparently noninvasive ductal and lobular carcinomas produced axillary metastases, and minimally invasive carcinomas produced them in 15 per cent. As axillary lymph nodes were not removed in all cases, these represent minimal figures.

Table 12–4. PROGNOSIS FOR RECURRENCE AND SURVIVAL AFTER RADICAL MASTECTOMY BASED UPON THE NUMBER OF AXILLARY LYMPH NODES WITH METASTASES (EFSCH 1940 TO 1965)*

Number of Axillary Metastases	Number of Cases	Survival		Relative Survival		Local Recurrence (%)	Overall Recurrence (%)
		5 Years	10 Years	5 Years	10 Years		
None	332	70	52	82	74	11	27
Any	456	41	22	47	30	36	67
1–2	171	52	34	60	46	21	52
3–4	71	51	27	58	38	38	66
5–6	49	41	22	47	30	49	74
7–8	38	24	11	28	14	47	87
9–10	32	38	21	42	26	47	66
11–12	20	26	0	31	0	40	85
13–15	23	30	4	34	6	52	83
15–20	23	22	8	24	9	39	87
21+	29	7	0	8	0	59	90

Note: The presence of metastases in axillary lymph nodes and the number of involved nodes are the most important and sensitive pathologic indicators of prognosis following surgical treatment of mammary carcinoma. Although the present convention is to identify three prognostic groups, i.e., patients with no metastases, those with one to three and those with four or more metastases, it is clear that prognosis progressively deteriorates as the number of involved nodes increases.

*After 5 to 24 years of observation.

recurrence, and total treatment failure correlate precisely with the total number of nodes that contain metastases. Wilson and coworkers (1984) confirmed this relationship in a national survey by the American College of Surgeons with over 20,000 cases.

The convention at present is to report results separately for patients with zero, one to three, or four or more involved axillary lymph nodes. Fisher and coworkers (1975b) reported 10 year surgical failure rates after radical mastectomy in 24 per cent of cases without metastases, in 76 per cent of cases with any metastases, in 64.5 per cent of cases with one to three involved axillary lymph nodes, and in 86.2 per cent of those with four or more involved axillary lymph nodes. Disease-free survival after mastectomies at MCW shows the influence of quantitative nodal involvement according to this convention (Fig. 12–7).

An observation deserving attention is that the number of axillary lymph nodes with metastases correlates not only with the probability of recurrence but also with the speed of recurrence. Patients with extensive involvement of regional nodes not only are more likely to have recurrence but also are more likely to have it sooner than others. Figure 12–8 plots the declining disease-free survival of the author's patients with recurrence after radical mastectomy according to nodal status. Patients with 11 or more diseased lymph nodes had rapid recurrence with a median disease-free survival (DFS) of only 10 months. The median DFS improved to 16 months in patients with 5 to 10 positive nodes, to 22 months in those with one to four positive nodes, and to a median of 26 months in patients with no histologic evidence of metastases. This can be interpreted to mean that tumors productive of extensive metastases had a faster median doubling time than did tumors with less metastatic potential. Alternatively, if the median tumor growth rates in all nodal categories are equivalent, it might be assumed that tumors that required longest to regrow to a detectable size had least residual tumor mass after surgery and, by inference, that residual tumor burden after surgery is directly related to the extensiveness of nodal metastasis.

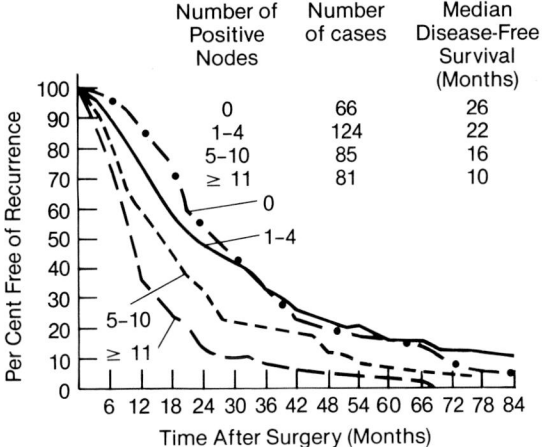

Figure 12–8. The disease-free survivals of patients with recurrence after radical mastectomy indicate that recurrences are more rapid in patients with large numbers of involved lymph nodes. These curves can be interpreted to mean that patients with the fewest nodes involved have the least residual tumor burden after radical mastectomy, or that cancers with the greatest metastatic ability have the most rapid growth rates.

SIZE, CONTAINMENT, AND LEVEL OF AXILLARY METASTASES

Further features of axillary invasion that are attended by an unfavorable prognosis include the presence of gross rather than microscopic metastases (Attiyen et al., 1977), invasion of extranodal tissues (Mambo and Gallager, 1977), involvement of nodes at the apex of the axilla (Table 12–5) (Haagensen, 1971; Donegan, 1972), and the absence of sinus histiocytosis in axillary nodes (Hunter et al., 1975). Nevertheless, each of these is of less importance than the total number of nodes involved. The 1983 version of the TNM classification acknowledges the importance of both the num-

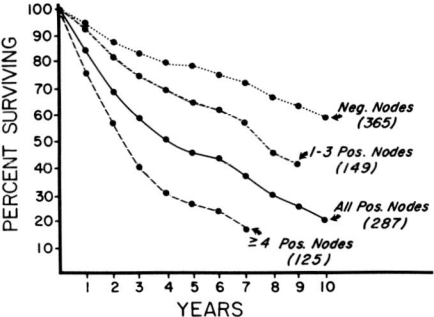

Figure 12–7. Disease-free survival after radical or modified mastectomy is strongly influenced by the number of nodes that contain metastases. The standard categories for node counts are shown, but they represent a simplification of this relationship. Numbers in parentheses are total numbers of cases.

Table 12–5. RECURRENCE AND SURVIVAL AFTER RADICAL MASTECTOMY ACCORDING TO THE HIGHEST LEVEL OF AXILLARY LYMPH NODES WITH METASTASES (EFSCH, 1940 TO 1965)

Axillary Level*	Number of Cases	10 Year Survival (%)	10 Year Relative Survival (%)	Local Recurrence (%)	Overall Recurrence (%)
I (Low)	93	29	42	28	50
II (Mid)	129	32	43	33	64
III (High)	177	10	13	45	80

Note: the highest level of involved axillary nodes divided according to the convention of Berg (1955) is of prognostic importance. At least 80 per cent of patients with metastases in the high axillary lymph nodes experience treatment failure. Little difference prognostically, however, can be appreciated between involvement of low nodes only and that of midaxillary nodes. This observation argues for dichotomizing axillary involvement between high node involvement (proximal to the medial border of the pectoralis minor muscle) versus involvement at lower levels.

*Axillary levels: Lateral and inferior to the pectoralis minor muscle (low, or Level I), behind the pectoralis minor (mid, or Level II) and medial and superior to the pectoralis minor muscle (high, or Level III).

ber and the size of metastases in axillary lymph nodes.

TOTAL AXILLARY NODES REMOVED

Fisher and Slack (1970) could find no correlation between the absolute number of lymph nodes removed from the axilla and the outcome of treatment, an observation that appears to minimize the importance of a complete axillary dissection. The same is true for axillary dissections at Ellis Fischel State Cancer Hospital (EFSCH), where, regardless of the total number of nodes reported in surgical specimens, the prognoses of patients with equivalent numbers of metastases remain unchanged (Fig. 12–9). It should be remembered, however, that in both studies the extent of dissection was equal in all cases (Levels I to III), and the difference in total count resulted not from the extent of dissection but from the pathologists' diligence or the patients' anatomy, so no conclusions can be reached about the completeness of dissection. This observation does mean, however, that the absolute number of involved nodes, not the proportion of all nodes that are positive, is the important factor.

ROTTER'S NODES

Kay (1965) found Rotter's nodes (interpectoral lymph nodes) in 65 per cent of radical mastectomy specimens, but their involvement by metastases did not influence the outcome of treatment independently of axillary nodal status. Cody and associates (1984) found Rotter's nodes to be involved in only 0.5 per cent of cases with negative axillary lymph nodes and considered unexcised nodes at this location of little consequence in cases of early breast cancer treated with modified mastectomy.

EXTENT OF AXILLARY DISSECTION FOR STAGING

The extent of axillary dissection necessary for adequate pathologic staging is the subject of debate, specifically regarding the procedure

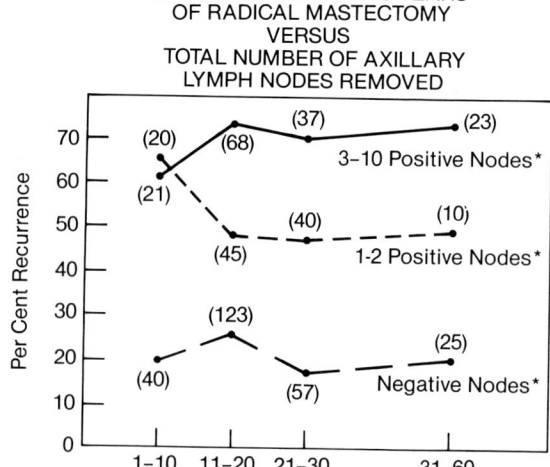

*No significant differences

Figure 12–9. Cases of invasive carcinoma of the breast treated with radical mastectomy at EFSCH demonstrating that the prognosis of patients based on the number of axillary nodes that contain metastases is constant despite the total number of lymph nodes examined. Parentheses indicate number of cases.

necessary to detect nodal metastases reliably if they are present. Davies and coworkers (1980) found that lymph node sampling missed 42 per cent of cases in which metastases were present and was clearly an inadequate procedure. Removing the pectoral nodes with the axillary tail of the breast still missed 14 per cent. Fisher and colleagues (1981) recommended removal of at least 10 nodes, but other authors have considered three or four adequate (Forrest et al., 1982). The fact is that dissections ordinarily are based on anatomic boundaries rather than nodal tallies during the operation. Most investigations of this problem are based on staged removals of axillary levels or tagged nodal boundaries during mastectomy. The findings at each level are compared with the completed total dissection. Pigott and coworkers (1984) investigated 72 cases with metastases in this manner and found that a Level I dissection (i.e., lateral to the pectoralis minor muscle) missed 25 per cent of positive axillae (50 per cent if the primary tumor was located medially and 20 per cent if it was located laterally), but the error was reduced to 1.4 per cent if nodes were removed from both Levels I and II (i.e., both lateral to and behind the pectoralis minor muscle). Tumor size had no influence of these results. Other investigators have performed similar studies and obtained different results (Table 12–6), leading to different conclusions about the adequacy of a Level I dissection. In a careful study, Danforth and coworkers (1986) confirmed Pigott and colleagues' results and attributed the discrepancies of other authors to imprecise technique with misallocations of nodes between Levels I and II. Overall accuracy varies with the proportion of the total population that is truly without metastases. As this proportion grows, the false negative error diminishes.

It appears that "skip" metastases do occur in the axilla to a greater or lesser degree, and that errors in detection can be made acceptably small by dissection of axillary Levels I and II. This should be the minimum for staging of invasive cancers. Obviously, for the most reliable detection and for the truest count of total metastases, tissues must be removed from all three axillary levels. Not only do abbreviated dissections compromise reliable detection, but in addition the total count of positive nodes will be limited by the total number of nodes removed, a hazard particularly present in lymph node samplings. The pathologic comparability of cases having different degrees of axillary dissection is at best imperfect and at worst highly questionable.

INTERNAL MAMMARY NODES

The internal mammary (IM) lymph nodes are not regularly available for histologic examination, but information from survey biopsies and therapeutic excisions has established their prognostic importance. Untreated metastases at this site are associated with a negligible 10 year survival of 5 per cent (Donegan, 1977). Haagensen (1971) sampled these nodes as part of his "triple biopsy" procedure and observed a similar poor outcome when metastases were present (14 per cent 10 year survival). Rather than having a mastectomy, such patients were referred for palliative irradiation (Haagensen, 1971). Of interest is the fact that metastases limited to the internal mammary nodes infer a prognosis similar to that when only axillary lymph node metastases are present, whereas when both groups are invaded, the outlook is substantially poorer (Caceres, 1967; Bucalossi et al., 1971; Urban and Marjani, 1971). For example, 56 per cent of Caceres's patients with only IM metastases and 52 per cent with only axillary metastases survived 5 years after extended mastectomies, but only 24 per cent with dual involvement did so. No more than 10 per cent of patients with involvement of both groups of nodes survived 10 years.

From the standpoint of staging it is of interest that IM nodes are positive in 8.9 per cent of cases when axillary lymph nodes are nega-

Table 12–6. ACCURACY OF AXILLARY NODE DISSECTION IN IDENTIFYING METASTASES

Reference	Cases (+)	Level I	Level I & II
Danforth et al. (1986)	65	71%	97%
Smith et al. (1977)	304	73%	90%
Pigott et al. (1984)	72	75%	99%
Schwartz (1986)	127	87%	98%
Boova et al. (1982)	80	91%	99%
Rosen et al. (1983)	281	98%	100%

The accuracy of a Level I (low) axillary lymph node dissection is shown according to various investigators. When the axilla contains metastases, failure to find them ranges from 3.4 per cent to 29 per cent. The overall error depends on the proportion of truly negative axillae. A Level I dissection is generally considered inadequate for staging. There is better agreement that a Level I & II dissection provides satisfactory accuracy.

tive (Table 12–7) and in up to 26 per cent when the primary tumor is medial. If the purpose of an axillary dissection is to identify patients with any nodal metastases, this fact alone would account for a false negative rate of almost 10 per cent.

SUPRACLAVICULAR NODES

Metastases in supraclavicular lymph nodes signal a particularly unfavorable outlook. This level is ordinarily reached only after extensive invasion of the axillary or internal mammary lymph nodes and almost always implies wider dissemination (Fentiman et al., 1986). Papaioannou and Urban (1964) reported that none of 28 patients with positive scalene lymph node biopsies lived more than 1 year without disease.

TUMOR SIZE

Whether measured by the clinician or the pathologist, the gross size (diameter) of invasive primary tumors rivals nodal metastasis in prognostic importance, accounting for the prominence of these two features in staging.

Table 12–7. FREQUENCY OF INTERNAL MAMMARY NODE (IM) BUT NO AXILLARY NODE (Ax) METASTASES BY LOCATION OF PRIMARY TUMOR

Source	Medial Primary		Lateral Primary	
	Number	IM+ (%)	Number	IM+ (%)
Handley and Thackray (1948)	17	17.6	33	3.0
Andreassen et al. (1954)	37	10.8	63	0.0
Wyatt et al. (1955)	27	25.9	33	0.0
Handley et al. (1956)	55	20.0	2	0.0
Caceres (1959)	89	4.5	118	1.7
Pavrovsky et al. (1969)	70	8.6	0	0.0
Urban and Marjani (1971)	267	13.1	34	2.9
Bucalossi et al. (1971)	570	5.8	621*	2.7
Livingston and Arlen (1974)	97	10.3	296	2.7
International Cooperative Study (Lacour et al., 1976)	630	5.2	796	3.4
Valagussa et al. (1978)	110*	6.4	197	4.1
Total	1969	7.6	2193	2.9

*Includes central lesions.
Internal mammary nodes contain metastases in 8.9 per cent of cases when axillary nodes do not, and this may range as high as 25.9 per cent for medial primaries. To this degree axillary lymph node dissection is inadequate as a means of detecting patients with nodal metastases.
From Morrow, M., and Foster, R. S., Jr.: Staging of breast cancer. A new rationale for internal mammary node biopsy. Arch. Surg., 116:748, 1981. Reprinted with permission.

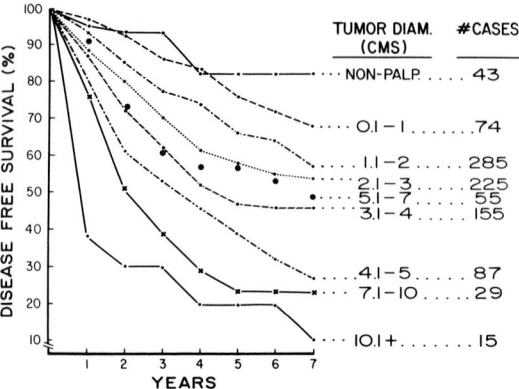

Figure 12–10. Survival after primary treatment is directly related to the maximum diameter of the primary tumor (cases treated at MCW). Only the small 5 to 7 cm category, shown with unconnected dots, is out of sequence. This simple relationship provides a strong impetus for diagnosis of tumors at their smallest size.

The two are closely related. When no other feature than tumor size is considered, there is a direct correlation between increasing diameter and deterioration in disease-free survival after treatment (Fig. 12–10). The explanation for this is the direct relationship between increasing tumor size and the probability that metastases will be present in axillary lymph nodes (Fig. 12–11) (Haagensen and Bodian, 1984). When tumors are 1.0 cm or less in diameter, 26 per cent already have metastasized to the axilla, and the probability rises to near certainty (78 per cent) for tumors over 10 cm in diameter. The figure also shows that the mean number of positive nodes in cases with involvement does not rise, as might be expected if the migration of tumor cells were progressive. Although tumor size and nodal metastases are obviously related, they also influence prognosis independently. As is shown in Figure 12–12, survival at any tumor size is influenced by axillary status. The influence of tumor size is most obvious when lymph nodes contain metastases.

Influences on Prognosis Other than Anatomic Extent of Tumor

A number of features of mammary carcinoma other than the anatomic extent have an important influence on prognosis. Inconsistencies

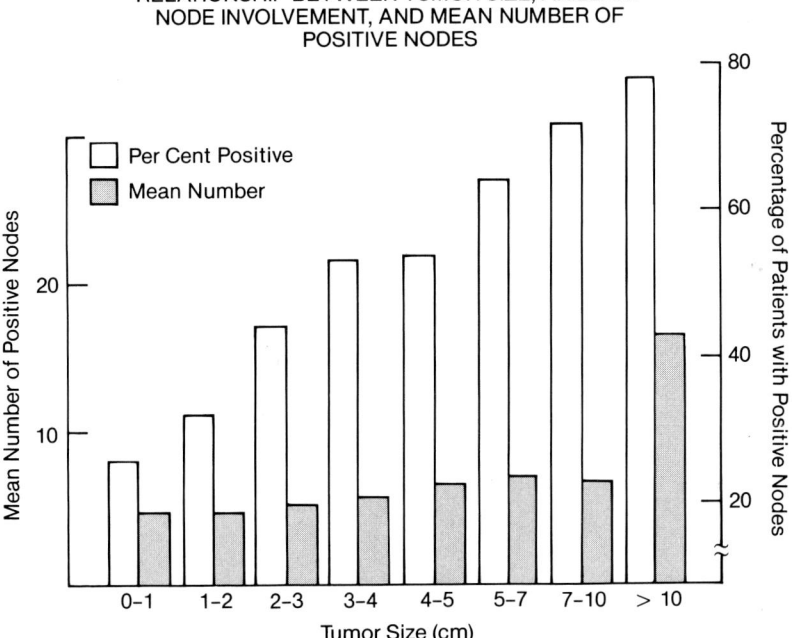

Figure 12–11. As tumor size increases, so does the frequency of histologically confirmed axillary metastases. Tumors 1 cm or less in diameter still have metastases in 27 per cent of cases. For uncertain reasons the mean number of positive nodes in an involved axilla is virtually the same for small tumors as for large ones up to 10 cm in diameter. Cases used in this analysis are the same as those in Figure 12–10.

within stage categories can be attributed in part to these neglected characteristics.

One of the more important influences is the histology of the primary tumor. The majority of invasive carcinomas tend to be pleomorphic histologically, but some relatively pure special types occur and are associated with a favorable prognosis. Mucinous, tubular (Grade I ductal), infiltrating comedo, and infiltrating papillary carcinomas are in this category. Unfortunately, they constitute less than 15 per cent of all carcinomas of the breast. The 5 year survival associated with these special types ranges from 63 to 83 per cent, according to McDivitt and coworkers (1968), compared with a 54 per cent survival associated with infiltrating ductal car-

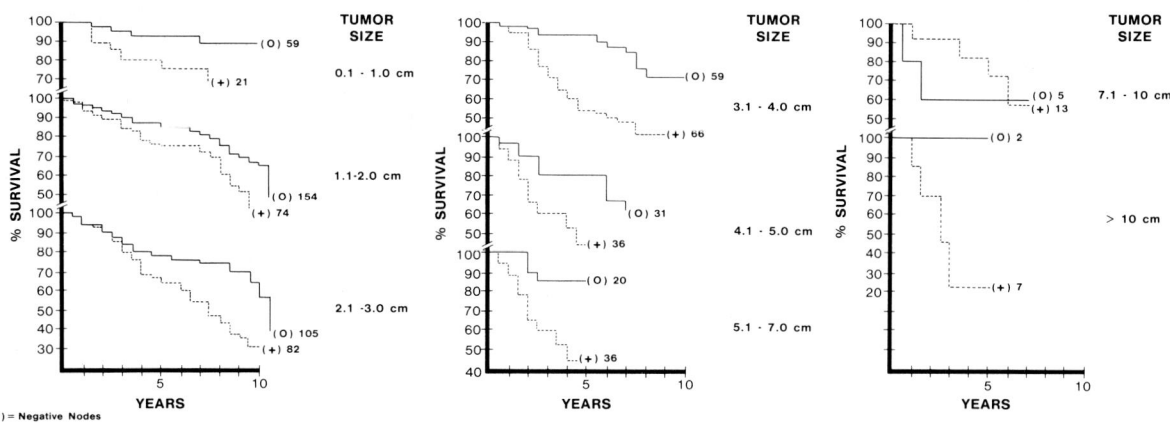

Figure 12–12. Survival after mastectomy is influenced by both tumor size and nodal involvement. For all tumor sizes, the presence of axillary node metastases reduces the prospects for survival. Although increasing tumor size does not influence prognosis in cases without nodal metastases, it does in cases with nodal metastases. Thus, a large tumor with involved nodes entails a poorer prognosis than a small one with involved nodes. As this is difficult to explain on the basis of quantitative nodal involvement (see Figure 12–11), it may relate to increasing hematogenous dissemination.

cinoma of the usual variety. Adair and colleagues (1974) reported favorable survival rates many years after treatment. The less aggressive behavior of these cancers is associated with reduced metastatic potential rather than with small size.

Histologic grade is also important. Tumors often vary throughout in this regard and permit only an average assessment. Fisher and associates (1975a) graded breast carcinomas on nuclear features and tubule formation and found that 70 per cent were poorly differentiated (Grade III); only 2.5 per cent were well differentiated (Grade I). Poorly differentiated carcinomas, based on low nuclear grade, were frequently associated with early treatment failures. The 1983 TNM classification categorizes information on the histologic type and grade of mammary carcinomas according to the outline shown in Table 12–8.

The biologic and metabolic characteristics of mammary carcinomas are of interest prognostically. patients with slowly growing cancers (prolonged gross doubling times) have a more favorable course than those with rapidly growing cancers (Kusama et al., 1972; Pearlman, 1976). Rapid growth is reflected in a high mitotic index, high thymidine labeling, and aneuploidy (see Chapter 9). The presence of estrogen receptor protein is associated with later recurrence and longer survival after surgical resection than occur with its absence (Knight et al., 1977; Gapinski and Donegan, 1980; Tomin and Donegan, 1987). Tumors that lack this protein contain excessive glycolytic enzymes, display rapid growth, and have a poor prognosis (Savlov et al., 1974). Myers and associates (1978) documented a relationship between elevated carcinoembryonic antigen (CEA) and poor prognosis. The frequency of elevation increased with clinical and pathologic stage, and these elevations were associated with recurrence and high death rates.

Carcinomas located medially within the breast metastasize more readily to internal mammary nodes and are singled out by some physicians for special treatment because of this. Whether cancers so situated have a poorer prognosis than others is uncertain. The experience with radical mastectomy at EFSCH reflects a slightly poorer survival of patients with inner quadrant primary tumors at 5 and 10 years than of patients with primary tumors in the outer quadrants of the breast (Table 12–9). This difference was not apparent when inner quadrant lesions were treated with extended mastectomy by Sugarbaker or with postoperative irradiation by Handley (Donegan, 1970). Neither Fisher and coworkers (1985b) nor Veronesi and Valagussa (1981) were able to find a significant difference in prognosis on the basis of the location of tumors medially and laterally.

The characteristics of the host may influence the clinical course of cancer. One such characteristic is age. It is commonly observed that

Table 12–8. HISTOPATHOLOGY OF CARCINOMA (AJC–UICC TNM, 1977) WITH PROGNOSES

	Number of Cases	Relative Survival (years)		
		5	10	15
Histologic Type of Cancer				
Cancer, NOS*				
Ductal				
Intraductal (in situ)				
Invasive with predominant intraductal component				
Invasive, NOS*				
Comedo	66	84%	77%	74%
Inflammatory				
Medullary with lymphocytic infiltrate	62	69%	68%	65%
Mucinous (colloid)	37	76%	72%	62%
Papillary	18	89%	65%	65%
Scirrhous				
Tubular				
Other				
Specify				
Lobular				
In situ				
Invasive with predominant in situ component				
Invasive	126	57%	42%	37%
Nipple				
Paget's disease, NOS*				
Paget's disease with intraductal carcinoma				
Paget's disease with invasive ductal carcinoma				
Other: Specify				
Histologic Grade				
GX Cannot be assessed				
G1 Well differentiated				
G2 Moderately well differentiated	245	80%	64%	56%
G3–G4 Poorly to very poorly differentiated	696	50%	39%	33%

Note: The 1983 TNM system includes histopathologic classification and grading of carcinomas according to the outline in this table.
*Not Otherwise Specified.
Data from Adair, F., et al.: long-term follow-up of breast cancer patients: The 30-year report. Cancer, 33:1145, 1975, Used with permission.

Table 12–9. RESULTS OF RADICAL MASTECTOMY ACCORDING TO LOCATION OF PRIMARY CARCINOMA

Quadrant	Number	Relative Survival (%) 5 Year	Relative Survival (%) 10 Year	Local Recurrence (%)
Upper outer	369	64	50	25
Lower outer	86	63	45	28
Upper inner	114	58	44	32
Lower inner	42	50	40	21
Central	129	62	59	18
Diffuse	37	41	19	65

Note: The prognosis of patients with carcinomas located in the inner quadrants of the breast at EFSCH was slightly less favorable than that of patients with laterally situated tumors. Local recurrence, however, was not appreciably different. No patients were treated with postoperative radiation.

young women have a relatively poor prognosis. This was the case for operable cases at EFSCH after survivals were corrected for the higher intercurrent mortality rates of the aged. The poorer prognosis is associated with a higher frequency of axillary lymph node metastases (Table 12–10). In all stages, Host and Lund (1986) found poorer survival for young patients (< 35 years old) and for older ones as well (> 75 years old) and speculated that the patients in the older group may have received less aggressive treatment. In Milwaukee the author found that older patients were treated with less complete surgery and less often with adjuvant therapy (Donegan, 1983). Sinus histiocytosis within regional lymph nodes can be interpreted as an immunologic response and is associated by some authors with a favorable prognosis (Black et al., 1975). Also of potential immunologic significance is the association of a high pretreatment circulating lymphocyte count with early clinical stage and favorable prognosis (Riesco, 1970; Papatestas et al., 1976; Lee, 1984). Patients at EFSCH who had axillary metastases and who were without recurrence for at least 5 years after radical mastectomy had significantly higher mean pretreatment lymphocyte counts than did patients with recurrence. Eosinophil, polyphononuclear leukocytes, and monocyte counts did not share this association. Meyer (1970) suggested that the reduction of circulating lymphocytes that follows postoperative irradiation reflects damage to cellular immunity. An unfavorable hormonal milieu may also promote tumor growth. Overweight patients have not only a greater risk for cancer of the breast but also a greater likelihood of recurrence after mastectomy (deWaard, 1975; Donegan et al., 1978). Tartter and coworkers (1981) found that a high serum cholesterol level potentiated this effect and possibly incriminated a high fat diet.

The variables that influence the clinical course of mammary carcinoma appear to be legion. The anatomic extent of disease (stage) is a highly useful guide to prognosis, but biologic and metabolic characteristics are important. Unfortunately, staging is always based on incomplete information and has the further limitation of being prognostically valid only for groups rather than for individual cases. In

Table 12–10. AGE VERSUS SURVIVAL AFTER RADICAL MASTECTOMY FOR MAMMARY CARCINOMA (EFSCH, 1940 to 1958)*

Age	Total	With Positive Axillary Lymph Nodes (%)	5 Year Survivors Number	5 Year Survivors Per Cent of Total	Per Cent of Gen. Pop. Expected to Survive 5 Years†	Corrected Survival‡ (%)
20–29	3	100.0	0	0.0	100.0	0.0
30–39	38	84.2	16	42.1	99.4	42.4
40–49	106	63.5	59	55.7	98.0	56.8
50–59	143	60.0	79	55.2	95.2	58.0
60–69	211	47.9	124	58.8	90.4	65.0
70–79	179	53.1	92	51.4	73.1	70.3
80–89	24	50.0	8	33.3	48.8	66.9

Note: The survival of elderly patients after surgical treatment of mammary carcinoma is lowered by deaths due to intercurrent disease. If survivals are corrected for age, the prognosis of younger patients is less favorable than that of the elderly.

*Age-specific survival after radical mastectomy corrected for natural mortality is directly correlated with age but falls short of statistical significance.

†Calculated for the average in each age category from the Missouri Life Tables: 1949–51. United States Department of Health, Education and Welfare.

‡Corrected for natural mortality by method derived from Abbott's formula. Finney, D. J.: Probit Analysis. 2nd Ed. Cambridge Press, 1962, p. 88.

many respects the clinical behavior of breast carcinoma poses a formidable challenge to those who wish to understand it better.

Untreated Cancer of the Breast

The clinical course of mammary cancer when the disease is untreated, or the natural history, provides a baseline against which to assess the value of therapy. At present almost all cases are treated in some fashion so that most information on this point stems from the 19th and early 20th centuries. Patients with cancers too advanced for treatment when surgical removal was the only recourse (oophorectomy was not used until 1896, and irradiation was not generally available before 1916), those who refused treatment, and those who were institutionalized in terminal stages of disease have provided information. At least seven authors have published works on this subject since 1926 (Greenwood, 1926; Daland, 1927; Forber, 1931; Nathanson and Welch, 1936; Wade, 1946; Phillips 1959; Bloom et al., 1962). Bloom and coworkers estimated that in slightly more than 5 per cent of cases in England seen between 1950 and 1962 the patients were untreated, and an additional 60 per cent were treated only by endocrine therapy or chemotherapy.

Bloom (1968) reviewed earlier reports as well as 250 cases from the cancer charity ward of the Middlesex Hospital, which operated between 1792 and 1933, and from the Royal Marsden Hospital of London. The 1728 collected cases had a mean survival of 39.9 months and a median survival of 2.5 years. Absolute survivals reported from the different sources varied from 12 to 22 per cent at 5 years, from 3.6 to 6.6 per cent at 10 years, and from 0.8 to 3.8 per cent at 15 years.

None of Bloom's own series of 250 patients had surgery or irradiation during their lives, and all were autopsied to prove the presence of cancer. Some lived many years without specific treatment; the 5, 10, and 15 year absolute survival rates were 18 per cent, 3.6 per cent, and 0.8 per cent, respectively. The median survival was 2.7 years, and not until 19 years after the onset of disease had the last patient died. Survivorship was inversely correlated with age and appeared definitely related to the histologic grade of tumor, with median survivals of 47.3 months for Grade I, 39.2 months for Grade II, and 22 months for Grade III cancers. A spontaneous regression was not recorded in any of the cases, and 95 per cent of the patients died as a direct result of their cancer, only 5 per cent of intercurrent disease. It is worthy to note that 73 per cent of the patients had marked ulceration of the breast prior to death; in 21 per cent it was so extensive that it sometimes destroyed the breast and chest wall and exposed the pleura.

In seeking to assess the impact of radical surgery on the natural history of untreated breast cancer, it can be observed that radical mastectomy results in a 55 to 65 per cent 5 year survival rate overall, whereas for untreated cases the rate is only about 20 per cent. This favorable comparison must be viewed in light of the biases that promote it. It is likely that the data pertaining to untreated cases are weighted with rapidly progressive cancers. Many women with slowly growing cancers may have escaped documentation by dying of other causes before seeking consultation. Second, selection operates in favor of mastectomy, as women with rapidly progressing tumors that quickly become inoperable are not chosen for mastectomy. Finally, untreated cases were collected from a time when expected survival was considerably less than it is today. To address this problem, Henderson and Cannelos (1980) compared cases treated with radical mastectomy at Johns Hopkins Hospital between 1889 and 1931 with Bloom's untreated cases seen between 1805 and 1933 and found no more than a modest 12 per cent improvement in survival with surgery. A personal review of the records of Halsted's first 50 cases treated with radical mastectomy between 1889 and 1894, calculating actuarial survival from first symptom (as in the untreated cases) revealed that the 5 and 10 year survivals of Halsted's patients were 40.4 per cent and 32.3 per cent (Fig. 12–13). This suggests that Halsted doubled 5 year survival and increased 10 year survival tenfold, a substantial improvement.

Sixty-four per cent of 2618 patients reviewed at EFSCH were treated with radical surgery. Computing survival for all cases from the first symptom, patients treated with radical surgery fared better than those treated with all other palliative measures by about 25 per cent at 5 years (Fig. 12–14). If it is assumed that the opportunity for surgical intervention was present at some point in all cases, it is possible to conclude that surgical intervention had a favorable influence.

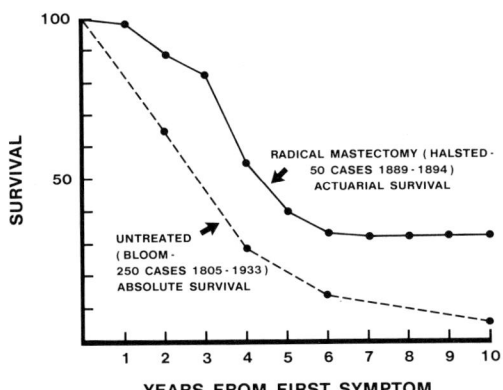

Figure 12–13. This comparison between the survival of Halstead's first 50 cases treated with radical mastectomy and Bloom's untreated cases of breast cancer, plotted from first symptom in both series, suggests that radical mastectomy was associated with an improved prognosis. The long follow-up of Bloom's cases pemitted computation of absolute survival as opposed to actuarial survival in those treated surgically. The untreated cases span a broad period that encompassed the introduction of radical surgery.

The 945 patients who had unsuccessful radical surgery at EFSCH fared no poorer than those who had none, suggesting that although surgery may fail to cure, when it is unsuccessful it has no detrimental influence on the patient's course. In fact, the patients with treatment failures fared somewhat better in their early years than did patients who were not surgical candidates, although at 10 years the survival was comparable.

When surgery fails to cure, it can still permanently eliminate cancer from the chest wall. In no more than 43 per cent of radical mastectomy failures at EFSCH was cancer present in the surgical area at the time of death.

Noninvasive (In Situ) Carcinoma (TNM Stage TIS)

The American College of Surgeons' National Survey of 1978 found that 1.9 per cent of 16,894 cases of breast cancer were noninvasive. The mean age of all patients with in situ carcinomas was 54.3 years (Bedwani et al., 1981).

It is widely accepted that invasive carcinoma of the breast is the result of progression within the mammary ducts from epithelial hyperplasia to atypical epithelial hyperplasia and then to noninvasive carcinoma, which subsequently becomes invasive (Gallager and Martin, 1969). The period of transit in the noninvasive form is probably variable, but it is estimated to average 6 years. This is the difference in average ages of patients with in situ and invasive carcinomas and is also the average interval

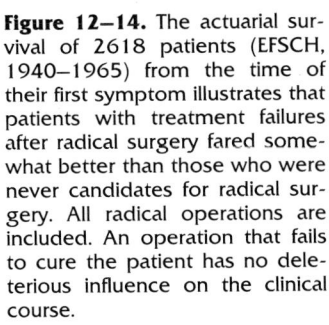

Figure 12–14. The actuarial survival of 2618 patients (EFSCH, 1940–1965) from the time of their first symptom illustrates that patients with treatment failures after radical surgery fared somewhat better than those who were never candidates for radical surgery. All radical operations are included. An operation that fails to cure the patient has no deleterious influence on the clinical course.

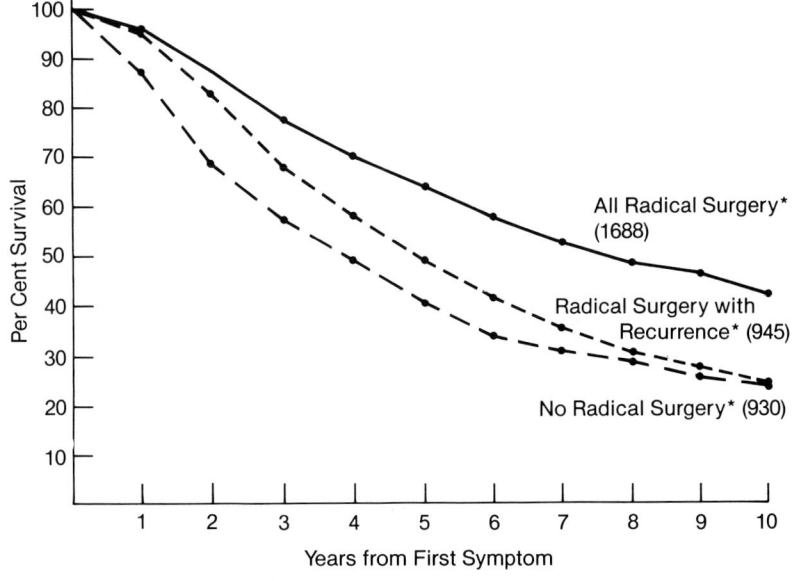

*Radical Surgery: Standard, Extended, or Modified Radical Mastectomy

between local excision of in situ carcinoma and the time that it recurs as invasive carcinoma.

Two histologic types of noninvasive carcinoma are recognized, ductal carcinoma in situ (DCIS) and lobular carcinoma in situ (LCIS). Both are characterized by a high likelihood of multicentricity (40 to 70 per cent), by occasionally being associated with occult invasion, and by a small risk of nodal metastasis. In 38 patients with a biopsy diagnosis of DCIS subsequently treated by mastectomy, Carter and Smith (1977) found that 18 per cent had occult invasion within the breast and 10.5 per cent had nodal metastases. In 49 cases of LCIS, 6 per cent had occult invasion and one patient (2 per cent) had a nodal metastasis. Even when no sign of invasion can be found on subserial analysis of the entire breast, DCIS produces nodal metastases in approximately 2 per cent of cases and LCIS in less than 1 per cent, without doubt the result of undiscovered sites of microinvasion (Ozello and Sanpitak, 1970; Schwartz et al., 1980; Tinnemans et al., 1986).

The term "minimal" breast cancer, coined by Gallager and Martin (1971) to identify a group of breast cancers with similarly good prognosis and perhaps to identify candidates for conservative treatment, included LCIS and DCIS as well as invasive carcinomas 0.5 cm or less in diameter. However, since invasive carcinoma even of less than 1.0 cm in diameter produces axillary metastases in up to 24 per cent of cases and consequently has a distinctly poorer prognosis, it is apparent that tumor size alone is not an adequate definition. Five year survivals with no evidence of disease for invasive carcinomas 1 cm or less in diameter is similar to that for in situ carcinoma only if axillary nodes are negative (Bedwani et al., 1981). For this reason, the concept of minimal breast cancer remains vague and has not had wide utility.

Diagnosis of in situ carcinoma by frozen section is fraught with difficulty, and it is best to await paraffin sections. Rosen and coworkers (1979) reviewed 129 frozen section or permanent section diagnosis of in situ carcinoma and found that of 46 diagnosed by frozen section, seven (15 per cent) were later found to be invasive on paraffin sections. The remaining 83 cases (64 per cent) had been diagnosed as atypia or benign on frozen section. DCIS was more often recognized on frozen section than was LCIS.

The two forms of in situ carcinoma have biologic behaviors as different as their histologies, and these peculiarities, with their therapeutic implications, are discussed in the following sections.

LOBULAR CARCINOMA IN SITU

Lobular carcinoma in situ is less frequent than ductal carcinoma in situ and predominates in premenopausal women (Fig. 12–15). It arises as a distinctive lesion in the lobules of the breast and is believed by most authorities to be the precursor of invasive lobular carcinoma. Its history is complicated. Early in this century it was identified by Ewing as being a benign lesion; in 1941 it was claimed by both Muir (1941) and Foote and Stewart (1941) to be a form of preinvasive carcinoma, with Muir it was considered acinar carcinoma and Foote and Stewart LCIS; now its nature is controversial. Some authors doubt its malignancy, preferring to use the term lobular neoplasia rather than lobular carcinoma (Haagensen et al., 1983). As breasts that contain this lesion and remain untreated more often develop invasive ductal carcinoma than the expected invasive lobular carcinoma, there is support for considering it a histologic marker of high risk rather than the source of subsequent cancers (Rosen et al., 1978). On the other hand, LCIS can usually be found in breasts with typical invasive lobular carcinoma. This lesion is more often multicentric than any other (60 to 90 per cent), and when found in one breast is present in the second breast as well in at least 40 per cent of cases (Donegan and Perez-Mesa, 1972). Axillary metastases are rare if no site

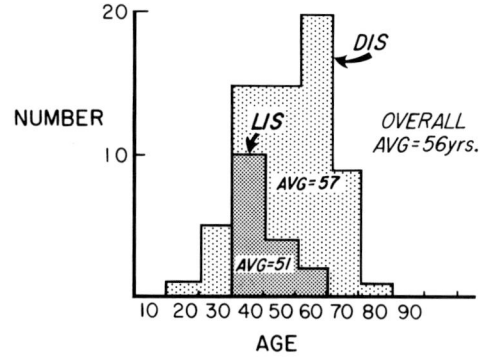

Figure 12–15. The age distribution of patients with noninvasive carcinoma of the breast at MCW demonstrates that lobular carcinoma in situ (LIS) occurs in a younger population than does ductal carcinoma in situ (DIS). Most cases of LIS occur in premenopausal women.

of invasion is found. In 1980, Rosen found four cases in the literature.

If untreated, 25 to 35 per cent of women with LCIS develop subsequent cancers of the breast, nine times the expected frequency, and deaths due to breast carcinoma are 11 times greater than expected (Rosen et al., 1978). The unique problem is that the risk of cancer is shared almost equally between the two breasts. McDivitt and colleagues (1967) projected the 20 year cumulative risk of subsequent cancers to be 35 per cent for the ipsilateral breast and 25 per cent for the contralateral breast. The risk is of long duration; these cancers appear over the course of 21 to 31 years. Although the absolute risk varies with the duration of follow-up, it is well confirmed that the risk is high for both breasts (Table 12–11). No good indicators exist to identify women who will be affected, but breast cancer in a close relative does increase the risk (Haagensen et al., 1978). LCIS associated with an invasive cancer implies the same high risk for the second breast as when it occurs alone.

The bilateral risk creates a dilemma for treatment, and controversy continues to exist about proper management. Appropriate treatment for the involved breast would seem equally appropriate for the opposite breast. Total mastectomy is regularly curative for LCIS, and bilateral mastectomy with reconstruction is a logical choice, but there is reluctance to use this drastic approach in view of the relatively innocuous nature of the lesion, the fact that a minority of patients will have future cancers, and the long interval before subsequent cancers arise. A cosmetic compromise is bilateral subcutaneous mastectomies with prosthetic implants (Blevins, 1981), but this does not remove all breast tissue and has not been proved effective in reducing the patient's risk (Klamer et al., 1983; Eldar et al., 1984). An approach advocated at some centers is total mastectomy on the involved side and an elective biopsy of the contralateral breast in an effort to detect contralateral cancers early (Rosen et al., 1981). A strong rationale for mastectomy is the fact than 4 per cent of women in whom a biopsy shows only LCIS will have an unsuspected invasive cancer found in the mastectomy specimen (Rosen et al., 1979). The elective biopsy is performed in the upper periareolar area as this is the most frequent distribution of LCIS (Lambird and Shelley, 1969). If LCIS is found in the other breast, it is also removed. Sixty-four per cent of the women treated at Memorial Hospital, New York City, with this policy retained the opposite breast, and the death rate was less than in a previous series in which contralateral biopsy was not used. It is of interest, however, that as many patients with a negative contralateral biopsy subsequently developed in situ or invasive carcinoma (17.2 per cent) as did those with no biopsy (17.6 per cent).

An alternative method of management that has more recently become accepted is close observation with periodic physical examinations and mammograms, the objective being to detect any subsequent cancer in either breast early and in a curable stage (Haagensen et al., 1978; Powers et al., 1980; Lattes, 1980; Hutter, 1984). For those not wishing the complete protection of bilateral total mastectomies and who understand that some risk is involved with any lesser approach, the presumably somewhat higher risk inherent in observation alone may be an acceptable plan. The surveillance is permanent, with conscientious monthly BSE, palpation every 6 months, and mammograms every 6 to 12 months. The success of this increasingly popular alternative is uncertain. Despite a well-structured outpatient department, Davis and Baird (1984) found the follow-up of 80 women with LCIS in the first breast suboptimal, with six of eight (75 per

Table 12–11. RISK OF INVASIVE CANCER SUBSEQUENT TO LOBULAR CARCINOMA IN SITU

Reference	Average Follow-up (yrs)	Ipsilateral		Contralateral		Overall Risk of Invasive Breast Cancer (X expected)
		Total Number	Per Cent	Total Number	Per Cent	
Rosen et al. (1978)	24	99	18%	96	14%	9×
Andersen (1977)	16	44	20%	44	9%	11.9×
Haagensen et al. (1978)	14	192	10%	204	9%	7.2×
Wheeler et al. (1974)	18	25	4%	32	9%	3.7×

The risk of developing invasive breast cancer subsequent to a biopsy diagnosis of lobular carcinoma in situ is high, reaching 25 to 35 per cent, and the risk is shared almost equally between the two breasts.

cent) subsequent cancers of the second breast detected in a late stage (i.e., T2 or greater).

On the other hand, Haagensen reported that of 285 patients with LCIS managed conservatively for an average of 16 years, during which 19 per cent developed breast cancer, only 4.5 per cent died of it or developed dissemination (Haagensen, 1986).

Recommendations for management of LCIS are difficult in view of the wide variation of practice. In making a decision a complete explanation to the patient of options with the risks and benefits of each is particularly important.

DUCTAL CARCINOMA IN SITU

This lesion arises from ducts outside the lobules. It can spread into the lobules, however, and this is termed "cancerization" of the lobule when it occurs. DCIS is found most often during biopsy of a mass, which in many instances is not itself malignant (Von Rueden and Wilson, 1984). Nipple discharge and mammographic changes (microcalcifications) also lead to its discovery, but mammograms can be falsely negative in up to 50 per cent of cases (Sunshine et al., 1985).

In most reports, DCIS is more frequent than LCIS, but the two lesions can occur together in a few cases. Like LCIS, DCIS is often multicentric but perhaps somewhat less so; additional foci are found in other quadrants of the breast in about 40 per cent of cases (Schwartz et al., 1980). Unlike LCIS, subsequent contralateral breast cancer after DCIS in one is no higher than usual and is equally divided between in situ and invasive cancers (Webber et al., 1981). Also unlike LCIS, recurrence after local excision alone is virtually always in the treated breast.

Lagios and coworkers (1982) found occult invasion in 6 to 21 per cent of cases of DCIS, with involvement of the nipple in 20 per cent. In three quarters of these cases, involvement of the nipple was not recognized clinically. Occult invasion, multicentricity, and axillary lymph node metastasis increase with the extent of the tumor. This group studied 53 cases of DCIS treated with mastectomy using serial subgross methods and found 21 per cent with occult invasion, all confined to tumors 26 mm or larger. Multicentricity was present in 54 per cent of lesions 26 mm or larger versus in only 14 per cent of smaller ones, and one case of nodal metastasis (2 per cent) was associated with a tumor 160 mm in diameter.

The treatment of DCIS has been structured on its known multicentricity, the threat of overlooked invasive cancer within the breast, and the occasional presence of nodal metastasis. The surgical response to these concerns would mandate a total mastectomy with axillary dissection, at least of the low nodes. It might be assumed that nodal metastases, should they exist, would be few and confined to the lower level, although there are no data to confirm this. In reality it appears that surgical practice varies with circumstances. In a survey of 468 cases of in situ carcinomas by the Michigan Cancer Foundation Registry treated between 1973 and 1978, total mastectomy with axillary dissection was the most popular operation for unilateral cases, but for elderly patients and for bilateral in situ cancers, total mastectomies predominated (Albert et al., 1982). Sunshine and coworkers (1985) reviewed 112 cases of in situ carcinoma in the Oregon Cancer Data Program and found the most frequent operation for DCIS to be total mastectomy and low axillary dissection. Rosen and colleagues also recommended total mastectomy with low axillary dissection.

Cure rates are not as favorable for DCIS as for LCIS. Rosner and associates (1980), reporting on a national survey of 323 patients with in situ cancer, found 5 year disease-free survival and recurrence for DCIS to be 63.8 per cent and 10.4 per cent, respectively, whereas for LCIS the rates were 83.5 per cent and 2.5 per cent. In black patients, recurrence of DCIS was significantly higher than for white patients (21.3 per cent versus 9.3 per cent).

Information on treatment with local excision alone is scant. DCIS is not as easily overlooked on biopsy as is LCIS. The information available suggests that recurrence can be expected to occur almost always in the treated breast and in up to 40 per cent of cases. These recurrences will often be invasive and constitute a threat to cure (Table 12–12). Seven of Page and colleagues' 28 patients (25 per cent) treated with local excision had breast recurrence after a median period of 6 years, and four (14 per cent) developed distant metastases desite further local treatment. Lagios and coworkers believed that excision alone is appropriate only for small, radiologically demonstrable lesions less than 25 mm in diameter that were completely excised from breasts and that were easily followed for recurrence, and then only if patients were aware of the risks involved with this nonstandard method of treatment. Rosner and colleagues (1980), however,

Table 12–12. LOCAL RECURRENCE AFTER LOCAL EXCISION OF DUCTAL CARCINOMA IN SITU (DCIS)

Reference	Number of Cases	Breast Recurrence		Follow-up Duration
		Number	**Per Cent**	
Local Excision Alone				
Haagensen et al. (1971)	11	8	73%	≤ 120 months
Farrow (1970)	25	5	20%	12–96 months
Betsill et al. (1978)	25	7†	28%	116 months average
Page et al. (1982)	28	7‡	28%	180 months
Lagios et al. (1982)	20	3*	15%	44 months average
Fisher et al. (1986)	22	5§	23%	39 months average
Local Excision Plus Breast Irradiation				
Fisher et al. (1986b)	29	2§	7%	39 months average
Recht et al. (1985)	40	4 ‖	10%	44 months median
Montague (1984)	34	1 (ax)	3%	3–17 yr
Zafrani et al. (1984)	54	3	6%	55 months median (1985 update)

*All ipsilateral; 2 in situ, 1 invasive.
†All ipsilateral; 1 in situ, 6 invasive.
‡All ipsilateral; all invasive (4 have distant metastases following retreatment).
§All ipsilateral (1 recurrence after treatment).
‖ All ipsilateral; 2 DCIS, 2 invasive.

Recurrence is frequent after local excision alone, may be invasive or in situ, and almost always is in the ipsilateral breast (in contrast to lobular carcinoma in situ).
Irradiation reduces the rate of recurrence in the breast, but salvage mastectomy is not always curative.

reporting on a national survey of 323 patients with in situ carcinoma, found treatment of DCIS with wedge excision as effective as more radical procedures; their results showed 66.7 per cent disease-free survival and 6.7 per cent recurrence in 15 cases versus 66.7 per cent and 11.1 per cent, respectively, with total mastectomy and low axillary dissection in 18 cases.

Although local excision alone may be considered inadequate treatment, its combination with irradiation of the breast is being explored, as clearly invasive cancers can be treated effectively in this manner. Whereas Schnitt and associates (1984) believed that invasive cancers with prominent DCIS components were poorly controlled by primary irradiation, other authors do not agree. Table 12–12 shows early results with this approach. Recht et al. (1985) collected 40 patients with DCIS from two centers who were treated between 1976 and 1983 with local excision and irradiation with a median follow-up of 40 months. Irradiation to the breast was 4600 to 5000 rad. Twenty-six patients had a boost of 1000 to 2000 rad to the site of excision, seven had irradiation to regional nodes, and 13 had an initial axillary dissection in which no positive nodes were found. Four patients had local recurrence at 17, 19, 35, and 63 months later, for a cumulative 5-year rate of 10 per cent. These four patients were treated with mastectomy with no further recurrence. Because there were no distant failures and the cosmetic results were good, the authors considered this to be a viable method of treatment. They would not insist on irradiating regional nodes, would consider axillary dissection only for large tumors, and be hesitant to treat patients with diffuse microcalcifications in the breast or central tumors with nipple discharge.

Fisher and colleagues (1986a) found 78 cases of DCIS that had been treated on a prospective randomized protocol of wide local excision versus total mastectomy designed for invasive cancers. After a mean observation period of 39 months, 14 per cent of the patients treated with local excision had recurrence in the breast at or close to the site of the original lesion, 4 to 53 months after treatment. Those who had received irradiation to the breast appeared to have reduced recurrence rates. Breast recurrence was seen in 23 per cent of unirradiated breasts but in only 7 per cent of irradiated breasts. These figures are virtually identical to the recurrence rates observed for cases of invasive carcinoma treated similarly. Four of the recurrences were invasive and three were in situ; after salvage mastectomy, one patient (4 per cent) had further recurrence, not significantly higher than the recurrence rate observed for DCIS after initial total mastectomy (2 per cent).

To investigate the relative advantage of breast irradiation, a randomized treatment protocol for DCIS has been initiated by the National Surgical Adjuvant Breast Project, in which patients have an axillary dissection, and if no metastases are found, they are placed in randomized groups for wide local tumor excision with or without irradiation of the breast. This is the first randomized study of primary irradiation for this lesion and results should be of considerable interest.

The experience with wide local excision and irradiation of the breast for DCIS is still limited, and an accurate comparison with mastectomy and low axillary dissection suffers from the lack of a controlled randomized study. Initial local control generally appears to be less effective than with mastectomy, but salvage mastectomy for failures when necessary may improve the comparability of end results. With this assumption, breast conservation is being made available as an alternative to mastectomy for DCIS.

NONINVASIVE CARCINOMA AT THE MEDICAL COLLEGE OF WISCONSIN

Between 1967 and 1979, noninvasive carcinomas at the Medical College of Wisconsin constituted 5.3 per cent of all breast cancers. This figure reached 9.5 per cent in the second year of a local American Cancer Society–National Cancer Institute (ACS-NCI) screening project, reflecting the effort at early diagnosis. In a review of 79 cases seen through 1979, 80 per cent of patients had DCIS, 15 per cent had LCIS, and 5 per cent had both DCIS and LCIS. No patient with LCIS was older than 65 years, and the average age (51 years) was 6 years younger than that of patients with DCIS. Five per cent of all patients had bilateral simultaneous cancers, and 12 per cent of the remainder developed a second primary tumor after an average follow-up of 3.9 years, amounting to 3.1 per cent per year or about three times the expected rate. Most cases of LCIS were treated with total mastectomy, whereas modified mastectomy was used for most of DCIS.

The 5 year survival rate for all cases was 89 per cent, and 10 year survival rate was 81 per cent. No patients died of their cancers, but four patients had recurrence, all cases of DCIS. One patient had a subcutaneous recurrence of DCIS near the scar 2 months after a simple mastectomy. It was treated with local excision, and the patient was alive and well 9 years 7 months later. This case illustrates the hazard of incomplete removal of mammary tissue. The second patient had recurrence in the axilla 26 months after a simple mastectomy for DCIS combined with LCIS. An axillary dissection yielded two nodal metastases, and the patient was free of recurrence 6 years 7 months later. This represents a 1.3 per cent rate of axillary metastasis, which is in agreement with the literature. Two other patients developed lytic lesions in bones consistent with metastases. One was treated with irradiation for symptomatic relief and was alive 6 years later; the other died of heart disease 7 years later, and no autopsy was performed.

The author's experience with elective contralateral biopsy in these cases has been unimpressive for intercepting subsequent primary tumors. Of the 74 cases with the second breast at risk, 52 cases were observed, and three patients or 6 per cent, developed cancer. Seven other patients had prophylactic mastectomies in which occult cancers were found in two, or 29 per cent. Elective biopsies in 15 cases yielded occult cancers in two patients or 13 per cent, and yet two of the 13 cases (17 per cent) with negative elective biopsies subsequently developed cancer in the second breast. So, despite elective mastectomies and elective biopsies with a yield of 18 per cent occult histologic cancers (4 of 22), the 13 cases with negative elective biopsies developed clinical cancers more often than did the 52 observed cases. It must be concluded that at least a remarkable 27.3 per cent of the second breasts were destined to develop cancers or that more cancers were detected histologically than would become evident clinically. Furthermore, elective biopsies missed as many occult cancers as were found, and the risk of second primary tumors was not reduced.

Early Invasive Carcinoma (cTNM Stages I and II)

These "early" stages of invasive cancer have constituted 75 to 80 per cent of the author's cases. They represent potentially curable patients and the largest group requiring treatment decisions.

RADICAL MASTECTOMY

The radical mastectomy of Halsted has been largely abandoned for treatment of early breast cancer. It is still used for some locally advanced cancers, notably those with direct involvement of the pectoralis major muscle or extensive axillary lymph node involvement. Currently, less than 4 per cent of all operations for cancer in the United States are radical mastectomies (Wilson et al., 1984), but the operation is of interest historically and as a point of departure for more recent operations.

Halsted's "complete" mastectomy was first mentioned in the surgical literature in 1891 within the text of an article in the Johns Hopkins Hospital Report entitled "The treatment of wounds with especial reference to the value of the blood clot in the management of dead spaces." Halsted had performed 13 such operations and had narrowed the large skin defect by means of a purse-string suture, allowing the remaining wound to granulate through an overlying blood clot. Between 1889 and 1894 Halsted performed 50 such mastectomies and reported his experience in the same year (1894) that Meyer of New York reported a similar operation developed independently in 1891.

These operations removed the entire breast with the overlying skin, the pectoralis major muscle, and the axillary contents in one piece (Fig. 12–16). They differed in that Halsted dissected the breast and muscles from the chest wall first, leaving the axilla until last, whereas Meyer proceeded in the reverse order. In addition, Halsted (1912) removed a large quantity of skin, ultimately using skin grafts to close the wound and simply divided the pectoralis minor muscle, whereas Meyer closed the wound primarily by removing less skin with the specimen, and he also removed the pectoralis minor muscle. Each subsequently modified his skin incision, and Halsted adopted Meyer's practice of removing the pectoralis minor muscle. Later surgeons developed a variety of incisions, and Raffl (1952) introduced suction catheters for skin flap decompression.

The "radical" mastectomy, as this operation came to be known, was adopted enthusiastically in the United States and abroad. The operation resulted in an immediate and dramatic reduction in chest wall recurrences, which were at this time as high as 82 per cent after lesser operations. Little evidence can be

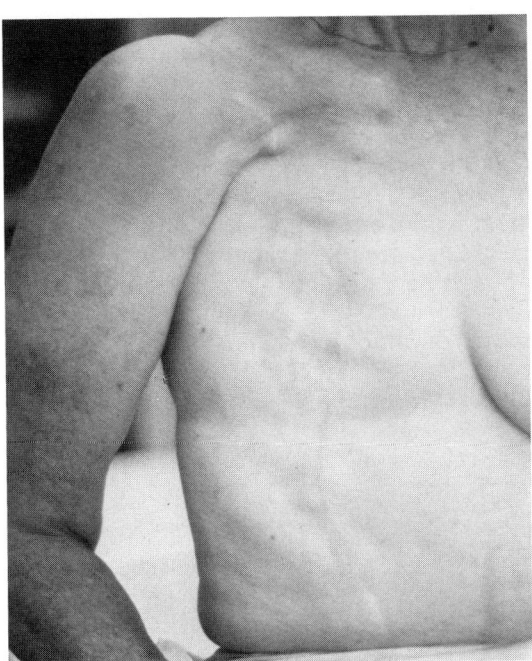

Figure 12–16. A typical Halstead type radical mastectomy with vertical incision reaching to the shoulder, removal of the pectoralis muscles, and removal of a large amount of skin with the breast, necessitating closure with a split thickness skin graft. This results in obvious deformity that is difficult to correct with a prosthesis or a surgical reconstruction of the breast.

found, however, that it provided better survival than lesser operations. On the contrary, a number of surgeons subsequently reviewed their experience to find that survival rates after Halsted's "complete" operation were, in fact, inferior to those after less extensive operations (Matas, 1898; Greenough et al., 1907). These disappointing results stemmed from an initial tendency to reserve Halsted's operation for relatively advanced cases and its ambitious application to cases that might formerly have been considered inoperable. Accurate comparisons with earlier operations were hampered by the absence of staging and of randomized trials.

In ensuing decades, two notable trends served to improve results: (1) diagnosis of breast cancer at increasingly earlier stages; and (2) selective use of the operation. The scholarly work of Haagensen helped to confine radical surgery only to those cases for which it promised cure. This selectivity, however, created the paradox of constant improvement in the results of treatment in the presence of undiminished overall death rates. McWhirter (Page, 1948) and Smithers and associates

(1952) commented on this illusion, which is now recognized as "stage shift," to wit, as surgery is confined to increasingly favorable cases with better results, more favorable ones are perforce referred for irradiation or nonsurgical therapy, with the result that both surgical and nonsurgical therapies appear to yield improved results without any overall increase in cures. For example, assume that cases of cancer are divided into three stages and that Stages I and II are customarily treated with surgery, with observed survival rates of 75 per cent (3 of 4) and 50 per cent (2 of 4), and Stage III is treated with irradiation, with a survival rate of 25 per cent (1 of 4). The surgical "cures" are, therefore, 5 of 8 (63 per cent), and irradiation cures are 1 of 4 (25 per cent). Cures overall are 6 of 12, or 50 per cent. If surgery is then restricted only to Stage I cases, surgical cures become 75 per cent and irradiation curves become 3 of 8, or 37.5 per cent. The apparent progress on both fronts is achieved without improving the overall cure rate of 50 per cent.

After 1903, the radical mastectomy was often supplemented with postoperative irradiation, particularly if axillary lymph nodes contained metastases or if primary tumors were situated in the medial hemisphere of the breast, where they were likely to have produced metastases to the internal mammary nodes. Later, other surgical adjuvants were introduced, so that the operation constituted the sole treatment only in particularly favorable cases.

Modern experience with radical mastectomy has been reported from many centers. Fisher and associates (1975b) reported the 5 and 10 year results with 370 cases collected from 23 medical centers in the United States after 1958. All were treated with radical mastectomy alone and represented a spectrum of practice throughout the country. Recurrence was observed in 49.5 per cent of these patients during the 10 year period. Radical mastectomy failed to cure 76.1 per cent of patients with axillary metastases and almost regularly failed (86.2 per cent) if more than three nodes contained metastases. Recurrence was surprisingly high (24.1 per cent) when axillary lymph nodes were free of metastases. These disappointing long-term results illustrate the limitations of local therapy even of this extent and the high likelihood of treatment failure when cancer is found in regional lymph nodes.

Schottenfeld and associates (1976) reported 5 and 10 year survival rates after radical mastectomy combined with selective postoperative irradiation according to the 1972 TNM clinical classification. These figures were, respectively: Stage I, 95.6 per cent and 90.9 per cent; Stage II, 71.8 per cent and 57.1 per cent; and Stage III, 53 per cent and 33.9 per cent.

Much experience with radical mastectomy was accumulated at EFSCH between 1940 and 1970, when it was the principal method of treating operable cases of breast cancer. By 1965, 2621 cases of breast cancer had been seen, of which 1291 were treated with Halsted's operation. The operations were performed by numerous surgeons and surgical residents and included many improvements in anesthesia, surgical technique, and postoperative care. Overall, an average of 3 hr 48 minutes was required to perform the operation, during which 1.3 units of whole blood (average) were transfused. Hospital deaths were recorded in 1.2 per cent of cases, most often from pulmonary emboli, myocardial infarctions, and cerebrovascular accidents.

The indications for the operation fluctuated considerably during these years. It was at times performed in the presence of locally advanced cancer with the intention of giving the benefit of a doubtful chance for cure, and on occasion it was used for palliation. Rarely was it supplemented with postoperative irradiation.

Recurrence, relative survival, and local treatment failure rates are shown in Figures 12–17 to 12–19 as a function of several features of the disease. Because the population was elderly (average age, 63.8 years) survival rates were age-corrected and reported as relative survivals, that is, observed survival ÷ expected survival of Missourians of similar sex and age × 100. From these data it is evident that a large number of variables pertaining to both the tumor and the patient can be correlated with end results. It is likewise evident that success is not ensured in any stage, and in no situation is freedom from local recurrence a certainty. When used for nondisseminated Columbia Stage D cancers, the operation failed to cure 86 per cent, and at least 50 per cent of patients were not permanently freed of disease on the chest wall (Table 12–13). Ultimate survival approached that reported for untreated cancer of the breast.

In 1984, Haagensen and Bodian reported their personal experience with the Halstead radical mastectomy, involving 1036 patients with a follow-up of 47 years. All of the patients with carcinoma of the central and inner portions of the breast had prophylactic radiother-

12 • Staging and Primary Treatment   367

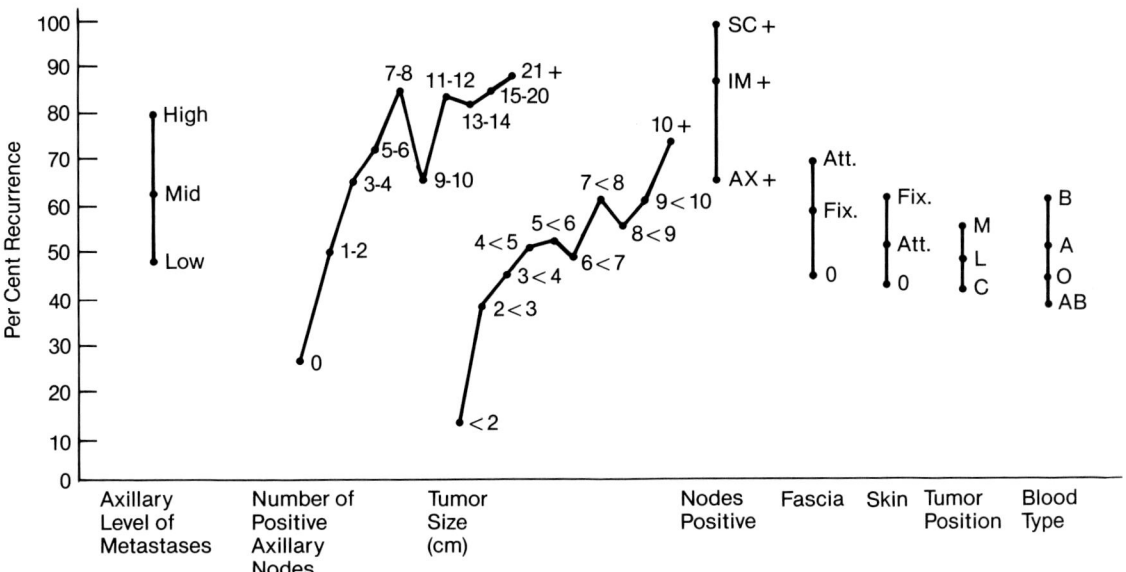

Figure 12–17. Treatment failure after radical mastectomy (i.e., recurrence after 5 to 24 years of observation), is correlated with the presence, number, and level of axillary metastases, the size of the primary tumor, the sites of regional node involvement, fixation of the primary tumor to fascia and skin, the position in the breast, and the patient's blood type. Recurrence occurred in more than 90 per cent of cases when 21 or more axillary lymph nodes were diseased and was virtually certain if supraclavicular metastases were present.

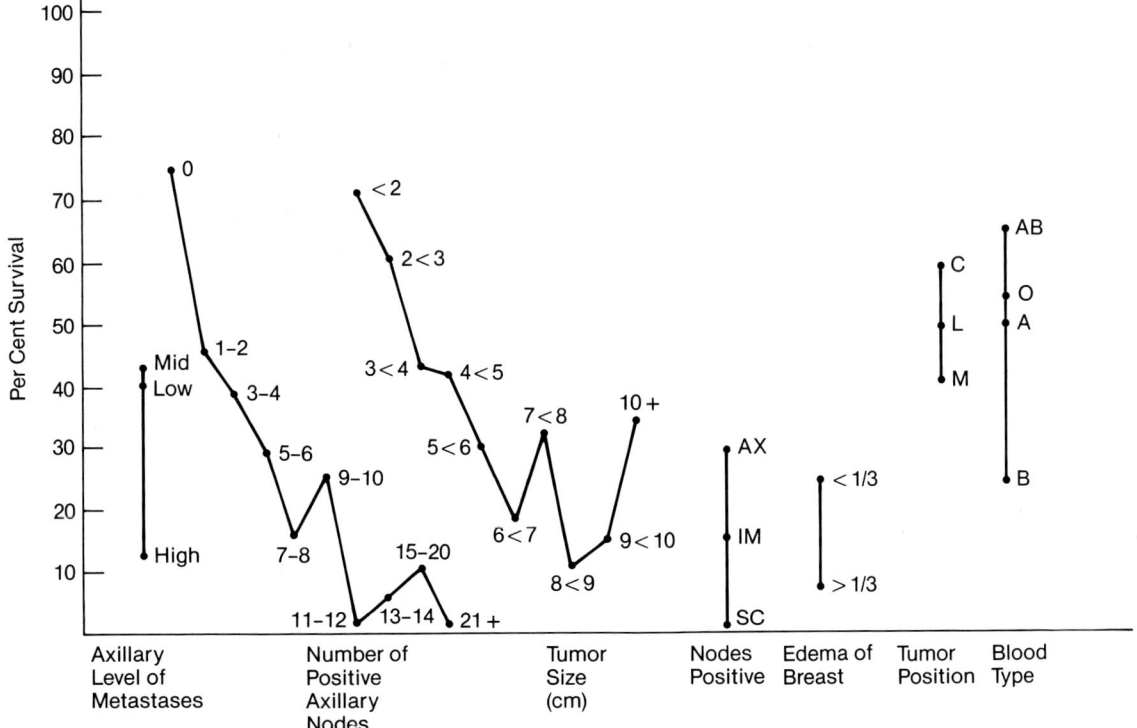

Figure 12–18. Ten year relative survival of 801 patients after radical mastectomy at EFSCH was most highly correlated with the number of axillary nodes that contained metastases and with the size of the primary tumor. Unfavorable characteristics were metastases in high axillary nodes, supraclavicular metastases, edema of more than one third of the breast, primaries located in the medial portion of the breast, and blood type B. Little prognostic differential was observed between metastases in the middle and the lower portions of the axilla.

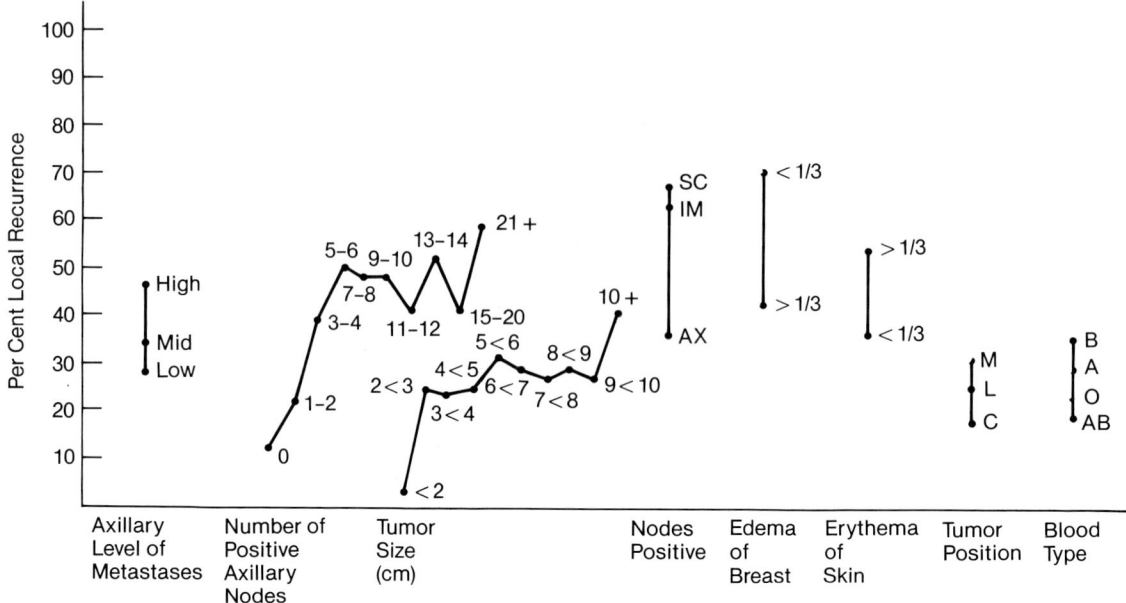

Figure 12–19. Local recurrence after 5 to 24 years of observation is illustrated acccording to a number of selected variables. Metastases in high axillary nodes, many axillary metastases, metastases in supraclavicular nodes, edema of more than one third of the breast, erythema of the skin of the breast, medial position of the tumor in the breast, and blood type B were most highly correlated with local recurrence. Tumor position M stands for medial hemisphere, L for lateral hemisphere, and C for central.

apy to the internal mammary region following this operation if the axillary nodes revealed metastases. The study began in 1935 and when, after 20 years, it was found that only 28.2 per cent of 85 patients with Columbia Stage C carcinomas remained alive for 10 years, further operations were limited to Columbia clinical Stages A and B, and the study continued to 1975. The 10 year survival of 727 patients with clinical Stage A was 80 per cent and of 208 with clinical Stage B was 50 per cent. Ten year local recurrence was 4.3 per cent in Stage A and 13.4 per cent with Stage B. The axillary dissection was meticulous in these cases, and none of the patients in Clinical Stage A developed axillary recurrence during follow-up. Despite the fact that 72 per cent of 208 Stage B patients had axillary metastases, only one patient developed axillary recurrence, a tribute to the therapeutic value of a meticulous axillary dissection. Local recurrence on the chest wall was correlated with the number of histologically involved axillary lymph nodes, rising to 21.9 per cent in patients with eight or more involved nodes in Stage A and 42.2 per cent in patients with eight or more involved nodes in Stage B. The extent of nodal involvement also influenced 10 year survival in both clinical stages. Haagensen reported edema of the arm in only 5 per cent of the patients when the

Table 12–13. RECURRENCE AND SURVIVAL AFTER RADIAL MASTECTOMY BY CLINICAL STAGE OVER 5 TO 24 YEARS OF OBSERVATION

Columbia Clinical Stage	Number of Cases	Local Recurrence (%)	Distant Recurrence (%)	Total Recurrence (%)	Relative Survival (%)	
					5 Year	10 Year
A	318	16	34	35	77	70
B	243	27	54	55	57	43
C	130	35	58	59	52	30
D	86	50	81	86	22	7

Note: The results of radical mastectomy for unilateral carcinoma of the breast at EFSCH are shown according to the Columbia clinical stage. Progression from stages A to D is accompanied by a progressive rise of local recurrence and of treatment failure and a decline of relative survival.

operation was "well done" and wound healing was uncomplicated.

After being the standard of treatment for eight decades, radical mastectomy has now been compared in prospective trials with most therapeutic alternatives and found to offer no advantage in early stages of the disease. The most prominent examples of these trials are discussed in the sections that follow.

Extended Radical Mastectomy

The internal mammary lymph node chain constitutes one of the primary routes of lymphatic drainage from the breast and frequently is the seat of metastatic disease. This anatomic fact and its possible contribution to treatment failure and local recurrence formerly induced many surgeons to include resection of the internal mammary nodes. Other surgeons ambitiously pursued metastatic disease to secondary nodal areas, the supraclavicular and mediastinal groups. These versions of the radical mastectomy became known as extended radical mastectomies. For the reasons that are given later, these operations now are rarely used.

Halsted was aware of the anatomic shortcomings of his original operation, and for a period he extended its scope, as did Meyer (1905), who frequently dissected the supraclavicular nodes. Halsted reported in 1898 to the American Surgical Association, "Our present method of operating for the cure of breast cancer is even more radical than it was at the time of the writer's first publication on this subject. The supraclavicular area is almost invariably cleaned out. I fail to see why the neck involvement in itself is more serious than the axillary. The neck can be cleaned out just as thoroughly as the axilla." At this time Halsted had performed 53 primary supraclavicular dissections and 14 secondary dissections after supraclavicular nodes had become involved clinically. The mediastinum had also been dissected. "Dr. Bloodgood, Instructor in Surgery, has on the necks of two patients done as many as three operations on each for glandular involvement and apparently saved his patients. In one of the cases he entered the mediastinum from above to remove a cancerous gland and had to excise a piece of the innominate vein. Dr. H. W. Cushing, my House Surgeon, has in three instances cleaned out the anterior mediastinum on one side for recurrent cancer. It is likely, I think, that we shall in the near future remove the mediastinal content at some of our primary operations." Halsted subsequently ceased to pursue supraclavicular dissections.

In 1918, interest was renewed in extra-axillary routes of lymphatic drainage from the breast. In this year W.S. Handley in London reported diagnostic biopsies of internal mammary nodes during five mastectomies and subsequently implanted intercostal radium tubes at the time of mastectomy, reporting 77 cases in 1927 (Handley, 1927).

In 1933, Prudente in Brazil added interscapulothoracic amputation and supraclavicular dissection to mastectomy for cases of mammary cancer with fixed axillary and mobile supraclavicular adenopathy. Two of 12 patients (17 per cent) were cured for prolonged periods but neither had supraclavicular metastases.

R.S. Handley and Thackray called attention to the less obvious internal mammary nodes with their report in 1949 of internal mammary lymph node biopsies in 50 unselected cases of mammary carcinoma. Metastases were found in 38 per cent of the cases, ostensibly making them incurable with radical mastectomy. More than half (51.6 per cent) of inner quadrant lesions associated with positive axillary nodes had metastases to the internal mammary nodes. This information spurred efforts to treat these nodes effectively, either with surgical removal or with postoperative irradiation.

Margottini and Bucalossi of Rome are credited with first practicing internal mammary node dissection as a routine part of radical mastectomy, which they began in 1948 (Margottini and Bucalossi, 1949). In 1950, Dahl-Iversen, and colleagues in Denmark, who had already appended supraclavicular dissections to their radical mastectomies, added internal mammary dissection and culminated their efforts in 1952 with dissection of both internal mammary and supraclavicular nodes (Dahl-Iverson, 1963). After 1951, Urban, Sugarbaker, and others in the United States began removing the internal mammary chain and an overlying portion of the chest wall en bloc with the radical mastectomy specimen. This became the most widely practiced version of the extended operation. The most ambitious practitioner of the early period was Wangensteen (1949, 1950, 1956; Wagensteen et al., 1957), who began performing a two-stage "super-radical" mastectomy, removing the specimen in four parts: (1) breast and axillary contents, (2) internal mammary artery and vein with accompanying lymph node chain, (3) upper mediastinal lymph nodes, and (4) low supraclavicular lymph nodes. The procedure was subsequently reduced to one stage with a decrease in mortality from 12.5 to 3.6 per cent and then abandoned.

It is plain that medial (or central) location of the primary tumor in the breast and the presence of metastases in axillary lymph nodes are the two most important determinants of internal mammary lymph node metastases. The published data of eight surgeons relative to these two variables, totalling 2742 cases, are summarized in Figure 12–20. Primary tumors located in the central (subareolar) area of the breast and medial quadrants metastasized to the internal mammary nodes in 28 per cent of cases, and lateral primary tumors did so in 18 per cent. When axillary metastases were present, the frequency of internal mammary metastases from centromedial lesions reached 50 per cent, versus 25 per cent for lateral lesions.

In the absence of axillary lymph node metastases, the frequency of involvement from medial and lateral primary tumors was 13 per cent and 4 per cent, respectively. Handley's and Sugarbaker's data suggest that metastases to these nodes also can be correlated with clinical stage (9 to 16 per cent in Columbia Clinical Classification (CCC) Stage A, 19 to 26 per cent in CCC Stage B, and 28 to 42 per cent in CCC Stage C), and the author's data relate it with tumor size (20 per cent if less than 2.0 cm and 33 per cent if greater than 5 cm (Donegan, 1972). On the basis of these observations, some surgeons thought that resection of internal mammary nodes was indicated with all mastectomies. Other surgeons confined dissections to lesions with the highest frequency of parasternal metastases, those located centromedially in the breast (Urban and Marjani, 1971).

This operation did not increase the small mortality rate associated with the standard radical mastectomy. No deaths resulted from 30 operations at EFSCH. Sugarbaker had one death in 262 cases (0.4 per cent) (Donegan, 1970).

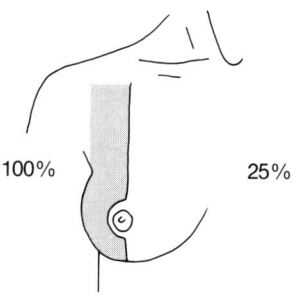

Lateral Primary with Axillary Metastasis

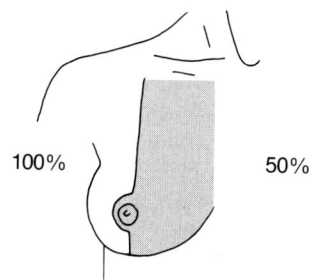

Central or Medial Primary with Axillary Metastasis

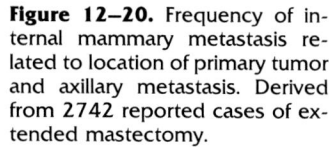

Figure 12–20. Frequency of internal mammary metastasis related to location of primary tumor and axillary metastasis. Derived from 2742 reported cases of extended mastectomy.

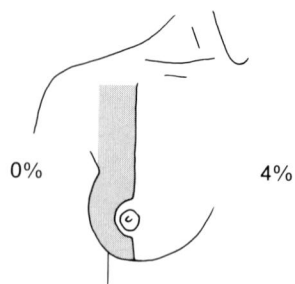

Lateral Primary Without Axillary Metastasis

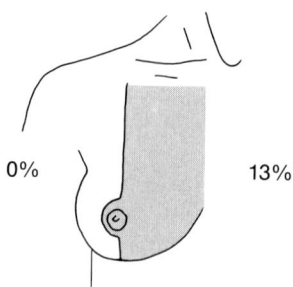

Central or Medial Primary Without Axillary Metastasis

Extended mastectomies varied in scope and technique. The principal issues were whether removal of the parasternal lymph nodes (1) improved disease control on the chest wall, and (2) improved the chances of cure. With respect to the former, it is known that metastases in internal mammary nodes enlarge and appear as parasternal recurrences in only 10 per cent of cases in which they are left untreated (Donegan, 1977). If their removal were to prevent this entirely, a 3 per cent reduction in recurrences at this site (0.1 × 30 per cent) would result, or, if used selectively for cases with medial lesions, a somewhat greater reduction would occur. If recurrence at this site were destined to be the first evidence of treatment failure, a small improvement might be seen in disease-free survival. Urban and Marjani (1971) did, in fact, find a reduction in parasternal chest wall recurrences when their extended operations, performed mostly for medial lesions, were matched with radical mastectomies performed at Memorial Hospital, New York City. Five year disease-free survival, as predicted, was improved when the axilla contained metastases, but overall survival was not improved. Unfortunately, the extended procedure was often supplemented with irradiation, and the time periods were asynchronous.

The first randomized clinical trial compared Dahl-Iversen's extended mastectomy (dissection of both the internal mammary and supraclavicular nodes) with McWhirter's technique of simple mastectomy and postoperative irradiation of all regional lymph nodes. The groups were composed of 335 and 331 patients, and no significant differences were found in crude survival, disease-free survival, or local recurrence (Kaae and Johansen, 1969). Irradiating the peripheral lymph nodes appeared as efficacious as removing them.

The most recent trial, conducted as a cooperative venture between five cancer centers in Lima, Villejuif (France), Rome, Milan, and Warsaw, randomized 1580 cases of T1, T2, T3a, N0, and N1 cancers between radical mastectomy (RM) and radical mastectomy with internal mammary node dissection (IMD); no irradiation was given in any case (Lacour et al., 1976). After 5 years of observation, the survival rates of the two groups were statistically indistinguishable: 69 per cent for RM and 72 per cent for IMD. Survival seemed to be better with IMD in the subgroup of small (T1, T2) medial tumors with axillary metastases (71 per cent for IMD versus 52 per cent for RM), but the statistical method for determining this was invalid, and it was balanced by an unexplained advantage for RM if tumors of similar size were lateral with normal axillary nodes (87 per cent versus 78 per cent). In 1983, Lacour and coworkers reported the 10 year results of this study using the four centers that continued follow-up (Lima, Villejuif, Milan, and Warsaw) (1453 cases) and found such variation in results between centers that no reliable differences in survival or disease-free survival could be identified either overall or in any subgroup (Lacour et al., 1983). Veronesi and Valagussa (1981) concluded the same in a separate report of the 737 cases accrued for the study at Milan (60.7 per cent and 57 per cent 10 year survivals for RM and for IMD, respectively). Of interest was that local-regional recurrences were similar at all sites in the two groups except parasternally, where, as predicted, internal mammary dissection reduced them to 0.3 per cent from an already trivial 3.7 per cent after radical mastectomy. In only nine cases were parasternal recurrences unassociated with other metastases, and four of these were permanently controlled with irradiation.

It may be concluded that the surgical removal of internal mammary lymph nodes does not contribute to cure. It does result in a trivial reduction of parasternal recurrences, but this is an infrequent problem and irradiation is as effective.

Total Mastectomy with Axillary Lymph Node Dissection (Modified Radical Mastectomy)

The term "modified radical mastectomy," or more precisely, total mastectomy and axillary lymph node dissection, refers to operations that spare the pectoralis major muscle while removing en bloc the breast and axillary contents (Fig. 12–21). In the mid-1970s this became the most popular operation for early stages of breast cancer in the United States, and it remains the most viable alternative for women not suited for or desirous of a breast sparing approach.

This operation leaves the patient with a more cosmetic result than does the standard radical operation. The pectoralis major muscle

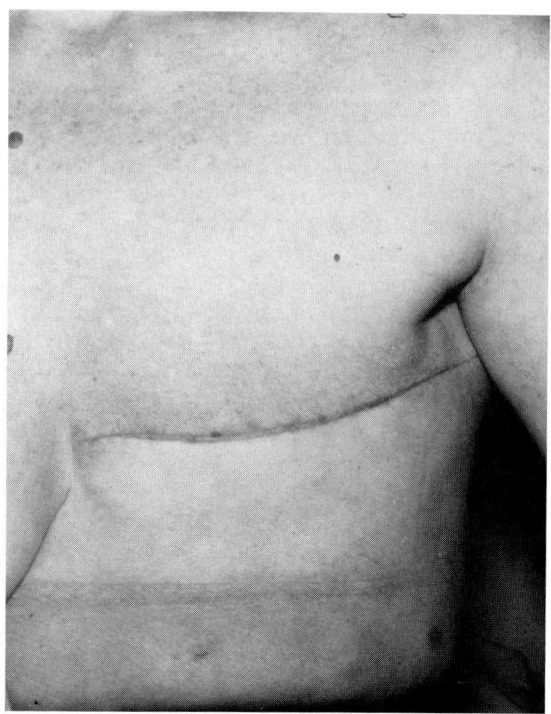

Figure 12–21. This figure illustrates the results of a modified radical mastectomy. The pectoralis major muscle has been preserved, and the incisional scar is cosmetically positioned.

accounts for much of the normal contour and softness of the anterior chest wall; its preservation eliminates the hollow inferior to the clavicle and the skeletonized appearance of the chest wall so obvious after a radical mastectomy. The patient is left with a stronger arm, and reconstruction of the breast is greatly facilitated.

The operation is not feasible in the presence of extensive axillary metastases, but attachment of a primary tumor to muscle is not a contraindication. When extension to muscle is discovered during surgery, the involved area can be removed with a margin without sacrificing the muscle entirely.

The author's unpublished studies with intramammary injection of vital dyes prior to mastectomy indicate that the lymphatics that traverse the pectoralis major muscle accompany branches of the thoracoacromial vessels and the lateral perforating intercostal vessels. In early cases, lymphatic spread of cancer through these routes is embolic, and there would seem to be no greater chance of directly transecting cancer in these lymphatics than in lymphatics draining to the internal mammary nodes, which are routinely cut. Removal of Rotter's nodes with the modified operation is compromised by the need to preserve the nutrient vessels and nerves to the pectoralis major muscle to which they are closely apposed; otherwise, if the pectoralis minor muscle is divided, a thorough dissection to the apex of the axilla can be accomplished.

The two forms of modified radical mastectomy can be distinguished: the Patey and the Scanlon operations, in which dissection of the axilla is complete (Levels I, II, and III), and the Auchincloss-Madden operation, with partial dissection of the axilla (Levels I and II).

TOTAL MASTECTOMY WITH LEVEL I, II, AND III AXILLARY DISSECTION

The Patey operation was developed by Patey at the Middlesex Hospital, London, in 1932 and was adopted in 1936 by R.S. Handley, who wrote extensively about it (Patey, 1967; Handley, 1974). The technique has been illustrated by Handley (1972). "The incision begins as a circle two inches clear of the edge of the tumor and is either enlarged by incisions toward the coracoid process and xiphisternum or by transverse incision. The flaps are thin but not actually devoid of fat and are cut back to the midline, the clavicle, the latissimus dorsi and one inch caudad to the breast. The breast is then dissected off the pectoralis major, the pectoral fascia being removed as completely as possible . . . the dissection proceeding from the medial to the lateral side" (Handley and Thackray, 1962). A complete axillary dissection is accomplished in continuity, "taking care to preserve the thoraco-acromial artery and the lateral anterior thoracic nerve which accompanies it," to preserve "the continued viability and function of the pectoralis major muscle." "In the removal of the pectoralis minor muscle," Handley (1972) points out, "the medial anterior thoracic nerve which penetrates it is necessarily sacrificed. Paralysis of the lateral portion of the pectoralis major results, and therefore . . . [this portion of the pectoralis major muscle] can be justifiably removed with the specimen." Handley completed the operation with survey biopsies of the internal mammary nodes, and if these, or "more than a few" axillary nodes, contained metastases, irradiation followed the operation.

Results reported with this operation have been comparable to those achieved with the standard radical operation, although no randomized trial has compared the two (Patey, 1967; Handley, 1969; Lesnick and Papatestas, 1974). Handley's 10 year crude survival rates were reported by Haagensen in 1974 as 63 per cent for CCC Stage A and 37 per cent for Stage B. Although Haagensen considered them inferior to his own results with radical mastectomy (70 per cent for Stage A and 43 per cent for Stage B), the differences were small.

In 1968 Handley permitted the author to personally review his cases, and 597 treated with the Patey operation were abstracted and staged retrospectively from the clinical records (Donegan et al., 1970). The operative mortality for the series was 0.2 per cent. The number of cases was reduced to 545 by excluding patients with noninvasive cancers, male patients, and women who were pregnant, who had a previous or simultaneous cancer, or who had any treatment other than postoperative irradiation. Of these 49.2 per cent had axillary metastases, and 10.2 per cent had metastases in the internal mammary nodes. The results, shown in Table 12–14, compare favorably with those achieved with the radical mastectomy. Local control for at least 5 years was achieved by the Patey operation in 84 per cent, versus 81 per cent for radical mastectomy, suggesting that preservation of the pectoralis major muscle did not engender local recurrence.

The operation designed by Scanlon is a technical improvement over the Patey operation, as it permits a full axillary node dissection without paralyzing the lateral portion of the pectoralis major muscle. Instead of removing the pectoralis minor muscle, the muscle is divided from its origin on the ribs and lifted up with the pectoralis major muscle, thereby preserving the medial anterior thoracic nerves while providing access to the apical nodes at Level III (Scanlon and Coprini, 1975). This is the operation preferred at present by the author.

TOTAL MASTECTOMY WITH LEVEL I AND II AXILLARY DISSECTION

The Auchincloss-Madden version of the modified radical mastectomy differs from the Patey operation in not removing the pectoralis minor muscle or the lymph nodes at the apex of the axilla. The dissection of the axilla is limited to Levels I and II. The justification for this approach is simply that 98.5 per cent of cases with metastases will be detected with a dissection of this extent, and that removal of high axillary nodes rarely cures if metastases are present in them. In 204 carefully cleared radical mastectomy specimens, Auchincloss found 107 in which metastases were present in axillary nodes. Seventy-one of these 107 patients (66 per cent) had not been cured by the operation. Exclusion of five patients who died of intercurrent disease left 31 patients living 8 to 10 years later, only four of whom had metastases in apical nodes. Theoretically, only 2 per cent of all patients (4 of 204) may have benefited from removal of apical nodes. Pickren and associates (1965) reviewed these same specimens with serial sections and found only one additional high node with occult tumor, leaving the results essentially unchanged.

Table 12–14. THE AUTHOR'S INDEPENDENT REVIEW OF PATEY MODIFIED RADICAL MASTECTOMIES PERFORMED BY R. S. HANDLEY (LONDON)

Clinical Stage	Number of Cases	Relative Survival (%)		5 Year Local Recurrence (%)
		5 Years	10 Years	
CCC A	337	83	79	10
B	175	72	48	24
C	27	51	46	34
Pathologic Stage				
Ax −	275	90	82	5
Ax +	264	67	48	27
IM +	56	48	18	45

Note: the cases of R. S. Handley treated by modified radical mastectomy with selective postoperative irradiation are shown staged clinically and pathologically. These results compare favorably with those for other forms of local treatment.
CCC, Columbia Clinical Classification.

As described by Auchincloss, the operation consists of a wide removal of the breast followed by an en bloc dissection of the axilla in the following manner. "The fascial investment of the pectoralis major muscle is stripped from the muscle around its lateral edge and, staying in the same plane, with the muscle retracted medially, the fascia covering the pectoralis minor muscle is similarly stripped in order to remove interpectoral nodes. The dissection is then carried upward along the edge of the minor muscle and somewhat posterior to it until the axillary vein is encountered. This is the high point of the axillary dissection and is suitably tagged for later pathological identification. It usually lies approximately 3.0 cm below the clavicle. From this point on, the dissection is performed exactly as would be done in a standard radical mastectomy" (Auchincloss, 1963). Madden (1965) supplemented the axillary dissection with discontinuous removal of nodal tissues from selected sites along the axillary vessels. Dissection around the pectoralis minor muscle should avoid damage to the medial anterior thoracic nerve that penetrates or courses lateral to the muscle.

Two randomized trials have compared modified mastectomy with radical mastectomy. Both have used the modified with axillary dissection limited to Levels I and II and have found similar results for both operations, thereby justifying adoption of the more limited, and less deforming, modified mastectomy. The first, in Manchester, England, concerned 534 patients with TNM Stage I and II cancers randomized between 1969 and 1976. No treatment but surgery was given until treatment failure was evident. After a median follow-up of 5 years, the 10 year actuarial results indicated no significant differences in survival, disease-free survival, local recurrence, or freedom from distant metastasis between the two treatments (Turner et al., 1981). The second study, performed at the University of Alabama between 1975 and 1978, involved 311 patients (Maddox et al., 1983) with TNM Stages I, II, and IIIa. As randomization was by the patient's year of birth, assignment was not binded, and those found to have positive axillary nodes received adjuvant chemotherapy. After a median of 5.5 years, no differences were seen in survival or disease-free survival. However, a trend was noted for increased local recurence after modified mastectomy. In 1979, a consensus meeting at the National Cancer Institute concluded that toal mastectomy and axillary dissection should replace the Halsted radical mastectomy as the treatment standard (NIH Consensus Development Panel, 1979).

MODIFIED MASTECTOMY AT MEDICAL COLLEGE OF WISCONSIN (MCW)

Experience with modified mastectomy at the Medical College of Wisconsin between the years 1969 and 1979 is in accord with randomized trials. In an analysis of invasive carcinoma in TNM Stages I, II, and III survival rates and survival free of recurrence (DFS) were not significantly different between radical and modified radical mastectomies (Figs. 12–22 and 12–23). Nor were significant differences found when comparisons were made by TNM stage or by axillary nodal count (Figs. 12–24 to 12–27). Local-regional recurrence increased with time but did not differ overall or when analyzed by stage or by axillary nodal status (Figs. 12–28 to 12–30). After both operations, patients were treated with irradiation or with adjuvant chemotherapy according to the inclinations of attending physicians.

The modified mastectomies were almost equally divided between Auchincloss and Patey types, and these two operations performed equally well (Figs. 12–31 to 12–33) in all categories except one. Local-regional recurrence was significantly higher after the Auchincloss operation in patients with four or more axillary nodes involved (Fig. 12–34), and further investigation found that it was because of a higher frequency of recurrence in the axilla (Table 12–15). It would appear that the more abbreviated axillary dissection was not as effective in controlling disease in the axilla when it was extensively involved. Therefore, it is the author's opinion that, to control this problem, a full axillary dissection (Levels I to III) should be performed if there is clinical evidence of axillary adenopathy prior to surgery.

Among the physical liabilities of modified mastectomy are numbness and paresthesias of the anterior chest and axilla, with phantom breast syndrome in some patients, failure to acquire full shoulder motion in an occasional patient, and ipsilateral arm edema of varying degrees in 8 per cent of patients (Donegan, 1970; Staps et al., 1985).

Text continued on page 381

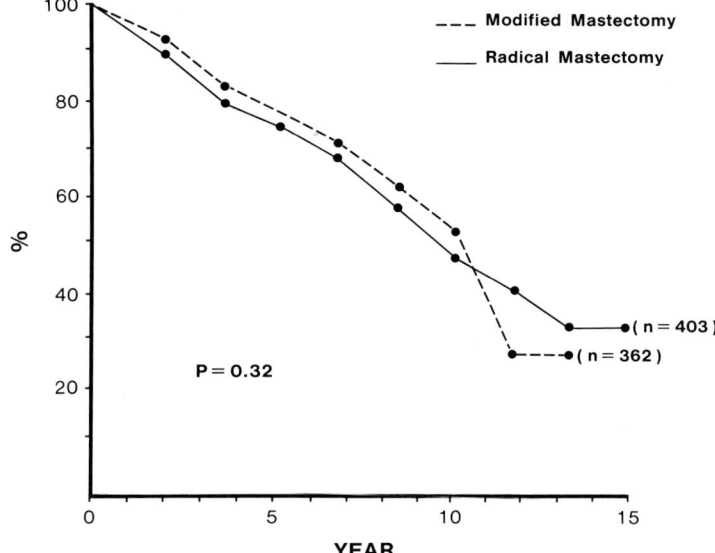

Figure 12–22. Modified and radical mastectomies performed at MCW between 1967 and 1979 resulted in survival rates that were indistinguishable. Irradiation and adjuvant chemotherapy were used selectively.

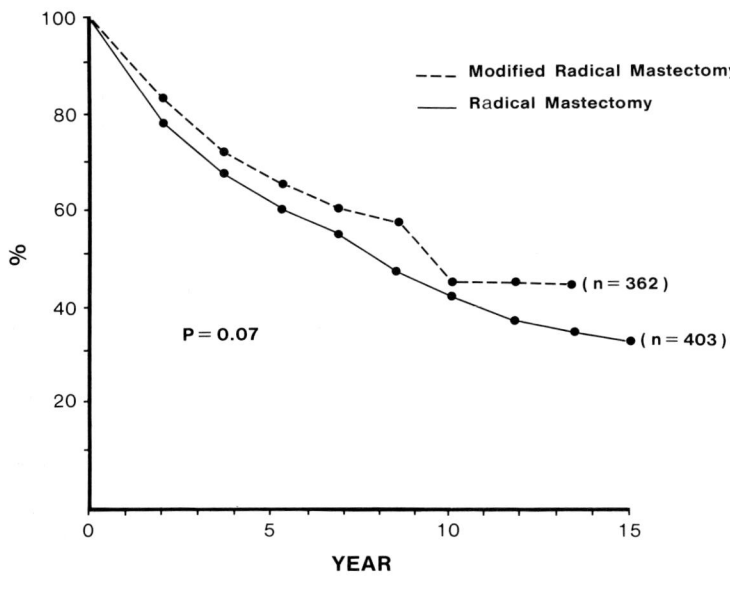

Figure 12–23. Modified and radical mastectomies at MCW between 1967 and 1979 produced disease-free survival rates that were not significantly different. The slight advantage for modified mastectomies may relate to the fact that more favorable cases were selected for this operation during its introduction.

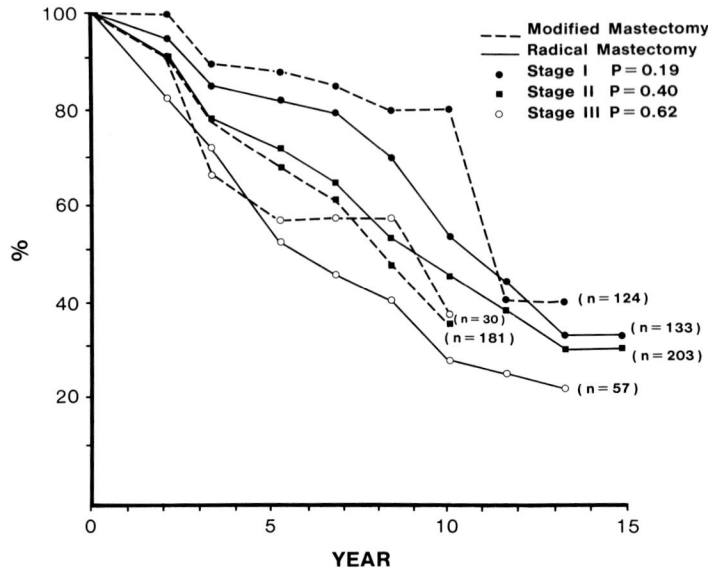

Figure 12–24. No significant difference in survival is evident between modified and radical mastectomies at MCW when compared by TNM clinical stage. Total cases are shown in parentheses.

Figure 12–25. Disease-free survival after modified and radical mastectomies at MCW between 1967 and 1979 showed no significant differences when compared within similar TNM clinical stages.

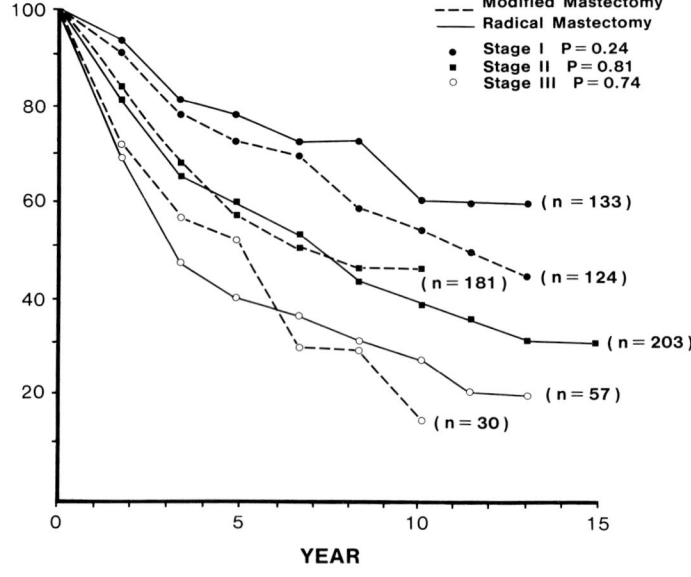

Figure 12–26. Radical and modified mastectomies performed at MCW provided similar survivals when compared by pathologic node category (no nodal metastases and 1 to 3 positive lymph nodes).

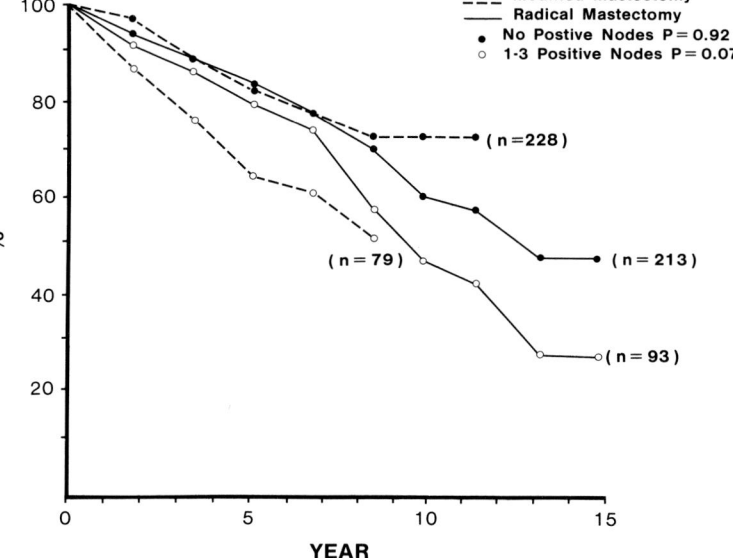

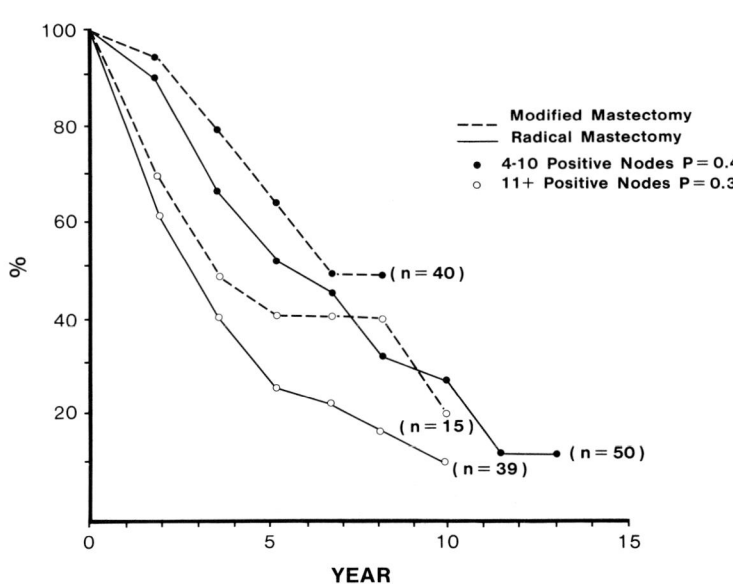

Figure 12–27. Modified and radical mastectomies performed at MCW between 1967 and 1979 resulted in no significant difference in survival when compared by nodal categories (4 to 10 positive nodes and 11 or more positive nodes). During this period modified mastectomy became the predominant method of surgical treatment, postoperative irradiation declined, and adjuvant chemotherapy increased.

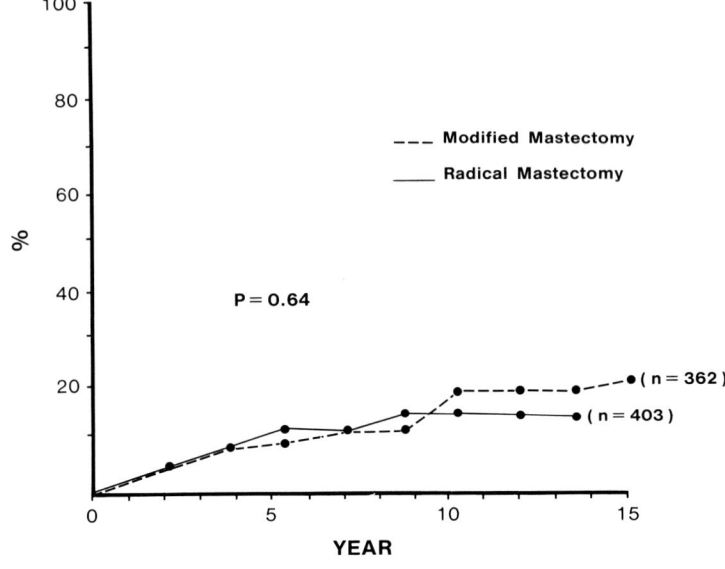

Figure 12–28. Overall cumulative local-regional recurrence for cases treated with modified versus radical mastectomy at MCW during the 12 years prior to 1979. No significant difference is present.

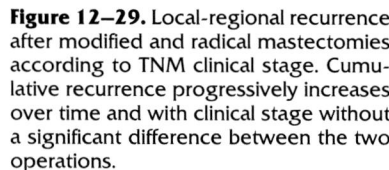

Figure 12–29. Local-regional recurrence after modified and radical mastectomies according to TNM clinical stage. Cumulative recurrence progressively increases over time and with clinical stage without a significant difference between the two operations.

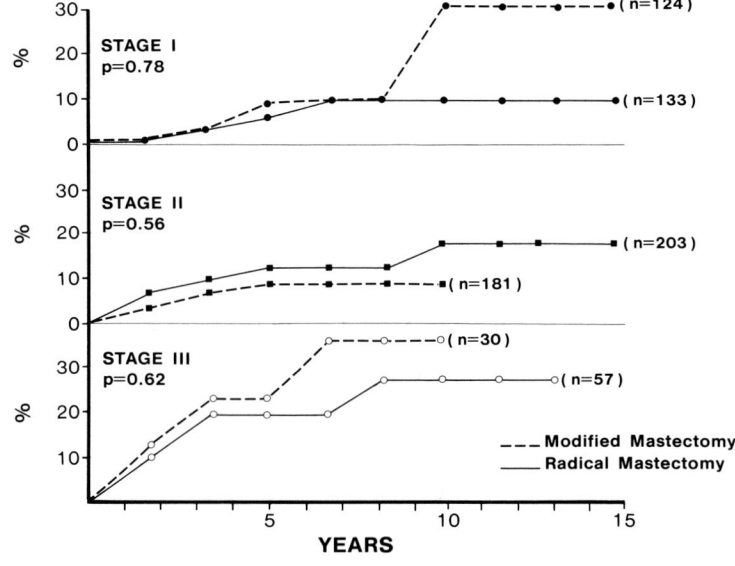

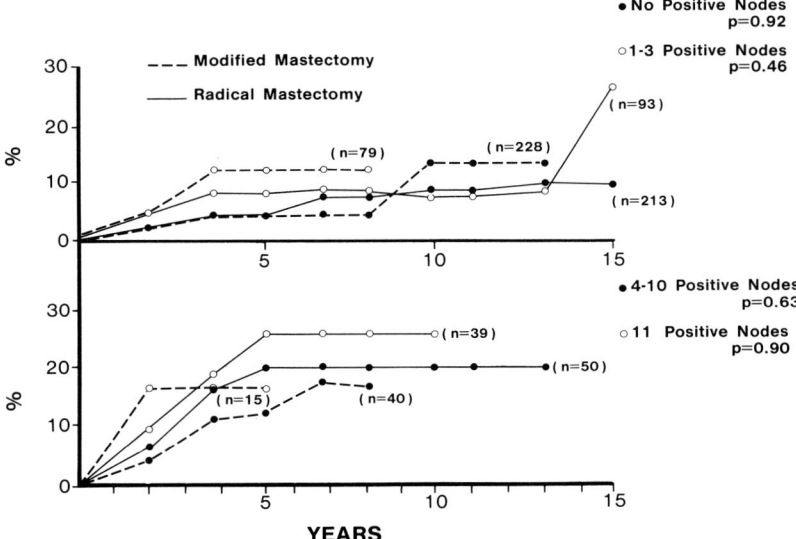

Figure 12–30. Cumulative local-regional recurrence by quantitative axillary nodal involvement. Recurrence increases progressively with increasing nodal involvement but without a significant difference between the two operations.

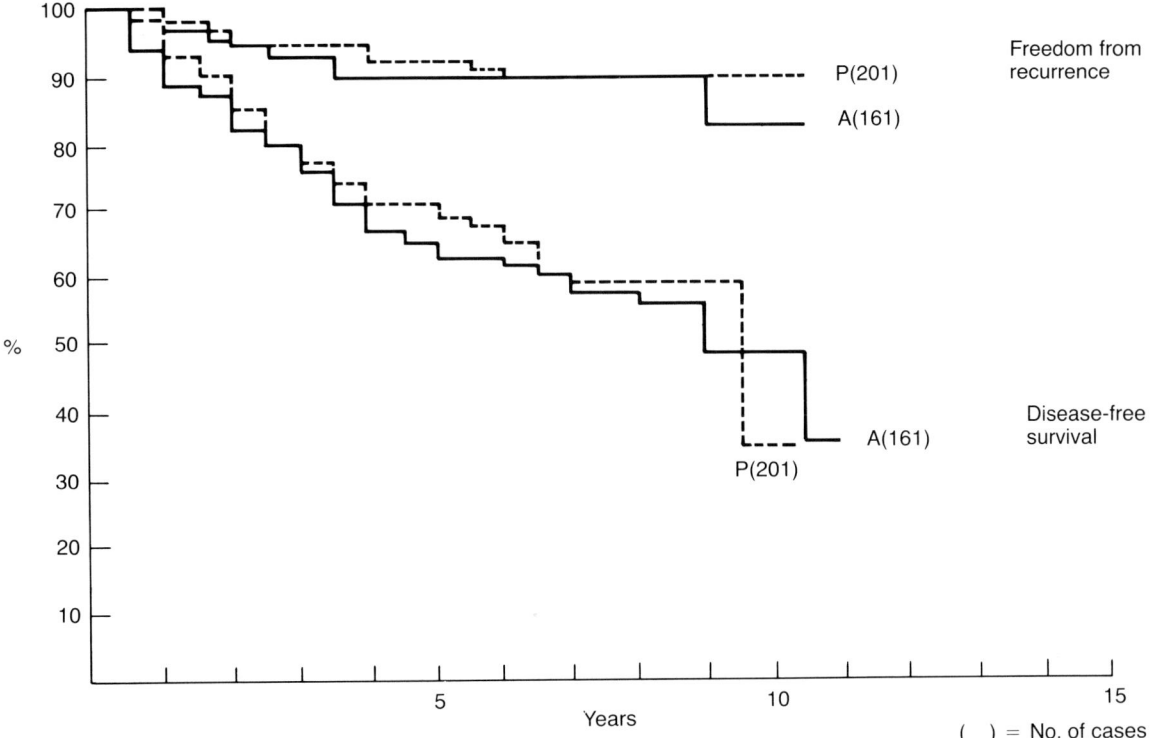

Figure 12–31. Modified mastectomies performed at MCW were almost equally divided between Auchincloss (A) and Patey (P) types. The operations differ only in the extent of axillary dissection. Patey mastectomies remove all levels of axillary nodes, whereas Auchincloss operations remove only levels I and II. Freedom from recurrence and disease-free survival were indistinguishable.

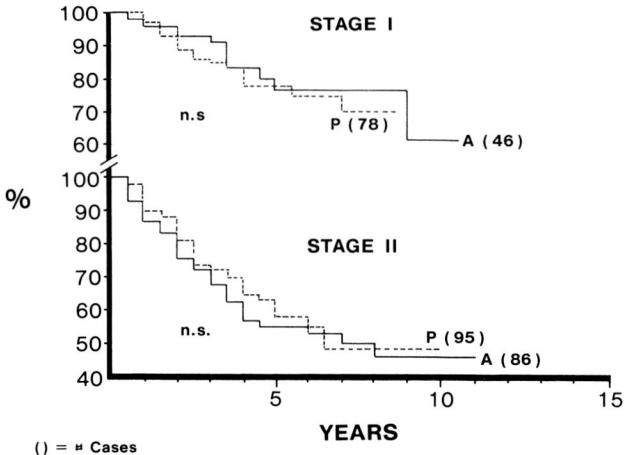

Figure 12–32. Disease-free survival by TNM clinical stage for Auchincloss (A) versus Patey (P) modified mastectomies. Approximately 80 per cent of patients with Stage I disease were alive and well after 5 years versus 60 per cent of those with Stage II disease, with no significant difference between the operations.

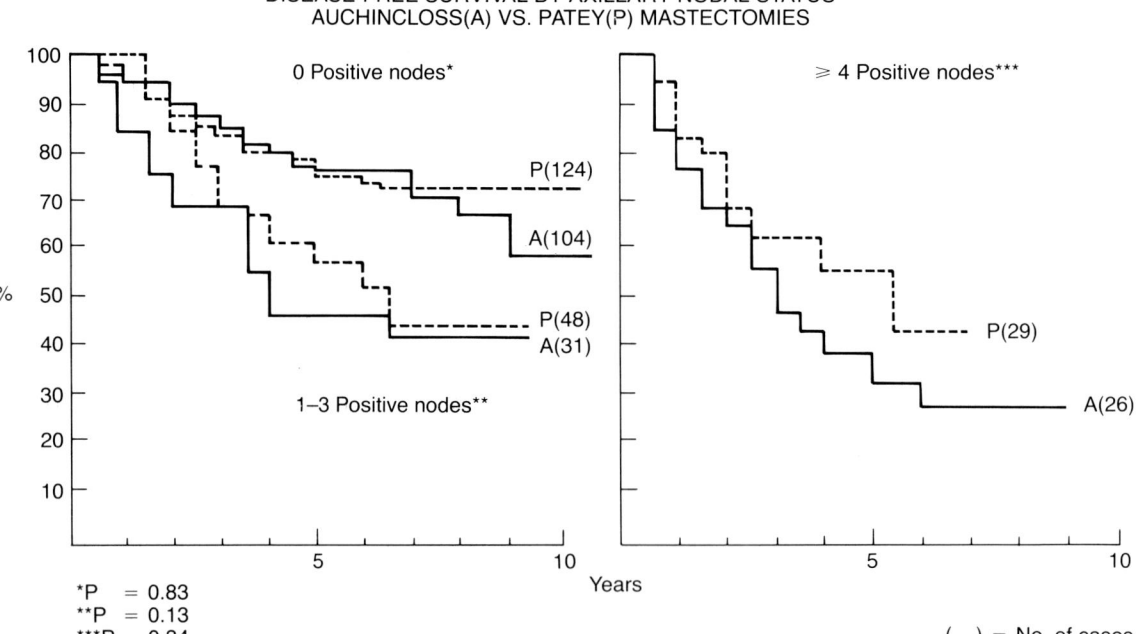

Figure 12–33. Disease-free survival declines with increasing numbers of histologically verified axillary lymph node metastases without a significant difference in results between Auchincloss (A) versus Patey (P) modified mastectomies.

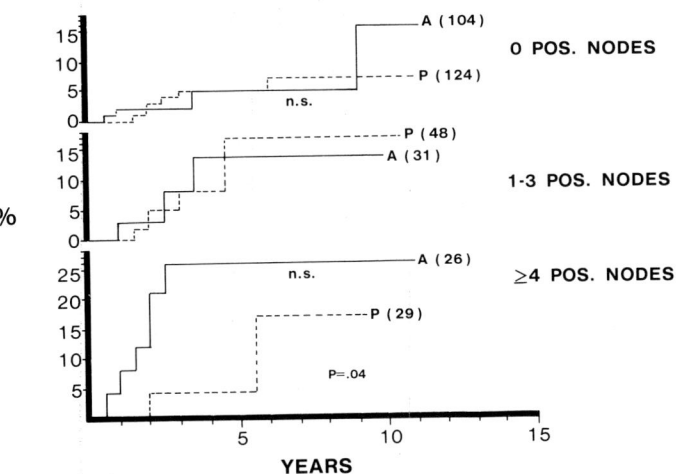

Figure 12–34. Local regional recurrence is higher after an Auchincloss modified mastectomy when four or more nodes are involved by metastases, principally because of more frequent recurrences in the axilla. This operation entails an incomplete axillary dissection.

Total (Simple) Mastectomy

"Total" has replaced the term "simple" mastectomy to emphasize the objective of completely removing all mammary tissue, something that earlier simple mastectomies often failed to do (Holleb et al., 1965). The procedure for simple removal requires flap development as extensive as for a radical operation plus removal of most of the lower axillary tissues (Level I) in order to encompass the axillary tail of the breast.

Table 12–15. LOCAL-REGIONAL RECURRENCE

Operation	Site		
	Skin	Axilla	Supraclavicular
Auchincloss Modification	10 (56%)	5 (28%)	3 (17%)
Patey Modification	13 (68%)	1 (5%)	5 (26%)
Radical Mastectomy	36 (70%)	7 (13%)	9 (17%)

These figures pertain to sites of local-regional recurrence in patients with four or more axillary nodal metastases. Recurrence in the axilla is high when an incomplete axillary lymph node dissection is performed in the presence of extensive nodal involvement. The Auchincloss modified mastectomy removes nodes from only axillary Levels I and II, whereas the Patey modification and the radical mastectomy remove nodes from all three levels. A complete nodal dissection should be performed in the presence of a clinically positive axilla to avoid this problem.

A number of surgeons have maintained that removal of the breast alone, with or without postoperative irradiation, is appropriate treatment for clinically localized (Stage I) breast cancer (Grace and Moitrier, 1936; McWhirter, 1964; Crile, 1975; Meyer et al., 1978) and have published favorable results with selected cases treated in this fashion. Total mastectomy without supplemental irradiation for apparently localized cancers poses the question of whether temporary neglect of occult metastases in regional nodes influences the chance of cure. Total mastectomy combined with irradiation of regional lymph nodes is radical in concept and simply raises the issue of whether irradiation of nodes is the equal of surgical removal (Bond, 1967).

In 1971, the National Surgical Adjuvant Breast Project (NSABP) initiated a prospective randomized clinical trial to address the issues raised by total mastectomy. Patients with early cancers confined to the breast (clinical Stage I, but without regard to size) were randomized for treatment with radical mastectomy, total mastectomy alone, or total mastectomy combined with postoperative irradiation to regional lymph nodes (axillary, internal mammary, and supraclavicular). Patients treated initially with total mastectomy alone had an axillary dissection if isolated axillary metastases became apparent. They were not considered treatment failures unless cancer subsequently reappeared.

Beyond being an empirical comparison of three treatment alternatives, certain conceptual questions were involved: (1) If the breast is removed in all cases, are clinically occult metastases in axillary lymph nodes managed as successfully with irradiation as with surgical removal? (2) Does the preservation of clinically uninvolved regional lymph nodes benefit the patient? (3) If occult axillary metastases are not removed initially en bloc with the breast, can they be removed at a later date if they become clinically enlarged without compromising cure?

Patients who presented initially with clinically involved axillary lymph nodes (Stage II) were randomized for treatment with either radical mastectomy (surgical removal of axillary nodes) or total mastectomy and irradiation to axillary and other regional nodes. By September 1974, 1765 patients had entered the study, and in 1985 a report on 1665 eligible patients was made after an average follow-up of 126 months (Fisher et al., 1985b). No significant difference was evident at this time in disease-free survival, distant metastasis, or cumulative survival between the three treatment options for clinical Stage I breast cancer. Irradiation reduced regional recurrence but did not improve survival. Eighteen per cent of patients initially treated with total mastectomy alone required subsequent axillary dissection for progressive metastases, as late as 112.6 months after mastectomy (Table 12–16). More than half (71 per cent) of those who required a subsequent axillary dissection had a further treatment failure, identifying them as a high risk group. As it is known that 40 per cent of clinical Stage I cases have occult axillary metastases, it is of interest that so few had early tumor progression at this site. It was not reported how many had progression in the axilla after recurrence elsewhere, however, so whether some regional metastases lie permanently dormant remains uncertain. Noteworthy was a negligible (1.4 per cent) recurrence rate in the axilla after complete axillary dissection in the radical mastectomy group. Also of interest was the failure of regional irrradiation, which included the internal mammary nodes, to improve survival.

The two treatment options in Stage II were equally efficacious in terms of survival and disease-free survival. Surgery was more effective than irradiation for controlling clinically enlarged axillary metastases and almost equally effective for control of occult axillary metastases in Stage I. Local and supraclavicular recurrences were lowest in both Stages I and II when treatment included irradiation.

This study, more convincingly than any other, casts doubt on the contribution to cure of prophylactic removal or irradiation of regional lymph nodes. It would appear that the case for lymph node dissection must be made on the usefulness of the nodes for pathologic staging and for preventing the progressive growth of regional metastases, two not inconsequential considerations. The study also failed

Table 12–16. RECURRENCES, NATIONAL SURGICAL ADJUVANT BREAST PROJECT, B-04, FEBRUARY 1986

	AX –			AX +	
	RM	TMR	TM	RM	TMR
Total Number	362	352	365	292	294
I Local	5%	1.4%	7.1%	7.9%	2.7%
II Regional			18% ←Ax. Salvage*		
Axillary	1.4%	3.1%	1.4%	1.0%	10.5%
Supraclavicular	1.1%	0.3%	2.7%	5.1%	0
Parasternal	0	0	0	0	0
III Distant	27.1%	32.7%	30.1%	37.1%	40.8%

*3 to 117 months; 71% subsequent failure.

This table shows sites of recurrence after radical mastectomy (RM), total mastectomy and regional irradiation (TMR), and total mastectomy alone (TM) according to the NSABP B-04 protocol. Regional recurrence in the axilla as the first sign of failure appeared in 18 per cent of patients treated with total mastectomy alone. After an axillary lymph node dissection in these cases, total axillary failures do not exceed 1.4 per cent, equivalent to a prophylactic axillary dissection as performed in the RM cases and somewhat better than the 3.1 per cent seen after axillary irradiation. Axillary failures were substantially fewer after radical mastectomy (1 per cent) for clinically involved nodes than after total mastectomy and irradiation of the axilla (10.5 per cent). Supraclavicular recurrences were few in all categories and no parasternal recurrences were recognized. Distant dissemination was constant despite variations in the method of primary treatment. This study demonstrated that prophylactic removal or irradiation of axillary lymph nodes did not influence the probability of cure.

to confirm that preservation of regional nodes retards dissemination of the tumor, as might be expected if they made a significant contribution to immunologic host defense.

The results of the International Multicenter Trial of the Cancer Research Campaign coordinated at King's College Hospital in London is also of particular interest with respect to the use of total mastectomy. In this study, 2268 patients in Manchester clinical Stages I and II (i.e., TNM T1 or T2, N0 or N1, M0) were randomized between May 1970 and April 1975 for treatment with total mastectomy followed in randomly selected cases by irrradiation to the skin flaps and the axillary, supraclavicular, and internal mammary nodes (Murray et al., 1976). After 5 years, patients with Stage I cancers had identical survival rates and freedom from dissemination whether or not they received postoperative irradiation. The same was true for patients with Stage II cancers. The point of greatest interest was that patients in both Stage I and Stage II had significantly higher frequencies of regional and local recurrence if irradiation was not used. Local recrudescence was most common in the axilla (observed in 70 per cent of cases alone or in combination), followed by the chest wall (observed in 35 per cent of cases alone or in combination). Although patients with local and regional recurrence had a poor prognosis, 70 per cent of the local recurrences were successfully controlled by additional treatment. This study further illustrates that treatment (in this case irradiation) of metastases in regional lymph nodes does prevent their progressive growth but has a negligible impact upon survival and dissemination. These results were confirmed by a similar trial with 1022 patients in Manchester, England (Lythgoe and Palmer, 1982). One third of Clinical Stage I patients treated only with total mastectomy had progression in the axilla, and 38 per cent had local recurrence.

It would appear that total mastectomy alone is insufficient to provide optimum local-regional control of invasive breast cancer, principally because of frequent progression of cancer in the axilla. As neglected cancer in axillary nodes progresses during the patient's remaining lifetime in a substantial number of cases, regional control is best achieved by treating it initially and sparing the patient, as far as possible, repeated subsequent bouts of treatment. Surgical removal and irradiation are equally effective for controlling occult axillary metastases and apparently are equally undistinguished in preventing dissemination in Stages I and II. The advantage of axillary dissection is that it also provides staging information important for accurately determining prognosis and deciding for adjuvant therapy. If delayed treatment of clinically inapparent metastases in regional lymph nodes by either method enhances or jeopardizes chances for cure, it is not apparent in clinical trials to date.

Total mastectomy results in anesthesia of the skin of the anterior chest. Arm edema is not expected unless irradiation of regional nodes is added, in which case it may be seen eventually in 5 per cent or fewer of patients. Treatment with total mastectomy and irradiation has the advantage of being relatively simple from the surgical standpoint, and it may be all that can be tolerated by some fragile patients, but it combines the most cosmetically objectional aspect of surgery (i.e., removal of the breast) with all of the liabilities of irradiation and provides no nodal staging.

Partial Mastectomy

Excision of primary cancers without sacrifice of the entire breast has been referred to variously as local excision, tumorectomy, lumpectomy, or tylectomy (from the Greek word for lump). Other terms implying the inclusion of overlying skin include quadrantectomy, extended tylectomy, wedge resection, and segmental mastectomy.

The issue of partial mastectomy centers on the multicentric origin of breast cancer. There is no doubt that microscopic foci of cancer often remain behind. Subserial sections of mastectomy specimens have shown foci of cancer in quadrants remote from the clinical primary tumor in 40 to 50 per cent of cases (Qualheim and Gall, 1957; Gallager and Martin, 1969; Fisher et al., 1975a; Tinnemans et al., 1986). Rosen and associates (1975) found residual cancer in either the breast, the regional lymph nodes, or both in 63 per cent of 203 mastectomy specimens after "simulated" partial mastectomies. Tumor size was important, as residua were found in the breast in 26 per cent if the excised primary tumor was less than 2 cm in diameter and in 38 per cent if it was larger.

The expectation is that irradiation can usually control residual microscopic cancer, but if it does not, the residual breast can be removed subsequently if needed without compromising cure. It is also expected that women will seek consultation earlier if they do not have to fear loss of the breast and that this will result in an overall gain in salvage. Partial mastectomy finds further support in a logical paradox: It is illogical to advocate total removal of the clinically involved breast for fear of leaving microscopic cancer and not also insist on removal of the opposite member, in which occult microscopic cancer is also often found, albeit less frequently.

In the 19th century, when tumors were large and irradiation was not available, local excisions regularly failed to cure. Even recent experience with local excision continues to confirm an unacceptably high frequency of recurrence in the breast, particularly if surgical margins are not tumor-free (Lagios et al., 1983; Tagert et al., 1985). By contrast, the results reported now with local excision followed by irradiation compare favorably with more extensive surgical procedures. Supportive historical reference is often made to the early works of Keynes with interstitial implants after local tumor excision (Keynes, 1932). Peters (1970) observed after a review at the Princess Margaret Hospital that the extent of resection appeared to have little influence on local tumor control or survival provided it was accompanied by comprehensive irradiation.

Prospective randomized trials of partial mastectomy have established the credibility of this form of treatment. Atkins and coworkers (1972) at Guys Hospital, London, began the first in 1961. Patients with Manchester clinical Stage I or Stage II (T1 or T2, N0 or N1) cancers were randomized to treatment with either "extended tylectomy" (no assessment of margins histologically) or classic radical mastectomy. Both operations were followed by comprehensive irradiation to regional lymph nodes, and the residual breast of those treated with tylectomy was also irradiated. Patients received doses of irradiation not exceeding 2700 rad to the apex of the axilla or 3800 rad to the remaining breast, which by current standards are not considered adequate. Early in the trial, patients also received thiotepa. One hundred and seven Stage I cases and 81 Stage II cases were treated and observed for up to 10 years. A significantly higher rate of local recurrence attended local excision in both Stage I and Stage II. Half of the local recurrences after local excision and irradiation occurred in the axilla or supraclavicular areas, but another quarter occurred in the parenchyma (7 per cent) and skin (22 per cent) of the breast. Although the survival of Stage I cases did not differ between the two treatments, the survival of Stage II patients treated with the simpler surgery was significantly less.

This study demonstrated that local and regional control of mammary carcinoma was poor if only low doses of irradiation were used. Furthermore, poor local regional control in the presence of axillary adenopathy appeared to invite dissemination and death. Because Stage I survival had not suffered in the initial trial, the investigators continued with a second series of 252 Stage I (T1 to T3a, N0 to N1a) cases, and this time conservative treatment resulted not only in poor local control but also in poor survival (Hayward, 1983). Thus, the results in Stage I were inconsistent, and this study remains unique in suggesting that poor local control results in poor survival.

In the Milan trial, which followed in Italy between 1973 and 1980, high dose irradiation was combined with wider excision. Seven hundred and one patients with small localized tumors (TNM Stage I) were randomized between radical mastectomy (later switched to modified mastectomy) or quadrantectomy (no assessment of surgical margins) plus full axillary dissection (Levels I to III) followed by 5000 rad of irradiation to the breast only and a 1000 rad boost to the area of excision. This was called the QUART treatment (*QU*adrentectomy, *A*xillary dissection, and *R*adio-*T*herapy). Adjuvant therapy was inconsistent: initially patients with axillary metastases were randomized for observation or to receive postoperative irradiation to internal mammary and supraclavicular nodes to see if this helped. After 1976, this was changed to cyclophosphamide, methotrexate, and 5-fluorouracil (CMF) adjuvant chemotherapy (12 cycles) for all patients with pathologically involved axillary lymph nodes, about 26 per cent of the total. It can be conjectured that in each of the two primary treatment groups, about 20 patients received nodal irradiation, 52 received adjuvant chemotherapy, and 278 received no adjuvant therapy. Survival and disease-free survival through 10 years have been statistically indistinguishable between the groups overall and when separated by axillary nodal status (Veronesi et al., 1985). Recurrence of tumor in the irradiated breast (4 per cent) has been somewhat higher than chest wall recurrence after mastectomy (2 per cent), and primary tumors in the second breast have also been slightly more numerous after QUART, but

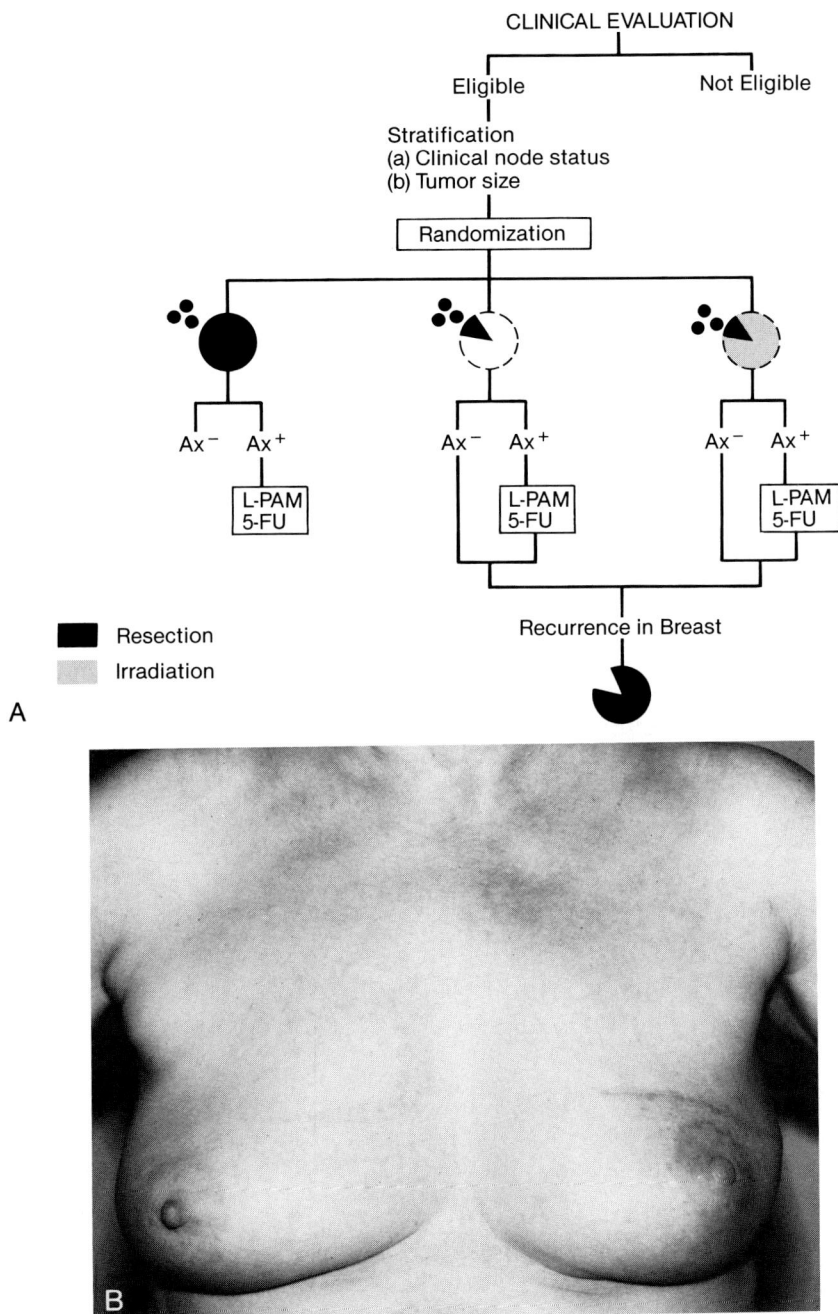

Figure 12–35. *A,* Protocol for B-06 of the NSABP (tumor ≤ 4 cm; axillary nodes ≤ 2 cm) concerned with partial mastectomy. Circles represent the breast; the smaller spheres represent axillary lymph nodes; the blackened areas represent surgical removal; and diagonal cross hatches represent radiation therapy. The axillary lymph nodes are removed in all cases, and metastases are an indication for adjuvant chemotherapy. The objective is to determine whether untreated microscopic foci of cancer in the residual breast have a deleterious influence on the patient's clinical course and, if so, whether they are best treated by irradiation or removal. If the initial treatment is segmental mastectomy, local recurrence is treated with total removal of the breast. L-PAM, L-phenylalanine mustard; 5-FU, 5-fluorouracil. *B,* Patient's appearance after segmental mastectomy, axillary dissection, and breast irradiation for a tumor of the upper outer quadrant of the left breast. The axillary incision, which is transverse, is hidden in the front view. The breast is reduced slightly in size and the nipple is elevated, but the cosmetic results are good.

not statistically. Cosmetic results are said to be good or better in 67 per cent.

The NSABP in the United States extended this approach to TNM Stage I and small (≤4 cm) Stage II tumors in a large randomized trial (protocol B-06) involved 2163 patients conducted between 1976 and 1983. Comparison was with modified mastectomy, and there were important variations (Fig. 12–35A) (Fisher et al., 1985a). The tumor was excised with little skin and only widely enough to achieve histologically tumor free margins ("segmentectomy"), no boost of irradiation was given to supplement the 5000 rad to the whole breast, and axillary dissection was not always complete, Levels I and II being acceptable (Fig. 12–35B). But, perhaps more importantly, to determine the natural history of multicentric cancer, the study included one arm in which the breast treated with segmentectomy was not irradiated. All patients with axillary metastases received adjuvant chemotherapy. After a mean follow-up of 39 months, 5 year survival and survival free of dissemination were not different in the three treatment arms, but disease-free survival after segmentectomy and irradiation was better than with total mastectomy (Fig. 12–36). Regional failures were comparable, as were rates for primary tumors in the second breast (Table 12–17). Failures in the irradiated breast were few (8 per cent); without irradiation, however, they reached 28 per cent at 5 years. In unirradiated patients with axillary metastases, they were much higher (36 per cent) (Fig. 12–37). A subsequent report placed breast recurrences at 6 per cent in irradiated and 24 per cent in unirradiated patients (Fisher et al., 1986b). Almost all (95 per cent) of these recurrences were in mammary parenchyma, and all were at or close to the site of excision, suggesting incomplete removal of extensions of the primary tumor despite surgical margins that were considered histologically tumor-free. Tumor size had no relationship to the frequency of breast recurrence. In contrast to the Guy's Hospital trial, high local failures in the unirradiated breast did not result in increased dissemination. This study documents that tumorectomy for TNM Stage I and small Stage II tumors provides survival equal to that of mastectomy, but that irradiation of the residual breast is necessary if optimum local control is to be achieved initially.

A small randomized trial of local excision and irradiation versus mastectomy at the Insti-

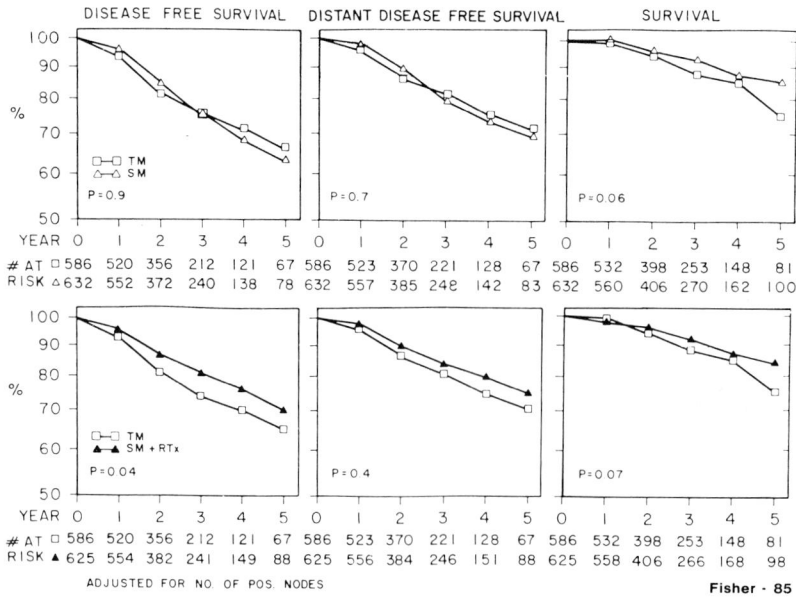

Figure 12–36. Shown are the results of the NSABP's protocol B-06 after a mean of 39 months of follow-up. This study compared total mastectomy (TM) with segmental mastectomy (SM) and with segmental mastectomy plus irradiation of the breast (SM + RT). All patients had axillary dissection, and those with metastases received adjuvant chemotherapy. The three methods of management produced equivalent survival and freedom from dissemination. Disease-free survival after segmental mastectomy and irradiation of the breast was superior to that of total mastectomy. (Reproduced by permission from Fisher, B., et al.: N. Engl. J. Med., *312*:665, 1985.)

Table 12–17. SITES OF RECURRENCE AFTER TOTAL MASTECTOMY AND AFTER SEGMENTAL MASTECTOMY WITH AND WITHOUT BREAST IRRADIATION (NSABP B–06), MAY 1985

	TM + AD	SM + AD	SM + AD + RT
Local	6.8%	5.9%*	0.8%*
Regional	3.8%	5.3%	3.5%
(AX)	1.4%	3.1%	1.1%
(IM)	0.3%	0.2%	0%
(SC)	1.7%	1.3%	2.1%
Distant	14%	15.5%	14.5%
Second Breast	2.5%	3.3%	2.9%

*Secondary failures.

Sites of tumor recurrence are shown for NSABP segmental mastectomy protocol B-06. An isolated breast recurrence according to this protocol was not counted as a local failure unless there was subsequent chest wall recurrence after salvage mastectomy. The figures in parentheses refer to such chest wall recurrences and they do not exceed that observed after initial total mastectomy. After a mean 39 months of follow-up, sites of recurrence and the frequency of cancer in the second breast have not varied between the treatment groups.

TM, Total mastectomy; AD, axillary dissection; RT, breast irradiation; SM, segmental mastectomy, AX, axilla; IM, internal mammary; SC, supraclavicular.

tute Gustave-Roussy in Villejuif, France (Sarrazin et al., 1984), used only Level I axillary dissection for patients with histologically negative nodes. It supported conservative treatment, and a small extension study involving 72 patients with positive axillary nodes treated conservatively found no improved survival or disease-free survival from adding nodal irradiation. The investigators noted that irradiation of a completely dissected axilla had the disadvantage of increasing brachial plexopathy and arm edema.

In 1979, the United States National Cancer Institute began a randomized study of very limited gross tumor excision, lumpectomy (margins not necessarily tumor-free) plus breast irradiation versus total mastectomy. All patients have an axillary dissection, and those with nodal metastases receive adjuvant chemotherapy. Patients treated conservatively have a boost of either interstitial or electron beam irradiation to the tumor bed, and selected patients have regional node irradiation. As of the end of December 1984, 175 patients had been entered and 23 had recurrence (Findlay et al., 1985).

Although preservation of the breast is the principal appeal of this approach, it must be appreciated that this goal is not always possible to achieve. Seven per cent of the patients of Prosnitz and associates (1983) required mastectomies because of local recurrence. In one series, mastectomies were necessitated in 4 per cent of cured cases by undesirable local effects of irradiation (Durand and Pilleron, 1977). Breast edema (usually transient) followed by progressive breast shrinkage has been the most frequent and obvious side effect (Clarke et al.,

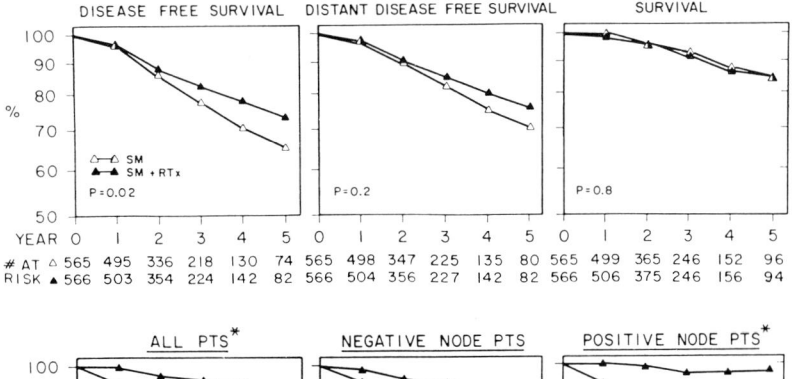
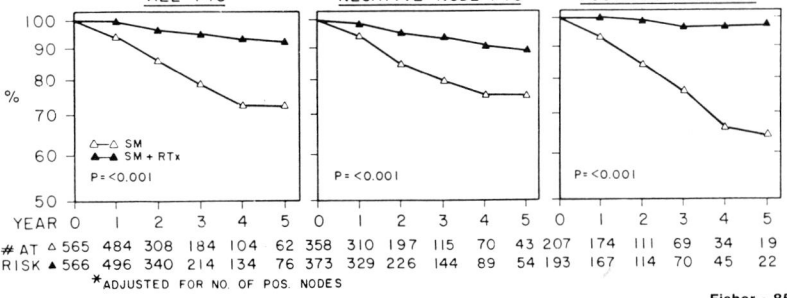

Figure 12–37. Shown are the initial results of the NSABP protocol B-06 study of segmental mastectomy. Survival was equivalent whether or not segmental mastectomy was followed by irradiation of the breast, but disease-free survival was improved when irradiation was used (upper row of figure). Recurrence in the breast was considerably higher when irradiation to the breast did not follow segmental mastectomy. This is true for those both with and without axillary nodal metastases. Breast recurrence reached 38 per cent in the latter. Recurrence in the breast was less frequent when irradiation of the breast was combined with systemic adjuvant chemotherapy (lower row of figure). (Reproduced by permission from Fisher, B., et al.: N. Engl. J. Med., *312*:665, 1985.)

1982) (Fig. 12–38). Infrequent complications include irradiation pneumonitis, rib fractures, arm edema, skin ulceration, or pleural effusions in about 10 per cent of patients (Prosnitz et al., 1983). Secondary neoplasia is a potential long-term risk. Radiation-induced cancers are estimated at 1.5 per cent based on retrospective experience with postmastectomy irradiation (Ferguson et al., 1982). Parts of the opposite breast are exposed to 200 to 2000 rad, but Montague (1984) found no evidence for increased cancer in the second breast.

Patients at high risk for recurrence in the breast are those (1) with lymphatic extension within the breast (Fisher et al., 1986b), (2) with inadequate irradiation to the breast, (3) with gross residual cancer, and, according to one authority, (4) with a substantial amount of intraductal carcinoma (Schnitt et al., 1984).

An important question is whether recurrence in the breast can be treated effectively with a "salvage mastectomy." Those with such a recurrence are obviously a selected group, having no simultaneous recurrence elsewhere and being technically suitable for mastectomy. It has been observed that breast recurrence has a better prognosis than nodal or dermal recurrence and that the disease-free survival from initial treatment of patients with solitary breast recurrence is not diminished if they can be rendered disease-free by a salvage mastectomy (Clarke et al., 1985). Several authors have reported a 50 per cent 5-year survival after salvage operations (Vilcoq et al., 1981, Kurtz et al., 1983; Harris et al., 1984).

Local excision plus irradiation is a viable alternative to mastectomy for many but not all patients. It is preferable when the anticipated cosmetic results are superior to mastectomy with reconstruction and when irradiation is acceptable to the patient. The surgeon must be skilled with the technique, as must the radiotherapist, to produce an optimum cosmetic result. Patients are not candidates who are pregnant, who have a large tumor in a small breast, who have had previous irradiation to the chest, who have multiple or poorly defined primary tumors, or who have gross residual cancer (unless it can be removed). Bilateral or central primary tumors do not constitute contraindications, but experience is limited and the technical aspects are more difficult.

It is not yet settled whether an irradiation boost to the tumor bed is helpful after tumor excision with free margins, but the fact that when it is not used, most breast recurrences are at or near the excision site, suggests that it may be helpful. Practice varies considerably regarding regional nodal irradiation.

SUMMARY

Currently, the two most popular treatment options for Stage I and II invasive carcinomas

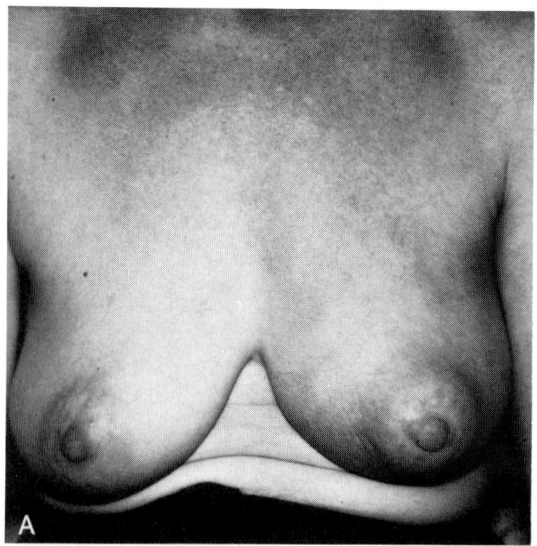 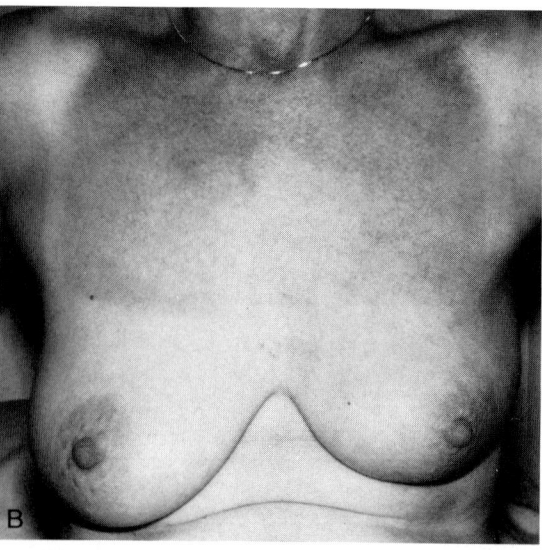

Figure 12–38. Progressive retraction of the breast is a frequent sequel of irradiation. A, The appearance of the left breast shortly following segmental mastectomy and irradiation. Mild edema is present, but the size approximates that of the right breast. B, The appearance 2.5 years later; there has been obvious shrinkage of the treated breast.

in the United States are (1) total mastectomy with axillary dissection and (2) tumor excision, axillary dissection, and breast irradiation. The former is more generally applicable, but the latter has cosmetic appeal. Neither is simple or without liabilities. The author's experience has been that, after a complete explanation of the advantages and disadvantages of each, somewhat more than half of all patients who are suitable for either method choose breast conserving treatment.

Locally Regionally Advanced Breast Carcinoma (cTNM Stage III)

Advanced local-regional breast carcinoma (Stage III) is a broad category both clinically and prognostically that ordinarily includes from 10 to 15 per cent of patients seen in most medical centers. Patients with large tumors (more than 5 cm in diameter) or with involved axillary lymph nodes that have become attached to each other or to surrounding tissues are categorized as TNM Stage IIIa, and those with more advanced disease (i.e., skin ulceration, fixation to the chest wall, edema, or satellite nodules) and patients with involved infraclavicular, internal mammary, and supraclavicular nodes or axillary involvement extensive enough to cause edema of the arm are designated as having Stage IIIb. Cases of inflammatory carcinoma are identified separately. Failure of some authors to do this complicates the comparison of Stage III cases.

From the therapeutic standpoint, Stage IIIa is technically operable and for the most part can be managed surgically as Stage II cases. Stage IIIb, with some exceptions, is technically inoperable. Treatment is largely palliative, and the type of local treatment is dictated by individual circumstances. By definition, Stage III breast cancer does not include patients with evidence of distant metastases, but the poor results of local and regional treatment in most cases indicates that the majority of these patients have occult distant micrometastases at the outset, and treatment requires a combination of aggressive local-regional and systemic therapy.

The clinical and prognostic heterogeneity of Stage III breast cancer and its relative infrequency hampers the accomplishment of randomized prospective controlled studies. Most investigations have been pilot studies of treatment strategies using multimodality therapy with emphasis on new drug combinations and radiation therapy combined with mastectomy in selected cases. Initial chemotherapy, with or without hormones, to halt the progress of occult dissemination and reduce the obvious local and regional involvement is the focus of current interest.

The results at the Medical College of Wisconsin with 123 cases of Stage III breast cancer during a period when surgery or irradiation was the primary intervention is shown in Figure 12–39. Overall 5 year disease-free survival was slightly more than 40 per cent and at 10 years, only 20 per cent of patients were cured. Stage IIIa cases, however, which were largely composed of patients with large tumors, many being sufficiently indolent that they had failed to metastasize to regional lymph nodes, fared considerably better than Stage IIIb cases. Inflammatory carcinoma had a prognosis during this period that was markedly inferior to other stage III cases. Similar to earlier stages of breast cancer, the prognosis in Stage III was dependent on the presence and number of nodal metastases (Fig. 12–40). Patients without nodal metastases had a 5 year disease-free survival of 65 per cent and this was largely maintained at 10 years. The dominant influence of axillary nodal involvement in Stage III was also observed by Fracchia and coworkers (1980); in the absence of nodal metastases, 82

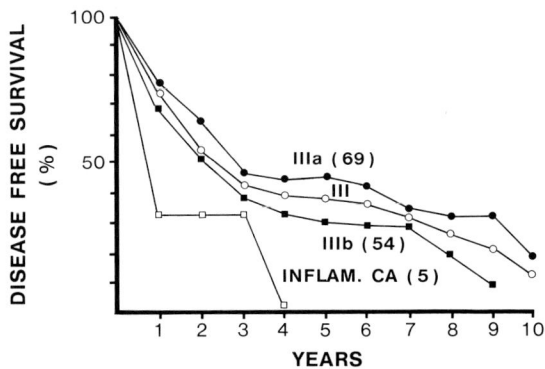

Figure 12–39. Disease-free survival of TNM stage III carcinoma of the breast treated at MCW with inflammatory carcinoma indicated separately. Survival is approximately 40 per cent at 5 years. The prognosis of Stage IIIa is superior to Stage IIIb.

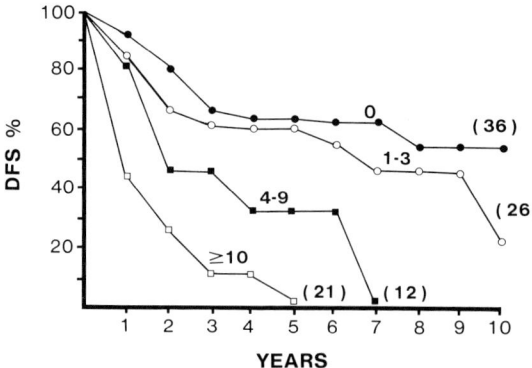

Figure 12–40. The number of involved axillary lymph nodes influences disease-free survival of surgically treated Stage III breast cancer. Despite the advanced clinical stage, patients without axillary metastases are a highly favorable group, with a 5 year survival of 65 per cent.

per cent of all patients were alive at 5 five years and 75 per cent at 10 years, and grave local signs (as identified by Haagensen) did not influence the survival rate of patients with negative nodes. Identification of this favorable group is a strong argument for initial surgical intervention in technically operable cases.

LOCAL-REGIONAL TREATMENT

Retrospective reviews of multimodality treatment with surgery and irradiation for Stage III have suffered from selection bias and lack of uniform follow-up. Patients for whom mastectomy was selected as initial treatment and followed by irradiation likely had less severe local advancement, whereas unresectable cases were treated initially with irradiation. When irradiation was used initially, patients who subsequently had mastectomy were selected because of their good response to irradiation and failure to develop dissemination.

Bedwinek and colleagues (1982) found a marked improvement in local control when surgery was used in combination with irradiation, but this analysis was not free of the foregoing biases. Fletcher and coworkers (1980) emphasized the importance of surgically removing gross tumor when possible to improve the results with local-regional irradiation, reporting a local-regional failure rate of only 15 per cent in Stage III patients, excluding inflammatory cancer, even without chemotherapy. Arnold and Lesnick (1979) reported the results of radical mastectomy in 229 patients with Stage III breast cancers and found actuarial survival of 33 per cent at 5 years and 22 per cent at 10 years. Treatment with preoperative or postoperative irradiation therapy did not lead to survival superior to that of mastectomy alone. Ninety per cent of the patients had recurrence, predominantly systemic, within 10 years, and the results were similar whether irradiation was given preoperatively or postoperatively.

Rao and associates (1982) reported that in Stage III patients treated with radiation therapy, the local failure rate and the 5 year disease-free survival were influenced by the size of the primary tumor and the nodal status. These rates were unaffected by grave local signs. Patients with large tumors (more than 8 cm) had a local failure rate of 76 per cent, and those with gross adenopathy had regional failure in 58 per cent. Thus, radiation alone was not able to control residual gross disease. No influence of tumor size or nodal involvement was noted when patients received a combination of radiation therapy and mastectomy.

In an analysis of 108 consecutive patients with Stage III breast cancer, Balawajder and colleagues (1983) found that radiation followed by mastectomy improved 5 year local control (80 per cent) but did not alter the probability of remaining free from metastatic disease. Minimum tumor doses of 6000 rad were recommended.

Townsend and coworkers (1985) sought to reduce the incidence of local recurrence in patients with locally-regionally advanced breast cancer with a combination of initial radiation followed by total mastectomy. Radiation consisted of 4500 to 5000 rad to the breast, chest wall, and regional lymph nodes over 5 weeks. Fifty-three patients were so treated and followed from 3 to 134 months. Twenty-two patients (41 per cent) developed wound complications. Recurrences were seen in six of the 53 patients (11 per cent). Although a significant reduction appeared to occur in local recurrences, there was rapid development of distal dissemination.

Although the combination of surgery and radiation therapy may increase local control, it would not be expected to influence preexisting occult distant metastases nor to influence survival or overall failure rates. Systemic therapy might influence both, hence its recent emphasis.

SYSTEMIC THERAPY

In one of the first prospective trials of systemic chemotherapy, DeLena and colleagues (1978) demonstrated that the addition of systemic chemotherapy with doxorubicin hydrochloride (Adriamycin) and vincristine both before and after irradiation improved relapse-free survival and total survival compared with historical controls. Still, local treatment failure was observed in 37.5 per cent of the patients. This lead to a rare randomized study of Stage III patients in which local irradiation and mastectomy were found equally efficacious in producing local control in operable cases if preceded by systemic chemotherapy (DeLena et al., 1981). In this study, 132 women with operable Stage III carcinoma (not inflammatory) who had no involvement of supraclavicular nodes received three cycles of Adriamycin plus vincristine and then were randomized for (1) radical (or modified) mastectomy or (2) radiation therapy to the breast and regional nodes (6000 rad over 6 weeks). Local treatment was followed by continued chemotherapy to a cumulative dose of 500 mg/m^2 of Adriamycin. In excess of 79 per cent of patients responded to initial chemotherapy. There was no significant difference between the two treatment groups in terms of patterns of treatment failure, median duration of response, and total survival. Local-regional control was achieved in 50 per cent of both groups at 3 years after treatment ended, and survival was a similar 51.7 per cent and 49.1 per cent at 4 years. The study did not address whether the combination of surgery and irradiation would improve local control.

Shanta and coworkers (1985) treated 521 patients with Stage III breast cancer who were unsuitable for initial surgery. Most of the patients treated earlier had preoperative irradiation followed by radical mastectomy, whereas 109 patients treated between 1976 and 1978 received preoperative concomitant chemotherapy and irradiation and then a Patey modified mastectomy. Tumors became resectable in 68 per cent and 77 per cent of the two groups. All premenopausal patients had a bilateral oophorectomy. Chemotherapy included methotrexate, fluorouracil, and Endoxan. Five year survival without disease was 45 per cent in the earlier group, in contrast to 64.6 per cent in the group that received systemic chemotherapy. The authors concluded that preoperative chemotherapy added to radiation distinctly improved the survival of these patients, but the effect was almost entirely in the cases with positive nodes. Hery and colleagues in France (1986) also used induction chemotherapy with three cycles of cyclophosphamide, Adriamycin (doxorubicin hydrochloride), fluorouracil, and vincristine (CAFV) followed by local-regional irradiation and then maintenance chemotherapy to treat 25 patients. Responses of 50 per cent or more were observed in 86 per cent of the breast lesions and in 80 per cent of cases of adenopathy. Local recurrences occurred in 24 per cent of the patients, and the survival rate of 4 years was a favorable 55 per cent.

Hortobagyi and coworkers (1983) reported a high rate of complete remission in Stage III cases managed with initial systemic therapy with 5-fluorouracil, Adriamycin, and cyclophosphamide (FAC) plus bacille Calmette-Guérin (BCG). This was followed by simple mastectomy or radiotherapy, or a combination of the two, and then continued chemotherapy. Ninety-four per cent of patients were rendered disease-free, but treatment compliance was poor, and only 32 of 52 patients (62 per cent) completed the full 2 years of treatment. After a median follow-up of 60 months, local recurrences were observed in 21 per cent of patients, and 55 per cent of patients were alive at 5 years.

Aisner and associates (1982) treated 27 patients with inoperable bulky primary tumors initially with three to four courses of chemotherapy (CAF with and without vincristine and prednisone). Seventy-four per cent of patients responded with tumor reduction; 4 per cent had a complete response. Thirty-six per cent of the patients had local recurrence, and after 3 years, 42 per cent of patients with noninflammatory Stage IIIb tumors were alive, approximately what is generally expected.

Papaioannou and associates (1983) conducted a trial of initial systemic combination chemoendocrine therapy followed by mastectomy with complete axillary dissection and then randomized the patients to local-regional irradiation followed by 10 additional cycles of chemotherapy and antiestrogen. They encountered numerous complications of chemotherapy, including one death, and reported that local disease control was not enhanced by the addition of irradiation.

Loprinzi and coworkers (1984) reported a pilot study using initial surgery to remove gross disease followed by radiation and non–cross-resistant alternating chemotherapy regimens. Patients had Stages IIIa and IIIb and inflammatory carcinomas. Thirty-two women were treated with initial surgery followed by two courses of induction chemotherapy with CMF ± prednisone ± tamoxifen. Local-regional radiotherapy followed and then randomization to maintenance chemotherapy with the earlier regimen, alternating with Adriamycin or vincristine ± tamoxifen. After a follow-up of 19 to 70 months, the 3 year survival was 65 per cent; median disease-free survival time was 29.5 months. Cardiotoxicity was seen in 25 per cent of the patients, and this high frequency was thought to be attributable to the combination of Adriamycin and radiotherapy.

SUMMARY

Systemic therapy is a regular feature of therapy for Stage III breast cancer. Patients with operable disease who fit this category will often receive systemic therapy as a postoperative adjuvant because of nodal metastases. In cases that are clearly inoperable, its use initially is a logical development. Tumor response can be evaluated, a considerable number of patients are converted to an operable status, and the development of dissemination may be delayed with a modest improvement in disease-free and observed survival (Olson, 1986). Radiation is currently the mainstay of local-regional treatment in nonoperable cases and can be made technically and probably biologically more effective by the surgical elimination of gross disease either beforehand or afterward in selected cases. The combination of surgery and irradiation appears to improve the prospects for local-regional control. It has little detectable effect on distant failure, which depends for its control on effective systemic therapy.

Inflammatory Carcinoma

The signs and symptoms of inflammatory carcinoma have been discussed in Chapter 6. This variant is considered separately here because of its distinctive nature and the special challenge it presents to effective treatment; this tumor is staged according to extent, as is any other, although it is given special distinction in the TNM staging system.

Dermal lymphatic invasion is the pathologic hallmark for inflammatory carcinoma. Most clinicians, however, still accept the classic clinical signs of diffuse redness, edema, heat, and general enlargement and induration of the breast as satisfying the diagnosis. Reports in the literature include cases with appropriate clinical signs, whether or not dermal lymphatic invasion is documented. Inflammatory carcinoma is generally found in TNM Stages IIIb and IV, and the tumors may be of various histologic types. Emphasis on involvement of dermal lymphatics has created some confusion about defining the entity, as cases can be found in which this is present without typical clinical signs, in which it is present with clinical signs, and in which it is not found when the clinical signs are present. Many authors omit the first category (dermal lymphatic involvement without clinical signs) from clinical reports. Ellis and Teitelbaum (1974) could document no instance of dermal lymphatic invasion in eight patients with inflammatory carcinoma who had lived for 5 years after mastectomy and emphasized the key importance of this finding. However, Lucas and Perez-Mesa (1978) found that the prognosis was poor in all three circumstances, although perhaps slightly less so when clinical signs were absent (Fig. 12–41). Therefore, in the presence of typical clinical signs, the presence or absence of dermal lymphatic invasion appears to have no influence on prognosis. It now appears that the more reliable histologic feature of inflammatory carcinoma is the regular presence of extensive lymphatic involvement within the breast, which may or

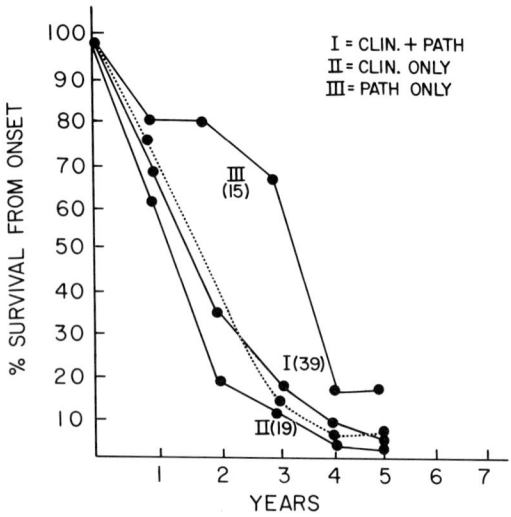

Figure 12–41. The survival of patients with typical clinical signs of inflammatory carcinoma (CLIN) is equally poor whether or not dermal lymphatic invasion can be demonstrated histologically (PATH). Patients with dermal lymphatic invasion but without a characteristic clinical picture have a prognosis that is slightly more favorable. (From Lucas, F. V., and Perez-Mesa, M.: Inflammatory carcinoma of the breast. Cancer, 41:1595, 1978. Reprinted with permission.)

may not have reached the dermis (Gallager, 1984).

The results with mastectomy for inflammatory carcinoma are so poor that this tumor has been considered inoperable since the early decades of this century (Lee and Tannenbaum, 1925). Haagensen (1971) reported that none of 20 patients treated with radical mastectomy were cured, and 50 per cent had recurrence on the chest wall. As a consequence, irradiation has been the preferred treatment, but still with little success in permanent control. The work of Chu and associates (1980) is representative, in which a 6 per cent 10 year disease-free survival followed irradiation with 69 per cent chest wall recurrence. The combination of mastectomy and irradiation has achieved minimal improvement (Bozzetti et al., 1981).

It is plain that micrometastases are present regularly at distant sites even when gross metastases are not, and this problem, which guarantees failure, is not addressed by local treatment. Typical results prior to 1965 are seen in the author's experience at EFSCH. Fifty-one patients with this diagnosis were seen prior to 1965. These cases represented approximately 2 per cent of all mammary carcinomas, a proportion generally reported in the literature. All were women, with ages ranging from 33 to 86 years; the average, 57 years, was slightly lower than the mean age of patients with noninflammatory cancers (61 years). In no instance was pregnancy associated. The condition was bilateral and simultaneous in two patients (4 per cent). Unilateral disease was marginally more frequent in the right breast (27 cases) than in the left (22 cases), although the eventual involvement of both breasts as the disease progressed was not uncommon. Barber and coworkers (1961) reported that 18.9 per cent of cases at the Mayo Clinic eventually involved both breasts.

Patients endured their symptoms for a median of 3 months before seeking medical attention. Physical findings included characteristic signs of inflammation: 31 per cent of the patients had increased heat, 88 per cent had edema, 84 per cent had erythema, and 75 per cent reported swelling of the breast. Twenty-four per cent demonstrated all of the foregoing, and 53 per cent reported pain in the breast. Forty-two patients (82 per cent) had axillary adenopathy, and 42 per cent had enlarged supraclavicular lymph nodes. Five patients had been treated with antibiotics for presumed inflammation, and one was treated with excision and drainage for a suspected abscess. Admission white blood cell counts varied from 3900 cells/cm^3 to a high of 12,300 cells/cm^3. Dermal lymphatic invasion was demonstrated in 64 per cent of the 22 patients who had biopsies of the skin. All had histologic diagnoses except three, who were untreated and who died of clinical cancer within 4 to 7 months. In one case, the primary tumor was a medullary carcinoma. One patient had Paget's cells in the epidermis of the nipple.

Seven patients for various reasons received no treatment during the entire course of the disease. These individuals survived a median duration of 6.5 months, ranging from 4 to 36 months. Two long-term survivors (33 and 36 months) raised the mean survival to 14.3 months. All forms of treatment, both local and systemic, were associated with median survivals (13.5 to 41.5 months) superior to those with no treatment, but with mean survivals only slightly increased by 6 months. The patients who had preoperative radiotherapy followed by radical mastectomy enjoyed an interval from their first sign of disease until death that was no longer than those treated with radiotherapy alone, and it was not possible to determine whether the combination provided more permanent local control of cancer than irradiation. One patient treated solely with irradiation was the only 5 year survivor. Systemic therapy with hormones, endocrine ablation, or single-drug chemotherapy did not result in a longer mean clinical course (19.6 months) than did local treatment alone (19.8 months).

Current strategy is a multimodality approach, using intensive multiagent systemic chemotherapy combined with local-regional irradiation and, in selected cases, mastectomy to rid the patient of residual gross or microscopic tumor. The success of this "neochemotherapy" in producing tumor reduction has in some centers reawakened interest in adding mastectomy to irradiation, or sometimes using it as the sole local treatment (Wiseman et al., 1982; Morris, 1983; Israel et al., 1986). Chemotherapy is begun initially and continued after local treatment is completed and typically consists of customary regimens of CAF, CMF, CFP, FAC, and CAFVP (CAFV plus prednisone). Some reduction in tumor mass is achieved in more than 90 per cent of cases, with complete responses ranging from 20 per cent to 72 per cent. After one to three cycles, or after optimum regression, irradiation is begun. If tumor regression is particularly marked with chemotherapy, mastectomy may replace irradiation, but in most instances it is reserved for cases clearly rendered operable in an attempt to achieve more effective local control than might be expected with irradiation alone. Its proper role is yet to be determined. The results achieved with various combinations of multimodality therapy are shown in Table 12–18. Projected survivals are noticeably improved over those that have followed local therapy alone, and local control is also possibly more effective.

At the Medical College of Wisconsin the author and B. Padrta reviewed 27 cases of inflammatory breast cancer treated since 1968. Ages ranged from 27 to 80 years with a median of 47; 30 per cent of the patients were less than 40 years old. One had bilateral involvement at the time of diagnosis. The median duration of symptoms was 6 weeks, and 22 per cent had been treated with antibiotics before diagnosis. The axilla was clinically involved in 73 per cent, and five of the patients already had metastases in bones, lung, or liver. Dermal lymphatic invasion was found in 65 per cent of skin biopsies. Estrogen receptors were measured in 13 cases and only four (33 per cent) were positive. Two of six cases had positive progesterone receptors. The overall survival of the 27 patients was 29 per cent at 5 years.

The 22 cases without dissemination had a 5 year survival of 39 per cent. Among these, a clinically negative axilla or the presence of a distinct breast mass were good prognostic signs, with 5 year survivals of 58 per cent and 52 per cent, respectively. As expected, dermal lymphatic invasion had no influence on prognosis. Initial treatment in all cases except one included irradiation or mastectomy or both, and most received combination chemotherapy. No influence of mastectomy on survival could be appreciated. Fifteen patients received chemotherapy as a component of initial treatment with a 5 year survival of 43 per cent, compared with one of 33 per cent for those who did not. The 5 year survival was 48 per cent for ten cases in which chemotherapy preceded surgery or irradiation.

A clear improvement in survival at this time, in contrast to earlier experience, is evident. It may be that cases are being found earlier, or that all patients now receive combination chemotherapy, if not as an adjuvant, then later in the course of treatment. Evaluation of treatment is difficult because inflammatory carcinoma is not entirely homogeneous prognostically. Patients with involvement of the breast alone have more favorable courses than those with regional node involvement, and the latter do better than patients with distant metastases (McBride and Hortobagyi, 1985; Sherry et al., 1985). Patients with a discrete mass in the breast likewise have a better prognosis than those without a mass (Hagelberg et al., 1984). Younger patients (less than 50 years old) seem to have a poorer prognosis than older patients (Fastenberg et al., 1985). From the therapeutic standpoint, patients whose tumors undergo complete or partial regression on chemotherapy appear to have a more favorable course than those with no response or progression (Fastenberg et al., 1985).

Other authors have found that these tumors often contain estrogen receptors. Sherry and coworkers (1985) reported them positive in 78

Table 12–18. RESULTS WITH TREATMENT OF NONDISSEMINATED INFLAMMATORY CARCINOMA

Reference	Years of Treatment	Total Cases	Dermal Lymphatic Invasion	Treatment	Median Survival	5 Year Survival	DFS	Local Recurrence
Barker et al. (1980)	1948–1972	69	Unknown	RT ± C				46%
McBride and Hortobagyi (1985)	1954–1981	81	Unknown	RT or S ± C		26%		
Chu et al. (1980)	1960–1977	62	27%	RT alone	18 months	14%	6%	69%
Hagelberg et al. (1984)	1969–1980	24	100%	C ± RT ± S	26 months	29%		
Knight et al. (1986)	1974–1982	18	72%	C + RT → S	23 months			29%
Fastenberg et al. (1985)	1973–1981	63	25%	C ± RT ± S	43 months	40%	31%	31%
Sherry et al. (1985)	1976–1983	11	"Most"	C ± RT ± S	27 months	60%		
Israel et al. (1986)	1978–1983	24	Unknown	C → S → C (Trial)	46 months	60%	45%	29%

C, Chemotherapy; S, mastectomy; RT, radiotherapy; DFS, disease-free survival; I, Immunotherapy

Five-year survival and freedom from recurrence of patients with inflammatory carcinoma of the breast has been improved by the addition of systemic combination chemotherapy to local treatment. Local recurrence may also have been reduced by the use of mastectomy in selected cases, but this is less certain.

per cent of nine cases and Hagelberg and colleagues (1984) in 57 per cent of seven cases. Consequently, hormonal therapy as a systemic adjuvant (tamoxifen is usually used) or for palliation is often effective, as may be endocrine ablation.

Conventional forms of palliative therapy provide useful rates of regression in cases of inflammatory carcinoma. Radiotherapy produces objective regressions in the majority (81.3 per cent) of cases in which it is used. Hormonal and endocrine therapy are also of value. One of six (17 per cent) of the author's patients responded to castration, 18 per cent of 11 patients responded to androgens, and one of seven patients (14 per cent) responded to estrogens.

Stage IV (M1)

All of these patients have clinically evident distant metastases that may involve one or more organ systems. Local management is for palliation only; strategy depends on the patient's general condition and the circumstances of the local and regional tumor. Regardless of how obvious the tumor is, a biopsy diagnosis is important in all instances before treatment is initiated. One objective of treatment is to control progressive disease on the chest wall in a manner that will not interfere with systemic therapy and possibly will enhance it. Radical surgery is not the therapy of choice, and resection should be relegated to that which will expedite radiation or systemic treatment. The simplest surgery is best so that potential complications are avoided. Small tumors are removed for diagnosis, estrogen and progesterone receptor assay, and elimination of gross disease. If removal of a large tumor will simplify the physics of irradiation, this can usually be performed with a simple mastectomy. Axillary dissection for extensive and fixed axillary involvement is not a useful procedure. When surgery is not successful in clearing all disease, irradiation to the axilla must be added, and the combination at this site risks considerable morbidity.

Wilson and coworkers' report (1984) on the National Survey of the American College of Surgeons on breast cancer indicated that a surprisingly high proportion of women with initial distant dissemination (50.5 per cent) had a modified or radical mastectomy. Many of these cases were possibly those in which a postoperative bone scan demonstrated metastases after the initial surgery was completed. Appropriate preoperative staging can eliminate this problem; local control can often be achieved with irradiation in these cases rather than adding the burden of a mastectomy to the patient's tribulations.

In a review of 40 cases with distant metastases at the Medical College of Wisconsin between 1967 and 1979, it was found that only 60 per cent of these patients survived for 1 year, 25 per cent for 3 years, and only 5.7 per cent for 5 years. The average age was 64 years, somewhat higher than the 59 years of patients generally first appearing with breast cancer. More than half of these patients (53 per cent) were managed with biopsy or segmentectomy followed by local-regional irradiation or systemic therapy. An additional six patients (15 per cent) were managed with a palliative simple mastectomy. The remainder (32.5 per cent) had a total removal of the breast with a variable extent of axillary lymph node dissection. It was not possible to determine the success of local-regional control achieved by the different procedures during the patient's remaining lifetime, nor is information readily available on this point. Survival was not enhanced by the more radical surgical procedures. Younger patients and those with more favorable cases had more extensive surgery, which may have accounted for a slightly higher 1 year survival (73.6 per cent versus 52 per cent) but 2 and 3 year survivals were virtually identical (42 per cent versus 37 per cent and 26.2 per cent versus 26.4 per cent, respectively). Palliation is a complicated task, and palliative surgery should be performed in consultation with other professionals who will be managing the patient so that a coherent plan is followed. It should enhance rather than interfere with other methods of treatment. When indicated, operations should not transect gross tumor and should be performed in a manner that will ensure prompt healing.

SUMMARY

Despite all combinations of local treatment, the ultimate risk of treatment failure correlates more closely with the stage of the disease at the time of treatment than with the particular form of treatment. Thus, the extent of disease must be considered the major, perhaps the ultimate, determinant of prognosis. Because, under controlled conditions, several therapeutic alternatives have appeared to provide virtually identical end results in terms of survival and ultimate dissemination of the disease, control within the field of treatment with least morbidity may, in fact, be the most meaningful end result of local treatment.

REFERENCES

Adair, F., Berg, J., Joubert, L., et al.: Long-term follow-up of breast cancer patients: The 30-year report. Cancer, 33:1145, 1974.

Aisner, J., Morris, D., Elias, E. G., et al.: Mastectomy as an adjuvant to chemotherapy for locally advanced or metastatic breast cancer. Arch. Surg., 117:882, 1982.

Albert, S., Belle, S., Eckert, D., et al.: Current surgical management of in situ cancer of the female breast. J. Surg. Oncol., 20:99, 1982.

Andersen, J. A.: Lobular carcinoma in situ of the breast. An approach to rational treatment. Cancer, 39:2597, 1977.

Andreassen, M., Dahl-Iverson, E., and Sorenson, B.: Glandular metastases in carcinoma of the breast: Results of a more radical operation. Lancet, 1:176, 1954.

Arnold, D. J., and Lesnick, G. J.: Survival following mastectomy for stage III breast cancer. Am. J. Surg., 137:362, 1979.

Atkins, H., Hayward, J. L., Klugman, D. J., et al.: Treatment of early breast cancer: A report after ten years of a clinical trial. Br. Med. J., 2:423, 1972.

Attiyeh, F. F., Jensen, M., Huvos, A. G., et al.: Axillary micrometastasis and macrometastasis in carcinoma of the breast. Surg. Gynecol. Obste., 144:839, 1977.

Auchincloss, H.: Significance of location and number of axillary metastases in carcinoma of the breast: A justification for a conservative operation. Ann. Surg., 158:37, 1963.

Auchincloss, H.: Modified radical mastectomy: Why not? Am. J. Surg., 119:506, 1970.

Baker, R. R., Holmes, E. R., Alderson, P. O., et al.: An evaluation of bone scans as screening procedures for occult metastases in primary breast cancer. Am Surg., 186:363, 1977.

Balawajder, I., Antich, P. P., and Boland, J.: An analysis of the role of radiotherapy alone and in combination with chemotherapy and surgery in the management of advanced breast carcinoma. Cancer, 51:574, 1983.

Barber, K. W., Jr., Dockerty, M. B., and Clagett, O. T.: Inflammatory carcinoma of the breast. Surg. Gynecol. Obstet., 112:406, 1961.

Barker, J. L., Montague, E. D., and Peters, L. J.: Clinical experience with irradiation of inflammatory carcinoma of the breast with and without elective chemotherapy. Cancer, 44:625, 1980.

Beadle, F. G., and Harris, R. J.: The role of postoperative radiotherapy in the treatment of operable breast cancer. Breast Cancer Res. Treat., 4:159, 1984.

Bedwani, R., Vana, J., Rosner, D., et al.: Management and survival of female patients with "minimal" breast cancer: As observed in the long-term and short-term surveys of the American College of Surgeons. Cancer, 47:2769, 1981.

Bedwinek, J., Rao, D. V., Perez, C., et al.: Stage III and localized stage IV breast cancer: Irradiation alone vs irradiation plus surgery. Int. J. Radiation Oncol. Biol. Phys., 8:31, 1982.

Berg, J. W.: The significance of axillary node levels in the study of breast carcinoma. Cancer, 8:776, 1955.

Berndt, H., and Titze, U.: TNM clinical stage classification of breast cancer. Int. J. Cancer, 4:837, 1969.

Betsill, W. L., Rosen, P. P., Lieberman, P. H., et al.: Intraductal carcinoma. Long-term follow-up after treatment by biopsy alone. J.A.M.A., 239:1863, 1978.

Black, M. M., Barclay, T. H. C., and Hankey, B. F.: Prognosis in breast cancer utilizing histology characteristics of the primary tumor. cancer, 36:2048, 1975.

Blevins, P. K.: Subcutaneous mastectomy and breast replacement: Its role in the treatment of benign, premalignant, and malignant breast disease. Am. Surgeon, 47:281, 1981.

Bloom, H. J. G.: The natural history of untreated breast cancer. Ann. N.Y. Acad. Sci., 114:747, 1964.

Bloom, H. J. G.: Survival of women with untreated breast cancer—past and present. In Forrest, A. P. M., and Kunkler, P. B. (Eds.): Prognostic Factors in Breast Cancer. Baltimore, Williams & Wilkins, 1968, p. 3.

Bloom, H. J. G., Richardson, W. W., and Harries, E. J.: Natural history of untreated breast cancer (1805–1933). Comparison of untreated and treated cases according to histological grade of malignancy. Br. Med. J., 2:213, 1962.

Bond, W. H.: The influence of various treatments of survival rates in cancer of the breast. In Jarrett, A. A. (Ed.): The Treatment of Carcinoma of the Breast. Amsterdam, Excerpta Medica Foundation, 1967, p 24.

Boova, R. S., Bonanni, R., and Rosato, F. E.: Patterns of axillary nodal involvement in breast cancer. Predictability of level one dissection. Ann. Surg., 196:642, 1982.

Bozzetti, F., Saccozzi, R., DeLena, M., et al.: Inflammatory cancer of the breast: Analysis of 14 cases. J. Surg. Oncol., 18:355, 1981.

Bucalossi, P., Veronesi, U., Zinge, L., et al.: Enlarged mastectomy for breast. AJR, 111:119, 1971.

Cahan, W. G., and Castro, E. B.: Significance of a solitary lung shadow in patients with breast cancer. Ann. Surg., 181:137, 1975.

Caceres, E.: An evaluation of radical mastectomy and extended radical mastectomy for cancer of the breast. Surg. Gynecol. Obstet., 125:337, 1967.

Caceres, E.: Incidence of metastases in the internal mammary chain in operable cancer of the breast. Surg. Gynecol. Obstet., 108:715, 1959.

Carter, D., and Smith, R. L.: Carcinoma in situ of the breast. Cancer, 40:1189, 1977.

Casey, J. J., Stempel, B. G., Scanlon, E. F., et al.: The solitary pulmonary nodule in the patient with breast cancer. Surgery, 96:801, 1984.

Castagna, J., Benfield, J. R., Yamada, H., et al.: The reliability of liver scans and function tests in detecting metastases. Surg. Gynecol. Obstet., 134:463, 1972.

Charkes, N. D., Malmud, L. S., Caswell, T., et al.: Preoperative bone scans. Use in women with early breast cancer. J.A.M.A., 233:516, 1975.

Chu, A. M., Wood, W. C., and Doucette, J. A.: Inflammatory breast carcinoma treated by radical radiotherapy. Cancer, 45:2730, 1980.

Citrin, D. L., Furnival, C. M., Bessent, R. G., et al.: Radioactive technetium phosphate bone scanning in preoperative assessment and follow-up study of patients with primary cancer of the breast. Surg. Gynecol. Obstet., *143*:360, 1976.

Clarke, D., Martinez, A., Cox, R. S., et al.: Breast edema following staging axillary node dissection in patients with breast carcinoma treated by radical radiotherapy. Cancer, *49*:2295, 1982.

Clarke, D. H., Le, M. G., Sarrazin, D., et al.: Analysis of local-regional relapses in patients with early breast cancers treated by excision and radiotherapy: Experience of the Institut Gustave-Roussy. Int. J. Radiation Oncol. Biol. Phys., *11*:137, 1985.

Cody, H. S., III, Egeli, R. A., and Urban, J. A.: Rotter's node metastases. Therapeutic and prognostic considerations in early breast carcinoma. Ann. Surg., *199*:266, 1984.

Committee on Clinical Stage Classification and Applied Statistics: Malignant tumours of the breast, clinical stage classification and presentation of results. Int. Union Against Cancer, *17*:544, 1961.

Crile, G., Jr.: Results of conservative treatment of breast cancer at ten and 15 years. Ann. Surg., *181*:26, 1975.

Cutler, S. J.: Classification and extent of disease in breast cancer. Semin. Oncol., *1*:91, 1974.

Cutler, S. J., Asire, A. J., and Taylor, S. G., III: Classification of patients with disseminated cancer of the breast. Cancer, *24*:861, 1969.

Dahl-Iversen, E.: An extended radical operation for carcinoma of the breast. Reflections and results. J. R. Coll. Surg. Edinb., *8*:81, 1963.

Dahl-Iversen, E., and Tobiassen, T.: Radical mastectomy with parasternal and supraclavicular dissection for mammary carcinoma. Ann. Surg., *170*:889, 1969.

Daland, E. M.: Untreated cancer of the breast. Surg. Gynecol. Obstet., *44*:264, 1927.

Danforth, D. N., Jr., Findlay, P. A., McDonald, H. D., et al.: Complete axillary lymph node dissection for stage I-II carcinoma of the breast. J. Clin. Oncol., *4*:655, 1986.

Davies, G. C., Millis, R. R., and Hayward, J. L.: Assessment of axillary lymph node status. Ann. Surg., *192*:148, 1980.

Davis, N., and Baird, R. M.: Breast cancer in association with lobular carcinoma in situ. Clinicopathologic review and treatment recommendation. Am. J. Surg., *147*:641, 1984.

De Lena, M., Varini, M., Zucali, R., et al.: Multimodal treatment for locally advanced breast cancer. Results of chemotherapy-radiotherapy versus chemotherapy-surgery. Cancer Clin. Trials, *4*:229, 1981.

De Lena, M., Zucali, R., Viganotti, G., et al.: Combined chemotherapy-radiotherapy approach in locally advanced (TIIIb-TIVMO) breast cancer. Cancer Chemother. Pharmacol., *1*:53, 1978.

deWaard, F.: Breast cancer incidence and nutritional status with particular reference to body weight and height. Cancer Res., *35*:3351, 1975.

DiStefano, A., Tashima, C. K., Yap, H. Y., et al.: Bone marrow metastases without cortical bone involvement in breast cancer patients. Cancer, *44*:196, 1979.

Donegan, W. L., Sugarbaker, E. D., Handley, R. S., and Watson, F. R.: The Management of Primary Operable Breast Cancer. A Comparison of Time-Mortality Factors After Standard, Extended, and Modified Radical Mastectomy. Sixth National Cancer Conference Proceedings. Philadelphia, J. B. Lippincott Co., 1970, pp. 135–143.

Donegan, W. L.: Patterns and prognosis of advanced breast carcinoma. Missouri Med., *67*:853, 858, 1970.

Donegan, W. L.: Mastectomy in the primary management of invasive mammary carcinoma. *In* Hardy, J. D. (Ed.): Advances in Surgery. Vol. 6. Chicago, Year Book Medical Publishers, 1972, p. 1.

Donegan, W. L.: The influence of untreated internal mammary metastases upon the course of mammary cancer. Cancer, *39*(2):533, 1977.

Donegan, W. L.: Treatment of breast cancer in the elderly. *In* Yancik, R., et al. (Eds.): Perspectives on Prevention and Treatment of Cancer in the Elderly. New York, Raven Press, 1983, p. 83.

Donegan, W. L., Hartz, A. J., and Rimm, A. A.: The association of body weight with recurrent cancer of the breast. Cancer, *41*:1590, 1978.

Donegan, W. L., and Perez-Mesa, C. M.: Lobular carcinoma—an indication for elective biopsy of the second breast. Ann. Surg., *176*:178, 1972.

Durand, J. C., and Pilleron, J. P.: Cancer of the breast, limited excision followed by radiation. Therapy and results in 150 cases treated at the Curie Foundation, 1960 to 1970. Bull. Cancer (Paris), 64:611, 1977.

Eldar, S., Meguid, M. M., and Beatty, J. D.: Cancer of the breast after prophylactic subcutaneous mastectomy. Am. J. Surg., *148*:692, 1984.

El-Domeiri, A. A., and Shroff, S.: Role of preoperative bone scan in carcinoma of the breast. Surg. Gynecol. Obstet., *142*:722, 1976.

Ellis, D. L., and Teitelbaum, S. L.: Inflammatory carcinoma of the breast: A pathologic definition. Cancer, *33*:1045, 1974.

Farrow, J. H.: The James Ewing Lecture. Current concepts in the detection and treatment of the earliest of the early breast cancers. Cancers, *25*:468, 1970.

Fastenberg, N. A., Buzdar, A. U., Montague, E. D., et al.: Management of inflammatory carcinoma of the breast. A combined modality approach. Am. J. Clin. Oncol., *8*:134, 1985.

Felix, E. L., Bagley, D. H., Sindelar, W. F., et al.: The value of the liver scan in preoperative screening of patients with malignancies. Cancer, *38*:1137, 1976.

Fentiman, I. S., Lavelle, M. A., Caplan, D., et al.: The significance of supraclavicular fossa node recurrence after radical mastectomy. Cancer, *57*:908, 1986.

Ferguson, D. J., Meier, P., Karrison, T., et al.: Staging of breast cancer and survival rates. No assessment based on 50 years of experience with radical mastectomy. J.A.M.A., *248*:1337, 1982.

Findlay, P. A., Lippman, M. E., Danforth, D., Jr., et al.: Mastectomy versus radiotherapy as treatment for stage I-II breast cancer: A prospective randomized trial at the National Cancer Institute. World J. Surg., *9*:671, 1985.

Fisher, B., and Slack, N. H.: Number of lymph nodes examined and the prognosis of breast carcinoma. Surg. Gynecol. Obstet., *131*:79, 1970.

Fisher, B., Redmond, C., Fisher, E. R., et al.: Ten-year results of a randomized clinical trail comparing radical mastectomy and total mastectomy with or without radiation. N. Engl. J. Med., *312*:674, 1985b.

Fisher, B., Bauer, M., Margolese, R., et al.: Five-year results of a randomized clinical trial comparing total mastectomy and segmental mastectomy with or without radiation in the treatment of breast cancer. N. Engl. J. Med., *312*:665, 1985a.

Fisher, B., Slack, N., Katrych, D., et al.: Ten year follow-up results of patients with carcinoma of the breast in a cooperative clinical trial evaluating surgical adjuvant chemotherapy. Surg. Gynecol. Obstet., *140*:528, 1975b.

Fisher, B., Wolmark, N., Bauer, M., et al.: The accuracy of clinical nodal staging and of limited axillary dissection as a determinant of histologic nodal status in carcinoma of the breast. Surg. Gynecol. Obstet., *152*:765, 1981.

Fisher, E. R., Gregorio, R. M., Fisher, B., et al.: The pathology of invasive breast cancer. A syllabus derived from findings of the National Surgical Adjuvant Breast Project (Protocol No. 4). Cancer, *36*:1, 1975a.

Fisher, E. R., Sass, R., Fisher, B., et al.: Pathologic findings from the National Surgical Adjuvant Breast Project (Protocol 6) I. Intraductal carcinoma (DCIS). Cancer, *57*:197, 1986a.

Fisher, E. R., Sass, R., Fisher, B., et al.: Pathologic findings from the National Surgical Adjuvant Breast Project (Protocol 6). II. Relation of local breast recurrence to multicentricity. Cancer, *57*:1717, 1986b.

Fletcher, G. H., Montague, E. D., Tapley, N. D., et al.: Radiotherapy in the management of nondisseminated breast cancer. *In* Fletcher, G. H. (Ed.): Textbook of Radiotherapy. 3rd Ed. Philadelphia, Lea and Febiger, 1980, p. 527.

Foote, F. W., Jr., and Stewart, F. W.: Lobular carcinoma in situ. A rare form of mammary cancer. Am. J. Pathol., *17*:491, 1941.

Forber, J. E.: Incurable cancer. Ministry of Health Reports on Public Health and Medical Subjects, No. LXVI. London, His Majesty's Stationery Office, 1931.

Forrest, A. P. M., Stewart, H. J., Roberts, M. M., et al.: Simple mastectomy and axillary node sampling (pectoral node biopsy) in the management of primary breast cancer. Ann. Surg., *196*:371, 1982.

Francchia, A. A., Evans, J. F., and Eisenberg, B. L.: Stage III carcinoma of the breast. A detailed analysis. Ann. Surg., *192*:705, 1980.

Galasko, C. S. B.: The significance of occult skeletal metastases, detected by skeletal scintigraphy, in patients with otherwise apparently "early" mammary carcinoma. Br. J. Surg., *62*:694, 1975.

Gallager, H. S.: Pathologic types of breast cancer: Their prognoses. Cancer, *53*:623, 1984.

Gallager, H. S., and Martin, J. E.: The study of mammary carcinoma by mammography and a whole organ sectioning—early observations. Cancer, *23*:855, 1969.

Gallager, H. S., and Martin, J. E.: An orientation to the concept of minimal breast cancer. Cancer, *28*:1505, 1971.

Gapinski, P. V., and Donegan, W. L.: Estrogen receptors and breast cancer: Prognostic and therapeutic implications. Surgery, *88*:386, 1980.

Gibbons, J., Holleb, A. I., and Farrow, J. H.: An evaluation of routine preoperative skeletal survey for the patient with operable breast cancer. N.Y. State J. Med., *61*:4219, 1961.

Grace, E. J., and Moitrier, W., Jr.: Simple mastectomy with x-ray in the treatment of cancer of breast. N.Y. State J. Med., *26*:1, 1936.

Greenough, R. B., Simmons, C. C., and Barney, J. D.: The results of operations for cancer of the breast at the Massachusetts General Hospital from 1894 to 1904. Am. Surg. Assoc., *25*:80, 1907.

Greenwood, M.: The natural history of cancer. Ministry of Health Reports on Public Health and Medical Subjects, No. XXVI, London, His Majesty's Stationery Office, 1926.

Haagensen, C. D.: Diseases of the Breast. Philadelphia, W.B. Saunders, 1971, pp. 426, 582, 637, 642.

Haagensen, C. D.: Diseases of the Breast, 3rd Ed. Philadelphia, W. B. Saunders, 1986, p. 240.

Haagensen, C. D.: The choice of treatment of operable carcinoma of the breast. Surgery, *76*:685, 1974.

Haagensen, C. D., and Bodian, C.: A personal experience with Halsted's radical mastectomy. Ann. Surg., *199*:143, 1984.

Haagensen, C. D., and Stout, A. P.: Carcinoma of the breast; criteria for operability. Ann. Surg., *118*:859, 1032, 1943.

Haagensen, C. D., Cooley, E., Miller, E., et al.: Treatment of early mammary carcinoma. A cooperative international study. Ann. Surg., *170*:875, 1969.

Haagensen, C. D., Lane, N., and Bodian, C.: Coexisting lobular neoplasia and carcinoma of the breast. Cancer, *51*:1468, 1983.

Haagensen, C. D., Lane, N., Lattes, R., et al.: Lobular neoplasia (so-called lobular carcinoma in situ) of the breast. Cancer, *42*:737, 1978.

Hagelberg, R. S., Jolly, P. C., and Anderson, R. P.: Role of surgery in the treatment of inflammatory breast carcinoma. Am. J. Surg., *148*:125, 1984.

Halsted, W. S.: The results of operations for the cure of cancer of the breast performed at the Johns Hopkins Hospital from June 1889 to January 1894. Johns Hopkins Hosp. Rep., *4*:297, 1894–95.

Halsted, W. S.: A clinical and histological study of certain adenocarcinoma of the breast: And a brief consideration of the supraclavicular operation and of the results of operations for cancer of the breast from 1889–1898 at the Johns Hopkins Hospital. Trans. Am. Surg. Assoc., *16*:144, 1898.

Halsted, W. S.: Developments in the skin grafting operation for mammary carcinoma. Trans. Am. Surg. Assoc., *30*:287, 1912.

Handley, R. S.: A surgeon's view of the spread of breast cancer. Cancer, *24*:1231, 1969.

Handley, R. S.: Modified radical mastectomy. *In* Nora, P.F. (Ed.): Operative Surgery—Principles and Techniques. Philadelphia, Lea & Febiger, 1972, p. 198.

Handley, R. S.: Techniques of surgical treatment. *In* Atkins, H. (Ed.): The Treatment of Breast Cancer. Baltimore, University Park Press, 1974, p. 49.

Handley, R., Patey, D., and Hand, B.: Excision of the internal mammary chain in radical mastectomy. Results of 57 cases. Lancet, *1*:457, 1956.

Handley, R. S., and Thackray, A. C.: Conservative and radical mastectomy (Patey's operation). Ann. Surg., *157*:162, 1962.

Handley, R. S., and Thackray, S. G.: Internal mammary lymph chain in carcinoma of the breast. Study of 50 cases. Lancet, *2*:276, 1949.

Handley, W. S.: Parasternal invasion of thorax in breast cancer and its suppression by use of radium tubes as operative precaution. Surg. Gynecol. Obstet., *45*:721, 1927.

Harris, J. R., Recht, A., Amalric, R., et al.: Time course and prognosis of local recurrence following primary radiation therapy for early breast cancer. J. Clin. Oncol., *2*:37, 1984.

Hayward, J. L.: The Guy's hospital trials on breast conservation. *In* Harris, J. R., Hellman, S., and Silen, W. (Eds.): Conservative Management of Breast Cancer. New Surgical and Radiotherapeutic Techniques. Philadelphia, J. B. Lippincott, 1983, p. 77.

Henderson, I. C., and Canellos, G. P.: Cancer of the breast. The past decade. N. Engl. J. Med., *302*:17, 1980.

Hery, M., Namer, M., Moro, M., et al.: Conservative treatment (chemotherapy/radiotherapy) of locally advanced breast cancer. Cancer, *57*:1744, 1986.

Hoffman, H. C., and Marty, R.: Bone scanning. Its value in the preoperative evaluation of patients with suspicious breast masses. Am. J. Surg., 124:194, 1972.

Holleb, A. I., Montgomery, R., and Farrow, J. H.: Hazard of incomplete simple mastectomy. Surg. Gynecol. Obstet., 121:819, 1965.

Hortobagyi, G. N., Blumenschein, G. R., Spanos, W., et al.: Multimodal treatment of locoregionally advanced breast cancer. Cancer, 51:763, 1983.

Host, H., and Lund, E.: Age as a prognostic factor in breast cancer. Cancer, 57:2217, 1986.

Hunter, R. L., Ferguson, D. J., and Coppleson, L. W.: Survival with mammary cancer related to the interaction of germinal center hyperplasia and sinus histiocytosis in axillary and internal mammary lymph nodes. Cancer, 36:528, 1975.

Hutter, R. V. P.: The management of patients with lobular carcinoma in situ of the breast. Cancer, 53:798, 1984.

Ingle, J. N., Tormey, D. C., and Tan, H. K.: The bone marrow examination in breast cancer. Diagnostic considerations and clinical usefulness. Cancer, 41:670, 1978.

Israel, L., Breau, J. L., Goguel, B., et al.: Impact of post mastectomy irradiation on survival and recurrence rates. A retrospective study comparing 345 irradiated and 432 non irradiated patients between 1972 and 1984. Proceedings of ASCO 5:58, 1986.

Israel, L., Breau, J. L., and Morere, J. F.: Two years of high-dose cyclophosphamide and 5-fluorouracil followed by surgery after 3 months for acute inflammatory breast carcinomas. A phase II study of 25 cases with a median follow-up of 35 months. Cancer, 57:24, 1986.

Kaae, S., and Johansen, H.: Simple mastectomy plus postoperative irradiation by the method of McWhirter for mammary carcinoma. Ann. Surg., 170:805, 1969.

Kay, S.: Evaluation of Rotter's lymph nodes in radical mastectomy specimens as a guide to prognosis. Cancer, 18:1441, 1965.

Keynes, G.: Radium treatment of breast cancer. Br. J. Surg., 19:415, 1932.

Klamer, T. W., Donegan, W. L., and Max, M. H.: Breast tumor incidence in rats after partial mammary resection. Arch. Surg., 118:933, 1983.

Knight, C. D., Jr., Martin, J. K., Jr., Welch, J. S., et al.: Surgical considerations after chemotherapy and radiation therapy for inflammatory breast cancer. Surgery, 99:385, 1986.

Knight, W. A., III, Livingston, R., Gregory, E., et al.: Estrogen receptor as an independent prognostic factor for early recurrence in breast cancer. Cancer Res., 37:4669, 1977.

Komaki, R., Donegan, W. L., Manoli, R., et al.: Prognostic value of pretreatment bone scans in breast carcinoma. AJR, 132:877, 1979.

Kurtz, M. J., Spitalier, M. J., and Amalric, R.: Results of salvage surgery for local failure following conservative therapy of operable breast cancer. Front. Radiat. Ther. Oncol., 17:84, 1983.

Kusama, S., Spratt, J. S., Donegan, W. L., et al.: The gross rates of growth and human mammary carcinoma. Cancer, 30:594, 1972.

Lacour, J., Bucalossi, P., Caceres, E., et al.: Radical mastectomy versus radical mastectomy plus internal mammary dissection. Cancer, 37:206, 1976.

Lacour, J., Le, M., Caceres, E., et al.: Radical mastectomy versus radical mastectomy plus internal mammary dissection. Cancer, 51:1941, 1983.

Lagios, M. D., Richards, V. E., Rose, M. R., et al.: Segmental mastectomy without radiotherapy. Short-term follow-up. Cancer, 52:2173, 1983.

Lagios, M. D., Westdahl, P. R., Margolin, F. R., et al.: Duct carcinoma in situ. Relationship of extent of non-invasive disease to the frequency of occult invasion, multicentricity, lymph node metastases, and short-term treatment failures. Cancer, 50:1309, 1982.

Lambird, P. A., and Shelley, W. M.: The spatial distribution of lobular in situ mammary carcinoma. J.A.M.A., 210:689, 1969.

Lattes, R.: Lobular neoplasia (lobular carcinoma in situ) of the breast—a histological entity of controversial clinical significance. Pathol. Res. Pract., 166:415, 1980.

Lee, B. J., and Stubenbord, J. G.: Clinical index of malignancy for carcinoma of the breast. Surg. Gynecol. Obstet., 47:812, 1928.

Lee, B. J., and Tannenbaum, N. E.: Inflammatory carcinoma of the breast. Surg. Gynecol. Obstet., 75:580, 1925.

Lee, Y. T.: Delayed cutaneous hypersensitivity, lymphocyte count, and blood tests in patients with breast carcinoma. J. Surg. Oncol., 27:135, 1984.

Lesnick, G. J., and Papatestas, A.: Results of treatment of stage I and stage II primary carcinoma of the breast by modified radical mastectomy with preservation of the pectoralis major muscle (Patey's operation). Abstract for the XI International Cancer Congress, Florence, Italy, October 20–26, 1974.

Lewi, H. J., Roberts, M. M., Donaldson, A. A., et al.: The use of cerebral computer assisted tomography as a staging investigation of patients with carcinoma of the breast and malignant melanoma. Surg. Gynecol. Obstet., 151:385, 1980.

Livingston, S., and Arlen, M.: The extended extrapleural radical mastectomy. Ann. Surg., 179:260, 1974.

Loprinzi, C. L., Carbone, P. P., Tormey, D. C., et al.: Aggressive combined modality therapy for advanced local-regional breast carcinoma. J. Clin. Oncol., 2:157, 1984.

Lucas, F. V., and Perez-Mesa, C.: Inflammatory carcinoma of the breast. Cancer, 41:1595, 1978.

Lythgoe, P. J., and Palmer, K. M.: Manchester regional breast study—5 and 10 year results. Br. J. Surg., 69:693, 1982.

MacKay, E. N., and Sellers, A. H.: A clinical trial of TNM staging of breast cancer. Ontario, 1960–1962. Int. J. Cancer, 1:511, 1968.

Madden, J. L.: Modified radical mastectomy. Surg. Gynecol. Obstet., 121:1221, 1965.

Maddox, W. A., Carpenter, J. T., Laws, H. L., et al.: A randomized prospective trial of radical (Halsted) mastectomy versus modified radical mastectomy in 311 breast cancer patients. Ann. Surg., 198:207, 1983.

Mambo, N. C., and Gallager, H. S.: Carcinoma of the breast. The prognostic significance of extranodal extension of axillary disease. Cancer, 39:2280, 1977.

Margottini, M., and Bucalossi, P.: Le metastasi linfoghiandolari mammarie interne nel cancro della mammella. Oncologia, 23:70, 1949.

Matas, R.: Personal experience with remarks of the operative treatment of cancer of the breast—discussion. Trans. Am. Surg. Assoc., 16:144, 1898.

McBride, C. M., and Hortobagyi, G. N.: Primary inflammatory carcinoma of the female breast: Staging and treatment possibilities. Surgery, 98:792, 1985.

McDivitt, R. W., Hutter, R. V. P., Foote, F. W., Jr., et al.: In situ lobular carcinoma. A prospective follow-up study indicating cumulative patient risks. J.A.M.A., 201:96, 1967.

McDivitt, R. W., Stewart, F. W., and Berg, J. W.: Tumors of the breast. In Atlas of Tumor Pathology. Washington, D.C., Armed Forces Institute of Pathology, 1968.

McWhirter, R.: Should more radical treatment be attempted in breast cancer? Caldwell Lecture, 1963. AJR, 92:3, 1964.

Meyer, A. C., Smith, S. S., and Potter, M.: Carcinoma of the breast. A clinical study. Arch. Surg., 113:364, 1978.

Meyer, K. K.: Radiation-induced lymphocyte-immune deficiency. A factor in the increased visceral metastases and decreased hormonal responsiveness of breast cancer. Arch. Surg., 101:114, 1970.

Meyer, W.: An improved method of radical operation for carcinoma of the breast. N.Y. Med. Rec., 46:746, 1894.

Meyer, W.: Carcinoma of the breast: Ten years' experience with my method of radical operation. J.A.M.A., 45:297, 1905.

Montague, E. D.: Conservation surgery and radiation therapy in the treatment of operable breast cancer. Cancer, 53:700, 1984.

Morris, D. M.: Mastectomy in the management of patients with inflammatory breast cancer. J. Surg. Oncol., 23:255, 1983.

Morrow, M., and Foster, R. S., Jr.: Staging of breast cancer. A new rationale for internal mammary node biopsy. Arch. Surg., 116:748, 1981.

Muir, R.: The evolution of carcinoma of the mamma. J. Pathol. Bacteriol., 52:155, 1941.

Murray, J. G., Mitchell, J. S., Gresham, G. A.: Management of early cancer of the breast. Report on an international multicentre trial supported by the Cancer Research Campaign. Br. Med. J., 1:1035, 1976.

Muss, H. B., White, D. R., and Cowan, R. J.: Brain scanning in patients with recurrent breast cancer. Cancer, 38:1574, 1976.

Myers, R. E., Sutherland, D. J., et al.: Prognostic value of CEA in breast cancer patients (Abstract). Proc. Am. Assoc. Cancer Res. Am. Soc., 19:148, 1978.

Nathanson, I. T., and Welch, C. E.: Life expectancy and incidence of malignant disease: Carcinoma of the breast. Am. J. Cancer, 28:40, 1936.

NIH Consensus Development Panel: Treatment of primary breast cancer. N. Engl. J. Med., 301:340, 1979.

Olson, J. E.: Breast cancer: Stage III disease. Current Concepts Oncol., 8:17, 1986.

Ozello, L., and Sanpitak, P.: Epithelial-stromal junction in intraductal carcinoma of the breast. Cancer, 26:1186, 1970.

Page, D. L., Dupont, W. D., Rogers, L. W., et al.: Intraductal carcinoma of the breast: Follow-up after biopsy only. Cancer, 49:751, 1982.

Page, M.: President's address. Proc. R. Soc. Med., 41:121, 1948.

Palmer, M. K., Lythgoe, J. P., and Smith, A.: Prognostic factors in breast cancer. Br. J. Surg., 69:697, 1982.

Papaioannou, A. N., and Urban, J. A.: Scalene node biopsy in locally advanced primary breast cancer of questionable operability. Cancer, 17:1006, 1964.

Papaioannou, A., Lissaios, B., Vsilaros, S., et al.: Pre- and postoperative chemoendocrine treatment with or without postoperative radiotherapy for locally advanced breast cancer. Cancer, 51:1284, 1983.

Papatestas, A. E., Lesnick, G. J., Genkins, G., et al.: The prognostic significance of peripheral lymphocyte counts in patients with breast carcinoma. Cancer, 37:164, 1976.

Patey, D. H.: A review of 146 cases of carcinoma of the breast operated on between 1930 and 1943. Br. J. Cancer, 21:260, 1967.

Pavrovsky, J., Tersip, K., and Palecek, L.: Results of radical operation for mammary gland carcinoma with revision of the parasternal space. Int. Surg., 51:509, 1969.

Pearlman, A. W.: Breast cancer—influence of growth rate on prognosis and treatment evaluation. A study based on mastectomy scar recurrences. Cancer, 38:1826, 1976.

Pearlman, N. W., Guerra, O., and Fracchia, A. A.: Primary inoperable cancer of the breast. Surg. Gynecol. Obstet., 143:909, 1976.

Peters, M. V.: Radiation therapy in the management of breast cancer. Proceedings of the Sixth National Cancer Conference. Philadelphia, J. B. Lippincott, 1970, p. 163.

Peters, T. G., Donegan, W. L., and Burg, E. A.: Minimal breast cancer: A clinical appraisal. Ann. Surg., 186:704, 1977.

Phillips, A. J.: A comparison of related and untreated cases of cancer of the breast. Br. J. Cancer, 13:20, 1959.

Pickren, J. W., Rube, J., and Auchincloss, H., Jr.: Modification of conventional radical mastectomy: A detailed study of lymph node involvement and follow-up information to show its practicality. Cancer, 18:942, 1965.

Pigott, J., Nichols, R., Maddox, W. A., et al.: Metastases to the upper levels of the axillary nodes in carcinoma of the breast and its implications for nodal sampling procedures. Surg. Gynecol. Obstet., 158:255, 1984.

Portmann, U. V.: Clinical and pathologic criteria as a basis for classifying cases of primary cancer of the breast. Cleveland Clin. Q., 10:41, 1943.

Powers, R. W., O'Brien, P. H., and Kreutner, A., Jr.: Lobular carcinoma in situ. J. Surg. Gynecol., 13:269, 1980.

Prosnitz, L. R., Goldenberg, I. S., Harris, J. R., et al.: Radiotherapy for carcinoma of the breast instead of mastectomy. An update. Front. Radiat. Ther. Oncol., 17:69, 1983.

Prudente, A.: L'amputation inter-scapulo-mammothoracique (technique et resultats). J. Chir., 65:729, 1949.

Qualheim, R. E., and Gall, E. A.: Breast carcinomas with multiple sites of origin. Cancer, 10:460, 1957.

Raffl, A. B.: The use of negative pressure under skin flaps after radical mastectomy. Ann. Surg., 136:1048, 1952.

Rao, D. V., Bedwinek, J., Perez, C., et al.: Prognostic indicators in stage III and localized stage IV breast cancer. Cancer, 50:2037, 1982.

Recht, A., Danoff, B. S., Solin, L. J., et al.: Intraductal carcinoma of the breast: Results of treatment with excisional biopsy and irradiation. J. Clin. Oncol., 3:1339, 1985.

Ridell, B., and Landys, K.: Incidence and histopathology of metastases of mammary carcinoma in biopsies from the posterior iliac crest. Cancer, 44:1782, 1979.

Riesco, A.: Five-year cancer cure: Relation to total amount of peripheral lymphocytes and neurophils. Cancer, 25:135, 1970.

Robbins, G. F., Knapper, W. H., Barrie, J., et al.: Metastatic bone disease developing in patients with potentially curable breast cancer. Cancer, 29:1702, 1972.

Rosen, P. P., Fracchia, A. A., Urban, J. A., et al.: "Residual" mammary carcinoma following simulated partial mastectomy. Cancer, 35:739, 1975.

Rosen, P. P.: Axillary lymph node metastases in patients with occult noninvasive breast carcinoma. Cancer, 46:1298, 1980.

Rosen, P. P., Braun, D. W., Jr., Lyngholm, B., et al.: Lobular carcinoma in situ of the breast: Preliminary results of treatment by ipsilateral mastectomy and contralateral breast biopsy. Cancer, 47:813, 1981.

Rosen, P. P., Lesser, M. L., Kinne, D. W., et al.:

Discontinuous or "skip" metastases in breast carcinoma. Analysis of 1228 axillary dissections. Ann. Surg., 197:276, 1983.

Rosen, P. P., Lieberman, P. H., Braun, D. W., Jr., et al.: Lobular carcinoma in situ of the breast. Detailed analysis of 99 patients with average follow-up of 24 years. Am. J. Surg. Pathol., 2:225, 1978.

Rosen, P. P., Saigo, P. E., Braun, D. W., Jr., et al.: Occult axillary lymph node metastases form breast cancers with intramammary lymphatic tumor emboli. Am. J. Surg. Pathol., 6:639, 1982.

Rosen, P. P., Senie, R., Schottenfeld, D., et al.: Noninvasive breast carcinoma. Frequency of unsuspected invasion and implications of treatment. Ann. Surg., 189:377, 1979.

Rosner, D., Bedwani, R. N., Vana, J., et al.: Noninvasive breast carcinoma. Results of a national survey by the American College of Surgeons. Ann. Surg., 192:139, 1980.

Sarrazin, D., Le, M., Rouesse, J., et al: Conservative treatment versus mastectomy in breast cancer tumors with microscopic diameter of 20 millimeters or less. The experience of the Institut Gustave-Roussy. Cancer, 53:1209, 1984.

Savlov, E. D., Wittliff, J. L., Hilf, R., et al.: Correlations between certain biochemical properties of breast cancer and response to therapy: A preliminary report. Cancer, 33:303, 1974.

Scanlon, E. F., and Caprini, J. A.: Modified radical mastectomy. Cancer, 35:710, 1975.

Schnitt, S. J., Connolly, J. L., Harris, J. R., et al.: Pathologic predictors of early local recurrence in stage I and II breast cancer treated by primary radiation therapy. Cancer, 53:1049, 1984.

Schottenfeld, D., Nash, A. G., Robbins, G. F., et al.: Ten-year results of the treatment of primary operable breast carcinoma. A study of 304 patients evaluated by the TNM system. Cancer, 38:1001, 1976.

Schwartz, G. F., D'Ugo, D. M., and Rosenberg, A. L.: Extent of axillary dissection preceding irradiation for carcinoma of the breast. Arch Surg. 121:1395–1398, 1986.

Schwartz, G. F., Feig, S. A., Rosenberg, A. L., et al.: Staging and treatment of clinically occult breast cancer. Cancer, 53:1379, 1984.

Schwartz, G. F., Patchefsky, A. S., Feig, S. A., et al.: Clinically occult breast cancer. Multicentricity and implications for treatment. Ann. Surg., 191:8, 1980.

Sears, H. F., Gerber, F. H., Sturtz, D. L., et al.: Liver scan and carcinoma of the breast. Surg. Gynecol. Obstet., 140:409, 1975.

Shanta, V., Krishnamurthi, S., Sastry, D. V. L.N., et al.: Multimodal approach in the therapy of stage III female breast cancer. J. Surg. Oncol., 28:134, 1985.

Sherry, M. M., Johnson, D. H., Page, D. L., et al.: Inflammatory carcinoma of the breast. Clinical review and summary of the Vanderbilt experience with multimodality therapy. Am. J. Med., 79:355, 1985.

Sklaroff, R. B., and Sklaroff, D. M.: Bone metastases from breast cancer at the time of radical mastectomy as detected by bone scan. Eight-year follow-up. Cancer, 38:107, 1976.

Smith, J. A., III, Gamez-Araujo, J., Gallagher, H. S., et al.: Carcinoma of the breast. Analysis of total lymph node involvement versus level of metastasis. Cancer, 39:527, 1977.

Smithers, D. W., Rigby-Jones, P., Galton, D. A. G., et al.: Cancer of the breast: A review. Br. J. Radiol. (Suppl. No. 4), 1, 1952.

Staps, T., Hoogenhout, J., and Wobbes, T.: Phantom breast sensations following mastectomy. Cancer, 56:2898, 1985.

Steinthal, C. F.: Zue Dauerheilung des Brustkrebses. Beitr. z klin. Chir., 47:226, 1905.

Stocks, L. H., and Patterson, F. M. S.: Inflammatory carcinoma of the breast. Surg. Gynecol. Obstet., 143:885, 1976.

Sugarbaker, P. H., Beard, J. O., and Drum, D. E.: Detection of hepatic metastases from cancer of the breast. Am. J. Surg., 133:531, 1977.

Sunshine, J. A., Moseley, H. S., Fletcher, W. S., et al.: Breast carcinoma in situ. A retrospective review of 112 cases with a minimum 10 year follow-up. Am. J. Surg., 150:44, 1985.

Tagert, R., Bratherton, D., Hartley, L., et al.: Partial mastectomy alone in early breast cancer. Br. Med. J., 290:434, 1985.

Tartter, P. I., Papatestas, A. E., Iannovich, L., et al.: Cholesterol and obesity as prognostic factors in breast cancer. Cancer, 47:2222, 1981.

Tinnemans, J. G. M., Wobbes, T., van der Sluis, R. F., et al.: Multicentricity in nonpalpable breast carcinomas and its implications for treatment. Am. J. Surg., 151:334, 1986.

Tomin, R., and Donegan, W. L.: Screening for recurrent breast cancers—Its effectiveness and prognostic value. J. Clin. Oncol., 5(1):62–67, 1987.

Townsend, C. M., Abston, S., and Fish, J. C.: Surgical adjuvant treatment of locally advanced breast cancer. Ann. Surg., 201:604, 1985.

Turner, L., Swindell, R., Bell, W. G. T., et al.: Radical versus modified radical mastectomy for breast cancer. Ann. R. Coll. Surg. Engl., 63:239, 1981.

UICC Committee on Clinical Stage Classification and Applied Statistics: Malignant tumours of the breast, clinical stage classification and presentation of results. Int. Union Against Cancer, 17:544, 1961.

Urban, J. A., and Marjani, M. A.: Significance of internal mammary lymph node metastases in breast cancer. AJR, 111:130, 1971.

Valagussa, P., Bonadonna, P., and Veronesi, U.: Patterns of relapse and survival following radical mastectomy: Analysis of 716 consecutive patients. Cancer, 41:1170, 1978.

Veronesi, U., and Valagussa, P.: Inefficacy of internal mammary nodes dissection in breast cancer surgery. Cancer, 47:170, 1981.

Veronesi, U., Cascinelli, N., Bufalino, R., et al.: Risk of internal mammary lymph node metastases and its relevance on prognosis of breast cancer patients. Ann. Surg., 198:681, 1983.

Veronesi, U., Zucali, R., and Del Vecchio, M.: Conservative treatment of breast cancer with the QU.A.R.T. Technique. World J. Surg., 9:676, 1985.

Vilcoq, J. R., Calle, R., Stacey, P., et al.: The outcome of treatment by tumorectomy and radiotherapy of patients with operable breast cancer. Int. J. Radiation Oncol. Biol. Phys., 7:1327, 1981.

Von Rueden, D. G., and Wilson, R. E.: Intraductal carcinoma of the breast. Surg. Gynecol. Obstet., 158:105, 1984.

Wade, P.: Untreated carcinoma of breast: Comparison with results of treatment of advanced breast carcinoma. Br. J. Radiol., 19:272, 1946.

Wangensteen, O. H.: Remarks upon a more radical operation for breast cancer. Ann. Surg., 130:315, 1949.

Wangensteen, O. H.: Further experiences with a cervicoaxillary mediastinal dissection for cancer of the breast. Ann. Surg., 132:839, 1950.

Wangensteen, O. H.: Another look at super-radical operation for breast cancer. Surgery, 41:857, 1957.

Wangensteen, O. H., Lewis, F. J., and Arhelger, S. W.: The extended or super-radical mastectomy for carcinoma of the breast. Surg. Clin. North Am., 36:1051, 1956.

Webber, B. L., Heise, H., Neifeld, J. P., et al.: Risk of subsequent contralateral breast carcinoma in a population of patients with in-situ breast carcinoma. Cancer, 47:2928, 1981.

Wheeler, J. E., Enterline, H. T., Roseman, J. M., et al.: Lobular carcinoma in situ of the breast. Cancer, 34:554, 1974.

Wiener, S. N., and Sachs, S. H.: An assessment of routine liver scanning in patients with breast cancer. Arch. Surg., 113:126, 1978.

Wilson, R. E., Donegan, W. L., Mettlin, C., et al.: The 1982 national survey of carcinoma of the breast in the United States by the American College of Surgeons. Surg. Gynecol. Obstet., 159:309, 1984.

Windeyer, B. W.: Cancer of the breast. AJR, 62:345, 1949.

Wiseman, C., Jessup, J. M., Smith, T. L., et al.: Inflammatory breast cancer treated with surgery, chemotherapy and allogeneic tumor cell/BCG immunotherapy. Cancer, 49:1266, 1982.

Wyatt, J., Sugarbaker, E., and Stanton, M.: Involvement of internal mammary lymph nodes in carcinoma of the breast. Am. J. Pathol., 31:143, 1955.

Young, J. O., Sadowsky, N. L., Young, J. W., et al.: Mammography of women with suspicious breast lumps. Arch. Surg., 121:807, 1986.

Yorkshire Breast Cancer Group: Critical assessment of the clinical TNM system in breast cancer. Br. Med. J., 281:134, 1980.

Zafrani, B., Fourquet, A., Vilcoq, J. R., et al.: Conservative management of intraductal breast carcinoma with tumorectomy and radiation therapy (Abstract). Int. J. Radiation Oncol. Biol. Phys., 10(Suppl. 2):140, 1984.

Zeman, R. K., Paushter, D. M., Schiebler, M. L., et al.: Hepatic imaging: Current status. Radiol. Clin. North Am., 23:473, 1985.

Zippin, C.: Comparison of the International and American systems for the staging of breast cancer. JNCI, 36:53, 1966.

CHAPTER 13

JOHN S. SPRATT
WILLIAM L. DONEGAN

Surgical Management

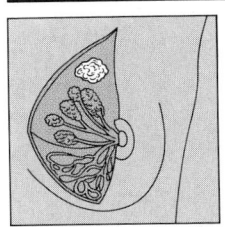

The natural history of mammary cancer is influenced in favor of the host by a variety of surgical procedures. Certain minor procedures are requisite for diagnosis. Therapeutic procedures include (1) removal of the breast entirely or in part, (2) removal of regional site, principally the axillary lymph nodes, and (3) a variety of other operations, including ovariectomy, adrenalectomy, skin grafting, tube thoracostomy, skeletal fixation, and venous access. This chapter discusses a number of these operations with their indications and potential complications.

Biopsy

The presence of a palpable mass and the presence of a suspicious lesion on mammography are the two principal indications for biopsy. Less frequently, chronic encrustations of the nipple suggestive of Paget's disease, chronic nipple discharge, erythema and edema of mammary skin, and cutaneous retraction, which can all occur in association with an impalpable cancer, are indications for biopsy. A course of action for the patient and her physician based on the presence of abnormal findings is contained in the flow diagram in Figure 13–1. The efficacy of this approach requires very close collaboration among diagnostic radiologist, surgeon, and pathologist.

Tissue samples from large masses are easily obtained for histologic diagnosis with the Tru-Cut Disposable Biopsy Needle, 6 inch cannula, 20 mm specimen notch (catalogue number 2N-2704, Travenol Laboratories, Inc., Deerfield, Illinois). The instructions contained on the package in which the needle comes should be followed explicitly. *After* all the pertinent physical findings requisite for proper clinical staging have been recorded, the biopsy is performed. The use of needle biopsy is restricted to tumors larger than 2 cm in diameter that are not deeply seated within the breast. Using the needle on small and mobile lesions increases the chance of obtaining a false negative examination with delay in diagnosis.

The technique for use of the needle is shown in Figure 13–2. If the diagnosis of cancer is not made by the pathologist, an open biopsy is required. Open biopsy is performed in those cases that do not meet the criteria set forth for needle biopsy.

Incisions for mammary biopsy vary with the location of the tumor and the clinical diagnosis and should lie within the bounds of a subsequent operation if one is required. Consideration is given to the subsequent cosmetic appearance. Least obvious scars develop with incisions that follow the lines of cutaneous tension. In the skin of the protuberant breast these lines are concentric, with the nipple at the center, that is, they parallel the circular margin of the areola. The most cosmetic incision therefore is circumareolar. In the presence of skin redness, edema, or suspected skin involvement, a sample of skin should be submitted for biopsy.

Of more importance than appearance, however, is the securing of a representative tissue sample. An incisional biopsy of large lesions is satisfactory. For small lesions, excisional biopsies are performed with a margin of normal tissue. Occasionally small tumors palpable preoperatively and lesions seen only on mammograms cannot be distinguished through the open wound. Special techniques are helpful in localizing them for removal (Chapter 6). If the suspicion of cancer was great enough to merit biopsy in the first place, the surgeon is obligated to remove accurately the tissue giving

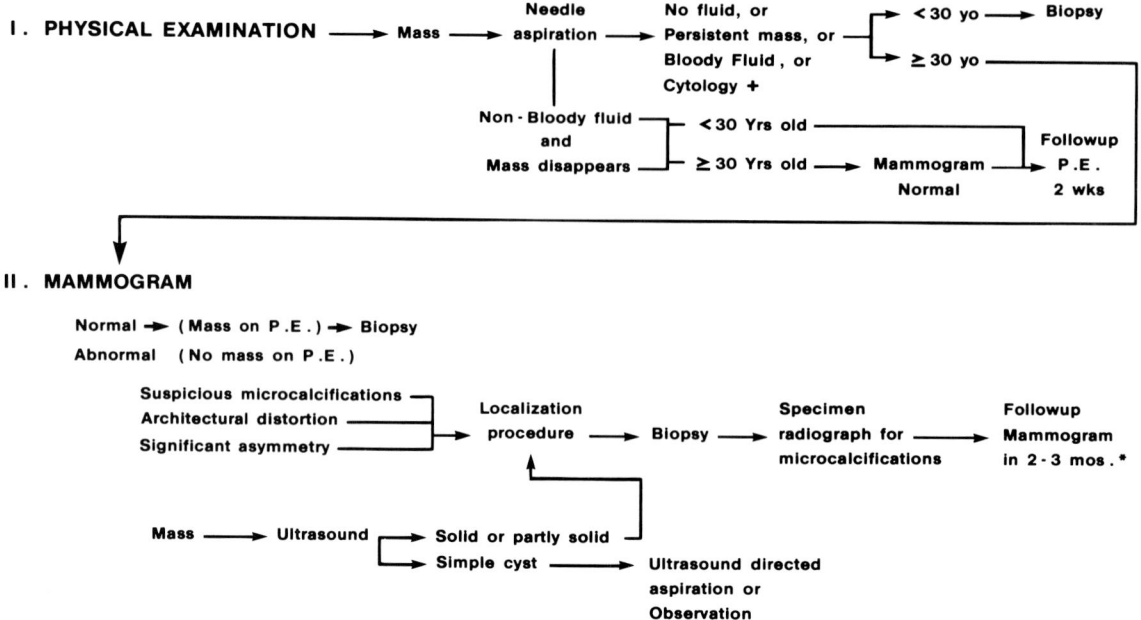

Figure 13–1. Suggested course of action for most frequent abnormal findings on physical examination and mammography.

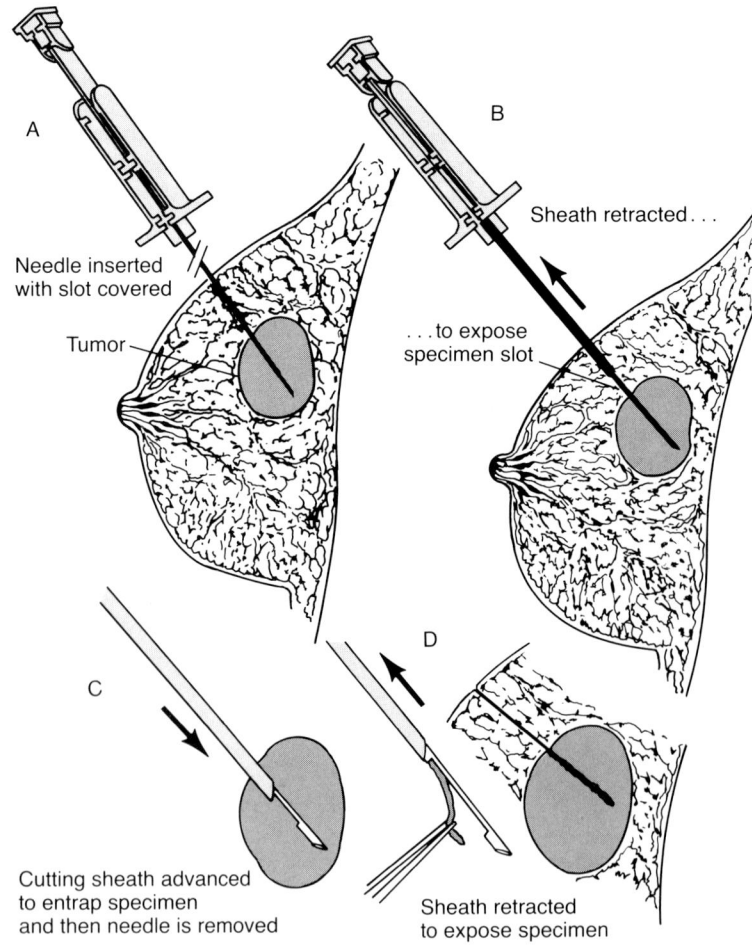

Figure 13–2. The biopsy is taken under local anesthesia. A small incision, the width of the needle shaft, is made, and the shaft is inserted into the breast until the needle passes into the mass that is to be biopsied. The sheath is then retracted to expose the specimen slot, after which it is advanced to shear the specimen from surrounding tissues. An an alternative technique, the needle shaft is advanced into the breast until its tip meets the mass. The obturator alone is advanced into the mass, and the sheath is then slipped forward over it to entrap the specimen. The needle is removed, and gentle pressure is applied on the biopsy site for hemostasis. The specimen is delivered by retracting the sheath of the needle and picking it from the slot or washing it into a specimen dish with a bit of saline. Its size is adequate for a frozen section examination and for permanent sections but not for quantitative sex steroid analysis.

rise to the suspicion. After the skin incision is made, bracketing the area of breast to be biopsied with stay sutures (2-0 Dexon on a large cutting needle) simplifies subsequent dissection.

The pathologist may have to cut the breast tissue into slices several millimeters thick to locate a small, occult neoplasm. With a cryostat, frozen sections of excellent quality that can be cut and stained quickly. If the pathologist is not absolutely certain of the diagnosis of cancer, then the surgeon must await permanent histologic sections. This delay does not affect the prognosis adversely.

Technical points of value include exposure by an adequate incision and wide wound margin retraction. Mammary parenchyma is tough, and ligatures placed about bleeding points with a medium sized cutting needle ensure hemostasis. Electrocautery is adequate for small bleeders. After securing complete hemostasis, drains are not necessary. The technique for open biopsy is shown in Figure 13–3 (see later discussion). A padded dressing secured with elastoplast reduces motion and discomfort in the biopsied breast, as does wearing a brassiere for several days. The elastoplast must not be stretched too taut to avoid traction skin burns. No more than one third of allowable elasticity should be used.

An aliquot of all biopsy specimens should be submitted for estrogen and progesterone receptor assays. The critical steps for submission are given in Table 13–1.

Beatty and coworkers (1983) provide a study on the relation between nosocomial wound infections after mastectomy and premastectomy biopsy. Their overall clean wound infection rate was 8.2 per cent among 294 patients, but this varied considerably according to the type and time of premastectomy biopsy. The lowest infection rates (3.2 per cent) were obtained after needle aspiration biopsy. With mastectomy immediately after open biopsy and frozen section ("one step"), the rate rose to 5.3 per cent. With a mastectomy following an open biopsy ("two step") the infection rate rose to 12.4 per cent. Whenever a 4 to 7 day interval elapsed between open biopsy and mastectomy, the rate of wound infection rose to its highest level (23.0 per cent). Their conclusions were that the longer the delay between

Table 13–1. HANDLING OF TUMOR BIOPSY SPECIMEN FOR STEROID RECEPTOR ANALYSIS

1. Receptor assays may be performed on primary tumors or metastatic lesions of all types. If both are submitted, specimens must be identified separately.

2. Receptors are heat labile. A biopsy specimen should be tansferred from the operation site on ice in an appropriate container (see number 5) on ice and handled at room temperature as little as possible. If the biopsy specimen is taken as part of the frozen section at diagnosis, keep it frozen. Also, if the specimen is to come from the mastectomy specimen, the removed breast should be delivered to pathology. The pathologist must excise promptly an aliquot of cancer to be placed on ice and sent directly for hormone receptor assays.

3. Specimen must be transported and stored dry. Hypertonic saline solutions will interfere with some of the assay methods. *Formalin destroys receptors.* Sterility is not important.

4. Amount of material required is about 0.3 to 0.5 cm^3 of solid tumor, trimmed of excess fat, necrotic, and connective tissues. These constituents add undersirable elements to the binding reaction. If weighing more than 0.4 g, the pathologist should divide the specimen into suitable portions before freezing. (Extra specimens are used for backup.) Assays should not be performed on specimens for which no histologic confirmation is made.

5. Specimens may be frozen in the cryostat, ultrafreezer, or liquid nitrogen. Store and transport dry, preferably in a clean plastic container. Use waterproof marking pen to identify container. Do not use tapes and stickers that are easily detached at low temperatures. Do not include identifying slips in containers if they will be in contact with the specimen. If sent to the Hormone Receptor Laboratory by commercial carrier, the specimen must be packed with sufficient dry ice to last until delivery.

6. Accompanying papers must Include the following:
    a. Patient's name, sex, age, hospital, and accession or admission number
    b. Surgery date and surgery number
    c. Requesting physician's name
    d. Pathologist's name
    e. Kinds of assays requested
    f. Billing address

7. Also submit other information regarding patient's history, especially regarding any previous hormone therapy that might influence steroid receptor levels. Pregnancy status must be stated for the same reason.

8. Mark outside clearly: BIOLOGICAL SPECIMEN; REFRIGERATE IMMEDIATELY; RUSH.

(Courtesy of James L. Wittliff, M.D.)

open biopsy and mastectomy, the higher was the risk of infection. With the lowest infection rate being associated with needle biopsies, they argued for the more frequent use of the needle to obtain histologic diagnosis. The authors have not experienced such high rates of infection.

Surgical Technique and Hormone Receptors

Because the results of estrogen and progesterone receptor assays of breast cancer are considered in the selection of adjuvant therapy routines, the surgeon's care in handling of tissues is important. Bridges and colleagues (1983) compared the hormone receptor values of tumor tissue removed by biopsy and frozen section with tumor tissue obtained after mastectomies. No difference in receptor values were found if removed tissue was kept cold and frozen rapidly. Assay values on biopsy specimens were consistent with the values on resected tissue, precluding the need for separate biopsies solely for hormone receptor assays. Cutting cautery kills tissue and should not be used to obtain specimens (Rosenthal, 1979).

Lymph node biopsy has been restricted to the removal for diagnosis of palpably enlarged lymph nodes in the axilla when no primary cancer in the breast can be found and to the removal of palpable supraclavicular and contralateral axillary lymph nodes when needed for staging.

Occasionally, the surgeon will encounter a mammary abscess and may be inclined to place a drain and discontinue the operation. It is well to remember that such abscesses may be cancers with a necrotic center or an infection associated with a cancer. Rather than being content with drainage alone, the surgeon should always secure a representative biopsy of the wall of the abscess.

Technique for Surgical Biopsy of the Breast

(Figure 13–3)

Indications for surgical biopsy of the breast are discussed in Chapter 6. Here the technique is shown for excisional biopsy of a small palpable tumor mass. The procedure is performed using full sterile precautions with the patient under light sedation. The thorax is elevated on the side to be biopsied using folded sheets and the arm lies to the side on an arm board (Fig. 13–3A). Ten milligrams of diazepam is administered by slow intravenous injection and ordinarily provides suitable sedation. Useful incisions are shown in Figure 13–3B. These are ordinarily placed directly over the tumor mass and follow the skin lines except in the lower hemisphere of the breast. The proposed incision is marked and a local anesthetic is injected into the dermis (Fig. 13–3C). It is not necessary to fill the subcutaneous tissues, although a regional block into the breast tissue around the tumor may be helpful. An incision is made and after a pause to secure dermal and subcutaneous bleeders, it is extended directly down to the tumor mass (Fig. 13–3D). The mass, secured with a Z stitch of 2-0 silk to be used as a tenaculum, is dissected sharply away from the surrounding tissues (Fig. 13–3E). No subcutaneous tissue is removed. At this point, if the tumor is large, only an incisional biopsy may be performed to confirm the diagnosis of cancer. However, if the diagnosis of cancer is not made, the entire mass is removed (Fig. 13–3F). The specimen is placed immediately in crushed ice for transport to the pathologist for frozen section examination. The latter is necessary to determine if an analysis for hormone receptors is appropriate. The biopsy specimen must come from within breast tissue, not subcutaneous tissues, to merit analysis. Closure of the breast tissue defect is not performed, but hemostasis must be absolute. The subcutaneous tissue is closed with interrupted absorbable sutures (Fig. 13–3G). A running subcuticular closure of the skin is performed with a fine absorbable suture followed by Steristrips and a light dressing (Fig. 13–3H). Insert A-B-C shows a cross section of the closure of subcutaneous tissues and skin.

Total Mastectomy

Total mastectomy is an operation that removes the entire mammary gland. It is indicated for sarcomas of the breast and may be used for lobular carcinoma in situ as an alternative to close observation. The incision encompasses the areola. The resection of skin farther than 4 cm from each margin of a palpable tumor achieves nothing therapeutically (Donegan et al., 1966). Resection of all of the skin of the

13 • Surgical Management 407

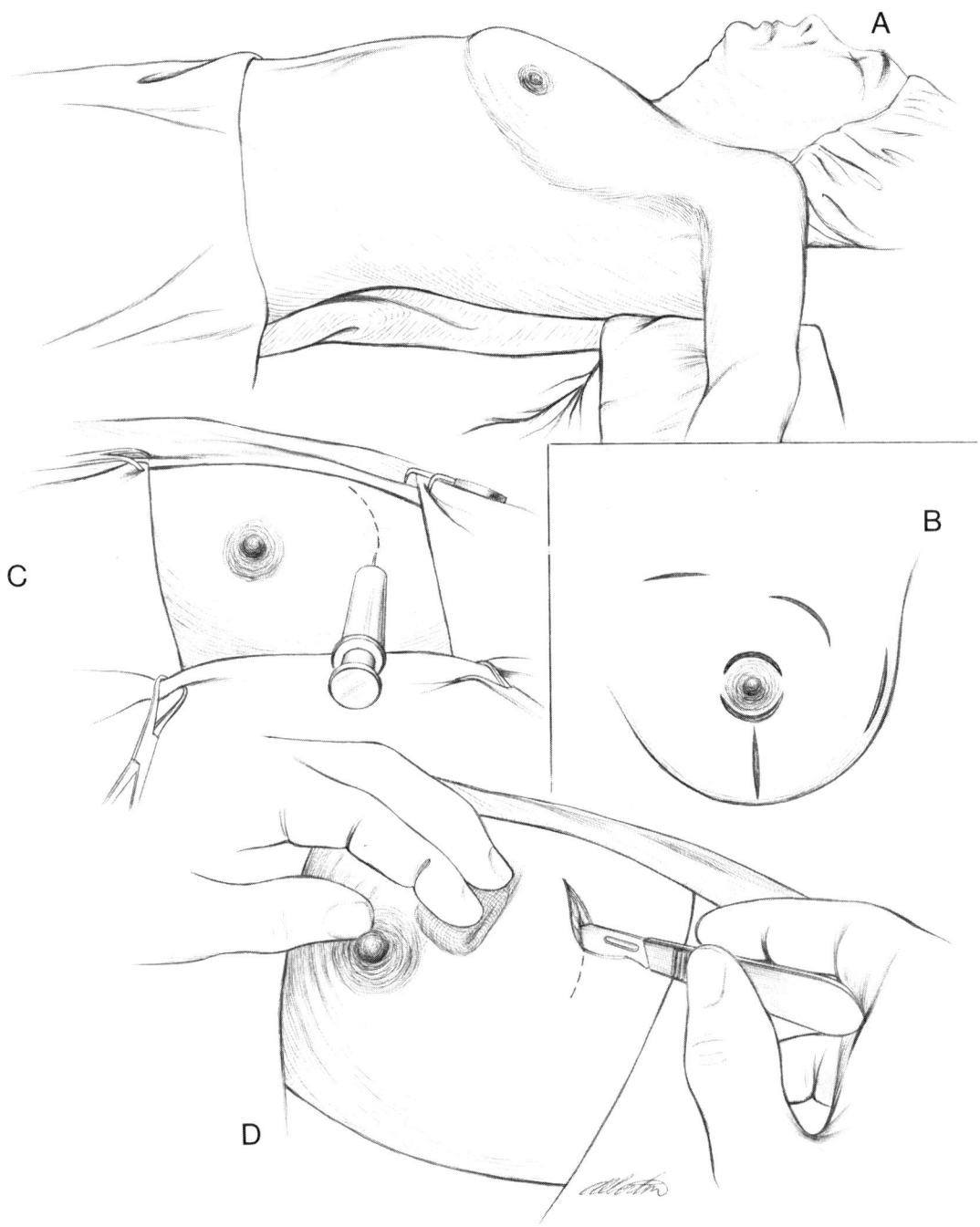

Figure 13–3. *A* to *H*, Technique for surgical biopsy of the breast. See text for details.
Illustration continued on following page

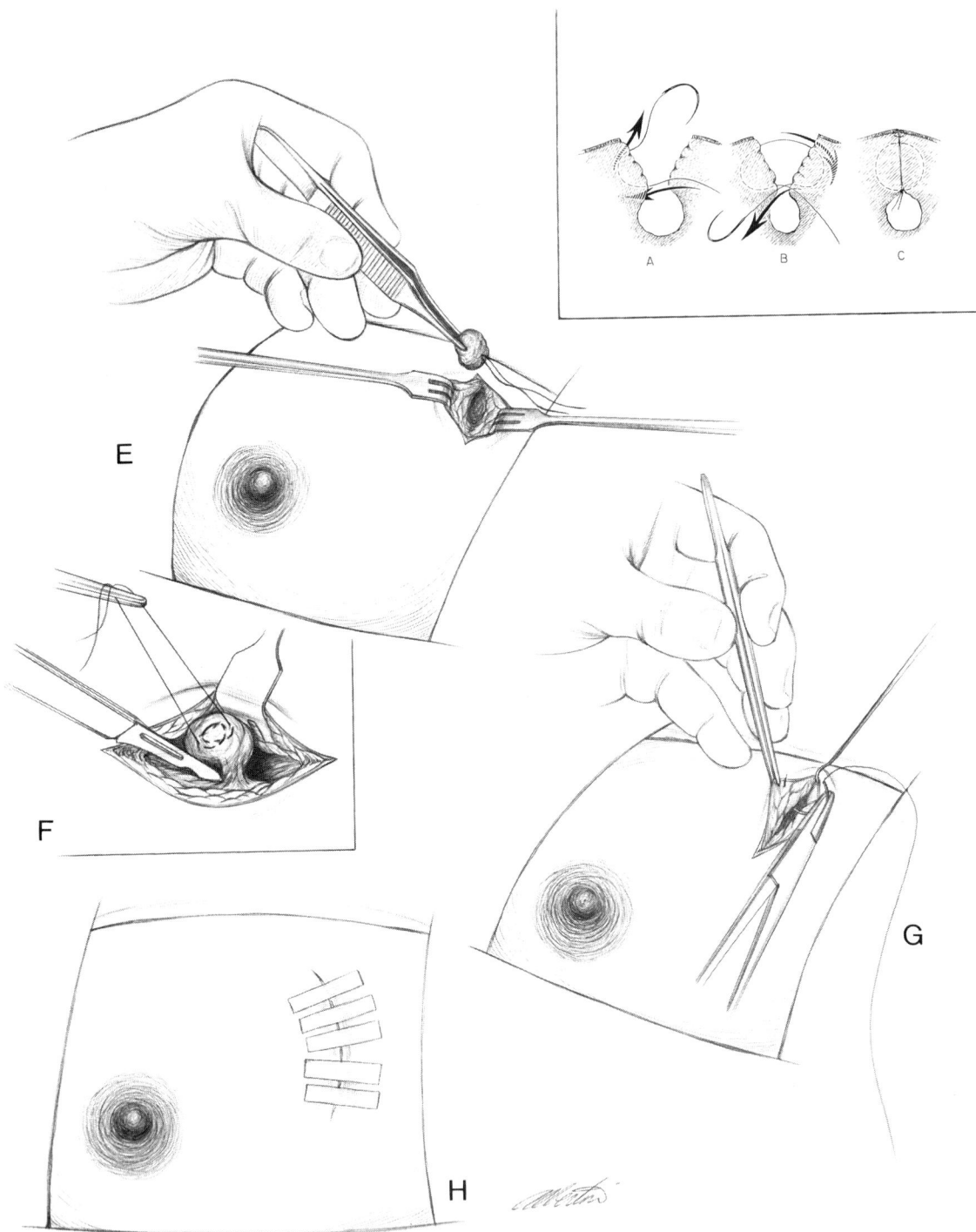

Figure 13–3 Continued

protuberant breast, as was once done for radical mastectomy is unnecessary.

The direction of the incision, transverse or diagonal, is determined by the location of the neoplasm. Cutaneous flaps are then elevated to the periphery of the gland in a nearly avascular plane over the superficial layer of the superficial fascia. The periphery of the breast can be estimated in advance by marking the skin with a sterile marking pencil along the clavicle to the midline of the sternum. The line goes down the midline of the sternum to the upper portion of the rectus abdominis muscle. It then extends laterally to the anterior edge of the latissimus dorsi muscle, cephalad along this edge to the axilla, and across the axilla, and then follows the deltopectoral groove to the clavicle. The flaps should never be elevated beyond the extent of the breast unless the surgeon has some specific reason for doing so. Infiltration of the entire subcutaneous space to be dissected with 1:400,000 epinephrine in saline before flap elevation greatly reduces blood loss.

When the subfascial plane is established near the clavicle, the plane is dissected under the mammary gland, including the deep pectoral fascia. The axilla is not entered. Medial and lateral suction catheters are placed beneath the flaps. The catheters go to continuous suction. They are removed when drainage is scant, on about the fifth to seventh postoperative day. The axilla is a skin area with a high endogenous bacterial count; for this reason, the drains should exit low on the chest.

The skin edges are approximated with subcutaneous sutures of 3-0 chromic catgut or an equivalent strength absorbable suture and with sutures or staples to the skin. The sutures must make the wound airtight to make the suction drainage effective.

Skin Graft

Skin grafting is infrequently needed today. Skin defects can usually be closed with flaps, providing a more cosmetic and stable cover. If the amount of skin removed prevents a primary closure, a graft may be necessary. Small defects can be closed with a defatted full thickness graft trimmed from a redundant portion of flap. The suction catheters are placed as before, and the margins of the cutaneous flaps are sutured to the underlying muscle to make the space between the flaps airtight. The skin graft is placed on the defect and sutured to the margin with interrupted silk sutures that are not cut.

At the completion of the suturing, the long tails of these sutures are tied firmly over a bulky gauze dressing holding a shaped piece of Telfa (gauze) against the graft. This gauze mold holds the graft firmly pressed to the chest wall, making a circumferential pressure dressing unnecessary. By the fifth postoperative day, the sutures can be cut and the dressing removed. The surface of the graft can be covered by a light dressing or can be left exposed if protected from abrasion.

For a split-thickness skin graft, the entire circumference of one thigh from below the knee to the groin is prepared. The thigh is draped separately with a wrapping of the foot and leg to leave the entire lower extremity mobile. Grafts are then cut with a Brown Electro-Dermatome with the micrometer scale set on 15. A thinner cutting can be made, but rarely less than 12 one thousandth of an inch.

The grafts should be cut only from the anterior and lateral thigh. A donor site on the inner thigh can be a source of considerable morbidity. Infection is more likely to occur near the perineum, and it is more difficult to treat. The surface of a donor site on the medial thigh frequently cannot be kept dry and free from abrasion by the other thigh.

Fine bacteriostatic-impregnated gauze or Telfa is applied to the raw donor site after capillary oozing has ceased and the donor site has been blotted dry. This is held in place with a circumferential dressing applied immediately. The dressing is removed down to the fine gauze or Telfa several days later, and the surface is dried thoroughly under a heat lamp. The fine mesh gauze or Telfa is then left undisturbed until it falls off spontaneously in about 2 weeks.

If infections develop, they should be treated expeditiously by wet to dry dressings and antibiotics to prevent the partial-thickness skin loss from being converted to a full-thickness loss by invasive infection.

Total Mastectomy and Axillary Lymph Node Dissection (Modified Radical Mastectomy)

Modified radical mastectomy is also known as total mastectomy with axillary lymph node dissection. With a low (Level I) lymph node dissection, this operation is appropriate and effective therapy for ductal carcinoma in situ. For invasive carcinomas, the lymph node dissection encompasses at least Levels I and II, and if lymph nodes are involved clinically, Level III as well. Even with the more complete axillary dissection, a clean removal of Rotter's lymph nodes lying along the course of the thoracoacromial vessels between the two pectoral muscles is not achieved.

Patey, Handley, Madden, and Auchincloss popularized the modified radical mastectomy. In 1976, it replaced the Halsted radical mastectomy as the most frequently used operation for early breast cancer in the United States (Wilson et al., 1984). The operation removes the breast and axillary lymph nodes, but not the pectoralis major muscle. The pectoralis minor muscle may be removed, divided, or left intact. The Patey variation removes the pectoralis minor muscle and thereby destroys the medial anterior thoracic nerve, which frequently runs through it, paralyzing the lateral part of the pectoralis major muscle. This is a cosmetic disadvantage. By dividing the muscle at its origin rather than removing it, the Level III axillary nodes can be removed, preserving the anterior pectoral nerves (medial and lateral) and the thoracoacromial vessels.

The Scanlon type of modified radical mastectomy appropriate for invasive cancers is shown in Figure 13–4. In this operation, the pectoralis minor muscle is divided distal to the medial anterior thoracic nerve to preserve all innervation to the pectoralis major muscle and prevent atrophy (Scanlon and Caprini, 1975). In selected cases a tumorectomy and axillary dissection followed by irradiation to the residual breast may be considered as an alternative to this operation (Fig. 13–4A to N).

An alternative approach to axillary dissection now preferred by one of the authors (J.S.S.) is described in Chapter 2. When the breast has been reflected laterally, exposing the entire anterior surface of the pectoralis major muscle, the avascular natural cleavage existing between the clavicular and sternal portions of the pectoralis major muscle is opened for its entire length. If any interpectoral or Rotter's nodes are present, they can be seen or they will lie in the fat about the nerves and vessels traversing the space between the pectoralis muscles. The lymph node–bearing fat may be dissected away from the nerves, leaving them intact. Then, the pectoralis minor muscle may be transected at its origin on the chest wall, leaving just enough muscle on the ribs to hold sutures when the pectoralis minor muscle is sutured back to its origin at the completion of the axillary dissection. The divided pectoralis minor muscle is then rotated cephalad on its intact insertion. This tends to stretch out and expose the multiple muscular nerve branches going to both major and minor pectoralis muscles. Through the excellent exposure by this technique, a complete axillary lymph node dissection may now be performed, teasing fat and fascia away from nerves to ensure good function of the pectoral muscles without the atrophy that accompanies denervation.

SEROMAS AND LYMPHOCELES

Seromas and lymphoceles under the skin flaps and axillary area can be a vexing problem after mastectomy with axillary dissection. At the lateral margin of an axillary dissection, the tissue containing most of the afferent lymphatics from the upper extremity have been transected. These open lymphatics spill their lymph into the wound. This spillage can be prevented in part during regional lymph node dissections by clamping and ligating the bundles of fatty areolar tissue containing most of the afferent lymphatics (Spratt et al., 1965). In the axilla, this is the areolar tissue and fascia about the axillary vein at the lateral extent of the axilla. This fatty areolar tissue can be ligated laterally with occlusion of many of the afferent conduits. Motion of an extremity generates an increased flow of lymph. The upper extremity may be kept at rest for about 5 days postoperatively to reduce the flow of lymph before beginning active exercises. These measures assist in preventing axillary fluid collections that may delay wound healing (Lotze et al., 1981). Seromas and lymphoceles were seen in 53 per cent of mastectomy patients at the Medical College of Wisconsin, and some persisted for many months. They can be reduced by using suction catheters until daily drainage is minimal. Wound drainage immediately after mastectomy consists of blood and serum, but it gradually becomes straw-colored and predominantly lymph fluid from severed lymphatics. The fluid may accumulate if suction catheters are discontinued before drainage is minimal. This problem is likely to occur in women with a large amount of suction drainage, and its

Text continued on page 419

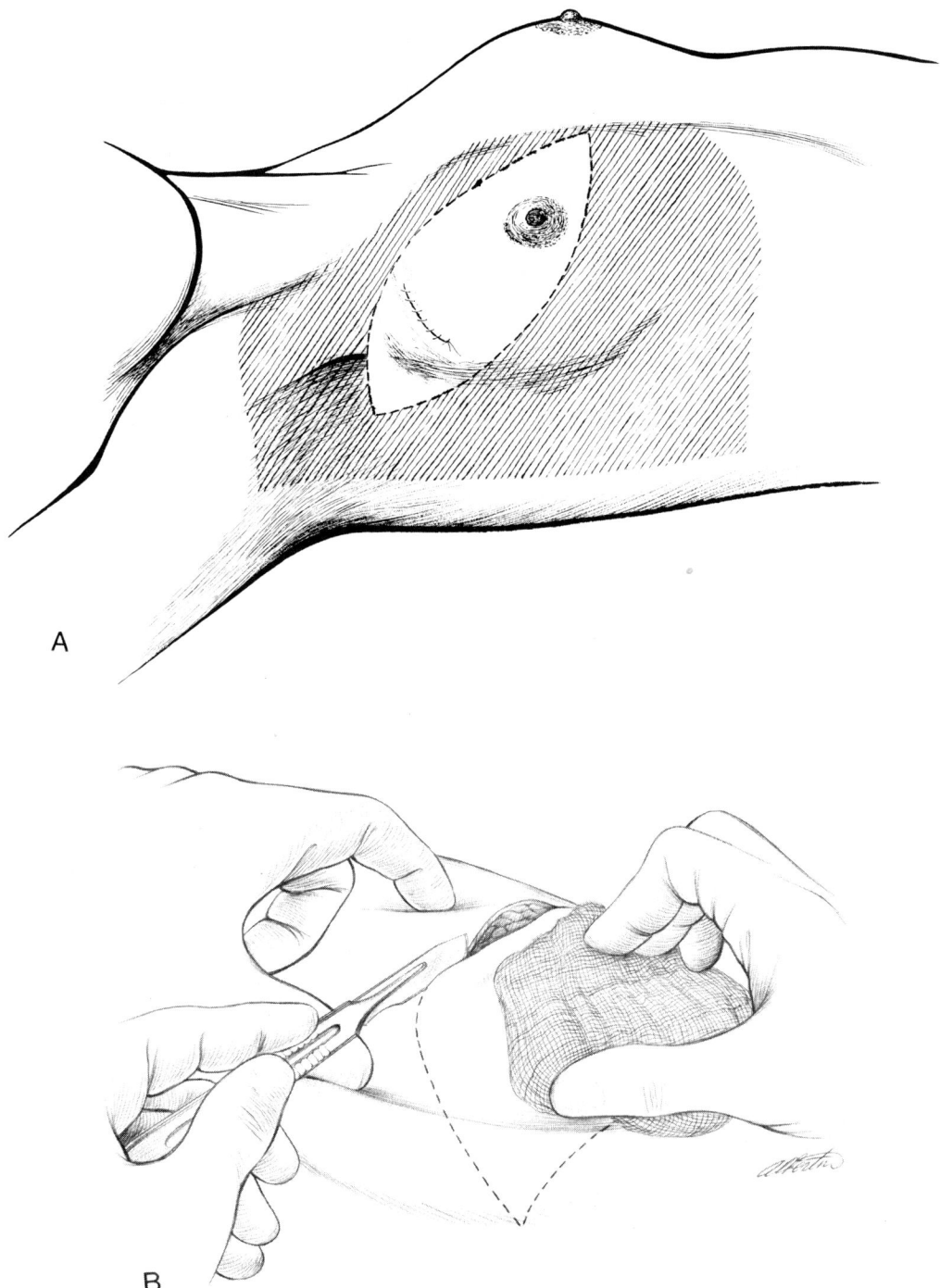

Figure 13–4. *A*, The area of anticipated skin flap dissection is shown shaded and is encompassed by a line at the midline of the sternum, along the inferior border of the clavicle, following the course of the cephalic vein in the deltopectoral groove, across the axillary fold, along the latissimus dorsi laterally, and rejoining the midline inferiorly along the course of a line two fingerbreadths below the inframammary fold. A diagonal incision is fashioned, which reaches the midline anteriorly and to the lateral edge of the breast laterally. It encompasses the nipple, the tumor site, and any previous biopsy incisions. The upper and lower lines of the incision are deliberately made of equal length by measuring with a silk ligature so that the incision can be closed smoothly and without corrugations.

B, The initial incision is made just through the skin so that the underlying fatty tissue bulges but is not incised.

Illustration continued on following page

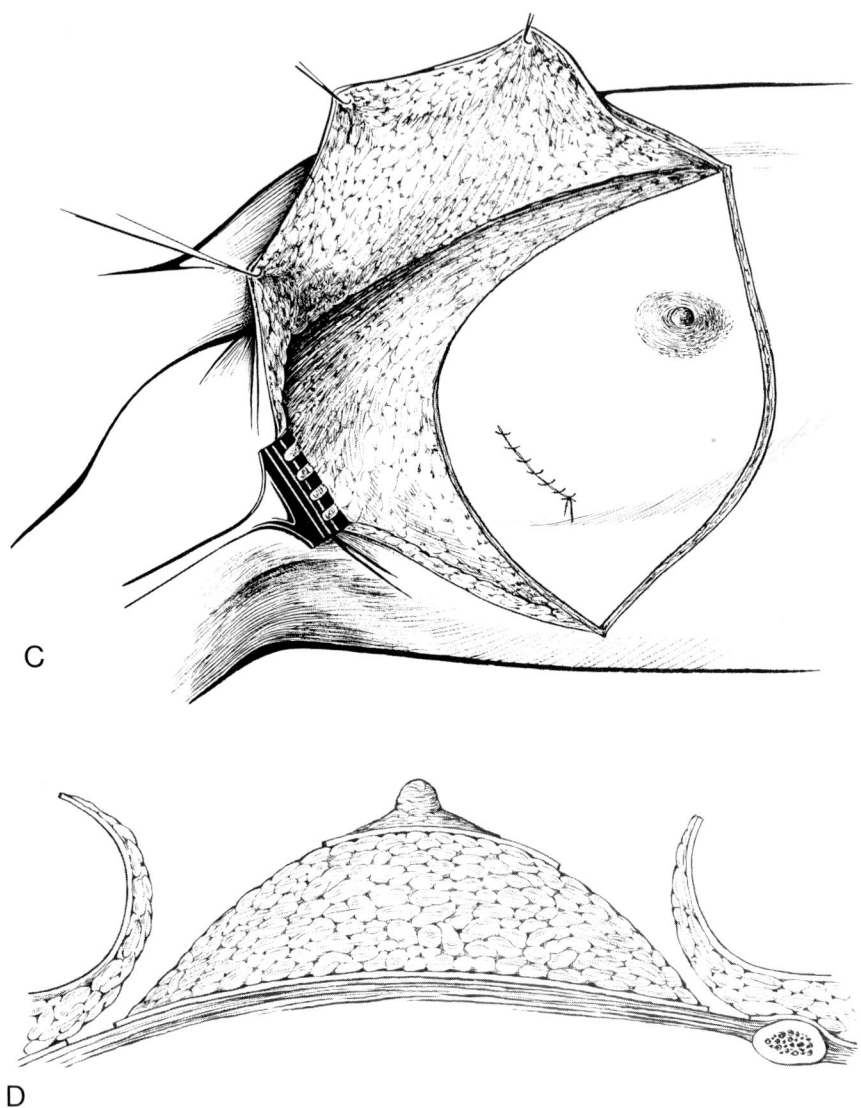

Figure 13–4 *Continued C* and *D*, Superior and inferior skin flaps are raised, the former up to the lower border of the clavicle and the deltopectoral groove and the latter to the border previously marked. Flaps are relatively thin so that no breast tissue remains on the flaps. They are retracted with skin hooks to avoid damaging and devitalizing the fatty tissue and are raised smoothly and with gentle tapering toward the base so that the blood supply from the periphery is not interrupted.

Illustration continued on opposite page

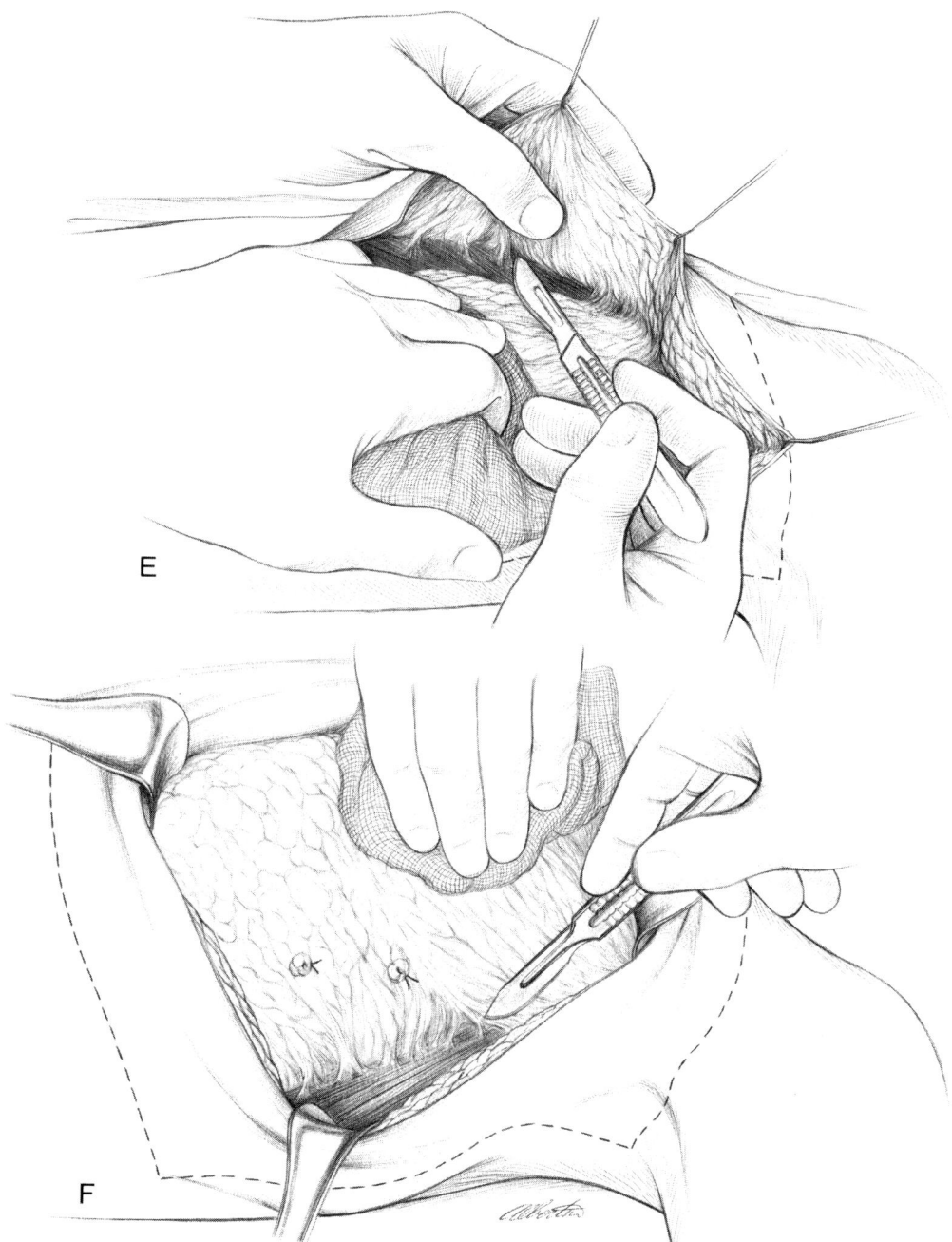

Figure 13–4 *Continued E*, At the free margin of the flap, approximately 0.5 cm or less of subcutaneous fat is left on the flap and this gradually thickens as the dissection proceeds toward the periphery until full thickness is reached at the lateral boundary. An important technique for continuous monitoring of flap thickness is for the surgeon's left hand to be placed behind the flap directly opposite the dissecting scalpel as shown here. An assistant's hand retracts the specimen. In this figure the medial flap has been raised to the midline of the sternum.

F, The lateral flap is raised to the anterior border of the latissimus dorsi muscle. Lateral perforating vessels are secured with ligatures in the process. The distal end of the latissimus is exposed to the limit of the lower flap. Toward the axilla it is exposed until its tendinous portion becomes evident or to the level of the border of the pectoralis major muscle. In the process the axillary flap is elevated from the underlying tissues. If the intercostobrachial nerve is to be preserved, the dissection toward the axilla is more limited in order to avoid accidental damage to the nerve.

Illustration continued on following page

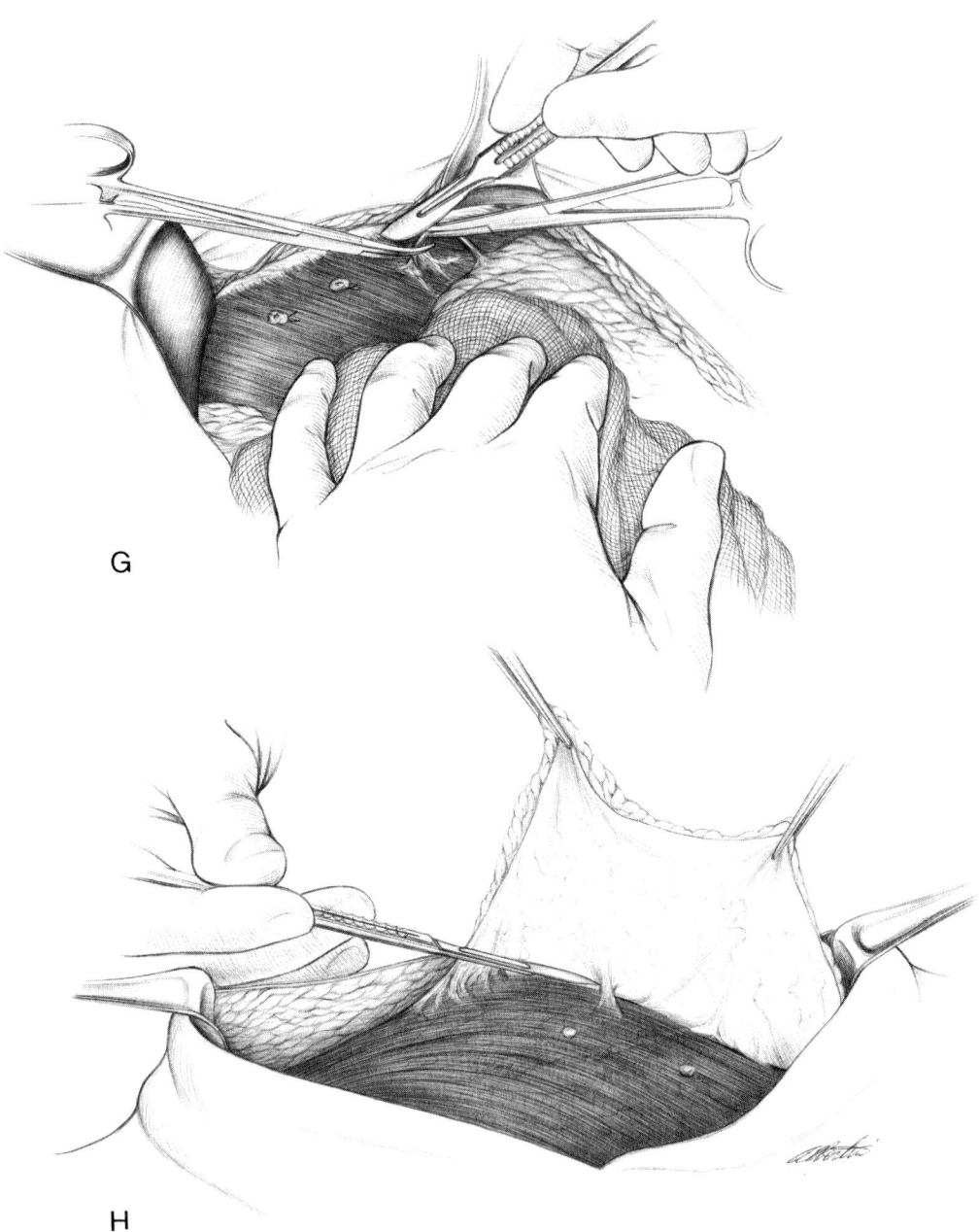

Figure 13–4 Continued G, Turning back to the medial side of the chest, the breast and deep pectoral fascia are elevated off the pectoralis major muscle and the dissection proceeds from medial to lateral, securing the anterior perforating vessel in the process with clamps and ligatures of absorbable suture.

H, Here the deep fascia is shown raised off the pectoralis major muscle and the dissection approaching its lateral border. At the lower end, beyond the insertion of the pectoralis major, the deep fascia of the upper abdominal muscles is left intact and only the overlying tissues are included with the specimen.

Illustration continued on opposite page

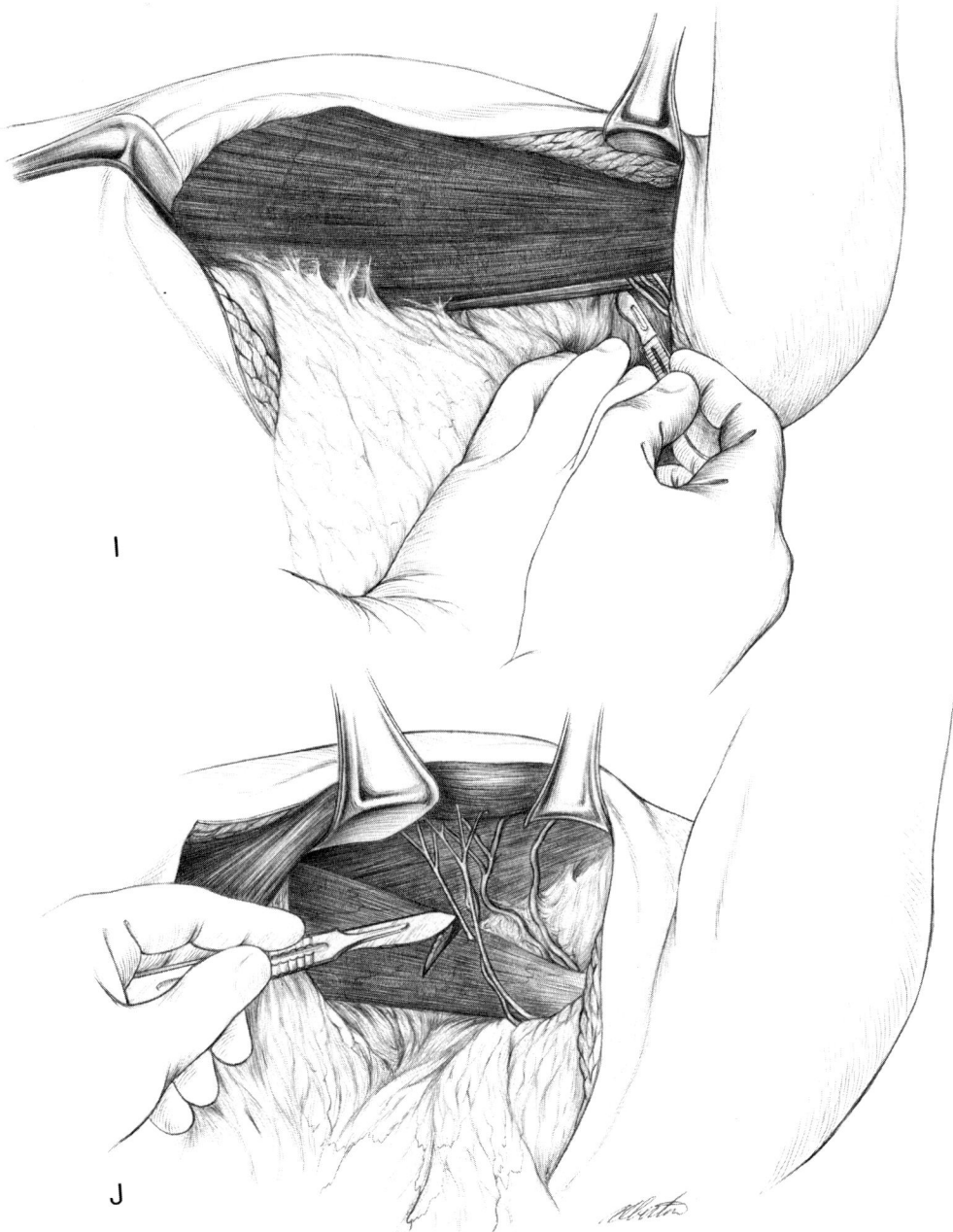

Figure 13–4 *Continued I*, The specimen is gradually dissected from the lateral margin of the pectoralis major muscle and the shoulder is extended to relax this muscle so that the pectoralis minor can be exposed. The border of the pectoralis minor muscle is cleaned, taking care to preserve the medial anterior thoracic nerve (and accompanying vessels) that innervates the lateral portion of the pectoralis major muscle. These structures are shown here just superior to the scalpel. At this point the axillary vein is exposed and traced medially to the point at which it disappears under the pectoralis minor muscle. An alternative approach to the axillary dissection is described in Chapter 1.

J, With the pectoralis major muscle retracted, the pectoralis minor muscle is divided distal to the medial anterior thoracic nerve and its branches, which course lateral to, and frequently through, the substance of the pectoralis minor muscle. More deeply in the wound arising medial to the pectoralis minor muscle and spreading on the posterior side of the pectoralis major are seen the lateral anterior thoracic nerve and the accompanying thoracoacromial vessels. These vessels and nerves are also protected during the dissection. Along their course lie Rotter's interpectoral lymph nodes in fat. These nodes may be removed by carefully defatting the nerves and vessels traversing the space between pectoralis minor and pectoralis major muscles.

Illustration continued on following page

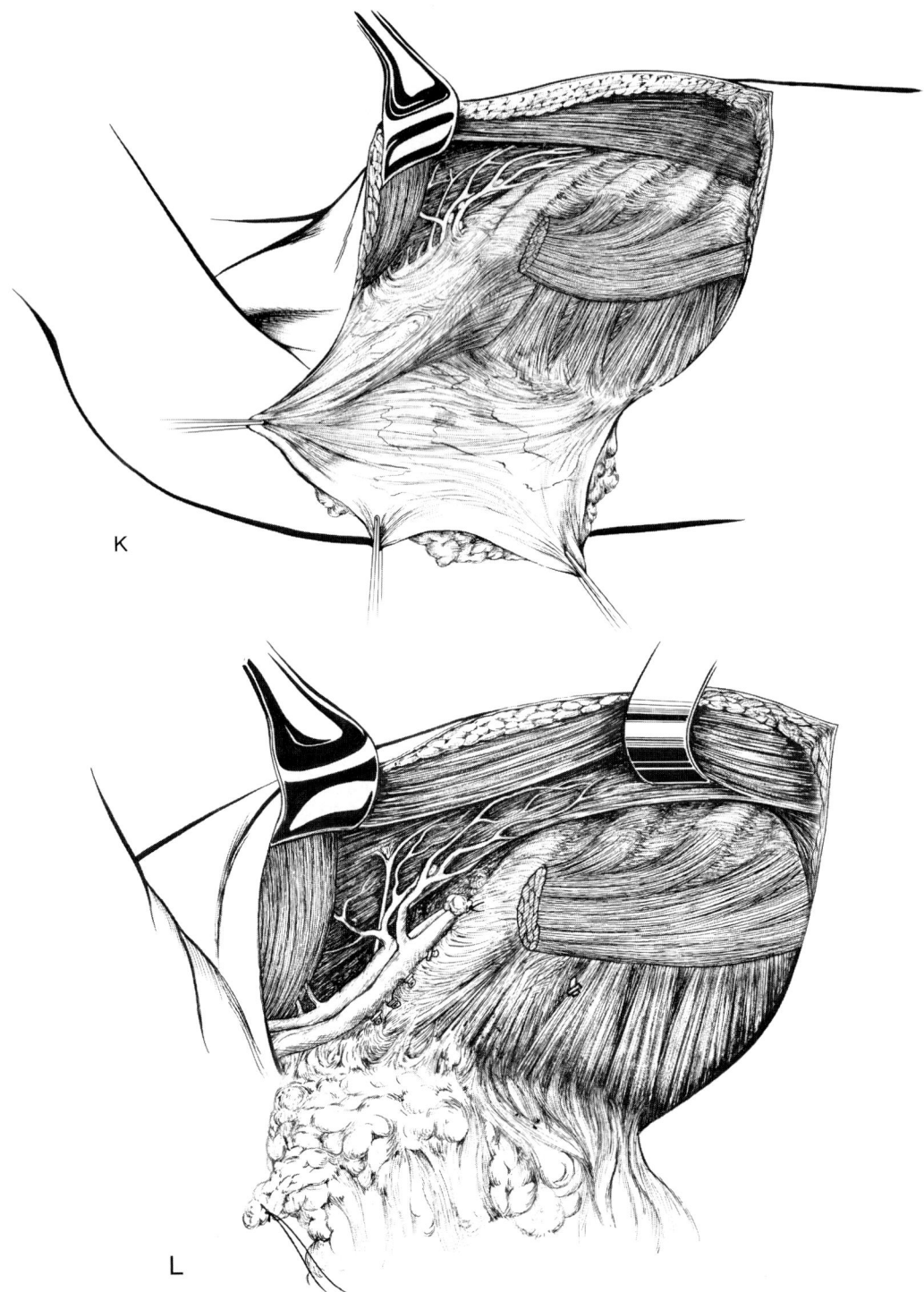

Figure 13-4 Continued *K*, With the pectoralis minor muscle divided, the upper portion is retracted on its origin and the axillary vein is exposed. The entire contents of the axilla to its apex, where the axillary vein crosses the first rib, can be cleaned of fatty node-bearing tissue.

L, Dissection of the axilla proceeds from medial to lateral with the tissues of the apex marked with a ligature for the orientation of the pathologist. Branches of the axillary vein coursing into the specimen are divided between hemoclips; the ligated apical lymphatics, still in continuity with the axillary contents, are shown laterally. The preserved lateral anterior thoracic nerve and the thoracoacromial vessels are shown spreading on the underside of the pectoralis major muscle. Some of Rotter's nodes are also visible. In this case the intercostobrachial nerve appearing at the second intercostal space has been sacrificed and is shown secured by a clip. Three to four centimeters more lateral, the surgeon can anticipate encountering the long thoracic nerve, which will appear in fatty tissues just off the chest wall and will course inferiorly and superiorly crossing deep to the axillary artery and vein.

Illustration continued on opposite page

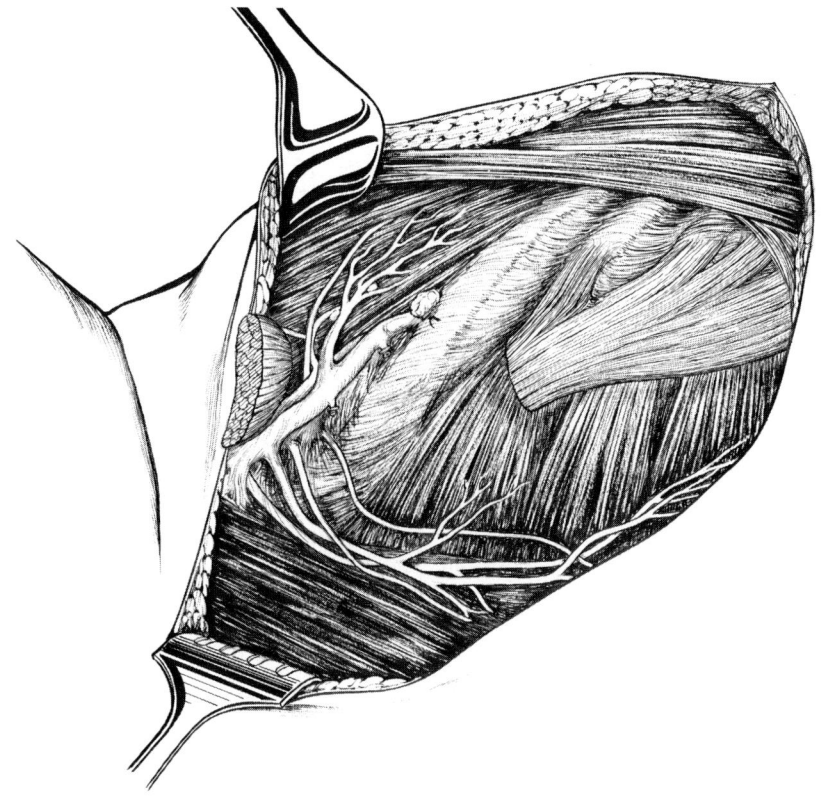

M

Figure 13–4 *Continued M,* The axillary tissues are dissected off the chest wall and finally off the border of the latissimus dorsi muscle, preserving in the process the long thoracic nerve, shown here lying along the serratus anterior muscle, as well as more lateral to it the thoracodorsal nerve, which innervates the latissimus dorsi accompanying the thoracodorsal vessels. It should be appreciated that this nerve appears from beneath the axillary vein and crosses laterally usually superficial to the thoracodorsal vessels. Both the long thoracic nerve and the thoracodorsal nerve arise from the brachial plexus. The intercostobrachial nerve, which crosses the axilla from medial to lateral superficial to other structures, has not been preserved in this case. It is not necessary to reconstitute the pectoralis minor muscle. Although it can be done, shortening of the muscle makes it a difficult task. One of us (JSS) does resuture an innervated muscle to the chest wall, believing that a contracted mass of muscle may be confused as a recurrence of tumor. Also, with healing it may resume its normal musculoskeletal function.

Illustration continued on following page

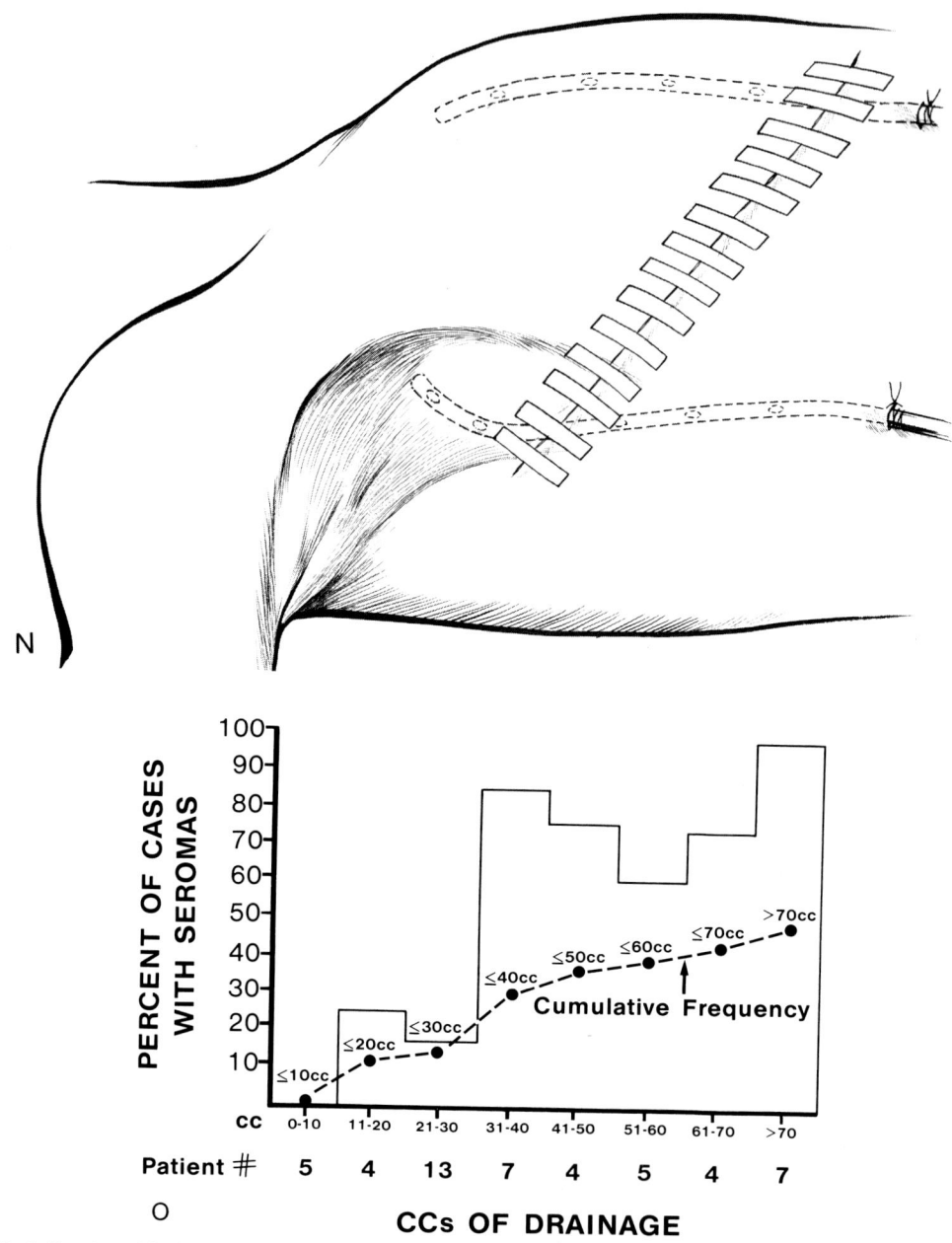

Figure 13–4 Continued N, Medial and lateral closed suction catheters have been placed in the wound and the incision is closed with absorbable sutures to the subcutaneous tissues followed by a continuous subcuticular suture of absorbable fine suture and Steri-strips. Alternatively, skin clips may be used in place of the subcuticular layer. A light dressing is applied to the incision and the catheter exit sites. A small pad in the axilla stabilizes the skin. The arm is not restricted. Drainage from the suction catheters is measured separately, and each is removed when the drainage has fallen to less than 30 cc per 24 hours. Earlier removal is followed by a high frequency of seroma formation. This operation results in anesthesia on the anterior chest throughout most of the area of the skin flaps as well as in the axilla and inner side of the arm. This can result in troublesome paresthesia. Approximately 8 per cent of patients ultimately develop some lymphedema of the ipsilateral arm, although this is rarely marked and an appropriate postoperatve educational program can contribute to prevention of lymphedema.

O, The frequency of seroma formation after drainage catheter removal is directly related to the 24-hour drainage volume immediately prior to removal. This is based on experience with 49 patients treated with modified mastectomy at the Medical College of Wisconsin. (O, From Tadych, K., and Donegan, W. L.: Postmastectomy seromas and wound drainage. Surg. Gynecol. Obstet., *165*:483, 1987. By permission of SURGERY, GYNECOLOGY & OBSTETRICS.)

frequency is directly related to the total amount of drainage in the 24 hr immediately prior to discontinuing suction drainage. If the total is less than 10 ml, no fluid accumulation is seen. If the amount is 25 ml, the frequency of accumulation is 6 per cent. With larger amounts, the rate is 100 per cent if over 75 ml is drained (Fig. 13–4*O*). Seromas can often be managed simply by percutaneous aspirations until accumulation stops, but this may require repeated office visits for prolonged periods. In some cases, a serosa-lined pocket develops that seems to prevent resolution. In protracted cases, open drainage with a small Penrose drain inserted into the most dependent part of the pocket through a stab wound will hasten resolution and usually is the solution to the problem. This requires that the patient be responsible for frequent dressing changes and temporarily refrain from abducting her arm. Reinsertion of closed suction drains has no advantage and often fails. If contamination of the fluid occurs during aspirations, it may result in infection and abscess formation and force open drainage. Resolution can be anticipated as the severed lymphatics that produce the fluid eventually close. Use of tetracycline as a sclerotic to treat or prevent this problem has not had uniform success (McCarthy et al., 1986).

Segmental Mastectomy and Axillary Lymph Node Dissection

SEGMENTAL MASTECTOMY

Tumorectomy, segmental mastectomy, lumpectomy, and tylectomy are all synonyms for a therapeutic procedure in which a primary tumor is removed from the breast with a margin of tissue, preferably with a margin histologically free of cancer, and with concern for producing an acceptable cosmetic result. It may be employed for TNM Stage I or II carcinomas of the breast as an alternative to total mastectomy and axillary dissection when the situation permits, and it is followed by irradiation to the residual breast, now free of all gross cancer. Postoperative axillary radiotherapy is not required when a complete axillary dissection is done. If used, it will increase the chances of lymphedema. Survival and disease-free survival are comparable to those of modified mastectomy in similar circumstances. Tumors should be 4.0 cm or less in diameter but may be slightly larger, and there should be no more than limited clinical involvement of the axilla. The following are generally considered contraindications: (1) poorly defined primary tumor; (2) multiple primary tumors; (3) large primary tumor in a small breast so that removal would leave a distorted breast; (4) pregnancy; and (5) previous irradiation to the chest. Centrally located tumors with direct involvement of the nipple requiring its removal and poorly differentiated tumors (poor nuclear grade) with a significant intraductal component currently are relative contraindications (Schnitt et al., 1984). Figure 13–5*A* to *H* illustrate the technique for this procedure.

Axillary Lymph Node Dissection

Axillary lymph node dissection permits pathologic evaluation of lymph nodes. This information is necessary for accurate assessment of prognosis and a decision for systemic adjuvant therapy. It accompanies tumorectomy in preparation for radiotherapy as treatment of the breast. After a thorough axillary dissection, axillary recurrence is unlikely; thus irradiation of the axilla is both unnecessary and undesirable. The procedure is illustrated in Figure 13–5*I* to *T*.

Standard or "Halsted" Radical Mastectomy

Until the mid-1970s, radical mastectomy was the standard treatment for mammary cancer. By 1982, only 3.6 per cent of primary operations for breast cancer in the United States were radical mastectomies. However, this operation is preferred over a modified mastectomy for locally advanced tumors, when a primary tumor extensively involves the pectoralis major muscle, or when a primary tumor is associated with extensive gross axillary metastases.

The patient is positioned eccentrically on the operating table with the side on which the mastectomy is to be performed adjacent to the

Text continued on page 433

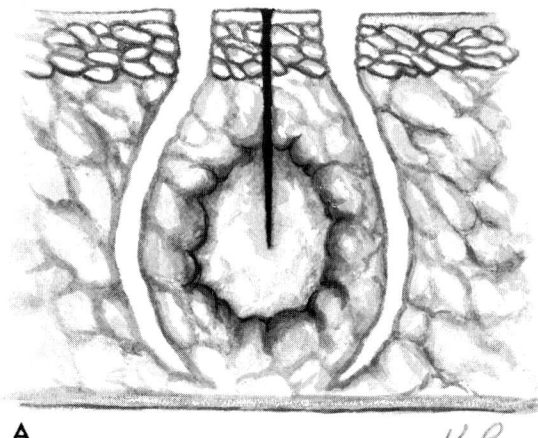

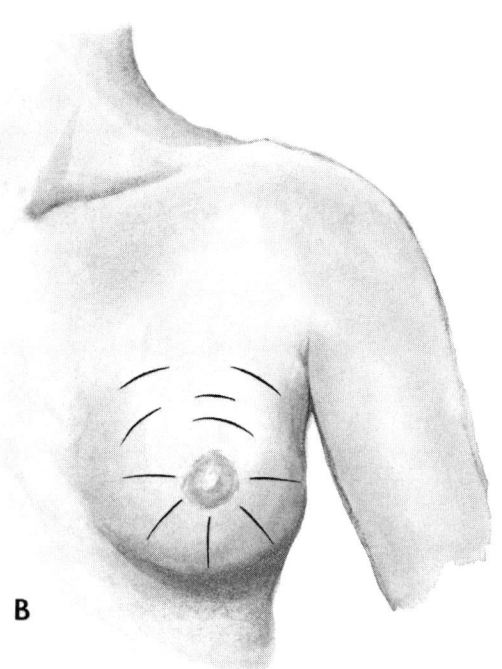

Figure 13–5. *A*, Schematic cross section of the technique for therapeutically excising a primary tumor mass that has been previously biopsied. The incisional biopsy tract is shown extending as a vertical line from the skin into the tumor. A modest amount of skin and subcutaneous tissue is removed around the biopsy incision. At the junction between subcutaneous tissue and breast tissue the excision is widened to encompass the tumor mass with a margin of normal tissue that is palpably and visibly uninvolved. The excision extends to, but not necessarily through, the deep pectoral fascia. If the tumor is small and has not previously been biopsied, this procedure can be performed as both an excisional biopsy and a therapeutic removal of the primary tumor. In this case no skin is removed. Immediate examination by a pathologist to ensure that all margins are free of neoplasm is desirable. If margins are not free, a wider removal may be possible. If not, removal of the breast may be more effective than radiotherapy.

B, Incisions for tumorectomy that generally produce the best cosmetic result. In the upper hemisphere of the breast they are transverse and curvilinear, following the skin lines. For deep-lying central tumors a para-areolar incision may be used. Radial incisions in the lower hemisphere of the breast preserve the distance between the nipple and the inframammary fold and prevent downward displacement of the nipple. The incision for a tumorectomy is kept separate from that of an axillary dissection.

Illustration continued on opposite page

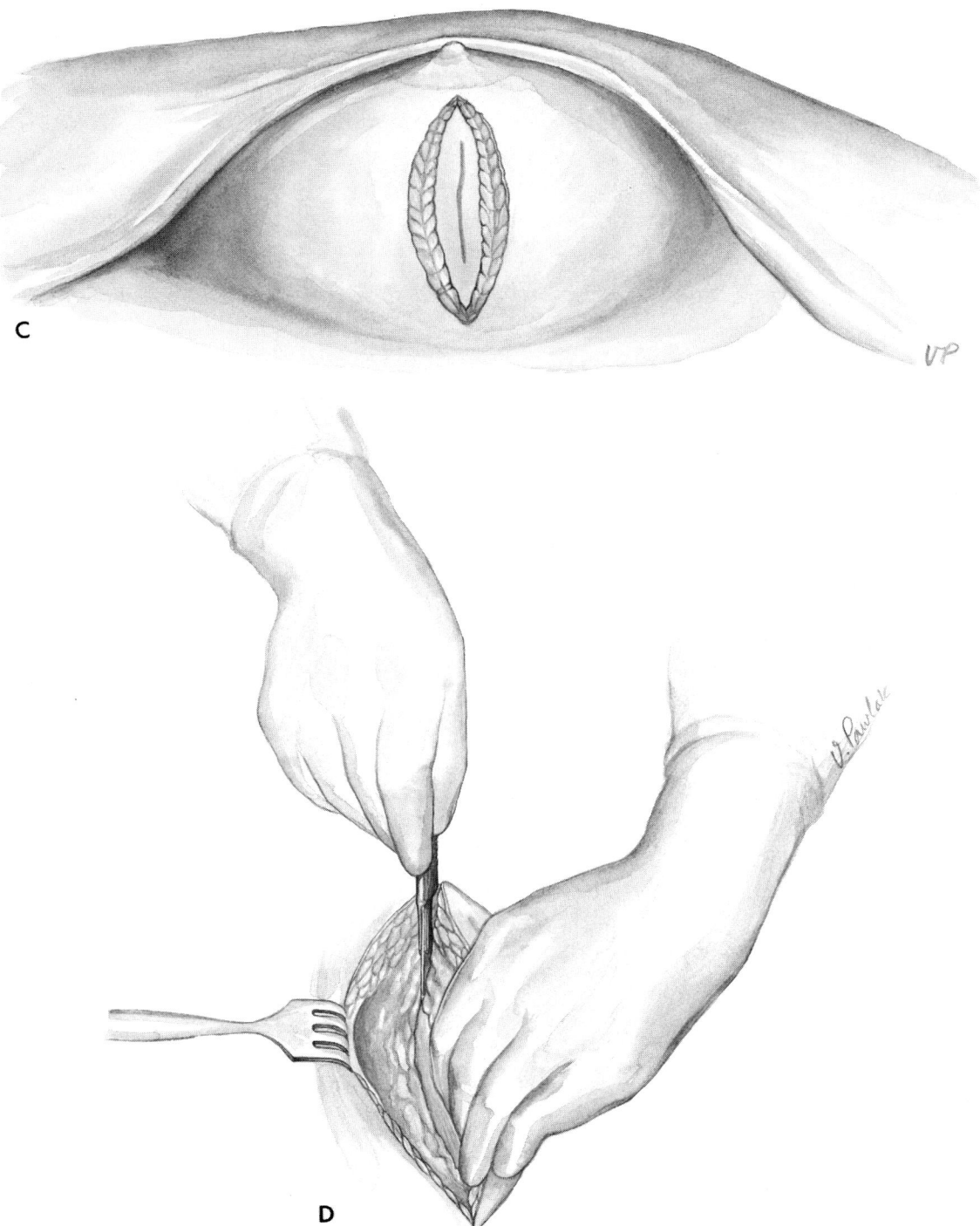

Figure 13–5 *Continued C,* Tumorectomy and axillary dissection are usually performed at the same operation, and the breast and axilla are prepared simultaneously. Tumorectomy is performed first, and during this part of the procedure the area of the axillary dissection is draped out of the field and is exposed later. This figure shows the initial incision around a previous biopsy incision. If estrogen and progesterone receptors were not obtained initially, the residual tumor in the breast may be assayed at this time. The initial incision extends around the previous biopsy incision and partially or totally through the subcutaneous tissue. Care is taken not to encounter the tumor mass or to break into the previous biopsy cavity. This tumor was in the lateral portion of the breast and a radial excision was therefore performed. When possible, the incision avoids the areola.

D, Once through the subcutaneous tissue, the incision is widened to ensure a tumor-free margin and carried down to the pectoral fascia on one side. At this level the deep margin is developed either deep to or superficial to the pectoral fascia.

Illustration continued on following page

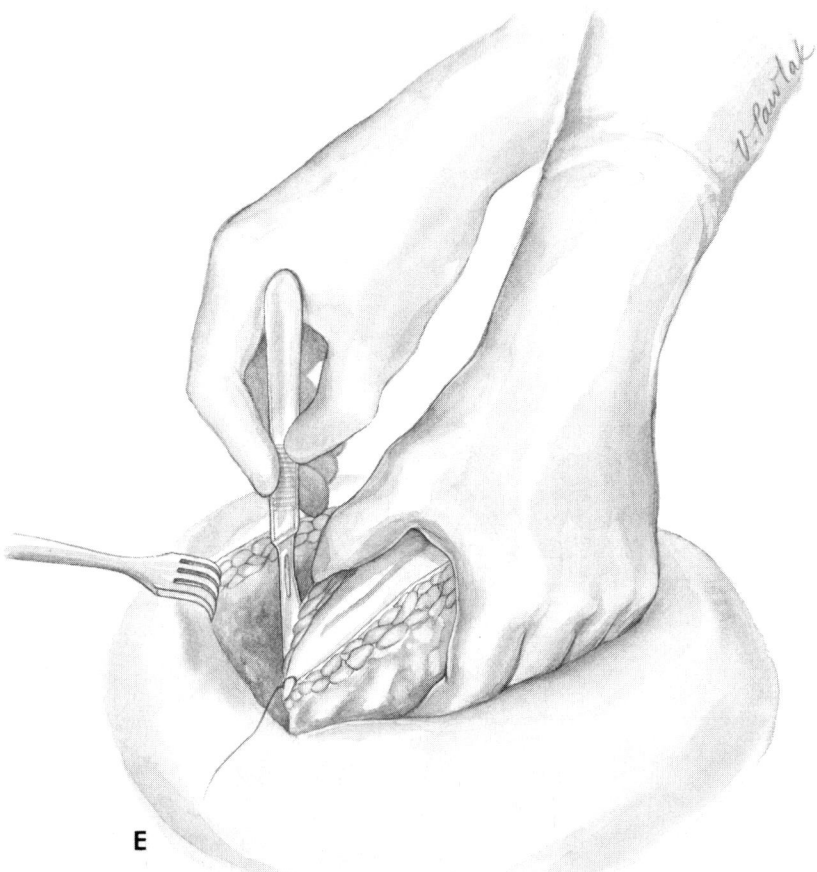

Figure 13–5 *Continued E,* When the deep margin of the dissection has been developed on one side of the involved area, fingers of the left hand are inserted beneath the tumor, lifting it, and using the thumb and tips of the fingers to identify a normal margin on the opposite side, which is then dissected. Silk sutures are placed at the margins of the specimen to identify its lateral and superior margins for the pathologist. The pathologist examines the specimen immediately and informs the surgeon whether margins are inadequate so that an additional margin of tissue can be removed if necessary at this point.

Illustration continued on opposite page

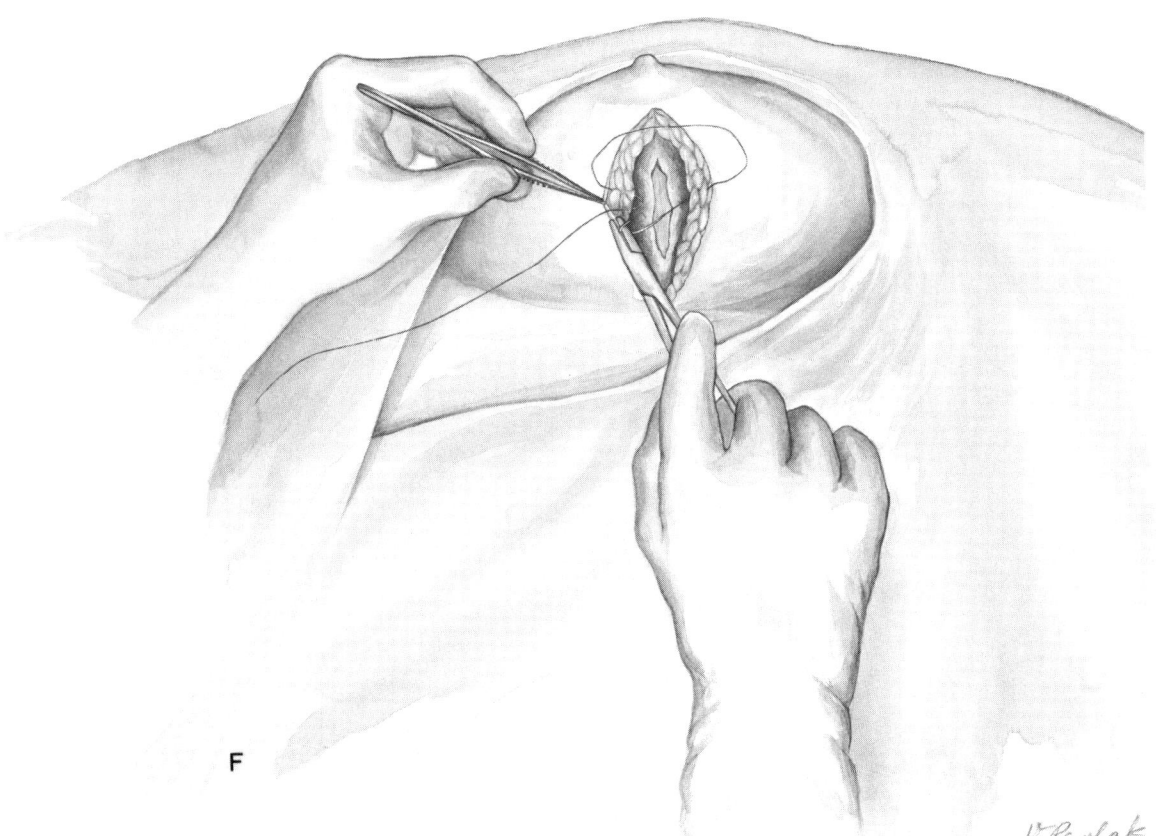

Figure 13–5 *Continued F,* The wound is shown after excision is complete. A portion of the deep fascia has been removed at the bottom of the wound with the specimen. It is not only unnecessary but undesirable to approximate breast tissue if the approximation distorts the contour of the breast. After meticulous hemostasis, it is unnecessary to use drains. The closure involves only the subcutaneous tissue and skin. The underlying cavity fills with serum, which is eventually absorbed and replaced with scar. The subcutaneous layer is closed with interrupted inverted sutures of 3–0 chromic catgut.

Illustration continued on following page

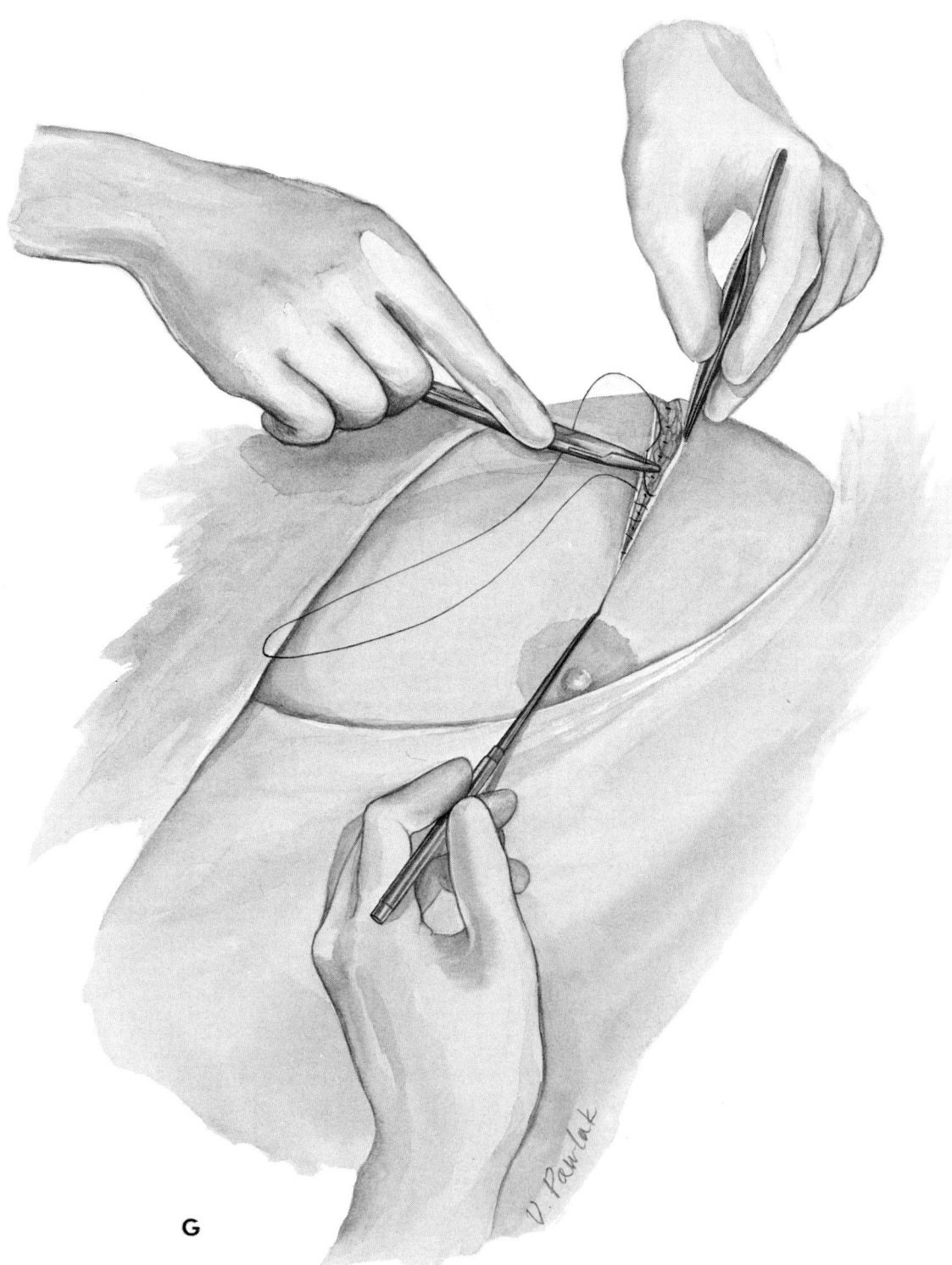

Figure 13–5 *Continued G,* After closure of the subcutaneous tissues the skin is closed with a running subcuticular suture of 4–0 absorbable suture. A skin hook at one or both ends is used to provide tension and facilitate suturing.
Illustration continued on opposite page

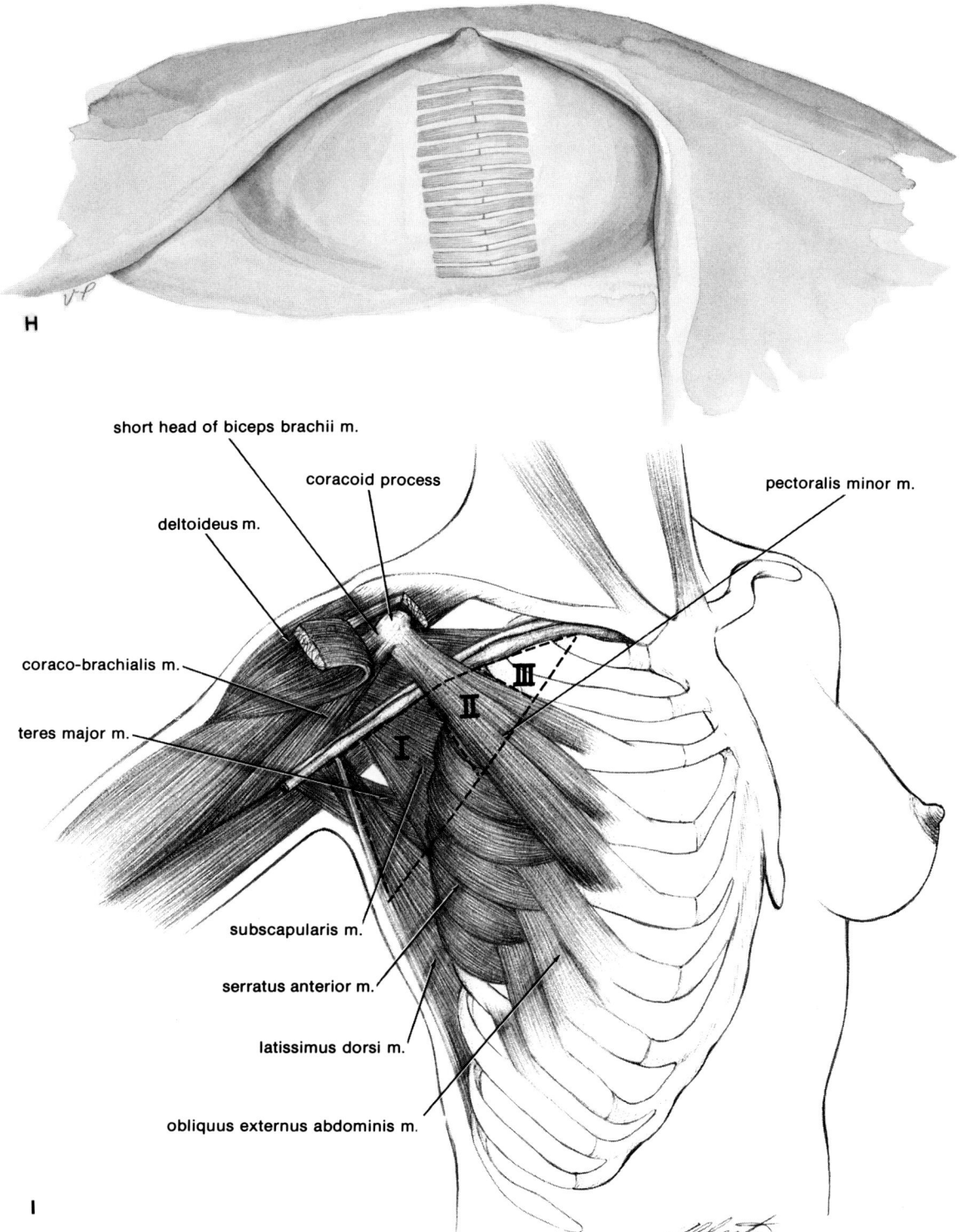

Figure 13–5. *Continued H,* Closure is completed by applying benzoin to the skin followed by Steri-strips, which are left in place for 7 to 8 days. Induration at the site of excision will persist for 3 to 4 months as a result of the healing reaction. The tissue subsequently softens. An axillary dissection immediately follows this procedure. When it is completed, a light dressing is applied, and the patient wears a brassiere for several days to provide support for the breast and improve comfort.

I, The axillary nodes are divided into three groups depending upon their position relative to the pectoralis minor muscle. Level I consists of those lateral to this muscle, Level II those behind it, and Level III those medial to it. The surgeon's operative notes should carefully specify whether nodes from Levels I and II or Levels I, II, and III were removed. The following figures illustrate an axillary dissection that removes nodes from Levels I and II. The illustrations in Chapter 1 and Figure 13–4*I* to *N* show the technique for preserving innervated pectoralis minor and major muscles, allowing for contiguous removal of Levels I, II, and III.

Illustration continued on following page

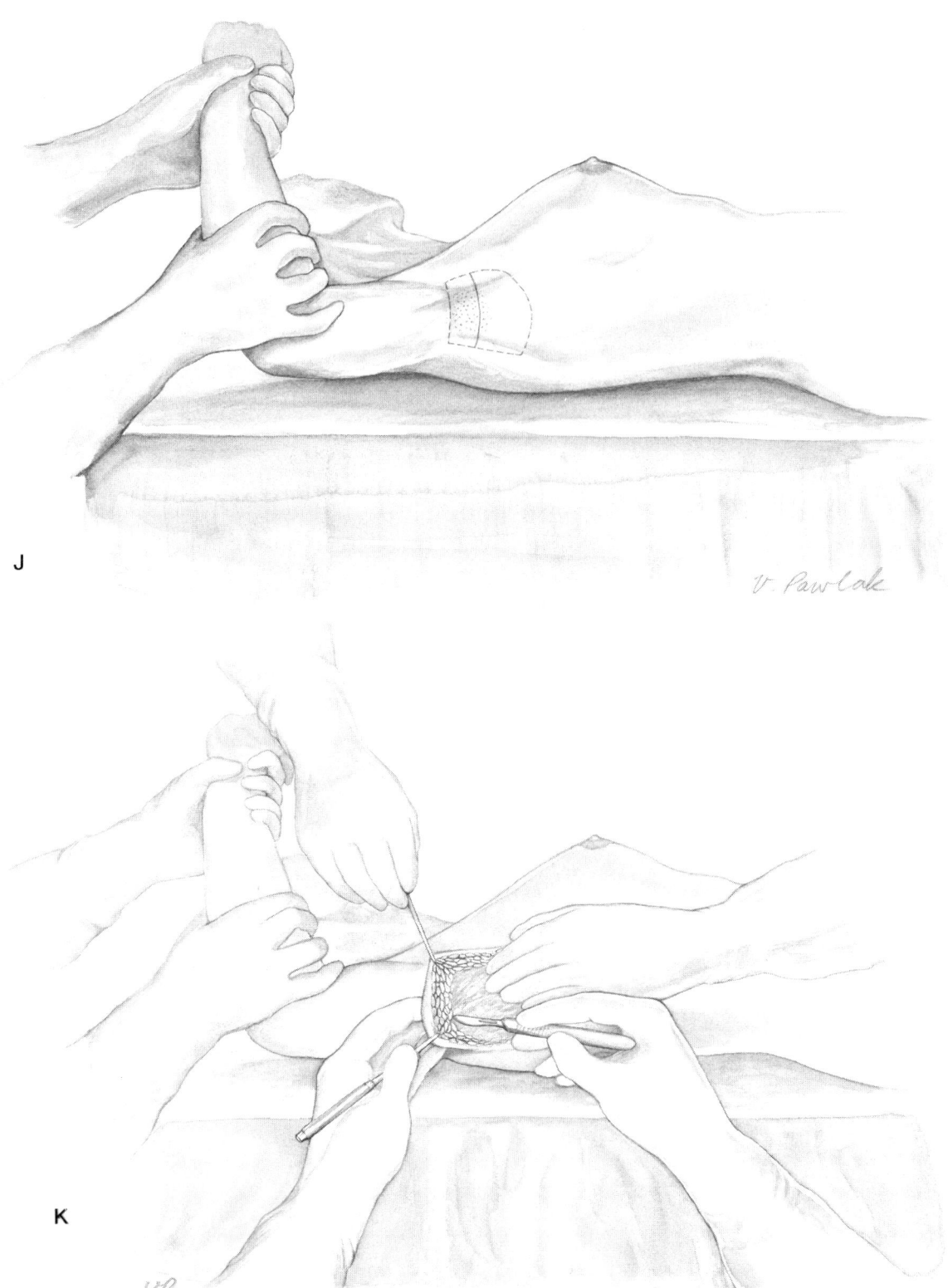

Figure 13–5 *Continued J,* The incision for an axillary dissection is made transversely in the skin lines two fingerbreadths below the axillary fold and extends from the border of the pectoralis major muscle to the latissimus dorsi muscle. The incision is ordinarily just within the hairline. The extent of flap development is shown by the dotted line in the figure.

K, The initial incision extends through the skin and subcutaneous tissue, and flap development is at the level of the axillary fascia. Flaps are developed with sharp dissection using skin hooks to retract the skin edges. Uniform thickness of the flap is ensured by keeping the fingers of the surgeon's retracting hand exactly opposite the dissecting scalpel. The lower flap is thicker and tapers gradually toward the chest wall.

Illustration continued on opposite page

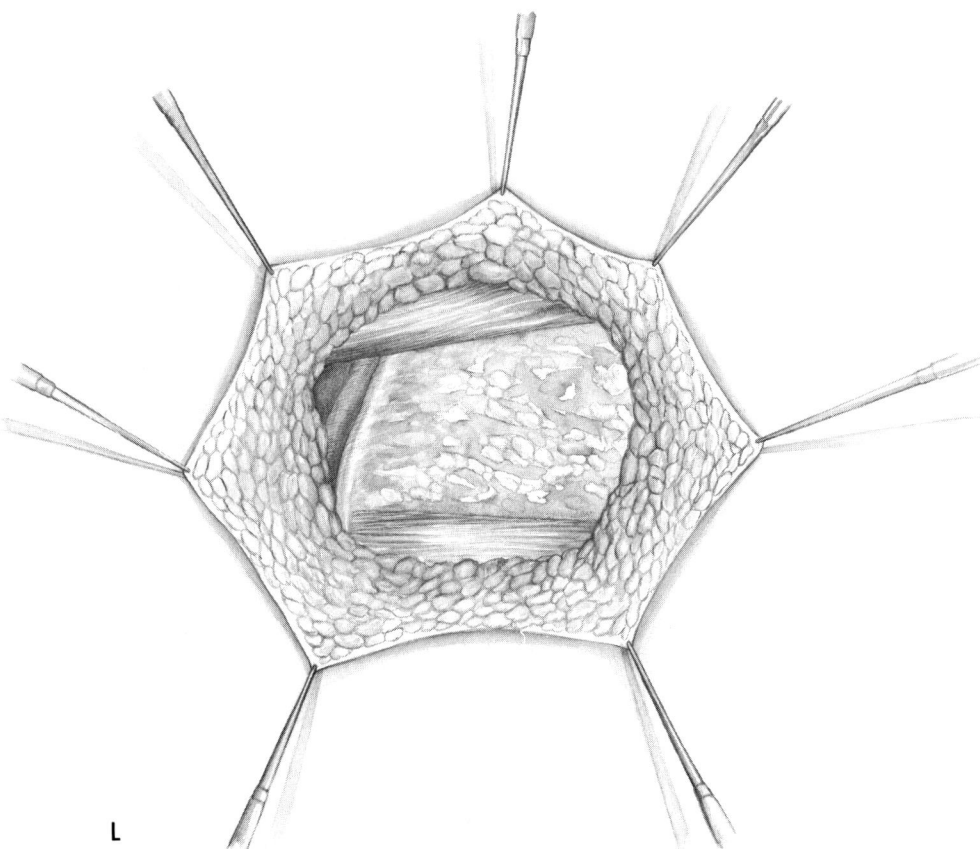

Figure 13–5 Continued *L*, With the skin flaps elevated, the anterior border of the dissection exposes the lateral border of the pectoralis major muscle. Posteriorly, the latissimus dorsi muscle is exposed and superiorly, the axillary vein.

Illustration continued on following page

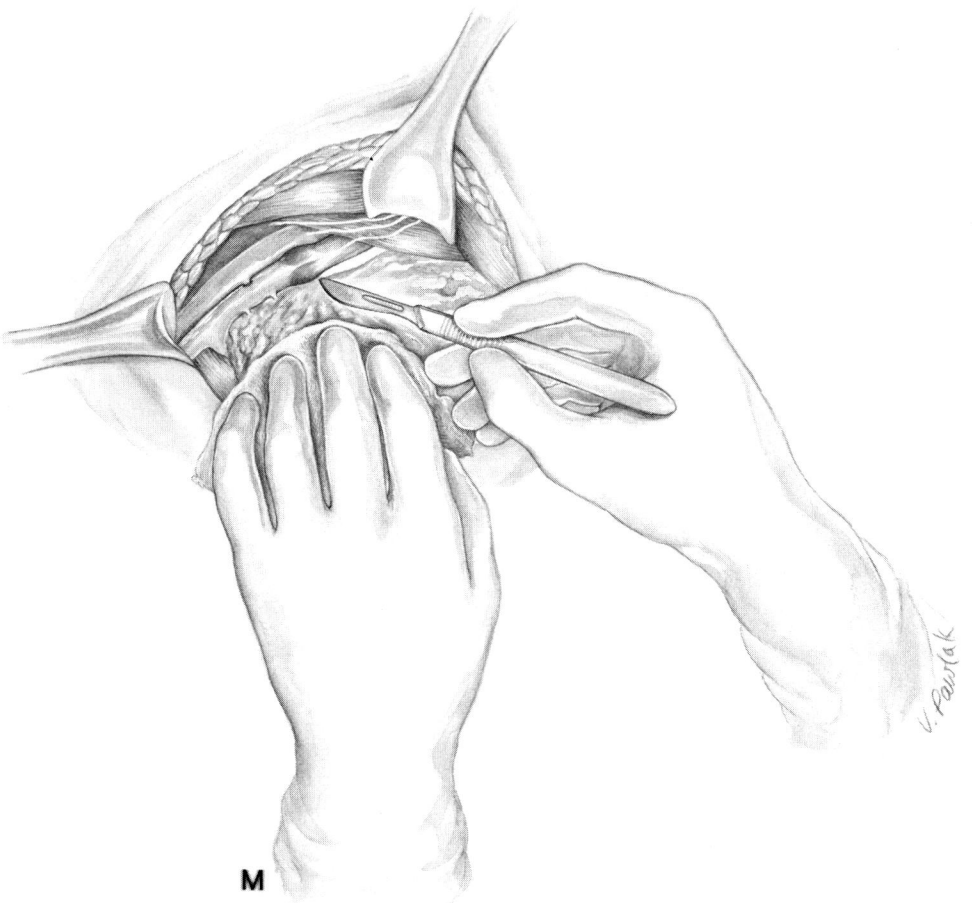

Figure 13–5 *Continued M*, The lateral border of the pectoralis major muscle is cleaned superiorly and retracted to expose the lateral border of the pectoralis minor. Crossing the latter will be found the medial anterior thoracic nerve and its accompanying vessels. These are preserved to maintain innervation to the lateral third of the pectoralis major muscle. These vessels are traced deeply and followed to their origin from the axillary vein, which is then cleaned from medial to lateral, the inferior tributaries being divided between hemoclips.

Illustration continued on opposite page

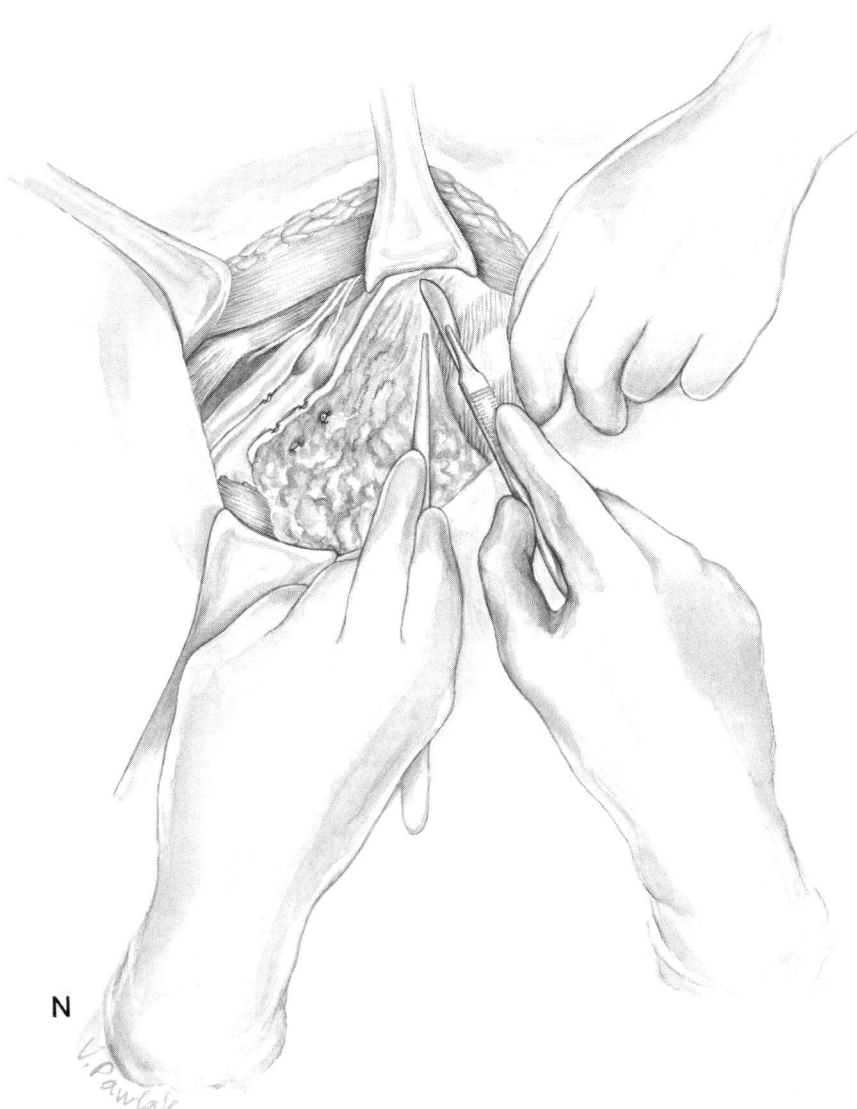

Figure 13–5 *Continued N*, With the shoulder flexed, adducted, and internally rotated, the pectoral muscles are relaxed, allowing them to be retracted medially and upward, exposing the axillary contents to the level of the medial border of the pectoralis minor muscle. This permits the surgeon to remove all Level II lymph nodes as well as those at axillary Level I. Here the surgeon has reached the apex of the dissection. This point is marked with a silk ligature for orientation for the pathologist. All of the fatty tissues and lymph nodes of the axilla from this point laterally and inferior to the axillary vein are dissected off the chest wall as the specimen. The next major structure to be encountered is the intercostobrachial nerve, which appears with accompanying vessels in the second intercostal space. Although it is not routine to spare this nerve, the advantage of doing so, when possible, is that sensation is preserved to the inner side of the upper arm (Temple and Ketcham, 1985). The nerve also serves as a landmark, indicating that the long thoracic nerve to the serratus anterior muscle will be encountered only 2 to 3 cm further laterally.

Illustration continued on following page

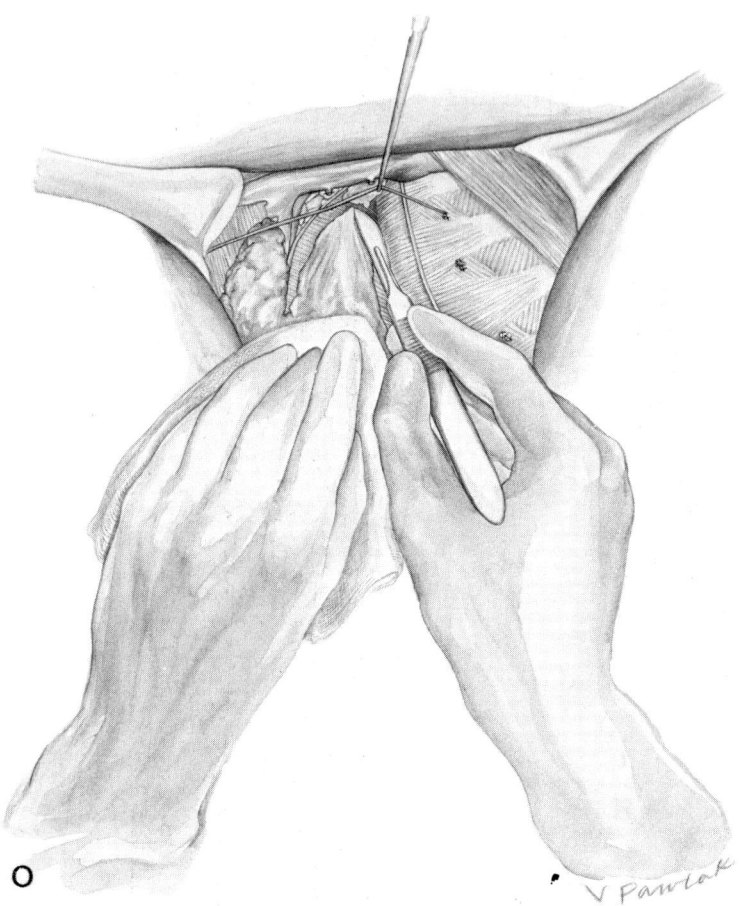

Figure 13–5 *Continued O,* Here the intercostobrachial nerve has been traced and preserved, as has the long thoracic nerve. Dissection is never performed medial to the latter, as this will destroy the small slips that innervate the serratus anterior muscle. The dissection proceeds lateral to it until the fascia of the subscapularis muscle is incised. The thoracodorsal nerve, which curves laterally in the fatty tissues, is identified, and the node-bearing tissue inferior to the axillary vein, between the long thoracic nerve medially and the thoracodorsal nerve laterally, is dissected off the fascia of the subscapularis muscle from above downward en bloc with the specimen.

Illustration continued on opposite page

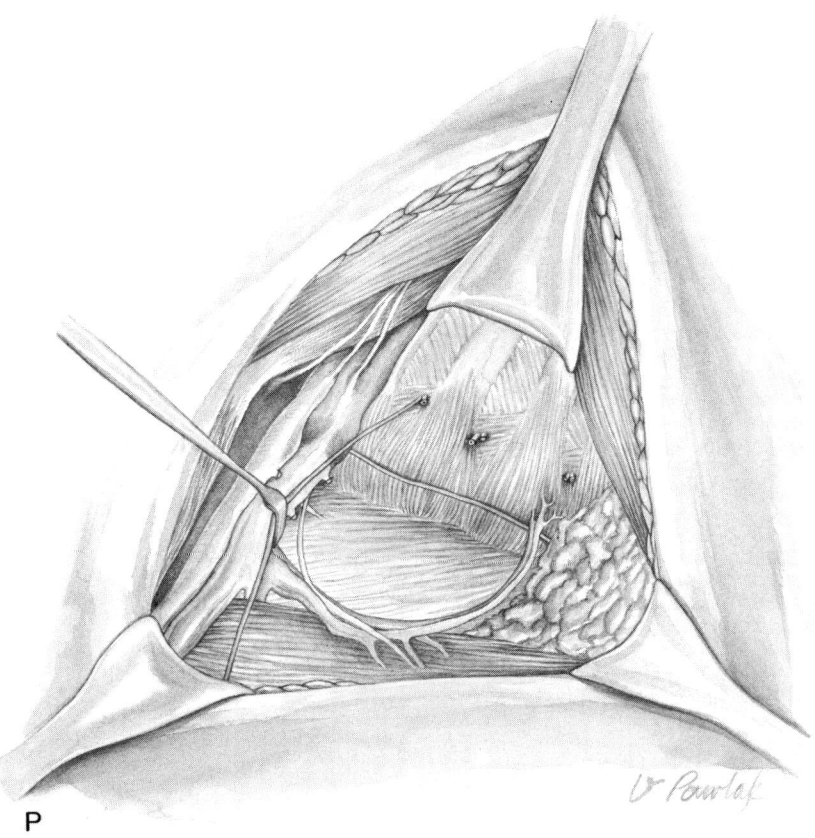

Figure 13-5 *Continued P*, Here the node-bearing tissue has been removed both medial and lateral to the thoracodorsal vessels and detached and removed from the fat and breast tissues attached to it inferiorly. Noteworthy is that the thoracodorsal nerve, after joining the vessels of the same name, crosses superficial to them laterally to innervate the latissimus dorsi, a point that should be kept in mind during the dissection. Furthermore, the nerve to the subscapularis muscle, shown here just beneath the axillary vein, will sometimes be encountered while removing the specimen from the fascia of this muscle and should be preserved. Also noteworthy is that the thoracodorsal vessels divide into branches supplying the latissimus dorsi and those coursing medially into the chest wall. There is no need to interrupt either in the dissection. Damage to the long thoracic nerve produces an unsightly "winged" scapula (Fig. 13–5*T*). Damage to the thoracodorsal nerve paralyzes the latissimus dorsi muscle, which extends, adducts, and internally rotates the humerus, making it difficult for the patient to reach to her back. A single closed suction drain is placed in the incision, looping gently forward inferior to the axillary vein. It should not impinge on the vein. It exits through a stab wound 8 to 10 cm inferior to the base of the lower flap. Irrigation of the wound with warm saline removes loose fat and tissue particles.

Illustration continued on following page

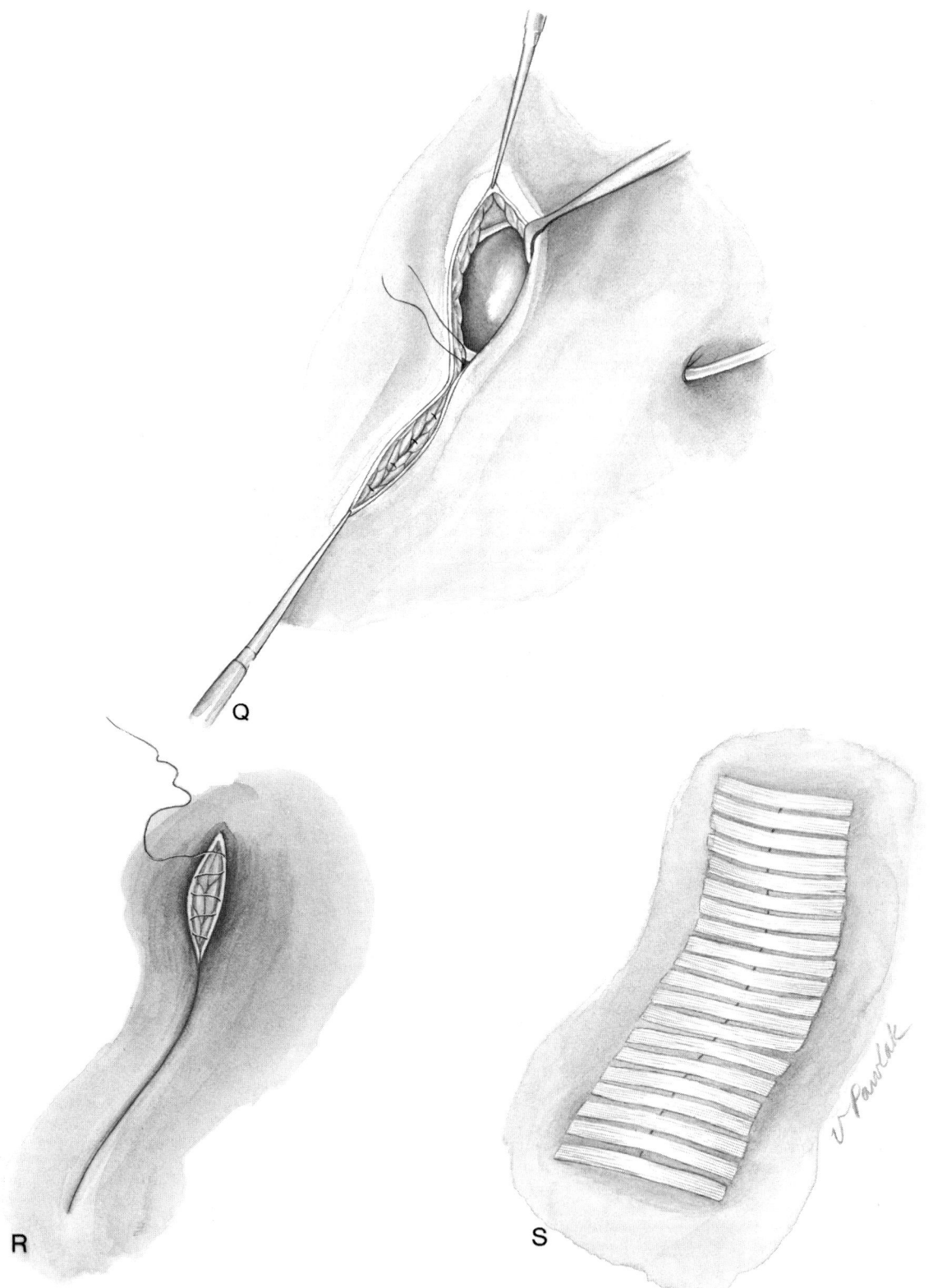

Figure 13–5 *Continued Q,* The incision is closed with interrupted 3–0 catgut or Dexon sutures to the subcutaneous tissue. Here the closed suction drain is shown in place.

R, Closure of the skin is accomplished with a continuous subcuticular 4–0 absorbable suture.

S, The skin closure is completed with application of Steri-strips and a light dressing. The drain is left in place until 24-hour drainage is less than 30 cc. No arm exercises are begun until the drains are out. Steri-strips are removed on the tenth or twelfth postoperative day.

Illustration continued on opposite page

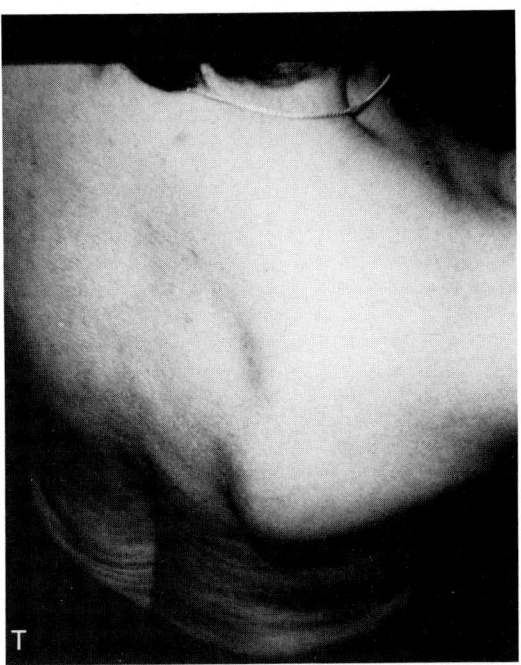

Figure 13–5 Continued T, A "winged" scapula, resulting from damage to the long thoracic nerve with paralysis of the serratus anterior muscle.

edge of the table. The ipsilateral arm is not used for intravenous medications; it is abducted and placed on an arm extension of the operating table. A folded sheet is placed under the ipsilateral shoulder. The entire anterior thorax, the abdomen above the umbilicus, and the ipsilateral axilla, shoulder, and upper extremity to the elbow are prepared antiseptically. The field is then draped with a sterile surface over the arm extension of the operating table and about the forearm to allow mobility of the upper extremity. The balance of the field is draped to put a dry double thickness about the periphery of the mastectomy field.

The basic incision is the same as for a total mastectomy. The flaps are elevated as for the total mastectomy to the periphery of the dissection. This periphery is delineated laterally and medially by two parallel lines, one running down the anterior margin of the latissimus dorsi muscle and one down the midline of the sternum. The superior margin connects with a line running along the sternoclavicular joint, the clavicle, and the deltopectoral groove and across the axillary fold to the insertion of the latissimus dorsi muscle in the humerus.

The inferior delineation runs straight between the medial and lateral boundaries of the dissection at the level of the epigastrium (4 cm below the inframammary fold). The cutaneous flaps are elevated just above the superficial layer of superficial fascia only to the limits of the dissection. The superficial and deep layers of superficial fascia and the panniculus between them are then transected along the anatomic margins described earlier to delineate the extent of the resection (Fig. 13–6A). Irregularities or unevenness in the fat left on the deep surface of the cutaneous flaps is thought to be a factor contributing to flap necrosis and serous effusions (Say and Donegan, 1974).

The dissection is directed next toward exposure of the insertion of the pectoralis major muscle. This insertion is transected in its tendinous portion, and the few vessels encountered are clamped and tied. The muscle belly is then dissected away from the cephalic vein; the vessels and nerves entering the superior margin and deep surface of the muscle are transected and ligated. The clavipectoral fascia is then incised near the coracoid process, and the insertion of the pectoralis minor muscle is transected (Fig. 13–6B,C). If this muscle is folded inferiorly, its blood and nerve supplies are also identified for ligation.

The dissection of the axilla is technically much simpler to perform if the pectoral muscles are transected next at their origin, permitting the entire specimen to fall laterally, and thus placing traction on the axillary fascia. The panniculus lying between the layers of superficial pectoral fascia is reflected medially and superiorly with incisions delineating the origin of the pectoralis major muscle.

The muscle is first detached from the clavicle. A tunnel can then be established medially between the deep surface of the muscle and the anterior chest wall. Some surgeons choose to remove only the sternal portion of the muscle, splitting it in the direction of its fibers and leaving the clavicular portion intact. The sternal origin of the muscle containing the anterior perforating vessels from the intercostal and internal mammary vessels can then be held between the fingers for the accurate placement of another row of clamps.

The muscular stump adjacent to the thoracic wall is suture ligated to occlude the perforating vessels. When a deep-lying lower inner quadrant cancer is present, the lower portion of the muscular origin is transected deep to the rectus sheath, and the sheath is included with the resection.

An avascular plane is present deep to the

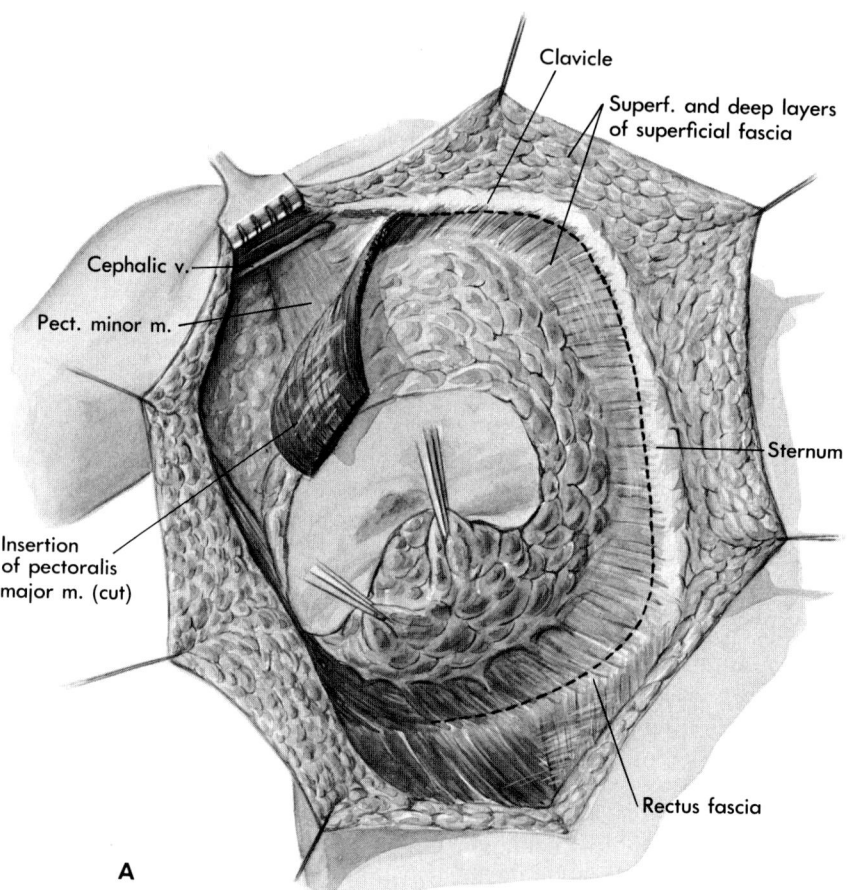

Figure 13–6. *A,* The incision for mastectomy requires a margin of 4 cm of skin in all directions around the palpable margin of the cancer, including the areola. Cutaneous flaps are elevated in a relatively avascular plane between the dermis and the superficial layer of superficial fascia to the midline of the sternum, the clavicle, the deltopectoral groove containing the cephalic vein, the insertion of the pectoralis major muscle, the latissimus dorsi muscle, and across the lower thorax at the level of the rectus sheath. At this periphery, the superficial and deep layers of superficial fascia and the panniculus between them is incised down to the underlying deep fascia and muscles.

Illustration continued on opposite page

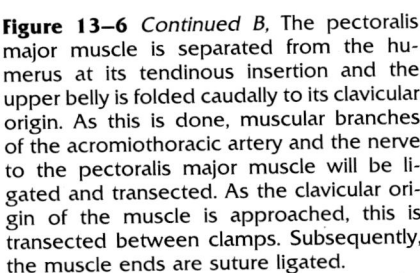

Figure 13-6 *Continued B,* The pectoralis major muscle is separated from the humerus at its tendinous insertion and the upper belly is folded caudally to its clavicular origin. As this is done, muscular branches of the acromiothoracic artery and the nerve to the pectoralis major muscle will be ligated and transected. As the clavicular origin of the muscle is approached, this is transected between clamps. Subsequently, the muscle ends are suture ligated.

C, The clavipectoral fascia overlying the pectoralis minor muscle is incised. Subsequently, the muscle will be transected near the coracoid process. As it is folded caudally, its blood and nerve supply are similarly ligated and transected. The fascia is separated from the thoracic wall medially, and the origins of the pectoralis minor muscle on the third, fourth, and fifth ribs are identified and transected.

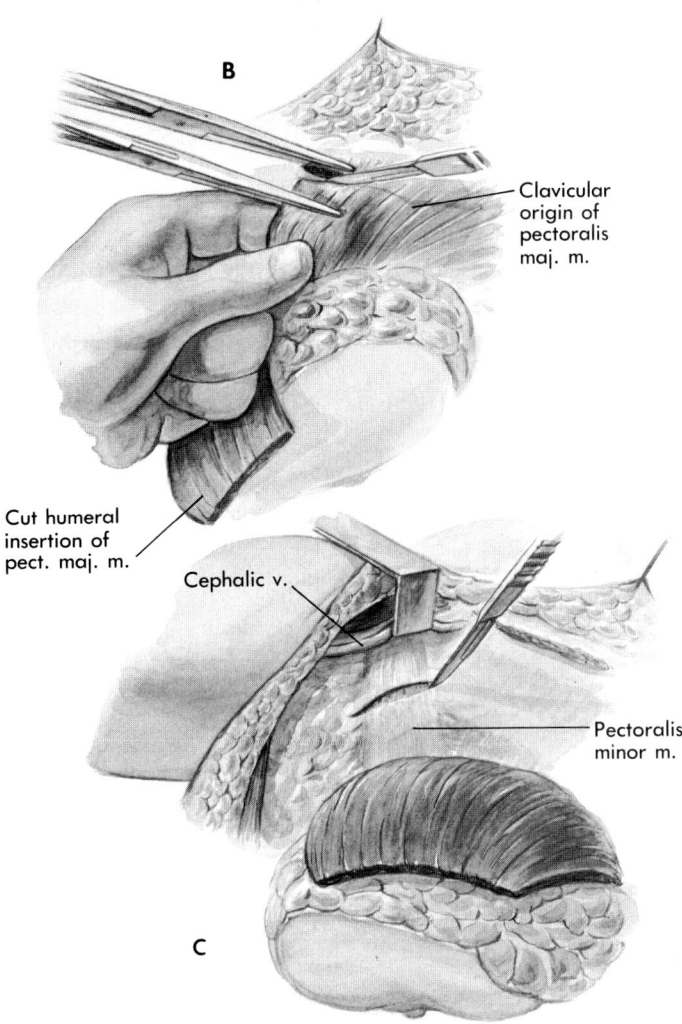

pectoralis major muscle. The plane is laid open by reflecting the thin fascia on the ribs, intercostal muscles, and serratus anterior muscle. The thin slips of pectoralis minor muscle arising from the anterolateral portions of the third to fifth ribs will be encountered. These slips are transected, mobilizing the specimen.

After subfascial detachment of the specimen from the portions of the serratus anterior and latissimus dorsi muscles caudal to the insertion of their nerves, the mobile portion of the specimen is wrapped in a sterile towel. As it falls laterally to expose the axilla, it may be laid next to the patient on the edge of the operating table.

The fascia enveloping the axillary vein and artery is now under tension. The vascular sheath is incised along the superior margin of the axillary vein and is reflected caudally. Individual venous tributaries are clamped and ligated as they enter the vein. The sheath is reflected from the anterior and inferior surface of the vein from beneath the clavicle medially to the latissimus dorsi muscle laterally (Fig. 13-7).

Medially, the fascia adjacent to the intercostal muscles is reflected laterally as far posteriorly as possible near the apex of the axilla. Appearing through this fascia, and coming down posterior to the medial end of the axillary vein from the brachial plexus, is the nerve to the serratus anterior muscle. The fascia overlying the nerve is incised, and the nerve is dissected free of the axillary contents from its point of first appearance beneath the axillary vein to its arborizing insertion into the muscle.

Appearing from beneath the axillary vein at a more lateral point is the nerve to the latissimus dorsi muscle. This passes through the axillary fat and may be removed with the

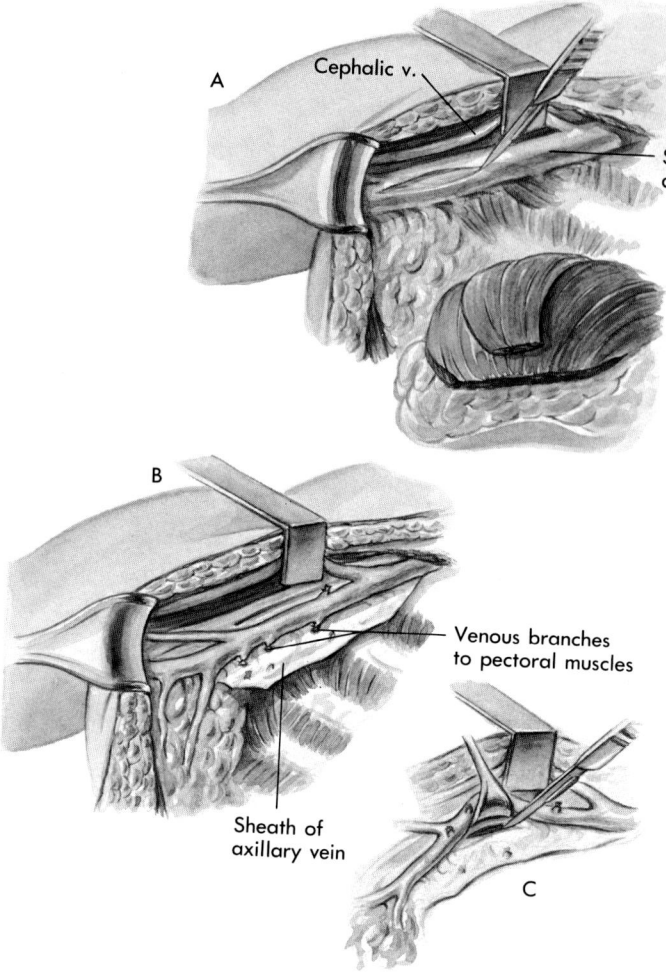

Figure 13–7. *A*, The sheath of the axillary vein is incised near its upper margin and is reflected inferiorly off the vein. As the sheath is reflected, individual venous branches are ligated and transected on the venous side of the sheath. *B*, This reflection is carried out over the entire length of the axillary vein from the clavicle to the tendon of the latissimus dorsi muscle. *C*, The thin sheath of the vein is transected a second time along the dorsal caudal surface of the vein to continue the en bloc mobilization of the axillary contents.

axillary contents. However, it is now customary to preserve this nerve to maintain full function of the arm (Fig. 13–8).

Laterally, the axillary fat containing the lymph cord from the arm is transected over the tendon of the latissimus dorsi muscle. This is then reflected medially until the subscapularis muscle is identified. The fascia is stripped away from this muscle as deep into the posterior axilla as possible. Caution is exercised to avoid injury to the nerve to the subscapularis muscle close to the axillary vein.

On completion of the preceding dissection, the axillary contents are mobilized except for a generally avascular fascial connection dorsal to the axillary vein. This connection is transected, and the axillary contents are swept inferiorly. Only a few fascial and vascular connections dorsally along the anterior margin of the latissimus dorsi muscle remain to be cut before the specimen is removed (Fig. 13–9).

The principles of wound closure are the same as those outlined for total mastectomy. One point seems worth emphasizing: The surgeon will frequently adduct the arm against the thorax to get laxity and length in the cutaneous flaps. This facilitates closure *but*, if the axillary flap has not adhered solidly to the thorax, the flap will tent up across the empty axilla the first time the arm is abducted and elevated. A serous effusion or lymph effusion from the open lymphatics of the upper extremity fills the space and results in morbidity. If the axillary skin does heal with a taut closure, scar contractures across the axilla are likely to occur. A better practice is to close the incision with the arm abducted, making certain that the cutaneous flap does not tent across a large axillary dead space.

INFECTIONS

With attention to aseptic technique and care to avoid devitalizing the skin flaps, infections

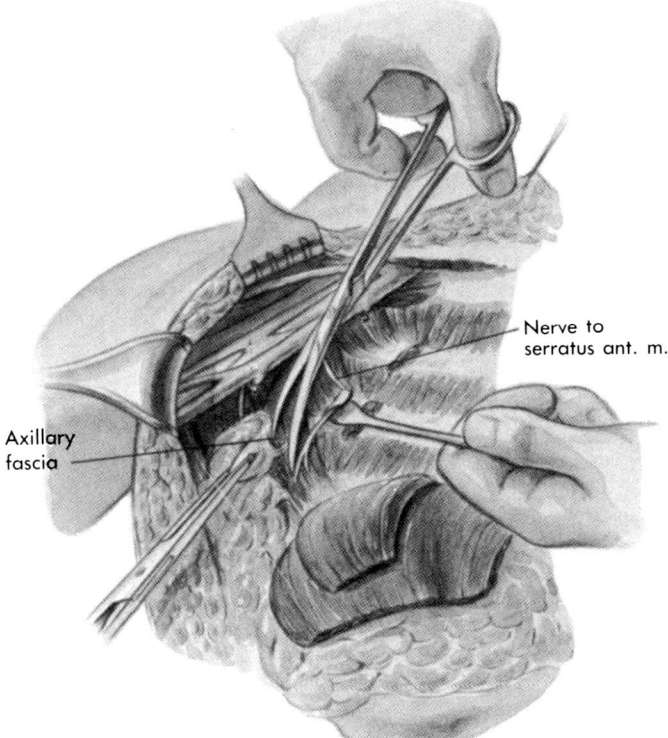

Figure 13–8. As the fascia is dissected away from the under surface of the axillary vein and from the intercostal muscles, the nerves to the latissimus dorsi and serratus anterior muscles will be seen. The more medial nerve to the serratus anterior muscle is dissected away from the axillary fascia throughout its length from the axillary vein to the insertion into the muscle. The nerve to the latissimus dorsi is transected twice, once beneath the vein and once adjacent to the muscle.

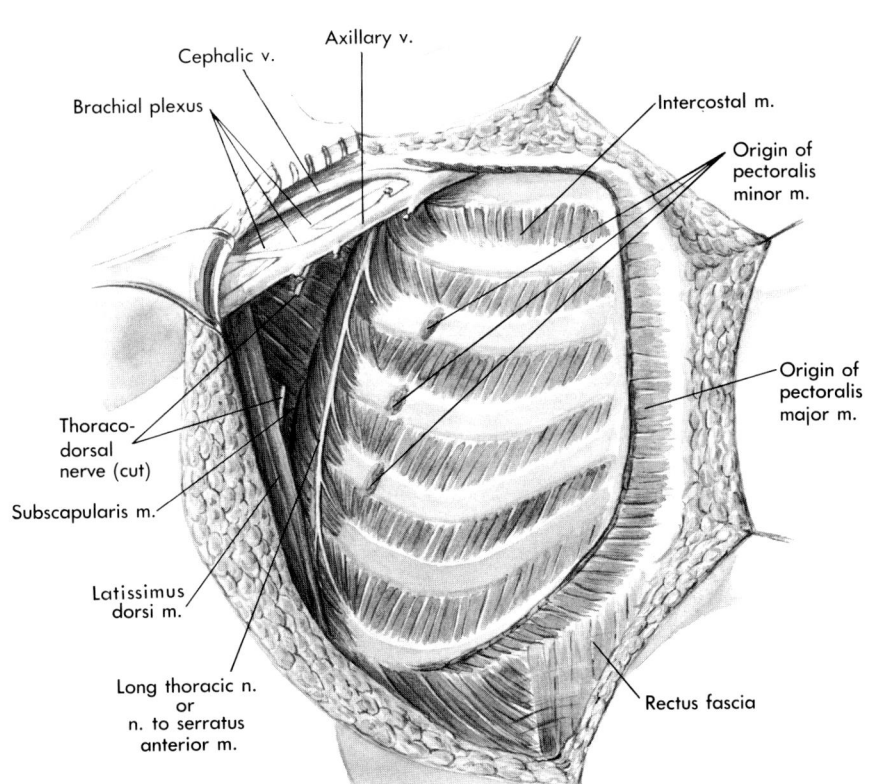

Figure 13–9. Appearance of the surgical defect existing after completion of a radical mastectomy.

after mastectomy are infrequent. When they do occur, they are usually due to skin contaminants, notably *Staphylococcus aureus*. Prompt antibiotic therapy is necessary to avoid progressive loss of the skin flaps. They cause little discomfort because the skin is anesthetic and begin with erythema of the skin edges, which can quickly progress to necrosis of the flap and dehiscence of the mastectomy closure. At the first signs of erythema, treatment with antibiotics is begun. Wound disruption and the collection of pus beneath the flaps requires wet dressings and dependent drainage. This is best accomplished by placing a Penrose drain through a stab incision at the most dependent portion of the lower skin flap. Suction drains are discontinued. With use of moist saline dressings, dependent open drainage, and antibiotics, serious infections can be brought rapidly under control with minimal loss of skin flaps.

NEUROPATHY OF THE ARM AFTER MASTECTOMY

A temporary sensory and motor neuropraxia of the upper extremity can follow mastectomy. It is immediate, in a sleeve distribution, and of varying severity. Weakness is seen in all motions of the shoulder, arm, and fingers, and the patient complains of tingling and dysesthesia throughout this distribution. The problem may result from stretching of the brachial plexus during the operation. For this reason, pulling on the arm during skin preparation, retraction of the brachial plexus during dissection, and vigorous manipulation of the shoulder should be avoided. Patients can be reassured it is a temporary condition. Three patients seen by one of the authors (W.L.D.) received physical therapy, and all recovered completely after several weeks.

Additional complications associated with mastectomy, including phantom breast syndrome, are discussed in the literature (Jamison et al., 1979; Aitken and Minton, 1983).

Internal Mammary Dissection

Recognition that the lymph node chain accompanying the internal mammary vessels is a frequent site of metastasis once led to use of en bloc dissection of the internal mammary lymph chain with radical mastectomy. This operation is seldom used today. Controlled studies have indicated that although it may reduce parasternal recurrences slightly, it achieves no increase in cure or survival rates (Veronesi and Valagussa, 1981; Lacour et al., 1983). Radiotherapy is equally effective in reducing parasternal recurrences in cases at high risk for this problem. It is discussed here because reports occasionally still refer to its use (Noguchi et al., 1982).

The basic steps of the radical mastectomy are unchanged, with the exception of detaching the origin of the pectoralis major muscle. The origin from the clavicle is taken or preserved as before, according to the surgeon's preference, down to the first intercostal space. The intercostal muscles are incised in this space from the sternum laterally for several centimeters. The thin muscle is spread to demonstrate the internal mammary artery and vein. These are ligated with 2-0 silk or Dexon and are transected.

A similar maneuver is performed in the fifth intercostal space just along the upper margin of the cartilage of the sixth rib. Deep to the belly of the pectoralis major muscle, a tunnel is established digitally just lateral to the origin of the muscle. A Lebsche knife is then inserted into the first interspace, tapped to midsternum, directed down the middle of the sternum until the fifth interspace is reached, and then turned into this space.

The chondral portions of the second, third, fourth, and fifth ribs just lateral to the origin of the pectoralis major muscle along the previously established tunnel are then transected. The intercostal arteries and veins along the lower margin of each rib are individually clamped and suture ligated. Throughout this dissection, the underlying pleura is incised and included with a block of chest wall. At the completion of this step, the entire internal mammary lymph node chain adherent to the under surface of the resected chest wall will have been mobilized to be included en bloc with the dissection (Fig. 13–10).

One of the suction catheters is placed through a stab incision in the caudal end of the medial cutaneous flap. The catheter is then placed into the thoracic wall defect with the tip of the catheter running to the first rib. The closure is made airtight. The medial catheter is placed for continuous suction (Fig. 13–11). Neither a prosthetic material to repair the

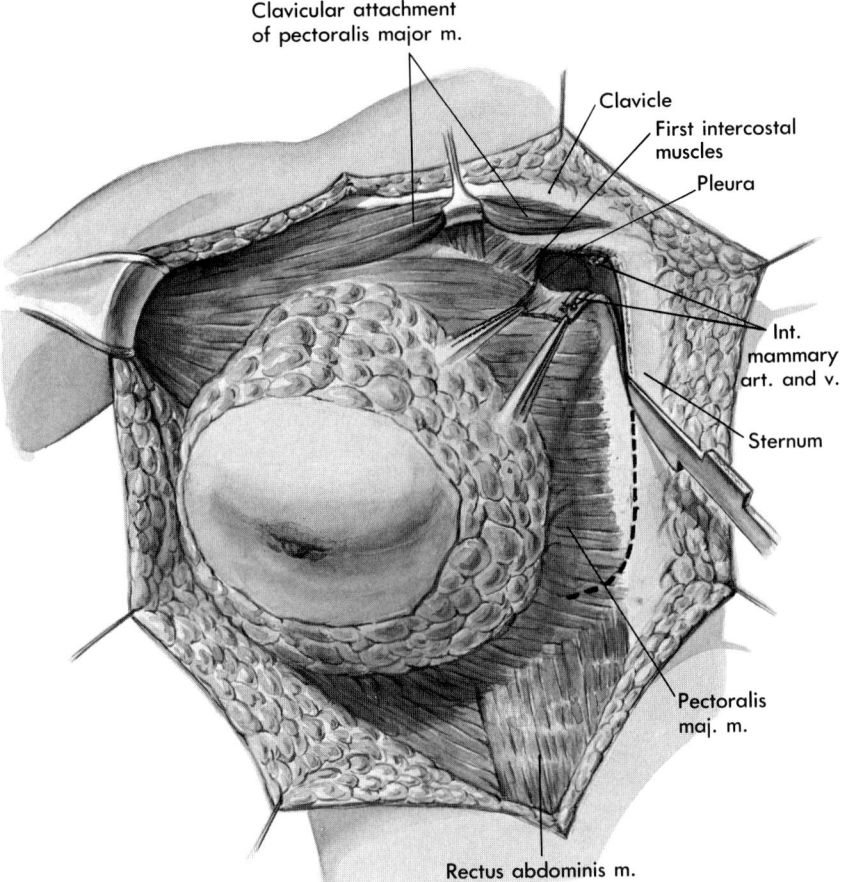

Figure 13–10. When the internal mammary lymph node chain is to be resected, the medial end of the clavicular attachment of pectoralis major muscle is either retracted superiorly and preserved along with the remaining clavicular head of the muscle, as in this illustration, or is reflected inferiorly along with the detached clavicular origin of the muscle. The intercostal muscles are then incised along the upper margin of the first interspace, and the internal mammary artery and vein are ligated and transected near the upper margin of the interspace. A similar maneuver is performed through the intercostal muscles at the lower margin of the fifth interspace. The Lebsche sternal cutting knife is then inserted into the interspace and is tapped to about midsternum and is then directed inferiorly down the midline, turning laterally into the fifth interspace. A tunnel is established by blunt digital dissection deep to the pectoralis major muscle and just lateral to its sternal insertion. The second, third, fourth and fifth ribs and the intervening intercostal muscles are then transected in this tunnel with either straight bone cutting forceps or heavy scissors. The pleura and the underlying areolar tissues are taken with this segment of thoracic wall.

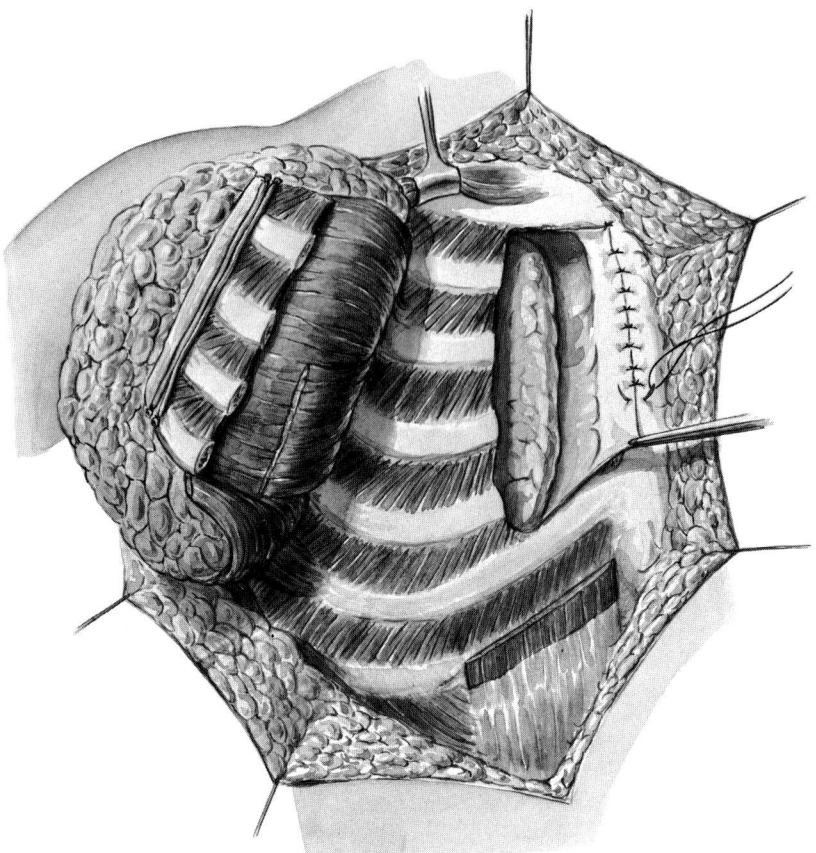

Figure 13–11. The defect persisting in the thoracic wall and pleura is closed by suturing the pleura to the thoracic wall around the periphery. Holes are made in the rib ends and sternum and sutures of No. 1 chromic catgut are passed through the holes. These are tied across the defect with the chest wall compressed medially to reduce the size of the defect. A suction catheter is then placed through a stab wound in the lower medial flap with the tip of the catheter lying in the upper end of the defect. The medial flap is then pulled across the defect and is sutured firmly to the intercostal muscles on the lateral side of the defect. Endotracheal anesthesia is always employed and the lungs are kept near full inflation as the defect is closed. The medial catheter is placed immediately on suction. A separate chest tube through the lateral thoracic wall leading to water-sealed drainage has not been necessary in our experience.

thoracic wall defect nor a separate chest tube attached to water-sealed drainage is necessary (Sugarbaker, 1964).

A catheter is also placed under the lateral cutaneous flap. Primary closure is with interrupted subcutaneous sutures and sutures to the skin. The closure should be airtight with respect to the negative pressure created by the suction catheters so that no leakage occurs.

BIOPSY OF THE INTERNAL MAMMARY NODES

It may be desirable for staging purposes to perform a biopsy of the internal mammary lymph nodes. If the primary tumor lies medially in the breast, the internal mammary nodes contain metastases in up to 26 per cent of cases when the axilla is uninvolved (Morrow and Foster, 1981). As the prognostic implications are similar to those for axillary metastases, these patients are candidates for systemic chemotherapy. Suitable cases are patients who would be eligible for adjuvant therapy and who have an invasive medial primary tumor with a clinically negative axilla. An internal mammary node biopsy can be performed at the end of a total mastectomy or a segmental mastectomy. No extra skin incision is required in either case, as the segmental mastectomy will be located medially in suitable candidates. The first and second intercostal spaces are the most likely to be involved. The fibers of the pectoralis major muscle at the intercostal space are separated bluntly to expose the intercostal muscles about 1 cm lateral to the border of the sternum, avoiding the perforating vessels in the process. Using a small self-retaining retractor to maintain exposure, the intercostal muscles are divided sharply but carefully with a scalpel until the fatty node-bearing tissue surrounding the internal mammary vessels is exposed. If the nodes are involved grossly, this may be apparent immediately; otherwise, the fatty tissue is gently stripped from around the vessels, taking care not to injure the latter or to penetrate the pleura, which lies directly beneath. A small forceps and gentle teasing is often sufficient for this. If the vessels are injured, they can be elevated with a small right angle clamp, the field cleared with a sucker, and the vessels secured with hemoclips. It is not possible to reapproximate the intercostal muscles, and the fibers of the pectoralis major muscle become reapproximated naturally without sutures. A chest x-ray is obtained postoperatively if there is any question about the pleura having been violated. Immediate frozen section is neither necessary nor desirable.

Blood Transfusions

Any blood transfusion carries marginal risks of sensitization, reaction, and disease transmission. In addition, increasing evidence suggests that blood transfusions impair cell-mediated immunity and macrophage migration. Blood tranfusions are additive to the immunosuppression associated with surgery. The immunosuppressive effect of whole blood is even so profound that its use has been shown to enhance allograft survivorship of transplanted primary cadaver kidneys (Fuller et al., 1982). Whether this enhances the ability of residual cancer cells to survive is questionable. These effects encourage surgical techniques that minimize both blood loss and the need for transfusions (Waymack et al., 1986). Francis and Shenton (1981) reported studies on Wistar albino female rats in which lymphocyte reactivity fell significantly after allogeneic transfusion but not after saline infusion or syngeneic transfusions. They reported that when lymphocyte reactivity was low, an inoculum of methylcholanthrene-induced (MC 7) sarcoma underwent a significant increase in tumor growth (Francis and Shenton, 1981).

Burrows and Tartter (1982) reported that among 122 patients who had undergone curative operations for primary adenocarcinomas of the colon and rectum, at every follow-up interval past the 6 month postoperative contact, the probability of recurrence was significantly greater in persons who underwent perioperative transfusions. The stage of cancer case distribution between transfused and nontransfused patients was not different. The more favorable state for the nontransfused persisted in groups receiving postoperative adjuvant therapy. The effect was not altered by the time at which the transfusion occurred (before, during, or after the operation).

Whether perioperative blood transfusion affects prognosis for patients with breast cancer remains an unresolved point. With careful anatomic surgical dissection, blood loss can certainly be kept at a minimum so that transfusions should be required infrequently. Tartter and coworkers (1985) reviewed the possible detrimental significance of these transfusions. Their inquiry evolved from the reported immunosuppressive effect and longer graft survival in renal transplant patients who receive blood transfusions. They compared the disease-free survival following mastectomy in patients who had received perioperative transfusions and those who had none (169 patients operated on between 1964 and 1972). The two groups were stated to be comparable with respect to age, stage, discharge hemoglobin, and type of mastectomy. The cumulative 5 year disease-free survival in the transfused patients was 51 per cent, ($p = 0.02$). Blood loss was also considered, and the authors observed only a 7 per cent difference. Survivorship at 1 year was only 77 per cent for those receiving transfusions, compared with 94 per cent for the untransfused.

On the other hand, Foster and colleagues (1984) conducted a similar study on 226 patients undergoing mastectomy and were unable to confirm any adverse effect on prognosis as a result of perioperative transfusions. Whether transfusions do or do not exert an immunosuppressive effect that reduces survivorship on persons undergoing mastectomy for breast cancer, therefore, remains unresolved. More detailed case stratification might show an effect in some subsets, but these studies are yet to be done. The generalization stands, however, that no blood should be given without a clear indication.

Until the question as to whether transfusions induce sufficient immunosuppression to enhance the virulence of a cancer is firmly resolved, cancer patients should be given only packed washed or washed frozen red cells for the urgent correction of anemia (Gantt, 1981). Moderate blood volume loss at operation can always be corrected with electrolyte solutions. Iron supplements in the postsurgical recuperative period can assist in the reconstitution of hemoglobin mass. The price in terms of real cost, transfusion morbidity, and tumor enhancing immune suppression may all be vastly reduced by avoiding transfusions. As previously noted, most blood loss occurs during the elevation of the skin flaps. This can be greatly lessened by infiltrating the subcutaneous plane to be dissected with 1:400,000 epinephrine in saline (1 ml or 1:1000 epinephrine diluted in 400 ml of normal saline solution) and by careful dissection.

LABORATORY PHLEBOTOMIES AND BLOOD LOSS

Paradoxically, the phlebotomies for diagnostic laboratory tests may result in enough blood loss to induce anemia in adults, contributing to transfusion requirements. Smoller and Kruskall (1986) reported that patients in intensive care units with arterial lines may have an average of 944.0 ml of phlebotomy blood loss per day! Among 36 patients evaluated, blood loss from phlebotomies contributed to the need for transfusions in 17 patients. Smoller and Kruskall suggested that the cumulative volume of blood loss from phlebotomies should be recorded and that blood-conserving collection procedures should be implemented, such as the use of pediatric sample tubes for adults and batching the requests for laboratory tests. Capillary tube samples drawn by finger stick can often replace the need for phlebotomy. Obviously, justification should exist for ordering all laboratory tests, particularly those requiring phlebotomies.

Inflammatory Cancer

Although mastectomy is not considered effective solo treatment for inflammatory cancer, nevertheless there is a place for selected surgery for this entity. It starts with the biopsy. Skin is not routinely biopsied for most breast masses. However, it should be biopsied and examined histologically when reddened or edematous skin or skin otherwise suspected of containing cancer is present. Inflammatory cancer in particular is confirmed by the microscopic observation of cancer cells in the dermal lymphatics. However, dermal lymphatic invasion may not be present universally. Hormone receptors should also be determined.

Recent studies support the more frequent use of mastectomy in selected situations (Morris, 1983). Whenever significant local tumor mass exists after treatment by either chemotherapy or radiotherapy, a mastectomy is tailored to remove this mass. The benefit is probably greater when used after a chemotherapeutic response, avoiding the morbidity of the protracted administration of 6000 to 8000 rad to a wide field. Radiotherapy is reserved for patients who do not respond to chemotherapy.

Surgical removal of advanced breast cancers after reduction by chemotherapy is feasible and may enhance the response of micrometastases to additional chemotherapy. Aisner and coworkers (1982) reported on a series of 27 patients having bulky primary tumors (15 of the 21 had overt metastases and 13 had inflammatory cancers). After three to four courses of chemotherapy, 24 patients were considered operable and 22 underwent mastectomy. Eighteen underwent primary closure of the skin without grafting. Only eight patients had recurred locally at the time of the report. In five patients, metastases responded to further chemotherapy. Perloff and Lesnick (1982) reported similar benefit from coordinated surgical ablation of advanced primary cancers in conjunction with chemotherapy.

Rehabilitation and Prevention of Lymphedema

Rehabilitation is a function of attitude as well as of performance. Attitude is a product of many variables, covering such widely divergent areas as the patient's informational and psychologic background; socioeconomic variables relating to family and associates; physician-patient relationship, which must include the systematic discussion of attitudes and information needed to motivate and encourage the patient and to alleviate anxieties; and the relationship of the patient with all supportive groups within and outside the medical setting.

The American Cancer Society has greatly enhanced the rehabilitation of the postmastectomy patient with its Reach to Recovery Program. The nurse's important role in postmastectomy care and rehabilitation is discussed fully in Chapter 20. It is important to emphasize that *active* and not passive or isometric exercises should begin as soon as drainage ceases. Any patient who does not rapidly develop a complete range of shoulder joint motion should be referred to physical therapy for a sustained program.

A major problem that still occasionally develops in breast cancer patients is chronic lymphedema. The prevention of this problem necessitates a clear understanding of the pathophysiology and anatomy in lymphedema, both acute and chronic, and an appreciation of the factors that predispose to it.

Anatomy and Pathophysiology in Lymphedema

LYMPHATIC SYSTEM

The lymphatic system consists of two major portions: (1) a complex system of intercommunicating capillaries and vessels, which conducts lymph from the periphery and empties it centrally into the venous system, and (2) the lymph nodes, which are interspersed along the lymphatic channels and serve various functions, including filtration, lymphocyte production, and antibody production. Lymph nodes tend to cluster in fatty tissue near the bifurcation of great veins. There is also a need to distinguish the tissue fluid circulating in the tissue spaces (between the cells) from the lymph, which is the fluid contained within lymphatic vessels. Lymph circulates through the skin (and other tissues of the body) via a system of closed vessels (Gray, 1939; Butcher and Hoover, 1955; Ruszynyak et al., 1960). The cutaneous lymphatic circulation arises in the subepithelial region of the dermis as a superficial plexus of capillaries with blindly ending papillae extending upward toward the epidermis. This plexus is valveless and is continuous over the entire surface of the body, although it normally drains only a small area. There are no lymphatic vessels in the epidermis per se. The subepithelial plexus is connected by oblique and vertical trunks to a system of larger lymphatic vessels in the subdermal region. The walls of the vessels of the superficial or subepithelial capillary plexus are composed of endothelium alone. There is no differentiation of adventitia or formation of muscular coats around these vessels.

The subdermal plexus of lymphatics is a system of collecting radicles containing valves to ensure a unidirectional flow of the lymph. Lymph flows from the subdermal plexus into a subcutaneous plexus, the major lymph trunks conducting fluid from the periphery. In addition to valves, the vessels of the subcutaneous plexus contain a muscular layer that converts the process of lymph drainage at this level from a completely passive one into a partially active one. It is this system of lymphatic vessels in the subcutaneous tissue that carries the lymph to the regional nodes. There is a system of deep lymphatics (that is, deep to the muscular fascia) that is much less extensive than the superficial system. This deep system drains the large muscular compartments, but the largest portion of the deep drainage by volume comes from the joints and the synovial tissues. Lymphatics are sparse within the muscles themselves. There are relatively few channels passing through the deep fascia connecting the superficial system and the deep system. Flow through the channels connecting these two systems is normally from the deep system to the superficial system (the opposite of the normal venous drainage). The most significant connection between the two systems is at the level of the regional lymph nodes, where both join to form a common trunk. Thus, each system (superficial and deep) functions independently of the other in the usual circumstances.

Even though the vessels in the subcutaneous system branch and reanastomose with each other, their caliber remains approximately the size of a 27 gauge needle, seldom increasing as they proceed toward the regional lymph nodes. Valves with paired cusps are placed regularly in this system. Distal to each valve is a small constriction, and proximal to each valve a small dilatation of the lumen is present.

Because the lymph channels of the subcutaneous system form a network by their method of anastomosing and branching, bypass channels for any particular lymph node or group of lymph nodes exist. Thus, lymph may bypass nodes and continue on to the next higher node or group of lymph nodes.

As a result of the valvular structure of the main lymph channels, flow of lymph in a unidirectional fashion is maintained. Retrograde lymphatic metastases occur only when proximal lymphatics are blocked and become dilated to a degree that makes the valves incompetent.

The lymphatic system (nodes and vessels) is a continuum of channels without specific anatomic demarcation. For convenience of description, lymph nodes have been artificially and arbitrarily divided into groups that are named by their anatomic surrounding. This grouping gives the impression of specific and discontinuous lymph node groups, each draining certain anatomic regions and structures. It must be kept in mind, however, that the lymphatic system is composed of a network of interconnecting vessels that form a continuous chain of channels with interspersed nodes. Certain organs and certain anatomic regions are drained by lymphatics that usually end in specific nodes. However, the continuum of the lymphatic system makes the division of lymph nodes into groups an artificial one imposed by the descriptive need of the anatomist.

Conditions are created for the development of lymphedema in the upper extremity whenever the major lymph conduits in the axilla are ablated by surgical removal, irradiation, or the uncontrolled progression of tumor. The prevention of lymphedema requires an understanding of prophylactic measures, the recovery process, and the adverse and often permanent changes that occur in an extremity allowed to accumulate and retain an excess of edema fluid.

These predisposing conditions for lymphedema are explained by Starling's hypothesis regarding the factors affecting the movement of water between the blood and tissue spaces (Fig. 13–12). As indicated by the protein content of thoracic duct lymph, a considerable fraction of plasma protein normally enters tissue spaces. With injury, infection, capillary rupture, or obstruction to outflow of lymph or venous blood and with arteriolar dilation from heat and exercise, protein leakage into the tissues may accelerate. The greater the protein content in tissue fluids, the greater is the osmotic pressure drawing more water into tissue spaces. The concomitant stretching of skin and subcutaneous tissues reduces the hydrostatic pressure produced by their normal turgor. Even after edema fluid is removed, this turgor may remain reduced, increasing susceptibility to reaccumulation of edema.

A useful program requires a coordinated

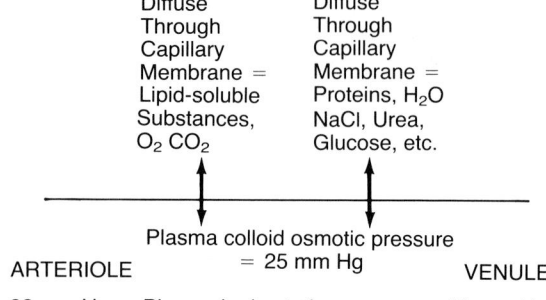

Figure 13–12. Diagram of factors considered in the Starling hypothesis. Considerable variation in the recorded pressure may exist. (U. of L. Medical Illustrations No. 13685–1.) (Adapted from Stillwell, G. K.: Treatment of postmastectomy lymphedema. Mod. Treat., 6:396, 1959.)

application of elevation of the affected region, massage, and moderate active exercise. Treatment of edema requires external elastic support and administration of antibiotics if any sign of associated infection exists. Treatment must also include careful patient education concerning the pathophysiology and consequences of lymphedema, the importance of elevation and active exercises, the need to protect the extremity from trauma and infections, the undesirable consequences of local or general overheating, and the limitations on excessive use. The most effective lymph reducing exercise is active exercise of an extremity elevated to take advantage of gravity. Massage of an elevated extremity working peripherally to centrally is helpful. Lymphedema pumps are beneficial, but overvigorous use may rupture the already reduced number of lymphatics.

REGENERATION OF LYMPHATICS

Ju and coworkers (1954) concluded that radical mastectomy reduced the lymph flow from the upper extremity by 40 per cent. They based their conclusions on the clearance of radioiodinated human serum albumin (RISA) injected subcutaneously. Serial studies showed that the RISA clearance improved with time but never returned to normal.

This improvement in clearance evolves parallel with the regeneration of lymphatics. Reichert (1926), Butcher and Hoover (1955), and Howard and colleagues (1964) have all demonstrated this regeneration after transection. Butcher and Hoover showed bridging of superficial lymphatics across linear incisions by the fifteenth day after incision with healing per primam. Infection, delay in wound healing, irradiation, and the persistence of cancer can all delay or permanently prevent bridging of lymphatics across a wound. Faced with such a variable process, the only questions that really count in assessing function are the following: Are there enough lymphatics to clear the extremity of lymph, and what can be done to assist them in doing so and to avoid overloading their capacity by stimulating increased lymph production?

QUANTITATING LYMPHEDEMA

The degree of lymphedema has been "staged" by past reviewers. These stages are based on the volume increase with respect to the contralateral or unaffected arm. Tracy and coworkers (1961) considered that an increase in volume of less than 150 ml is insignificant, 150 to 600 ml is slight, 400 to 750 ml is moderate, and greater than 750 ml is severe.

Stillwell (1969) based his classification on the percentage of volume increase. He regarded an increase of less than 10 per cent as insignificant, an increase of 11 to 20 per cent as slight, an increase of 41 to 80 per cent as marked, and an increase of greater than 80 per cent as severe. Periodic circumferential measurements of the arm at standard sites can be used to detect and evaluate the course of edema (15 cm distal to the acromion and 15 cm distal to the olecranon are convenient sites; measurements 15 cm proximal and distal to the elbow are also used).

However, any increase is to be avoided, and this preventive process must begin when a person with breast cancer is first seen. The patient must understand the pathophysiology of lymphedema because it is the patient who must follow a lifelong program of preventive care and who must understand the urgency of expeditious treatment if lymphedema develops, no matter how "insignificant" or "slight." Untreated "slight" lymphedema is a precondition for progression to moderate, marked, and finally severe lymphedema. Retention of any lymphedema brings about progressive and irreversible changes.

NATURE AND EFFECT OF EDEMA FLUID

Untreated lymphedema inexorably progresses from reversible pitting lymphedema through phases of subcutaneous fibrosis to produce a nonpitting edema by forming permanent fibrokeratotic skin changes called elephantiasis. The emphasis has to be placed on the "inexorable progress." This progress may be very subtle, but once the fibrosis occurs, it is permanent. However, the fibrosis may increase each time unorganized lymph reaccumulates in the extremity and is allowed to remain for even short periods. Excess protein containing lymph in an extremity is "organized" by the fibroblasts, leaving *permanent* fibrosis and producing a fibrokeratotic extremity.

Thompson (1967) provided a comprehensive review of the surgical operations used for chronic fibrokeratotic lymphedema of the extremity and of their results. More recently omental transfer and the physiologically appealing technique of lymphaticovenous anastomosis in the arm have been added (Savage, 1985). Both have had their successes and failures.

Kinmonth (1982) cites a personal communication from Mowlem (1955), who observed that even after pedicle grafts were brought into a lymphedematous extremity past a point of lymphatic obstruction the lymphatic system still retained an incompetence and was incapable of recovery. Thus, many combinations of pedicle grafts have been tried and abandoned. Lymphaticovenous anastomoses often fail for the same reason. The buried dermis flap seems to be the only operation associated with any sustained benefit. This operation is not described here because of the infrequency of its need. A careful review of indications, technique, and postoperative management should be reviewed in Kinmonth's book (1982) if it is thought that an extremity is too far advanced for physiologic control of the edema.

Treves (1957) showed that the combination of irradiation of the axilla and axillary dissection increases the prevalence of lymphedema in the upper extremity and should be avoided. Lymphedema after modified radical mastectomy in the absence of irradiation occurs in less than 10 per cent of cases, and in most of these it is mild. The frequency is no higher after segmental mastectomy and axillary dissection if irradiation is confined to the breast.

A late complication of chronic lymphedema is lymphangiosarcoma. This tumor arises from the endothelium in chronic lymphedema and usually is manifested as multiple macular or papular purple lesions of the extremity. Results of treatment have been uniformly poor. The risk of this complication further emphasizes the need for a coordinated program to prevent chronic lymphedema (Peterson, 1969).

In conclusion, debilitating fibrokeratotic lymphedema of the upper extremity is a major but generally preventable complication of ablative therapy of the axillary contents by surgical dissection or radiotherapy, particularly when the two are used in combination. Recurrent cancer in the axilla and supraclavicular area is particularly likely to produce the condition. In the absence of recurrent cancer, the condition should be prevented if possible or kept to an insignificant degree by applying the principles discussed in this section. Preparation requires preoperative counselling regarding the possibility of this problem, education in its prevention, and surveillance through the lifelong follow-up of the patient. Extremity measurements, expeditious treatment of lymphangitis and lymphedema, and reinforcement of patient education become an integral part of this process during follow-up.

Nerve Entrapment and Radiation Neuropathy

A collateral complication of lymphedema if it is allowed to develop is nerve entrapment (Ganel et al., 1979). These entrapments may contribute to some of the disabling symptoms associated with lymphedema. Entrapments occur most frequently in the brachial plexus and in the carpal tunnel. Entrapment symptoms must be differentiated from radiation neuropathy. Surgical scarring alone in the axilla does not produce brachial plexus neuropathy (Say and Donegan, 1974). The late effects of radiotherapy add to the risk of neuropathy of the brachial plexus (Kogelnik and Karcher, 1977).

Surgical decompression in a radiotherapeutic field or in the presence of recidivated cancer is of little value. For persistence of carpal tunnel syndrome after effective management of the lymphedema, decompression may occasionally be helpful. All sources of metabolic neuropathy should be excluded and managed first. Microvascular damage to the nerve trunks themselves secondary to the irradiation may account for the persistence of symptoms even when the scar about a nerve can be removed or divided successfully.

Irradiation and Surgery

The cancer surgeon is aware that operations in and around heavily irradiated tissues are frequently difficult to perform and that the resulting wounds are susceptible to necrosis and delayed healing. Likewise, scarred fields of major surgical procedures exhibit a reduced tolerance to radiotherapy. In both instances, the most important variables are the time-dose factors, amount of irradiation, and the location and size of the treatment ports. Single doses of 2000 rads (R) completely inhibit the regeneration of both blood and lymph capillaries in wounded mammalian tissue, but capillary regeneration can occur normally in wounded tissue receiving less than a 1000 R single dose (Van den Brenk, 1956, 1957). Any tissue receiving more than a 1000 R single dose is subject to necrosis. Protracted time-dose schedules reduce but do not eliminate these radiobiologic effects.

Tissue "tolerance" is a general term used to define the maximum dosage a tissue can receive over a given period of time without subsequent necrosis. For most tissues, tolerance is about 6000 to 8000 R over 5 to 8 weeks. Surgical operations performed in any tissue treated to "tolerance" will be complicated by the obliteration of tissue planes, a markedly decreased capacity for primary wound healing, a susceptibility to necrosis from the trauma of surgery, and the risk of infection (Spratt and Sala, 1962).

Does the Substitution of Axillary Irradiation for Axillary Dissection Prevent Lymphedema?

One of the arguments for the substitution of radiotherapy of the axilla instead of axillary dissection is that lymphedema is avoided. This is not true, according to the report of Tough (1968). He reported on 573 cases treated by simple mastectomy followed by radical radiotherapy and followed for at least 5 years. Of his patients, 100 (17 per cent) had developed lymphedema during this period. Lymphedema risk was related to clinical stage and the recidivation of cancer in the axilla. However, 30 cases of lymphedema (5 per cent) developed during this period without any sign of cancer recidivation.

Wound Healing in Irradiated Tissue

When the irradiation involves soft tissue that can be replaced by the contractional approximation of adjacent normal tissues, the irradiated area is slowly replaced by the ingrowth of vasculature and scar from adjacent nonirradiated tissue (Spratt et al., 1961). When the field of treatment is very large or lies on a rigid surface, such as the chest wall, this contractional healing cannot occur. Such an area remains a scar of decreased vascularity indefinitely and never becomes as tolerant as normal tissue to injury. With minor trauma these scars are subject to progressive necrosis, often requiring excision and full-thickness coverage with pedicle grafts.

After mastectomy, the chest and axilla are greatly reduced in soft tissue content. The radiotherapist must deal with thin skin over a bony surface beneath which lies normal lung that is quite sensitive to injury by irradiation. Intervening muscles, when preserved and irradiated, are subject to radiation fibromyositis and contracture. These factors influence the field shape, the beam direction, and time-dose factors for postoperative irradiation. Routine pre- or postoperative therapy to the breast and adjacent lymph node–bearing areas fails to improve survival (Paterson and Russell, 1959; Borgstrom and Lindgren, 1962; Butcher et al., 1964; Oeser and Albrecht, 1964).

Oophorectomy

Oophorectomy is of value for palliative endocrine therapy of premenopausal women. The role of oophorectomy in the therapy of mammary carcinomatosis is well established, but any value of prophylactic oophorectomy is unproved (Tengrup et al., 1986).

Experience with therapeutic oophorectomy varies (Lee, 1971; Peetz et al., 1981). Overall objective response rates that last over 6 months occur in 20 to 48 per cent, depending on selection of patients. Factors associated with a better response include the premenopausal state, a long disease-free interval after mastectomy, blood types B and AB, symptomatic recurrent disease limited to bone, and the presence of metastases and corpus luteum in the removed ovaries. Estrogen receptor protein in tumor tissue is associated with a high probability of response to castration. Objective response for any period is associated with an improved survival rate over that in nonresponders. The antiestrogen tamoxifen has produced response rates equal to those of oophorectomy in premenopausal women and can be tried initially, but oophorectomy remains effective as a subsequent therapy whether or not the patient responds to tamoxifen (Planting et al., 1985; Ingle et al., 1986).

If the lung contains metastases extensive enough to cause dyspnea at rest, or if extensive hepatic metastases can be proved, the patient is not a candidate for oophorectomy. Patients with negative estrogen and progesterone receptors also are not candidates.

An evolving indication for oophorectomy is a prior response to tamoxifen. Sawka and coworkers (1986) evaluated the effect of oophorectomy in premenopausal women with metastatic breast cancer whose cancers either did not respond to tamoxifen or whose cancers initially responded and then failed. In the failed group, only 2 of 14 assessable patients (14 per cent) remained stable after oophorectomy, whereas in 12 patients (86 per cent) the disease progressed. With initial resonse to tamoxifen followed by escape and then oophorectomy, 9 of 15 (60 per cent) responded to oophorectomy. Serial monitoring of follicle stimulating hormone, prolactin, and estradiol levels in the studied population argued against a "medical ovariectomy" effect of tamoxifen. The effect seems to be primarily on the tumor, and when failure to respond to tamoxifen occurs, oophorectomy may be indicated.

The keys to keeping safe such simple surgical procedures as the bilateral removal of normal ovaries are adequate exposure, a knowledge of the regional anatomy, and an unremitting attention to the details of asepsis, hemostasis, and gentleness with living tissues. In using this operation for mammary cancer, the surgeon must also consider preoperatively the extent of the cancer and the potential tolerance to general anesthesia.

The operation can be performed through low midline incision, cutting the rectus fascia down to the pubis, or through a more cosmetic Pfannenstiel incision. The bladder, previously emptied by sterile catheterization during the preoperative preparation, is identified and reflected inferiorly as the peritoneum is opened. Laparotomy gauzes are placed to cover the subcutaneous fat, and a self-retaining retractor is inserted.

The operating table is tilted 15 degrees head down, and the intestines are packed superiorly out of the pelvic cavity and held there with the center blade of the retractor. The ovary is grasped with a Babcock clamp, and the mesovarium is perforated through its transparent center and clamped in two parts wide of the ovary itself. The bundles, containing the ovarian artery on the lateral side and the ligament of the ovary on the medial side, are transected and suture ligated with heavy silk after the ovary is removed. By staying close to the ovary with good visibility, risks to the ureters are minimized. If adhesions or the patient's anatomy requires removal of the fallopian tubes, the distal portion of the infundibulopelvic ligament is carefully encompassed by incising the peritoneum on either side of it and passing a right angle clamp beneath, being careful not to include the nearby ureter, which can usually be visualized. The ligament is ligated with heavy silk and also suture ligated, then divided. The ovarian tube and ovarian ligament are clamped at the juncture with the uterus, divided, and suture ligated with silk. With the major vessels and ligaments thus secured, the remaining tissue attached to the specimen is carefully transected with scissors and the tube and ovary are delivered en bloc. With hemostasis complete, the bowel is replaced in the pelvis, and the incision is closed using stout interrupted nonabsorbable suture for the musculofascial layers and a fine synthetic suture for the skin. A dry sterile dressing is applied. Blood loss is minimal with this technique. Postoperatively, nasogastric decompression is usually not necessary.

Hospital mortality rate is low (0.5 per cent) in well selected patients, although in some series it has reached 4 per cent, owing to rapid progression of extensive metastases in liver, lungs, or brain (Puga et al., 1976; Peetz et al., 1981).

Adrenalectomy

Adrenalectomy is not performed as often as formerly because its benefit can be approximated by medical adrenal ablation with the combination of aminoglutethimide (Cytadren) and hydrocortisone. Some patients who are good candidates for adrenal ablation, however, find the side effects of aminoglutethimide (e.g., rash, nausea and vomiting, hypotension) intolerable and are best treated with surgical adrenalectomy. High levels of tumor estrogen and progesterone receptors and previous benefit from oophorectomy are good predictors of a positive response.

Although the role of adrenalectomy has been reduced, it has not been eliminated by the availability of endocrine suppressive drugs (Nemoto et al., 1984). Nemoto and colleagues conducted a randomized study on 51 patients with breast cancer. They concluded that both tamoxifen and adrenalectomy were effective and that this effectiveness was retained in crossovers. That is, patients who failed on tamoxifen would still respond to adrenalectomy, and vice versa. The initial response was superior with adrenalectomy. The lack of initial response to either adrenalectomy or tamoxifen does not rule out response to the other. Kiang and associates (1980) made similar observations with respect to tamoxifen and hypophysectomy.

With adrenalectomy, the preoperative preparation and postoperative care of the patient are critical to success. It is important not only that replacement therapy be begun before operation but also that its maintenance be ensured afterward. Patients of known unreliability and those who are not within easy reach of medical attention are poor candidates for total adrenalectomy.

Maintenance is almost always possible with cortisone acetate, 25 mg twice a day, and a salt intake of 3.0 g per day; the salt intake is accomplished by instructing the patient to salt all food liberally. Rarely, a patient will require fludrocortisone acetate (Florinef) to maintain electrolyte balance, and this can be given as 0.05 to 0.1 mg daily. A replacement schedule that has proved satisfactory is given in Table 13–2.

During the follow-up period, the physician should be alert to symptoms of extreme weakness, nausea and vomiting, elevated temperature, rapid weight loss, or hypotension, which usually indicate adrenal insufficiency. Stressful situations may require a temporary additional

Table 13–2. REPLACEMENT SCHEDULE FOR BILATERAL TOTAL ADRENALECTOMY*

Day	Medication	Route
Day before operation	50 mg cortisone twice or 100 mg hydrocortisone sodium succinate (Solu-Cortef) at 6 P.M.	Orally Intramuscularly
Day of operation	100 mg Solu-Cortef prior to operation, 100 mg during surgery and 50 mg every 4 hr thereafter	Intramuscularly
1st postoperative day	100 mg Solu-Cortef every 8 hr	Intramuscularly
2nd postoperative day	50 mg Solu-Cortef every 6 hr	Intramuscularly
3rd postoperative day	50 mg Solu-Cortef every 12 hr	Intramuscularly
4th postoperative day	25 mg Solu-Cortef every 8 hr or 25 mg cortisone every 8 hr	Intramuscularly Orally
5th postoperative day	25 mg cortisone every 12 hr	Orally
Maintenance	25 mg cortisone twice a day	Orally

*Diet to include 3.0 NaCl daily.

intake of cortisone, and acute crises may require hospitalization with intensive therapy, including intravenous saline and increased corticosteroids. After adrenalectomy, patients wear a medical alert bracelet as a precaution and carry a card stating their need for cortisone and identifying their physician.

PROCEDURE FOR ADRENALECTOMY

The adrenal glands can be removed through an anterior or a posterior approach. The anterior approach is advantageous because (1) both adrenals can be removed through a single incision with the patient supine, (2) the abdomen can be explored through this incision to assay the extent of neoplastic disease, and (3) the ovaries can be removed through the same incision. With the proper instruments and experience, both adrenals can be removed quickly (Figs. 13–13 and 13–14). The posterior approach offers less risk of ileus and perhaps a faster recovery.

The average anesthetic time for bilateral adrenalectomies performed through the anterior approach is 3 hours. Dissection techniques

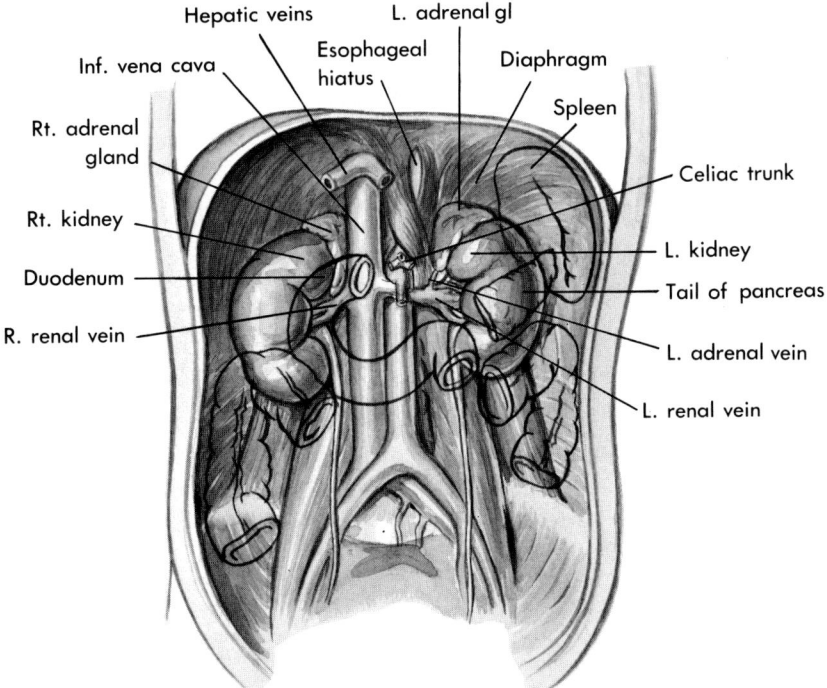

Figure 13–13. The relationship of the adrenal glands to other abdominal organs and the vena cava can be appreciated in this perspective.

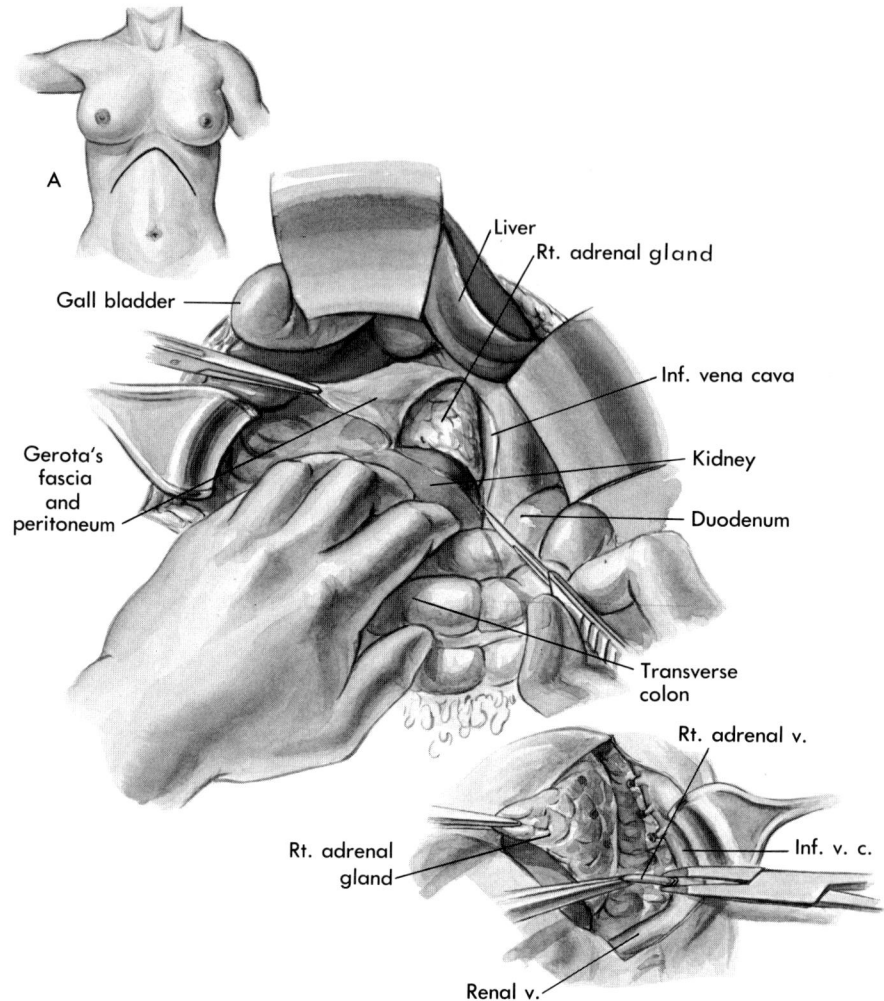

Figure 13–14. Either a transverse incision parallel to and about 1 inch below the costal margins (A) or preferably a high straight transverse incision can be used to approach the adrenals. If the ovaries are also to be removed, a single vertical midline incision is advantageous.
  The right adrenal is taken first. The hepatic flexure of the colon is reflected inferiorly and the duodenum is reflected medially. The kidney is manually retracted caudally. The flap of Gerota's fascia is incised and elevated lateral to the vena cava and above the upper pole of the kidney. The fatty areolar tissue investing the adrenal and kidney is teased away from the vena cava down to and along the upper margin of the right renal vein. As this is done, the veins and arteries bridging across to the adrenal gland will be encountered. These are doubly occluded with hemoclips and transected between the clips as they are identified. Occasionally a vein leaves the adrenal from its upper pole and this must be dissected under direct vision. With the above complete, the gland can be bluntly and sharply dissected from its bed without further concern over significant hemorrhage.

should keep blood loss to a minimum, avoiding the use of transfusions if at all possible. The key to an easy operation is the availability of dissection instruments 8 to 12 inches in length, including a 10 inch forceps for the placement of hemoclips on the adrenal blood vessels.

The incision extends transversely across the upper abdomen from one anterior axillary line to the other. Alternatively, a vertical midline incision can be used. The right adrenal usually is removed first. The hepatic flexure of the colon is reflected inferiorly. The peritoneum overlying the vena cava alongside the second (descending) part of the duodenum is incised, and the duodenum is reflected medially as with the standard Kocher maneuver. The peritoneal incision is extended laterally over the upper pole of the right kidney, and the right-angled flap is turned laterally and superiorly, exposing the fatty areolar tissue containing the adrenal gland. This tissue is gently teased away from the vena cava and the right renal vein.

The dark yellow appearance of the adrenal gland is quite distinct and different from the retroperitoneal fat. When the margin is identified, it is teased away from the renal vein and vena cava very gently so as to make the adrenal blood vessels apparent, particularly the large short vein that enters the vena cava. These are individually secured with two hemoclips and transected between the clips.

The medial margin is very intimately attached to the vena cava and frequently extends behind the great vein. When the medial margin has been dissected around the upper pole of the gland, the remaining bed is avascular and the adrenal gland is removed by blunt and sharp dissection (Fig. 13–14).

On the left side, the adrenal is approached by incising the peritoneum lying lateral to the descending colon and the splenic flexure. The retroperitoneal space is entered and the colon, mesocolon, and pancreas are reflected off the left kidney until the area above the pole and adjacent to the aorta is accessible. If the retroperitoneal fat is probed gently, the adrenal gland will be found; its vasculature is identified and transected and the gland is removed. The largest vein on this side enters the renal vein (Figs. 13–15 and 13–16).

Both adrenal fossae are inspected for hemostasis before the abdomen is closed. The peritoneal incisions for exposure of the adrenal fossae are left open. The abdominal incision is closed with continuous 0 absorbable suture to the peritoneum, interrupted nonabsorbable figure-of-eight sutures or continuous nonabsorbable sutures to the musculofascial layers, and staples or sutures to the skin.

Bilateral adrenalectomies can also be performed through bilateral posterior lumbar incisions. This approach has the advantage of minimal postoperative ileus. There are situations in which the posterior approach is probably both easier and safer than the anterior approach. Examples include patients who have had abdominal procedures in the past that are likely to be associated with extensive adhesions in the upper abdomen, abdominal carcinomatosis with or without ascites, and obesity or anatomic deformity that would compromise exposure by the anterior approach. If the ovaries are present, they must be removed via another approach.

To remove the adrenals by the posterior approach, the patient is placed in the "jackknife" position (Egdahl and Melby, 1972). The incisions extend from the iliac crest to the tenth rib and run 6 to 7 cm lateral to the midvertebral line (Fig. 13–17). The twelfth rib is freed from its periosteal sheath and is resected. The twelfth intercostal nerve is identified during this dissection and is preserved. Damage to it produces a belt-like distribution of paresthesia. The transversalis fascia and renal fascia are then incised to expose the kidney. The pleura is reflected away from the diaphragm without being opened. The pleura is held cephalad with a retractor while the diaphragm is opened for digital exploration of the suprarenal space. The adrenal gland is then dissected from its areolar attachments from above downward. As it is further dissected from its bed, the last attachments medially are its vascular attachments. Arteries and veins as they are encountered are occluded proximally and distally with hemoclips and transected. The incision is then closed in layers without drainage. The technique on each side is identical.

Malignant Effusions

Effusions secondary to neoplasia arise as a result of imbalances in fluid flow through the cavity. Whether fluid accumulates depends on the factors in Starling's equation:

$$F = K(P_{cap} - P_{if}) - (\pi_{cap} - \pi_{if})$$

where F = fluid movement, K = filtration coefficient in ml/sec/cm^2/cm of water, P_{cap} = capillary hydrostatic pressure, P_{if} = pericapil-

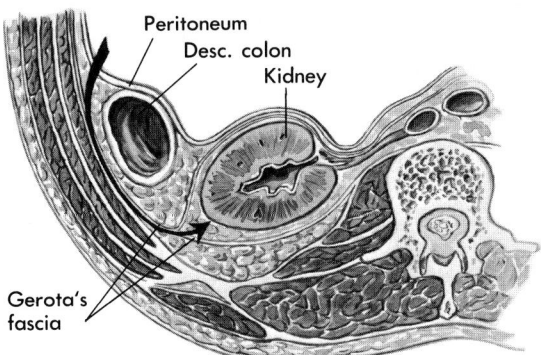

Figure 13–15. The preferred approach to the left adrenal gland is through the retroperitoneal space lateral to the descending colon and into Gerota's fascia. The peritoneum lateral to the upper descending colon is incised for 6 to 8 inches. The colon is reflected medially and the retroperitoneal space is laid open down to the kidney.

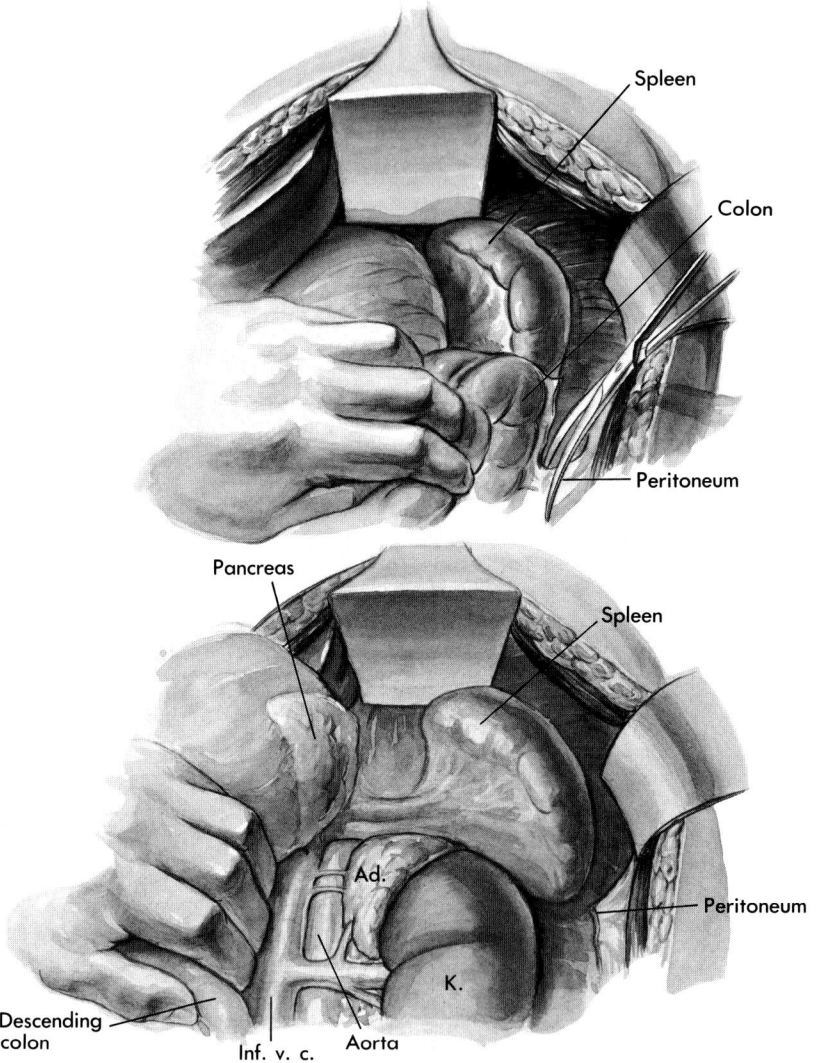

Figure 13–16. The steps described in Figure 13–13 are being carried out in this illustration. The left adrenal gland is more accessible than the right. The vasculature is transected between hemoclips as previously described.

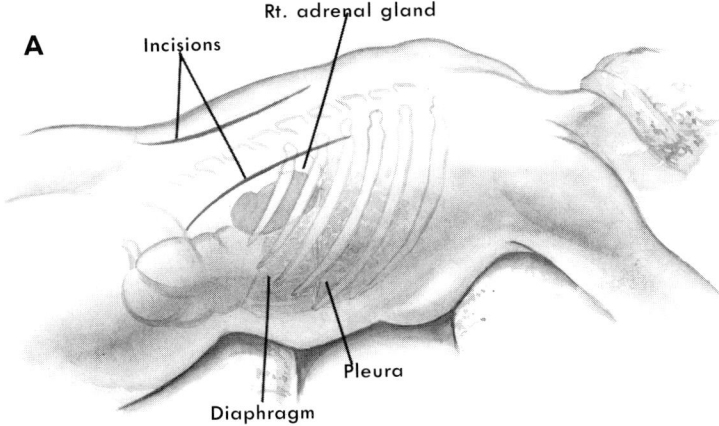
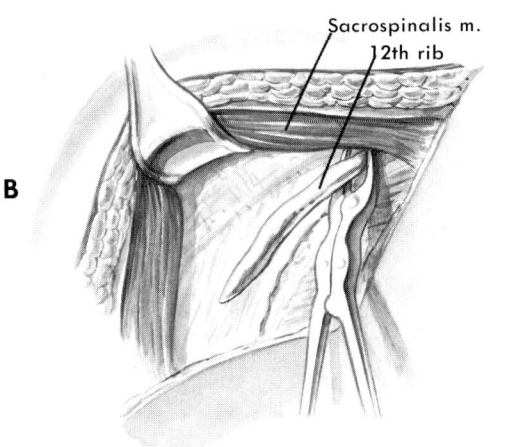
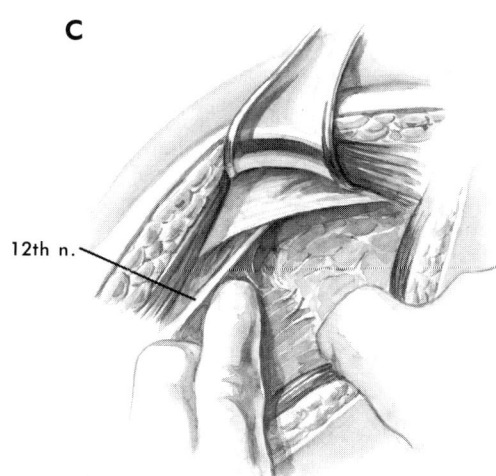

Figure 13–17. The posterior surgical approach for removal of the adrenal glands is illustrated in these figures. Indications for adrenalectomy and for the posterior approach are discussed in the text.

A, General endotracheal anesthesia is induced in the supine position and the patient is then turned and placed in the prone "jackknife" position. The patient's knees are slightly flexed to prevent venous stagnation, and supports are placed under the shoulders and hips to permit effective ventilation. The center of the operating table is elevated in order to flatten the normal lumbar curve. A curvilinear incision is made approximately 5 cm. lateral to the spinous processes of the vertebrae, extending from the level of the 10th rib to the level of the superior border of the posterior iliac crest.

B, The incision is extended through the subcutaneous tissues and through the posterior lamella of the lumbodorsal fascia medial to the border of the latissimus dorsi muscle. This exposes the sacrospinalis muscle on the medial side of the wound. The sacrospinalis muscle is perforated by small blood vessels and posterior lumbar nerves, which must be secured and divided. The sacrospinalis muscle is retracted medially, and the 12th rib is resected subperiosteally, taking care not to enter the subadjacent pleural cavity.

C, The middle lamella of the lumbodorsal fascia is divided in the direction of the incision, and the pleural reflection is pushed superiorly out of harm's way. The quadratus lumborum muscle is evident laterally.

Illustration continued on following page

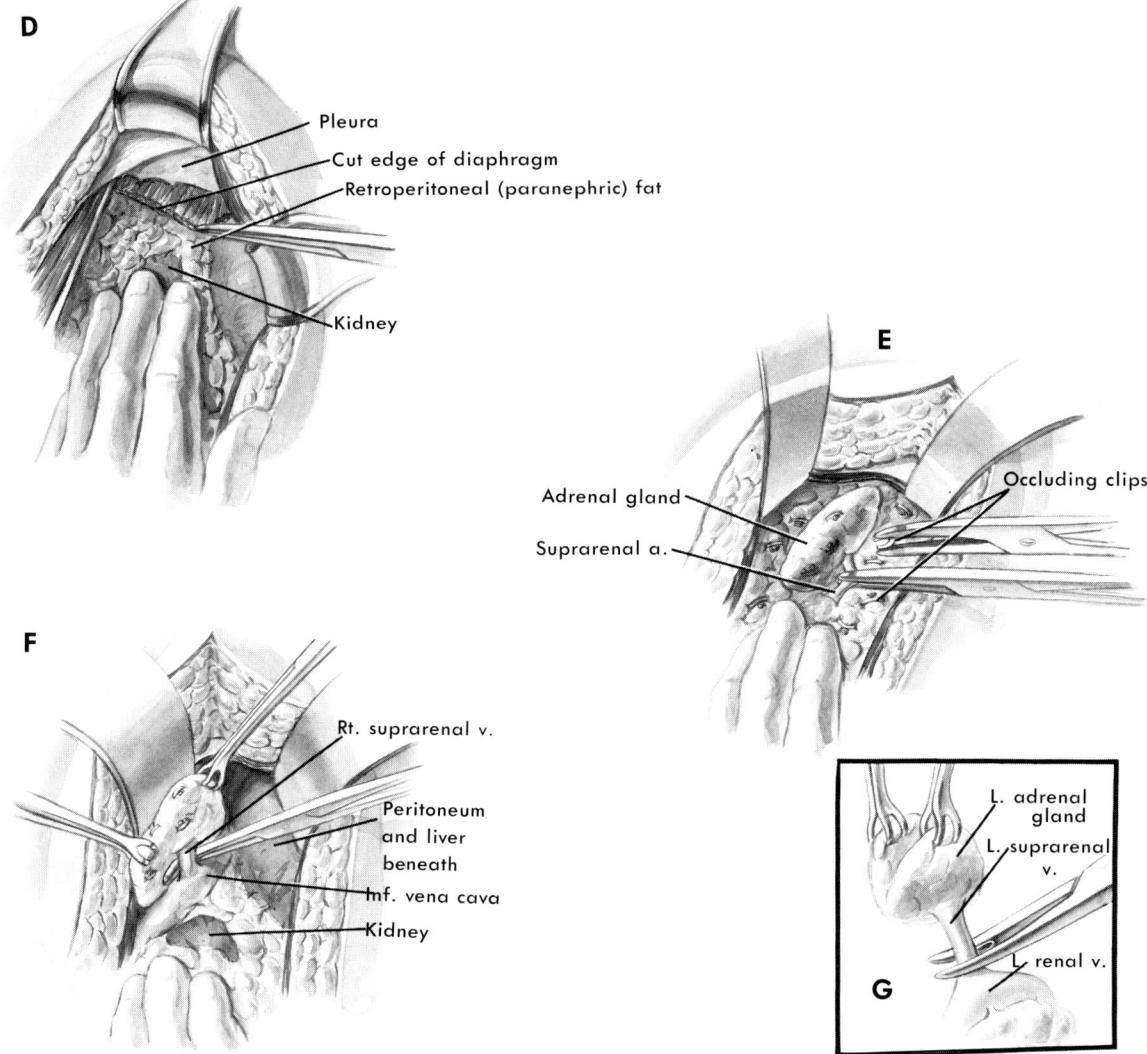

Figure 13–17 *Continued* D, The transversalis fascia, the lower fibers of the diaphragm, and the posterior layer of Gerota's fascia are divided, and the perinephric fat is separated to expose the kidney. The kidney is manually depressed to facilitate exposure of the adrenal gland.

E, Within the fatty tissues at the superior pole of the kidney (and closely applied to the inferior vena cava on the right side), the adrenal gland is easily distinguished from the surrounding fat by its bright golden color. With gentle dissection the adrenal is mobilized from the surrounding fat, while the multiple small vessels that enter it are secured with metal clips. This greatly facilitates the dissection. The arteries are small and multiple, whereas the adrenal vein is usually large and solitary.

F, The adrenal vein is carefully isolated. The vein of the left adrenal enters the renal vein, while that of the right adrenal is considerably shorter and enters the inferior vena cava directly. It is important to secure the vein prior to dividing it. Substantial bleeding follows accidental division of the right adrenal vein and blind attempts to control it are ill-advised, as they can result in damage to the vena cava with even more profuse bleeding. If heavy bleeding occurs, local digital compression of the vena cava or a period of packing will usually permit the field to be cleared long enough for the vessel to be secured precisely.

G, The adrenal vein is secured with metal clips prior to its division, and it is transected several millimeters from the clip in order to leave a secure cuff of vessel. The adrenal gland must be removed in its entirety, as must any accessory adrenal tissue that may be found in the operative field.

When the operation is completed on one side, moist gauze is placed in the wound, and it is covered while the operation is performed on the second side. At the end of the operation, both wounds are inspected for hemostasis and irrigated with saline. The incisions are closed in layers using stout, nonabsorbable, interrupted sutures and no drains. The skin is closed with interrupted sutures of fine nylon, and a dressing is applied. The sutures are not removed for two weeks, since earlier removal can result in separation of the skin edges. If the pleura is opened during the dissection, the lung is reexpanded by placing a suction catheter into the pleural cavity through a defect and withdrawing it as the pleura is closed. An indwelling chest tube with water-sealed drainage is ordinarily not necessary. Patients tolerate adrenalectomy by the posterior approach very well; postoperative ileus is minimal, and recovery is rapid.

lary or interstitial fluid hydrostatic pressure, π_{cap} = plasma protein osmotic pressure, and π_{if} = pericapillary protein osmotic pressure.

The Starling phenomenon was illustrated in Figure 13–12 (Starling, 1898; Memon and Zawadzki, 1981).

Neoplasms on serosal surfaces create the exudation of fluid high in protein and cellular content. Neoplasms may also plug lymphatic routes of absorption essential for the removal of protein and particulate components of an exudate and venous routes of fluid resorption. Viable cancer cells float free in malignant effusions and may be counted, cultured in tissue culture, and categorized histologically. A fluid sample of any effusate should be sent for protein, electrolyte, and cancer specific marker analyses. When open exposure of the serosal surface associated with the effusion is available, a biopsy of the serosal surface should be obtained.

The development of serous effusions with breast cancer is a late and ominous occurrence. Confirmation of the nature and composition of the effusion is an essential first step and the extensive literature on management has been reduced to what the authors consider workable approaches.

PLEURAL EFFUSIONS

The development of pleural effusions is a frequent event in the advanced phases of mammary carcinoma. The morbidity of effusion can be greatly aggravated by the method of management. A typical sequence of events is to receive a patient who has had several thoracenteses with a needle for diagnosis and repeated drainage. The drainage is always incomplete and frequently is complicated by a pneumothorax, resulting in partial or complete collapse of the lung. The lung becomes entrapped quickly in a fibrinous or cancerous peel, and the patient has needlessly lost pulmonary capacity. This complication is preventable by expeditious treatment of all pleural effusions developing with mammary cancer. If specific systemic therapy has failed to control the effusion and the patient is symptomatic, or if the diagnosis is not established, patients with effusions are admitted to the hospital. Thoracentesis is performed with a No. 28 trocar at the most dependent part of the effusion. Tubing of 24F size with extra holes cut in it is passed through this trocar, and the trocar is removed. In lieu of the trocar, a short intercostal incision may be made for insertion of the chest tube under direct vision. Pleural biopsies may be obtained simultaneously. In either instance, the procedure is best done in an adequately equipped operating room under local anesthesia with standby airway and support capabilities. An immediate postoperative chest radiograph is taken to check the position of the tube. The tube is sutured to the skin and is placed to water-sealed drainage. As soon as the fluid is removed, a sclerosing agent in diluent is instilled into the pleural cavity through the thoracostomy tube. Agents that have proved useful are listed in Table 13–3. All act by producing a sterile adhesive serositis that obliterates the pleural cavity and prevents reaccumulation of the effusion. The tube is clamped for 2 hr, during which time the patient is encouraged to move about in ways that enhance a uniform distribution of the medication throughout the pleural cavity. It is then unclamped and left to water-sealed drainage, with the use of suction, until all effusion has drained and the lung is fully expanded. This will have occurred and the water column will have stopped oscillating within 24 to 48 hr. The tube is removed, and the incision is

Table 13–3. EFFECTIVE AGENTS FOR INTRAPLEURAL THERAPY OF MALIGNANT PLEURAL EFFUSIONS IN CONJUNCTION WITH CLOSED THORACOSTOMY DRAINAGE*

Agent	Dose	Total Volume†	Response	Reference
Nitrogen mustard	0.4 mg/kg up to 20 mg total	40 ml	87%	Anderson et al. (1974)
Quinacrine	200–400 mg	20 ml	70%	Borja and Pugh (1973)
Tetracycline	500 mg	80 ml	88%	Bayly et al. (1978)
Bleomycin	60–120 mg	100 ml	67%	Paladine et al. (1976)

*Temporary nausea and vomiting are expected side effects of treatment with intrapleural nitrogen mustard. Since leukopenia can be expected, it is best not to use it in conjunction with systemic chemotherapy. This disadvantage is not present with tetracycline, bleomycin, and quinacrine, but not infrequently fever may occur, and bleomycin administration may produce a rash.

†The medication is dissolved in normal saline solution.

dressed immediately with a pressure dressing containing petrolatum gauze.

Borja and Pugh (1973) reported a series managed as just described and compared the results to multiple needle thoracenteses with small doses of Atabrine. With the tube thoracostomy, the response rate was 70 per cent, and with multiple needle thoracenteses, it was 67 per cent. However, the multiple small dose method took longer, did not provide immediate relief from the effusion, and from earlier experience it is known that hydropneumothorax and trapped lung are more frequent. Fever and moderate pain controlled by analgesics were the main forms of toxicity noted. One patient with very extensive intrapleural neoplasm died acutely. Atabrine is no longer available commercially, but other serosal irritants have been used.

A useful review of the technique of tube thoracostomy and the agents that have been used for intrapleural therapy, including isotopes and talc poudrage, is provided by Greenwald and coworkers (1978). Fentiman and colleagues (1983) reported a randomized trial on 46 patients comparing intracavitary mustine and talc. They concluded that the early use of intracavitary talc was most effective. Their approach, carried out under general anesthesia, consisted of complete drainage of the fluid with an intercostal cannula. A thorascope was passed to assess the intrapleural extent of metastases. A second intercostal cannula was then inserted, through which talc was insufflated using a Stanford Code insufflator. This was continued until talc came freely from the second cannula. Two intercostal catheters were left in place, attached to water-seal drainage to ensure full expansion of the lungs. If any intrapleural fluid or air remained on postoperative chest radiographs, the catheters were attached to suction. A similar drainage and expansion procedure was followed for mustine, but the drug was given through one of the catheters in 50 ml of saline. Drainage was delayed for 2 hr to allow time for absorption of the mustine. The talc routine gave clearly superior results with less immediate morbidity and fewer late recurrences of the effusion. Fentiman et al. (1983) convincingly argue for this very active approach.

Unless the patient has severe cardiac or renal disease, tuberculosis, or an acute febrile illness associated with the effusion, it is not necessary to prove the presence of malignant cells in the effusion before using intrapleural therapy. The development of pleural effusions is a very frequent event in the natural history of advanced mammary cancer and occurs about four times as often on the side of the involved breast as on the opposite side, presumably owing to direct penetration of the chest wall by infiltrating cancer.

When the effusion first develops, malignant cells may not be identified even with cell block. They can often be obtained with pleural biopsies. A sample of fluid is always submitted for protein analysis, cell count, cell block, and bacterial culture, but the surgeon is justified in using intracavitary chemotherapy on the basis of the most probable cause of the effusion, that is, mammary cancer. This has resulted in the early and effective control of pleural effusions.

PERICARDIAL EFFUSION

Persistent pericardial effusion is a complication of both pericardial metastasis and radiotherapy and may require surgical intervention. Dubir and Warren (1984) recommend drainage through an upper midline abdominal incision extending from the xiphisternal junction caudally for about 10 cm. The incision extends through the linea alba into the peritoneal cavity. The left lobe of the liver is reflected inferiorly, and the fat over the central tendon of the diaphragm left of the triangular ligament is reflected away. Two stay sutures are placed in the diaphragm in the area of the window and an incision is made between them for entry into the pericardium. Pericardial fluid is taken for analysis as required. The pericardium may be explored with the finger, and a biopsy specimen of the pericardium may be taken if needed. To prevent the pericardial window from closing, the edges of the pericardium and the peritoneum at the edges of the window are approximated with a continuous, locked, nonabsorbable suture. The needle should be passed from pericardium to peritoneum to avoid injury to the heart. The abdominal incision is then closed in layers. This effectively ensures continual drainage of pericardial fluid into the peritoneal cavity, reducing the chances that the pericardial effusion will recur. Dubix and Warren reported the use of this technique of nine patients without mortality or recurrence of the effusion.

Orthopedic Procedures

Mammary cancer has the capacity to produce skeletal metastases resulting in pathologic fractures. The diversity of fracture types would require considerable length to discuss management in detail. Suffice it to say that isolated long bone fractures from metastatic mammary cancer occurring in women who are still in good general physical condition and who otherwise could reasonably expect a period of symptom-free survival should be stabilized promptly by standard orthopedic surgical techniques, including open reduction of the pathologic fracture site when necessary. These fractures have a surprising capacity to heal. Even if healing is too incomplete to tolerate weight bearing, the person with the fracture is immediately more comfortable with proper treatment (Fig. 13–18).

The spontaneous collapse of vertebrae containing metastases is frequent and occasionally is complicated by compression of the spinal cord. Prompt evaluation of the level of the compression and decompression laminectomy are occasionally required in these cases. To be

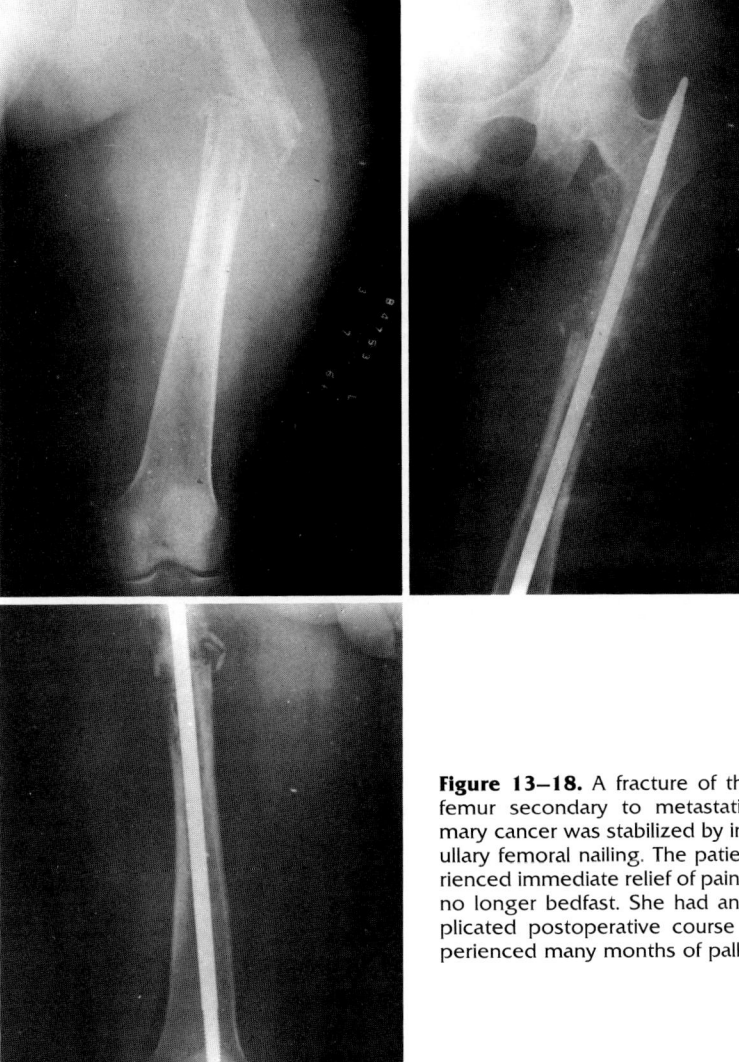

Figure 13–18. A fracture of the upper femur secondary to metastatic mammary cancer was stabilized by intramedullary femoral nailing. The patient experienced immediate relief of pain and was no longer bedfast. She had an uncomplicated postoperative course and experienced many months of palliation.

effective, the operation must be done as soon as the diagnosis is established. These vertebral metastases may be multiple and may progress after any form of therapy. Ultimately, the entire verteral column may become extensively decalcified and may be associated with multiple fractures. These cases often benefit from back braces or cervical support collars, both prophylactically and therapeutically. With braces, ambulation may be maintained for longer periods. An additional discussion of the management of metastases of neurosurgical significance are to be found in Chapter 25.

One therapeutic decision that occasionally has to be made is whether or not to stabilize weight-bearing long bones with metastases. Knutson and Spratt (1970) reviewed this question. The total incidence of long bone metastasis secondary to mammary cancer was 3.45 per cent, with 90 per cent of the metastases involving the femur. Among those cases with femoral metastases, 75 per cent had metastases in other bones. This high prevalence is based entirely on radiographic survey and antedates the availability of radionuclide scans for the diagnosis of skeletal metastases. With radionuclide scanning the prevalence of metastases in multiple bones would be expected to be higher.

Knutson and Spratt's patients were followed to the end of life, and 42.4 per cent of them developed a fracture of the femur. Neither fracture nor internal fixation affected survival. However, over 50 per cent who would otherwise have been bedfast were able to ambulate as a result of the internal fixation. Without internal fixation, only 2.6 per cent ever walked again. Lytic lesions of weight-bearing long bones, particularly if painful, should be considered for prophylactic internal fixation.

The pain attending isolated skeletal metastases in the absence of fracture is most effectively treated by palliative irradiation therapy. When the cancer is so diffuse as to respond no longer to radiotherapy or hormonal or chemical therapy, the patient is usually in a preterminal state. At this point, the diffuseness of the cancer generally precludes the effective use of neurolytic procedures for the control of pain. The treating physician must rely on opiates and tranquilizing drugs or titrated intravenous opiates to quiet the terminal anguish. As with all other mortal diseases, there is a definite loneliness that foreshadows death, and the sympathetic, positive familiarity of a good physician can do much to ameliorate its severity.

Hepatic Metastases

Metastasis to the liver from breast cancer is an ominous occurrence, and prognosis is poor. Fewer than 20 per cent of patients survive for more than 1 year after the diagnosis of hepatic metastases.

The treatment of hepatic metastases from breast cancer that are refractory to systemic therapy by hepatic infusional chemotherapy has largely been ineffective. Whenever hepatic artery infusional therapy is to be attempted, the drugs most effective in systemic treatment offer the best choice for reduction in hepatic metastases. When no agent has had a significant systemic effect, Wallace and coworkers (1984) recommend vinblastin (Velban), cisplatin, or a combination of the two. Variable percentages of partial responses but no complete remissions have been reported. None of the reported studies provide controls. Thus, the true impact of treatment is not known. The role of hepatic artery embolization in the management of breast cancer metastatic to the liver remains unknown.

The resection of hepatic metastases from carcinoma of the breast with patient benefit is possible only occasionally. The surgical techniques for the safe resection of large parts of the liver or total resection with a replacement transplant are now well developed. Hepatic involvement with breast cancer metastases so extensive as to require a total hepatic resection and transplant is generally associated with generalized mammary carcinomatosis and would have to be regarded as experimental. On the other hand, there are scattered case reports of limited metastases from mammary cancer that have been removed by subtotal hepatectomies. Foster (1978) found only five such cases in a large survey. The only operative death occurred after resection of a large solitary metastasis of the left lateral hepatic segment becoming manifest 17 years after mastectomy. Three patients died 6, 8, and 19 months after liver resection. One was alive 3 months after resection with known residual cancer. Thus, the experience with breast cancer is limited and probably will remain so. However, an occasional patient with limited metastasis associated with a less aggressive pattern of behavior may be benefitted by resection.

Angioaccess

The surgeon is frequently called upon to provide a safe, infection-free conduit to a major vein for chemotherapy, nutrients, and other supportive medications (i.e., angioaccess). He or she is also called upon to manage the complications of the angioaccess devices and of the medications delivered through them that may produce local tissue destruction. As a generalization, when considering the placement of angioaccess devices, the surgeon must determine the location of past and potential future radiotherapy treatment ports and avoid these areas as a prevention against tissue necrosis. The great veins of the neck and axilla most frequently appear in radiotherapy ports in breast cancer care. They often are also in the fields of surgical dissection and chest wall tumor recurrence. Veins in the upper extremity on the sides of mastectomies or axillary radiotherapy should also be avoided because of the risk of lymphedema. These restrictions obviously limit access, and careful planning becomes necessary. Except for these limitations with breast cancer, the techniques and their complications are well described elsewhere and are not specific to the problems of breast cancer (Raaf, 1984).

Extravasation of Chemotherapeutic Drugs

The surgical management of vesicant drug extravasations has been evaluated only partially. The resulting ulcers develop slowly over 7 to 10 days and may continue to enlarge for several months. Secondary complications occur when nerves, tendons, and joints are involved. In a review of the literature and controlled animal study, Loth (1986) observed that the frequency of this problem ranges from 0.5 to 6.0 per cent. Prompt surgical debridement of extravasations was found to reduce ulcer size, expedite healing, and reduce secondary complications. Excision and grafting for chronic ulcers has been successful.

Summary

In this chapter a variety of surgical techniques for mastectomy and endocrine gland ablation, the management of pathologic fractures and effusions, and less frequent procedures are reviewed. With their judicious use, many persons can be cured and many others can be given long periods of symptom-free survival. With attention to (1) proper indications and contraindications for surgery, (2) surgical detail, and (3) good supportive care, very few patients will be made worse.

REFERENCES

Aisner, J., Morris, D., Elias, G., et al.: Mastectomy as an adjuvant to chemotherapy for locally advanced or metastatic breast cancer. Arch. Surg., 17:882, 1982.

Aitken, D. R., and Minton, J. P.: Complications associated with mastectomy. Surg. Clin. North Am., 63:1331, 1983.

Anderson, C. B., Philpott, G. W., and Ferguson, T. B.: The treatment of malignant pleural effusions. Cancer, 33:916, 1974.

Auchincloss, H.: Significance of location and number of axillary metastases in carcinoma of the breast; a justification for a conservative operation. Ann. Surg., 158:37, 1963.

Bayly, T. C., Kisner, D. L., Sybert, A., et al.: Tetracycline and quinacrine in the control of malignant pleural effusions. Cancer, 41:1188, 1978.

Beatty, J. D., Robinson, G. V., Zaia, J. A., et al.: A prospective analysis of nosocomial wound infection after mastectomy. Arch. Surg., 118:1421, 1983.

Borgstrom, S., and Lindgren, M.: Preoperative roentgen therapy of cancer of the breast: Preliminary communication. Acta Radiol., 58:9, 1962.

Borja, E. R., and Pugh, R. P.: Single-dose quinacrine (Atabrine) and thoracostomy in the control of pleural effusions in patients with neoplastic diseases. Cancer, 31:899, 1973.

Bridges, K. G., Keshgegian A. A., Kumar, H. A. M., et al.: Influence of surgical technique on estrogen and progesterone determinations in breast cancer. Cancer, 51:2317, 1983.

Burrows, L., and Tartter, P.: Effect of blood transfusions on colonic malignancy recurrence rate. Lancet, 2:662, 1982.

Butcher, H. R., and Hoover, A. L.: Abnormalities of human superficial cutaneous lymphatics associated with stasis ulcers, lymphedema, scar and cutaneous autografts. Ann. Surg., 142:663, 1955.

Butcher, H. R., Jr., Seaman, W., Eckert, C., et al.: An assessment of radical mastectomy and postoperative irradiation therapy in the treatment of mammary cancer. Cancer, 17:480, 1964.

Daly, J. M., Lawson, M., Speier, A., et al.: Angioaccess in cancer patients. Curr. Probl. Cancer, 5(9):1, 1981.

Donegan, W. L., Perez-Mesa, C. M., and Watson, F. R.: A biostatistical study of locally recurrent breast carcinoma. Surg. Gynecol. Obstet., 122:529, 1966.

Dubir, R., and Warren, S. E.: Drainage of pericardial effusion using the peritoneal and pericardial window technique. Surg. Gynecol. Obstet., 159:485, 1984.

Egdahl, R. H., and Melby, J. C.: Bilateral adrenalectomy for metastatic breast cancer. Hosp. Pract., August 1972, p. 79.

Fentiman, I. S., Rubens, R. D., and Hayward, J. L.: Control of pleural effusions in patients with breast cancer. Cancer, 52:737, 1983.

Foster, J. H.: Survival after liver resection for secondary tumors. Am. J. Surg., 135:389, 1978.

Foster, R. S., Jr., Foster, J. C., and Costanza, M. C.: Blood transfusions and survival after surgery for breast cancer. Arch. Surg., 119:1138, 1984.

Francis, D. M. A., and Shenton, B. K.: Blood transfusion and tumor growth: Evidence from laboratory animals. Lancet, 2:871, 1981.

Fuller, T. C., Burroughs, J. C., Delmonico, F. L., et al.: Influence of frozen blood transfusions on renal allograft survival. Transplant. Proc., 14:293, 1982.

Ganel, A., Engel, J., Sala, M., et al.: Nerve entrapments associated with post mastectomy lymphedema. Cancer, 44:2254, 1979.

Gantt, C. L.: Red blood cells from cancer patients. Lancet, 2:363, 1981.

Gray, J. H.: The relation of lymphatic vessels to the spread of cancer. Br. J. Surg., 26:462, 1939.

Greenwald, D. W., Phillips, C., and Bennett, J. M.: Management of malignant pleural effusion. J. Surg. Oncol., 10:361, 1978.

Haagensen, C. D.: Diseases of the Breast. Philadelphia, W. B. Saunders Co., 1971.

Handley, R. S.: Modified radical mastectomy. In Nora, P. (Ed.): Operative Surgery. Philadelphia, Lea & Febiger, 1972, p. 198.

Handley, R. S.: The technique and results of conservative radical mastectomy (Patey's operation). Prog. Clin. Cancer, 1:462, 1965.

Howard, J. M., Danese, C., and Laine, J. B.: Experimental lymphatic anatomosis. J. Cardiovasc. Surg., 5:694, 1964.

Ingle, J. N., Krook, J. E., Green, S. J., et al.: Randomized trial of bilateral oophorectomy versus tamoxifen in premenopausal women with metastatic breast cancer. J. Clin. Oncol., 4:178, 1986.

Jamison, K., Wellisch, D. K., Katz, R. L., et al.: Phantom breast syndrome. Arch. Surg., 114:93, 1979.

Ju, D. M. C., Blakemore, A., Stevenson, T. W.: A lymphatic function test. Surg. Forum, 5:607, 1954.

Kiang, D. T., Frenning, D. H., Vosika, G. J., et al.: Comparison of tamoxifen and hypophysectomy in breast cancer treatment. Cancer, 45:1322, 1980.

Kinmonth, J. B.: The Lymphatics: Lymphography and Diseases of the Chyle and Lymph Systems. London, Edward Arnold, 1982.

Knutson, C. O., and Spratt, J. S., Jr.: The natural history and management of mammary cancer metastatic to the femur. Cancer, 26:1199, 1970.

Kogelnick, H. S., and Karcher, K. H.: Radiobiological considerations of late effects arising from radiotherapy. Proceedings of an International Symposium on the Radiobiological Research Needed for the Improvement of Radiotherapy (Nov. 22–26, 1976). Proceedings Series, International Atomic Energy Agency, Vienna, 1977.

LaCour, J., Le, M., Caceres E., et al.: Radical mastectomy versus radical mastectomy plus internal mammary dissection. Cancer, 51:1941, 1983.

Lee, Y. T.: The ABO blood groups and results of therapeutic oophorectomy for advanced carcinoma of the breast. Surg. Gynecol. Obstet., 132:871, 1971.

Loth, T. S.: Minimal surgical debridement for the treatment of chemotherapeutic agent-induced skin extravasations. Cancer Treat. Rep., 70:401, 1986.

Lotze, M. T., Duncan, M. A., Gerber, L. H., et al.: Early versus delayed shoulder motion following axillary dissection. Ann. Surg., 193:288, 1981.

McCarthy, P. M., Martin, J. R., Jr., Wells, D. C., et al.: An aborted, prospective, randomized trial of sclerotherapy for prolonged drainage after mastectomy. Surg. Gynecol. Obstet., 162:418, 1986.

Madden, J. L.: Modified radical mastectomy. Surg. Gynecol. Obstet., 121:1221, 1965.

Memon, A., and Zawadzki, Z. A.: Malignant effusions: Diagnostic evaluation and therapeutic strategy. Curr. Prob. Cancer, 5(8):1, 1981.

Morris, D. M.: Mastectomy in the management of patients with inflammatory cancer. J. Surg. Oncol., 23:255, 1983.

Morrow, M., and Foster, R. S., Jr.: Staging of breast cancer. A new rationale for internal mammary node biopsy. Arch. Surg., 116:748, 1981.

Mowlem, R.: Personal communication. Cited in Kinmonth, J. H.: The Lymphatics: Lymphography and Diseases of the Chyle and Lymph systems. London, Edward Arnold, 1982.

Nemoto, T., Patel, J., Rosner, D., et al.: Tamoxifen (Nolvadex) versus adrenelectomy in metastatic breast cancer. Cancer, 53:1333, 1984.

Noguchi, M., Sakuma, H., Matsuba, A., et al.: A new method of extended radical mastectomy permitting complete resection of the internal mammary lymph nodes. Breast, 8:26, 1982.

Oeser, H., and Albrecht, A.: Wert und Ergebnisse der zusatzlichen Strahlenwendung bei chirurgisch behandeltem Mammakarzinom. Fortschr. Geb. Rontgenstr. Nuklearmed., 101:410, 1964.

Paladine, W., Cunningham, T. J., Sponzo, R., et al.: Intracavitary bleomycin in the management of malignant effusions. Cancer, 38:1903, 1976.

Paterson, R., and Russell, M. H.: Clinical trials in malignant disease. III. Breast cancer: Evaluation of postoperative radiotherapy. J. Fac. Radiol., 10:175, 1959.

Patey, D. H., and Dyson, W. H.: The prognosis of carcinoma of the breast in relation to the type of operation performed. Br. J. Cancer, 2:7, 1948.

Peetz, M. E., Awrich, A. E., Moseley, H. S., et al.: Results of oophorectomy by menstrual and estrogen receptor states in patients with metastatic breast cancer. Am. J. Surg., 141:554, 1981.

Perloff, M., and Lesnick, G. J.: Chemotherapy before and after mastectomy in Stage III breast cancer. Arch. Surg., 117:879, 1982.

Peterson, L. F. A.: Surgical Treatment of Lymphedema and Treatment of Lymphangiosarcoma. Mod. Treat., 6:413, 1959.

Planting, A. S. T., Figusch, J. A., Wijst, J. B., et al.: Tamoxifen therapy in premenopausal women with breast cancer. Cancer Treat. Rep., 69:363, 1985.

Puga, F. J., Welch, J. S., and Bisel, H. F.: Therapeutic oophorectomy in disseminated carcinoma of the breast. Arch. Surg., 111:877, 1976.

Raaf, J. H.: Vascular access in chemotherapy. In Waltzer, W. C., and Rapaport, F. T. (Eds.): Angioaccess: Principles and Practices. New York, Grune & Stratton, 1984, p. 161.

Reichert, F. L.: The regeneration of lymphatics. Arch. Surg., 13:871, 1926.

Rosenthal, L. J.: Discrepant estrogen receptor protein levels according to surgical technique. Am. J. Surg., 138:680, 1979.

Ruszynyak, I., Mihaly, F., and Szabo, G.: Lymphatics and lymph circulation. New York, Pergamon Press, 1960.

Saltzstein, S. L.: Histologic diagnosis of breast carcinoma with the Silverman needle biopsy. Surgery, 48:366, 1960.

Savage, R. C.: The surgical management of lymphedema. Surg. Gynecol. Obstet., 160:283, 1985.

Sawka, C. A., Pritchard, K. I., Paterson, A. H., et al.:

Role and mechanism of action of Tamoxifen in premenopausal women with metastatic breast carcinoma. Cancer Res., 46:3152, 1986.

Say, C. C., and Donegan, W. L.: A biostatistical evaluation of complications from mastectomy. Surg. Gynecol. Obstet., 138:370, 1974.

Scanlon, E. F., and Caprini, J. A.: Modified radical mastectomy. Cancer, 35:710, 1975.

Schnitt, S. J., Connolly, J. L., Harris, J. R., et al.: Pathologic predictors of early local recurrence in stage I and II breast cancer treated by primary radiation therapy. Cancer, 53:1049, 1984.

Smoller, B. R., and Kruskall, M. S.: Phlebotomy for diagnostic laboratory tests in adults. Patterns of use and effect on transfusion requirements. N. Engl. J. Med., 314:1233, 1986.

Spratt, J. S., Heinbecker, P., and Saltzstein, S. L.: The influence of succinylsulfathiazole (sulfasuxidine) upon the response of canine small intestine to irradiation. Cancer, 14:862, 1961.

Spratt, J. S., Jr., and Sala, J. M.: The healing of wounds within irradiated tissue. Mo. Med., 59:409, 1962.

Spratt, J. S., Jr., Shieber, W., and Dillard, B. M.: Anatomy and Surgical Technique of Groin Dissection. St. Louis, C. V. Mosby, 1965.

Starling, E. H.: On absorption of fluid from connective tissue spaces. J. Physiol., 19:312, 1898.

Stillwell, G. K.: Treatment of postmastectomy lymphedema. Mod. Treat., 6:396, 1959.

Sugarbaker, E. D.: Extended radical mastectomy. J.A.M.A., 178:96, 1964.

Tadych, K., and Donegan, W. L.: Postmastectomy seromas and wound drainage. Surg. Gynecol. Obstet., 165:483, 1987.

Tartter, P. I., Burrows, L., Papatestas, A. E., et al.: Perioperative blood transfusion has prognostic significance for breast cancer. Surgery, 97:225, 1985.

Temple, W. J., and Ketcham, A. S.: Preservation of the intercostobrachial nerve during axillary dissection for breast cancer. Am. J. Surg., 150:585, 1985.

Tengrup, I., Nittby, L. T., and Landberg, T.: Prophylactic oophorectomy in the treatment of carcinoma of the breast. Surg. Gynecol. Obstet., 162:209, 1986.

Thompson, N.: The surgical treatment of chronic lymphedema of the extremities. Surg. Clin. North Am., 47:445, 1967.

Tough, I. C. K.: Oedema of the arm after simple mastectomy and radiotherapy for breast cancer. J. R. Coll. Surg. Edinb., 13:312, 1968.

Tracy, G. D., Reeve, T. S., Fitzsimons, E., et al.: Observations on the swollen arm after radical mastectomy. N.Z. J. Surg., 30:204, 1961.

Treves, N.: Evaluation of the etiological factors of lymphedema following radical mastectomy. Cancer, 10:444, 1957.

Van den Brenk, H. A. S.: Studies in restorative growth processes in mammalian wound healing. Br. J. Surg., 43:525, 1956.

Van den Brenk, H. A. S.: The effect of ionizing radiation on the regeneration and behavior of mammalian lymphatics; in vivo studies in Sandison-Clark chambers. AJR, 78:837, 1957.

Veronesi, U., and Valagussa, P.: Inefficacy of internal mammary node dissection in breast cancer surgery. Cancer, 47:170, 1981.

Wallace, S., Charnsangavey, C., Corvasco, C. H., et al.: Percutaneous transcatheter infusion and infarction in the treatment of human cancer. I. Curr. Probl. Cancer, 8:40, 1984.

Waymack, J. P., Rapien, J., Garnett, D., et al.: Effect on transfusions on immune function in a traumatized animal model. Arch. Surg., 121:50, 1986.

Wilson, R. E., Donegan, W. L., Mettlin, C., et al.: The 1982 national survey of breast cancer in the United States by the American College of Surgeons. Surg. Gynecol. Obstet., 159:309, 1984.

CHAPTER 14

J. FRANK WILSON
JAMES D. COX

Definitive, Adjuvant, and Palliative Radiation Therapy for Mammary Cancer

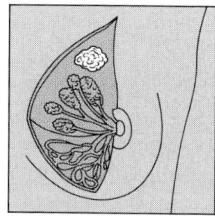

The remarkable speed with which ionizing radiation was recognized as a highly potent agent against breast cancer shortly after the discovery of x-rays in 1895 was fortuitous (Hodges, 1964). By 1905, the first radiologic textbooks recommended radiation therapy for locally advanced, unresectable primary breast carcinoma or for patients who categorically refused surgery. Despite this early application, subsequent progress toward definition of the optimal role of irradiation in breast cancer management was achieved slowly. Medical opinion concerning acceptable treatment options changed little until the Halstedian precepts of "en bloc" surgical dissection were successfully challenged in a series of modern clinical trials. First tentative attempts to exploit more fully the powerful new technique as an adjuvant to radical mastectomy did not even occur until the 1930s. The lack of good quality, highly controllable radiation delivery systems until the late 1950s, hampered investigators, and it took nearly another 20 years to fully recognize the regularity with which irradiation is capable of eradicating cancer cell aggregates depending on their size and the radiation doses employed (Fletcher, 1985).

Although it is now generally accepted that radiation doses of 45 to 50 grays (Gy) (1 Gy = 100 rad) are sufficient to eliminate subclinical deposits of cancer cells 90 to 95 per cent of the time (Fletcher, 1974), gross tumor masses are likely to be controlled only when substantially higher doses are administered (Arriagada et al., 1985) (see Table 14–4). Primary or metastatic masses a few centimeters in diameter or larger are likely to require doses that approach or even exceed the radiation tolerance of normal tissues in the area. Therefore, therapeutic ratio is enhanced when irradiation must contend only with microscopic disease. In this circumstance, moderately intense, well-tolerated doses of irradiation yield a high probability of tumor control, yet the incidence of associated late treatment sequelae will be minimal or nil. Practical applications of these fundamental radiobiologic principles in current strategies for optimal use of irradiation in the management of breast carcinoma will be apparent in the following discussion.

The value of irradiation as a preoperative or postoperative adjunct to mastectomy has been the subject of intense controversy extending over the past half century. It is ironic that while this debate continues, a strong trend favoring so-called definitive or primary radiation therapy for cancer of the breast has developed. This particular treatment represents the ultimate extension of the radiobiologic principles just mentioned, as with this approach all gross tumor is excised from the breast prior to administering irradiation to doses appropriate for subclinical residuae. In this manner, not only is a high rate of tumor control achieved, but in addition maximal esthetic and functional preservation is afforded the patient.

Skillfully applied radiation therapy has an increasingly indispensable role in the management of many cases of breast cancer, depending on multiple clinicopathologic factors, including the stage of disease, histopathologic findings, extent of surgery, and the patient's preferences. These and other factors must be weighed carefully in each case to select patients for treatment and to correctly tailor the irradiation to the individual needs. The following discussion will review the rationale and results of the currently recommended uses of radiation therapy in the management of patients with breast cancer.

Conservative Surgery and Definitive Irradiation

The seemingly new concept of treating breast cancer with limited surgery followed by irradiation can actually be traced to its origins in the work of a few early pioneers. Although the British surgeon Keynes (1929) reported gratifying results of extensive radium needle implantations of the breast and nodal areas with occasional tumorectomy, this particular approach was never widely practiced and ultimately was abandoned. It was, more precisely, the explorations of several individuals working with external beam irradiation in Europe and Canada that, by the late 1960s, demonstrated the curative potential of conservative therapy for breast cancer (Baclesse, 1959; Risannen, 1969; Peters, 1976). Aided by rapid technologic development in radiation therapy delivery systems, many other groups then began to expand the clinical experience. This has resulted since 1970 in the publication of numerous persuasive series that sophisticated radiation therapy in combination with limited surgery can be regarded as a treatment of choice in favorable cases of breast carcinoma. Retrospective series reported since 1980, which reflect the large worldwide experience with this definitive irradiation for Stages I and II breast cancer, are summarized in Table 14–1. These results are remarkable for the consistent demonstration of high local-regional control rates and corresponding survival figures, which are comparable to those reported in mastectomy series.

In 1976, Peters reported the results of a matched pair study involving 217 clinical Stage I patients treated with wide excision and irradiation from 1939 to 1969. When compared with patients matched for age and primary tumor size who were treated with radical mastectomy and postoperative irradiation, survival rates up to 30 years showed no dependence on the method of treatment (Fig. 14–1). Prospective randomized trials comparing mastectomy versus conservative surgery plus irradiation have also been completed or currently are in progress. To date, these studies confirm the

Table 14–1. RESULTS OF CONSERVATIVE SURGERY AND DEFINITIVE IRRADIATION FOR STAGE I AND II BREAST CANCER

Author	Number of Patients	Clinical Stage	Local Recurrence Rate (%)	5 Year Disease-Free Survival (%)	10 Year Disease-Free Survival (%)
Pierquin et al. (1986)*	72	T1	8	—	72
	167	T2	13	—	64
Danoff et al. (1985)	104	I	5	82 (at 4 yr)	—
	80	II		70	—
Montague (1984)	134	I	6	85	78
	157	II	5	78	73
Chu et al. (1984b)	64	I	8	93	—
	82	II	17	73	—
Calle et al. (1982)*	87	T1	12 (at 10 yr)	—	84
	56	T2-T3		—	68
Amalric et al. (1983)	274	T1 + T2	12 (at 10 yr)	85	75
Clark et al. (1982)*	680	I + II	8–12	83	71
Hellman et al. (1980)	58	I	5	96	—
	118	II	7	68	—

*Results obtained without axillary dissection.

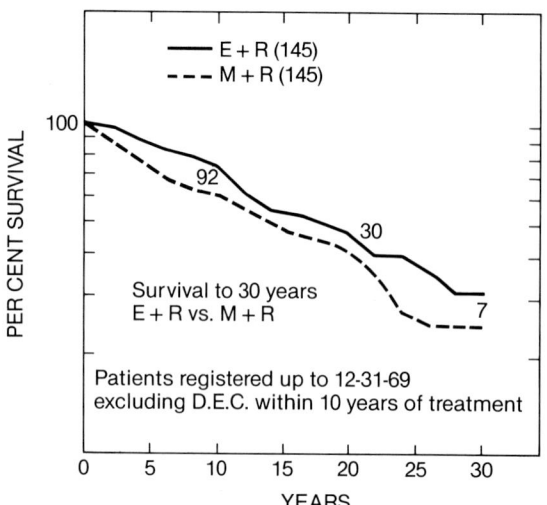

Figure 14–1. Survival rates up to 30 years for 145 patients with clinical stage I breast cancer treated with local excision and irradiation (E + R) compared with rates observed in patients matched for age and size of primary who were treated with mastectomy and irradiation (M + R). (From Peters, M. V.: Cutting the "Gordian Knot" in early breast cancer. Ann. R. Coll. Phys. Surg. (Canada), 8:186–192, 1976. Reprinted with permission.)

equivalence of the two treatment methods and are summarized in Table 14–2. Excluded from this tabulation are the early Guy's Hospital trials (Hayward, 1974), which employed too low radiation doses (30 Gy in 2 weeks; 38 Gy in 3 weeks) to provide adequate local or regional control of disease in the patients treated with wide excision and irradiation; as a result there was excessive mortality in this group.

This retrospective and prospective evidence validates treatment of selected cases of mammary carcinoma by tumor excision followed by irradiation. Breast-sparing therapy is not, however, a panacea for all women with breast cancer. The most suitable candidates are those patients with small primary tumors (< 4 cm) and no more than limited clinical involvement of axillary lymph nodes. Larger primary lesions may also be considered for this therapy, particularly if the patient has large breasts. Associated inflammatory changes or tumor extension to the skin or chest wall precludes conservative therapy. Other relative selection factors considered in the identification of patients eligible for the conservative therapy have been presented elsewhere (Wilson, 1983; Lichter, 1986) and will not be reviewed in detail here. However, since preservation of the breast in a near normal status is a major treatment aim, several management principles deserve emphasis. Patients' best interests are always served when all physicians involved in their care evaluate the patient prior to any intervention.

Whether wide local excision (tylectomy), segmental resection, or some other surgical approach is used to extirpate the primary mass from the breast, the goals of esthetic and functional preservation must be borne in mind. Optimally, the operation removes the mass along with a narrow margin of normal breast tissue without producing unattractive deformity of the breast remnant. Particular care must be taken if the breast is small to avoid excessive distortion. Use of the smallest possible incisions with respect for normal skin lines, resulting in minimal skin loss, contributes to obtaining the best esthetic results.

Dissection of the lateral axilla (Levels II and III) prior to the irradiation is usually recommended for determination of axillary lymph node status to establish prognosis and to select patients for adjuvant chemotherapy. It is noteworthy, however, that the good results in several of the series in Table 14–2 were achieved without surgical assessment of the axilla or use of chemotherapy. In these series, axillary

Table 14–2. RESULTS OF RECENT RANDOMIZED TRIALS COMPARING MASTECTOMY VERSUS CONSERVATIVE SURGERY PLUS IRRADIATION

Author/(Inst.)	Number	Stage	5 Year Disease-Free Survival	
			Conservative	*Mastectomy*
Findlay et al. (NCI) (1985)	197	T1 T2 N0 N1	No differences (median follow-up, 32 months)	
Veronesi et al. (Milan) (1985)	701	T1 N0	85%	82.5%
Fisher et al. (NSABP) (1985)	1843	Stage I + II <4 cm	81.4% (N−) 57.5% (N+)	72.9% (N−) 57.9% (N+)
Sarrazin et al. (IGR) (1984)	179	T1 T2 N0 N1	95%	91%

lymph node recurrences rarely developed following axillary irradiation alone. For example, in the Creteil series (Otmezguine et al., 1980; Pierquin et al., 1980), only 7 of 156 clinical Stage I and II patients treated with definitive irradiation without axillary dissection developed nodal recurrence within 5 years. In six of these seven patients, simultaneous recurrence in the breast was also detected.

Although complete axillary dissection provides a somewhat more accurate assessment than the limited dissection, it is associated with a greater risk of complications. Clarke and associates (1982) noted a 79 per cent incidence of breast lymphedema after staging axillary dissection and breast irradiation. In contrast, Rose and colleagues (1983) observed only occasional mild breast edema and no arm complications following low axillary dissections that stopped short of the axillary vein. As available adjuvant chemotherapy is of unproved benefit except for premenopausal women with one to three positive axillary nodes, the requirement of complete dissection in postmenopausal women is particularly questionable. The risk-benefit ratio of complete versus limited axillary dissection will no doubt be the focus of future study and debate.

Once adequate healing has occurred, usually 10 to 14 days following the surgical procedures, radiation therapy is begun. The remaining breast is usually irradiated via opposed medial and lateral tangential portals, which parallel the arc of the chest wall at depth and encompass a thin volume of the underlying lung. The margins of these fields are carefully matched with those of the supplementary fields, if any, used to irradiate the peripheral nodal regions. A total dose to the target areas of 45 to 50 Gy in 5 to 5½ weeks is administered. A booster dose of an additional 15 to 20 Gy directed to the operative bed in the breast is then administered either with electron beam irradiation or by temporary interstitial implantation of radioactive sources (iridium-192).

Boosting of either type has usually been employed in the single institution series cited in Table 14–1. Supporting theoretical arguments for this dose augmentation are that any residual tumor cell aggregates are most likely to be in close proximity to the surgical bed and may be relatively protected by hypoxic conditions in the area. Although a local recurrence rate of only 7.7 per cent without boosting was observed in the National Surgical Adjuvant Breast Project (NSABP) trial (Fisher et al., 1985), surgical margins in the patients in the single institution series frequently have not been as complete as in this group study. Therefore, until prospective studies that test the merits of boosting are conducted, the practice should continue routinely, especially when there is the least doubt concerning the adequacy of the tumor removal.

Esthetically satisfactory end results of conservative therapy for early stage breast cancer have been observed in all series. Observer-based evaluations reveal excellent results in 75 to 82 per cent of patients, satisfactory results in another 13 to 22 per cent, and unsatisfactory results in no more than 5 per cent of patients thus treated (Pierquin et al., 1980; Ray et al., 1983; Clarke et al., 1983). Moreover, patient self-evaluation of the outcome indicates that most women are satisfied with the posttherapeutic status of the breast and consistently rate the results higher than physicians do (Patterson et al., 1985). Somewhat inferior esthetic results and a higher rate of complications are reported in patients who also receive multiagent chemotherapy. However, this negative effect is not so serious that the combination is contraindicated when systemic therapy is required (Danoff et al, 1983; Ray et al., 1984). On the contrary, evidence from the ongoing National Cancer Institute (NCI) trial (Lippman et al., 1984) demonstrates that comprehensive irradiation does not significantly interfere with the patient's ability to tolerate optimal doses of systemic chemotherapy.

Irradiation as an Adjunct to Mastectomy

POSTOPERATIVE IRRADIATION

Numerous retrospective and prospective studies have demonstrated that adequate irradiation following total, modified radical, or radical mastectomy for breast carcinoma significantly reduces the incidence of subsequent local and regional recurrence (Paterson and Russell, 1959; Host and Brennhovd, 1977; Wallgren et al., 1980; Fisher et al., 1985). This major advantage is readily provided by employing any of several acceptable treatment techniques to administer radiation doses of 45 to 50 Gy to the regional lymphatics or tissues of the chest wall according to the patient's needs. Elective irradiation to moderate doses of this order have been shown to prevent recurrence in all but 5 to 10 per cent of patients at risk for such recurrences (Montague and Fletcher, 1985).

Although such postoperative irradiation is nearly innocuous in terms of troublesome late radiation sequelae, judicious selection of patients at high risk for postoperative recurrences is indicated to restrict radiotherapy to those most likely to be benefited. Irradiation directed to the apical axillary, supraclavicular, and internal mammary lymph nodes is usually advised for patients with histologically positive axillary nodes or those whose primary tumor was located centrally or in the medial quadrants of the breast, regardless of the axillary nodal status. Indications for extending the irradiation to the chest wall include findings of a large breast mass (> 5 cm), tumor extension to the skin or chest wall, and dense axillary lymph node involvement ($> 4+$), all of which are associated with an increased incidence of local recurrence. Postoperative irradiation is also indicated when surgical margins are suspected or are known to have been inadequate. Toonkel and coworkers (1982b) have argued for broadening the indications for routinely irradiating the chest wall based on their observation of a statistically significant improvement ($p = 0.009$) in 5 and 10 year survival rates in Stage II and III patients when the chest wall was irradiated in addition to the peripheral lymphatics.

Whether the improved local and regional control of breast carcinoma achieved by adjunctive postoperative irradiation is also accompanied by any survival benefit remains highly controversial. Several randomized trials showing no enhancement of survival with the addition of irradiation are often cited as evidence that it does not (Paterson and Russell, 1959; Fisher et al., 1970; Cancer Research Campaign, 1976). However, these studies are representative of many early trials involving radiotherapy, which, when subjected to critical review, have been found deficient with respect to the radiation dosages or tehniques employed. It is particularly doubtful that the internal mammary lymph nodes of patients irradiated in these trials received what is now considered to be an adequate radiation dose (Fletcher and Montague, 1978).

Until appropriately designed clinical trials with the statistical ability to demonstrate small but significant survival differences are conducted, the medical community cannot afford to ignore the existing evidence that carefully planned postoperative irradiation results in improved survival for some patients. Host and Brennhovd (1977) conducted a randomized study to measure the value of postoperative irradiation after radical mastectomy. Patients with histologically proved axillary metastases treated with megavoltage beams using adequate portals had a significantly better survival than patients who were not irradiated (Fig. 14–3). In the Stockholm Breast Cancer Trial,

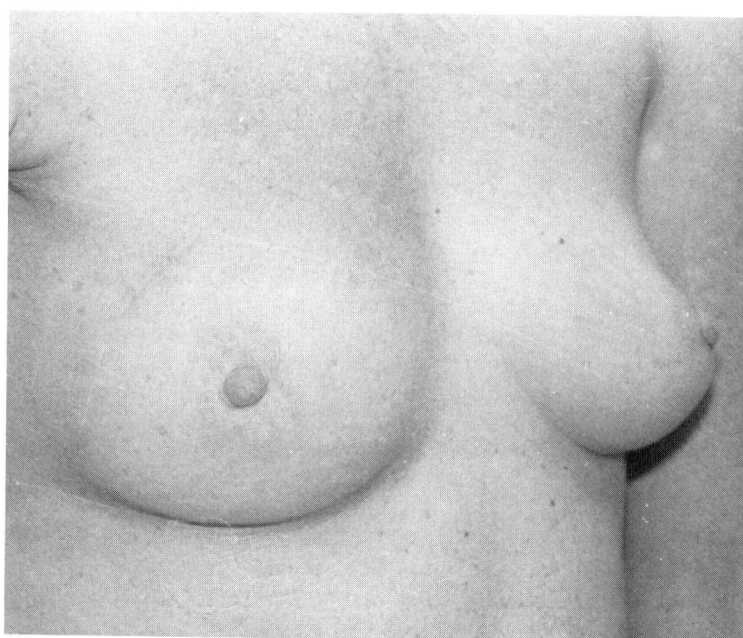

Figure 14–2. Esthetic results at 3 years in a 55 year old woman treated by excisional biopsy, external beam irradiation (5000 cGy), and boost by electron beam (1000 cGy) for a T1N0M0 (UOQ right breast).

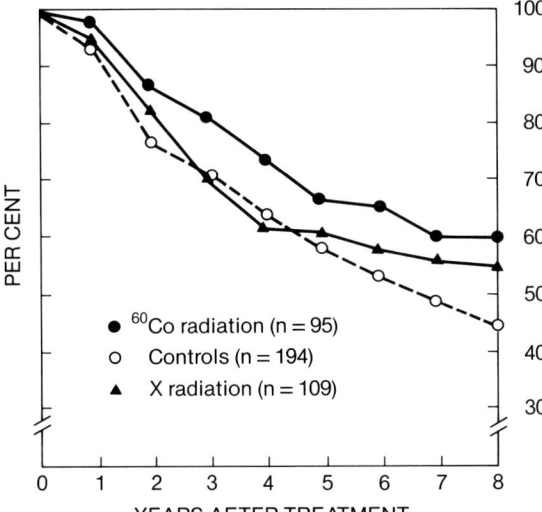

Figure 14–3. Disease-free survival in patients with histologically positive axillary nodes receiving postoperative irradiation. When the curves are analyzed over their entirety by the log rank test, there is a significant statistical advantage (P = 0.014) for the patients irradiated with cobalt-60. No survival advantage was detected in those treated with kilovoltage. (From Host, H., and Brennhovd, I. O.: The effect of post-operative radiotherapy in breast cancer. Int. J. Radiation Oncol. Biol. Phys., 2:1061, 1977. Reprinted with permission.)

preoperative irradiation was compared to mastectomy alone or mastectomy followed by postoperative irradiation (Wallgren et al., 1980). Both preoperative and postoperative irradiation significantly reduced the incidence of local and regional recurrence, and disease-free survival was better with either radiation regimen than following surgery alone. The difference was statistically significant for preoperative but not for postoperative irradiation. This seeming discrepancy was later attributed to differences in the radiation techniques employed in the study, which resulted in underdosage of the internal mammary nodes in patients treated postoperatively (Strender et al., 1981). Finally, retrospective review of experience with over 1400 patients treated at M. D. Anderson Hospital, Houston Texas, demonstrated nearly identical 10 year survival rates in patients who received either mastectomy alone or mastectomy followed by postoperative irradiation (Rodger et al., 1983; Montague and Fletcher, 1985). However, only 14 per cent of the patients who had surgery only versus 71 per cent of those treated with postoperative irradiation had histologically proved axillary metastases. As survival rates in any series are invariably inversely proportional to the percentage of patients with involved lymph nodes, the data strongly suggest that the addition of irradiation was often curative.

PREOPERATIVE IRRADIATION

Adequate preoperative irradiation will convert a significant proportion of borderline resectable primary breast masses to a status of full resectability, although this approach is now seldom considered. Moreover, dramatic reduction in the expected incidence of axillary lymph node involvement and of extranodal tumor extension is observed following preoperative irradiation (Table 14–3). One argument raised against preoperative irradiation is that it would, in fact, obscure the accuracy of prognostication based on assessment of axillary lymph node status and interfere with patient selection for adjuvant chemotherapy.

Retrospective and prospective studies of irradiation administered as a preoperative adjunct to radical mastectomy demonstrate that it is at least as effective in this instance as postoperative irradiation in securing local and regional control of breast cancer (Rodger et al., 1983; Wallgren et al., 1980). In the Swedish trial (Wallgren and associates 1980) compared preoperative or postoperative irradiation to radical mastectomy alone. Patients irradiated preoperatively had a significantly better survival ($p = 0.03$) than those treated with surgery alone. Patients with tumors located in the medial quadrants of the breast appeared to benefit most from the preoperative irradiation, suggesting that the improvement related to adequate irradiation of the internal mammary lymph nodes. Whether any of the theoretical advantages of preoperative irradiation were realized, including potential reduction in the release of viable malignant clonogens into the systemic circulation during surgical manipulation, have not been clarified by this or any other trial to date.

Radiation Therapy of Local-Regional Recurrences

Evidence that the development of apparently isolated local-regional recurrence of breast carcinoma following mastectomy almost inexorably heralds the subsequent appearance of systemic metastases should not deter imple-

Table 14-3. INCIDENCE OF AXILLARY LYMPH NODE METASTASES AND EXTRANODAL TUMOR EXTENSION FOLLOWING PREOPERATIVE IRRADIATION

Author	Clinical Axillary Status	Incidence of Histologically Positive Nodes		Incidence of Extranodal Tumor	
		Surgery Only	With Preoperative Radiation	Surgery Only	With Preoperative Radiation
Wallgren (1978)	—	37% (238/638)	21% (65/306)	52%	19%
Rodger (1983)	N−	44% (396/895)	12% (10/87)		
	N+	64% (711/324)	35% (124/355)	10%	5%

mentation of aggressive radiation therapy for such disease. Major palliation for the duration of the patient's remaining life can be secured frequently enough to justify its routine use. The lower ultimate incidence of local-regional symptoms following aggressive irradiation suggests that it may be justified even for patients with asymptomatic local-regional recurrences who already have identifiable distant metastases (Bedwinek et al., 1983). Overall, only about one fourth of patients who develop local-regional recurrence will survive 10 years. However, significantly better long-term survival rates are observed in patients in whom the recurrences are controlled by irradiation compared with patients who have uncontrolled disease (Chu et al., 1984a,b; Chen et al., 1985) (Fig. 14-4).

Although in some subsets of patients local control rates as high as 78 per cent with a corresponding 5 year disease-free survival rate of 48 per cent have been reported following irradiation of local-regional recurrences, even this modest success rate is highly dependent on a favorable case mix and the adequacy of the irradiation (Chen et al., 1985). Overall, however, not more than half of all patients with chest wall recurrences come to medical attention at an early enough stage of disease evolution to be treated successfully or in fact have their disease controlled. Because the majority of patients with locally progressive disease ultimately develop directly related severe functional compromise, this finding underscores the necessity of an aggressive approach (Bedwinek et al., 1981a). Most failures following irradiation can be attributed to the administration of inadequate radiation doses or failure to use large enough fields to encompass the areas of gross involvement with wide margins. Routinely irradiating the peripheral lymphatics in addition to the chest wall for local

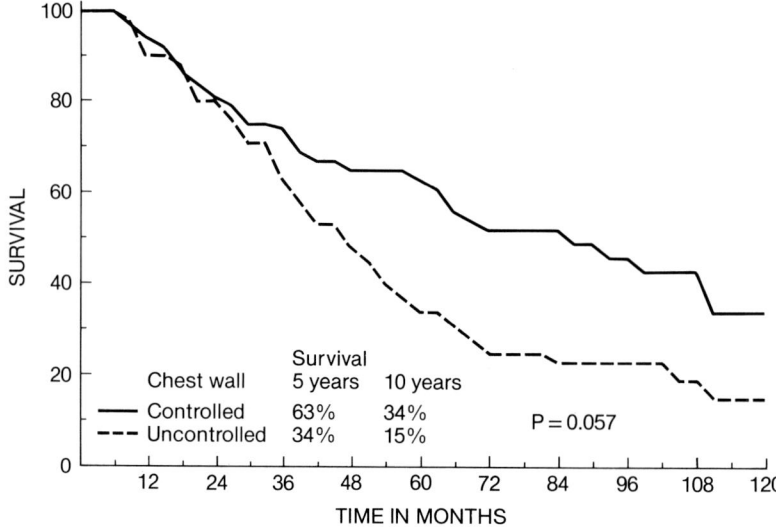

Figure 14-4. Five and 10 year survival of 106 patients treated at M. D. Anderson Hospital between January 1956 and December 1981 for chest wall recurrence of carcinoma of the breast. The survival rates of patients whose chest wall recurrences were controlled by irradiation are compared with those who failed treatment. (From Chen, K., et al.: Results of irradiation in the treatment of locoregional breast cancer recurrence. Cancer, 56:1269, 1985. Reprinted with permission.)

recurrences results in improved long-term survival (Toonkel et al., 1983). Local control rates will be inversely proportional to the number and size of the recurrences treated. Doses of at least 6000 rad are required to control recurrent masses that are 1 to 3 cm in diameter (Bedwinek et al., 1981a). For more voluminous cancers, doses must be pushed upward to the limits of normal tissue tolerance. Factors associated with poorer prognosis despite appropriate irradiation include simultaneous nodal and chest wall recurrence, advanced initial disease stage and a short disease-free interval from the time of initial therapy (Patanaphan et al., 1984). The argument for *elective* postoperative irradiation in patients at high risk for local-regional recurrences is reinforced when the difficulties encountered in controlling such disease once it is allowed to become clinically apparent are considered.

Radiation Therapy of Locally Advanced Breast Carcinoma

Locally advanced carcinomas of the breast (AJC-UICC Stages III and IV), which are judged inoperable by the criteria established by Haagensen and Stout in 1943, pose a complex management problem. Occult distant metastases, which eventually become manifest in most, if not all, patients with these stages of disease, impose a poor prognosis. Therefore, a major therapeutic aim in such cases is to provide patients with the treatment that will result in the highest probability of freedom from symptomatic local-regional disease for the duration of their remaining life. To maintain a satisfactory quality of life, distressing treatment sequelae must at the same time be kept to a minimum.

Because this staging designation includes patients with both technically resectable and categorically unresectable local-regional disease, this status is the principal factor influencing treatment recommendations. The radiobiologic principles mentioned in this chapter's introductory remarks come into play.

Radical radiation therapy has long been the treatment of choice for technically unresectable lesions, resulting in reported local tumor control rates usually in the range of 35 to 70 per cent. Corresponding 5 year survival figures usually in the 10 to 30 per cent range have been reported. Arriagada and coworkers (1985) have analyzed the results of treating 463 patients with breast cancer with radiation therapy alone. This emphasizes the dependency of the success rate of such therapy on two factors: tumor size and tumor dose (Table 14–4). The radiation dosage to the tumor emerged as the most significant independent factor, able to produce up to tenfold increase in the probability of local tumor control compared with a twofold decrease for tumor size. The point is that for tumor masses of the size usually dealt with (> 5 cm in diameter) in the locally advanced categories, radiation doses likely to result in tumor control must be at such a high level that a significant incidence of severe treatment-related sequelae can be expected. For example, Spanos and colleagues (1980) reported a 24 per cent incidence of late soft tissue necrosis and severe fibrosis in patients treated to doses in excess of 8000 rad who lived long enough to develop these difficulties.

Technically resectable advanced breast cancer is, therefore, approached more effectively if excisional biopsy or simple mastectomy with or without axillary dissection is performed prior to irradiation (Bedwinek et al., 1982; Harris et al., 1983; Chu et al., 1984a). If the chest wall and regional lymphatics are rendered free of gross tumor by these procedures, radiation doses less associated with normal tissue damage are effective in securing freedom from progressive disease in these areas. In one report involving 132 patients, simple mastectomy and axillary dissection followed by 50 Gy in 5 weeks resulted in local-regional control in 87 per cent of patients (Montague and Fletcher, 1985).

Table 14–4. THREE YEAR LOCAL CONTROL RATES FOLLOWING RADIATION THERAPY ALONE FOR PRIMARY BREAST CARCINOMAS ACCORDING TO TOTAL RADIATION DOSE AND TUMOR SIZE

Tumor Dose (Gy)	Tumor Size			
	4 cm	6 cm	8 cm	> 8 cm
> 40–50	25%	24%	5%	0%
> 50–60	59%	46%	36%	17%
> 60–70	—	—	28%	21%
> 70–80	81%	71%	61%	36%
> 80	100%	66%	79%	50%

Modified from Arriagada, R., et al.: Int. J. Radiation Oncol. Biol. Phys., 11:1751, 1985.

The role of systemic chemotherapy in the management of patients with locally advanced, clinically nondisseminated carcinoma of the breast has not been fully defined. Adjunctive chemohormonal therapy did not result in improved relapse-free or overall survival in a recently reported prospective trial (Schaake-Koning et al., 1985).

Radiation Therapy of Distant Metastases

A large proportion of patients with cancer of the breast develop distant metastases, which produce distressing symptoms and eventually become life-threatening. Radiation therapy is the most effective means of providing symptomatic relief. Such treatment is not undertaken with the express purpose of increasing duration of survival, although, in the individual patient, eradication of a tumor that is impinging on a vital structure may prolong life. Two of the most common sites of distant metastasis are the skeletal system and the central nervous system. Data are available that permit realistic expectation of the beneficial effects of radiation therapy.

SKELETAL METASTASIS

Prospective studies of radiation therapy for skeletal metastasis have been conducted by the Radiation Therapy Oncology Group (RTOG) (Tang et al., 1982). In these studies, patients with metastases from tumors arising in many different anatomic sites and, consequently, with many different histopathologic diagnoses, were treated in a consistent manner. The vast majority of patients had metastases from carcinomas of the breast, lung, and prostate.

Approximately 1000 patients were studied. The results showed that 90 per cent of patients who had moderate to severe pain experienced some relief, and over one half had complete disappearance of pain. Results were the same whether there were solitary or multiple sites of symptomatic metastases. Metastases in pelvic bones required a longer time for maximum relief of symptoms compared with other sites of involvement. Patients with carcinomas of the breast and prostate experienced relief of pain more frequently than those with carcinomas of the lung and other malignant tumors; they also experienced a longer period of symptomatic relief.

The aim of palliative irradiation is to provide the most rapid, complete, and durable relief of symptoms possible. A brief course of treatment is desirable so that the patient is inconvenienced as little as possible. It is important that there be few short-term side effects, and it is imperative to have a very low risk of late sequelae. However, duration of the palliation depends on administration of a total dose of radiation sufficient to eradicate the tumor, or at least reduce it, to the smallest number of clonogenic cells compatible with a low probably of adverse effects. In practice, palliative courses of radiation therapy last 2 to 3 weeks. In special circumstances, it can be advantageous to treat for longer or shorter periods.

At the extreme of short courses of palliative radiation therapy are single treatments. They are, in general, associated with a more rapid relief of symptoms, but the length of the palliation is less. The presence of multiple symptomatic skeletal metastases may justify consideration of half-body irradiation with a single administration. This is an old approach that has returned to favor (Salazar et al., 1981). Upper half-body irradiation is associated with moderate acute symptoms that can be prevented by hydration, corticosteroids, and antiemetics; thus, it requires hospitalization. Radiation pneumonitis may result if the single dose is excessive. Somewhat higher doses may be given with middle and lower half-body irradiation. Doses used with half-body treatments are approximately two to four times those used in a course of fractionated radiation therapy (i.e., 6 to 10 Gy versus 2.5 to 4 Gy). Pain relief occurs with approximately the same frequency as with fractionated radiation therapy.

METASTASIS TO THE CENTRAL NERVOUS SYSTEM

Carcinoma of the breast may compromise the central nervous system in several ways. The most common problem is metastasis to the parenchyma of the brain, but involvement of the vertebrae with secondary pressure on the spinal cord or nerve roots, extradural metastasis, leptomeningeal carcinomatosis, and even intramedullary metastasis may be observed.

The RTOG has undertaken large-scale, prospective trials of palliative irradiation for brain metastases. The investigators have documented the effectiveness of radiation therapy in relieving symptoms (Borgelt et al., 1981). Table 14–5 shows the frequency with which palliation of specific neurologic symptoms is achieved. Complete relief is achieved in 35 to 72 per cent, and some benefit is derived from radiation therapy in 65 to 85 per cent of patients. Seizure, both major motor and focal in type, as well as headache, are most consistently relieved, but substantial benefit is seen in the majority of patients with any of the common symptoms.

Back pain and neurologic symptoms and signs may herald the onset of paraplegia caused by metastases from carcinoma of the breast. Myelography can demonstrate the level of the block, and computed tomography usually shows whether the impingement on the spinal cord is the result of an extradural tumor or due to vertebral collapse and mechanical compromise. In the former case, immediate institution of radiation therapy may alleviate neurologic symptoms without need for decompressive laminectomy. If there is mechanical compromise, laminectomy is usually necessary. Paraplegia that is completely established can still be reversed, but the longer the period of complete paralysis, the lower the probability of reversing it.

Carcinomatous meningitis is rarely treated effectively with radiation therapy alone. However, irradiation of the base of the skull can reverse distressing cranial nerve abnormalities, and cranial irradiation may be combined with intrathecal administration of cytotoxic chemotherapeutic agents to achieve palliation.

Table 14–5. RELIEF BY RADIATION THERAPY OF SPECIFIC NEUROLOGIC SYMPTOMS FROM BRAIN METASTASIS

Symptom	Number of Patients	Per Cent Complete Relief	Per Cent Overall Relief (Complete and Partial)
Seizures	327	72	85
Headache	982	60	82
Impaired mentation	780	44	70
Cerebellar dysfunction	477	45	69
Motor loss	910	35	67
Cranial nerve symptoms	459	42	65

THORACIC METASTASES

Intrathoracic spread of mammary cancer is not rare. Secondary involvement of the mediastinum following metastasis to the internal mammary nodes is perhaps far more common than previously appreciated. Hemoptysis, dyspnea, and even superior vena caval obstruction may occur. Each of these symptoms is somewhat consistently reversed by mediastinal irradiation. Pleural effusion, however, cannot be palliated with radiation therapy because it would be necessary to deliver high doses to the entire pleura, which secondarily would produce radiation pneumonitis and scarring, with possibly greater pulmonary compromise than that resulting from the effusion.

HEPATIC METASTASES

The only indication for palliative irradiation of patients with hepatic metastases from cancer is pain. There is little, if any, benefit to be derived from irradiation for abnormal hepatic function or hepatomegaly, but pain resulting from stretching of the capsule of the liver may be relieved in over half the patients treated (Borgelt et al., 1981).

Side Effects of Radiation Therapy

There is a low probability of adverse effects from radiation therapy for carcinoma of the breast. The skin of the breast irradiated following excisional biopsy, or that of the chest wall following mastectomy, frequently will show a gradual reddening during the third and fourth week of treatment. Unless there is a specific need to have a maximal dose of radiations at the surface, most techniques for irradiating the breast or chest wall produce dry desquamation but infrequently cause a moist reaction. In patients with locally advanced mammary tumors with involvement of the skin or inflammatory changes, it may be necessary to have a maximal effect on the surface. Moist desquamation will result and then will heal in a predictable manner in the weeks following completion of irradiation.

Late cutaneous sequelae from radiation therapy include hypochromia, atrophy, and telangiectasia, usually confined to those regions that required a maximal dose to the surface of the skin. Patients who receive irradiation to the site of the original tumor by means of interstitial implantation of the radioactive sources or by high energy electron beam may have late sequelae confined to the skin surrounding the scar from the excision.

Because it is impossible to irradiate the entire thickness of the chest wall without irradiating the adjacent anterior portion of the lung, scarring may be demonstrable in chest radiographs months or years after treatment. Similarly, irradiation of the internal mammary and supraclavicular regions may result in pulmonary effects. Infrequently, symptomatic radiation pneumonitis may occur, manifested by cough, fever, and dyspnea. Symptomatic treatment is indicated until the inflammatory changes resolve, which they will do spontaneously over a period of several weeks. In the rare case of severe symptoms, corticosteroids may be indicated.

Effects on other organs are so infrequent as to be well beyond the scope of this chapter. The interested reader is referred to review articles on the subject (Rubin, 1984; Cox et al., 1986). It is worth mentioning that a variety of cytotoxic drugs may enhance the side-effects of ionizing radiations. Most notable are doxorubicin, dactinomycin, and methotrexate. Both acute and late sequelae may be accentuated by the simultaneous administration of such drugs and radiation therapy. In general, there is little interaction with regard to effects on normal tissues when there is at least a 2-week interval between the administration of drugs and ionizing radiations.

It is well recognized that ionizing radiations are carcinogenic. This fact has been emphasized by some authors as an argument for avoiding radiation therapy in the management of patients with cancer of the breast. However, data derived from whole-body exposures to radiations far different in character from the high energy photons and electrons used in the treatment of patients with cancer have little bearing on the risk of carcinogenesis following therapeutic applications of carefully focused radiations. There is no evidence, for example, that radiation therapy increases the already substantial risk of development of carcinoma in the contralateral breast. There are case reports suggesting that sarcomas arising in the chest wall result from prior irradiation, but the frequency is so low as to approximate the risk of lymphangiosarcoma arising in the chronically lymphedematous arm after axillary dissection. Studies such as that of Ferguson and associates (1984), which describe late effects of primitive treatments (conventional x-rays of 1.5 and 3 mm of copper half-value layer administered over 3 to 5 months), have little if any relevance to contemporary radiation therapy. Conclusions from these experiences are no more valid than those from surgery prior to antibiotics and modern anesthesia.

Summary

The role of radiation therapy has shifted from surgical adjuvant therapy to definitive management in an effort to preserve esthetics and function. Postoperative irradiation is important in selected patients who have undergone mastectomy, and preoperative irradiation deserves further investigation. Aggressive, thorough local-regional irradiation for postoperative recurrence has proved to be more beneficial than highly localized irradiation. Combinations of surgery, chemotherapy, and radiation therapy are indicated in patients with locally advanced cancer of the breast. A high proportion of patients with distant metastases benefit from palliative irradiation. The side effects of radiation therapy are predictable and relatively mild, and a large proportion of all patients with mammary cancer profit from the use of this technique.

REFERENCES

Amalric, R., Santamaria, F., Robert, F., et al.: Conservation therapy of operable breast cancer—results at five, ten, and fifteen years in 2216 consecutive cases. *In* Harris, J., Hellman, S., and Silen, W. (Eds.): Conservative Management of Breast Cancer, New Surgical and Radiotherapeutic Techniques. Philadelphia, J. B. Lippincott, 1983, p. 15.

Arriagada, R., Mouriesse, H., Sarrazin, D., et al.: Radiotherapy alone in breast cancer. I. Analysis of tumor parameters, tumor dose, and local control: The experience of the Gustave-Roussy Institute and The Princess Margaret Hospital. Int. J. Radiation Oncol. Biol. Phys., 11:1751, 1985.

Baclesse, P.: Roentgentherapy alone in cancer of the breast. Acta Un. Int. Cancre, 15:1023, 1959.

Bedwinek, J. M., Fineberg, B., Lee, J., et al.: Analysis of failures following local treatment of isolated local-regional recurrence of breast cancer. Int. J. Radiation Oncol. Biol. Phys., 7:581, 1981a.

Bedwinek, J. M., Lee, J., Fineberg, B., et al.: Prognostic indicators in patients with isolated local-regional recurrence of breast cancer. Cancer, 47:2232, 1981b.

Bedwinek, J. M., Munro, D., and Fineberg, B.: Local-regional treatment of patients with simultaneous local-regional recurrence and distant metastases following mastectomy. Am. J. Clin. Oncol., 6:295, 1983.

Bedwinek, J., Venkata, R., Perez, C., et al.: Stage III and localized Stage IV breast cancer: Irradiation alone vs. irradiation plus surgery. Int. J. Radiation Oncol. Biol. Phys., 8:31–36, 1982.

Borgelt, B. B., Belber, R., Brady, L. W., et al.: The palliation of helpatic metastases: Results of the Radiation Therapy Oncology Group. Int. J. Radiation Oncol. Biol. Phys., 7:587, 1981.

Borgelt, B., Belber, R., Kramer, S., et al.: The palliation of brain metastases: Final results of the first two studies by the Radiation Therapy Oncology Group. Int. J. Radiation Oncol. Biol. Phys., 6:1, 1980.

Calle, R., Vilcoq, J. R., Pilleron, J. P., et al.: Conservative treatment of operable breast carcinoma by irradiation with or without limited surgery—ten-year results. In Harris, J., Hellman, S., and Silen, W. (Eds.): Conservative Management of Breast Cancer, New Surgical and Radiotherapeutic Techniques. Philadelphia, J. B. Lippincott, 1983, p. 3.

Cancer Research Campaign: Management of early cancer of the breast. Report on an international multicentre trial supported by the Cancer Research Campaign. Br. Med. J., 1:1035, 1976.

Chen, K. K., Montague, E. D., and Oswald, M. J., Results of irradiation in the treatment of locoregional breast cancer recurrence. Cancer, 56:1269, 1985.

Chu, A. M., Cope, O., Doucette, J., et al.: Non-metastatic locally advanced cancer of the breast treated with irradiation. Int. J. Radiation Oncol. Biol. Phys., 10:2299, 1984a.

Chu, A. M., Cope, O., Russo, R., et al.: Patterns of local-regional recurrence and results in Stages I and II breast cancer treated by irradiation following limited surgery. Am. J. Clin. Oncol., 7:221, 1984b.

Clark, R. M., Wilkinson, R. H., Mahoney, L. J., et al.: Breast cancer: A 21 year experience with conservative surgery and radiation, Int. J. Radiation Oncol. Biol. Phys., 8:967, 1982.

Clarke, D., Martinez, A., and Cox, R. S.: Analysis of cosmetic results and complications in patients with Stage I and II breast cancer treated by biopsy and irradiation. Int. J. Radiation Oncol. Biol. Phys., 9:1807, 1983.

Clarke, D., Martinez, A., Cox, R. S., et al.: Breast edema following staging axillary node dissection in patients with breast carcinoma treated by radical radiotherapy. Cancer, 49:2295, 1982.

Cox, J. D., Byhardt, R. W., Wilson, J. F., et al.: Complications of radiation therapy and factors in their prevention. World J. Surg., 10:171, 1986.

Danoff, B. F., Goodman, R. L., Glick, J. H., et al.: The effect of adjuvant chemotherapy on cosmesis and complications in patients with breast cancer treated by definitive irradiation. Int. J. Radiation Oncol. Biol. Phys., 9:1625, 1983.

Danoff, B. F., Pajak, T. F., Solin, L. J., et al.: Excisional biopsy, axillary node dissection and definitive radiotherapy for stage I and II breast cancer. Int. J. Radiation Oncol. Biol. Phys., 11:479, 1985.

Ferguson, D. J., Sutton, H. G., Jr., and Dawson, P. J.: Late effects of adjuvant radiotherapy for breast cancer. Cancer, 54:2319, 1984.

Findlay, P. A., Lippmann, M., Danforth, D., et al.: A randomized trial comparing mastectomy to radiotherapy in the treatment of Stage I-II breast cancer: A preliminary report. Proc. ASCO, 4:60, 1985.

Fisher, B., Bauer, M., Margolese, R., et al.: Five-year results of a randomized clinical trial comparing total mastectomy and segmental mastectomy with or without radiation in the treatment of breast cancer. N. Engl. J. Med., 312:665, 1985.

Fisher, B., Slack, N., Cavanaugh, R. J., et al.: Postoperative radiotherapy in the treatment of breast cancer. Results of the NSABP clinical trial. Ann. Surg., 172:711–732, 1970.

Fletcher, G. H.: Clinical dose response curve of subclinical aggregates of epithelial cells and its practical application in the management of human cancer. In Friedman, M. (Ed.): Biological and Clinical Basis of Radiosensitivity. Springfield, Ill., Charles C Thomas, 1974, p 485.

Fletcher, G. H.: The enigma of breast cancer. In Ames, F. C., Blumenschein, G. R., and Montague, E. D. (Eds.): Current Controversies in Breast Cancer. Austin, University of Texas Press, 1984, p. 139.

Fletcher, G. H., and Montague, E. D.: Does adequate irradiation of the internal mammary chain and supraclavicular nodes improve survival rates? Int. J. Radiation Oncol. Biol. Phys., 4:481, 1978.

Fletcher, G. H.: History of irradiation in the primary management of apparently regionally confined breast cancer. Int. J. Radiation Oncol. Biol. Phys., 11:2133, 1985.

Haagensen, C. D., and Stout, A. P.: Carcinoma of the breast: Criteria of operability. Ann. Surg., 118:859, 1943.

Hayward, J.: The conservative treatment of early breast cancer. Cancer, 33:593, 1974.

Hellman, S., Harris, J. R., and Levene, M. B.: Radiation therapy of early carcinoma of the breast without mastectomy. Cancer, 46:988, 1980.

Hodges, P. C.: The Life and Times of Emil H. Grubbe. Chicago, The University of Chicago Press, 1964.

Host, H., and Brennhovd, I. O.: The effect of postoperative radiotherapy in breast cancer. Int. J. Radiation Oncol. Biol. Phys., 2:1061, 1977.

Keynes, G.: The treatment of primary carcinoma of the breast with radium. Acta Radiol., 10:293, 1929.

Lichter, A.: The treatment of breast cancer without mastectomy. Current status and future perspectives. Postgrad. Med., 79(8):93–102, 1986.

Lippman, M. E., Lichter, A. S., Edwards, B. K., et al.: The impact of primary irradiation treatment of localized breast cancer on the ability to administer systemic adjuvant chemotherapy. J. Clin. Oncol., 2:21, 1984.

Montague, E. D.: Conservation surgery and radiation therapy in the treatment of operable breast cancer. Cancer, 53:700, 1984.

Montague, E. D., and Fletcher, G. H.: Local regional effectiveness of surgery and radiation in the treatment of breast cancer. Cancer, 55:2266, 1985.

Otmezguine, Y., Martin, M., LeBourgeois, J. P., et al.: Etude des recidives parmi 202 cancereuses du sein traitees conservativement par radiotherapie. J. Eur. Radiother., 3:115, 1980.

Patanaphan, V., Salazar, O. M., and Poussin-Rosillo, H.: Prognosticators in recurrent breast cancer. Cancer, 54:228, 1984.

Paterson, R., and Russell, M. H.: Clinical trials in malignant disease. III. Breast cancer: Evaluation of postoperative radiotherapy. Clin. Radiol., 10:175, 1959.

Patterson, M. P., Pezner, R. D., Hill, L. R., et al.: Patient self-evaluation of cosmetic outcome of breast-preserving cancer treatment. Int. J. Radiation Oncol. Biol. Phys., 11:1849, 1985.

Peters, M. V.: Cutting the "Gordian knot" in early breast cancer. Ann. R. Coll. Phys. Surg. (Can.), 8:186, 1976.

Pierquin, B., Raynal, M., Otmezguine, Y., et al.: Le traitement conservateur des cancers du sein. Presse Med., 15:375, 1986.

Pierquin, B., Owen, R., Maylin, C., et al.: Radical radiation therapy of breast cancer. Int. J. Radiation Oncol. Biol. Phys., 6:17, 1979.

Ray, G. R., and Fish, V. J.: Biopsy and definitive radiation therapy in stage I and II adenocarcinoma of the female breast: Analysis of cosmesis and the role of electron beam supplementation. Int. J. Radiation Oncol. Biol. Phys., 9:813, 1983.

Ray, G. R., Fish, V. J., Marmor, J. B., et al.: Impact of adjuvant chemotherapy on cosmesis and complications in stages I and II carcinoma of the breast treated by biopsy and radiation therapy. Int. J. Radiation Oncol. Biol. Phys., 10:837, 1983.

Rissanen, P. M.: A comparison of conservative and radical surgery combined with radiotherapy in the treatment of stage I carcinoma of the breast. Eur. J. Radiol., 42:423, 1969.

Rodger, A., Montague, E., and Fletcher, G.: Preoperative or postoperative irradiation as adjunctive treatment with radical mastectomy in breast cancer. Cancer, 51:1388–1392, 1983.

Rose, C. M., Botnick, L., Weinstein, M., et al.: Axillary sampling in the definitive treatment of breast cancer by radiation therapy and lumpectomy. Int. J. Radiation Oncol. Biol. Phys., 9:339–344, 1983.

Rubin, P.: The Franz Buschke Lecture. Late effects of chemotherapy and radiation therapy. A new hypothesis. Int. J. Radiation Oncol. Biol. Phys., 10:5, 1984.

Salazar, O. M., Rubin, P., Hendrickson, F. R., et al.: Single-dose half-body irradiation for the palliation of multiple bone metastases from solid tumors: A preliminary report. Int. J. Radiation Oncol. Biol. Phys., 7:773, 1981.

Sarrazin, D., Le, M., Rouesse, J., et al.: Conservative treatment versus mastectomy in breast cancer tumors with macroscopic diameter of 20 millimeters or less. Cancer, 53:1209, 1984.

Schaake-Koning, C., van der Linden, E. H., Hart, G., et al.: Adjuvant chemo-and hormonal therapy in locally advanced breast cancer: A randomized clinical study. Int. J. Radiation Oncol. Biol. Phys., 11:1759, 1985.

Spanos, W. J., Montague, E. D., and Fletcher, G. H.: Late complications of radiation only for advanced breast cancer. Int. J. Radiation Oncol. Biol. Phys., 6:1473, 1980.

Strender, L. E., Wallgren, A., Arndt, J., et al.: Adjuvant radiotherapy in operable breast cancer: Correlation between dose in internal mammary nodes and prognosis. Int. J. Radiation Oncol. Biol. Phys., 7:1319, 1981.

Tang, D., Gillick, L., and Hendrickson, F. R.: The palliation of symptomatic osseous metastases. Final results of the study by the Radiation Therapy Oncology Group. Cancer, 50:893, 1982.

Toonkel, L. M., Fix, I., Jacobson, L. H., et al.: The significance of local recurrence of carcinoma of the breast. Int. J. Radiation Oncol. Biol. Phys., 9:33, 1983.

Toonkel, L. M., Fix, I., Jacobson, L. H., et al.: Postoperative radiation therapy for carcinoma of the breast: Improved results with elective irradiation of the chest wall. Int. J. Radiation Oncol. Biol. Phys., 8:977, 1982b.

Veronesi, U., Zucali, R., and Del Vecchio, M.: Conservative treatment of breast cancer with the Q.U.A.R.T. technique. World J. Surg., 9:676, 1985.

Wallgren, A., Arner, O., Bergstrom, J., et al.: The value of preoperative radiotherapy in operable mammary carcinoma. Int. J. Radiation Oncol. Biol. Phys., 6:287, 1980.

Wilson, J. F.: Breast cancer treatment—current status, 3. Simple excision with irradiation. Postgrad. Med., 74:151, 1983.

CHAPTER 15

J. SEEGER
J. C. ALLEGRA

Chemotherapy of Breast Cancer

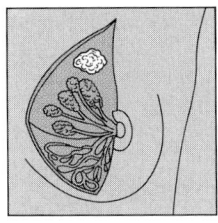

Breast cancer was diagnosed in approximately 119,000 women in the United States in 1985. For the same year, it was predicted that 38,400 women would die as a result of this disease (Silverberg, 1985). It can, however, be stated that despite these grim statistics, intensive public education with an emphasis on breast self-examination and mammography has led to an increasing number of new cases being diagnosed at an earlier stage. In fact, the majority of women now come to medical attention with Stage I operable breast cancer, which is not only highly curable but also amenable to breast-preserving, less radical surgery. Despite this earlier detection, breast cancer still accounts for 18 per cent of all cancer deaths in women. It is the leading cause of death in women aged 35 to 54 years old and second to cardiovascular disease in older women (Logan, 1975).

Mortality and incidence rates vary throughout the world, with England and Wales ranking first, and the United States ranking fourteenth (Bourke, 1983). In some countries with high rates, the incidence of breast cancer in the 50 to 54 year old age group drops slightly, possibly related to alterations in the hormonal environment associated with menopause. In countries with low rates, such as Japan (ranking number 48), immigrants to higher risk countries approach the adopted country's incidence by the second generation. This phenomenon supports the hypothesis that environmental factors (such as diet) are important in the etiology of breast cancer.

Since breast cancer is such a common disease in women (1 in 12 affected in the United States), it is not surprising that there exists a long list of potential risk factors. These include unopposed ovarian cycling, decreased parity, and some categories of benign breast disorders. However, family history of breast cancer and a previous history of breast cancer are now considered to be the two most important risk factors.

Staging

Staging, the process of grouping patients according to extent of disease, facilitates analysis of natural history, prognosis, and subsequent treatment impact. In breast cancer, staging is extremely important as, to a large extent, it dictates treatment decisions in adjuvant therapy in Stage I versus Stage II disease. Clinical staging is determined by initial physical examination, laboratory evaluation, and diagnostic radiographs. Pathologic confirmation of the primary tumor is required, as well as analysis of the axillary nodes. This leads to a final pathologic stage on which treatment is now based. Of interest, clinical examination of the axilla is notoriously inaccurate, with up to 40 per cent of clinically negative nodes containing tumor cells (Fisher, et al., 1981) and a significant proportion of clinically positive axillary nodes being found to not contain tumor.

Several staging systems for breast cancer exist, but the most universally used is accepted by both the Union Internationale Contre le Cancer (UICC) and the American Joint Commission on Cancer Staging and End Results Reporting (AJCC). This system describes the tumor by TNM classification; a summary is presented in the accompanying table (Beahrs and Myers, 1983).

TNM TUMOR CLASSIFICATION

Clinical Staging
T   Primary tumor
T0 No evidence of primary tumor
T1 Tumor 2 cm or less in greatest dimension
    T1a No fixation to underlying pectoral fascia or muscle
    T1b Fixation to underlying pectoral fascia or muscle
        i   tumor <0.5 cm
        ii tumor >0.5 <1.0 cm
        iii tumor >1.0 <2.0 cm
T2 Tumor more than 2 cm but not more than 5 cm in greatest dimension
    T2a No fixation to underlying pectoral fascia or muscle
    T2b Fixation to underlying pectoral fascia or muscle
T3 Tumor more than 5 cm in greatest dimension
    T3a No fixation to underlying pectoral fascia or muscle
    T3b Fixation to underlying pectoral fascia or muscle
T4 Tumor of any size with direct extension to chest wall or skin (Chest wall includes ribs, intercostal muscles, and serratus anterior muscle, but not pectoral muscle.)
    T4a Fixation to chest wall
    T4b Edema (or "peau d'orange"), ulceration of the skin of the breast, or satellite skin nodules confined to the same breast
    T4c Both of the above
N   Regional lymph nodes
N0 Homolateral axillary lymph nodes not considered to contain growth
N1 Movable homolateral axillary nodes considered to contain growth
N2 Homolateral axillary nodes considered to contain growth and fixed to one another or to other structures
N3 Homolateral supraclavicular or infraclavicular nodes considered to contain growth or edema of the arm

Pathologic Staging
Lymph Nodes Status
N0 No evidence of homolaterally axillary lymph node metastasis
N1 Metastasis to movable homolateral axillary nodes not fixed to one another or to other structure
N1a Micrometastasis <0.2 cm in lymph node(s)
N1b Gross metastasis in lymph node(s)
    I   Metastasis more than 0.2 cm but less than 2.0 cm in one to three lymph nodes
    II Metastasis more than 0.2 cm but less than 2.0 cm in four or more lymph nodes
    III Extension of metastasis beyond the lymph node capsule (less than 2.0 cm in dimension)
    IV Metastasis in lymph node 2.0 cm or more in dimension
N2 Metastasis to homolateral axillary lymph nodes that are fixed to one another or to other structures
N3 Metastasis to homolateral supraclavicular or infraclavicular lymph node(s)

Metastatic Disease
M   Distant metastasis
M0 No (known) distant metastasis
M1 Distant metastasis present, specify site

Postsurgical Resection Pathologic Staging

Stage	T	N	M
Stage I	T1a or T1b	N0 or N1a	M0
Stage II	T0	N1b	M0
	T1a or T1b	N1b	M0
	T2a or T2b	N0, N1a or N1b	M0
Stage III	T1a or T1b	N2	M0
	T2a or T2b	N2	M0
	T3a or T3b	N0, N1 or N2	M0
Stage IV	T4	any N	any M
	any T	N3	any M
	any T	any N	M1

Dimpling of the skin, nipple retraction, or any other skin changes except those in T4b may occur in T1, T2, or T3 without changing the classification.

After clinical staging, pathologic examination is performed on either a segmental mastectomy specimen containing the primary cancer and at least Level I and Level II axillary nodes or on a formal modified radical mastectomy specimen with all levels of axillary lymph nodes. Lymph node status, description of metastatic disease, and postsurgical resection pathologic staging can be categorized as shown in the table.

Accurate staging is critical to processing data regarding the natural history of breast cancer. Furthermore, all breast cancer clinical trials require pathologic staging and are referred to here by the Stage I to IV system. It is important to note that some of the clinical trials summarized in this chapter do not adhere strictly to this described staging system. The National Surgical Adjuvant Breast Project (NSABP), for example, puts greater emphasis on lymph nodes status. In the NSABP clinical trials, patients are classed as Stage I or Stage II as a function of having negative or positive axillary lymph nodes, independent of tumor size. In these trials, a patient with a $T_2N_0M_0$ lesion would be a Stage I patient, and a patient with a $T_{1a}N_{1a}M_0$ lesion would be Stage II.

These staging systems are also crucial to the design of clinical trials, especially in the consideration of risk and benefit to patients. Contrast lymph node negative, Stage I patients, who have a high cure rate following mastectomy (>80 per cent), with lymph node positive Stage II patients, of whom only a minority are cured by mastectomy (≅25 to 35 per cent). It is obvious that potential benefit is much greater in Stage II patients than in Stage I patients, and this great difference in potential benefit would alter the risks allowed to these patient groups. This accounts for the large number of adjuvant therapy trials in Stage II patients compared with the small number of studies in Stage I patients and also accounts for the difference in potential toxicity of therapy in Stage II patients compared with Stage I trials, which are characterized by less toxic therapy.

Systemic Therapy of Metastatic Disease (Stage IV)

Metastatic breast cancer currently is not curable and, indeed, the vast majority of patients with this stage of disease die of the effects of growing tumor. It is important to note, however, that although it is not curable, metastatic breast cancer is very treatable and is one of the most responsive solid tumors to cytotoxic chemotherapy. It is also true that patients whose tumors respond to therapy not only have increased survival but also have an improved quality of life. Typically, a patient will receive either hormonal or cytotoxic agents and, if response occurs, years of palliation associated with prolonged survival and an improved quality of life can be expected. Eventually, however, resistance develops, tumor progresses, and therapy must be altered. Continuing this sequence requires potentially more toxic drugs, and response rate and response duration both decrease.

One of the greatest impacts on breast cancer therapy has been identification of and the ability to measure estrogen receptors (ER) in tissue (Jensen et al., 1967, 1971) (see Chapter 17). Observation of the biologic behavior as a function of ER leads to the following correlates. Of all primary breast cancers, 60 per cent are ER positive (Allegra et al., 1980); however, the frequency of ER positivity and the concentration of receptors are higher in postmenopausal than in premenopausal women. Estrogen receptor positive carcinomas have a longer disease-free survival, longer overall survival, and longer overall survival independent of lymph node status (Hahnel et al., 1979). The frequency of ER positive breast cancer also increases with the age of patients, as does the actual concentration of receptor protein in tumors.

The ER status has been correlated to cell replication activity through measurement of the thymidine labeling index (TLI). In vivo, breast cancer cells are exposed briefly to tritiated thymidine, and those cells that are actively replicating nuclear DNA are labeled. A high TLI reflects a rapid rate of cell replication and a more biologically aggressive tumor (Silvestrini et al., 1979). Meyers and colleagues (1977) measured both ER and TLI in 63 primary invasive breast carcinomas and reported an association of high TLI and absent ER. More recently, TLI has been shown to correlate inversely with ER concentration but directly with tumor size and mitotic activity (Silvestrini et al., 1985). From data of this type, it is convenient to divide breast cancer into two subsets, hormone dependent (ER positive) and hormone independent (ER negative). Hormone dependent tumors are slower growing and have fewer cells in the S phase than their hormone independent counterparts. Hormone independent tumors have a high degree of aneuploidy and are frequently characterized by both high nuclear and histopathologic tumor grade.

It is generally agreed that approximately 60 per cent of patients with ER positive carcinomas can be expected to respond to endocrine therapy (Morgan et al., 1976). and, most important, ER negative tumors do not respond in any significant way to hormonal manipulation. Controversy, however, surrounds predicting responses to chemotherapy on the basis of ER status. Lippman and coworkers (1978) reported a retrospective study that correlated a low or absent estrogen receptor value with a greater chance for response to chemotherapy. Theoretically ER negative tumors with a higher TLI and growth rate responded better to cytotoxic drugs. Many similar evaluations followed, some contradictory, showing a higher response rate to chemotherapy in ER positive patients (Kiang et al., 1978). In a controlled study of 36 patients with previously untreated advanced breast cancer, all of whom received the same regimen of cyclophosphamide, methotrexate, and 5-fluorouracil (CMF), a better response (88 per cent) was seen in the ER positive group versus 35 per cent in the ER negative group (Chang et al.,

1981). Cautious interpretation is warranted because ER positive patients are known to have both longer disease-free survival and longer overall survival, which may be independent of treatment. To further complicate matters, data from the NSABP, which were presented at the NIH Consensus (1985) Development Conference on Adjuvant Treatment of breast cancer, suggest that the beneficial effects of adjuvant chemotherapy treatment in NSABP trials is most evident in patients whose tumors lack ER or have poor nuclear grade. Although the relationship between receptor status plus response to chemotherapy treatment is not nearly as clear-cut as the relationship between ER and hormonal therapy, it does warrant continued clinical investigation.

Single Agents in Advanced Breast Cancer

Since the initial evaluation of chemotherapy in humans in 1942, virtually every promising new drug developed has been tested in breast cancer. Various classes of active antineoplastic agents are summarized in Table 15–1.

The most extensively studied and most active alkylating agent is cyclophosphamide; however, significant activity exists in virtually all of the alkylating agents. The antimetabolites also have considerable activity in human breast cancer, with 5-fluorouracil (5-FU) and methotrexate being the two drugs used most widely in this category. Activity has also been demonstrated for the vinca alkaloids, with vincristine being used in multiple combination chemotherapy treatment regimens and with vinblastine being effective when used as a 5 day infusion (Yap et al., 1980).

Doxorubicin hydrochloride (Adriamycin), an anthracycline antibiotic, is the most active single agent in advanced breast cancer. Response rates of up to 50 per cent in previously untreated patients have been reported (Ahmann et al., 1974). In patients failing combined chemotherapy, a salvage response rate of 30 per cent can be achieved with Adriamycin (Tormey, 1975). The standard dose for advanced breast cancer is 60 to 75 mg/m² every 3 weeks intravenously, but more recently schedules have been varied to minimize side effects and extend the population receiving Adriamycin. As an example, in some patients an infusion of 60 mg/m² over 24 to 96 hr may eliminate nausea and vomiting without compromising therapeutic effect (Legha et al., 1982), and in patients with prohibitive cardiac history, a weekly low dose Adriamycin schedule of 10 mg/m² has been proposed to limit cardiotoxicity (Chlebowski et al., 1979b). The success with Adriamycin as a single agent has fostered many Adriamycin-based combinations regimens and new efforts to develop anthracycline analogues. Several analogues are being tested in Phase II trials in search of equal or improved efficacy with less toxicity than Adriamycin (Bonfante et al., 1985). At the present time, no analogue is close to being commercially available in the United States.

The low response rates and the short durations of remission that imply rapid development of drug resistance have led clinicians

Table 15–1. SINGLE AGENT ACTIVITY IN BREAST CANCER

	Number of Responders	Total	Per Cent
Alkylating Agents			
Cyclophosphamide	182	529	34
L-Phenylalanine mustard	20	86	23
Nitrogen mustard	32	92	35
Chlorambucil	11	54	20
Thio-tepa	48	162	30
Antimetabolites			
5-Fluorouracil	324	1263	26
Methotrexate	120	356	34
Arabinosyl cytosine	6	64	9
Hydroxyurea	2	16	12
Mitotic Inhibitors			
Vincristine	47	226	20
Vinblastine	19	95	20
Antitumor Antibiotics			
Adriamycin (doxorubicin hydrochloride)	67	193	35
Actinomycin D	5	44	11
Mitomycin C	23	60	38
Bleomycin	0	8	0
Mithramycin	5	32	16
Miscellaneous			
BCNU	16	76	21
CCNU	18	155	12
Methyl-CCNU (MeCCNU)	2	33	6
Hexamethylmelamine	11	39	28
Imidazole carboxamide	2	29	7
Procarbazine	1	21	5
6-Thioguanine	1	23	5

BCNU, Bischlorethylnitrosurea; CCNU, N-(2-chloroethyl)-N'-cyclohexyl-N-nitrosourea.
Modified from Carter, S. K.: Integration of chemotherapy into combination modality treatment of solid tumors. Cancer Treat. Rev., 3:141, 1976.

away from the use of single agent therapy in breast cancer. The availability of many active drugs has been instrumental in the development of combination chemotherapy treatment regimens with their potential additive or synergistic effects.

Combination Chemotherapy in Breast Cancer

With such a diversity of drugs that are active as single agents in advanced breast cancer, combinations of drugs with independent mechanisms of action and nonoverlapping toxicities are possible. The first investigator to apply these concepts in advanced breast cancer was Greenspan as early as 1963. He combined cytotoxic and hormonal agents in a five-drug regimen and reported a 50 per cent response rate (Greenspan, 1966).

The five drug combination reported by Cooper in 1969 has become the most famous and most extensively studied. The drugs consisted of cyclophosphamide, methotrexate, 5-FU, vincristine, and prednisone (CMFVP). Doses and schedules are listed in Table 15–2. The initial abstract reported a 90 per cent complete remission rate in 60 patients refractory to hormone therapy (Cooper, 1969). Several cooperative groups adopted the CMFVP regimen with modifications of dose or schedule or both. Between 1972 and 1974, 11 different studies were reported with response rates of 20 to 70 per cent. Although no study was able to reproduce Cooper's initial reported response of 90 per cent, combining drugs has greatly improved results over those achieved with single agents. Randomized trials comparing single drugs to various combinations confirmed the benefit of multidrug therapy (Table 15–3). Two cooperative groups have compared CMFVP given on a continuous versus intermittent schedule, with results favoring the continuous regimen (Smalley et al., 1973; Broder and Torney, 1974).

The CMFVP regimen was tested by clinical trials that removed drugs one at a time to see if response was affected. Of all the permutations studied, the combination of cyclophosphamide, methotrexate, and 5-FU (CMF) can reproducibly achieve a 50 per cent response rate, and this has become the standard combination chemotherapy treatment program for advanced breast cancer (Fisher et al., 1975a).

Because Adriamycin remains the most active drug against breast cancer, Adriamycin-based programs are also prevalent (Blum and Carter, 1974). Table 15–4 shows that Adriamycin alone and CMFVP are equally efficacious. The Adriamycin-treated patients achieved responses earlier and had a somewhat shorter duration of response.

Table 15–2. COMMON CYCLOPHOSPHAMIDE- AND ADRIAMYCIN-BASED CHEMOTHERAPY REGIMENS

Cyclophosphamide-Based Regimens	
CMFVP (Cooper, 1969)	
C = Cyclophosphamide	2 mg/kg/day orally
M = Methotrexate	0.7 mg/kg/wk intravenously × 8 wk
F = 5-Fluorouracil	12 mg/kg/day × 4, then 500 mg/wk intravenously
V = Vincristine	0.035 mg/kg/wk intravenously
P = Prednisone	0.75 mg/kg/day orally
CMF (DeLena et al., 1975)	
C = Cyclophosphamide	100 mg/m²/day orally on days 1–14
M = Methotrexate	30–40 mg/m² intravenously on days 1 and 8 every 28 days
F = 5-Fluorouracil	400–600 mg/m² intravenously on days 1 and 8 every 28 days
CFP (Broder and Tormey, 1974)	
C = Cyclophosphamide	150 mg/m²/day orally × 5
F = 5-Fluorouracil	300 mg/m² day intravenously × 5 q 6 wk
P = Prednisone	30 mg/day × 7
Adriamycin-Based Regimens	
FAC (Blumenschein et al., 1974)	
F = 5-Fluorouracil	500 mg/m² intravenously on days 1 and 8
A = Adriamycin (doxorubicin hydrochloride)	50 mg/m² intravenously on day 1 every 28 days
C = Cyclophosphamide	500 mg/m² intravenously on day 1
ACMF (Kennealey et al., 1978)	
A = Adriamycin	40 mg/m² on day 21
C = Cyclophosphamide	1000 mg/m² on day 1
M = Methotrexate	30 mg/m² on days 21, 28, and 35
F = 5-Fluorouracil	400–600 mg/m² on days 21, 28, and 35. Repeat cycle q 6 wk
AC (Salmon and Jones, 1974)	
A = Adriamycin	40 mg/m²
C = Cyclophosphamide	200 mg/m² on days 3 to 6. Repeat cycle q 21 days

Table 15–3. SINGLE AGENTS VERSUS COMBINATION CHEMOTHERAPY

Drugs	Number of Patients	Response (Per Cent)	Median Response (Months)	Reference
L-PAM (6 mg/m^2/day × 5) versus	91	21	3.3	Canellos et al. (1976)
CMF	93	53	6.3	
Cyclophosphamide versus	27	25	7.0	Mouridsen et al. (1977)
CMFVP	28	63	13.0	
Cyclophosphamide versus	49	55	5.5	Rubens et al. (1975)
CMF + Velban	50	62	7.0	

L-PAM, L-Phenylalanine mustard.

Many adriamycin-based combinations, such as 5-FU, Adriamycin, and cyclophosphamide (FAC), Adriamycin and cyclophosphamide (AC), and Adriamycin plus CMF (ACMF), have been used extensively. These regimens are listed in Table 15–2. No advantage in response rates appears to exist for a combination of more than three drugs because more myelosuppression requires reduced dosage (Muss et al., 1977). It is generally accepted that for standard community care in the absence of investigational protocols, CMF and FAC programs offer a 50 per cent chance of response.

One combination that has neither cyclophosphamide nor Adriamycin should be mentioned. Biochemical experiments suggest that the antitumor effects of methotrexate and 5-FU are enhanced by giving these agents in sequence. Theoretically, methotrexate changes the intracellular phosphorylation, causing 5-FU to accumulate intracellularly and ultimately increasing tumor kill. In clinical studies, patients receive methotrexate 200 mg/m^2 intravenously followed in 1 hr by 5-FU (600 mg/m^2 intravenously on days 1 and 8 every 28 days). Leucovorin rescue (10 mg/m^2 every 6 hr × 6) is begun orally 24 hr after each methotrexate dose. Gewirtz and Cadman (1981) reported a response in 11 of 17 patients so treated. Other investigators have seen similar responses with lower doses of methotrexate (100 mg/m^2) administered in the same sequence with 5-FU (Plotkin et al., 1985). This regimen is attractive because it can be used in patients no longer able to receive Adriamycin and in those with little bone marrow reserve. Further clinical trials are in progress to determine the optimal interval between methotrexate and 5-FU administration.

For the first time with Adriamycin-based combinations, complete remissions ranging from 10 to 25 per cent have been reported. Achieving a complete remission is a necessary first step in attempting cure. With various Adriamycin-based regimens, Legha and co-

Table 15–4. SINGLE AGENTS SEQUENTIALLY VERSUS COMBINATION CHEMOTHERAPY

	Number of Patients	Response (Per Cent)	Median Duration (Months)	Reference
5-FU, Cyclophosphamide, Vincristine versus	30	53	—	Baker et al. (1974)
CFV	46	43	6.0	
5-FU, Methotrexate, Cyclophosphamide Vincristine, Prednisone versus	34	18	4.0	Smalley et al. (1976)
CMFVP continuous versus	35	46	7.0	
CMFVP intermittent	33	27	8.5	
Adriamycin versus		55	5.0	Hoogstraten and George (1974)
CMFVP continuous versus	200 total	65	13.5	
CMFVP intermittent		59	9.0	SWOG
Adriamycin versus	20	45	—	Ahmann et al. (1975)
CFP	28	43	—	

5-FU, 5-Fluorouracil.

workers (1979) were able to achieve complete remission in 116 patients with advanced breast cancer. The median duration of remission was 17 months, but tumors tended to recur in sites of prior known disease while the patients were on maintenance therapy. It was concluded that even with complete disappearance of all disease clinically, only a small fraction of tumor cells were killed. Thus evolved studies designed with sequential noncross-resistant combinations.

Exposing tumor cells to alternating combinations of drugs would, theoretically, delay the development of resistant populations of cells and prolong survival. Two major studies have been done alternating Adriamycin-based regimens with cyclophosphamide-based drugs (Abeloff and Ettinger, 1977; Brambilla et al., 1978). Neither has shown improvements in response, complete response, duration of response, or survival over a fixed combination used until disease progression. These results may indicate early development of resistant tumor cells independent of drug exposure.

Chemotherapy Combined with Immunotherapy

Immunotherapy in advanced breast cancer has not been extensively studied and remains open for research development. In theory, various stimulants of the immune system are administered to generate antibodies against malignant cells. Levamisole, a synthetic anthelmintic agent, in vitro stimulates phagocytosis, lymphoblast transformation, and delayed hypersensitivity reactions without having any direct cytotoxic properties.

Two randomized clinical trials have reported longer survival in patients treated with chemotherapy plus levamisole compared with those who had chemotherapy alone (Klefstrom et al., 1981; Stephens et al., 1981). But small patient numbers in these trials and other numerous trials reporting no benefit or deleterious effects (Samal et al., 1984) leave the issue in doubt.

Bacille Calmette-Guérin (BCG) vaccine has been shown to have antitumor effects in animal models, but the mechanism of action has not been established. Sensitized lymphocytes may release cytotoxic lymphokines that affect tumor cells but not normal cells. The largest study showing survival benefit in Stage IV breast cancer treated with chemotherapy plus intradermal BCG has been criticized for not having randomized patients (Gutterman, 1976).

Future research in immunotherapy of breast cancer will involve investigating monoclonal antibodies with selective cytotoxicity for breast cancer cells (LeMaistre et al., 1984).

Combination Chemotherapy and Hormonal Therapy

Combination cytotoxic drugs improved response rates in breast cancer so dramatically that clinical studies are at present exploring the effects of adding hormonal maneuvers to cytotoxic combinations. The rationale is attractive, as mechanisms of action and toxicity are so varied. It has been observed that previous failure with hormone therapy does not compromise the subsequent results of cytotoxic therapy. Patients who progress with chemotherapy likewise also are eligible for hormonal manipulation if previous attempts have not been exhausted, again without compromising response.

Another observation that makes cytotoxic plus hormonal therapy attractive is the heterogeneity of cell populations in a tumor. Even with high positivity for estrogen receptors, a proportion of cells are refractory to hormonal therapy. Estrogen receptor negative tumors, even with the majority of cells lacking estrogen receptor, also contain some hormonally sensitive cells. Furthermore, it has been observed in the laboratory that human breast cancer cells can be inhibited by the antiestrogen compound tamoxifen and stimulated by estradiol administration (Lippman et al., 1976).

A model has been designed using the knowledge of tumor heterogeneity for ER and the pharmacologic ability to synchronize and stimulate ER plus cells followed by cell cycle–specific cytotoxic agents to kill rapidly dividing cells. Allegra and colleagues (1982) reported a Phase II trial of combination chemotherapy and hormonal therapy based on this model. Patients received tamoxifen to arrest the ER positive cells for 10 days, followed by conjugated estrogens (Premarin) to rescue and stimulate growth for four days. Then the cytotoxic drug methotrexate (200 mg/m^2 intravenously) was administered, followed in 1 hr by 5-FU (600 mg/m^2 intravenously). Leucovorin rescue was given 24 hr later at 10 mg/m^2 orally every 6 hr for six doses. The cycle is then repeated every 18 days. Both patients with ER positive and patients with ER negative tumors were treated.

The overall response rate was 72 per cent with a complete response rate of 56 per cent. Complete responses were seen in lung, visceral, and bone dominant metastases and responses were seen in both premenopausal and postmenopausal patients. Toxicity was minimal. The scientific lesson learned from this study may help in the transition from partial remission to complete remission to cure in advanced breast cancer (Allegra, 1983).

New Chemotherapeutic Agents in Breast Cancer

The search for more effective, less toxic drugs active in breast cancer continues. Because Adriamycin is the most active single agent, new anthracycline analogues are being synthesized and tested in clinical trials. As in the ongoing randomized study by Bonfante and colleagues (1975), several new drugs such as 4'epi-Adriamycin and 4-demethoxy-daunorubicin are compared to Adriamycin with respect to response, myelosuppression, and cardiotoxicity.

The most extensively tested anthracycline analogue, an anthraquinone, which is being processed to be released from investigational status by the Food and Drug Administration, is mitoxantrone (dihydroxyanthracenedione or DHAD). Several trials have confirmed its efficacy in advanced breast cancer with minimal toxicity (Coleman et al., 1984; Cornfleet et al., 1984). In a randomized crossover study of mitoxantrone versus Adriamycin, response rates, duration of response, and survival were equivalent. Quality of life assessment suggested less (nonhematologic) toxicity, such as alopecia, nausea, vomiting, and mucositis, as well as less cardiomyopathy (Henderson and Dukhart, 1984). These encouraging initial results led to substituting mitoxantrone for Adriamycin in established combination regimens (Bishop et al., 1984). Preliminary reports show equal response rates (50 per cent) but less alopecia and cardiotoxicity with mitoxantrone (Bennett et al., 1984). If this experience is universally confirmed, mitoxantrone will be an excellent addition to the growing list of agents active in breast cancer.

Prednimustine is another promising new oral agent that is active against breast cancer. The drug is an ester of chlorambucil and prednisolone, designed to use the steroid moiety as a carrier across the cell membrane to deliver the cytotoxic moiety in higher doses with fewer side-effects (Harrap et al., 1977). Activity in multiple hematogenous and solid tumors, especially those responsive to chlorambucil alone, has been observed in humans (Pommatau et al., 1977). Lober and colleagues (1983) reported a Phase III trial of prednimustine compared to chlorambucil and prednisolone given individually. The treatment resulted in a higher response rate and less pancytopenia in the prednimustine group (Lober et al., 1983). In the future, randomized trials will be designed to compare prednimustine with other alkalating agents active in breast cancer.

Toxicity

Chemotherapy affects every organ and tissue in the body to a varying degree. Because chemotherapy is aimed at rapidly dividing cells and cannot selectively distinguish malignant from normal cells, toxicity is expected. Familiarity with side-effects is necessary in planning treatment to maximize the therapeutic index.

Bone marrow is a common tissue affected by chemotherapy, requiring frequent monitoring of blood counts to adjust the dose and schedule of drug administration. Granulocytes, with a half-life of 6 hr, are usually affected first. If the absolute granulocyte count is suppressed to 1000 leukocytes mm^3, the patient is at risk for sepsis from endogenous organisms and must receive prophylactic broad-spectrum antibiotics for any febrile episodes. Recovery time is a function of agent, dose, rate of metabolism, and degree of myelosuppression. Platelets (half-life, 5 to 7 days) are usually the next cell line suppressed, but thrombocytopenia is rarely the dose-limiting factor. Severe anemia is not a significant factor because of the long half-life of red blood cells (120 days) and the ease of replacement (Hoagland, 1982).

Skin changes can range from minor hyperpigmentation with 5-FU and bleomycin, to total alopecia occurring predominantly with Adriamycin and high dose cyclophosphamide, to severe extravasation reactions produced by vesicants such as vincristine, Adriamycin, and mitomycin C. The radiation recall phenomenon is an exacerbation of normal skin reaction to radiation in tissues previously or concurrently exposed to Adriamycin or actinomycin C.

Cardiotoxicity, although not common, can be refractory, progressive, and fatal if it occurs. Adriamycin is the major offender. Acute electrocardiographic abnormalities can be demonstrated during and immediately after administration. Various arrhythmias and nonspecific ST-T wave changes are evident with monitoring and usually are reversible. Adriamycin also causes a cumulative, dose-dependent cardiomyopathy. The risk increases greatly after a total life-time dose of 550 mg/m^2, with other factors such as age, underlying heart disease, cyclophosphamide therapy, and prior mediastinal irradiation also contributing. Attempts to avoid this devastating complication include monitoring cardiac function with Muga scans or endomyocardial biopsies and research to develop analogues with similar efficacy and less cardiotoxicity (Von Hoff et al., 1982).

Pulmonary toxicity from chemotherapy is manifested as a dry cough and exertional dyspnea, which can progress to fatal pulmonary insufficiency. Classic interstitial fibrosis is found histologically. Bleomycin is the drug most often implicated. Risk factors include age, previous thoracic irradiation, and cumulative drug dose of 500 units. There is no known effective therapy except prevention. Pulmonary function tests may be useful to document early damage. Bischlorethylnitrosourea (BCNU) has been incriminated in pulmonary toxicity when doses exceed 1400 mg/m^2 (Ginsberg and Comis, 1982).

Awareness of potential hypersensitivity reactions is necessary for preparedness for emergencies if chemotherapy is administered in the outpatient setting. L-Asparaginase has been associated with a 1 per cent mortality rate from anaphylaxis. Bleomycin, even in doses of 1 unit, can produce a severe reaction with high fever, hypotension, and profound circulatory collapse. For unknown reasons, patients with lymphoma are at greater risk for such a bleomycin reaction. Cisplatin, Adriamycin, and cyclophosphamide have been reported to cause immediate and severe allergic reactions (Weiss, 1982).

Gastrointestinal side-effects are the most clinically significant to the patient. Nausea and vomiting, aside from being psychologically distressing, contribute to malnutrition and dehydration. Much clinical effort has been spent to develop more effective antiemetic regimens. Metochlorpropamide (Reglan), an effective antiemetic agent specifically for cisplatin-induced nausea, has improved patient tolerance. Other agents that are also strongly emetogenic include Adriamycin, cyclophosphamide, L-phenylalanine mustard (Alkeran), all commonly used in breast cancer therapy. Because of the rapid turnover of the cells lining the gastrointestinal tract, they are also subject to chemotherapy effects manifested clinically as mucositis and diarrhea (Mitchell and Schein, 1982).

The list of potential and newly reported toxicities of chemotherapy is growing as clinical use broadens. Some effects that physicians consider minor inconveniences may be of more consequence to the patient. Sex hormone and steroid administration with Cushing's syndrome or masculinization can be particularly distressing. Chemically induced menopause is often part of therapy. The most common complaints of women on adjuvant chemotherapy are weight gain and malaise, which can affect compliance. The risk of second malignancies after curative adjuvant chemotherapy remains an unknown factor and will only be resolved after many more years of observation. Some authors reported the benefits of chemotherapy to exceed the observed risk of leukemia after adjuvant chemotherapy (Rockette et al., 1985). The physician who administers chemotherapic agents must manage the minor as well as the potentially life-threatening toxicities (Perry and Yarbro, 1984).

Beyond understanding the importance of the therapeutic-toxic ratio, the clinician must also consider the goal of therapy. Adjuvant therapy is directed at improving disease-free survival and ultimately curing patients, with minimal acute and long-term toxicity. The psychosocial and economic impact of chemotherapy must be placed on the balance with physical toxicity.

Stage III Breast Cancer

Stage III breast cancer is locally advanced, either because of a large bulky primary tumor, or because extensive nodal involvement but without distant metastasis. This group of patients carries a poor prognosis.

It is clear that even radical surgery as a single treatment method cannot cure locally advanced breast cancer. Of 122 patients treated with radical mastectomy, 49 per cent had recurrence locally at 5 years and only 1 per cent were alive at 5 years free of disease (Haagensen and Stout, 1943). Radiation therapy as a single method seemed to improve local control but not survival (Baclesse, 1949). It was also learned that radiotherapy was more effective at local control when bulky tumor was excised and radiation was administered in doses greater than 6000 rad (Balawajder et al., 1983). With technical advances in radiotherapy allowing high doses delivered either by megavoltage external beam or interstitial implantation, local control improved to approximately 75 per cent recurrence-free at 5 years (Bruckman et al., 1979).

By the middle to late 1970s, adjuvant chemotherapy had been added to the armamentarium in an attempt to improve survival. Results are encouraging. Bruckman and coworkers (1979) reported a 4 year relapse-free survival rate of 51 per cent in patients receiving adjuvant chemotherapy, versus 29 per cent for controls.

These clinical data suggest that radiotherapy or surgery, or both, is necessary for local control but chemotherapy is necessary to control subclinical metastases probably present at the time of diagnosis, which, if left untreated, will eventually be manifested as advanced disease. However, combinations and schedules to optimize local control and survival are still being explored. DeLena and colleagues (1975) designed a randomized trial to compare mastectomy versus radiation as a local-regional method, with both groups receiving aggressive chemotherapy before and after. After 3 years, there was no difference in the two treatment groups in treatment failure, duration of response, or survival, but a 5 year update showed a significant survival advantage in the group who received surgery.

A theoretical argument can be made for preoperative chemotherapy in Stage III breast cancer. Micrometastases with accelerated growth rate may be enhanced in the perioperative period, and treatment of systemic disease is often delayed for up to 4 weeks by a mastectomy. Administering preoperative chemotherapy also may serve as an early, and simple, in vivo test of tumor chemosensitivity (Papaioannou, 1985). Some investigators have applied these theories by using induction chemotherapy followed by local radiation. If residual tumor mass is still present, debulking is accomplished by mastectomy. Chemotherapy then resumes. With this approach, Hu and coworkers (1985) reported 100 per cent local-regional control and 87 per cent relapse-free survival after 3 years. Hortobagyi and colleagues (1983) advocate an Adriamycin-based regimen (FAC) followed by local therapy (simple mastectomy or radiotherapy, or both) followed by a cyclophosphamide-based regimen (CMF) to complete 2 years of treatment. At five years, 40 per cent of patients remained free of disease.

As with advanced breast cancer, immunotherapy and hormonal therapy have been added to the treatment for Stage III breast cancer. Grohn and coworkers (1984) found the addition of immunotherapy very toxic when administered with surgery, radiotherapy, and chemotherapy. The concepts of synchronization and stimulation of ER positive cells using hormonal manipulation followed by cytotoxic drugs are also being applied. A similar schema of hormones and cytotoxic drugs described by Allegra and colleagues (1982) (see *Combination Chemotherapy and Hormonal Therapy* earlier in this chapter) is being used at the National Cancer Institute (Lippman et al., 1985). The induction chemotherapy includes even more aggressive cytotoxic agents (Adriamycin and cyclophosphamide) followed by radiation with or without surgery, and then 6 more months of chemotherapy. Early reports show therapy to be well tolerated. The complete response rate was 46 per cent with 10 complete responses confirmed pathologically. Excellent local palliation and encouraging systemic disease control were suggested.

In summary, the clinical emphasis for Stage III breast cancer patients is aggressive multimethod therapy usually with a sandwich approach of systemic-local and regional-systemic therapy. Because the ultimate measure of efficacy is the 10 to 20 year relapse-free survival, clinical trials are still too early to conclude that any approach is superior.

Stage II Breast Cancer

Stage II breast cancer (pathologically positive axillary nodes) has been the target of extensive clinical trials and controversy for the last 10 years. Prognosis is directly related to histologic involvement of axillary lymph nodes and can be further subdivided by extent of involvement, with a distinctly poorer prognosis associated with four or more positive nodes, regardless of the total number removed at dissection. After radical mastectomy, patients with histologically positive nodes have a 10 year survival of 25 to 48 per cent, as reported by major surgical investigators (Devita 1982). Survival for one to three positive nodes ranged from 34 to 63 per cent and from 16 to 27 per cent for four or more positive nodes. The goal of adjuvant therapy is to augment the effectiveness of surgery by killing any remaining breast cancer cells, which, if effective, should translate into an increased disease-free interval and potential cure.

Understanding the biologic behavior of cancer has come full circle since the 2nd century A.D. when Galen considered cancer a systemic disease caused by excess black bile and therefore not surgically approachable. This theory prevailed until the 18th century, when several revolutionary surgeons observed a seemingly orderly fashion of dissemination via the axillary glands, which, if excised early enough, may lead to cure. The era of radical surgery and en bloc dissection was solidified by Halsted, who reported cures in breast cancer patients treated with such methods (Halsted, 1907).

But laboratory studies suggested otherwise. In 1869, Ashworth observed circulating malignant cells in the blood. This hematogenous dissemination was confirmed and found to be markedly increased by manipulation or trauma of the primary tumor. Theoretically, effective antitumor drugs administered postsurgically would kill these cells and prevent dissemination. And, indeed, this was demonstrated in vitro by Martin (1959) with a mouse model. Thus evolved the current concepts of breast cancer as a systemic disease.

By the early 1960s, several trials began using a single alkylating agent triethylenethiophosphoramide (thiotepa) in the immediate postoperative period in women with resectable breast cancer. The rationale of adjuvant chemotherapy was to prevent implantation of hematogenously disseminated cells and eradicate subclinical metastasis. The cooperative group of the National Surgical Adjuvant Breast Project (NSABP) designed a prospective randomized trial of brief, low dose thiotepa versus placebo. At 10 years, a statistically significant survival benefit was seen in treated postmenopausal women with four or more positive nodes (Fisher, 1968). Another clinical trial initiated by Donegan and coworkers in 1963 extended surgical adjuvant thiotepa postoperatively for 1 year. The most recent update after a median of over 15 years follow-up showed significant survival benefit in patients with negative axillary nodes, but neutral or detrimental effect in patients with 1 to 3 positive nodes and four or more positive nodes, respectively (Donegan and Kardinal, 1985).

The European experience with intensive, postoperative chemotherapy given as a brief course compared with no therapy demonstrated benefit for the treated group. Nissen-Meyer and colleagues (1979) reported a multicenter randomized trial from Scandinavia in which women were treated with cyclophosphamide for 6 days after mastectomy. Although there was no stratification for nodal status, after 10 years' follow-up a small but significant reduction was seen in recurrence and death (Nissen-Meyer et al., 1978). One interesting piece of statistical data was that this benefit was lost if therapy was delayed more than 3 weeks postoperatively.

These early single agent trials are summarized in Table 15–5. Results were encouraging but skepticism remained owing to lack of stratification and variation in surgical, radiotherapeutic, or hormonal manipulations of patients studied.

In vitro studies are contributing new information regarding the biologic behavior of breast cancer that is being applied in clinical trials. For example, it was demonstrated that breast cancer cells are capable of metastasizing via the blood and lymphatics interchangeably even before they have amassed a size large enough for clinical detection. Instead of just killing breast cancer cells released by surgical manipulation, adjuvant therapy must also kill established but microscopic metastases within the body. But these micrometastasis are known to have a higher growth fraction, which should be more sensitive to cytotoxic therapy. Much has been learned about cell cycle kinetics and metabolism of malignant cells. Tumor cells replicate by four distinct phases of growth, and various cytotoxic drugs are active in different phases. By combining multiple drugs that are tumoricidal at different metabolic stages in replication, it is hoped that cell kill will be maximized and drug resistance overcome.

Subsequent clinical trials applied this better understanding of tumor biology and were well

Table 15–5. EARLY SINGLE AGENT TRIALS FOR SURGICAL ADJUVANT THERAPY

Study	Drug	Conclusion	Reference
NSABP (1958)	Thiotepa versus placebo	Premenopausal women with 4+ nodes benefited	Fisher (1975b)
Donegan (1966)	Thiotepa versus no therapy	Relapse-free survival advantage in node negative patients	Donegan (1974)
NSABP (1972)	L-PAM versus placebo	Premenopausal women 1–3+ nodes benefited	Fisher et al. (1980)
Nissen-Meyer (1965)	Cyclophosphamide versus no therapy	Longer overall survival in treated group at 12 years	Nissen-Meyer (1979)

NSABP, National Surgical Adjuvant Breast Project.
L-PAM, L-Phenylalanine mustard.

controlled, with greater patient stratification. The first major trial conducted by the NSABP, Protocol B-05, entered patients with Stage II breast cancer treated with radical or modified radical mastectomy and stratified by age and degree of nodal involvement. Patients received either L-phenylalanine mustard (L-PAM) for 5 days orally every 6 weeks for 2 years or placebo. Disease-free survival was significantly improved in the treated group, with greatest benefit for premenopausal women.

From this initial study, data were integrated into the design of another clinical trial, B-07. All parameters of eligibility and stratification were the same, but this study compared L-PAM alone to L-PAM plus 5-FU. At 5 years, there was a slight benefit for women treated with two drugs over those treated with one, but the most statistically significant improvement was in postmenopausal women with four or more positive nodes. These two NSABP trials and subsequent B-08 and B-09 protocols are summarized in Table 15-6.

In 1973, the Milan, Italy, Instituto Nationale Tumori began an adjuvant program for operable breast cancer. The first program was to test the ability of combination chemotherapy to affect micrometastases based on a known active drug combination for advanced disease, CMF (Bonadonna et al., 1976). Treated patients, after radical mastectomy, received CMF on days 1 and 8 of a 28 day cycle for 12 cycles. Annual analysis of relapse-free survival showed significant benefit for the treated group (64 per cent versus 48 per cent for controls) at 5 years (Rossi et al., 1980). Statistically, benefit was seen in premenopausal women with one to three positive nodes. Subsequent protocols comparing 12 cycles of therapy with six cycles showed equal efficacy (Tancini et al., 1979). Although a shorter length of treatment did not affect the survival advantage, reduction in dose did. When patients received less than 75 per cent of the optimal dose of drugs, significant reductions in relapse-free survival and overall survival were seen (Bonadonna et

Table 15–6. NSABP ADJUVANT CHEMOTHERAPY FOR OPERABLE BREAST CANCER

NSABP Protocol	Drugs	Relapse-Free Survival (Per Cent)	Conclusion	Reference
B-05	L-PAM versus Placebo	55 / 44	Benefit greatest in premenopausal women with 1–3+ nodes	Fisher et al. (1980)
B-07	L-PAM versus L-PAM + 5-FU	50 / 54	Benefit first seen in postmenopausal women with 4+ nodes	Fisher et al. (1977)
B-08	L-PAM + 5-FU versus L-PAM, 5-FU, MTX	74 / 70	No increased benefit 2 versus 3 drugs	Fisher et al. (1980)
B-09	L-PAM + 5-FU versus L-PAM + 5-FU + Tamoxifen	74.8 / 80.1	Superior relapse-free survival in women ≥ 50 years with any node + ER > 10 fmol/mg	Fisher et al. (1980)

NSABP, National Surgical Adjuvant Breast Project.
L-PAM, L-Phenylalanine mustard; 5-FU, 5-fluorouracil; MTX, methotrexate; ER, estrogen receptor.

al., 1979). Because many older, postmenopausal women required dose reduction for hematologic toxicity, this was postulated as a major factor in the failure of adjuvant CMF therapy in postmenopausal women.

Another cooperative group, the Southwest Oncology Group Study, compared CMFVP to L-PAM in the adjuvant setting. Not only was improved, relapse-free survival seen in the group treated with combination chemotherapy, but in addition, postmenopausal women benefited as well (Glucksberg et al., 1979).

The same concept of noncross-resistant combinations of drugs developed regarding advanced breast cancer has been applied in the adjuvant situation. Table 15–7 reviews the results of a study with CMFP for six cycles followed by AV for four cycles. This study could not demonstrate any benefit from what has been termed late intensification chemotherapy. The NSABP is now investigating intensification therapy as designed in the ongoing B-15 and B-16 protocols.

Adriamycin-based adjuvant regimens have been less popular owing to the lower therapeutic-toxic ratio. Investigators from M.D. Anderson Hospital, Houston, however, have studied FAC adjuvant chemotherapy and also showed improved survival in postmenopausal as well as premenopausal women (Buzdar et al., 1984).

Stage I Breast Cancer

Stage I (lymph node negative) breast cancer has such a high surgical cure rate that adjuvant therapy has not been investigated aggressively. Approximately 20 per cent of women with Stage I breast cancer will eventually develop disseminated disease and die, supporting the in vitro evidence that breast cancer can disseminate before it is detectable clinically. The chemotherapist has an obligation to those 20 per cent of patients to investigate adjuvant benefits. Tolerance for toxicity should be low as the potential benefit will be to a small number of patients.

The NSABP currently has two active protocols for Stage I breast cancer. One is designed for ER negative patients using low toxicity cytotoxic drugs. The other study, designed for ER positive women, is a randomized study of tamoxifen verses placebo. This is the initial step to determining if there is any role for adjuvant therapy for Stage I breast cancer. Referral for participation in these protocols is encouraged, and treatment of Stage I breast cancer outside of a protocol is discouraged.

Chemohormonal Adjuvant Therapy

Most major clinical trials have demonstrated benefit from adjuvant chemotherapy only for the subset of premenopausal women. Since the late 1970s, determination of estrogen receptor status has become routine, allowing further stratification of those patients who might benefit from adjuvant hormonal manipulation. The major drug studied is tamoxifen (Nolvadex), a synthetic nonsteroidal antiestrogen.

Table 15–7. CMF-BASED ADJUVANT CHEMOTHERAPY FOR OPERABLE BREAST CANCER

Drugs	Relapse-Free Survival (Per Cent)	Conclusion	Reference
CMF × 12 cycles versus no therapy	64 48	Benefit in women with 1–3+ nodes, premenopausal only	Bonadonna et al. (1976)
CMF × 12 cycles versus CMF × 6 cycles	46 54.8	No significant difference in 6 versus 12 cycles	Tancini et al. (1979)
CMFVP versus L-PAM	47 26	Premenopausal and postmenopausal benefits regardless of nodal status	Glucksberg et al. (1979)
CMFP × 6 cycles + AV × 4 cycles versus CMF	46.4 55	No significant benefit seen by late intensive chemotherapy	Bonadonna et al. (1985)

Table 15–8. ADJUVANT TRIALS STAGE II BREAST CANCER WITH TAMOXIFEN

Study Regimen	Relapse-Free Survival (Per Cent)	Overall Survival (Per Cent)	Conclusion	Reference
Mastectomy + radiotherapy versus	40	51	Subset of patients with 100 fmol/mg ER benefited from adjuvant tamoxifen	Mouridsen et al. (1985)
Mastectomy + Radiotherapy + Tamoxifen × 1 yr	44	51		
No therapy versus	42	77	No survival advantage in any treatment subset after 3 years	Taylor et al. (1984) (ECOG)
Full dose CMFP versus	42	74		
CMFP + Tamoxifen	55	73		
Prednisone and 5-fluorouracil (PF) versus	74		Superior relapse-free survival in women ≥50 years, any node +, ER ≥ 10 fmol/mg	Fisher et al. (1981)
PF + Tamoxifen (B-09)	80			
No treatment versus	79	88	Modest improvement in relapse-free survival premenopausal and postmenopausal women	Baum et al. (1983)
Tamoxifen	85	90		

Table 15–8 summarizes some large clinical trials and their conclusions regarding benefits seen with adjuvant tamoxifen. Uniformly, advantage in relapse-free survival was seen except in the Eastern Cooperative Oncology Group Study (ECOG), in which, after 3 years' follow-up, benefits became statistically insignificant (Taylor et al., 1985). These trials used standard tamoxifen doses of 20 to 30 mg daily for a duration of 1 to 2 years.

Because of the long natural history of breast cancer, which can relapse 10 to 20 years after primary resection, some investigators have recommended continuous prolonged therapy with tamoxifen for up to 4 years. Tamoxifen has been proved to be well tolerated and without excessive side-effects at constant blood levels for more than 4 years (Tormey and Jorday, 1984). The ongoing NSABP trials are incorporating these data into the design of B-14 and B-16 adjuvant trials in women who are estrogen receptor positive. It will be necessary to follow these trials for 5 to 10 years before the impact of adjuvant hormonal therapy on overall survival can be determined.

Summary on Adjuvant Therapy for Operable Breast Cancer

Despite extensive clinical studies and data generated from treating breast cancer in the adjuvant setting, questions are still unanswered. It has not been resolved if adjuvant therapy merely delays relapse or truly improves overall survival. The National Institute of Health Consensus Development Conference (1985) reviewed updated trials and published recommendations regarding adjuvant chemotherapy for breast cancer (U.S. Department of Health and Human Services, 1985). Recommendations for patients treated outside the context of a clinical trial by standard community care include the following:

1. Premenopausal women with positive axillary lymph nodes: combination drugs in optimal doses and schedules as described by efficacious major clinical trial.

2. Postmenopausal women with positive nodes who are ER positive: tamoxifen. Recommendations for ER negative women are still unclear, but tamoxifen is recommended in women with four or more positive nodes.

Routine use of adjuvant systemic chemotherapy in Stage I (lymph node negative) breast cancer is not advised. Physicians are strongly urged to participate in controlled clinical trials by enrolling eligible patients. Only in this manner can current standard community care be improved on and ultimately improve the prognosis for operable breast cancer.

REFERENCES

Abeloff, M. D., and Ettinger, D. S.: Treatment of metastatic breast cancer with Adriamycin-cyclophosphamide induction followed by alternating combination therapy. Cancer Treat. Rep., 61:1685, 1977.

Ahmann, D. L., Bisel, H. F., Edmonson, J. H., et al.: An analysis of a multiple-drug program in the treatment of patients with advanced breast cancer utilizing 5-fluorouracil, Cytoxan, prednisone with or without vincristine. Cancer, 36:1925, 1975.

Ahmann, D. L., Bisel, H. F., Eagan, R. T., et al.: Controlled evaluation of Adriamycin (NSC-123127) in patients with disseminated breast cancer. Cancer Chemother. Rep., 58:877, 1974.

Allegra, J. C.: Methotrexate and 5-fluorouracil following tamoxifen and Premarin in advanced breast cancer. Semin. Oncol., 10:23, 1983.

Allegra, J. C., Barlock, A., Juff, K. K., et al.: Changes in multiple or sequential estrogen receptor determinations in breast cancer. Cancer, 45:792, 1980.

Allegra, J. C., Woodcock, T. M., Richman, S. P., et al.: A phase II trial of tamoxifen, premarin, methotrexate and 5-fluorouracil in metastatic breast cancer. Breast Cancer Res. Treat., 2:93, 1982.

Anderson, D. E.: A genetic study of human breast cancer. JNCI, 48:1029, 1972.

Ashworth, T. R.: A case of cancer in which cells similar to those in the tumours were seen in the blood after death. Aust. Med. J., 14:146, 1869.

Baclesse, R.: Roentgen therapy as the sole method of treatment of cancer of the breast. AJR, 62:311, 1949.

Baker, L. H., Vaughn, C. B., Al-Sarref, M., et al.: Evaluation of combination vs. sequential cytotoxic chemotherapy in the treatment of advanced breast cancer. Cancer, 33:513, 1974.

Balawajder, I., Antich, P. P., and Boland, J.: An analysis of the role of radiotherapy alone and in combination with chemotherapy and surgery in the management of advanced breast carcinoma. Cancer, 51:574, 1983.

Baum, M., Brinkley, D. M., Dorsett, J. A., et al.: Controlled trial of tamoxifen as adjuvant agent in management of early breast cancer. Lancet, 1:257, 1983.

Beahrs, D. H., and Myers, M. H.: Manual for Staging of Cancer. Philadelphia, J.B. Lippincott, 1983, p. 127.

Bennett, J. M., Kremetz, E. T., Reisman, A., et al.: A randomized multicenter trial of cyclophosphamide, Novantrone, and 5-fluorouracil (CNF) versus cyclophosphamide, adriamycin, and 5-fluorouracil (CAF) in patients with metastatic breast cancer (Abstract). Proc. ASCO, 3:126, 1984.

Bishop, J., Hilcoat, B., Raghavan, D., et al.: Mitomycin C, Mitoxantrone in previously treated patients with advanced breast cancer (Abstract). Proc. ASCO, 3:116, 1984.

Blum, R. D., and Carter, S. K.: A new anticancer drug with significant clinical activity. Ann. Intern. Med., 80:249, 1974.

Blumenschein, G., Cardenas, J., Feireich, E., et al.: FAC chemotherapy for breast cancer. Proc. ASCO, 15:193, 1974.

Bonadonna, G., Brusamolino, E., Valagussa, P., et al.: Combination chemotherapy as an adjuvant treatment in operable breast cancer. N. Engl. J. Med., 294:405, 1976.

Bonadonna, G., Valagussa, P., Rossi, A., et al.: CMF adjuvant chemotherapy in operable breast cancer. In Jones, S. E., and Salmon, S. E. (Eds.): Adjuvant Therapy of Cancer II. New York, Grune & Stratton, 1979, p. 227.

Bonadonna, G., Valagussa, P., Rossi, A., et al.: Ten-year experience with CMF-based adjuvant chemotherapy in resectable breast cancer. Breast Cancer Res. Treat., 5:95, 1985.

Bonfante, V., Rossi, A., Brambilla, C., et al.: Comparative activity and toxicity of Adriamycin (ADM) and new anthracycline analogs in advanced breast cancer (Abstract). Proc. AACR 26:165, 1985.

Bourke, G. J.: The Epidemiology of Cancer. Philadelphia, Charles Press, 1983, p. 191.

Brambilla, C., Valagussa, P., and Bonadonna, G.: Sequential combination chemotherapy in advanced breast cancer. Cancer Chemother. Pharmacol., 1:35, 1978.

Broder, L. E., and Tormey, D. C.: Combination chemotherapy of carcinoma of the breast. Cancer Treat. Rev., 1:183, 1974.

Bruckman, J. E., Harris, J. R., Levene, M. B., et al.: Results of treating stage III carcinoma of the breast by primary radiation therapy. Cancer 43:985, 1979.

Buzdar, A. U., Smith, T. L., Blumenschein, G. R., et al.: Breast cancer adjuvant therapy trials of M.D. Anderson Hospital: Results of two studies. In Jones, S. E., and Salmon, S. E. (Eds.): Adjuvant Therapy of Cancer IV. Orlando, Fla., Grune & Stratton, 1984, p. 217.

Canellos, G. P., Pocock, S. J., Taylor, S. G., III, et al.: Combination chemotherapy for metastatic breast carcinoma. Prospective comparison of multiple drug therapy with L-phenylalanine mustard. Cancer, 38:1882, 1976.

Chang, J. C., and Wergowske, G.: Correlation of estrogen receptors and response to chemotherapy of cytoxan, methotrexate and 5-fluorouracil (CMF) in advanced breast cancer. Cancer, 48:2503, 1981.

Chlebowski, R. T., Irwin, L. E., Pugh, R. P., et al.: Survival of patients with metastatic breast cancer treated with either combination or sequential chemotherapy. Cancer Res., 39:4503, 1979a.

Chlebowski, R., Pugh, R., Paroly, W., et al.: Adriamycin on a weekly schedule: Clinically effective with low incidence of cardiotoxicity. Clin. Res., 27:53A, 1979b.

Coleman, R. E., Maisey, M. N., Knight, R. K., et al.: Mitoxantrone in advanced breast cancer—a phase II study with special attention to cardiotoxicity. Eur. J. Cancer Clin. Oncol., 20:771, 1984.

Cooper, R.: (Abstr) Proc. Am. AACR., 10:15, 1969.

Cornbleet, M. A., Stuart-Harris, R. C., Smith, I. E., et al.: Mitoxantrone for the treatment of advanced breast cancer: Single-agent therapy in previously untreated patients. Eur. J. Cancer Clin. Oncol. 20:1141, 1984.

DeLena, M., Brambilla, C., Morabito, A., et al.: Adriamycin plus vincristine compared to and combined with cyclophosphamide, methotrexate, and 5-fluorouracil for advanced breast cancer. Cancer 35:1108, 1975.

DeLena, M., Varini, M., and Zucali, R.: Multimodal treatment for locally advanced breast cancer. Cancer Clin. Trials, 4:229, 1981.

Devita, V. T., Hellman, S., and Rosenberg, S. A.: Cancer: Principles and Practice of Oncology. Philadelphia, J. B. Lippincott, 1982, p. 920.

Donegan, W. L.: Extended surgical adjuvant thiotepa for mammary carcinoma. Arch. Surg., 109:187, 1974.

Donegan, W. L., and Kardinal, C. G.: Long-term results of extended adjuvant thiotepa for operable breast cancer (Abstract). Proc. ASCO, 4:75, 1985.

Fisher, B., Ravdin, R. G., Ausman, R. K., et al.: Surgical adjuvant chemotherapy in cancer of the breast. Results of a decade of cooperative investigation. Ann. Surg., 168:337, 1968.

Fisher, B., Carbone, P. P., Economou, S. G., et al.: L-phenylalanine mustard (L-PAM) in the management of primary breast cancer: A report of early findings. N. Engl. J. Med., 292:117, 1975.

Fisher, B., Glass, A., Redmond, C., et al.: L-phenylalanine mustard (L-PAM) in the management of primary breast cancer: An update of earlier findings and a comparison with those utilizing L-PAM plus 5-fluorouracil (5-FU). Cancer, 39:2883, 1977.

Fisher, B., Redmond, C., Fisher, E. R., et al.: The contribution of recent NSABP clinical trials of primary breast cancer therapy to an understanding of tumor biology—an overview of findings. Cancer, 46:1009, 1980.

Fisher, B., Slack, N., Katrych, D., et al.: Ten-year follow up results of patients with carcinoma of the breast in a cooperative clinical trial evaluating surgical adjuvant chemotherapy. Surg. Gynecol. Obstet., 140:528, 1975b.

Fisher, B., Wolmark, N., Bauer, M., et al.: The accuracy of clinical nodal status in carcinoma of the breast. Surg. Gynecol. Obstet., 152:765, 1981.

Gewirtz, A. M., and Cadman, E.: Preliminary report on the efficacy of sequential methotrexate and 5-fluorouracil in advanced breast cancer. Cancer, 47:2552, 1981.

Ginsberg, S., and Comis, R. L.: The pulmonary toxicity of antineoplastic agents. Semin. Oncol., 9:34, 1982.

Glucksberg, H., Rivkin, S. E., and Rasmussen, S.: Adjuvant chemotherapy for stage II breast cancer: A comparison of CMFVP versus L-PAM. In Jones, S. E., and Salmon, S. E. (Eds.): Adjuvant Therapy of Cancer II. New York, Grune & Stratton, 1979, p. 261.

Greenspan, E. M.: Combination cytotoxic chemotherapy in advanced disseminated breast carcinoma. J. Mt. Sinai Hosp., 33:1, 1966.

Grohn, P., Heionen, E., Klefstrom, P., et al.: Adjuvant postoperative radiotherapy, chemotherapy, and immunotherapy in stage III breast cancer. Cancer, 54:670, 1984.

Gutterman, J. U., Mavligit, G. M., Hortobagyi, B. N., et al.: BCG immunotherapy of disseminated breast cancer and colorectal cancer. In Lamoreaux, G., Turcotte, R., and Portelance, V. (Eds.): BCG in Cancer Immunotherapy. New York, Grune & Stratton, 1976, pp 227–288.

Haagensen, C. D., and Stout, A. P.: Carcinoma of the breast: Criteria of operability. Ann. Surg., 118:859, 1943.

Hahnel, R., Woodings, T., and Vivian, A. B.: Prognostic value of estrogen-receptors in primary breast cancer. Cancer 44:671, 1979.

Halsted, W. S.: The results of radical operations for the cure of cancer of the breast. Ann. Surg., 46:1, 1907.

Harrap, K. R., Riches, P. G., Gilby, E. D., et al.: Studies on the toxicity and antitumor activity of prednimustine: A prednisolone ester of chlorambucil. Eur. J. Cancer, 13:873, 1977.

Henderson, I. C., and Dukhart, G.: A randomized trial comparing mitoxantrone with doxorubicin in patients with metastastic breast cancer (Abstract). Proc. ASCO, 3:120, 1984.

Hoagland, H. C.: Hematologic complications of chemotherapy. Sem. Oncol., 9:95, 1982.

Hoogstraten, B., and George, S.: Adriamycin and combination chemotherapy in breast cancer: A Southwest Oncology Group study. Proc. AACR, 15:70, 1974.

Hortobagyi, G. N., Blumenschein, G. R., Spanos, W., et al.: Multimodal treatment of locoregionally advanced breast cancer. Cancer, 51:763, 1983.

Hu, E., Stockdale, F. E., Carlson, R. W., et al.: Locally advanced breast cancer patients (T_3/T_4 or N_3) treated with a sandwich approach of chemotherapy, radiotherapy and chemotherapy. Proc. ASCO, 4:58, 1985.

Jensen, E. V., Block, G. E., Smith, S., et al.: Estrogen receptors and breast cancer response to adrenalectomy. Natl. Cancer Inst. Monogr., 34:55, 1971.

Jensen, E. V., DeSombre, E. R., and Jungblut, P. W.: Estrogen receptors in hormone-responsive tissues and tumors. In Wissler, R. W., Dae, T. L., and Wood, S., Jr.: Endogenous Factors Influencing Host-Tumor Balance. Chicago, University of Chicago Press, 1967, pp. 15–30.

Kennealey, G. T., Boston, B., Mitches, M. S., et al.: Combination chemotherapy for advanced breast cancer. Two regimens containing adriamycin. Cancer 42:27, 1978.

Kiang, D. T., and Kennedy, B. J.: Factors affecting estrogen receptors in breast cancer. Cancer, 40:1571, 1977.

Kiang, D. T., Grenning, D. H., Goldman, A. J., et al.: Estrogen receptors and responses to chemotherapy and hormonal therapy in advanced breast cancer. N. Engl. J. Med., 229:1330, 1978.

Klefstrom, P., Holsti, P., Grohn, P., et al.: Combination of levamisole immunotherapy with conventional treatments in breast cancer. In Terry, W. D., and Rosenberg, S. A. (Eds.): Immunotherapy of Human Cancer. New York, Elsevier, 1981.

Legha, S. S., Benjamin, R. S., Macray, B., et al.: Adriamycin therapy of continuous intravenous infusion in patients with metastatic breast cancer. Cancer, 49:1762, 1982.

Legha, S. S., Buzdar, A. U., Smith, T. L., et al.: Complete remissions in metastatic breast cancer treated with combination drug therapy. Ann. Intern. Med., 91:847, 1979.

LeMaistre, F., Edwards, D., Krolick, K., et al.: A monoclonal antibody–ricin. A chain conjugate with selective cytotoxicity for breast cancer cells (Abstract). Proc. ASCO, 3:57, 1984.

Lippman, M. E., Allegra, J. C., Thompson, E. B., et al.: The relationship between estrogen receptors and response rate to cytotoxic chemotherapy in metastatic breast cancer. N. Engl. J. Med., 298:1223, 1978.

Lippman, M., Bolan, G., and Huff, A. A.: The effects of estrogens and antiestrogens on hormone responsive human breast cancer in long-term tissue culture. Cancer Res., 36:4595, 1976.

Lippman, M., Sorace, R., Bagley, C., et al.: Effective systemic management of locally advanced breast cancer, (Abstract). Proc. ASCO, 4:65, 1985.

Lober, J., Mouridsen, H. T., Christiansen, I. E., et al.: A phase III trial comparing prednimustine (LEO 1031) to chlorambucil plus prednisolone in advanced breast cancer. Cancer, 52:1570, 1983.

Logan, W. P. D.: Cancer of the breast: No decline in mortality. WHO Chronicle, 29:462, 1975.

Martin, D. S.: An appraisal of chemotherapy as an adjuvant to surgery for cancer. Am. J. Surg., 97:685, 1959.

Meyers, J. S., Rao, B. R., Stevens, S. D., et al.: Low incidence of estrogen receptor in breast carcinomas with rapid rates of cellular replication. Cancer, 40:2290, 1977.

Mitchell, E. P., and Schein, P. S.: Gastrointestinal toxicity of chemotherapeutic agents. Sem. Oncol. 9:52, 1982.

Morgan, C. R., Jr., Schein, P. S., Wooley, P. V., et al.: Therapeutic use of tamoxifen in advanced breast cancer: Correlation with biochemical parameters. Cancer Treat. Rep., 60:1437, 1976.

Mouridsen, H. T., Brahm, T. P. M., and Rahbek, I.: Evaluation of single-drug versus multiple drug chemotherapy in the treatment of advanced breast cancer. Cancer Treat. Rep., 61:47, 1977.

Mouridsen, H. T., Rose, C., Thorpe, S. M., et al.: Adjuvant treatment with tamoxifen in postmenopausal patients with high risk breast cancer (Abstract). Proc. ASCO, 4:57, 1985.

Muss, H. B., White, D. R., Cooper, M. R., et al.: Combination chemotherapy in advanced breast cancer.

A randomized trial comparing a three- vs. five-drug program. Arch. Intern. Med., *137*:1711, 1977.

Nissen-Meyer, R., Kjellgren, K., Malmio, K., et al.: Surgical adjuvant chemotherapy: Results with one short course with cyclophosphamide after mastectomy for breast cancer. Cancer, *41*:2088, 1978.

Papaioannou, A. N.: Preoperative chemotherapy: Advantages and clinical application in Stage III breast cancer. Recent Results Cancer Res.,, *98*:67, 1985.

Perry, M. C., and Yarbro, J. W.: Toxicity of Chemotherapy. New York, Grune & Stratton, 1984.

Plotkin, D., Waugh, W., and Peng, J.: Sequential methotrexate-5-fluorouracil in advanced breast cancer (Abstract.) Proc. ASCO, *4*:62, 1985.

Pommatau, E., Mathé, G., Hoyat, M., et al.: A phase II clinical trial of prednimustine: Clinical screening cooperative group of E.O.R.T.C. Biomedicine, *27*:158, 1977.

Rockette, H., Bisher, B., Fisher, E., et al.: Leukemia following adjuvant chemotherapy for breast cancer (Abstract). Proc. ASCO, *4*:66, 1985.

Rossi, A., Bonadonna, G., Valagussa, P., et al.: CMF adjuvant program for breast cancer: Five-year results. Proc. AACR, *21*:404, 1980.

Rubens, R. D., Knight, R. K., and Kaywood, J. L.: Chemotherapy of advanced breast cancer: A controlled randomized trial of cyclophosphamide versus a 4 drug combination. Br. J. Cancer, *32*:730–1975.

Salmon, S., and Jones, S. Chemotherapy of advanced breast cancer with a combination of Adriamycin and cyclophosphamide. (Abstract.) Proc. AACR, *15*:90, 1974.

Samal, B. A., Foulkes, M. A., McDonald, B.: Levamisole probably shortens response and survival in CMFVP-maintained advanced breast cancer patients (Abstract). Proc. ASCO, *3*:126, 1984.

Silverberg, E.: Cancer statistics, 1985. CA, *35*:19, 1985.

Silverstrini, R., Daidone, M. G., and DiFronzo, G.: Relationship between proliferative activity and estrogen receptors in breast cancer. Cancer, *44*:665, 1979.

Silvestrini, R., Daidone, M. G., DiFronzo, G., et al.: Clinical importance of cell kinetics and its relation with conventional prognostic factors in breast cancer. Proc. ASCO, 1985.

Smalley, R. V., Murphy, S., Chan, Y. K., et al.: Comparison of two five drug regimes vs. sequential chemotherapy in metastatic breast carcinoma. Cancer Chemother. Rep., *57*:110, 1973.

Smalley, R. V., Murphy, S., Huguley, C. M., Jr. et al.: Combination vs. sequential 5 drug chemotherapy in metastatic cancer of the breast. Cancer Res., *36*:3911, 1976.

Stephens, E. J. W., Wood, H. F., and Mason, B.: The influence of levamisole on the survival of patients with end-stage mammary carcinoma treated with chemotherapy. *In* Terry, W. D., and Rosenberg, S. A. (Eds.): Immunotherapy of Human Cancer. New York, Elsevier, 1981.

Tancini, G., Bajetta, E., Marchini, S., et al.: Preliminary 3-year results of 12 versus 6 cycles of adjuvant CMF in premenopausal breast cancer. Cancer Clin. Trials 2:285, 1979.

Taylor, S. G., Kalish, L. A., Olson, J. E., et al.: Adjuvant CMFP versus CMFP plus tamoxifen versus observation alone in postmenopausal, node-positive breast cancer patients: three-year results of an Eastern Cooperative Oncology Group Study. J. Clin. Oncol., *3*:144, 1985.

Tormey, D. C.: Adriamycin in breast cancer: An overview of studies. Cancer Chemother. Rep., 6:319, 1975.

Tormey, D. C., and Jorday, V. C.: Long-term tamoxifen adjuvant therapy in node-positive breast cancer: a metabolic and pilot clinical study. Breast Cancer Res. Treat., *4*:297, 1984.

U.S. Department of Health and Human Services, Public Health Service, National Institutes of Health, Office of Medical Applications of Research: Adjuvant Chemotherapy for Breast Cancer. Vol. 5, no. 12, 1985.

Von Hoff, D. D., Rozencweig, M., and Piccart, M.: The cardiotoxicity of anticancer agents. Semin. Oncol., *9*:23, 1982.

Weiss, R. B.: Hypersensitivity reactions to cancer chemotherapy. Semin. Oncol., *9*:5, 1982.

Windhorst, D. (Ed.): Immunotherapy of Cancer: Present Status of Trials in Man. New York, Raven Press, 1978, p. 655.

Yap, H. Y., Blumenschein, G. R., Keating, M. J., et al.: Vinblastine given as continuous 5-day infusion in the treatment of refractory advanced breast carcinoma. Cancer Treat. Rep., *64*:277, 1980.

CHAPTER 16

RICKY J. BALLOU
MICHAEL T. TSENG
JOHN S. SPRATT

Chemosensitivity of Cultured Human Breast Cancer Cells

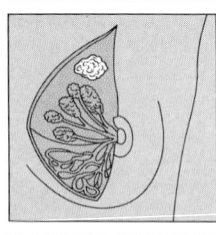

Breast cancer remains a major health problem in terms of both eventual mortality and the possibility of body disfigurement and morbidity from local-regional treatment. Despite improved surgical techniques, the recent introduction of powerful cytotoxic drugs, and the use of local or regional radiotherapy, the overall cure rate has not changed appreciably (Bonadonna and Valagussa, 1982). The prospect for long-term survival of patients with localized breast cancer is 70 per cent at best, and it is substantially poorer for those with regional nodal metastases (Fisher et al., 1972). Fewer than one half of all women who undergo surgical resection of a potentially curable breast lesion are so cured; conversely, a large proportion of these women will, over the next few years, be found to have metastatic disease (Valagussa et al., 1978). Although these patients have little likelihood of cure, excellent long-term control and palliation of the disease can be accomplished with currently available therapeutic techniques (e.g., chemotherapy, endocrine therapy, and radiotherapy). It has long been appreciated that mammary cancer is often hormone responsive. Procedures such as ovariectomy, adrenalectomy, and antihormonal therapy, have been attempted; the exact mechanisms of any therapeutic response are obscure, however, owing in part to the lack of appropriate experimental animal models. The advent of cell culturing technologies and highly defined cell lines has proved to be highly beneficial in the study of endocrine treatment of breast cancer.

The ability to observe cells and tissue in isolation became practical with the advancement of Harrison's "hanging drop" cover slip method in 1907. This led to the development of the culture flask with a unique side arm, enabling investigators to propagate and subculture their initial cell population (Carrel and Burrows, 1911). Carrel was one of the first investigators to recognize the value of cell culture as a means of investigating and possibly combating neoplastic diseases (Carrel and Burrows, 1911; Carrel, 1923). Wright and coworkers (1957) and DiPaolo and Dowd (1961) were pioneers in the use of a patient's own tumor tissue for in vitro prediction of drug sensitivity. This concept of heterogeneous treatment planning was fanned initially by favorable reports in advanced ovarian carcinomas (Limburg and Krahe, 1964). A plethora of in vitro methods has since been developed, including the clonogenic assay, introduced in the early 1970s by Park and colleagues (1971) and later expanded by Hamburger and Salmon (1977). All these procedures have a common end point, that of predicting the clinical responses of a patient to a specific treatment modality. In studying the in vitro growth characteristics of breast cancer biopsy tissue, breast atypias, normal breast tissue, breast fluid, and established breast tumor cell lines, Buehring and Williams (1976) noted that malignant breast cells generally divide more slowly than their nontransformed counterparts. Thymidine uptake of cultured human breast carcinoma also indicates a relatively low rate of proliferation compared with ovarian or lung carcinoma (Mattern et al., 1983). Successive passage of cells derived from normal tissue, solid tumors, or body fluid has yielded a large number of cell lines. These lines, in turn, have provided an opportunity to probe the structure and functional responses of cells in a controlled environment. In this chapter, breast cancer cells maintained in culture for biochemical characterization as well as for predictive tests will be examined.

Primary Cell Culture and Maintenance of Established Cell Lines

The commercial availability of synthetic cell culture media since the 1950s has made it possible for many researchers to develop in vitro screening procedures for the prediction of the response of an individual patient's tumor to specific anticancer drugs. These anticancer agents are often tested on cells grown in monolayer (anchorage-dependent) cultures, and the results most often are assessed according to (1) morphologic criteria (Wright et al., 1957; Lickiss et al., 1974; Homes and Little, 1974); (2) the degree of metabolic inhibition (DiPaolo and Dowd, 1961; Laszlo et al., 1958; Roper and Drewinko, 1976); or (3) inhibition of incorporation of radiolabeled precursors into DNA, RNA, and proteins (Livingston et al., 1974, 1980; Volm, 1981). Although the anchorage-dependent culture technique permits the growth of the heterogeneous cell population making up a solid tumor, the inability to discriminate those cells possessing unlimited capacity for division from those that are terminally differentiated has led to an increasing interest in the culturing of clones of cells in soft agar (Agrez et al., 1982; Alberts et al., 1982). In 1961, Till and McCulloch showed that a subpopulation composing less than 1 per cent of the spleen cells of normal mice can repopulate the hematopoietic tissues of lethally irradiated syngeneic recipients. Pike and Robinson (1970) reported the formation of cell colonies when cells were maintained in an anchorage-independent two-layer soft agar (clonogenic) system. This clonogenic cell growth technique was subsequently introduced into the in vitro chemosensitivity test system by Salmon and colleagues in 1978. The principal difference between this type of chemosensitivity test and others is the method of cell maintenance (Fig. 16–1).

Although the clonogenic assay permits determination of the reproductive potential of selected cell subpopulations within a given tumor, it is a laborious technique, plagued by extremely low plating efficiencies and relatively long incubation periods. In contrast, the anchorage-dependent cell cultures proliferate rapidly, preserve greater cellular heterogeneity of the tumors, and permit rapid and accurate quantification of results. Hence, in the authors' laboratory, the anchorage-dependent cell culture technique was chosen as the standard method, with the soft agar clonogenic assay being employed only when specimen size permitted the maintenance of parallel cultures. For experimentation, two established breast cancer cell lines (MCF-7 and MDA-MB-231), were obtained from the Mason Research Institute (Worcester, Mass.). These, along with

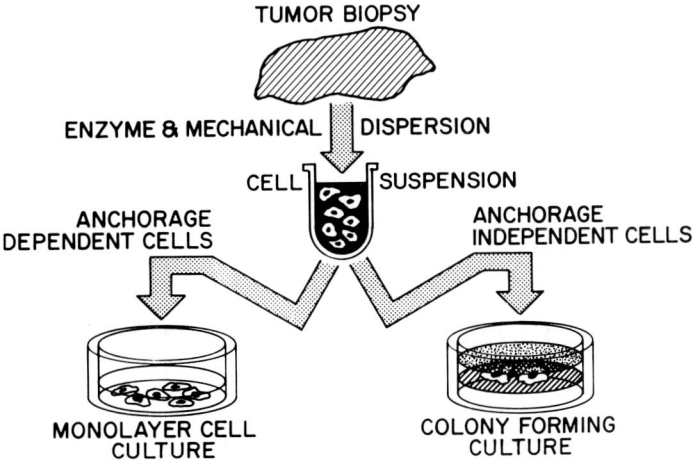

Figure 16–1. A comparison of two major cell culture techniques used for chemosensitivity testing. Anchorage-dependent cultures form a monolayer on the bottom of the dish. Anchorage-independent cultures form spherical colonies at the interphase of a semisolid and a solid agar basal layer.

several human breast biopsy specimens, were maintained in supplemented media (10 per cent fetal calf serum, 100 U/ml penicillin, 100 µg/ml streptomycin, 0.25 µg/ml fungizone, 1 µg/ml insulin, 2 µg/ml corticosterone, and 1 µg/ml prolactin) and were incubated at 37° C in a humidified 95 per cent air–5 per cent CO_2 atmosphere (Ballou et al., 1983).

Chemosensitivity of Breast Tissue in Primary Culture

The ability to determine the sensitivity of bacterial pathogens to antibiotics by in vitro methods has had a major impact on the selection of effective drug treatments for infectious diseases. As the selection of any agent(s) to be used in the treatment of advanced breast cancer currently is somewhat empirical, a similar benefit could be realized by the use of chemosensitivity screening procedures. The authors have tested biopsy samples from 13 randomly selected patients with advanced breast cancer against several agents currently used in clinical drug therapy. The number of agents tested was determined by the number of cultures that could be established from each sample. The authors' standard procedure measures the cell survival after 24 hr of continuous drug exposure. In one test, cells were plated in 24 well culture plates at a seeding density of 5×10^5 cells per well. Two or 3 days later, when the cells exhibited log phase growth, drug-containing media were introduced. As reported previously (Ballou et al., 1983; Safa et al., 1983), a single drug concentration (10^{-5}M) was selected, and triplicate wells were assigned to a given drug. A randomized table was used, with nontreated controls receiving only fresh media. Twenty-four hours later, the media were removed and the cultures were washed twice with minimum essential medium to remove any dead cells or cellular debris. Surviving cells were removed with the use of a trypsin-Versene mixture (M.A. Bioproducts, Walkersville, Mass.) and enumerated by use of an electronic cell counter. The percentage survival was normalized against the nontreated controls, which formed the basis for ranking drugs in order of cytotoxicity. The results were further analyzed by the Wilcoxan Rank Sum test (Wilcoxan and Wilcox, 1964) so that the statistical significance of differences could be determined. A tumor was designated as a responder to a drug if the drug showed a cytotoxic advantage at a p value of 0.05 or less. The results are summarized in Table 16–1. Of the 13 samples, only two exhibited a statistically significant response, whereas several showed a variable degree of growth inhibition. Two tumor samples, from patients EF and SR, were each significantly affected by two agents. However, in each case the agents were different. Tumor samples from patient EF were significantly sensitive at the 95 per cent confidence level to doxorubicin hydrochloride (Adriamycin) and at the 99 per cent confidence level to mitoxantrone, a new anticancer agent. Tumor samples from patient SR were significantly ($p < 0.05$) responsive to vinblastine and highly responsive ($p < 0.01$) to mitomycin C. Interestingly, SR tumor was not sensitive to Adriamycin, nor was EF tumor significantly sensitive to mitomycin C. The mean response of these tumors suggests a low level of sensitivity to these agents.

Results from other laboratories also indicate a limited response for those patients with advanced breast cancer. The experimental agent mitoxantrone had a pronounced effect on cell growth in the one biopsy sample in which it was used. The authors tested both mitoxantrone and another new agent, aclacinomycin-A, for their ability to inhibit cell growth in two human breast cancer cell lines. These results were compared to those of two established, clinically active agents, tamoxifen and Adriamycin. As can be seen in Table 16–2, both aclacinomycin-A and mitoxantrone were more effective than either tamoxifen or Adriamycin in inhibiting cell growth. It is important to emphasize that the MDA-MB-231 cell line is an estrogen receptor negative line, whereas the MCF-7 line is estrogen receptor positive. Therefore, tamoxifen would be expected to be more effective in the latter case. In addition to cell growth inhibition, DNA synthesis was also much more inhibited by aclacinomycin-A and mitoxantrone than it was by Adriamycin or tamoxifen. After 24 hours of treatment, mitoxantrone reduced DNA synthesis by 80 per cent or greater in the two cell lines, whereas aclacinomycin-A resulted in almost total inhibition of DNA synthesis. Adriamycin exhibited a 25 to 60 per cent inhibition in DNA synthesis, whereas tamoxifen produced a 15 to 30 per cent inhibition. Hence, in vitro

Table 16–1. CHEMOSENSITIVITY OF HUMAN BREAST CANCER CELLS IN PRIMARY CULTURE*

Drugs†	Initials of Patients													Mean Response
	EF	AL	LY	MF	MB	EG	JA	AH	SR	LC	MM	LH	CW	
Adriamycin	26.2‡	94.1	54.4	NT	63.0	74.1	100.2	NT	88.5	106.5	92.2	81.6	62.4	76.7 ± 23.7
Tamoxifen	37.8	41.2	NT	85.5	64.0	81.5	100.7	110.7	90.0	123.5	91.6	81.3	70.0	81.5 ± 25.6
5-Fluorouracil	92.8	104.5	94.6	100.4	58.0	NT	101.0	96.6	91.5	74.6	90.9	76.6	NT	86.5 ± 18.4
Mitomycin C	49.3	NT	53.9	NT	NT	NT	71.6	NT	70.7§	103.7	NT	NT	NT	69.8 ± 21.4
Methotrexate	50.1	NT	NT	NT	NT	97.6	101.1	96.2	97.8	NT	NT	NT	99.4	90.4 ± 19.8
Melphalan	88.9	NT	62.8	80.3	NT	NT	NT	NT	NT	NT	NT	NT	NT	77.3 ± 13.0
Vinblastine	NT	NT	NT	NT	NT	NT	NT	NT	80.4‡	89.5	NT	NT	NT	84.9 ± 6.4
Mitoxantrone	8.6§	NT	NT	NT	NT	NT	NT	NT	NT	NT	NT	NT	NT	—

*Chemosensitivity is defined as percentage of survival after 24 hr of continuous exposure to agents.
†All drugs were given at 10^{-5} M final concentration.
‡Chemosensitivity is significant at $p \leq 0.05$, Wilcoxan Rank Sum test.
§Chemosensitivity is significant at $p \leq 0.01$, Wilcoxan Rank Sum test.
NT, Not tested.

Table 16–2. CHEMOSENSITIVITY OF HUMAN BREAST CANCER CELL LINES*

Drugs†	Growth Inhibition		Thymidine Labeling	
	MCF-7	MDA-MB-231	MCF-7	MDA-MB-231
Tamoxifen	55.10	94.33	53.41	82.20
Adriamycin	51.33	55.01‡	60.30	76.66‡
Mitoxantrone	27.30‡§	41.66‡§	3.22‡	23.30‡§
Aclacinomycin-A	29.00‡§	32.33‡§	1.16‡	0.00‡§

*Chemosensitivity is defined as percentage of control values.
†All drugs were given at 10^{-5} M final concentration.
‡Drugs that are significantly more effective than tamoxifen.
§Drugs that are significantly more effective than Adriamycin.

chemosensitivity testing could eventually play a major role in improving the specificity of cancer chemotherapy by aiding in the selection of the agents to be used clinically. The tissue culture–chemosensitivity studies can also provide baseline data on new agents, which might be more effective than the agents currently approved for treatment.

Resistance

Human neoplasms are a heterogeneous group of proliferating cells whose behavior ranges from those that result in essentially no mortality (with proper treatment) to those that are fatal in a matter of months, regardless of treatment delivered. Tumors are heterogeneous not only in terms of histologic composition but also in terms of biochemically sensitive and resistant cell populations within the neoplastic cell mass. It has been documented that in human solid tumors as many as 15 to 30 per cent of the cells may initially be resistant to a single agent such as cis-platinum, and as many as 10 per cent may be resistant to a five drug combination (Ahmann, 1983). The average tumor that is detectable clinically consists of at least 10^9 cells (Speafica and Garattini, 1978). If this tumor was then treated with a chemical agent, an average of 150 to 300 million cells would be resistant to that agent, which would still be a substantial tumor burden. In addition to this initial drug resistance, cyclic treatment with single or combination drugs frequently resulted in the selection of variant mammalian cells that were resistant to specific drugs. Failure of chemotherapeutic treatment is a common and frustrating clinical problem, one not limited to breast cancer. This nonresponse is wide-ranging, and may extend to unrelated classes of drugs with which the patient has had no prior exposure. The appearance of chromosomes with expanded regions was reported by Biedler and Spengler (1976) in methotrexate-resistant Chinese hamster lung cell lines. Chromosomal abnormality in the unstable amplified state is manifested in paired extrachromosomal elements called double minute chromosome (Brown et al., 1983). The consequences of gene amplification are the overproduction of one or more proteins, which enable the cells to efflux antibiotics rapidly (George and Levy, 1983), and the ability to overcome selective pressures (Wahl et al., 1979; Beach and Palmiter, 1981; Rosann et al., 1982; Young et al., 1983; McConlogue, et al., 1984). Rath and coworkers (1984) examined the emergence of methotrexate-resistant 3TG cells and found that dehydrofolate reductase (DHFR)–amplified genes are generated by a selection process instead of being a distinct, preexisting subpopulation. Similar conclusions were reached when a transplantable murine breast tumor became resistant to melphalan, cis-platinum, and cyclophosphamide after repeated drug treatment (McMillan et al., 1985). Chromosomal abnormalities indicative of gene amplification have been observed in human Chinese hamster and mouse cell lines with high levels of acquired resistance to vincristine. One specific protein, V-19, is overproduced in these resistant cells (Schimke, 1984; Meyers et al., 1985). Regardless of whether resistant cells are preexisting or selected for, increased copies of DHFR genes have been observed clinically in leukemia (Cardman et al., 1984; Horns et al., 1984), in oat cell carcinoma of the lung (Curt et al., 1983), and in patients with ovarian adenocarcinoma (Trent et al., 1984) following treatment with methotrexate. It has been estimated that five-fold DHFR gene amplification may be sufficient to convey resistance to the conventional clinical dosage of methotrexate.

In addition to the perplexing problem of resistance is the phenomenon of "tumor evolution." Tumors from their inception are continually changing. As a tumor enlarges, alterations in the cell kinetics of the tumor population occur. The most probable explanation for this phenomenon is that as a tumor mass grows, the central core cells receive fewer and fewer nutrients; the tumor mass essentially outgrows its blood supply resulting in a progressive slowing down of cellular activity (Carter and Livingston, 1982). This concept is of clinical importance because most of the agents used to treat cancer have, as their mode of action, the ability to interfere with normal DNA synthesis. Therefore, cells that are mitotically active are more sensitive than are normal cells. In conjunction with this, smaller tumor foci have a greater proportion of their cells actively synthesizing DNA than larger tumor masses and, consequently, are more sensitive to chemotherapy (Griswold, 1975; Schabel, 1977; Skipper, 1978). A reduction of tumor mass by surgery, even when it is known that the procedure itself will be noncurative, has been shown to increase the rate of cell division in those cells remaining at the surgical margins. Consequently, these cells become more dangerous to the patient while at the same time becoming more sensitive to adjuvant chemotherapy. It must be remembered that chemosensitivity testing by in vitro methods uses tissue that has been removed radically from the tumor bulk. In addition, the tumor tissue actually used by the therapist may be from the primary tumor, whereas the chemotherapy may be applied to inhibit metastatic growths. Accordingly, these tumors may have different kinetic properties than did the original primary tumor. Therefore, from the oncologist's point of view, a tumor represents a "moving target"; in vitro screening must be viewed as a procedure in selecting the best antitumor agent for a particular patient at a specific time in the course of the disease.

Correlations Between Laboratory Tests and Clinical Responses

With the advent of cancer chemotherapy, it soon became apparent that drug sensitivity of a tumor could not be predicted from either clinical symptoms or from histologic examination. It has been recognized for many years that the experimental models previously used to study chemosensitivity (i.e., continuous cell lines and chemically induced tumors propagated in animals) have several limitations. As models for human cancer treatment, they provide data on the possible effects an agent may have on a specific type of tumor; however, they fail to give accurate data on the behavior of a specific individual's tumor to anticancer agents. Hence, a number of groups began to investigate the possibility of using the patient's own tumor material for in vitro drug sensitivity screening (Wright et al., 1957; DiPaolo and Dowd, 1961).

In 1964, Limburg and Krahe reported substantial improvements in the median survival time of patients with advanced ovarian carcinomas when treatment was based on results of in vitro testing. Over the next decade, disaggregated biopsy specimens containing either single cells, tissue explants, or tumor slices were used to establish suspension, monolayer, or organ cultures. Over the past 30 years, various procedures have been used to test the sensitivity of tumor cells to antitumor drugs prior to therapy. A number of methods use fresh tumor material and can be carried out in a few hours (Bickis et al., 1966; Kummer et al., 1970; Wüst and Matthes, 1970; Volm et al., 1979; Volm, 1981; Sondak et al., 1984). Others require culturing of the tumor cells for 1 to 3 days (Wright et al., 1957; Limburg and Krahe, 1964; Tanneberger and Bacigalupo, 1970; Homes and Little, 1974; Ebeling and Spitzbart, 1977; Dendy, 1980) or 2 to 4 weeks (Hamburger and Salmon, 1977; Salmon et al., 1978; Meyshens and Salmon, 1981; Von Huff et al., 1981), or even 2 to 3 months (Fujita et al., 1980; Shorthouse et al., 1980). However, none of the test methods described has acquired widespread clinical use, although certain procedures have achieved clinical importance in some medical and research centers (Limburg and Krahe, 1964; Salmon et al., 1978; Volm et al., 1979; Sondak et al., 1984).

The ideal chemosensitivity screening system must be simple, sensitive, specific, easily standardized, cheap, rapid, and flexible and must provide results that correlate with clinical data (Hamburger and Salmon, 1977). Therefore, the test of intermediate duration has a number of attractive features. For example, the degree of cytotoxicity can be measured by isotope uptake or cell counts, both techniques that can easily be automated. These techniques frequently use microtitration plates, which greatly simplifies the handling of 60 or 96 replicate cultures. With a large number of replicate cultures derived from a relatively small amount of tumor material, it is possible to produce dose-response curves over a large range of drug concentrations, to test a statistically acceptable number of replicates, and to test drug combinations in vitro.

From a clinical correlation standpoint, Dendy (1980) and Shorthouse and colleagues (1980) reported the results of drug sensitivity tests carried out under intermediate assay parameters that accurately predicated simulated clinical findings. When comparing cases in which the groups were correlated as to age distribution, clinical stage, and histologic grade, the patients treated according to results obtained from in vitro drug screening survived longer in the early months of treatment than did patients treated in accordance with empirical clinical selection. Therefore, there appears to be an interesting correlation between in vitro sensitivity measured by intermediate duration assays and clinical responses. Various investigators have shown that in vitro drug resistance correlates positively with in vivo resistance to drug treatment at or above the 90 per cent level, where in vitro sensitivity correlates with in vivo sensitivity in about 60 to 70 per cent of the cases (Homes and Little, 1974; Salmon et al., 1980; Sondak et al., 1984). Thus far, it seems reasonable to assume that in vitro drug screening serves mainly to eliminate ineffective agents from the treatment regimen.

Tissue-Specific Drug Delivery and Enhanced Therapeutic Efficacy

The idea of selective delivery of therapeutic agents by tissue-specific carriers was proposed in 1906 by Ehrlich. The selectivity of anticancer agents can be enhanced by binding the drug to carrier molecules. One recent development in the selective enhancement of drug uptake is the use of liposomes, which are closed, multilamellar, phospholipid spheres. They are internalized by endocytosis, and their contents are released by lysosomal action (Gregoriadis, 1978; Mayhew et al., 1978). This approach, however, does not yet qualify as a tumor-specific drug-delivery method. Although the existence of actual tumor-specific antigens remains an open question, the introduction of cell hybridization techniques for the production of monoclonal antibodies has stimulated a worldwide search for antibodies with specificity for cancer cells. In 1979, Herlyn and coworkers reported two monoclonal antibodies against human colorectal carcinoma. In 1982, Atkinson and associates reported on their use of monoclonal antibodies, generated by inoculating mice with colon cancer cell line SW-1116, to detect cancer in fixed, paraffin-embedded tissues by means of immunoperoxidase methods. The availability of a tumor-specific, monoclonal antibody would begin a new era in the immunochemotherapy of cancer. Investigators have already reported enhanced cytotoxicity by covalently linking antibodies to the toxins, to Adriamycin, and to melanotropin, to achieve the desirable local concentration and biologic response (Ruben and Dulbecco, 1974; Kitao and Hattori, 1977; Varga et al., 1977; Moolten et al., 1982).

Summary

In this chapter, the effect of several clinically used chemotherapeutic agents on established breast tumor cell lines and primary cultures of several breast cancers was assessed. As a rule, both the established cell lines and the primary cultures exhibit a high degree of drug resistance. Nevertheless, the use of cultured tumor biopsy specimens for in vitro chemosensitivity screening is advocated. The authors believe that until more effective drugs become available, it would be of benefit to incorporate the chemosensitivity test into the management strategy for patients with breast cancer. Hybridoma technology may make it possible to generate quantities of antibodies that specifically recognize various cancer tumors. If so, this covalent linking of drugs and antibodies may provide a method for the optimum delivery of drug in recurrent cancer. In view of this, the initial screening by some type of in vitro chemosensitivity tests can become even more important in the management of breast cancer.

REFERENCES

Agrez, M. V., Kovach, J. S., and Vert, R. W.: Human colorectal carcinoma: Patterns of sensitivity to chemotherapeutic agents in human stem cell assay. J. Surg. Oncol., 20:187, 1982.

Ahmann, F. R.: Chemotherapy and hormonal therapy of advanced breast cancer. In Feig, S. A., and McLelland, R. (Eds.): Breast Cancer—Current Diagnosis and

Treatment. New York, Masson Publishing, 1983, p. 533.
Alberts, D. S., Mackel, C., Pocelinko, R., et al.: Phase I clinical investigation of 9, 10-anthracenedicarboxaldehyde bis [(4,5-dihydro-1H-imidazol-2-yl)hydrazone] dihydrochloride with correlative *in vitro* human clonogenic assay. Cancer Res., *42*:1170, 1982.
Atkinson, B. F., Ernst, C. S., and Herlyn, M.: Gastrointestinal cancer-associated antigen in immunoperoxidase assay. Cancer Res., *42*:4820, 1982.
Ballou, R. J., Safa, A. R., and Tseng, M. T.: Response of 7,12-dimethylbenz-[a]anthracene-induced rat mammary tumors to tamoxifen, *in vitro*. Proc. Soc. Exp. Biol. Med., *173*:256, 1983.
Beach, L. R., and Palmiter, R. D.: Amplification of the methallothionein-I gene in cadmium-resistant mouse cells. Proc. Natl. Acad. Sci. USA, *78*:2110, 1981.
Bickis, I. J., Henderson, I. W., and Quastel, J. H.: Biochemical studies of human tumors. II. *In vitro* estimation of individual tumor sensitivity to anticancer agents. Cancer, *19*:103, 1966.
Biedler, J. L., and Spengler, B. A.: Metaphase chromosomes anomaly: Association with drug resistance and cell-specific products. Science, *191*:185, 1976.
Bonadonna, G., and Valagussa, P.: Adjuvant therapy of primary breast cancer. *In* Carter, S. K., Glatsten, E., and Livingston, R. B. (Eds.): Principles of Cancer Treatment. New York, McGraw-Hill, 1982, p. 315.
Brown, P. C., Johnston, R. N., and Schimke, R. T.: Approaches to the study of mechanisms of selecting gene amplification in cultured mammalian cells. *In* Gene Structure and Regulation in Development. New York, Alan R. Liss, 1983, p. 197.
Buehring, G. C., and Williams, R. P.: Growth rates of normal and abnormal human mammary epithelium in cell culture. Cancer Res., *36*:3742, 1976.
Cardman, M. D., Schornegal, J. H., Rivest, R. S., et al.: Resistance to methotrexate due to gene amplification in patients with acute leukemia. J. Clin. Oncol., *2*:16, 1984.
Carrel, A.: A method for physiological studies of tissues *in vitro*. J. Exp. Med., *38*:47, 1923.
Carrel, A., and Burrows, M. T.: Cultivation *in vitro* of malignant tumors. J. Exp. Med., *13*:571, 1911.
Carter, S. K., and Livingston, R.: Principles of cancer chemotherapy. *In* Carter, S. K., Glatstein, E., and Livingston, R. B. (Eds.): Principles of Cancer Treatment. New York, McGraw-Hill, 1982, p. 95.
Curt, G. A., Carney, D. M., Cowen, K. H., et al.: Unstable methotrexate resistance in human small-cell carcinoma associated with double minute chromosomes. N. Engl. J. Med., *308*:199, 1983.
Dendy, P. P.: The use of *in vitro* methods to predict tumor response to chemotherapy. Br. J. Cancer, *41* (Suppl. IV):195, 1980.
DiPaolo, J. A., and Dowd, J. E.: Evaluation of inhibition of human tumor tissue by cancer chemotherapeutic drugs with an *in vitro* test. JNCI, *27*:807, 1961.
Ebeling, K., and Spitzbart, H.: Zur Erfassung zytostatischer Effekte an Zellkulturen in vitro und deren gegenwärtige Bedeutung für eine individualisierte Tumorchemotherapie der fortgeschrittenen Ovarialkarzinoms. Zentralbl. Gynäekol., *99*:1041, 1977.
Ehrlich, P.: Collected Studies on Immunity. Vol. II. New York, John Wiley and Sons, 1906, p. 442.
Fisher, B., Saffer, E. A., and Fisher, E. R.: Studies concerning the regional lymph node in cancer. III. Response of regional lymph node cells from breast and colon cancer patients to PHA stimulation. Cancer, *30*:1202, 1972.
Fujita, M., Hayata, S., and Taguchi, T.: Relation of chemotherapy on human cancer xenografts in nude mice to clinical response in donor patients. J. Surg. Oncol., *15*:211, 1980.
George, A. M., and Levy, S. B.: Amplifiable resistance to tetracycline, chloramphenicol, and other antibiotics in *Escherichia coli:* Involvement of a nonplasmid-determined efflux of tetracyclines. J. Bacteriol., *155*:531, 1983.
Gregoriadis, G.: Liposomes in therapeutic and preventive medicine: The development of the drug carrier concept. Ann. N.Y. Acad. Sci., *308*:343, 1978.
Griswold, D. S.: The potential for murine tumor models in surgical adjuvant chemotherapy. Cancer Chemother. Rep., *5*:187, 1975.
Hamburger, A. W., and Salmon, E.: Primary bioassay of human tumor stem cells. Science, *197*:461, 1977.
Harrison, R. G.: Observations on the living developing nerve fiber. Proc. Soc. Exp. Biol. Med., *4*:140, 1907.
Herlyn, M., Steplexsi, Z., Herlyn, D., et al.: Colorectal carcinoma-specific antigen: Detection by means of monoclonal antibodies. Proc. Natl. Acad. Sci. USA, *76*:1438, 1979.
Homes, H. L., and Little, J. M.: Tissue culture microtest for predicting response of human cancer to chemotherapy. Lancet, *2*:985, 1974.
Horns, R. C., Dower, W. J., and Schimke, R. T.: Gene amplification in a leukemic patient treated with methotrexate. J. Clin. Oncol., *2*:1, 1984.
Kitao, T., and Hattori, K.: Concanavalin A as a carrier of daunomycin. Nature, *265*:81, 1977.
Kummer, H., Muhlenen, A., and Laissue, J.: Survival of labelled and non-labelled platelets in the lethally irradiated dog; an evaluation of the 51-chromate method. Helv. Med. Acta, *35*:226, 1970.
Laszlo, J., Stengle, J., Wright, K., et al.: Effects of chemotherapeutic agents on metabolism of human acute leukemia cells *in vitro*. Proc. Soc. Exp. Biol. Med., *97*:127, 1958.
Lickiss, J. N., Cane, K. A., and Baikie, A. G.: *In vitro* drug selection in antineoplastic chemotherapy. Eur. J. Cancer, *10*:809, 1974.
Limburg, H., and Krahe, M.: Die Züchtung von menschlichem Krebsgewebe in der Gewebekultur und seine Sensibilitätstestung gegen neuere Zytostatika. Deutsch. Med. Wschr., *89*:1938, 1964.
Livingston, R. B., Ambus, U., George, S. L., et al.: *In vitro* determination of thymidine-[^{3}H] labeling index in human solid tumors. Cancer Res., *34*:1376, 1974.
Livingston, R. B., Titus, G. A., and Heilbrum, L. H.: *In vitro* effects on DNA synthesis as a prediction of biologic effect from chemotherapy. Cancer Res., *40*:2209, 1980.
Mattern, J., Kaufmann, M., and Volm, M.: Short term assay using radioactive nucleic acid precursors. *In* Dendy, P., and Hill, B. (Eds.): Human Tumor Drug Sensitivity Testing *In Vitro*. New York, Academic Press, 1983, p. 57.
Mayhew, E., Papahadjopoulus, D., Rustum, T. M., et al.: Use of liposomes for the enhancement of the cytotoxic effect of cytosine-arabinoside. Ann. N.Y. Acad. Sci., *308*:371, 1978.
McConlogue, L., Gupta, A., Wu, M., et al.: Molecular cloning and expression of the mouse ornithine decarboxylase gene. Proc. Natl. Acad. Sci. USA, *81*:540, 1984.
McMillan, T. J., Stephens, T. C., and Steel, G. G.: Development of drug resistance in murine mammary tumors. Br. J. Cancer, *52*:823, 1985.
Meyers, M. B., Spengler, A., Chang, T. D., et al.: Gene amplification associated cytogenetic aberrations and

protein changes in vincristine resistant chinese hamster, mouse, and human cells. J. Cell Biol., *100*:588, 1985.

Meyshens, F. L., and Salmon, S. E.: Modulation of clonogenic human melanoma cells by follicle-stimulating hormone, melatonin, and nerve growth factor. Br. J. Cancer, *43*:111, 1981.

Moolten, F. L., Schreiber, B. M., and Zajdel, S. H.: Antibodies conjugated to protein cytotoxins as specific antitumor agents. Immunol. Rev., *62*:47, 1982.

Park, C. H., Bergsagel, D. E., and McCulloch, E. A.: Mouse myeloma tumor stem cells: A primary culture assay. JNCI, *46*:411, 1971.

Pike, B. R., and Robinson, W. A.: Human bone marrow colony growth in agar-gel. J. Cell. Physiol., *76*:77, 1970.

Rath, H., Tisty, T., and Schimke, R. T.: Rapid emergence of methotrexate resistance in cultured mouse cells. Cancer Res., *44*:3303, 1984.

Roper, P. R., and Drewinko, B.: Comparison of in vitro methods to determine drug induced cell lethality. Cancer Res., *36*:2182, 1976.

Rossana, E., Rao, L. G., and Johnson, L. F.: Thymidine synthesis over-production in 5-fluorodeoxyuridine-resistant mouse fibroblasts. Mol. Cell. Biol., *2*:1118, 1982.

Ruben, R. C., and Dulbecco, R.: Augmentation of cytotoxic drug action by antibodies directed at cell surfaces. Nature, *248*:81, 1974.

Safa, A. R., Tseng, M. T., and Ballou, R. J.: Sequential study of the influence of Adriamycin on cell proliferation and ultrastructure of cultured mammary tumor cells. Proc. Soc. Exp. Biol. Med., *174*:276, 1983.

Salmon, S. E., Alberts, D. S., Meyshens, F. L., et al.: Clinical correlations of *in vitro* drug sensitivity. In Salmon, S. E., (Ed.): Cloning of Human Tumor Stem Cells. New York, Alan R. Liss, 1980, p. 223.

Salmon, S. E., Hamburger, A. W., Soehnlen, B., et al.: Quantitation of different sensitivity of human tumor stem cells to anticancer drugs. N. Engl. J. Med., *298*:1321, 1978.

Schabel, F.: Surgical adjuvant chemotherapy of metastatic murine tumors. Cancer, *40*:558, 1977.

Schimke, R. T.: Gene amplification, drug resistance and cancer. Cancer Res., *44*:1735, 1984.

Shorthouse, A. J., Smyth, J. F., Steel, G. G., et al.: The human tumor xenograft: A valid model in experimental chemotherapy? Br. J. Surg., *67*:715, 1980.

Skipper, H. E.: Adjuvant chemotherapy. Cancer, *41*:936, 1978.

Sondak, V. K., Berelsen, C. A., Tanigawa, N., et al.: Clinical correlation with chemosensitivities measured in a rapid thymidine incorporation assay. Cancer Res., *44*:1725, 1984.

Speafica, F., and Garattini, S.: Chemotherapy of experimental metastasis. In Baldwin, R. W. (Ed.): Secondary Spread of Cancer. London, Academic Press, 1978, p. 101.

Tanneberger, S., and Bacigalupo, G.: Einige Erfahrungen mit individuellen zytostatischen Behandlung maligner Tumoren nach prätherapeutischer Zytostatika-Sensibilitätsprüfung in vitro. Arch. Geschwulstforsch. *35*:44, 1970.

Till, J. E., and McCulloch, E. A.: A direct measurement of the radiation sensitivity of normal mouse bone marrow cells. Radiation Res., *14*:213, 1961.

Trent, J. M., Buick, R. M., Olson, S., et al.: Cytologic support for gene amplification in methotrexate-resistant cells obtained from a patient with ovarian adenocarcinoma. J. Clin. Oncol., *2*:8, 1984.

Valagussa, P., Bonadonna, G., and Veronesi, U.: Patterns of relapse and survival following radical mastectomy. Analysis of 716 consecutive patients. Cancer, *41*:1170, 1978.

Varga, J. M., Asto, N., Lande, S., et al.: Melanotropin-daunomycin conjugate shows receptor-mediated cytotoxicity in cultured murine melanoma cells. Nature, *267*:56, 1977.

Volm, M.: *In vitro* short term test to determine the resistance of human tumors to chemotherapy. Cancer, *48*:2127, 1981.

Volm, M., Wayss, K., Kaufmann, M., et al.: Pretherapeutic detection of tumor resistance and the results of tumor chemotherapy. Eur. J. Cancer, *15*:983, 1979.

Von Hoff, D. D., Casper, J., Bradley, E., et al.: Association between human tumor colony-forming assay results and response of an individual patient's tumor to chemotherapy. Am. J. Med., *70*:1027, 1981.

Wahl, G. M., Padgett, R. A., and Stark, G. R.: Gene amplification causes overproduction of the first three enzymes of UMP synthesis in N-(phosphoacetyl-1-aspartate) resistant hamster cells. J. Biol. Chem., *254*:8679, 1979.

Wilcoxan, F., and Wilcox, R. A.: Methods for comparing more than two treatments. In Wilcoxan, F. (Ed.): Some Rapid Approximation Statistical Procedures. Lederle Laboratories, Pearl River, N.Y., 1964, p. 9.

Wright, J. C., Cobb, J. P., Gumport, S. L., et al.: Investigation of the relation between clinical and tissue culture response to chemotherapeutic agents on human cancer. N. Engl. J. Med., *257*:1207, 1957.

Wüst, G. P., and Matthes, K. J.: In vitro-Messung des Einbes von ^{3}H-Thymidin in Jensen Sarkom unter Cytostaticaeinwirkung mit Hilfe der Flüssigkeits-Szintillations-Spektrometrie. Z. Krebsforsch., *73*:204, 1970.

Young, A. P., and Ringold, G. M.: Mouse 3GT cells that overproduce glutamine synthetase. J. Biol. Chem., *258*:1126, 1983.

CHAPTER 17

CARL G. KARDINAL

Endocrine Therapy of Breast Cancer

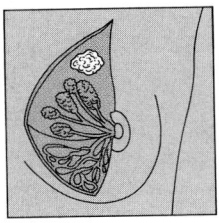

A quantum increase in the understanding of the endocrinology of breast cancer has occurred; as a result, revolutionary changes have taken place in endocrine therapy in recent years. In the previous edition of this book glimpses of these changes were noted, such as quantitative estrogen receptors and the use of antiestrogens, but the role of receptors in prognosis and the use of tamoxifen in the adjuvant setting had not yet been recognized. Luteinizing hormone releasing hormone (LHRH) agonists had not yet been introduced. The central themes were the classic issues of estrogens versus androgens and additive versus ablative therapy—issues that now seem to be of historic interest only.

During the 1970s, the trend was definitely shifting away from endocrine therapy for advanced breast cancer. Endocrine therapy was unreliable, producing only a 25 to 30 per cent objective response rate and requiring up to 6 to 8 weeks for the response to occur. Combination chemotherapy, on the other hand, induced objective responses in 60 to 70 per cent of unselected cases, and the onset of action was comparatively rapid. It seemed that during the 1980s chemotherapy might even replace hormonal therapy for the treatment of advanced breast cancer. However, the advances in chemotherapy that occurred during the 1970s have plateaued during the 1980s. Endocrine therapy, on the other hand, has advanced exponentially. These advances have required a reassessment of the role of endocrine therapy in the treatment of breast cancer as well as a reevaluation of the physician's approach to the patient. It seems that a second golden age of hormonal therapy is taking place, one based on an improved understanding of breast cancer biology.

The Endocrine Basis of Therapy

The normal development and function of the mammary gland depend on the coordinated action of several hormones: prolactin, estrogen, progesterone, adrenal corticosteroids, insulin, growth hormone, and thyroid hormone (Frantz and Wilson, 1985) (Fig. 17–1). Ductal growth is promoted by estrogen. Lobuloalveolar development is promoted by prolactin and progesterone; lactation is fostered by prolactin. Far and away the two most important hormones involved in mammary physiology, and presumably in mammary pathology, are estrogen and prolactin (Calandra et al., 1984).

ESTROGEN

Estrogen is a highly potent mammary mitogen. Currently all forms of endocrine manipulation for the treatment of breast cancer are directed toward inhibiting, ablating, or otherwise interfering with estrogen activity. However, in the stimulation of breast development, estrogen is ineffective by itself in the absence of the anterior pituitary hormones (Lyons et al., 1958). Estrogen increases growth hormone secretion, and together they promote ductal development (Frantz and Rabkin, 1965). Estrogen appears to inhibit prolactin and acts to regulate prolactin receptors in breast tissue (Frantz and Wilson, 1985).

Estrogen is the major stimulus for the growth of hormone-dependent breast cancer (Santen, 1982). The ovaries and the placenta are the principal sites of estrogen synthesis. However, estrogen is synthesized in multiple other areas, such as the adrenal gland, adipose tissue, and mammary tumors themselves (Miller et al., 1982; Siiteri, 1982). Estrogens

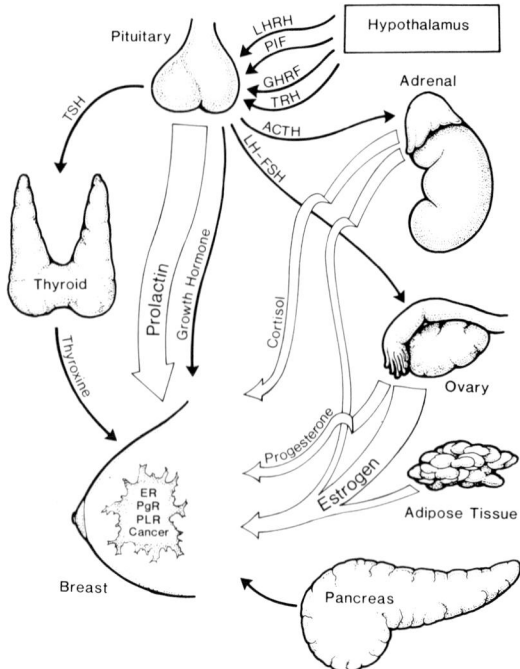

Figure 17–1. The endocrine basis of breast cancer therapy. Estrogen and prolactin are the dominant mitogens to normal breast tissue. However, the role of prolactin in human breast cancer is not yet established. Ductal growth is promoted by estrogen in the presence of growth hormone; lobular development is promoted by prolactin and progesterone. Estrogen is synthesized not only in the ovary but also in adrenal and adipose tissue. The roles of cortisol, thyroxine, and insulin are permissive rather than regulatory. LHRH, Luteinizing hormone releasing hormone; PIF, prolactin inhibitory factor; GHRF, growth hormone releasing factor; TRH, thyrotropin releasing hormone; ACTH, adrenocorticotropic hormone; LH, luteinizing hormone; FSH, follicle stimulating hormone; TSH, thyroid stimulating hormone; ER, estrogen receptor; PgR, progesterone receptor; PLR, prolactin receptor.

are synthesized by the aromatization of androgens via the enzyme aromatase (Fig. 17–2). Aromatase is the rate-limiting step in estrogen production. Consequently, there has been a concentrated effort to synthesize pharmacologic aromatase inhibitors as potential therapeutic agents for hormonally sensitive breast cancer. As already indicated, aromatase is not restricted to classic endocrine tissues, such as the ovary and the adrenal gland, but is also present in adipose tissue and the hypothalamus, and, in minor amounts, in muscle, fibroblasts, and even cancer tissue (Lipton et al., 1987). Estradiol is believed to stimulate breast growth (mitogenesis) by binding to cytoplasmic receptor, which then translocates to the cell nucleus, where the complex stimulates increase in RNA polymerase activity. As a result, RNA concentration and estrogen-induced protein levels increase, and the depleted cytoplasmic ER is resynthesized (Jordan et al., 1980).

PROLACTIN

Next to estrogen, prolactin is the most important hormone involved in breast development and function. Like estrogen, prolactin is a potent mitogen to breast tissue (Shiu and Friesen, 1980). In the absence of prolactin and growth hormone, estrogen alone is ineffective in inducing ductal development or other mammary growth. Conversely, prolactin requires estrogen as a stimulator of epithelial cell proliferation. As mentioned previously, along with progesterone, prolactin fosters lobuloalveolar development. Prolactin receptors are present in human mammary tissue and increase during pregnancy and lactation (Dhadly and Walker, 1983). High affinity receptors for prolactin have also been demonstrated in human breast cancer (Peyrat et al., 1984). Considering the known effect of prolactin on cell multiplication, this hormone could have a role in the development of breast tumors in humans. The prolactin analogues buserelin and pergolide do have direct growth inhibiting effects on human breast cancer cells in tissue culture (Wiznitzer and Benz, 1984). The potential clinical usefulness of buserelin will be discussed in the section later in this chapter. To date, however, prolactin has not been confirmed to have stimulating activity on human breast cancer.

OTHER HORMONES

The other hormones involved in the physiology of normal breast development and function all interact with estrogen or prolactin or both. *Progesterone* has no effect unless there is concomitant or preceding estrogen stimulation. Under these conditions, progesterone interacts with prolactin to promote lobuloalveolar development (Freeman and Topper, 1978). Growth hormone appears to synergize with prolactin to promote ductal development (Frantz and Wilson, 1985). Insulin and glucocorticoids appear to be necessary for most phases of breast growth and secretion but probably exert a permissive rather than a regulatory role (Shyamala, 1973; Topper and Oka, 1974).

Thyroid hormone does not appear to be essential for breast development or lactation,

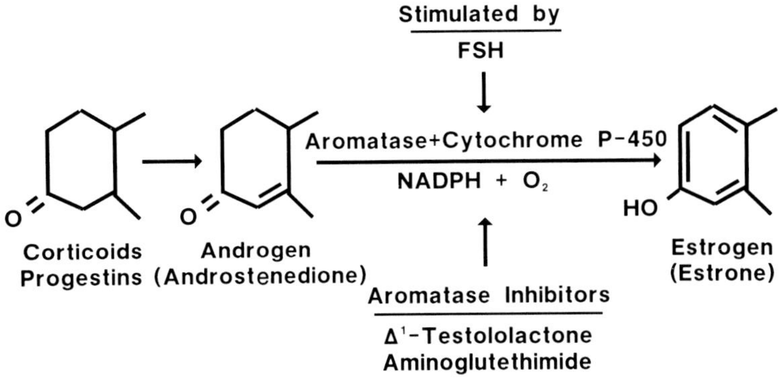

Figure 17–2. The synthesis of estrogen by the aromatization of androgens (androstenedione) via the enzyme aromatase. Aromatase is the rate-limiting step in estrogen synthesis and is the target of the drugs testololactone and aminoglutethimide.

although both processes may be adversely affected in states of thyroid hormone excess or deficiency (Cowie et al., 1980). It has been reported, however, that among women undergoing screening mammography, the prevalence of breast cancer was higher in women receiving thyroid hormone than in those who were not (Kapdi and Wolfe, 1976). This supposed increased risk could not be confirmed in two subsequent carefully performed studies (Shapiro et al., 1980; Hoffman et al., 1984). The final word seems to be that the use of thyroid supplements does not increase the risk of developing breast cancer.

Historical Aspects

By the late 19th century it was well recognized that the gonads influenced a variety of other tissues and that these influences could be altered by removal of the testes or ovaries. Hormones were not described as the chemical mediators of these responses until the 1920s (Rossof, 1980). Believing that younger women with advanced breast cancer had a poorer prognosis than older women, Schinzinger in 1889 asked, "whether it would be permissible to make the ladies old more quickly by removing their ovaries which would cause the mammary gland to atrophy and give the tumor the opportunity to be encapsulated in the shrinking tissue of the gland." Schinzinger further suggested that "in women who are still menstruating, one should first perform a castration before operating for breast cancer in order to prevent it from spreading locally or to stop a too rapid growth." Evidently Schinzinger never actually performed an oophorectomy for breast cancer, nor was he able to convince his German colleagues to do so.

It is unclear whether Beatson was aware of the writings of Schinzinger or whether he performed the first oophorectomy for breast cancer based purely on his own research. Beatson wrote his thesis for the doctor of medicine degree on the subject of lactation and was convinced that the ovary sent out influences "more subtle and more mysterious" than those from the nervous system. Regardless of the exact reason, Beatson performed the first therapeutic bilateral oophorectomy for the treatment of advanced breast cancer on June 15, 1895. The procedure was performed on a 33 year old woman with a locally recurrent breast cancer that had developed 5 to 6 months following a mastectomy. Beatson initially placed the patient on thyroid tablets, but as there was no change in the local area after 1 month he proceeded with the oophorectomy. Following the oophorectomy, the thyroid tablets were resumed to function as "a powerful lymphatic stimulant." Eight months after the operation "all vestiges of the previous cancerous disease had disappeared" (Beatson, 1896). The patient was thought to have been cured and indeed she did remain in remission 46 months before she relapsed and died of her disease. Interestingly, the use of thyroid hormone with oophorectomy continued until the 1970s, when the Cooperative Breast Cancer Group confirmed that the effects of surgical castration were not enhanced by the addition of thyroid hormone (O'Bryan, et al., 1974).

Following Beatson's initial report, oophorectomy became widely practiced, but after merely 10 years the procedure was largely abandoned, probably for the following reasons: (1) The procedure was not truly curative, as was initially hoped, and (2) irradiation castration came into use and was safer.

In 1902 Thompson reported on 80 cases treated with oophorectomy and noted the duration of response was 6 to 12 months. In 1905, Lett reviewed 99 cases and reported that the response rate in premenopausal women was 29.3 per cent. Surgical oophorectomy fell into disrepute and was ignored for nearly half a century, yet this was the first demonstration of an effective systemic treatment for cancer of any type (Yarbro, 1985).

By the early 1940s the structural framework was in place for the resurrection of endocrine therapy. The hormones testosterone and estrogen had been discovered, and their physiologic action had been described. But interestingly, it was not an endocrinologist but a urologist, Huggins, who sparked the revival (Kardinal, 1985). Huggins and associates (Huggins and Hodges, 1941; Huggins and Bergenstal, 1952) reported on the relationship between prostatic cancer, testosterone, and acid phosphatase and on the response of prostatic cancer to surgical orchiectomy, estrogens, and later adrenalectomy. For this work Huggins was awarded the Nobel prize in 1966.

Huggins' success with prostate cancer stimulated interest in castration for the treatment of advanced breast cancer. In 1945, Adair and colleagues reviewed 304 women castrated radiotherapeutically and 31 women castrated surgically, noting equal results. Rossof (1980) also reported good results in six cases of male breast cancer treated with surgical orchiectomy.

By 1948 the value of additive hormonal therapy in breast cancer using androgens or estrogens was recognized and was reported by Taylor and colleagues. Taylor also introduced the use of progestins in 1951 (Taylor and Morris, 1951). Thus, what might be considered the first golden age of hormonal therapy had begun. The Cooperative Breast Cancer Group, organized under the chairmanship of Albert Segaloff of the Ochsner Clinic, concerned itself with the evaluation of estrogens versus androgens, the role of thyroid hormone with oophorectomy, and the role of megestrol acetate in the adjuvant setting. Perhaps the most important contribution of this group of investigators was the establishment of objective criteria for the evaluation of response to treatment in patients with advanced breast cancer (Segaloff, 1966). With slight modification, these criteria were adopted by the International Union Against Cancer (Hayward et al., 1977) and remain in use today.

It was well established during the 1960s that the objective response rate to hormonal manipulation, whether additive or ablative, was no greater than 25 to 30 per cent, and that the median duration response was approximately 12 months. In 1969, Cooper reported to the American Association for Cancer Research an objective response rate of 80 per cent in hormonally refractory breast cancer to the five drug chemotherapeutic regimen of cyclophosphamide, methotrexate, 5-fluorouracil, vincristine, and prednisone. Response rates of this magnitude were unknown with hormonal therapy. The first golden age of hormonal therapy came to an abrupt end. Recent advances in the understanding of hormonal mechanisms seem to be ushering in a second golden age of hormonal therapy.

Principles of Hormonal Therapy

Approximately 130,000 new cases of breast cancer occur per year in the United States and 70 per cent of these patients will ultimately have recurrence and die of their disease (Baum, 1984). Rutgvist and coworkers (1984), in reviewing the data on 14,731 cases followed for 5 to 18 years from the Cancer Registry of Norway, have questioned whether or not breast cancer is a curable disease. They noted that the overall cured fraction (i.e., those subject to normal mortality risk) was 35 ± 1 per cent standard error. However, survival times fit a lognormal model, implying a continued late mortality. A summary of data by Rutgvist and colleagues is presented in Table 17–1. As can be seen, survival even in Stage I disease is poor, but the median survival time of Stage I patients whose cancers recur is

Table 17–1. LONG-TERM FOLLOW-UP OF BREAST CANCER PATIENTS DATA FROM THE CANCER REGISTRY OF NORWAY

Stage	Cured Fraction	Median Survival of Noncured Patients
I	54 ± 3%	7.6 years
II	27 ± 1%	3.4 years
III	19 ± 2%	2.1 years
IV	2 ± 1%	0.7 years

Data from Rutquist, L. E., et al.: Is breast cancer a curable disease? Cancer, 53:1793, 1984.

considerably longer (7.6 years) than patients with Stage IV disease (0.7 year), implying that patients with a low initial tumor burden are at risk for recurrence for considerably longer periods of time (Clark et al., 1987). The mortality rate for breast cancer might be even higher were it not for the fact that the median age at diagnosis is 59 years, and the median time to recurrence (in Stage I disease) is 7.6 years, indicating that a number of patients may die of intercurrent disease prior to the recurrence of their breast cancer (Lippman, 1985).

If Baum and Rutgvist and coworkers are correct that some 65 to 70 per cent of all cases of breast cancer will recur and ultimately cause death, and if there are 130,000 new cases per year in the United States, this will mean that approximately 91,000 of these patients will ultimately need further therapy in the adjuvant setting as well as for metastatic disease. It can also be concluded that since the response rate to endocrine therapy in unselected cases is 25 to 30 per cent, some 27,000 cases will respond to hormone treatment.

Once a breast cancer has recurred at a distant or even a local metastatic site, the disease is no longer curable by currently available methods. The goals of treatment change from cure to palliation of symptoms and prolongation of a useful, productive life. Advanced breast cancer clearly is a systemic disease and must be treated systemically. Currently the only effective systemic treatments available are endocrine therapy (additive and ablative) and cytotoxic chemotherapy. Perhaps in the near future biologic response modifiers, such as interferon or interleukin II, and monoclonal antibodies may play a role in the management of advanced breast cancer (Schlom et al., 1984; Kardinal, 1985).

The management of patients with advanced disease has undergone considerable change over the past two decades. In the 1960s, when chemotherapy was in its infancy, sequential hormone therapy was developed. During the 1970s, the selection of therapy for advanced breast cancer was still largely clinical (Segaloff, 1975). The use of hormonal receptors did not come into wide clinical use until the late 1970s and early 1980s. The clinical decision to use hormonal therapy versus chemotherapy was based on two major criteria: (1) the site of metastasis and the number of metastatic sites; and (2) the disease-free interval (Fig. 17–3 and Table 17–2).

Cutler and associates (1969) recognized that

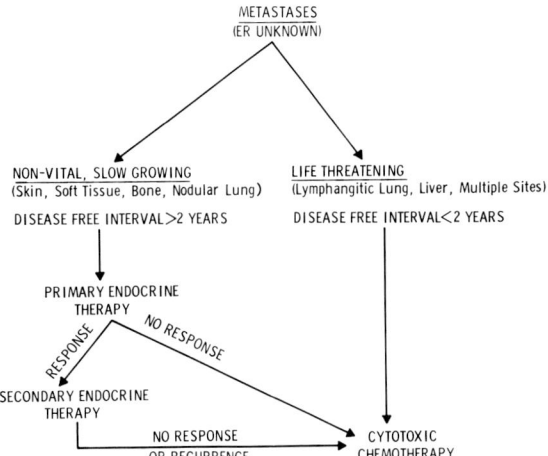

Figure 17–3. Clinical approach to the patient with advanced breast cancer when the receptor status is unknown. This was the standard approach to the patient in the 1970s, in the prereceptor era. This approach is still valid in the 1980s in patients whose receptor status is unknown.

there were certain metastatic sites that could be considered "dire," such as the liver, lymphangitic lung, and the central nervous system (Table 17–2). Skin, soft tissue, bone, and nodular lung metastases (unless multiple and bilateral) were associated with a better prognosis. From this it could be deduced that, if the patient did have multiple sites of metastasis or had a dire prognostic site involved, the clinician could not risk the 6 to 8 weeks necessary to determine if the patient would be one of the 25 to 30 per cent who would respond to hormones. Instead, the patient had to be treated directly with cytotoxic chemotherapy, with its more rapid onset of action and higher response rate.

The other important prognostic factor well recognized during the 1960s and 1970s was the

Table 17–2. THE EFFECT OF THE NUMBER OF METASTATIC SITES ON SURVIVAL

Number of Sites	Number of Cases	Median Survival
1	249	19 months
2*	200	13 months
3*	114	10 months
4*	51	6 months
"Dire"†	111	6 months

*Does not include a "dire" prognosis site.
†"Dire" = liver, peritoneum, brain, or spinal cord metastases.
Modified from Cutler, S. J., et al.: Classification of patients with disseminated cancer of the breast. Cancer, 24:861, 1969.

Table 17–3. THE EFFECT OF DISEASE-FREE INTERVAL ON SURVIVAL AFTER DISSEMINATION

Disease-Free Interval	Number of Cases	Median Survival After Dissemination
<1 year	135	7 months
1–2 years	142	7 months
2–5 years	208	15 months
5+ years	129	25 months

Modified from Cutler, S. J., et al.: Classification of patients with disseminated cancer of the breast. Cancer, 24:861, 1969.

disease-free interval (Cutler et al., 1969; Carter, 1972). Disease-free interval is defined as the time between the primary therapy and the development of recurrence. The greater the disease-free interval, the greater the survival after the development of metastases (Table 17–3). There is a direct relationship between the disease-free interval and hormonal responsiveness. Tumors with prolonged disease-free intervals are slower growing, more highly differentiated, and more likely to retain hormonal responsiveness (Rozencwieg and Heuson, 1975). Disease-free interval and the site and number of metastatic sites remain important predictors of hormonal responsiveness in patients whose receptor status is unknown.

Evaluating Hormonal Dependency: Estrogen and Progesterone Receptors

The pioneering work of Jensen and colleagues (1971), McGuire (1973), Wittliff (1974), and DeSombre and coworkers (1976) established the relationship between the presence of estrogen receptor (ER) in the cytosol of breast cancer tissue and response to hormonal manipulation. By the use of the ER alone and by restricting hormonal manipulation to those patients who are ER positive ($\geq$ 10 fmol/mg protein), the response rate to hormonal manipulation can be increased from between 25 and 30 per cent in unselected cases to 55 per cent in ER positive cases (Wittliff, 1984). The ER data from the NIH Consensus Development Conference on Steroid Receptors in Breast Cancer are summarized in Table 17–4. Interestingly, the response rates to additive

Table 17–4. RELATIONSHIP BETWEEN ESTROGEN RECEPTOR STATUS OF BREAST CANCER AND OBJECTIVE RESPONSE TO ENDOCRINE THERAPY

ER + (Responses/Total)	ER − (Responses/Total)
522/977 (53%)	36/567 (6%)

Data from the NIH Consensus Development Conference on Steroid Receptors in Breast Cancer.
Modified from Wittliff, J. L.: Steroid-hormone receptors in breast cancer. Cancer, 53:630, 1984.

(56 per cent) and ablative (55 per cent) forms of hormonal manipulation in ER positive cases are equivalent (Table 17–5) (McGuire et al., 1975). This probably reflects the fact that both additive and ablative therapy are designed to block estrogen production or action.

In 1975, Horwitz and colleagues hypothesized that the presence of progesterone receptor (PgR) in human breast cancer is a sensitive marker for predicting response to endocrine therapy. PgR was found in 56 per cent of tumors with ER, and in preliminary observation it was noted that only those tumors with PgR regressed after endocrine therapy. Horwitz and coworkers further postulated that because the synthesis of PgR is estrogen-dependent, the presence of PgR would indicate that the tumor was capable of synthesizing at least one end-product under estrogen regulation and remained endocrine responsive. This is basically true. Response rates in cases that are both ER and PgR positive is 78 per cent. From this it can be concluded, as Allegra (1984a) has done, that receptors are necessary for a tumor to be hormone dependent, but are not in themselves sufficient. The data regarding hormonal responsiveness and receptor status (ER+, PgR+; ER+, PgR−; ER−, PgR−) are summarized in Table 17–6 (Witt-

Table 17–5. RELATIONSHIP BETWEEN ESTROGEN RECEPTOR STATUS AND RESPONSE TO ADDITIVE AND ABLATIVE ENDOCRINE THERAPY

	ER + (Responses/Total)	ER − (Responses/Total)
Additive hormone treatment	59/105 (56%)	12/109 (11%)
Ablative endocrine therapy	59/107 (55%)	8/94 (8%)
Total	118/212 (56%)	20/203 (10%)

Modified from Wittliff, J. L.: Steroid-hormone receptors in breast cancer. Cancer, 53:630, 1984. After McGuire.

Table 17-6. RELATIONSHIP BETWEEN ESTROGEN (ER) AND PROGESTERONE (PgR) RECEPTOR STATUS AND RESPONSE TO ENDOCRINE THERAPY

ER+, PgR+	ER+, PgR-	ER-, PgR-	ER-, PgR+
135/174	55/164	16/165	5/11
78%	34%	10%	45%

Modified from Wittliff, J. L.: Steroid-hormone receptors in breast cancer. Cancer, 53:630, 1984.

liff, 1984). The ER-, PgR+ group, with its small numbers and relatively high hormonal response rate (45 per cent), may well be an artifact and reflect a false negative ER, possibly from improper specimen handling when the tissue is obtained (Bridges et al., 1983; Kiang and Kollander, 1987).

As might be anticipated, there is a quantitative relationship between estrogen receptor concentration in breast cancer tissue and response to endocrine therapy (Allegra, 1983b) (Table 17-7). The higher the ER, the more likely a response. There is also a striking difference in response when PgR is evaluated as a function of ER concentration (Osborne et al., 1980) (Table 17-8).

The difference in response by metastatic site to endocrine manipulation in ER positive tumors is not as great as might be anticipated (Allegra, 1983b) (Table 17-9). The old belief, which goes as far back as Beatson (1896), that visceral metastases respond poorly to endocrine manipulation, is not necessarily true. However, what is true is that patients with heavy tumor cell burdens in visceral sites may not be able to afford the 6 to 8 weeks required for the onset of an endocrine response. Patients with lower metastatic tumor cell burdens in visceral sites, however, may have good objective responses to hormonal manipulation.

Receptor status varies as a function of age (Allegra, 1984b) (Table 17-10) and thus with

Table 17-7. QUANTITATION OF ER AND RESPONSE TO ENDOCRINE THERAPY

ER (fmol/mg)	Primary Cancer	Metastatic Biopsy
0-10	9%	8%
10-50	50%	40%
100	83%	61%

Data from Allegra, J. C.: Methotrexate and 5-fluorouracil following tamoxifen and Premarin in advanced breast cancer. Semin. Oncol., 10(Suppl. 2):23, 1983a; and from Osborne, C. K., Yochmorwitz, M. G., Knight, W. A., et al.: The value of estrogen and progesterone receptors in the treatment of breast cancer. Cancer, 46:2884, 1980.

Table 17-8. RESPONSE TO ENDOCRINE THERAPY BY QUANTITATIVE ER VS QUALITATIVE PgR

ER (fmol/mg)	Response Rate
3-100	34%
>100	63%
PgR	
Negative (<5 fmol/mg)	31%
Positive (≥5 fmol/mg)	80%

Modified from Osborne, C. K., et al.: The value of estrogen and progesterone receptors in the treatment of breast cancer. Cancer, 46:2884, 1980.

menopausal status (Wittliff, 1984) (Table 17-11). The younger the patient, the more likely she is to be receptor negative and hormonally unresponsive. Conversely, the older the patient, the more likely she is to be receptor positive and to be hormonally responsive. This difference in receptor content by age and menopausal status is probably why premenopausal patients have a poorer prognosis than postmenopausal patients. However, when receptor content and nodal status are comparable, response rates and survival are equivalent in premenopausal and postmenopausal women.

CHANGES IN RECEPTORS

The percentage of ER positive and PgR positive cancers diminishes with progression of the malignancy (Nomura et al., 1985) (Table 17-12). Differences in the receptor content between the primary lesion and metastatic sites have been observed by several investigators (Brannan et al., 1979; Allegra et al., 1980; Hull et al., 1983). When changes in receptors occur, the change almost always is from the receptor positive state to the receptor negative state, implying tumor dedifferentiation. However, receptor negative to receptor positive

Table 17-9. OBJECTIVE RESPONSES TO ENDOCRINE THERAPY IN ER POSITIVE TUMORS BY DOMINANT SITE OF METASTATIC DISEASE

Skin	52%
Soft tissue	57%
Nodes	61%
Lung	62%
Liver	55%
Bone	50%
Bone marrow	67%
Central nervous system	0%

Modified from Allegra, J. C.: The use of steroid hormone receptors in breast cancer. In Margolese, R. (Ed.): Breast Cancer. New York, Churchill Livingstone, 1983, p. 187.

Table 17–10. THE RELATIONSHIP BETWEEN RECEPTOR STATUS AND AGE

Age (Years)	Per Cent ER+	Per Cent PgR+
40	44	31
40–49	48	36
50–59	53	42
60–69	58	36
70	69	29

Modified from Allegra, J. C.: In The Management of Breast Cancer Through Endocrine Therapies. Amsterdam, Excerpta Medica, 1984b, pp. 1–13.

changes have been reported (Rosen et al., 1977; Holdaway and Bowditch, 1983; Nomura et al., 1985).

The tumor dedifferentiation theory may not explain why receptor positive tumors tend to become receptor negative. Almost all patients with advanced breast cancer receive multiple types of treatment, such as chemotherapy and hormonal therapy, during the course of their disease. Some observed changes in receptor status may be induced by treatment (Table 17–13). It appears that hormonal therapy has a greater tendency to induce changes from ER positive to ER negative than does cytotoxic chemotherapy (Nomura et al., 1985), which implies that chemotherapy kills cells indiscriminately regardless of their receptor status, leaving the same proportion of ER positive and ER negative cells (Kardinal et al., 1986). However, hormonal therapy selectively interferes with ER positive cells. Allegra and coworkers (1980) have suggested that the observed conversion of ER positive tumors to ER negative status after treatment with tamoxifen may be due to the drug's occupying the ER receptor sites, causing artificially low ER determinations. This suggests that ER positive breast cancers that become ER negative after antiestrogen therapy may still respond to second line endocrine therapy.

Table 17–11. RELATIONSHIP OF RECEPTOR STATUS AND MENOPAUSAL STATE

Receptor Status	Premenopausal	Postmenopausal
ER+, PgR+	45%	63%
ER+, PgR−	12%	15%
ER−, PgR−	28%	17%
ER−, PgR+	15%	5%

Modified from Wittliff, J. L.: Steroid-hormone receptors in breast cancer. Cancer, 53:630, 1984.

Table 17–12. CHANGES IN RECEPTOR CONTENT WITH PROGRESSION OF DISEASE

	Per Cent ER+	Per Cent PgR+
Primary lesion	53.8%	26.3%
First relapse	56.5%	24.5%
Second relapse	39.0%	19.1%
Preterminal	20.0%	3.4%

Data from Nomura, Y., et al.: Changes of steroid hormone receptor content by chemotherapy and/or endocrine therapy in advanced breast cancer. Cancer, 55:546, 1985.

RECEPTORS AND BREAST CANCER BIOLOGY

Over the past several years, it has become apparent that the ER and PgR status of a breast cancer is an important prognostic indicator as well as an indicator of response to endocrine therapy (Gapinski and Donegan, 1980; Clark and McGuire 1983; McGuire and Clark, 1983). It has also been demonstrated that receptors correlate with the cellular turnover rates, nuclear grade, and the degree of histologic differentiation (Fisher et al., 1987). Meyer and colleagues (1977) demonstrated that tumors with low thymidine labeling indices (TLI) (i.e., low cellular replication rates), tended to be ER positive and conversely, those with a high TLI tended to be ER negative. Fisher and coworkers (1980b) and Parl and colleagues (1984) have demonstrated that ER positive tumors tend to be well differentiated and ER negative tumors tend to be poorly differentiated. It can be deduced from this that the more like normal breast tissue a breast cancer is (i.e., the better differentiated the tumor) the more likely the tumor is to be ER

Table 17–13. CHANGES IN ER CONTENT BY TREATMENT

Treatment	Per Cent ER+ Pretreatment	Per Cent ER+ Posttreatment
Antiestrogen	71%	43%
Adreno-oophorectomy	64%	25%
Chemotherapy	36%	32%
Chemoendocrine therapy	60%	28%
Between first and last treatment	63%	16%

Modified from Nomura Y., et al.: Change of steroid hormone receptor content by chemotherapy and/or endocrine therapy in advanced breast cancer. Cancer, 55:546, 1985.

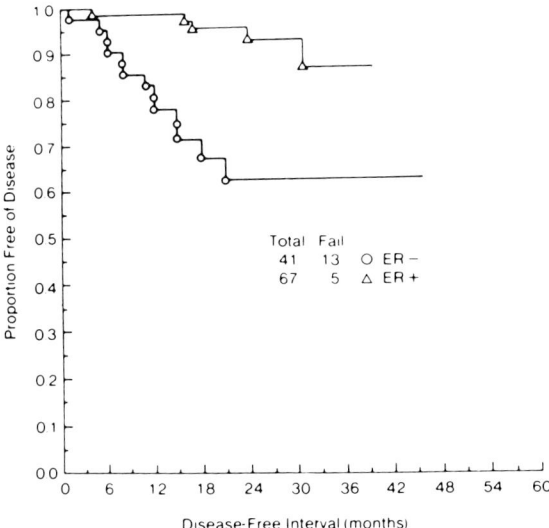

Figure 17–4. The relationship between disease-free interval and estrogen receptor status in patients with breast cancer not receiving adjuvant therapy. (From Allegra, J. C.: In Allegra, J. C. [Ed.]: The Management of Breast Cancer Through Endocrine Therapies. Amsterdam, Excerpta Medica, 1984, p. 8. Reprinted with permission.)

positive and hormonally responsive and the better the prognosis.

Allegra and colleagues (1979) and Knight and associates (1977) have also demonstrated that the ER status of the primary tumor is associated with the disease-free interval. ER positivity is associated with prolonged disease-free intervals, and ER negativity is associated with shortened disease-free intervals (Fig. 17–4). This association is independent of age, menopausal status (Fig. 17–5), tumor size (Fig. 17–6), or nodal status (Fig. 17–7). Thus, it appears that receptor status is an independent prognostic variable. Also, the purely clinical observation that tumors with prolonged disease-free intervals tend to retain their hormonal responsiveness has been confirmed by scientific data.

The role of progesterone receptors as a prognostic variable has been critically evaluated by Clark and associates (1983). They noted that when analyzed separately, the presence and quantity of either ER or PgR was positively correlated with disease-free survival (Fig. 17–8). However, the presence of PgR was more significant than ER for predicting time to recurrence (Fig. 17–9). When patients were divided into groups (ER+, PgR+; ER+, PgR−; ER−, PgR− [there were too few ER−, PgR+ to be evaluated]), disease-free survival for the ER+, PgR+ group was significantly better than for either the ER+,

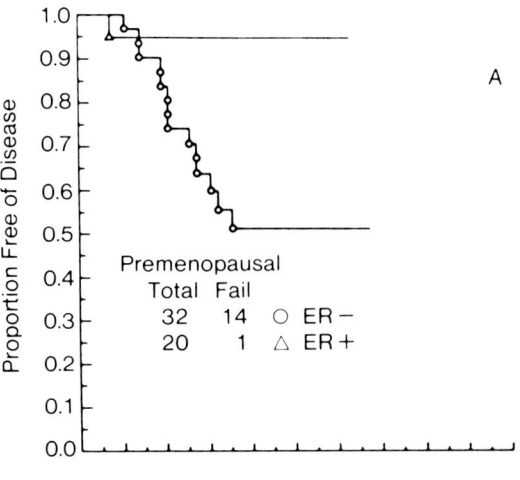

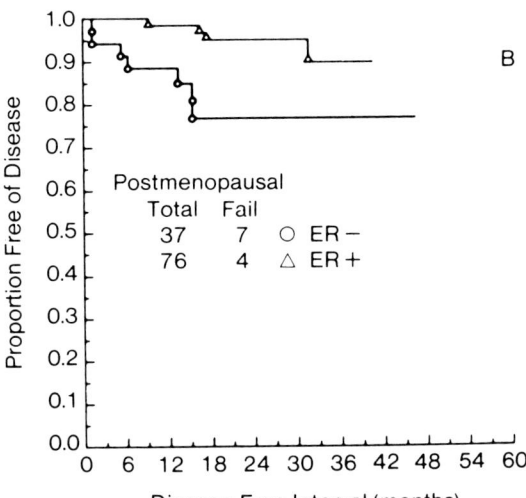

Figure 17–5. The relationship between disease-free interval, estrogen receptor status, and menopausal state in patients with breast cancer. (From Allegra, J. C.: In Allegra, J. C. [Ed.]: The Management of Breast Cancer Through Endocrine Therapies. Amsterdam, Excerpta Medica, 1984, p. 9. Reprinted with permission.)

PgR− or ER−, PgR− patients (Fig. 17–10). In addition, the disease-free survival of the Er+, PgR− group was only marginally better than that of the Er−, PgR− group.

Axillary nodal metastases are a critical prognostic variable, and patients with negative axillary nodes do considerably better than patients with any degree of axillary nodal involvement (Fisher et al, 1968; 1975; Bonadonna et al., 1976). (Tables 17–14 and 17–15). In addition, patients with one to three positive nodes have a better prognosis than those with more than four. Within the group with more

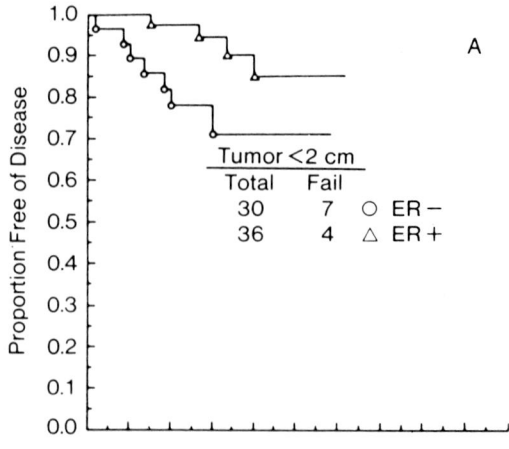

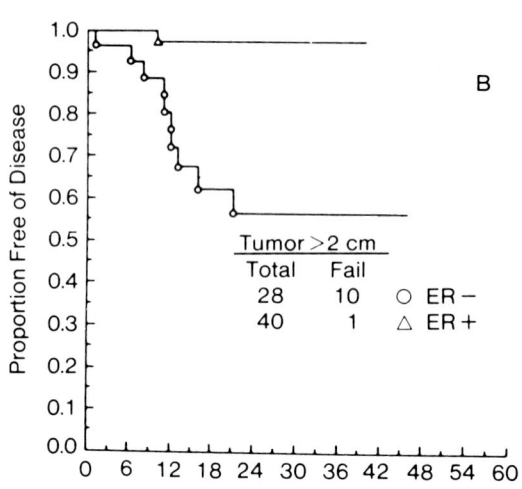

Figure 17–6. The relationship between disease-free interval, estrogen receptor status, and tumor size in patients with breast cancer. (From Allegra, J. C.: In Allegra, J. C. [Ed.]: The Management of Breast Cancer Through Endocrine Therapies. Amsterdam, Excerpta Medica, 1984, p. 10. Reprinted with permission.)

than four involved nodes, patients with four to six do better than those with 7 to 12, who in turn do better than those with more than 13 involved nodes (Fisher et al., 1983a) (Figs. 17–11 and 17–12).

Most investigators, such as Allegra and coworkers (1979) (Fig. 17–7) have confirmed that receptors constitute a variable independent of nodal status. This has been confirmed by Clark and McGuire (1983) in the United States, Hartviet and colleagues (1980) in Norway, and Croton and associates in Great Britain (1981) (Fig. 17–13). Patients who are receptor posi-

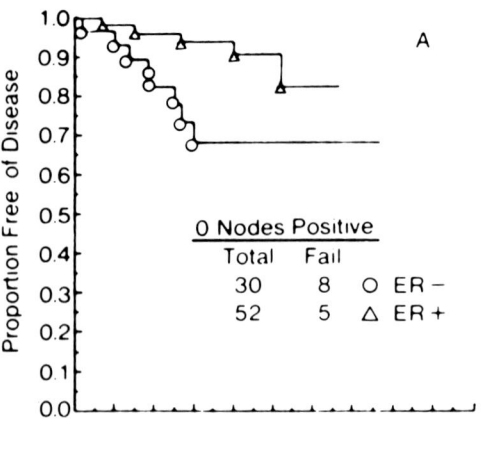

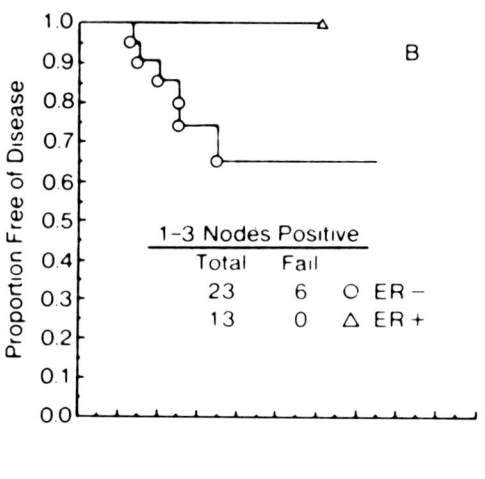

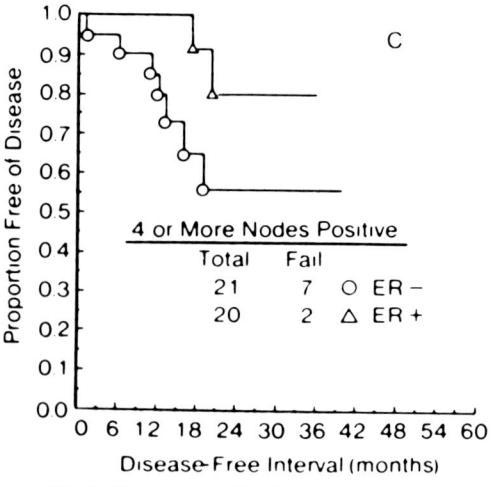

Figure 17–7. The relationship between disease-free interval, estrogen receptor status, and degree of axillary node involvement in patients with breast cancer. (From Allegra, J. C.: In Allegra, J. C. [Ed.]: The Management of Breast Cancer Through Endocrine Therapies. Amsterdam, Excerpta Medica, 1984, p. 11. Reprinted with permission.)

Figure 17-8. The relationship between disease-free survival and quantitative progesterone receptor levels. Patients with ≥50 fmol/mg (N = 41) have a significantly longer disease-free survival than patients with 5 to 49 fmol/mg (N = 68); each of these groups have longer disease-free periods than patients with < 5 fmol/mg (n = 41). (Reprinted by permission from Clark, G. M., et al.: Progesterone receptors as a prognostic factor in stage II breast cancer. N. Engl. J. Med., 309:1343, 1983.)

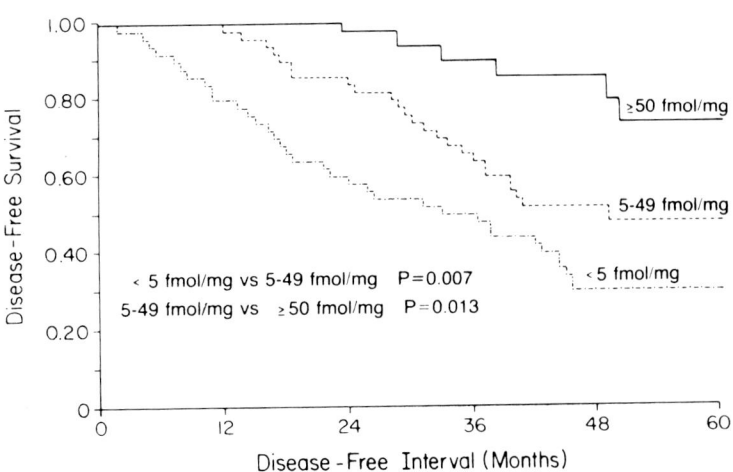

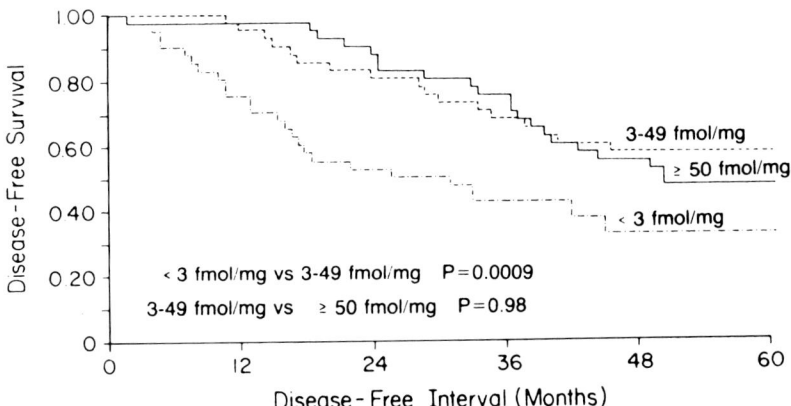

Figure 17-9. The relationship between disease-free survival and quantitative estrogen receptor levels. Patients with ER levels <3 fmol/mg (n = 45) had significantly shorter disease-free survival than those with moderate or high levels. However, there was no difference between patients with 3 to 49 fmol/mg (n = 82) and those with at least 50 fmol/mg (n = 62). (Reprinted with permission from Clark, G. M., et al.: Progesterone receptors as a prognostic factor in stage II breast cancer. N. Engl. J. Med., 309: 1343, 1983.)

Figure 17-10. Relationship between estrogen and progesterone receptor status and disease-free survival. Patients who are ER+ and PgR+ (n = 104) have a significantly longer disease-free survival than patients who are ER+ and PgR− (n = 39) or patients who are ER− and PgR− (n = 40). (Reprinted with permission from Clark, G. M., et al.: Progesterone receptors as a prognostic factor in stage II breast cancer. N. Engl. J. Med., 309:1343, 1983.)

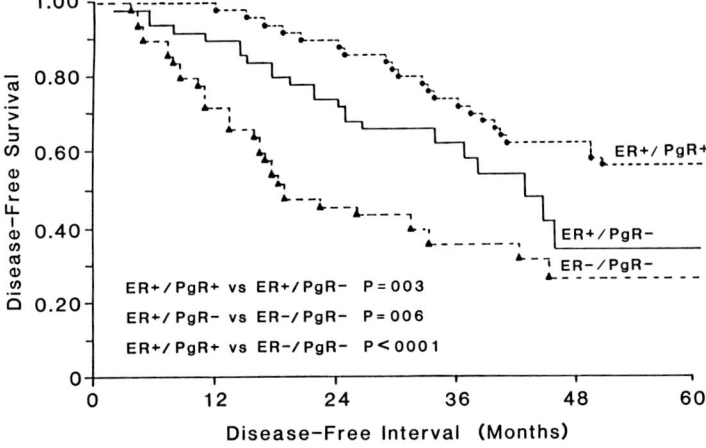

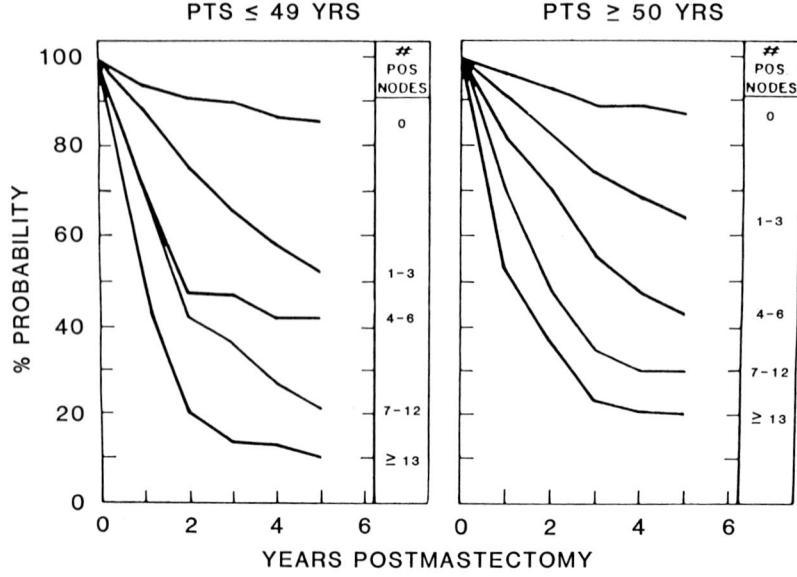

Figure 17–11. Disease-free survival relative to age and number of positive axillary nodes for patients (PTS) ≤ 49 years and ≥ 50 years. (From Fisher, B., et al.: Relation of number of positive axillary nodes to the prognosis of patients with primary breast cancer: An NSABP update. Cancer, 52:1551, 1983. Reprinted with permission.)

Figure 17–12. Absolute survival relative to age and number of positive nodes for patients (PTS) ≤ 49 years and ≥ 50 years. (From Fisher, B., et al.: Relation of number of positive axillary nodes to the prognosis of patients with primary breast cancer: An NSABP update. Cancer, 52:1551, 1983. Reprinted with permission.)

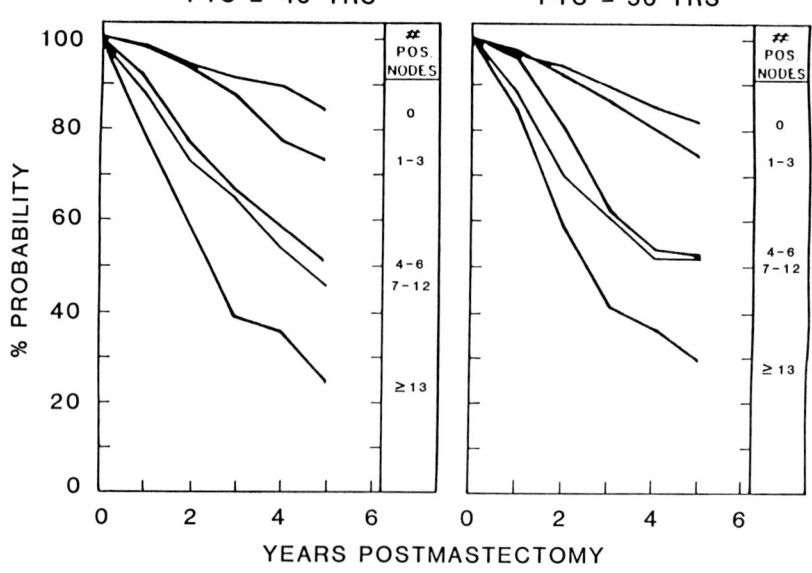

Table 17–14. TREATMENT FAILURE AFTER STANDARD RADICAL MASTECTOMY

	Number	Per Cent Treatment Failures			
		18 Months	3 Years	5 Years	10 Years
All Patients	370	19	—	39.7	49.5
Negative nodes	198	6	—	17.7	24.1
Positive nodes	172	35	—	71.0	76.1
Premenopausal					
Negative nodes	52	6	17	21.2	25.5
Positive nodes	60	50	61	70.0	76.3
1–3 nodes positive	24	13	—	45.8	56.6
≥4 nodes positive	36	64	82	86.1	88.9
Postmenopausal					
Negative nodes	146	8	15	16.4	23.6
Positive nodes	112	22	50	62.5	76.0
1–3 nodes positive	58	18	37	51.7	67.9
≥4 nodes positive	54	48	62	74.1	84.3

Adapted from Fisher, B., Ravdin, R. G., Ausman, R. K., et al.: Surgical adjuvant chemotherapy in cancer of the breast. Results of a decade of cooperative investigation. Ann. Surg., 163:337, 1968; Fisher, B., Slack, N., Katrych, D., et al.: Ten year follow-up results of patients with carcinoma of the breast in a cooperative clinical trial evaluating surgical adjuvant chemotherapy. Surg. Gynecol. Obstet., 140:528, 1975; and Fisher, B., Bauer, M., Wickerham, L., et al.: Relation of number of positive axillary nodes to the prognosis of patients with primary breast cancer. An NSABP update. Cancer, 52:1551, 1983a.

tive and node negative have the best prognosis, and patients who are receptor negative and node positive the poorest, with the states of receptor positive, node positive and receptor negative, node negative having an intermediate prognosis. It should be pointed out that these are not the findings of all investigators, particularly in Stage I patients. Crowe and associates (1982), in evaluating 510 Stage I patients, noted that in the postmenopausal group, ER positive patients had a better prognosis than those who were ER negative, but premenopausal ER positive patients had no prognostic advantage over the ER negative patients. Butler and colleagues (1985), evaluating 556 Stage I patients, documented no differences in disease-free interval or absolute survival between premenopausal or postmenopausal patients who were ER positive and those who were ER negative.

Another important observation is that receptor positive patients have a significantly better survival from the date of first recurrence than receptor negative patients (Godolphin et al., 1981; Kinne et al., 1981) (Fig. 17–14). In addition, within the receptor positive group, those whose quantitative ER value is the high-

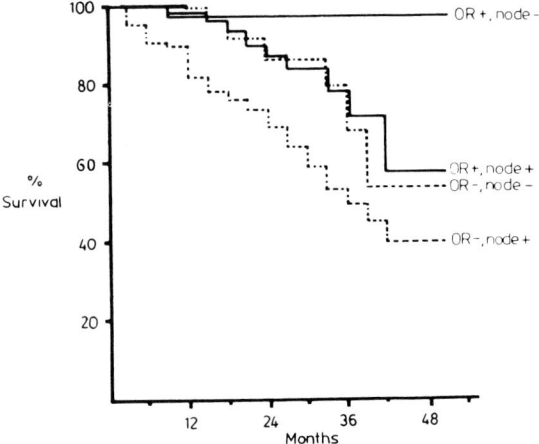

Figure 17–13. Absolute survival rates according to lymph node and estrogen receptor status. OR, Estrogen receptors. (From Croton, R., et al.: Oestrogen receptors and survival in early breast cancer. Br. Med. J., 283:1289, 1981. Reprinted with permission.)

Table 17–15. TREATMENT FAILURE AFTER STANDARD RADICAL MASTECTOMY IN 381 PATIENTS WITH AXILLARY NODE INVOLVEMENT

	Per Cent Treatment Failures			
	18 Months	3 Years	5 Years	10 Years
All patients with positive nodes	27.4	51.6	63.6	75.5
1–3 nodes positive	18.6	39.7	54.2	67.7
≥4 nodes positive	37.1	64.5	73.8	83.6
Survival rate	92.5	72.8	56.2	39.7

Modified from Bonadonna, G., et al.: *In* Breast Cancer: A Report to the Profession. National Cancer Institute, Bethesda, Md., 1976.

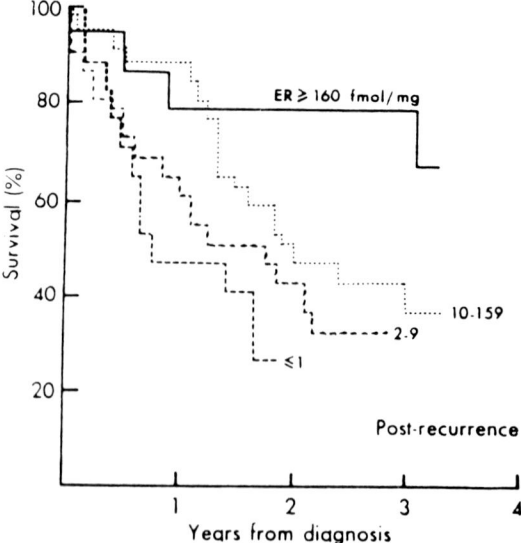

Figure 17–14. Survival from the date of first recurrence for breast cancer patients in four groups by estrogen receptor concentration. (From Godolphin, W., et al.: Estrogen receptor quantitation and staging as complementary prognostic indicators of breast cancer: A study of 583 patients. Int. J. Cancer, 28:677, 1981. Reprinted with permission.)

est ($\geq$160 fmol/mg) do better than those with lower levels of positivity (10 to 159 fmol/mg). After recurrence, the poorer prognosis in the receptor negative group may be due to the fact that ER negative patients are more likely than ER positive patients to develop visceral metastases, and ER positive tumors have a higher frequency of the more indolent osseous metastases (Qazi et al., 1984; Sherry et al., 1986).

CARCINOEMBRYONIC ANTIGEN (CEA)

The usefulness of the plasma CEA level in monitoring response to treatment, as a predictor of early relapse, and as a prognostic factor in colorectal cancer has been well documented (Kardinal and Bush, 1985). In the past few years, it has become apparent that the cytosolic concentration of CEA may have a similar usefulness in breast cancer (Duffy et al., 1983; Mansour et al., 1983). Schwartz and colleagues (1985) have demonstrated that the cytosolic CEA is related to pathologic stage and is independent of ER status, histologic differentiation, and other pathologic variables (Table 17–16). The CEA value may therefore provide information on some other biologic characteristic of breast cancer. Falkson and coworkers (1982) have demonstrated that in patients receiving postsurgical adjuvant chemotherapy, a rising CEA level is a more sensitive predictor of recurrence than is the lactic dehydrogenase or alkaline phosphatase level. Also, changes in the plasma CEA level during hormone therapy or chemotherapy reflect an increasing or decreasing tumor cell burden (Silva et al., 1982). However, the high cost of CEA assays and their relative insensitivity negate the routine use of CEA determinations in breast cancer patients (Loprinzi and Ahmann, 1986).

Ablative Hormonal Therapy

OOPHORECTOMY

Surgical castration remains the treatment of choice for hormonally responsive breast cancer in premenopausal women (Wells and Santen, 1984; Veronesi et al., 1987). As reviewed by Haas (1981), the overall response rate in unselected cases is 31 per cent (365 responders in 1163 patients), and the median response duration is 12 months, but responses lasting 25 years have been reported (Mecklenburg and Lipsett, 1973). As mentioned previously, the response rate can be increased to 55 per cent by restricting oophorectomy to ER positive patients and to 78 per cent by restricting the procedure to ER positive, PgR positive patients. Oophorectomy should not be performed in ER negative women as the response rate is less than 10 per cent. The contraindications to surgical castration are listed in Table 17–17.

Table 17–16. RELATIONSHIP OF CARCINOEMBRYONIC ANTIGEN (CEA) LEVEL TO STAGE

	CEA (ng/mg Cytosol Protein)		
	5	6–60	60
Stage I–II	10/20 (50.0%)	4/20 (20.0%)	6/20 (30.8%)
Stage III–IV	2/17 (11.8%)	6/17 (35.5%)	9/17 (52.9%)

Modified from Schwartz, M. R., et al.: Carcinoembryonic antigen and steroid receptors in the cytosol of carcinoma of the breast. Cancer, 55:2464, 1985.

Table 17–17. CONTRAINDICATIONS TO SURGICAL CASTRATION

Uncontrolled central nervous system metastases
Massive hepatic metastases
Pulmonary lymphangitic metastases or bloody pleural effusion
Uncontrolled hypercalcemia
Myelophthisic anemia
More than 1 year postmenopausal
ER negative receptor status

The traditional role of oophorectomy as the primary mode of endocrine therapy in premenopausal women is currently being challenged by the antiestrogen tamoxifen (Haas, 1981; Ingle et al., 1986; Buchanan et al., 1986). Response rates and response durations appear to be equivalent (Margreiter and Wiegele, 1984; Planting, et al., 1985). In fact, Pritchard and coworkers (1984) and Sawka and coworkers (1986) have stated that response to tamoxifen is a good predictor of response to oophorectomy. This implies that tamoxifen should be used as primary therapy and oophorectomy restricted to those patients who have previously responded to tamoxifen. That tamoxifen is a good predictor of response to oophorectomy could not be confirmed by the Southwest Oncology Group (Hoogstraten et al., 1982, 1984). In the Southwest Group Trial, none of 14 premenopausal patients who responded to tamoxifen responded to oophorectomy, whereas 5 of 22 patients who failed to respond to tamoxifen responded to oophorectomy with continued tamoxifen. In addition, Kalman and associates (1983) have reported response to oophorectomy after failure to respond to tamoxifen in a premenopausal patient. The use of tamoxifen in premenopausal patients will be discussed later in this chapter, in the section on *Additive Hormonal Therapy,* but in short, tamoxifen is not a substitute for surgical oophorectomy.

OOPHORECTOMY AND CHEMOTHERAPY

Attempts have been made to improve the response to oophorectomy by the addition of cytotoxic chemotherapy. Four prospective randomized trials have been performed, but each of these was done prior to the availability of estrogen or progesterone receptors (vanDyk and Falkson, 1971; Ahmann et al., 1977; Falkson et al., 1979; Rossof et al., 1982). In each of these trials the response rate was higher in patients treated with oophorectomy plus chemotherapy than in those undergoing oophorectomy alone, but the response did not exceed that reported for the use of chemotherapy alone. This series of reports is best considered uninterpretable in light of the current data on hormone receptor and combination chemotherapy.

RADIATION OOPHORECTOMY

The use of irradiation for castration of women with locally advanced and disseminated breast cancer began in the early 1920s, using a technique described by Halberstadter in 1905 (deCourmeller, 1922; Wintz, 1926; Ahlbom, 1930). The procedure was safe, and the results were equivalent to surgical castration (Adair et al., 1945; Diczfalusy et al., 1959). The reduction of estrogen production by radiotherapy is considerably slower than with surgery and may require 3 to 5 months to reach the basal level (Block et al., 1958). The argument that radiation oophorectomy is still indicated in patients who are too sick to undergo a surgical oophorectomy is not valid; it is hardly acceptable to wait 3 to 5 months for a therapeutic response, and alternative modes of therapy should be initiated. There are so many alternative modes of treatment available, such as tamoxifen, aminoglutethimide, and even cytotoxic chemotherapy, that there are few if any indications for radiation oophorectomy.

OOPHORECTOMY IN THE ADJUVANT SETTING

Prophylactic castration was originally proposed by Taylor in 1934. After 4 years, the results with 50 patients castrated therapeutically were sufficiently similar to those in 47 patients treated prophylactically that Taylor concluded that the production of artificial menopause was not advantageous (Taylor, 1939). However, numerous other investigators reported conflicting results with prophylactic oophorectomy, and the procedure continued to be practiced widely until the 1970s. In 1961, the National Surgical Adjuvant Breast Project (NSABP) initiated a prospective randomized trial of surgical oophorectomy as adjunct treatment to radical mastectomy for the treatment of operable breast cancer (Ravdin et al., 1970). A total of 699 patients were entered into the study. No significant differences were seen in recurrence or survival rates. When the data were interpreted in terms of the nodal status of the different treatment groups, still no differences were found. Nonetheless, there are two more recent studies, each of which show marginal improvement in late survival in the prophylactically oophorectomized group (Bryant and Weir, 1981; Meakin et al., 1983). In neither of these studies were hormonal receptor data available, and in neither were the results impressive enough to recommend that the procedure be adopted. Finally, in 1985 the Ludwig Breast Cancer Study Group reported the results of a study randomizing premenopausal women with Stage II breast cancer and four or more positive axillary nodes to adjuvant chemotherapy with cyclophosphamide, methotrexate, 5-fluorouracil, and prednisone (CMFP) versus CMFP plus oophorectomy (Ludwig Breast Cancer Study Group, 1985). No difference was found in disease-free or absolute survival, even in receptor positive cases. This study should lay the issue of adjuvant oophorectomy to rest.

ADRENALECTOMY AND HYPOPHYSECTOMY

Although adrenalectomy and hypophysectomy are effective modes of therapy in hormonally responsive breast cancer, they are seldom practiced today and are currently of historic interest only. Although the operative mortality rates associated with adrenalectomy and hypophysectomy are low, there is an appreciable morbidity associated with these procedures (Fracchia et al., 1967). These operations have been replaced by tamoxifen and the adrenal blocking agent aminoglutethimide (Wells and Santen, 1984), two simpler, less expensive, and safer means of suppressing estrogen levels.

Adrenalectomy became popular in the 1950s as a means of treatment of metastatic breast cancer in postmenopausal women or in premenopausal women who had previously responded to oophorectomy (Harris and Spratt, 1969). The procedure became possible in 1951 with the introduction of cortisone acetate for adrenal replacement. The first report of the efficacy of adrenalectomy for advanced breast cancer was by Huggins and Bergenstal in 1952.

Hypophysectomy was introduced by Luft and Olivecrona in 1953 as an alternative to adrenalectomy. Response rates of adrenalectomy and hypophysectomy proved to be equivalent, and the choice between the two procedures was really one of available expertise (McDonald, 1962). Because general surgeons were more readily available than neurosurgeons, adrenalectomy became the more popular procedure.

Santen and coworkers (1981) reported a prospective randomized clinical trial of surgical versus medical adrenalectomy using aminoglutethimide plus hydrocortisone. Ninety-six postmenopausal women were stratified by disease-free interval, site of dominant disease, and ER status. Estrogen levels decreased similarly in response to either treatment. No significant differences were seen in response rate, response by dominant site of metastatic disease, or response duration (Figs. 17–15 and

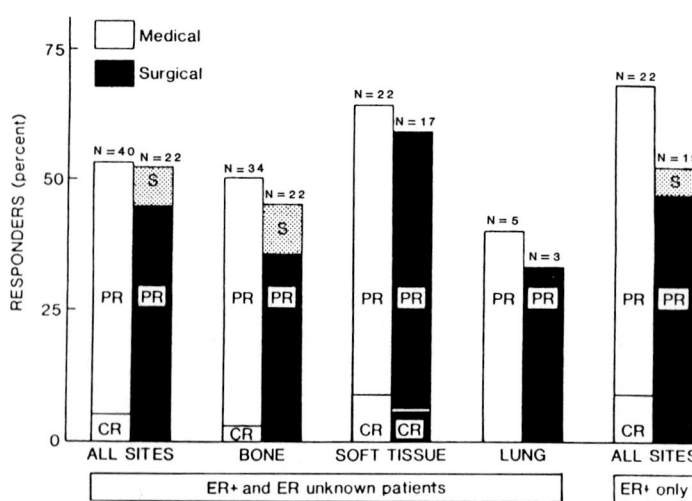

Figure 17–15. Percentage of patients with a response to treatment in medical adrenalectomy versus surgical adrenalectomy. Open bars represent patients treated with aminoglutethimide and hydrocortisone; solid or shaded bars represent patients treated with surgical adrenalectomy. CR, Complete response; PR, partial response; S, stable disease. (Reprinted with permission from Santen, R. J., et al.: A randomized trial comparing surgical adrenalectomy with aminoglutethimide plus hydrocortisone in women with advanced breast cancer. N. Engl. J. Med., 305:545, 1981.)

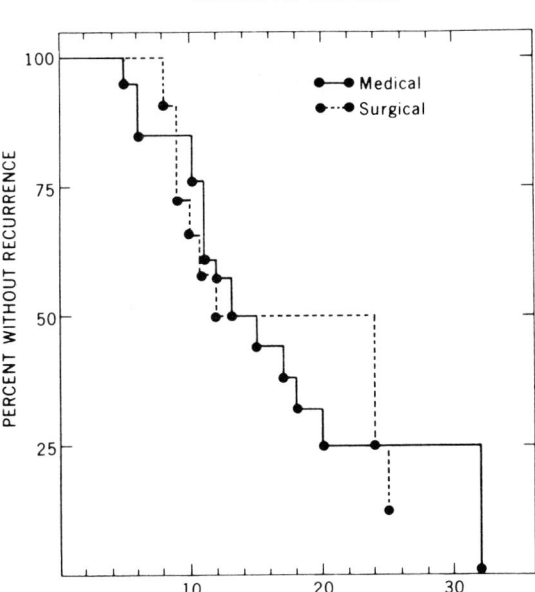

Figure 17–16. Life table analysis of the duration of response of patients treated by medical adrenalectomy with aminoglutethimide and hydrocortisone versus surgical adrenalectomy. (Reprinted with permission from Santen, R. J., et al.: A randomized trial comparing surgical adrenalectomy with aminoglutethimide plus hydrocortisone in women with advanced breast cancer. N. Engl. J. Med., 305:545, 1981.)

17–16). Santen and colleagues concluded that medical adrenalectomy with aminoglutethimide plus hydrocortisone can be logically chosen in place of surgical adrenalectomy.

Kiang and associates (1980) reported equivalent response rates and response duration in 26 patients randomized to hypophysectomy or to tamoxifen. Nemoto and colleagues (1984) reported equivalent response rates in 51 patients randomized to tamoxifen and adrenalectomy. The major ablative procedures, adrenalectomy and hypophysectomy, are now seldom used.

Additive Hormonal Therapy

Additive hormonal therapy has changed radically since the first edition of this book. Tamoxifen has emerged as the additive agent of choice, followed by megestrol acetate and aminoglutethimide (Ingle, 1984). Androgens and estrogens, which had traditionally been the mainstays of additive therapy, now play a secondary and even tertiary role. In postmenopausal patients, tamoxifen and aminoglutethimide have essentially replaced the major ablative procedures of adrenalectomy and hypophysectomy. However, oophorectomy remains the primary treatment of metastatic breast cancer in hormonally responsive premenopausal patients. In addition, a new group of drugs, the luteinizing hormone releasing hormone analogues (LHRH agonists) and danazol, are being evaluated on an investigational basis.

As a plateau has been reached in the response rates of advanced breast cancer to both cytotoxic and hormonal therapy, renewed interest has occurred in rates of response to a second hormonal therapy. It has been thought almost axiomatic that the best predictor of response to a second form of hormonal therapy is an initial response to a primary form of hormonal therapy. Although this statement appears to be true, its converse is not; that is, an initial failure to respond to primary hormonal therapy does not rule out a response to subsequent hormonal therapy. Wilson (1983) has reviewed in detail the response of breast cancer to secondary hormonal therapy. When there is a response to an initial form of hormonal therapy, the chance of responding to secondary therapy is approximately 55 per cent. However, as many as 30 per cent of patients with failure to initial therapy will respond to subsequent hormonal manipulation. Wilson's data are summarized in Table 17–18.

It is important to emphasize that response rates and response durations to all of the major forms of additive and ablative hormonal therapy are essentially the same: 75 to 78 per cent in ER+ PgR+; 33 per cent in ER+ PgR−; less than 10 per cent in ER−, PgR−; and 45 per cent in ER−, PgR+ (Tables 17–5 and 17–6). The significant differences lie in the side-effects and the morbidity of the treatment. In addition, the response rate in ER positive patients to various forms of hormonal manipulation by dominant site of metastatic disease (except for brain metastases) is equivalent, contrary to what was formerly believed (Table 17–9).

TAMOXIFEN

Tamoxifen (Nolvadex) is now the treatment of choice for postmenopausal women with hormonally dependent breast cancer (Manni et

Table 17–18. SECONDARY RESPONSE TO HORMONAL THERAPY AFTER RESPONSE OR FAILURE TO INITIAL HORMONAL THERAPY

First Treatment	Second Treatment	Number	Response to First Treatment	Response after First Response	Response after First Failure
Androgen	Tamoxifen	51	26 (51%)	18 (69%)	9 (36%)
Tamoxifen	Androgen	26	11 (42%)	4 (36%)	3 (20%)
Estrogen	Tamoxifen	25	12 (48%)	12 (100%)	8 (62%)
Tamoxifen	Estrogen	5	2 (40%)	2 (100%)	1 (33%)
Progestin	Tamoxifen	7	3 (58%)	2 (67%)	3 (75%)
Tamoxifen	Progestin	12	7 (58%)	1 (14%)	1 (20%)
Oophorectomy/ Adrenelectomy	Tamoxifen	18	8 (44%)	2 (25%)	0 (0%)
Hypophysectomy	Tamoxifen	16	12 (75%)	7 (58%)	0 (0%)
Tamoxifen	Hypophysectomy	58	26 (45%)	15 (58%)	8 (25%)
Tamoxifen	Aiminoglutethimide	91	41 (45%)	22 (54%)	16 (32%)
Aminoglutethimide	Tamoxifen	31	16 (52%)	5 (31%)	2 (13%)
	TOTALS	330	164 (50%)	90 (55%)	51 (31%)

Modified from Wilson, A. J.: Response in breast cancer to a second hormonal therapy. Rev. Endocrine-Related Cancer, *14*:5, 1983.

al., 1979; Ingle et al., 1981). Although oophorectomy remains the primary form of hormonal manipulation in premenopausal women, tamoxifen clearly is the secondary agent of choice (Pritchard et al., 1980; Manni and Pearson, 1980). Tamoxifen has achieved this status as it is effective, with 76 per cent objective responses in ER+, PgR+ cases, and because it is unusually safe and essentially devoid of side-effects (Bloom and Fishman, 1983; Lippman, 1983). The relative role of tamoxifen as primary or secondary hormonal therapy is outlined in Table 17–18.

Tamoxifen is a nonsteroidal antiestrogen that binds to estrogen receptor and forms an inert complex. Direct binding studies with radiolabeled tamoxifen have shown that the numbers of tamoxifen and estradiol binding sites are equivalent (Lippman et al., 1976). With increasing concentrations of tamoxifen, ^{3}H-estradiol is displaced from the estrogen receptor site. Because the action of tamoxifen requires binding with the estrogen receptor, it is ineffective in ER negative cases. A secondary effect of ths administration of tamoxifen is the initiation of cytoplasmic PgR synthesis.

The blockage of estrogen receptors by tamoxifen is a reproducible effect, but tamoxifen-induced regression in rat mammary carcinoma can be reversed by increasing prolactin output with perphenazine (Manni et al., 1977). This suggests that the tamoxifen-ER blockade is not irreversible. It is doubtful that tamoxifen is directly cytotoxic. The tamoxifen-ER complex renders the tumor cell unable to enter the cell cycle and reproduce; therefore, tamoxifen is cytostatic. The malignant cells are not destroyed even though their growth and replication are inhibited by the continued presence of the drug. When the drug has been cleared from a rat with mammary cancer, the normal cycling environment returns, the malignant cells are reactivated, and palpable tumors develop (Jordan et al., 1980). It can therefore be concluded that it clearly is desirable to maintain tamoxifen blood levels for prolonged periods of time to effectively suppress tumor growth (Jordan, 1983; Jordan et al., 1984).

The cytostatic rather than cytocidal properties of tamoxifen have been confirmed by Sutherland and colleagues (1983) and Osborne and coworkers (1983). These investigators demonstrated that tamoxifen acts as a cell cycle inhibitor with the cells accumulating in the G_0-G_1 phase of the cell cycle. However, the cells can be "rescued" from the tamoxifen cell cycle block with estrogen (Lippman and Bolan, 1975). This further confirms the reversibility of the ER-tamoxifen bond. This observation also forms the basis of cell synchronization induced by tamoxifen with "Premarin-priming" that has been used to clinical advantage by Allegra (1983*a*) and Bentz et al. (1987).

In postmenopausal patients, tamoxifen has little effect on circulating gonadotropin levels or on plasma concentrations of estrogens. However, in premenopausal patients, tamoxifen induces profound increases in plasma estradiol level and at high doses increases pituitary gonadotropin levels as well (Lippman, 1983). On this basis it might be anticipated that a lower response rate would occur in premenopausal women, but this has not been observed (Pritchard et al., 1980; Margreitar and Wiegele, 1984).

Tamoxifen Dose. In postmenopausal patients, tamoxifen does not have a significant dose-response curve. Responses to the standard dose of 10 mg twice daily are equivalent to those for 20 mg twice daily, and doses up to 90 mg daily have no advantage (Ingle, 1984). The appropriate dose of tamoxifen in premenopausal women is more difficult to recommend. Most studies have used 20 mg twice daily, but the response rates have been equivalent to those for 10 mg two or three times daily. Manni and Pearson (1980) evaluated tamoxifen in doses of 40 to 120 mg/day in premenopausal women with advanced breast cancer. They noted that although a dose of 40 mg/day was able to induce tumor regression, it was unable to completely suppress the menstrual cycle. Doses of 120 mg/day were more effective in suppression of menses but were not more effective in inducing an antitumor response.

Tamoxifen Flare. Tamoxifen flare was described in 1978 by Plotkin and coworkers. This curious phenomenon, characterized by increased bone or soft tissue pain and occasionally hypercalcemia, occurs in approximately 10 per cent of cases. When a flare occurs it develops in the first few weeks of therapy. Contrary to its manifestations, which may seem like progression, a flare generally heralds a response to treatment. Flares should be treated with analgesics or other symptomatic therapy, and full dose tamoxifen should be continued. Brooks and Lippman (1985) have proposed that the flare occurs because it takes several weeks for tamoxifen to reach therapeutic levels, and at lower concentrations the drug may be estrogenic and stimulatory, as has been noted in tissue culture.

Several cases of thromboembolic complications have been reported to have developed within 6 months of the initiation of tamoxifen therapy (Lipton et al., 1984). The frequency of this complication is unknown, but Enck and Rios (1984) have reported lowered functional antithrombin III levels in 42 per cent of a small group of patients on tamoxifen therapy. The other side-effects of tamoxifen are directly related to estrogen blockade, such as hot flashes, menstrual irregularities, and, rarely, dysfunctional uterine bleeding.

Adjuvant Tamoxifen in Stage II Breast Cancer. Over the past 10 years there has been considerable interest in the adjuvant use of tamoxifen. Most of the trials in the United States have included cytotoxic chemotherapy alone, although a recent NSABP trial evaluated cytotoxic chemotherapy with 5-fluorouracil and melphalan (L-PAM) with and without tamoxifen (Fisher et al., 1981, 1983b). The Eastern Cooperative Oncology Group reported a similar chemohormonal adjuvant study (Taylor et al., 1985.). The rationale for adjuvant therapy is illustrated in Tables 17–1, 17–14 and 17–15, as well as in Figures 17–11 to 17–13. These tables and figures illustrate the usefulness of axillary nodal status as well as receptor status in predicting recurrence in Stage I and Stage II breast cancer.

In Europe and Canada, there has been considerable interest in the use of tamoxifen alone as an adjuvant in Stage II breast cancer, particularly in postmenopausal patients (Baum et al., 1983, 1985; Ribeiro and Palmer, 1983; Rose et al., 1985; Pritchard, 1987). As tamoxifen is cytostatic rather than cytocidal, cells are still capable of replicating and must be suppressed for prolonged periods by continuous therapy (Jordan et al., 1984). This establishes the rationale for continuing adjuvant tamoxifen indefinitely. Although short-term tamoxifen has been essentially devoid of side-effects, the possible development of long-term complications from continuous antiestrogen therapy, such as osteoporosis, must be a concern (Gotfredsen et al., 1984).

Of the major tamoxifen adjuvant studies reported to date, one has demonstrated a prolongation in absolute survival. This is the Nolvadex Adjuvant Trial Organization (NATO) trial under the chairmanship of Michael Baum (Baum et al., 1985). The NATO trial began November 1, 1977, and was closed to patient entry on February 6, 1981. A total of 1285 women aged 75 years or younger were entered. Premenopausal women with positive axillary nodes and postmenopausal women with both positive and negative axillary nodes were randomized either to an untreated control group or to receive 10 mg of tamoxifen twice daily for 2 years. In 1983 NATO was able to report a significant improvement in the disease-free interval (Fig. 17–17) in the tamoxifen-treated group (Baum et al., 1983), and in 1985 a significant improvement was reported in absolute survival (Fig. 17–18) (Baum et al., 1985). There were 34 per cent fewer deaths in the tamoxifen-treated group than in the untreated controls. The benefit appeared to be independent of menopausal, nodal, or ER status. The NATO group admits that the fail-

520   17 • Endocrine Therapy of Breast Cancer

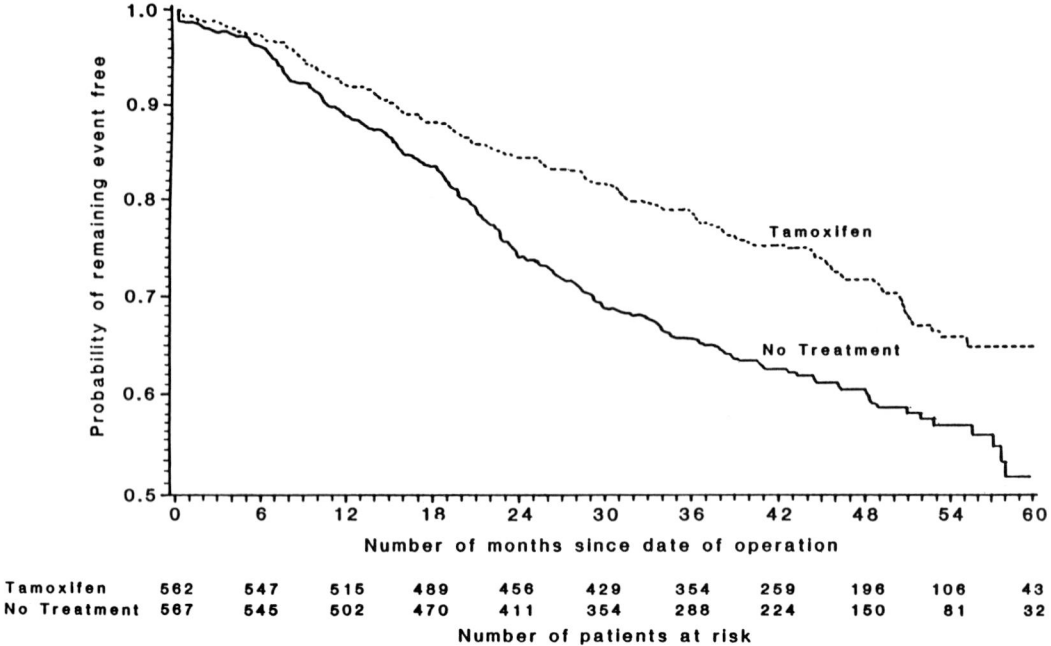

Figure 17–17. Results of the Nolvadex Adjuvant Trial Organization (1985) demonstrating prolonged disease free survival in breast cancer patients treated with adjuvant tamoxifen. (Modified from Baum, M., et al.: Controlled trial of tamoxifen as single adjuvant agent in the management of early breast cancer: Analysis at six years by Nolvadex Adjuvant Trial Organization. Lancet, 1:836, 1985. Used with permission.)

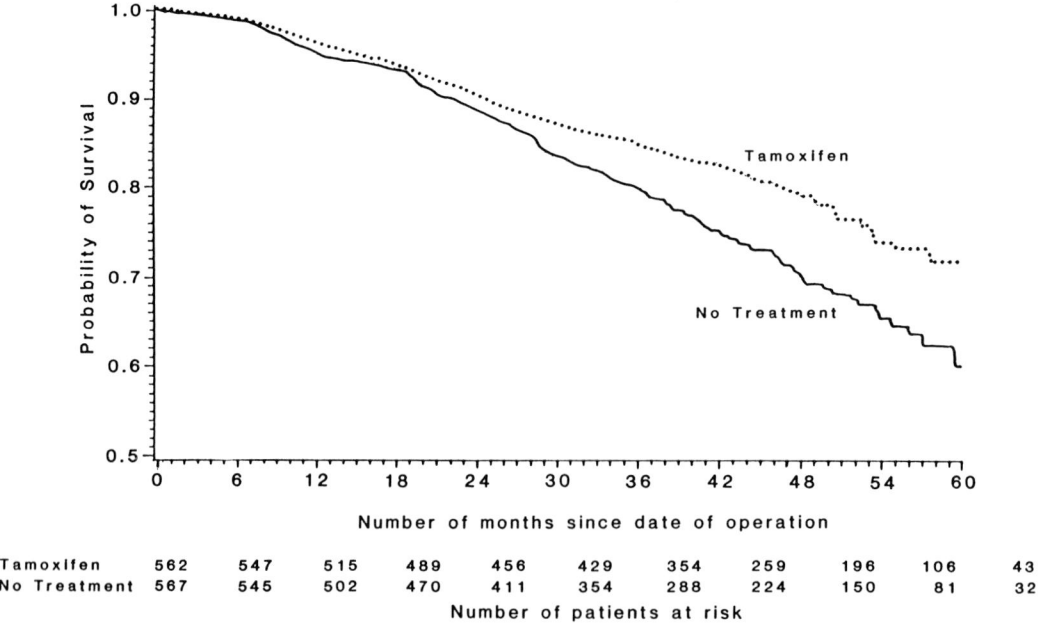

Figure 17–18. Results of the Nolvadex Adjuvant Trial Organization (1985) demonstrating prolonged absolute survival in breast cancer patients treated with adjuvant tamoxifen. (Modified from Baum, M., et al.: Controlled trial of tamoxifen as single adjuvant agent in the management of early breast cancer: Analysis at six years by Nolvadex Adjuvant Trial Organization. Lancet, 1:836, 1985. Used with permission.)

ure of the ER content to predict response to tamoxifen is "counterintuitive." Ribeiro and Palmer (1983), studying a small group of postmenopausal women with four or more positive nodes, in whom ER assays had not been performed, reported a striking survival advantage in the tamoxifen-treated group (Fig. 17–19). However, in two other major adjuvant studies randomizing patients to tamoxifen alone versus a no treatment control, benefit from tamoxifen therapy was restricted to ER positive patients (Pritchard et al., 1984; Rose et al., 1985). In fact, the Danish Breast Cancer Cooperative Group (Rose et al., 1985). noted a quantitative relationship between ER content and relapse-free survival (Fig. 17–20). In the Danish study, postmenopausal women with poor prognosis breast cancer (defined as positive axillary nodes, tumor ≥ 5 cm in diameter, or invasion of the skin or fascia) were randomized between postoperative radiation therapy (RT) or postoperative RT plus tamoxifen. There was no benefit from the addition of tamoxifen in patients with ER < 100 fmol/mg, but those with ER ≥ 100 fmol/mg had a significantly longer relapse-free survival.

The National Surgical Adjuvant Breast Project (NSABP) reported a clinical trial for the adjuvant therapy of Stage II breast cancer comparing chemotherapy with 5-fluorouracil and L-PAM (PF) versus PF and tamoxifen (PFT) (Fisher et al., 1981, 1983b). Patients 50 years of age or older with either one to three or more than three positive axillary nodes had a markedly longer disease-free survival with PFT than with PF. The effectiveness of PFT was related to the quantitative levels of both ER and PgR (Fig. 17–21). However, in women younger than 50 years old no difference was seen between PF and PFT regardless of receptor concentration (Fig. 17–22). In light of the European data it must be suspected that the benefit observed in the postmenopausal (≥ 50 years) group was from the tamoxifen alone rather than from the PFT combination. The NSABP initiated a clinical trial in September 1984, which should help answer this question (Fig. 17–23).

The National Institutes of Health convened a Consensus Development Conference on Adjuvant Chemotherapy for Breast Cancer on September 9–11, 1985. One of the major topics addressed by the Consensus panel was the role of endocrine treatment in the adjuvant therapy of breast cancer. After review of the available data, the following statement was issued: "Tamoxifen should now be regarded as standard therapy for postmenopausal patients with positive axillary lymph nodes and positive hormone receptor status." They also concluded that "a longer duration of adjuvant tamoxifen (at least 2 years) may be more effective than 1 year," and that there is "no evidence to suggest that a dose of tamoxifen of higher than 20 mg per day is indicated" (Consensus Conference, 1985).

PROGESTINS

The progestins have emerged as the clear second choice, after tamoxifen, in the additive hormonal therapy of endocrine responsive breast cancer in postmenopausal women. Their role in premenopausal women is not yet well defined. The allocation of progestins to sec-

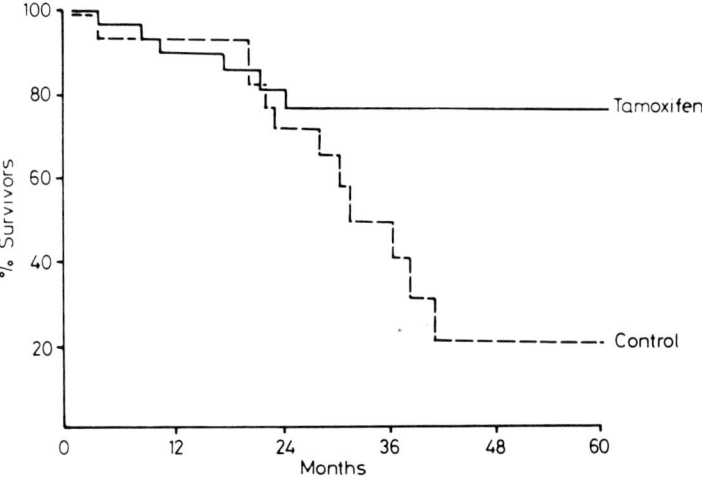

Figure 17–19. Absolute survival of postmenopausal women with four or more positive axillary lymph nodes (N = 67) treated with adjuvant tamoxifen as compared with a no treatment control group (N = 12). (From Ribeiro, G., and Palmer, M. K.: Adjuvant tamoxifen for operable carcinoma of the breast. Report of clinical trial by the Christel Hospital and Holt Radium Institute. Br. Med. J., 286:827, 1983. Reprinted with permission.)

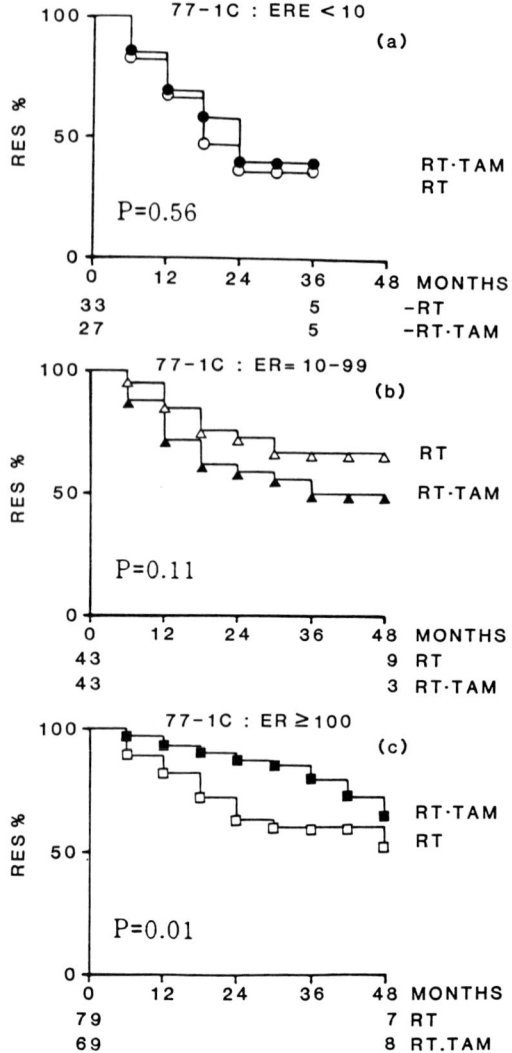

Figure 17–20. Recurrence-free survival (RFS) in relation to quantitative estrogen receptor (ER) assay (< 10 fmol/mg, 10 to 99 fmol/mg, ≥ 100 fmol/mg) and mode of adjuvant treatment in stage II breast cancer. RT, Radiation therapy; TAM, tamoxifen. (From Rose, C., et al.: Beneficial effect of adjuvant tamoxifen therapy in primary breast cancer in patients with high estrogen receptor values. Lancet, 1:16, 1985. Reprinted with permission.)

ond-line therapy may not be totally justified as response rates in ER+, PgR+ patients appear to be equivalent to those for tamoxifen (Morgan, 1985; Muss et al., 1985) (Fig. 17–24). However, recent data from Muss and coworkers (1987) have demonstrated that even though response rates are equivalent, the disease-free survival of patients treated initially with tamoxifen is significantly greater than that of those treated with megestrol acetate ($p = 0.009$). The side-effects of progestins, although minimal, may be slightly greater than those of tamoxifen (Ingle, 1984). Progestins may be associated with mild glucocorticoid action and weight gain (Gregory et al., 1985). Of the available progestins, megestrol acetate (Megace) is currently the drug of choice for its ease of administration, safety, and efficacy.

Progestins appear to have a direct cytotoxic action on human breast cancer cells in long-term tissue culture (Allegra and Kiefer, 1985). Progestins are also antiestrogenic and exhibit a general inhibitory effect on estrogen-induced protein synthesis. The antiestrogenic effect appears to be a result of a decrease in the concentration of cytoplasmic ER or its nuclear translocation, or both (Rochefort, 1984). Because of their antiestrogenic properties, progestins clearly are more active in receptor positive patients, and not surprisingly, PgR is the single best predictor of response (Blumenschein, 1983; Johnson et al., 1983).

The dose of megestrol acetate is 40 mg four times daily, although a single oral dose of 160 mg daily appears to be well tolerated and to have comparable therapeutic efficacy (Carpenter and Peterson, 1985). In contrast to tamoxifen, progestins may exhibit a dose-response curve. Cavilli and associates (1984) have reported a significantly higher response in women treated with medroxyprogesterone acetate (MPA) at a dose of 1000 mg intramuscularly daily, compared with those treated with 500 mg intramuscularly three times weekly. However, Pannuti and coworkers (1979) were not able to demonstrate a difference in response between doses of 1500 mg and 500 mg of MPA intramuscularly daily.

Hypercalcemic and pain flares have also been reported with megestrol acetate (Otteman and Long, 1984). Like tamoxifen flares, a megestrol flare may herald a response to treatment (Greenwald, 1983).

The relative response rates to progestational agents as primary or secondary therapy for metastatic breast cancer are illustrated in Table 17–18.

AMINOGLUTETHIMIDE

Aminoglutethimide (AG) was initially introduced in the 1960s as an anticonvulsant agent but was found to be a potent blocker of adrenal steroidogenesis (Cash et al., 1967). Of greater importance with reference to breast cancer, AG also blocks the aromatase system and via this mechanism blocks the peripheral conver-

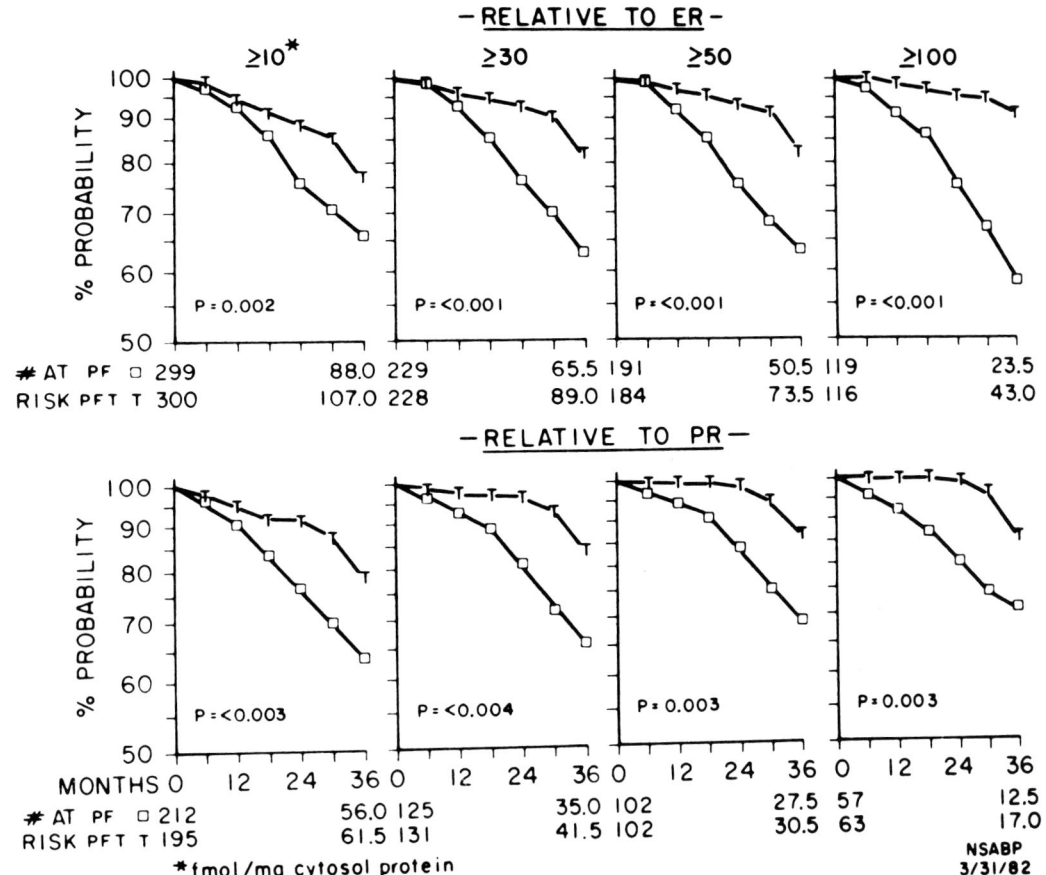

Figure 17–21. Disease-free survival in stage II breast cancer patients age 50 years or older treated with PF (L-PAM + 5-fluorouracil) versus PFT (PF + tamoxifen) relative to estrogen receptor (ER) and progesterone receptor (PR) concentration. (From Fisher, B., et al.: Influence of estrogen and progesterone receptor levels on the response to tamoxifen and chemotherapy in primary breast cancer. J. Clin. Oncol., 1:227, 1983. Copyright 1983 by American Society of Clinical Oncology. Reprinted with permission.)

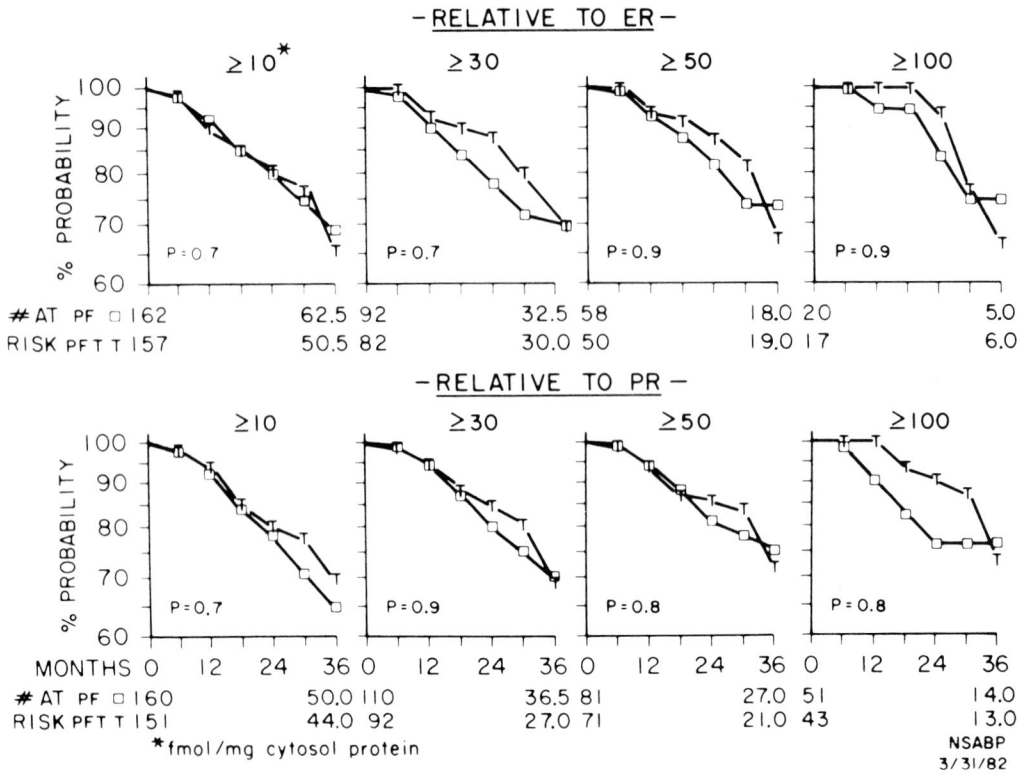

Figure 17–22. Disease-free survival in stage II breast cancer patients age 49 years or less treated with PF (L-PAM + 5-fluorouracil) versus PFT (PF + tamoxifen) relative to estrogen receptor (ER) and progesterone receptor (PR) concentration. (From Fisher, B., et al.: Influence of estrogen and progesterone receptor levels on the response to tamoxifen and chemotherapy in primary breast cancer. J. Clin. Oncol., *1*:227, 1983. Copyright 1983 by American Society of Clinical Oncology. Reprinted with permission.)

sion of androstenedione to estrone (Fig. 17–2). This effectively blocks estrogen production in adrenal tissue, adipose tissue, and breast cancer tissue as well (Miller et al., 1982; Siiteri, 1982). Samojlik and colleagues (1982) have noted that, in postmenopausal women with metastatic breast cancer who were treated with AG, plasma estrone levels declined 72 per cent and the urinary excretion of estrone fell 85 per cent over a 12 week period. Aminoglutethimide appears to be equally effective in inducing suppression of estrogen synthesis in postmenopausal and in premenopausal women who have had a prior oophorectomy. Because of this, AG has become of major importance in the treatment of premenopausal women with hormonally responsive breast cancer. AG has essentially replaced the need for surgical adrenalectomy and hypophysectomy in the treatment of advanced breast cancer (Santen et al., 1981) (Figs. 17–5 and 17–16).

Recommended dosage of AG is 250 mg twice daily for 14 days, increasing to four times a day thereafter; plus 100 mg of hydrocortisone (20 mg in the morning, 20 mg at 5 P.M., and 60 mg at bedtime) for 14 days and then 40 mg daily thereafter (10 mg in the morning, 10 mg at 5 P.M., and 20 mg at bedtime) (Lipton et al., 1982).

Because its side-effects are significantly greater than those of tamoxifen, megestrol acetate, or oophorectomy, AG has been relegated to a tertiary role in hormonal therapy. Acute toxicities occurring in the first 6 weeks include lethargy in 48 per cent, drug rash in 33 per cent, orthostatic hyotension with dizziness in 20 per cent, ataxia in 10 per cent, and drug fever in 2.5 per cent. After 6 weeks, even with continuous therapy, the side effects decline significantly: lethargy in 10 per cent, orthostatic hypotension and dizziness in 12 per cent, depression in 10 per cent, hypothyroidism in 5 per cent, and ataxia, blurred vision, nausea, or a combination of these in 2.5 per cent (Santen et al., 1981). Severe hematologic toxicity with leukopenia, thrombocytopenia,

NSABP PROTOCOL B-16

Adjuvant Therapy For Stage II Breast Cancer

AGE AND RECEPTOR CRITERIA

50-59 years with PgR ≥10 fm/mg
60-70 years – all patients

- Tamoxifen alone x 5 years
- Tamoxifen x 5 years + AC Q 21 days x 4 cycles
- Tamoxifen x 5 years + PF Q 6 wks x 17 cycles + Adriamycin Q 3 wks. (max. 300mg/m^2)

Figure 17-23. Schema of NSABP protocol B-16. This important study is designed to determine if the beneficial effect observed in receptor positive *postmenopausal* (≥50 years) stage II breast cancer patients by the addition of tamoxifen to PF (L-PAM + 5-fluorouracil) adjuvant chemotherapy (see Fig. 17–22) is from the tamoxifen alone (see Figs. 17–18 to 17–20 and 17–22) or from the combined chemohormonal therapy (PF + tamoxifen). A second question being asked is whether Adriamycin plus cyclophosphamide (AC) will enhance the effect of tamoxifen. This study opened for patient entry in September 1984.

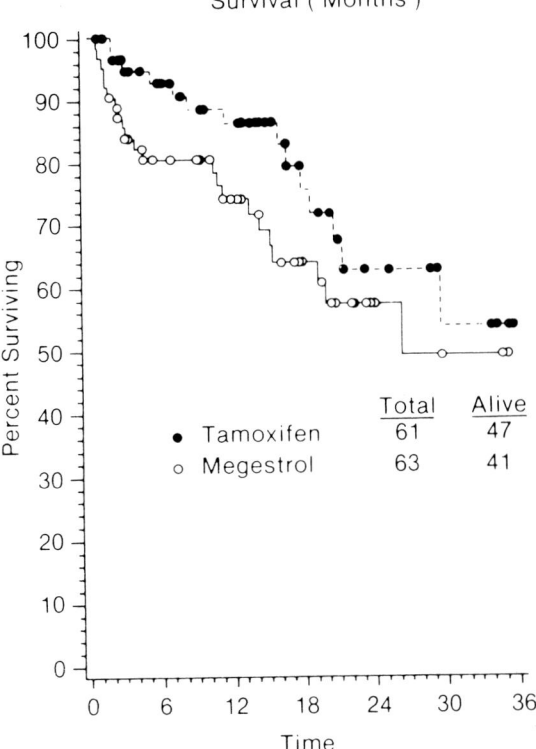

Figure 17–24. Even though there is a trend in favor of tamoxifen, as yet there is no definite survival advantage ($p=0.16$). (From Muss, H. B., et al.: Megestrol acetate versus tamoxifen in advanced breast cancer: A phase III trial of the Piedmont Oncology Association [POA]. Semin. Oncol., *12*(Suppl. 1):55, 1985. Reprinted with permission.) However, recent data (Muss, H. B., et al. 1987) have demonstrated a significantly greater disease-free survival for patients treated initially with tamoxifen ($p=0.009$).

or even pancytopenia may occur in up to 4 per cent of patients (Ingle, 1984).

An adjuvant study currently in progress at the Royal Marsden Hospital in England is comparing AG versus placebo therapy in postmenopausal patients with Stage II breast cancer. At this time the data are too preliminary to draw any conclusions (Coombes et al., 1984).

The relative efficacy of AG in the primary and secondary therapy of advanced breast cancer is shown in Table 17–18.

ESTROGENS

Prior to the introduction of tamoxifen, diethylstilbestrol (DES), a synthetic estrogen, was the hormonal treatment of choice in postmenopausal women with advanced breast cancer (Ingle et al., 1981). Large doses of estrogens gave the highest response rate and the most prolonged remissions (Kennedy, 1974). In postmenopausal women, the overall random response rate to estrogens is 36 per cent, but response increases with age and the number of years post menopause (Council on Drugs, 1960). The overall response rate to DES in ER positive tumors is 63 per cent. In general, the median duration of response to estrogen is 12 to 18 months, but responses of longer than 5 years have been documented.

The mechanism by which estrogens act on metastatic breast cancer is unknown. Tumor cells that contain ER bind estrogens with great affinity and specificity. High dose estrogen may flood the system and by mass action may actually be antiestrogenic. Hall (1974) proposed that tumor cells that respond to high dose estrogen may be more like than unlike normal cells, and massive doses of a normal differentiation-promoting substance might cause the tumor to mature, differentiate, and stop proliferating.

The most commonly used estrogen remains diethylstilbestrol, in the dosage of 5 mg three times daily. Other estrogen preparations that have been used are ethinyl estradiol, 3 mg daily, and conjugated equine estrogens, 30 mg daily.

Nausea is the most common early side-effect of DES. This may be avoided by increasing the dose in a stepwise fashion, that is, starting with 5 mg daily for 7 to 10 days, increasing to 5 mg twice a day for an additional 7 to 10 days, and then giving the full dosage of 5 mg three times daily. Vomiting, anorexia, and even diarrhea may occur, but the gastrointestinal side-effects of DES usually subside within 2 weeks. Increased nipple, areolar, and axillary pigmentation is frequent. Fluid retention occurs in about one third of cases and may aggravate or even precipitate congestive heart failure. The use of high-dose estrogens may be associated with thromboembolic phenomena.

Breakthrough or withdrawal uterine bleeding in postmenopausal women on estrogen therapy occurs in 40 per cent of patients. This is usually of little clinical significance and responds to cessation of treatment or abates spontaneously with continued therapy, but if persistent it may require dilation and curettage. Persistent uterine bleeding associated with estrogen therapy may signal the presence of an endometrial carcinoma.

Hypercalcemic flares occur in from 10 to 25 per cent of women with metastatic breast cancer treated with DES (Kennedy et al., 1953). For practical purposes, in breast cancer patients, spontaneous or induced hypercalcemia occurs only in association with osseous metastases. Induced hypercalcemia from any additive form of hormonal therapy seems to indicate that the tumor has retained its endocrine responsiveness and often heralds a response to continued hormonal treatment (Hall et al., 1963; Muggia and Heinemann, 1970).

Estrogen Rebound Regression. Patients who respond to estrogen therapy and who later escape from the therapeutic effect with progression of metastatic disease may respond to the sudden withdrawal of estrogens with another period of tumor regression. Rebound regression was originally described by Escher (1949) and occurs in up to 32 per cent of estrogen responders (Kaufman and Escher, 1961; Baker and Vaitkevicius, 1972). Patients who show a rebound response have a significantly longer disease-free interval before estrogen therapy than those who do not. The duration of rebound regression is usually 3 to 10 months, but Nestro and colleagues (1976) reported that the median duration was in excess of 18 months.

Case History (No. 63-31885, EFSCH)

In September 1963, a 66 year old black woman complained of a mass in the right breast of 1 month's duration. The entire right breast was found to be occupied by a mass that was hard and fixed to the skin. Axillary adenopathy was present on the side of the lesion, and the largest lymph node measured 1.5 × 2.0 cm. A needle biopsy of the breast mass revealed poorly differentiated adenocarcinoma. Because of the locally advanced stage of the lesion, the patient was not considered a candidate for mastectomy and was placed on diethylstilbestrol, 5 mg orally three times a day. She continued to take this medication for almost 2 years with symptomatic improvement and almost total regression of the primary neoplasm. In September 1965, the breast mass measured only 2.0 × 2.5 cm; however, progression was evident in the form of newly developing subcutaneous nodules in the involved breast, a 1 cm right supraclavicular lymph node, and a 1.5 cm hard lesion in the opposite breast. Stilbestrol was discontinued, and after 1 month all palpable lesions had diminished in size. Three months after suspending therapy, all masses, including the original one in the right breast, were absent, and the only evidence of residual disease was a 1.5 cm lymph node located in the right axilla. In November 1973 the patient was still free of disease. She died in March 1974 at the age of 77 years, almost 11 years after her initial treatment.

ANDROGENS

Androgens were the first additive agents to prove useful for the hormonal therapy of mammary cancer. Through the animal research of Lacassagne and Raynaud (1939) it became evident that testosterone could inhibit certain implantable and spontaneously occurring neoplasms. In London in the same year, Loeser (1939) reported two cases in which postoperative recurrence of mammary cancer had not reappeared for one and a half years after incidental androgen treatment directed toward menstrual problems. Ulrich (1939) in Paris noted marked shrinkage of breast tumors in two women who were receiving androgens. Fels (1944) in Argentina also noted favorable results in three women aged 34, 48, and 54 years who were treated with testosterone. Farrow and Woodward (1942) treated 33 patients with testosterone and first reported the rise of serum calcium level, which often is induced by androgens when bony metastases are present. Further experience with androgens established their palliative value in both premenopausal and postmenopausal women with disseminated disease.

The Cooperative Breast Cancer Group amassed considerable experience with androgenic agents. In 1964, this group reported the results of therapy in 564 postmenopausal women with metastatic mammary cancer treated with testosterone proprionate (Cooperative Breast Cancer Group, 1964). An overall objective regression rate of 21 per cent was observed. Based upon pre-ER data, the response of osseous metastases to androgens is equivalent to that for estrogens, 25 to 30 per cent, but the response rate of soft tissue metastases (breast, skin, nodes) to androgens (20 to 25 per cent) is significantly less than the 35 to 45 per cent reported for estrogens (Kennedy, 1974). Fewer than 18 per cent of visceral metastases respond to androgens (Kennedy, 1965). Because of the inferior response rate of visceral and soft tissue lesions, metastatic bone disease should be considered the primary indication for the use of androgens (Fig. 17–25).

Androgens display their antitumor effect in receptor positive patients with breast cancer by two mechanisms of action: (1) blocking of pituitary gonadotropin release and subsequent ovarian secretion of estrogen; and (2) an antiestrogenic effect (Rochefort, 1984).

Androgens exert their antiestrogenic effect by complex interactions with three receptors: ER, PgR, and androgen receptor (AR). Androgens in high doses are stimulating to human breast cancer cells in tissue culture, and this effect is mediated via the ER (Zava and McGuire, 1978). However, at lower doses, androgens compete with estradiol for the ER and are antiestrogenic. Androgens can also bind to PgR and may have progestin-like actions. Because the dosage of androgen required to give an antiestrogenic effect is in the range to saturate the AR but is too low to saturate the ER, it has been postulated that the therapeutic effect is mediated via the AR. This is verified, at least to some degree, by the observation that in tissue culture of rat mammary carcinomas and human breast cancer, antiandrogens such as cyproterone inhibit the antiestrogenic effect of androgens (Rochefort, 1984).

The subjective, hematopoietic, and anabolic effects of androgens are notable. Androgens stimulate erythropoiesis probably via erythropoietin (Kennedy, 1962). Patients treated with androgens may experience an increased sense of well-being, pain relief, increased appetite, and weight gain. According to Kennedy, however (1974), it is not unusual to observe continued progression of disease despite excellent symptomatic improvement.

The side-effects of androgens are predominantly those associated with the physiologic effects of male hormones, that is, virilization with frontal baldness, plethora, acne, hirsutism, fluid retention, and, less commonly, an increased libido and clitoral hypertrophy. The virilizing effects vary with the androgenic preparation used. They occur in more than 50 per cent of patients treated with testosterone propionate, in 35 to 40 per cent of patients treated with fluoxymesterone, and in none treated with testolactone. Unfortunately, the virilizing and therapeutic effects of androgens may not be totally separable; the objective response rate to testolactone is only 14 per cent (Volk et al., 1974). Androgens with a 17 α methyl substitution, such as fluoxymesterone and methyltestosterone, may cause reversible cholestatic jaundice and, rarely, a multifocal hepatocellular necrosis termed peliosis hepatis (Naeim et al., 1973; Bagheri and Boyer, 1974). Owing to large areas of cystic hemorrhagic necrosis, peliosis hepatis may cause an abnormal liver scan that can be confused with metastases.

Fluoxymesterone (Halotestin) has emerged as the androgen of choice because it is at least as potent as testosterone propionate, is less virilizing, and can be taken orally. The dosage for fluoxymesterone is 20 to 30 mg by mouth daily.

ADRENAL CORTICOSTEROIDS

There are only limited indications for the use of corticosteroids as single agents for metastatic breast cancer. Responses to corticosteroids are generally nonspecific, but temporary objective regression of tumor occurs in approximately 18 per cent of cases (Kelley, 1971). Specific tumor responses appear to be limited to premenopausal patients with a prior response to castration and to postmenopausal women with a prior response to other forms of additive therapy (Kennedy, 1965). Unlike the case with aminoglutethimide, the use of

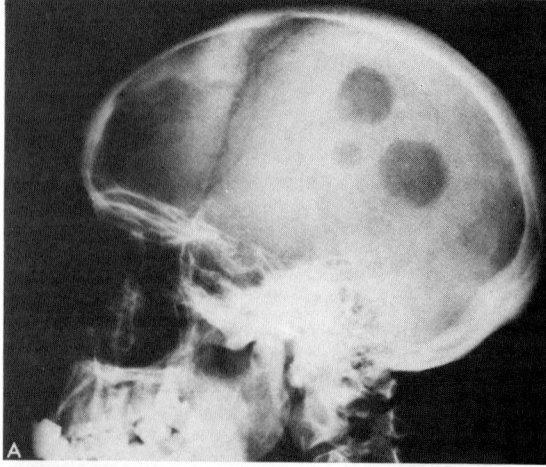
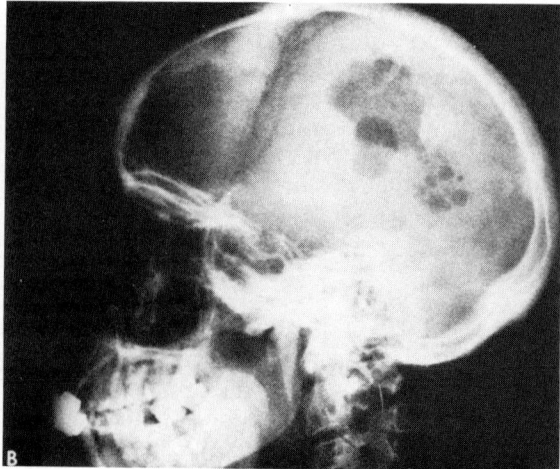
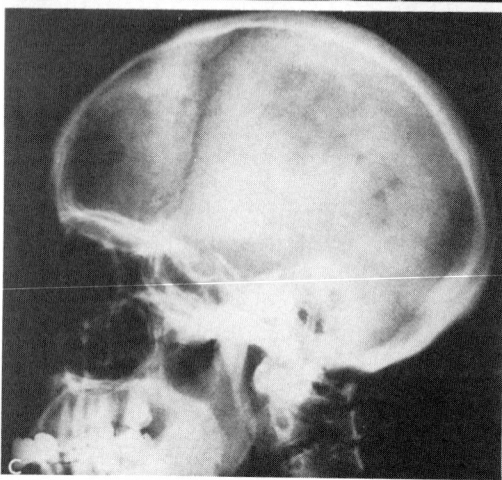

Figure 17–25. This 65 year old black woman had a right modified mastectomy in June 1975 for an invasive carcinoma of the right breast with axillary metastases, and she received postoperative irradiation. A, Sixteen months after her operation, lytic metastases became evident in the skull and pelvis. She was placed on diethylstilbestrol, 5 mg orally three times daily, and after 6.5 months x-rays showed a mixed response (B). The two most prominent lesions had enlarged, and small new ones appeared peripheral to them. The posterior defect had recalcified, but within it lytic areas suggested growth of estrogen-resistant clones of cells. Estrogens were discontinued and after a 1 month delay fluoxymesterone was begun at a dose of 10 mg twice daily. C, Three months later all lesions were recalcifying and eventually healed. This patient's tumor appeared to represent a mixed population of cells, some of which were sensitive to estrogens and others to androgens.

corticosteroids does not constitute a "medical adrenalectomy."

It has been proposed that corticosteroids may be helpful in the treatment of jaundice due to hepatic metastases and restricted lung function due to lymphangitic pulmonary metastases, but data are sparse. Corticosteroids are often used in combination with cytotoxic agents, but the contribution of corticosteroids to combination chemotherapy remains questionable.

Adrenal corticosteroids are particularly helpful in the medical management of brain or spinal cord metastases. For the acute management of increased intracranial pressure, a loading dose of dexamethasone, 8 mg intravenously, can be given followed by 4 mg intravenously or orally every 6 hours. The long-term use of daily high-dose dexamethasone can precipitate fluid and electrolyte imbalances and steroid myopathies. Hyperosmolar states can also develop in patients with a diabetic tendency. The dose of dexamethasone during radiation therapy for brain or spinal cord metastases should be maintained at 4 mg every 6 to 8 hours. Following completion of radiation therapy, the dexamethasone dosage should be tapered over a 2- to 3-week period (Kornblith et al., 1985).

Corticosteroids may be a useful adjunct in the management of patients with far advanced or preterminal disease, frequently causing euphoria, stimulating appetite, and decreasing pain (Schell, 1972). Schell demonstrated that narcotic requirements were often decreased. Subjective improvement occurs in as many as 75 per cent of the patients treated. Bruera and coworkers (1985) recently reported a randomized double-blind study of methylprednisolone versus placebo in terminally ill cancer patients and confirmed Schell's observations. Terminally ill cancer patients treated with 32 mg of methylprednisolone daily had decreased pain intensity, increased appetite, and increased sense of well-being over placebo-treated controls.

It is difficult to make dose recommendations as no dose-response data are available for breast cancer. Objective tumor regression has followed cortisone acetate, 100 to 400 mg daily, and prednisone, 30 to 250 mg daily. The lower doses may be as effective as the high doses (Gardner et al., 1962; Stoll, 1963). Euphoria can be produced by 20 to 40 mg of oral prednisone daily.

The side-effects of long-term corticosteroid administration are well known. These include sodium and fluid retention, aggravation or precipitation of diabetes mellitus, hypertension, hypokalemia, muscle weakness, peptic ulcer, defects of cell-mediated immunity, and overt Cushing's syndrome.

Newer Agents for Hormonal Manipulation

LHRH AGONISTS

In animals, chronic treatment with supraphysiologic doses of luteinizing hormone releasing hormone (LHRH) agonists causes (1) decreased gonadotrophin (FSH and LH) excretion, (2) decreased prolactin excretion, (3) decrease in plasma sex steroid concentration, (4) reduction in weight of secondary sexual organs, and (5) inhibition of the actions of the sex steroids at their target organs (Klijn et al., 1984). LHRH analogues, therefore, act directly or indirectly on the pituitary, the gonads, and the target organs of the sex steroids. Schally and coworkers (1984) have demonstrated significantly decreased tumor weight and volume in mouse and rat mammary cancers treated with D-Trp^6-LH-RH (decapeptyl). Currently, the LHRH analogues, buserelin, decapeptyl, and leuprolide, are in clinical trials. Leuprolide is now commercially available for the treatment of prostate cancer (Leuprolide Study Group, 1984). However, leuprolide also seems to have activity in premenopausal women with advanced breast cancer. Harvey and coworkers (1985) reported objective responses in 11 of 25 cases treated with leuprolide.

Preliminary data from Klijn and deJong (1982) and Klijn and coworkers (1984) on the use of buserelin for metastatic breast cancer in premenopausal women have been favorable. Eight of 17 patients had an objective response to buserelin alone or in combination with tamoxifen. One of the responders was ER negative, raising the question as to whether the response was mediated by the decrease in prolactin levels. Mathé and coworkers (1987), using Schally's "decapeptyl," have observed responses in both premenopausal and postmenopausal women with advanced breast cancer.

DANAZOL

Danazol (2,3-isoxazol-17α-ethinyl testosterone) has four important mechanisms of action: (1) inhibition of pituitary gonadotropin secretion, probably by inhibiting gonadotropin-releasing hormone, (2) inhibition of adrenal and gonadal steroidogenesis, (3) binding to androgen and progesterone receptors, and (4) binding to sex hormone binding globulin and corticosteroid binding globulin (Barbieri and Ryan, 1981). Danazol is relatively nontoxic and has been released by the FDA for the treatment of endometriosis and relief of the pain and nodularity associated with chronic cystic mastopathy (Ingle, 1984).

Peters and coworkers (1977) reported a 66 per cent objective response rate to danazol in the treatment of dimethylbenzanthracene (DMBA)-induced mammary cancers in rats. In doses of 100 to 200 mg three times daily (same dosage range as for treatment of chronic cystic mastopathy), Coombes and associates (1980) reported objective responses in 7 of 37 postmenopausal patients treated with danazol.

SOMATOSTATIN

Somatostatin inhibits growth hormone release, prolactin secretion, insulin and glucagon release, and pentagastrin-induced gastric secretion (Schally et al., 1986; Karashima and Schally, 1987). Somatostatin also inhibits other growth factors such as epidermal growth factor (EGF) and transforming growth factor beta (TGFβ). Somatostatin analogues possess significant antitumor activity in experimental tumors, including rat mammary carcinomas (Schally et al., 1987). Clinical trials of somatostatin analogues in human breast cancer will soon be initiated.

COMBINATION HORMONAL THERAPY

Numerous combinations of hormonal agents have been evaluated in the treatment of metastatic breast cancer: fluoxymesterone plus ethinyl estradiol, DES plus testosterone propionate, tamoxifen plus megestrol acetate, tamoxifen plus medroxyprogesterone acetate, tamoxifen plus DES, tamoxifen plus prednisone, tamoxifen plus AG, tamoxifen plus fluoxymesterone, medroxyprogesterone acetate plus AG, and ethinyl estradiol plus medroxyprogesterone acetate. The results of all of these studies can be summarized with the statement that the combinations failed to demonstrate an advantage over the use of single agent hormonal therapy. This is what would be anticipated as the mechanism of action of each of these agents is basically the same—inhibition of synthesis or action of estrogen. What is of more interest from a conceptual point of view are the preliminary studies of Klijn and coworkers (1984) using the antiestrogen tamoxifen with the antiprolactin drug buserelin, thus blocking the two major mitogenic hormones to the breast. Further studies with tamoxifen plus buserelin in a large series of patients would be of considerable interest.

COMBINATION CHEMOHORMONAL THERAPY

The rationale for the use of combination therapy with cytotoxic drugs and hormonal manipulation is based upon three assumptions: (1) tumors are heterogeneous (i.e., breast cancers are composed of various proportions of receptor positive and receptor negative cells); (2) there is a differential response between receptor positive and receptor negative cells to cytotoxic chemotherapy and hormonal therapy; and (3) neither chemotherapy nor hormonal therapy interferes with the action of the other form of treatment, so that response rates for combined therapy will be additive and not antagonistic. Unfortunately, these three assumptions may not be totally valid.

One limitation of the methods currently available for assaying ER and PgR in tissue cytosol is the inability to assess heterogeneity within the breast cancer itself (DeSombre et al., 1984). Various histologic methods to stain for ER have been attempted, but although they seem to confirm tissue heterogeneity with regard to ER, the results have been inconsistent with the cytosolic ER assays (DeSombre, 1982). King and colleagues (1982) have described the use of a specific monoclonal antibody to human breast cancer ER in lightly fixed and frozen sections of tissue. Interestingly, using this technique in ER rich breast cancer, all of the staining is restricted to the cell nuclei. This implies that ER may actually be a nuclear receptor rather than a cytoplasmic receptor, and there may well be a difference between what is cytosolic and what is truly cytoplasmic. Using a similar technique, Nenci (1984) was able to demonstrate that breast tumors rarely display homogeneous cell types, (i.e., they rarely are composed of only ER positive or only ER negative cells); almost all breast tumors prove to be composed of mixed receptor positive and receptor negative cell populations in variable proportions. Nenci (1984) also noted that positivity of 20 per cent of the cell population was sufficient to give a positive ER by cytosolic assay. These observations concerning cell heterogeneity in breast cancer seem clinically relevant and may explain why the probability of tumor regression after endocrine therapy correlates better with a quantitative than with a simply qualitative receptor assay.

Salmon (1984) asked, "Is the estrogen receptor expressed clonally in the human tumor clonogenic assay (HTCA) with some colonies positive and others negative, or is it expressed over time in all colonies that grow in HTCA (the latter being more consistent with ER as a differentiation antigen)?" Using the MCF-7 human breast cancer cell line, he was able to demonstrate that at the small cluster stage of growth, the proportion of ER positive cells was small and variable, and some ER negative clusters were present. However, ER positivity increased progressively with time, with the greatest positivity occurring at the colony stage of growth. Once the colony stage was reached, ER was expressed in 70 per cent of the cells in colonies, and none of the colonies was ER negative. These findings support the concept that ER is proliferation-differentiation dependent and that cells are not truly clonally ER positive or ER negative. Salmon (1984) went on to postulate that ER is expressed increasingly in transitional cells and end cells rather than in tumor stem cells. Therefore, endocrine therapy acts beyond the level of the tumor stem cell and will suppress, but not eradicate, breast cancer clones. In contrast, cytotoxic agents appear to kill cells in both stem cell and transitional cell compartments.

Salmon's observations seem to demonstrate that breast cancers may not actually be heterogeneous with reference to ER, but rather may be at different phases of cellular differentiation.

As discussed previously, receptor positive cells have a well-documented differential response to hormonal therapy. An important question is whether there is a differential response between receptor positive and receptor negative cells to cytotoxic chemotherapy, or whether chemotherapy kills ER positive and ER negative cells indiscriminately, as Salmon's (1984) HCTA tissue culture data seem to imply.

In 1978, Lippman and colleagues reported the analysis of a retrospective study of 70 patients with metastatic breast cancer treated with cytotoxic chemotherapy. Objective responses were seen in 34 of 45 (75 per cent) of ER negative (<10 fmol/mg) patients, but only 3 of 25 (12 per cent of ER positive ($\geq$ 10 fmol/mg) cases responded ($p=0.0001$). These data were so striking that it seemed that a differential response to chemotherapy for ER positive versus ER negative cells had been established. However, 6 months later, in another retrospective study, Kiang and associates (1978) reported the opposite finding. In women treated with chemotherapy, 24 of 28 (86 per cent) of ER positive patients responded, compared to 13 of 36 (36 per cent of ER negative patients ($p < 0.0001$). Clearly, there was a problem. Since then a variety of retrospective studies have been reported, some seeming to confirm that ER positive tumors respond better to chemotherapy (Mortimer et al., 1981; Paone et al., 1981), some confirming the original observation that ER positive tumors respond poorly to chemotherapy (Lippman and Allegra, 1980), and some reporting no difference in response to chemotherapy by ER status (Corle et al., 1984; Pouillart et al., 1982; Falkson et al., 1985). Because of a need to establish firmly whether or not there is a differential response rate to cytotoxic chemotherapy between ER positive and ER negative cells, the Cancer and Leukemia Group B (CALGB) performed a prospective randomized study from January 1980 to August 1982 (Kardinal et al., 1983; Perry et al., 1984). All of the patients were postmenopausal. They were stratified by ER status (< 7 or $\geq$ 7 fmol/mg) and site of dominant metastatic disease. Objective responses were observed in 26 of 37 ER negative patients (70 per cent) and in 20 of 40 ER positive patients (50 per cent) ($p = 0.07$). A differential response between ER positive and ER negative cells to cytotoxic chemotherapy cannot be confirmed. It seems that chemotherapy kills both types of cells indiscriminately. It can be concluded that, at least with reference to ER positive cells, chemotherapy and hormonal therapy are competing for the same cell population (Kardinal et al., 1986).

The third assumption necessary to propose an additive effect between chemotherapy and hormonal therapy is that there is no interference between the two types of treatment. The experimental data of Sutherland and coworkers (1983) and Osborne and colleagues (1983) have demonstrated that tamoxifen acts as a cell cycle inhibitor, arresting cells in the G_0-G_1 phase of the cell cycle. Drugs that are cell cycle–specific, such as methotrexate and 5-fluorouracil, require for a cytotoxic effect that the target cells be actively dividing. Even the cell cycle–nonspecific drugs, such as the alkylating agents and the antitumor antibiotics, are most effective in actively dividing cells. At least theoretically, tamoxifen has the potential to interfere with the effectiveness of cytotoxic drugs by interfering with cell replication. The interference by tamoxifen on chemotherapeutic effectiveness has not yet been confirmed in clinical chemohormonal trials.

To date, there are no convincing data that the simple addition of a hormonal agent such as tamoxifen to a standard chemotherapeutic regimen, such as CMF (cyclophosphamide, methotrexate, and 5-fluorouracil) or CAF (cyclophosphamide, Adriamycin, and 5-fluorouracil) has increased the response rate or duration of response over that of either regimen alone. Kardinal and associates (1983) reported a prospective randomized study of 246 postmenopausal patients with advanced cancer of the breast, stratified by ER receptor status and dominant site of metastatic disease, who were treated with CAF versus CAF plus tamoxifen (T-CAF). No difference in response rate or response duration to CAF or T-CAF was seen with respect to ER status or dominant site of metastatic disease. Two other studies evaluated tamoxifen alone versus tamoxifen plus CMF (Glick et al., 1980; Bezwoda, et al., 1982). In neither of these studies was the addition of CMF advantageous. Krook and associates (1985) also demonstrated no advantage in time to disease progression or survival by the addition of tamoxifen to CFP (cyclophosphamide, 5-fluorouracil, and prednisone) over the use of CFP alone. The failure to demonstrate an advantage to the simple addition of hormonal agents to cytotoxic chemotherapy does not rule out the possibility that the kinetic effects of tamoxifen might increase chemotherapeutic effectiveness. Preliminary data by Allegra (1983a) demonstrate that tumor cell synchronization by tamoxifen, then recruitment by equine estrogens (Premarin priming), may well enhance the response to cytotoxic chemotherapy.

Patient Management

The approach to the patient with metastatic breast cancer depends on three major factors: (1) the estrogen and progesterone receptor status, (2) the patient's menopausal status, and (3) the distribution of disease (Fig. 17–26). Clinical judgment involves the determination of how potentially life-threatening the disease is at the point when therapy is to be initiated. If the disease is immediately life-threatening, the patient should be treated directly with cytotoxic chemotherapy because of its more rapid onset of action, regardless of the receptor status. Potentially life-threatening circumstances include lymphangitic lung metastases and massive hepatic metastases. Central nervous system metastases, although life-threatening, respond to neither chemotherapy nor hormonal therapy. If the clinical situation is not life-threatening (i.e., if the patient can safely wait 6 to 8 weeks for the onset of action) and the tumor is ER positive, it is highly desirable to treat the patient with some form of hormonal manipulation. Hormonal therapy is preferred in the appropriate clinical setting, as the response rates are high in ER+, PgR+ patients and hormonal therapy is essentially free of side-effects, in contrast to cytotoxic chemotherapy.

After the judgment is made that the patient is a candidate for hormonal manipulation, how does the clinician decide which form of hormonal therapy is most appropriate for the individual patient? In addition, what sequence of hormonal agents should be followed, as the patient may respond not only to the primary form of hormonal manipulation but also to secondary and even tertiary forms of endocrine therapy?

Most forms of hormonal manipulation, additive or ablative, induce approximately the same overall response rate and response duration. Selection of the form of hormonal manipulation is based primarily on side-effects or other morbidity associated with the therapy, as graphically illustrated by Santen (1984) (Fig. 17–27). The relative side-effects of the various additive hormonal agents are outlined in Table 17–19. Currently used sequential approaches to hormonal manipulation in premenopausal and postmenopausal patients with advanced breast cancer are illustrated in Figure 17–26.

The therapist can be more liberal in the management of hormonal manipulation in the ER+, PgR+ patient because the response rate to therapy is very high (78 per cent) (Table

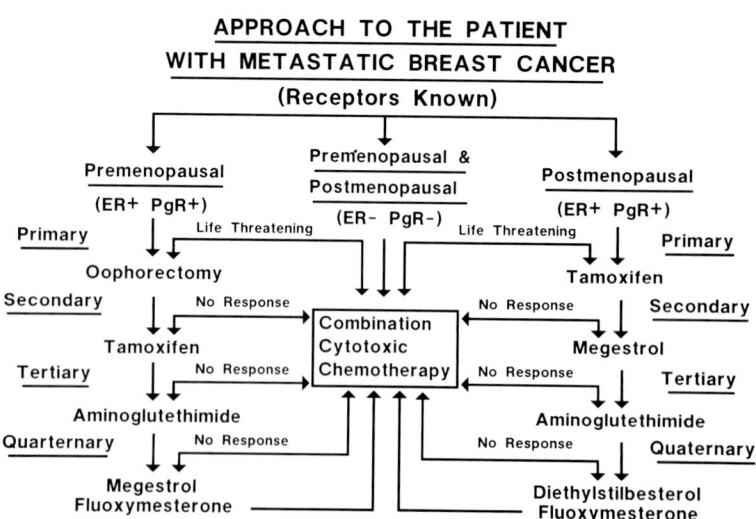

Figure 17–26. Diagram depicting a series of *clinical judgment* issues in patients with metastatic breast cancer (receptors known): (1) All ER− PgR− (pre- or postmenopausal) cases should be treated with chemotherapy, *but not* all ER+ PgR+ (those ER+ PgR+ with immediately life-threatening disease should receive chemotherapy initially). (2) The sequential approach to hormonal manipulation in premenopausal women differs from the approach for postmenopausal women. (3) A judgment must be made at each sequential step. For instance, if the patient fails to respond to primary hormone therapy, consideration should be given at this point to treating with chemotherapy. The same judgment must be made if the patient responds to primary hormone treatment but fails on secondary therapy, and in a like manner for tertiary and quaternary therapy. (4) ER+ PgR− and ER− PgR+, not depicted in the diagram, should be treated as ER+ PgR+ if the disease is indolent; if it is aggressive, patients should be treated as ER− PgR−

Figure 17–27. Considerations in choosing endocrine therapy. Hypox, Hypophysectomy; Adx, adrenalectomy; TAM, tamoxifen; AG, aminoglutethimide; Prog, progestins; E_2, estrogen; Andr, androgens; Gluc, glucocorticoids. (From Santen, R. J.: *In* Allegra, J. C. [Ed.]: Management of Breast Cancer Through Endocrine Therapies. Amsterdam, Excerpta Medica, 1984, p. 19. Reprinted with permission.)

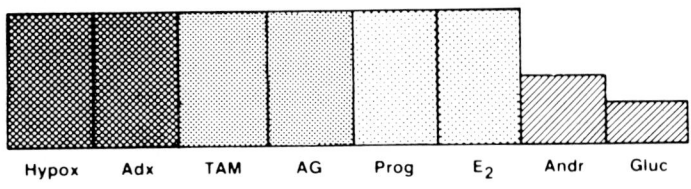

EFFICACY

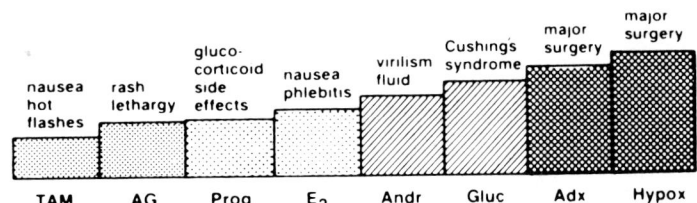

PROBLEMS WITH THERAPY

Table 17–19. RELATIVE SIDE-EFFECTS OF ADDITIVE HORMONAL AGENTS

	DES	Fluoxymesterone	Megestrol	Tamoxifen
Flushing	−	+ + +	−	+
Nausea	+ + +	+	+	+
Edema	+ + +	+	+	−
Congestive heart failure	+ + +	+	+	−
Frontal baldness	−	+	−	−
Weight gain	+	+	+ +	−
Flare	+ +	+	+	+
Urinary incontinence	+ +	−	−	−
Virilization	−	+ + +	−	−
Pigmentation	+ +	−	−	−
Vaginal bleeding	+ +	−	+	+
Thromboembolism	+ +	−	−	+

DES, Diethylstilbestrol.
Modified from Osborne, C. K.: Advanced Breast Cancer. Syracuse, N. Y., Bristol Laboratories Monograph, 1984.

17–6). That is, the physician may be more willing to take greater risk and to treat sicker patients. However, in patients who are ER+, PgR− or ER−, PgR+, whose response rates are only 30 to 40 per cent, much greater caution in patient selection must be used. In these cases, hormonal therapy should be restricted to patients with indolent disease, such as bone metastases, soft tissue metastases, and, possibly, nodular lung metastases. ER−, PgR− patients should not be treated with hormonal therapy, as response rates are consistently less than 10 per cent. The approach to the patient with metastatic breast cancer in whom the receptor status is unknown is illustrated in Figure 17–3.

REFERENCES

Adair F. E., Treves, N., Farrow, J. H., et al.: Clinical effects of surgical and x-ray castration in mammary cancer. J.A.M.A., *128*:161, 1945.

Ahlbom, H.: Castration by roentgen rays as auxilliary treatment in the treatment in the radiotherapy of cancer mammae at Radiumhemmet, Stockholm, Acta Radiol., *11*:614, 1930.

Ahmann, D. L., O'Connell, M. J., Hahn R. G., et al.: An evaluation of early or delayed adjuvant chemotherapy in premenopausal patients with advanced breast cancer undergoing oophorectomy. N. Engl. J. Med., *297*:356, 1977.

Allegra, J. C.: Methotrexate and 5-fluorouracil following tamoxifen and Premarin in advanced breast cancer. Semin. Oncol., *10*(Suppl. 2):23, 1983*a*.

Allegra, J. C.: The use of steroid hormone receptors in breast cancer. *In* Margolese, R. (Ed.): Breast Cancer. New York, Churchill Livingstone, 1983*b*, p. 187.

Allegra, J. C.: Mechanism of hormone response and resistance: Clinical studies. Rev. Endocrine-Related Cancer, Suppl. *14*:53, 1984*a*.

Allegra, J. C.: Role of hormone receptors in determining treatment of breast cancer. *In* The Management of Breast Cancer Through Endocrine Therapies. Amsterdam, Excerpta Medica, 1984*b*, pp. 1–13.

Allegra, J. C., and Kiefer, S. M.: Mechanisms of action of progestational agents. Semin. Oncol., *12*:(Suppl. 1): 3, 1985.

Allegra, J. C., Barlock, A., Huff, K. K., et al.: Changes in multiple or sequential estrogen receptor determinations in breast cancer. Cancer, *45*:792, 1980.

Allegra, J. C., Lippman, N. E., Simon, R., et al.: Association between steroid hormone receptor status and disease free interval in breast cancer. Cancer Treat. Rep., *63*:1271, 1979.

Bagheri, S. A., and Boyer, J. L.: Peliosis hepatis associated with androgenic-anabolic steroid therapy. Ann. Intern. Med., *81*:610, 1974.

Baker, L. H., and Vaitkevicius, V. K.: Reevaluation of rebound regression in disseminated carcinoma of the breast. Cancer, *29*:1268, 1972.

Barbieri, R. L., and Ryan, K. J.: Danazol: Endocrine pharmacology and therapeutic application. Am. J. Obstet. Gynecol., *141*:453, 1981.

Baum, M.: Does treatment influence the national history of breast cancer? Rev. Endocrine-Related Cancer, Suppl. *14*:193, 1984.

Baum, M., Brinkley, D. M., Dossett, J. A., et al.: Controlled trial of tamoxifen as adjuvant agent in management of early breast cancer: Interim analysis at four years by the Nolvadex Adjuvant Trial Organization. Lancet, *1*:257, 1983.

Baum, M., Brinkley, D. M., Dossett, J. A., et al.: Controlled trial of tamoxifen as single adjuvant agent in management of early breast cancer: Analysis at six years by Nolvadex Adjuvant Trial Organization. Lancet, *1*:836, 1985.

Beatson, G. T.: On the treatment of inoperable cases of carcinoma of the mamma: Suggestions for a new method of treatment with illustrative cases. Lancet, 2:104, 162, 1896.

Benz, C., Gandara, D., Miller, B., et al.: Chemoendocrine therapy with prolonged estrogen priming in advanced breast cancer: Endocrine pharmacokinetics and toxicity. Cancer Treat. Rep., *71*:283, 1987.

Bezwoda, W. R., Dorman, D., DeMoor, N. G., et al.: Treatment of metastatic breast cancer in estrogen receptor positive patients: A randomized trial comparing tamoxifen alone to tamoxifen plus CMF. Cancer, *50*:2747, 1982.

Block, G. E., Vial, A. B., and Pullen, F. W.: Estrogen excretion following operative and irradiation castration in cases of mammary cancer. Surgery, *43*:415, 1958.

Bloom, N. D., and Fishman, J. H.: Tamoxifen treatment failures in hormonally responsive breast cancers: Correlation with steroid receptors. Cancer, *51*:1190, 1983.

Blumenschein, G. R.: The role of progestins in the treatment of breast cancer. Semin. Oncol., *10*(Suppl. 4):7, 1983.

Bonadonna, G., Rossi, A., Valaguassa, P., et al.: Adjuvant chemotherapy trial with CMF. *In* Breast Cancer: A Report to the Profession 1976. Sponsored by the White House, National Cancer Institute, and the American Cancer Society, National Cancer Institute, Bethesda, Md., Meeting Abstract, 1976, p. 52.

Brannan, M. J., Donegan, W. L., and Appleby, D. E.: The variability of estrogen receptors in metastatic breast cancer. Am. J. Surg., *137*:260, 1979.

Bridges, K. G., Keshgegian, A. A., Kumar, H. A. M., et al.: Influences of surgical technique on estrogen and progesterone receptor determinations in breast cancer. Cancer, *51*:2317, 1983.

Brooks, B. J., and Lippman, M. E.: Tamoxifen flare in advanced endometrial carcinoma. J. Clin. Oncol., *3*:222, 1985.

Bruera, E., Roca, E., Cedars, L., et al.: Action of oral methylprednisolone in terminal cancer patients: a prospective randomized double-blind study. Cancer Treat. Rep., *69*:751, 1985.

Bryant, A. J. S., and Weir, J. A.: Prophylactic oophorectomy in operable instances of carcinoma of the breast. Surg. Gynecol. Obstet., *153*:660, 1981.

Buchanan, R. B., Blamly, R. W., Durrant, K. R., et al.: A randomized comparison of tamoxifen with surgical oophorectomy in premenopausal patients with advanced breast cancer. J. Clin. Oncol., *4*:1326, 1986.

Butler, J. A., Bretsky, S., Menendez-Botet, C., et al.: Estrogen receptor protein of breast cancer as a predictor of recurrence. Cancer, *55*:1178, 1985.

Calandra, R. S., Chaneau, E. H., Giaroli, A. R., et al.: Incidence of estrogen, progesterone, and prolactin receptors in human breast cancer. *In* Gurpide, E., Colandra, R., Levy, C., et al. (eds.): Hormones and Cancer. New York, Alan R. Liss, 1984, pp. 97–108.

Carpenter, J. T., and Peterson, L.: Use of megestrol acetate in advanced breast cancer on a single daily dose schedule. Semin. Oncol., *12*(Suppl.):40, 1985.

Carter, S. K.: Single and combination nonhormonal chemotherapy in breast cancer. Cancer, *30*:1543, 1972.

Cash, R., Brough, A. J., Cohen, M. N. P., et al.: Aminoglutethimide (Elipten-Ciba) as an inhibitor of adrenal steroidogenesis: Mechanism of action and therapeutic trial. J. Clin. Endocrinol. Metab., *27*:1239, 1967.

Cavilli, F., Goldhiroch, A., Jungi, F., et al.: Randomized trial of low- vs high-dose medroxyprogesterone acetate in the induction treatment of postmenopausal patients with advanced breast cancer. J. Clin. Oncol., *2*:414, 1984.

Clark, G. M., and McGuire, W. L.: Prognostic factors in primary breast cancer. Breast Cancer Res. Treat., *3*(Suppl. 1):69, 1983.

Clark, G. M., McGuire, W. L., Hubay, C. A., et al.: Progesterone receptors as a prognostic factor in stage II breast cancer. N. Engl. J. Med., *309*:1343, 1983.

Clark, G. M., Sledge, G. W., Jr., Osborne, C. K., et al.: Survival from first recurrence: Relative importance of prognostic factors in 1,015 breast cancer patients. J. Clin. Oncol., *5*:55, 1987.

Coombes, R. C., Chilvess, C., and Powles, T. S.: Adjuvant aminoglutethimide therapy for postmenopausal patients with primary breast cancer. Jones, S. E., and Salmon, S. E. (Eds.): *In* Adjuvant Therapy of Cancer IV. New York, Grune & Stratton, 1984, pp. 349–358.

Coombes, R. C., Dearnaley, D., Humphreys, J., et al.: Danazol treatment of advanced breast cancer. Cancer Treat. Rep., *64*:1073, 1980.

Consensus Conference: Adjuvant Chemotherapy for Breast Cancer. J.A.M.A., *254*:3461, 1985.

Cooper, R.: Combination chemotherapy in hormone resistant breast cancer (Abstract) Proc. Am. Assoc. Cancer Res., *10*:15, 1969.

Cooperative Breast Cancer Group: Testosterone propionate therapy in breast cancer. J.A.M.A., *188*:1069, 1964.

Corle, D. K., Sears, M. E., and Olson, K. B.: Relationship of quantitative estrogen-receptor level and clinical response to cytotoxic chemotherapy in advanced breast cancer: An extramural analysis. Cancer, *54*:1554, 1984.

Council on Drugs: Androgens and estrogens in the treatment of disseminated mammary carcinoma. J.A.M.A., *172*:1271, 1960.

Cowie, A. T., Forsyth, I. A., and Hart, I. C.: Hormonal Control of Lactation. Berlin, Springer-Verlag, 1980.

Croton, R., Cooke, T., Holt, S., et al.: Oestrogen receptors and survival in early breast cancer. Br. Med. J., *283*:1289, 1981.

Crowe, J. P., Hubay, C. A., Pearson, O. H., et al.: Estrogen receptor as a prognostic indicator for stage I breast cancer patients. Breast Cancer Res. Treat., *2*:171, 1982.

Cutler, S. J., Asire, A. J., and Taylor, S. G., III: Classification of patients with disseminated cancer of the breast. Cancer, *24*:861, 1969.

deCourmeller, F. V.: La radiotherapie indirecte, ou dirigée par les correlations organiques. Arch. Elect. Med., *32*:264, 1922.

DeSombre, E. R.: Breast cancer: Hormone receptors, prognosis and therapy. Clin. Oncol., *1*:191, 1982.

DeSombre, E. R., Greene, G. L., King, W. J., et al.: Estrogen receptors, antibodies and hormone dependent cancer. *In* Gurpide, E., Calandra, R., Levy, C., et al. (Eds.): Hormones and Cancer. Alan R. Liss, New York, 1984, pp. 1–22.

DeSombre, E. R., Kledzik, G., Marshall, S., et al.: Estrogen and prolactin receptor concentrations in rat mammary tumors and response to endocrine ablation. Cancer Res., *36*:354, 1976.

Dhadly, M. S., and Walker, R. A.: The localization of prolactin binding sites in human breast tissue. Int. J. Cancer, *31*:433, 1983.

Diczfalusy, E., Notter, G., Edsmyr, F., et al.: Estrogen excretion in breast cancer patients before and after ovarian irradiation and oophorectomy. J. Clin. Endocrinol., *19*:1230, 1959.

Duffy, M. J. O'Connell, M., O'Sullivan, F., et al.: CEA-like materials in cytosols from human breast carcinomas: Correlation with biochemical and pathologic parameters. Cancer, *51*:121, 1983.

Enck, R. E., and Rios, C. N.: Tamoxifen treatment of metastatic breast cancer and antithrombin III levels. Cancer, *53*:2607, 1984.

Escher, G. C.: Clinical improvement in inoperable breast carcinoma under steroid treatment. *In* Council of Pharmacy and Chemistry, American Medical Association: Proceedings of the First Conference on Steroid Hormone and Mammary Carcinoma. Chicago, American Medical Association, 1949, p 92.

Falkson, G., Falkson, H. C., Glidewell, O., et al.: Improved remission rates and remission duration in young women with metastatic breast cancer following combined oophorectomy and chemotherapy: A study by Cancer and Leukemia Group B. Cancer, *43*:2215, 1979.

Falkson, G., Gelman, R. S., Tormey, D. C., et al.: The Eastern Cooperative Oncology Group experience with cyclophosphamide, adriamycin, and 5-fluorouracil (CAF) in patients with metastatic breast cancer. Cancer, *56*:219, 1985.

Falkson, H. C., Falkson, G., Portugal, M. A., et al.: Carcinoembryonic antigen as a marker in patients with breast cancer receiving postsurgical adjuvant chemotherapy. Cancer, *49*:1859, 1982.

Farrow, J. H., and Woodward, H. Q.: Influence of androgenic and estrogen substances on the serum calcium in cases of skeletal metastases from mammary cancer. J.A.M.A., *118*:339, 1942.

Fels, E.: Treatment of breast cancer with testosterone propionate: Preliminary report. J. Clin. Endocrinol., *4*:121, 1944.

Fisher, B.: A commentary on the role of the surgeon in primary breast cancer. Breast Cancer Res. Treat., *1*:17, 1981.

Fisher, B., Bauer, M., Wickerham, L., et al.: Relation of number of positive axillary nodes to the prognosis of patients with primary breast cancer: An NSABP update. Cancer, *52*:1551, 1983a.

Fisher, B., Ravdin, R. G., Ausman, R. K., et al.: Surgical adjuvant chemotherapy in cancer of the breast: Results of a decade of cooperative investigation. Ann. Surg., *163*:337, 1968.

Fisher, B., Redmond, C., Brown, A., et al.: Treatment of primary breast cancer with chemotherapy and tamoxifen. N. Engl. J. Med., *305*:1, 1981.

Fisher, B., Redmond, C., Brown, A., et al.: Influence of estrogen and progesterone receptor levels on the response to tamoxifen and chemotherapy in primary breast cancer. J. Clin. Oncol., *1*:227, 1983b.

Fisher, B., Slack, N., Katrych, D., et al.: Ten year follow-up results of patients with carcinoma of the breast in a cooperative clinical trial evaluating surgical adjuvant chemotherapy. Surg. Gynecol. Obstet., *140*:528, 1975.

Fisher, E. R., Redmond, C. K., Liu, H., et al.: Correlation of estrogen receptor and pathologic characteristics of invasive breast cancer. Cancer, *45*:349, 1980*b*.

Fisher, E. R., Sass, R., and Fisher, B.: Pathologic findings from the National Surgical Adjuvant Breast Project: Correlations with concordant and discordant estrogen and progesterone receptors. Cancer, *59*:1554, 1987.

Fracchia, A. A., Randall, H. T., and Farrow, J. H.: The results of adrenalectomy in advanced breast cancer in 500 consecutive patients. Surg. Gynecol. Obstet., *125*:747, 1967.

Frantz, A. G., and Rabkin, K. J.: Effects of estrogen and sex difference on secretion of human growth hormone. J. Clin. Endocrinol. Metab., *25*:1470, 1965.

Frantz, A. G., and Wilson, J. D.: Endocrine disorders of the breast. In Wilson, J. D., and Foster, D. W. (Eds.). Williams Textbook of Endocrinology. Philadelphia, W.B. Saunders, 1985, pp. 402–421.

Freeman, C. S., and Topper, Y.: Progesterone is not essential to the differentiative potential of mammary epithelium in the male mouse. Endocrinology, *103*:186, 1978.

Gapinski, P. V., and Donegan, W. L.: Estrogen receptors and breast cancer: Prognostic and therapeutic implications. Surgery, *84*:386, 1980.

Gardner, B., Thomas, A. N., and Gordan G. S.: Antitumor efficacy of prednisone and sodium liothyronine in advanced breast cancer. Cancer, *15*:334, 1962.

Glick, J. H., Creech, R. H., Torri, S., et al.: Tamoxifen plus sequential CMF chemotherapy versus tamoxifen alone in postmenopausal patients with advanced breast cancer: A randomized trial. Cancer, *45*:735, 1980.

Godolphin, W., Elwood, J. M., and Spinelli, J. J.: Estrogen receptor quantitation and staging as complementary prognostic indicators in breast cancer: A study of 583 patients. Int. J. Cancer, *28*:677, 1981.

Gotfredsen, A., Christiansen, C., and Palshof, T.: The effect of tamoxifen on bone mineral content in premenopausal women with breast cancer. Cancer, *53*:853, 1984.

Greenwald, E. S.: Megestrol acetate flare. Cancer Treat. Rep., *67*:405, 1983.

Gregory, E. J., Cohen, S. L., Oines, D. W., et al.: Megestrol acetate therapy for breast cancer. J. Clin. Oncol., *3*:155, 1985.

Haas, H. A. D.: A trial of oophorectomy against Nolvadex (tamoxifen). Rev. Endocrine-Related Cancer, Suppl. *10*:27, 1981.

Hall, T. C.: Predictive tests in cancer. Br. J. Cancer, *30*:191, 1974.

Hall, T. C., Dederick, M. M., and Nevinny, H. B.: Prognostic value of hormonally induced hypercalcemia in breast cancer. Cancer Chemother. Rep., *30*:21, 1963.

Harris, H. S., and Spratt, J. S.: Bilateral adrenalectomy in metastatic mammary cancer. Cancer, *23*:145, 1969.

Hartviet, F., Maartmann-Moe, H., Stoa, K. F., et al.: Early recurrence of estrogen receptor negative breast carcinomas. Acta Chir. Scand., *146*:93, 1980.

Harvey, H. A., Lipton, A., Max, D. T., et al.: Medical castration produced by the GnRH analogue leuprolide to treat metastatic breast cancer. J. Clin. Oncol., *3*:1068, 1985.

Hayward, J. L., Carbone, P. D., Heuson, J. C., et al.: Assessment of response to therapy in advanced breast cancer. A project of the program on clinical oncology of the International Union Against Cancer, Geneva, Switzerland. Cancer, *39*:1289, 1977.

Hoffman, D. A., McConsey, W. M., Briston, L. A., et al.: Breast cancer in hypothyroid women using thyroid supplements. J.A.M.A., *251*:616, 1984.

Holdaway, I. M., and Bowditch, J. V.: Variation in receptor status between primary and metastatic breast cancer. Cancer, *52*:479, 1983.

Hoogstraten, B., Fletcher, W. S., Gad-el-Mawla, N., et al.: Tamoxifen and oophorectomy in the treatment of recurrent breast cancer. Cancer Res., *42*:4788, 1982.

Hoogstraten, B., Gad-el-Mawla, N., Maloney, T. R., et al.: Combined modality therapy for first recurrence of breast cancer: A Southwest Oncology Group Study. Cancer, *54*:228, 1984.

Horwitz, K. B., McGuire, W. L., Pearson, O. H., et al.: Predicting response to endocrine therapy in human breast cancer: a hypothesis. Science, *189*:726, 1975.

Huggins, C., and Bergenstal, D. M.: Inhibition of human mammary and prostatic cancer by adrenalectomy. Cancer Res., *12*:134, 1952.

Huggins, C., and Hodges, C. V.: Studies on prostatic cancer. Cancer Res., *1*:293, 1941.

Hull, D. F., Clark, G. M., Osborne, C. K., et al.: Multiple estrogen receptor assay in human breast cancer. Cancer Res., *43*:413, 1983.

Ingle, J. N.: Additive hormonal therapy in women with advanced breast cancer. Cancer, *53*:766, 1984.

Ingle, J. N., Ahmann, D. L., Green, S. J., et al.: Randomized clinical trial of diethylstilbestrol versus tamoxifen in postmenopausal women with advanced breast cancer. N. Engl. J. Med., *304*:16, 1981.

Ingle, J. N., Krook, J. E., Green, S. J., et al.: Randomized trial of bilateral oophorectomy versus tamoxifen in premenopausal women with metastatic breast cancer. J. Clin. Oncol., *4*:178, 1986.

Jensen, E. V., Block, G. E., Smith, S., et al.: Estrogen receptors and breast cancer: Response to adrenalectomy. Prediction of response in cancer therapy. Natl. Cancer. Inst. Monogr., *34*:55, 1971.

Johnson, P. A., Bonomi, P. D., Anderson, K. M., et al.: Progesterone receptor level as a predictor of response to megestrol acetate in advanced breast cancer: A retrospective study. Cancer Treat. Rep., *67*:717, 1983.

Jordan, V. C.: Laboratory studies to develop general principles for the adjuvant treatment of breast cancer with antiestrogen: Problems and potential for future clinical applications. Breast Cancer Res. Treat., *3*(Suppl. 1):73, 1983.

Jordan, V. C., Allen, K. E., and Dix, C. J.: Pharmacology of tamoxifen in laboratory animals. Cancer Treat. Rep., *64*:745, 1980.

Jordan, V. C., Mirecki, D. M., and Gottardis, M. M.: Continuous tamoxifen treatment prevents the appearance of mammary tumors in a model system. In Jones, S. E., and Salmon, S. E. (Eds.). Adjuvant Therapy of Cancer IV. Grune & Stratton, 1984, pp. 27–34.

Kalman, A. M., Thompson, N., and Vogel C. L.: Response to oophorectomy after tamoxifen failure in a premenopausal patient. Cancer Treat. Rep., *66*:1867, 1983.

Kapdi, C. C., and Wolfe, J. N.: Breast cancer: Relationship to thyroid supplements for hypothyroidism. J.A.M.A., *236*:1124, 1976.

Karashima, T., and Schally, A. V.: Inhibitory effects of somatostatin analogs on prolactin secretion in rats pretreated with estrogen or haloperidol (42518). Proc. Soc. Exp. Biol. Med., *185*:69, 1987.

Kardinal, C. G.: Cancer chemotherapy: Historical aspects and future considerations. Postgrad. Med., *77*:165, 1985.

Kardinal, C. G., and Bush, D. J.: Complications of

treatment for advanced colorectal cancer. In Ferrari, B. T., Ray, J. E., and Gathright, J. B. (Eds.): Complications of Colon and Rectal Surgery: Prevention and Management. Philadelphia, W.B. Saunders, 1985, pp. 267–300.

Kardinal, C. G., Perry, M. C., Korzun, A.H., et al.: Lack of differential response of estrogen receptor positive (ER+) vs. ER negative (ER−) breast cancer to Cytoxan® and Adriamycin® and 5-fluorouracil (CAF) chemotherapy (abstract). Proc. Am. Soc. Clin. Oncol., 5:74, 1986.

Kardinal, C. G., Perry, M. C., Weinberg, V., et al.: Chemoendocrine therapy vs. chemotherapy alone for advanced breast cancer in postmenopausal women: Preliminary report of a randomized study: Cancer and Leukemia Group B study 8081. Breast Cancer Res. Treat., 3:356, 1983.

Kaufman, R. J., and Escher, G.: Rebound regression in advanced mammary carcinoma. Surg. Gynecol. Obstet., 113:635, 1961.

Kelley, R. M.: Hormones and chemotherapy in breast cancer. Cancer, 28:1686, 1971.

Kennedy, B. J.: Stimulation of erythropoiesis by androgenic hormones. Ann. Intern. Med., 57:917, 1962.

Kennedy, B. J.: Hormonal therapy for advanced breast cancer. Cancer, 18:1551, 1965.

Kennedy, B. J.: Hormonal therapies in breast cancer. Semin. Oncol., 1:119, 1974.

Kennedy, B. J., Tibbetts, D. M., Nathanson, I. T., et al.: Hypercalcemia, a complication of hormone therapy of advanced breast cancer. Cancer Res., 13:445, 1953.

Kiang, D. T., and Kollander, R.: Breast cancers negative for estrogen receptor but positive for progesterone receptor, a true entity? J. Clin. Oncol., 5:662, 1987.

Kiang, D. T., Frenning, D. H., Goldman, A. I., et al.: Estrogen receptors and responses to chemotherapy and hormonal therapy in advanced breast cancer. N. Engl. J. Med., 299:1330, 1978.

Kiang, D. T., Frenning, D. H., Vosika, G. J., et al.: Comparison of tamoxifen and hypophysectomy in breast cancer treatment. Cancer, 5:1322, 1980.

King, W. J., Jensen, E. V., Miller, L., et al.: Immunocytochemical detection of estrogen receptor in frozen sections of human breast tumors with monoclonal antireceptor antibodies. Abstr. Endocrine. Soc., 1982, p. 258.

Kinne, D. W., Ashikari, R., Butler, A., et al.: Estrogen receptor protein in breast cancer as a predictor of recurrence. Cancer, 47:2364, 1981.

Klijn, J. G. M., and deJong, F. H.: Treatment with a luteinizing-hormone-releasing-hormone analogue (buserelin) in premenopausal patients with metastatic breast cancer. Lancet, 1:1213, 1982.

Klijn, J. G. M., deJong, F. H., Blankenstein, M. A., et al.: Anti-tumor and endocrine effects of chronic LHRH agonist treatment (buserelin) with or without tamoxifen in premenopausal metastatic breast cancer. Breast Cancer Res. Treat., 4:209, 1984.

Knight, W. A., Livingston, R. B., Gregory, E. J., et al.: Estrogen receptor as an independent prognostic factor for early recurrence in breast cancer. Cancer Res., 37:4669, 1977.

Kornblith, P. L., Walker, N. D., and Cassady, J. R.: Treatment of metastatic cancer. In DeVita, V. T., Hellman, S., and Rosenberg, S. A. (Eds.): Cancer: Principles and Practice of Oncology, 2nd ed. Philadelphia, J. B. Lippincott, 1985, p. 2101.

Krook, J. E., Ingle, J. N., Green, S. J., et al.: Randomized clinical trial of cyclophosphamide, 5FU, and prednisone with or without tamoxifen alone in postmenopausal women with advanced breast cancer. Cancer Treat. Rep., 69:355, 1985.

Lacassagne, A., and Raynaud, A.: Sur le mechanisme d'une action preventive de la testosterone sur le carcinome mammaire de la souris. Compt. Rend. Soc. Biol., 131:586, 1939.

Lett, H.: An analysis of 99 cases of inoperable breast cancer treated by oophorectomy. Lancet, 1:227, 1905.

Leuprolide Study Group: Leuprolides versus diethylstilbestrol for metastatic prostate cancer. N. Engl. J. Med., 311:1281, 1984.

Lippman, M. E.: Antiestrogen therapy of breast cancer. Semin. Oncol., 10(Suppl. 4):11, 1983.

Lippman, M. E.: Endocrine responsive cancers of man. In Wilson, J. D., and Foster, D. W. (Eds.): Williams Textbook of Endocrinology. Philadelphia, W.B. Saunders, 1985, pp. 1309–1326.

Lippman, M. E., and Allegra, J. C.: Quantitative estrogen receptor analyses. The response to endocrine and cytotoxic chemotherapy in human breast cancer and the disease-free interval. Cancer, 46:2829, 1980.

Lippman, M. E., and Bolan, G.: Oestrogen-responsive human breast cancer in long-term tissue culture. Nature (London), 256:592, 1975.

Lippman, M. E., Allegra, J. C., Thompson, E. B., et al.: The relation between estrogen receptors and response rate to cytotoxic chemotherapy in metastatic breast cancer. N. Engl. J. Med., 298:1223, 1978.

Lippman, M. E., Bolan, G., and Huff, K.: Interactions of antiestrogens with human breast cancer in longterm tissue culture. Cancer Treat. Rep., 60:1421, 1976.

Lipton, A., Harvey, H. A., and Hamilton, R. W.: Venous thrombosis as a side effect of tamoxifen treatment. Cancer Treat. Rep., 68:887, 1984.

Lipton, A., Harvey, H. A., Santen, R. J., et al.: A randomized trial of aminoglutethimide vs tamoxifen in metastatic breast cancer. Cancer, 50:2265, 1982.

Lipton, A., Santner, S. J., Santen, R. J., et al.: Aromatase activity in primary and metastatic human breast cancer. Cancer, 59:779, 1987.

Loeser, A.: Male hormone in the treatment of cancer of the breast. Acta Un. Int. Cancre, 4:375, 1939.

Loprinzi, C. L., and Ahmann, D. L.: Carcinoembryonic antigen: A routine test in patients with breast carcinoma? (Editorial). Arch. Intern. Med., 146:2125, 1986.

Ludwig Breast Cancer Study Group: Chemotherapy with or without oophorectomy in high-risk premenopausal patients with operable breast cancer. J. Clin. Oncol., 3:1059, 1985.

Luft, R., and Olivecrona, H.: Experiences with hypophysectomy in man. J. Neurosurg., 10:301, 1953.

Lyons, W. R., Li, C. H., and Johnson, R. E.: The hormonal control of mammary growth and lactation. Recent Prog. Horm. Res., 14:219, 1958.

Manni, A., and Pearson, D. H.: Antiestrogen-induced remissions in premenopausal women with stage IV breast cancer: Effects in ovarian function. Cancer Treat. Rep., 64:779, 1980.

Manni, A., Trujillo, J. E., Marshall, J. S., et al.: Antihormone treatment of stage IV breast cancer. Cancer, 43:444, 1979.

Manni, A., Trujillo, J. E., and Pearson, O. H.: Predominant role of prolactin in stimulating the growth of 7,12-dimethylbenz[a]-anthracene-induced rat mammary tumor. Cancer Res., 37:1216, 1977.

Mansour, E. G., Hastert, M., Park, C. H., et al.: Tissue and plasma carcinoembryonic antigen in early breast cancer. Cancer, 51:1243, 1983.

Margreiter, R., and Wiegele, J.: Tamoxifen (Nolvadex)

for premenopause patients with advanced breast cancer. Breast Cancer Res. Treat., 4:45, 1984.
Mathé, G., Keiling, R., Prévot, G., et al.: LH-RH agonist: Breast and prostate cancer. In Klijn, J. G. M., et al. (Eds.): Hormonal Manipulation of Cancer: Peptides, Growth Factors, and New (Anti) Steroidal Agents. New York, Raven Press, 1987, pp. 315–319.
McDonald, I.: Endocrine ablation in disseminated mammary carcinoma. Surg. Gynecol. Obstet., 115:215, 1962.
McGuire, W. L.: Estrogen receptors in human breast cancer. J. Clin. Invest., 52:73, 1973.
McGuire, W. L., and Clark, G. M.: The prognostic role of progesterone receptors in human breast cancer. Semin. Oncol., 10(Suppl. 4):2, 1983.
McGuire, W. L., Carbone, P. O., and Vollmer, E. P.: Estrogen Receptors in Human Breast Cancer. New York, Raven Press, 1975.
Meakin, J. W., Allt, W. E. C., Beals, F. A., et al.: Ovarian irradiation and prednisone following surgery and radiotherapy for carcinoma of the breast. Breast Cancer Res. Treat., 3(Suppl. 1):45, 1983.
Mecklenburg, R. S., and Lipsett, M. B.: Disappearance of metastatic breast cancer after oophorectomy. N. Engl. J. Med., 289:845, 1973.
Meyer, J. S., Rao, B. R., Stevens, S. C., et al.: Low incidence of estrogen receptor in breast carcinomas with rapid rates of cellular replication. Cancer, 40:2290, 1977.
Miller, W. R., Hawkins, R. A., and Forrest, A. P. M.: Significance of aromatase activity in human breast cancer. Cancer Res. (Suppl.) 42:3365s, 1982.
Morgan, L. R.: Megestrol acetate vs tamoxifen in advanced breast cancer in postmenopausal patients. Semin. Oncol., 12(Suppl. 1):43, 1985.
Mortimer, J., Reimer, R., Greenstreet, R., et al.: Influence of estrogen receptor status on response to combination chemotherapy for recurrent breast cancer. Cancer Treat. Rep., 65:763, 1981.
Muggia, F. M., and Heinemann, H. O.: Hypercalcemia associated with neoplastic disease. Ann. Intern. Med., 73:281, 1970.
Muss, H. B., Paschold, E. H., Black, W. R., et al.: Megestrol acetate vs tamoxifen in advanced breast cancer: A phase III trial of the Piedmont Oncology Association (POA). Semin. Oncol., 12(Suppl. 1):55, 1985.
Muss, H., Paschold, E., Black, W., et al.: Megestrol acetate (M) vs. tamoxifen (T) in advanced breast cancer (ABC): A five year report. (Abstract) Proceedings, American Society of Clinical Oncology, 5:55, 1987.
Naeim, F., Copper, P. H., and Semion, A. A.: Peliosis hepatis. Possible etiologic role of anabolic steroids. Arch. Pathol., 95:284, 1973.
Nemoto, T., Patel, J., Rosner, D., et al.: Tamoxifen (Nolvadex) versus adrenalectomy in metastatic breast cancer. Cancer, 53:1333, 1984.
Nenci, I.: Charting steroid-cell interactions in normal and neoplastic tissues. In Gurpide, E., Calandra, R., Levy, C., et al. (Eds.): Hormones and Cancer. New York, Alan R. Liss, 1984, pp. 23–26.
Nestro, R. W., Cady B., Oberfield, R. A., et al.: Rebound response after estrogen therapy for metastatic breast cancer. Cancer, 38:1834, 1976.
Nomura, Y., Tashiro, H., and Shinozuka, K.: Changes of steroid hormone receptor content by chemotherapy and/or endocrine therapy in advanced breast cancer. Cancer, 55:546, 1985.
O'Bryan, R. M., Gordon, G. S., Kelley, R. M., et al.: Does thyroid substance improve response of breast cancer to surgical castration? Cancer, 33:1082, 1974.
Osborne, C. K.: Advanced Breast Cancer: The Current Approach to Diagnosis and Treatment. Syracuse, N.Y., Bristol Laboratories Monograph, 1984.
Osborne, C. K., Boldt, D. H., Clark, G. M., et al.: Effects of tamoxifen on human breast cancer cell cycle kinetics: Accumulation of cells in early G1 phase. Cancer Res., 43:3583, 1983.
Osborne, C. K., Yochmorwitz, M. G., Knight, W. A., et al.: The value of estrogen and progesterone receptors in the treatment of breast cancer. Cancer, 46:2884, 1980.
Otteman, L. A., and Long, H. J.: Hypercalcemic flare with megestrol acetate. Cancer Treat. Rep., 68:1420, 1984.
Pannuti, F., Martoni, A., DiMarco, A. R., et al.: Prospective, randomized clinical trial of two different high dosages of medroxyprogesterone acetate (MAP) in the treatment of metastatic breast cancer. Eur. J. Cancer, 15:593, 1979.
Paone, J. F., Abeloff, M. D., Ettinger, D. S., et al.: The correlation of estrogen and progesterone receptor levels with response to chemotherapy for advanced carcinoma of the breast. Surg. Gynecol. Obstet., 152:70, 1981.
Parl, F. F., Schmidt, B. P., Dupont, W. D., et al.: Prognostic significance of estrogen receptor status in breast cancer in relation to tumor stage, axillary node metastasis and histologic grading. Cancer, 54:2237, 1984.
Perry, M. C., Kardinal, C. G., Weinberg, V., et al.: Chemotherapy compared to chemotherapy plus hormone therapy in the treatment of postmenopausal women with advanced breast cancer: An interim report. In Amers, F. C., Blumenschein, G. R., and Montague, E. D. (Eds.): Current Controversies in Breast Cancer. Austin, University of Texas Press, 1984, p. 477.
Peters, T. G., Lewis, J. D., Wilkinson, E. J., et al.: Danazol therapy in hormone-sensitive mammary carcinoma. Cancer, 40:2797, 1977.
Peyrat, J. P., Djiane, J., Kelly, P. A., et al.: Characterization of prolactin receptors in human breast cancer. Breast Cancer Res. Treat., 4:275, 1984.
Planting, A. S. T., Alexieva-Figusch, J., Blonk-v. d. Wijst, J., et al.: Tamoxifen therapy in premenopausal women with metastatic breast cancer. Cancer Treat. Rep., 69:363, 1985.
Plotkin, D., Lechner, J. J., Jung, W. E., et al.: Tamoxifen flare in advanced breast cancer. J.A.M.A., 240:2644, 1978.
Pouillart, P., Madgelenat, H., Jouve, M., et al.: Metastatic breast cancer: Prognostic significance and sensitivity to cytotoxic chemotherapy according to the results of the estradiol and progesterone receptor assay. Bull. Cancer (Paris), 69:461, 1982.
Pritchard, K. I.: Current status of adjuvant endocrine therapy for resectable breast cancer. Semin. Oncol., 14:23, 1987.
Pritchard, K. I., Meakin, J. W., Boyd, N. F., et al.: A randomized trial of adjuvant tamoxifen in postmenopausal women with axillary node positive breast cancer. In Jones, S. E., and Salmon, S. E. (Eds.): Adjuvant Therapy of Cancer IV. New York, Grune & Stratton, 1984, pp. 339–348.
Pritchard, K. I., Thompson, D. B., Myers, R. E., et al.: Tamoxifen therapy in premenopausal patients with metastatic breast cancer. Cancer Treat. Rep., 64:787, 1980.
Qazi, R., Chuang, J. L. C., and Drobyski, W.: Estrogen receptors and the pattern of relapse in breast cancer. Arch. Intern. Med., 144:2365, 1984.
Ravdin, R. G., Lewison, E. F., Slack, N. H., et al.: Results of a clinical trial concerning the worth of pro-

phylactic oophorectomy for breast cancer. Surg. Gynecol. Obstet., *131*:1055, 1970.

Ribeiro, G., and Palmer, M. K.: Adjuvant tamoxifen for operable carcinoma of the breast: report of clinical trial by the Christie Hospital and Holt Radium Institute. Br. Med. J., *286*:827, 1983.

Rochefort, H.: Biochemical basis of breast cancer treatment by androgens and progestins. *In* Gurpide, E., Calandra, R., Levy, C., et al. (Eds.): Hormones and Cancer. New York, Alan R. Liss, 1984. pp. 79–96.

Rose, C., Thorpe, S. M., Anderson, K. W., et al.: Beneficial effect of adjuvant tamoxifen therapy in primary breast cancer in patients with high oestrogen receptor values. Lancet, *1*:16, 1985.

Rosen, P. P., Menendez-Botet, C. J., Urbou, J. A., et al.: Estrogen receptor protein (ERP) in multiple tumor specimens form individual patients with breast cancer. Cancer, *39*:2194, 1977.

Rossof, A. H.: The early history of hormone manipulation in human cancer—an appreciation of Sir George Thomas Beatson. Rev. Endocrine-Related Cancer, Suppl. *6*:7, 1980.

Rossof, A. H., Gelman, R., and Creech, R. H.: Randomized evaluation of combination chemotherapy vs observation alone following response or stabilization after oophorectomy for metastatic breast cancer in premenopausal women. Am. J. Clin. Oncol., *5*:253, 1982.

Rozencwieg, M., and Heuson, J. C.: Breast cancer: Prognostic factors and clinical evaluation. *In* Staquet, M. S. (Eds.). Cancer Therapy: Prognostic Factors and Criteria of Response. New York, Raven Press, 1975, pp. 139–147.

Rutgvist, L. E., Wallgren, F., and Nilsson, B. O.: Is breast cancer a curable disease? A study of 14,731 women with breast cancer from the Cancer Registry of Norway. Cancer, *53*:1793, 1984.

Salmon, S. E.: In vitro observations in clonogenic assay and potential extrapolations to adjuvant therapy of cancer. *In* Jones, S. E., and Salmon, S. E. (Eds.): Adjuvant Therapy of Cancer IV. New York, Grune & Stratton, 1984, pp. 17–26.

Samojlik, E., Santen, R. J., Kirschner, M. A., et al.: Steroid hormone profiles in women treated with aminoglutethimide for metastatic carcinoma of the breast. Cancer Res., *42*:3349s, 1982.

Santen, R. J.: Introduction to the conference, Aromatase: New perspectives for breast cancer. Cancer Res., Suppl. *42*:3268s, 1982.

Santen, R. J.: Basic principles in choosing endocrine therapy. *In* Allegra, J. C. (Ed.): The Management of Breast Cancer Through Endocrine Therapies. Amsterdam, Excepta Medical, 1984, pp. 14–28.

Santen, R. J., Worgul, T. J., Samojlik, E., et al.: A randomized trial comparing surgical adrenalectomy with aminoglutethimide plus hydrocortisone in women with advanced breast cancer. N. Engl. J. Med., *305*:545, 1981.

Schally, A. V., Redding, T. W., and Comaru-Schally, A. M.: Inhibition of the growth of some hormone dependent tumors by D-Trp^6-LH-RH. Med. Oncol. Tumor Pharmacother., *1*:109, 1984.

Schally, A. V., Cai, R.-Z., Torres-Aleman, I., et al.: Endocrine, gastrointestinal and antitumor activity of somatostatin analogues. *In* Moody, T. W. (Ed.): Neural and Endocrine Peptides and Receptors. New York, Plenum Publishing Corp., 1986.

Schally, A. V., Redding, T. W., Cai, R.-Z., et al.: Somatostatin analogs in the treatment of various experimental tumors. *In* Klijn, J. G. M. (Ed.): Hormonal Manipulation of Cancer: Peptides, Growth Factors, and New (Anti-)Steroidal Agents. New York, Raven Press, 1987.

Schell, H. W.: Adrenal corticosteroid therapy in far-advanced cancer. Geriatrics, *27*:131, 1972.

Schinzinger, A. S.: Über carcinoma mammae. Beilage zum Centralblatt fur Chirurgie, *16*:55, 1889.

Schlom, J., Greimer, J., Hand, P. H., et al.: Monoclonal antibodies to breast cancer–associated antigens as potential reagents in the management of breast cancer. Cancer, *54*:2777, 1984.

Schwartz, M. R., Randolph, R. L., and Panko, W. B.: Carcinoembryonic antigen and steroid receptors in the cytosol of carcinoma of the breast: Relationship to pathologic and clinical features. Cancer, *55*:2464, 1985.

Segaloff, A.: Assessment of response to treatment by the Cooperative Breast Cancer Group. *In* Hayward, J. L., and Bulbrook, R. D. (eds.). Clinical Evaluation in Breast Cancer. New York, Academic Press, 1966, p. 125.

Segaloff, A.: Hormone treatment of breast cancer. J.A.M.A., *234*:1175, 1975.

Shapiro, S., Slone, D., Kaufman, D. W., et al.: Use of thyroid supplements in relation to the risk of breast cancer. J.A.M.A., *244*:1685, 1980.

Sherry, M. M., Greco, F. A., Johnson, D. H., et al.: Metastatic breast cancer confined to the skeletal system: An indolent disease. Am. J. Med., *81*:381, 1986.

Shiu, R. P. C., and Friesen, H. G.: Mechanism of action of prolactin in the control of mammary gland function. Ann. Rev. Physiol., *42*:83, 1980.

Shyamala, G.: Specific cytoplasmic glucocorticoid hormone receptors in lactating mammary glands. Biochemistry, *12*:3085, 1973.

Siiteri, P. K.: Review on studies of estrogen biosynthesis in the human. Cancer Res., Suppl. *42*:3269s, 1982.

Silva, J. S., Height, G. S., Haagensen, D. E., et al.: Quantitation of response to therapy in patients with metastatic breast carcinoma by serial analysis of plasma gross cystic disease fluid protein and carcinoembryonic antigen. Cancer, *49*:1236, 1982.

Stoll, B. A.: Corticosteroids in therapy of advanced mammary cancer. Br. Med. J., *2*:210, 1963.

Sutherland, R. L., Green, M. D., Hall, R. E., et al.: Tamoxifen induces accumulation of MCF7 human mammary carcinoma cells in the G_0/G_1 phase of the cell cycle. Eur. J. Cancer Oncol., *19*:615, 1983.

Taylor, G. W.: Artificial menopause in carcinoma of the breast. N. Engl. J. Med., *211*:1138, 1934.

Taylor, G. W.: Evaluation of ovarian sterilization for breast cancer. Surg. Gynecol. Obstet., *68*:452, 1939.

Taylor, S. G., III, and Morris, R. S.: Hormones in breast metastasis therapy. Med. Clin. North Am., *35*:51, 1951.

Taylor, S. G., III, Slaughter, D. P., Smejkal, W., et al.: The effect of sex hormones on advanced carcinoma of the breast. Cancer, *1*:604, 1948.

Taylor, S. G., IV, Kalish, L. A., Olson, J. E., et al.: Adjuvant CMFP versus CMFP plus tamoxifen versus observation alone in postmenopausal, node positive breast cancer patients: Three year results of an Eastern Cooperative Oncology Group Study. J. Clin. Oncol., *3*:144, 1985.

Thompson, A.: Analysis of cases in which oophorectomy was performed for inoperable carcinoma of the breast. Br. Med. J., *4*:1538, 1902.

Topper, Y. J., and Oka, T.: Some aspects of mammary gland development in the mature mouse. *In* Larson, B. L., and Smith, V. R. (Eds.): Lactation: A Comprehensive Treatise. New York, Academic Press, 1974, pp. 327–348.

Ulrich, P.: Testosterone (hormone male) et son role

possible dans le traitement de certains cancers du sein. Acta Un. Int. Cancre, *4*:377, 1939.

vanDyk, J. J., and Falkson, G.: Extended survival and remission rates in metastatic breast cancer. Cancer, *27*:300, 1971.

Veronesi, U., Cascinelli, N., Greco, M., et al.: A reappraisal of oophorectomy in carcinoma of the breast. Ann. Surg., *205*:18, 1981.

Volk, H., Deupree, R. H., Goldenberg, I. S., et al.: A dose response evaluation of delta-1-testololactone in advanced breast cancer. Cancer, *33*:9, 1974.

Wells, S. A., and Santen, R. J.: Ablative procedures in patients with metastatic breast carcinoma. Cancer, *53*:762, 1984.

Wilson, A. J.: Response in breast cancer to a second hormonal therapy. Rev. Endocrine-Related Cancer. *14*:5, 1983.

Wintz, H.: Experience in irradiation of breast cancer. Br. J. Radiol., *31*:100, 1926.

Wittliff, J. L.: Specific receptors of the steroid hormones in breast cancer. Semin. Oncol., *1*:109, 1974.

Wittliff, J. L.: Steroid-hormone receptors in breast cancer. Cancer, *53*:630, 1984.

Wiznitzer, I., and Benz, C.: Direct growth inhibiting effects of the prolactin antagonists burserelin and pergolide on human breast cancer (Abstract). Proc. Am. Assoc. Cancer. Res. *25*:208, 1984.

Yarbro, J. W.: Cancer research and the development of cancer centers. *In* Gross, S. C., and Garb, S. (Eds.): Cancer Treatment and Research in Humanistic Perspective. New York, Springer, 1985, pp. 3–15.

Zava, D. T., and McGuire, W. L.: Human breast cancer: Androgen action mediated via estrogen receptor. Science, *199*:787, 1978.

CHAPTER 18

MARC K. WALLACK
JERRY A. BASH

Immunology and Immunotherapy of Mammary Tumors

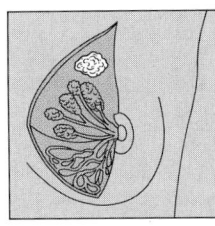

Although immunotherapy is often regarded as a new approach to cancer treatment, both theoretical tumor immunology and clinical immunotherapy originated independently near the turn of the present century (Ehrlich, 1909; Coley, 1891). The history of tumor immunology has been linked to that of specific immunotherapy by association with the dramatic success that antimicrobial immunity has had in prevention of infectious disease. Unfortunately, a comparison of tumor-specific antigens to microbial antigens reveals an inherent problem; tumor antigens are generally weakly immunogenic and often are identical to normal tissue components expressed during differentiation (Lennox, 1985). The original concept of immune surveillance (Ehrlich, 1909; Burnet, 1970; Thomas, 1959), which was based on the inherent ability of the immune system to recognize and eliminate tumor cells, has been difficult to confirm experimentally (Stutman, 1985). On the other hand, the relationship of an intact immune system to prevention of malignancy is being dramatically demonstrated in the current epidemic of Kaposi's sarcoma associated with acquired immune deficiency syndrome (AIDS) (Fahey et al., 1985). The pragmatic approach to immunotherapy is exemplified by the original work of Coley, in which a toxic mixture of bacteria was administered to patients with advanced cancer following the observation that concomitant infection sometimes resulted in regression (Coley, 1912). The molecular basis of this approach is now offering promise in the form of recombinant tumor necrosis factor (Old, 1985). Adoptive immunotherapy, the transfer of immune cells with antitumor reactivity into tumor-bearing hosts, has been successful in animals for many years. Only recently is this approach proving the ability of immunocytes to mediate regression of human tumors (Rosenberg et al., 1987).

Breast cancer offers one of the best examples of malignancy with immunologic implications. There are animal models in which tumor-associated antigens have been demonstrated and against which successful immunotherapeutic regimens have been developed. The human disease itself has a course of histopathologic development that strongly suggests participation of the host immune response. The availability of surgical specimens from lymph node dissection has provided much opportunity for relating reactive changes to prognosis of disease. For these reasons, breast cancer has been cited as a model for cancer immunology (Black et al., 1984).

Until recently, therapy of breast cancer has emphasized the three standard treatment methods of surgery, radiotherapy, and chemotherapy. These approaches, in a wide variety of combinations, have had variable success in other malignancies, but have had only limited progress in the treatment of breast cancer. The recent use of hormone therapy in the adjuvant setting has generated much excitement (see Chapter 17). However, even in light of the encouraging results with this approach, there is little evidence for a substantial improvement in the long-term survival of breast cancer patients (Urban, 1986).

It is therefore clear that different approaches

are needed. Immunotherapy, although a very old concept with a long history of promise and disappointment, has in recent years developed into a legitimate fourth treatment method, included under the classification of biologic response modification (Oldham, 1984). Within the last decade, both advances in basic biologic and genetic research and technical achievements in immunobiology have revolutionized this approach.

This chapter briefly reviews the history of immunologic studies of mammary tumor so as to place the most recent advances in immunobiology and immunotherapy in context. The immunology and immunotherapy of breast cancer have been reviewed comprehensively previously (Nathanson, 1977; Nauts, 1984; Black and Zachrau, 1987). This chapter therefore emphasizes the most recent, significant and representative contributions.

Immunobiology of Experimental Mammary Tumors

SPONTANEOUS MAMMARY TUMORS

The occurrence of spontaneous mammary tumors associated with immunosuppression lends support to the hypothesis of immune surveillance. Mice undergoing an induced graft versus host disease accompanied by profound immune suppression develop a high incidence of mammary carcinoma (Gartner et al., 1984).

One of the mechanisms that has been proposed for the escape of breast tumors from immune surveillance has been the status of the mammary gland as an immunologically privileged site (i.e., a site with local isolation from peripheral immune afferent or efferent arms of the immune response, or both). Much evidence exists from studies of tumor emergence or transplantation in the mouse mammary fat pad to support this theory. Mammary tumors implanted subcutaneously elicit a much more prompt immune response than do those transplanted into the mammary fat pad (Miller, 1985). A higher conversion of preneoplastic nodules to tumors occurs in situ (i.e., in the mammary fat pads) than in heterotopically transplanted nodules (Slemmer, 1972).

A group of spontaneous mammary carcinomas occurring in inbred Nottingham Wistar (Not-W) rats have been studied extensively with regard to the relationship of immunogenicity to tumor progression. Although induced resistance to rechallenge was found to be specific to the immunizing tumor, no relationship between tumor immunogenicity and latent period of development could be shown, and spontaneous regressions were not observed (Greager and Baldwin, 1966).

Traditionally, tumors with no known inducing agent have been classified as spontaneous, although many of the mammary adenocarcinomas that arise in mice of certain strains possess mouse mammary tumor virus antigens and should thus be considered virus-induced.

VIRUS-INDUCED MAMMARY TUMORS

The most extensive body of research performed with experimental mammary tumors has been in the mouse mammary tumor virus (MMTV) model, in which certain strains of mice have a predictably high incidence of mammary tumors arising from immunologically related endogenous viruses (Gross, 1947).

The MMTV model has recently been used to study the efficacy of active immunization with vaccines prepared from spontaneous mammary tumors in preventing the occurrence of spontaneous or virus-induced tumors in other mice. Vaccines prepared from cells of primary spontaneous mammary tumors of RIII/IMr, GR/Imr, C3H/Imr, A/Imr, and C3HfC57BL/Imr mice were used to immunize MMTV-free BALB/c/Imr and C57BL/Imr mice before challenge with MMTV from the respective strains. Mammary tumor vaccines from C3H protected mice from tumorigenesis by all four MMTVs and significantly enhanced development of A-MMTV-induced tumors. The need for viral antigens acting alone or in concert with cellular antigens was indicated by the failure of vaccines prepared from C3HfC57BL tumor cells free of C3H-MMTV to induce protection. A second set of experiments was conducted in which the same vaccines were used to immunize mice from the homologous strains that have a high incidence of spontaneous tumors from natural infection with MMTV. Tumorigenesis was not prevented in any of the strains, although delay of appearance was observed in RIII and GR mice (Girardi et al., 1985).

The phenomenon of virus augmentation of responses to tumor antigens that alone are weakly immunogenic has been described in many other virus–tumor cell combinations (Austin and Boone, 1979) and is a promising approach to active immunotherapy.

CARCINOGEN-INDUCED MAMMARY TUMORS

Carcinogen-induced mouse mammary adenocarcinomas have been extremely useful in studies of the influence of immune responses on tumor progression because they generally are immunogenic in the host of origin.

Dimethylbenzanthracene (DMBA)-induced adenocarcinomas are illustrative of these transplantable tumor lines. The D1-DMBA-3 and D1-DMBA-2 tumors have been used to study the cause and effect of tumor progression related to changes in lymphocyte subsets in the spleens of BALB/c mice. It has been shown that a relative increase in Lyt-2+ cells at the expense of Lyt-1+ cells occurs in the tumor infiltrating T cell populations and these T cells become less responsive to stimulation by both tumor-associated antigens and T cell mitogens during the course of tumor progression (Buessow et al., 1984).

DMBA-induced murine mammary tumors have been used in an attempt to demonstrate biologic markers that could discriminate between normal, preneoplastic, and neoplastic cells. Among a panel of monoclonal antibodies directed against these tumors, one of these reagents, AMT8, detected an antigen that was expressed in preneoplastic nodules and that could serve as a marker of early mammary tumorigenesis (Johnson et al., 1985).

Chemically induced mammary adenocarcinomas have been also studied extensively in rats (Kreider et al., 1976). One of these tumors, 113762A, has been particularly useful as it has been adapted to grow in ascites form and displays low immunogenicity and high frequency of spontaneous metastasis. A recently cloned variant of the 13762A tumor has been found to be significantly more immunogenic and susceptible to immune attack. Mice immunized with the cloned variant were resistant to the parental strain, and lymphocytes from these immunized mice were able to adoptively transfer specific immunity to the parental tumor (Kreider and Bartlett, 1985).

IMMUNOTHERAPY MODELS

Rodent models have been used extensively in preclinical testing of immunotherapeutic regimens. These have been reviewed extensively and evaluated in terms of their relevance to treatment of naturally occurring cancer in man (Kallman et al., 1985).

One of the central questions regarding active immunotherapy has been the relative importance of tumor immunogenicity in induction of resistance to tumor progression. Using spontaneous rat mammary adenocarcinomas SP4, SP15, and SP22 to study *Corynebacterium parvum* and bacille Calmette-Guérin (BCG) treatment of tumors inoculated in the mammary pad tissue, it was found that early intratumor inoculation of both of these bacterial adjuvants effectively caused regression of primary tumors and reduced incidence of regional lymph node metastases of the most immunogenic tumor but were ineffective in animals bearing the less immunogenic tumor lines (Greager and Baldwin, 1978).

Given the relative abundance of evidence relating the influence of the immune response on the progression of murine mammary adenocarcinomas, it has been proposed that those tumors of greatest metastatic potential may be able to effect immunosuppression (Buessow et al., 1984). Immunotherapeutic approaches might then include the use of agents that prevent tumor-induced immunosuppression. It has been demonstrated that a high positive correlation exists between levels of prostaglandin E production and the tumorigenicity and metastatic potential of a variety of murine tumors. Prostaglandin E in turn was associated with suppression of natural killer (NK) cell activity. When endogenous prostaglandin synthesis was inhibited by the addition of indomethacin to tumor cell cultures, the sensitivity to NK lysis was increased (Fulton and Heppner, 1985).

Mouse models have been invaluable in demonstrating the usefulness of combined therapeutic techniques against breast cancer. The value of intermittent chemotherapy after surgical resection of the primary tumor and the importance of dose and schedule of such chemotherapies are based on the need to avoid suppression of host antitumor immunity at a time when a low tumor burden makes for a more effective immune attack (Stolfi et al., 1974).

Perhaps the most dramatic illustration of the value of mouse models of immunotherapy is that provided by studies of adoptive immunotherapy with IL-2 and lymphokine activated killer (LAK) cells, which led to the application of this approach in clinical immunotherapy

(Rosenberg, 1986). The demonstration that primary explants of mouse mammary adenocarcinomas are lysed by human interleukin-2 stimulated syngeneic lymphocytes (Merluzzi et al., 1985) suggests that this approach to treatment of breast cancer may be successful in humans.

One of the most useful means of developing immunotherapeutic approaches to treatment of cancer has been provided by the technique of growing human tumors in immunodeficient, athymic "nude" mice. This method provides a means of assessing antitumor effects against human tumors in an in vivo model (Shorthouse et al., 1980). This technique, which has been especially useful in preclinical evaluation of monoclonal antibodies, was used to evaluate two monoclonal antibodies for their ability to inhibit human breast tumor growth. The conclusion from this study was that effective treatment of solid tumors by this means would require multiple monoclonal antibodies to circumvent the problems of low antigen density (Capone et al., 1984).

One very useful model for immunotherapy of breast cancer with monoclonal antibodies is based on a tumor-specific transplantation antigen of ascitic mouse mammary tumor of C3H/He mice (Nishioka et al., 1969; Takeuchi et al., 1969). The immunotherapeutic potential of monoclonal antibodies of different classes has recently been characterized in several in vitro and in vivo assays. Antibody of the gamma-2a class was most effective in protection against tumor challenge or when administered with tumor cells in a Winn assay. Histologic data coupled with the use of macrophage toxic agents suggest that antibody-dependent cell-mediated cytotoxicity with macrophage effector cells was the important mechanism (Seto et al., 1986).

Although purely in vitro assay for immunotherapeutic effector factors or cells cannot be considered true models, they have provided very useful preliminary screening assays. Because many human breast carcinoma lines have been established in culture, they have provided a useful means of analyzing toxic or growth inhibitory effects of monoclonal antibodies. A colony inhibition assay has been used to screen 85 cancer monoclonal antibodies conjugated to the A chain of the ricin molecule. This approach allowed identification of promising immunotherapeutic immunotoxins on the basis of their selective binding and toxicity to tumor cells rather than normal cells in culture (Bjorn et al., 1985).

As the availability of inbred strains allows more controlled studies in mice than in an outbred population, such as humans, the relevance of murine models has been criticized, and the use of outbred large animals, such as dogs, has been advocated. Dogs have proved useful as models for breast cancer in that spontaneous adenocarcinoma of the breast is observed not infrequently. Dogs with mammary adenocarcinoma were used to demonstrate the potential usefulness of extracorporeal immunoabsorption in *Staphylococcus aureus*–containing chambers. Using this model, reduction of tumor burden of the soft tissue nodule type was observed, but those tumors localized in the viscera were unaffected (Holohan et al., 1982). This procedure has produced some encouraging results in clinical trials, although the theoretical basis of the effect is controversial (Bertram, 1985).

SUMMARY

Animal models have been very useful in the study of the immunology and immunotherapy of mammary tumors. The mouse mammary tumor virus model has been particularly valuable in studying the development of mammary tumors in a controlled way and has resulted in both indirect and direct evidence for the role of a similar virus as one cause of human breast cancer. In addition to the MMTV model, a number of chemically induced mammary adenocarcinomas have been produced in mice and rats and shown to express tumor-associated antigens that play a role in the development and growth of these tumors in vivo. They have been used extensively to study the evolution of tumors from preneoplastic nodules and the relative immunologic privilege of the mammary fat pad. These models have also been of great value in preclinical evaluation of therapeutic regimens, which include both specific and nonspecific approaches. The nude mouse has proved to be of great value as a recipient of xenogeneic transplants of human breast tumors, which can then be tested for sensitivity to immunologic inhibition (e.g., by monoclonal antibodies conjugated to toxins, drugs, or radionuclides). Dog models have been useful in providing a large outbred animal for evaluation of surgical adjuvant therapeutic procedures, such as extracorporeal filtration.

Immunobiology of Human Breast Cancer

ANTIGENICITY

Immunologic Evidence for Human Mammary Tumor Virus. The mouse mammary tumor virus (MMTV) system (discussed earlier) has been an extremely useful model for studying tumor virus–host interaction although a human equivalent to MMTV has yet to be demonstrated directly. Nonetheless, there is an abundance of immunologic evidence associating MMTV-related antigens and human mammary tumors. First, it was observed that leukocytes of patients with breast cancer react with MMTV in leukocyte migration assays (Black et al., 1974). There have been several reports of antibodies to MMTV-related antigen in sera of patients with breast carcinoma (Day et al., 1981; Tomana et al., 1981). Further evidence for the existence of a MMTV-related antigen in human mammary tumors has been reported, and the antigen has been related to the major envelope glycoprotein of MMTV (Mesa-Tejada et al., 1978; Dion et al., 1980). Further study of this antigen has revealed its presence in metastatic lesions of human mammary tumors as well as in human breast carcinoma lines. Moreover, clonal derivatives of such lines have been shown to contain retrovirus particles that have antigenic cross-reactivity with gp52, the major external protein of MMTV (Keydar et al., 1982). These cross-reactive antigens have been characterized further as two glycosylated polypeptides with molecular weights of 68,000 and 60,000 daltons, the larger of which is present in the viral particles shed by human breast carcinoma lines (Segev et al., 1985). Further evidence for a human mammary tumor virus includes the demonstration of retrovirus-like particles with reverse transcriptase activity in human milk samples (Keydar, et al., 1978) and the detection of sequences related to the MMTV genome in the DNA of human mammary tumors (Callahan et al., 1982; May et al., 1983). MMTV gp52-related antigens have been detected on the surface of normal human lymphocytes (Lopez, 1986). By analogy with the mouse system in which MMTV-RNA has been associated with the expression of this antigen on a subset of B lymphocytes (Lopez et al., 1985), the DNA sequences that code for this molecule may function as a proto-oncogene with an important role in the growth or differentiation (or both) of cells of the bone marrow–derived lymphoid lineage.

Although final confirmation of the retrovirus causation of human breast cancer awaits more definitive studies, the existence of MMTV cross-reactive antigens provides a potentially useful marker for the diagnosis and perhaps the prognosis of breast cancer. Antibodies reactive with MMTV have been detected by several investigators in the sera of American women with breast cancer in higher percentages than in healthy women or patients with benign breast disease (Day et al., 1981; Tomana et al., 1981). On the other hand, less than 5.0 per cent of women from mainland China with breast cancer had MMTV-reactive antibodies in their sera (Day et al., 1981). This epidemiologic evidence underlines the phenomenon of multiple causation of cancers of similar types and suggests that the MMTV-associated marker may define a subset with poor prognosis. For example, the MMTV-related antigen that is expressed in metastatic lesions is present in increased incidence in Tunisian patients suffering from a rapidly progressive form of breast cancer known as *poussée evolutive* (Levine et al., 1984).

In addition to the serologic evidence for breast cancer-associated antigens related to MMTV, there is much evidence for similar antigens detected in assays for cell-mediated immunity. Many of the studies that have described MMTV-related breast cancer antigens on the basis of patient lymphocyte stimulation have used an assay based on direct inhibition of leukocyte migration by extracts from MMTV-infected mouse tissue (Black et al., 1974). This technique has the disadvantages of not being quantitative, of not being able to discriminate inhibition from toxicity, and of not being able to separate MMTV antigens from murine cellular components. A modification of the leukocyte inhibition technique in which an indirect (two-step) procedure is used to measure migration inhibition factor production has been successfully used with MMTV-antigens grown in feline tissue to document cellular responses to MMTV both by MMTV-tumor bearing mice and by leukocytes of human breast cancer patients (McCoy et al., 1984). Other studies of leukocyte migration inhibition may serve to identify a group of benign breast disease patients whose breast pathology is thought to be associated with a high risk for developing breast cancer (Cannon et al., 1982).

It is clear from the evidence cited earlier that both humoral and cell-mediated immune responses to MMTV-related antigens occur that are distinct from reactivity to antigens unrelated to virus. The role of these responses as well as the role of host responses to less well defined tumor-associated antigens in the progression of disease remains to be determined.

Other Breast Tumor-Associated Antigens (TAA). The existence of organ-specific neoantigens (ONA) in breast cancer has long been reported on the basis of serologic specificity of circulating antibodies such as the complement-dependent antibodies (Hindsley et al., 1979) or on the ability of crude tumor extracts to elicit delayed skin responses (Austin et al., 1982).

The search for tumor-specific antigens that preoccupied tumor immunologists in the past has been recently supplanted by the recognition that although many antigens exist in higher concentration on tumor cells than on normal cells, it is questionable that truly tumor-specific antigens exist (Lennox, 1985). The term tumor-associated antigens (TAA) has therefore been adopted as an operational definition that has become increasingly useful in diagnosis, staging, monitoring, and therapy. The identification and characterization of TAA have been revolutionized by the advent of hybridoma technology and the resultant proliferation of monoclonal antibodies that identify components associated with breast tumors. These reagents have been reviewed by Colcher and associates (1984) and Burchell and Taylor-Papadimitriou (1985). Only a few illustrative examples are therefore discussed here. They can generally be classified into those reagents that identify human breast cancer antigens that are not shared with other tumor or normal cells, those that are common to other adenocarcinomas, and those that are directed against normal breast tissue components that are present in increased amounts in breast tumors.

In the last 5 years several monoclonal antibodies have been developed that identify a wide variety of breast tumor antigens (Colcher et al., 1984; Burchell and Taylor-Papadimitriou, 1985). Monoclonal antibodies that identify epithelial components of the delipidated human milk fat globule membrane (Taylor-Papadimitriou, 1981; Hilkens et al., 1981), although not specific for a tumor antigen, have been shown to be valuable in diagnosis and prognosis of breast carcinoma (Wilkinson et al., 1984; Rasmussen et al., 1985). On the other hand, some monoclonal antibodies, such as 10-302 (Soule et al., 1983) bind to all tested breast carcinomas and a number of other human carcinomas but not to normal mammary epithelium or other normal tissues. Several monoclonal antibodies (Colcher et al., 1984) recognize common carcinoma antigens shared with several tumors in addition to breast cancer but are nonreactive with normal cells. Although murine monoclonal antibodies with selective reactivity to human breast cancer cells have been described (Papsidero et al., 1983; White et al., 1985), the antigens recognized by these reagents have not been characterized. A 43,000 dalton membrane glycoprotein present in breast tumor cells but not in normal cells has been characterized by immunoprecipitation with a monoclonal antibody (Edwards et al., 1986). This antigen was, however, not tumor-restricted in that it was found to be present in tumors of other histologic origins. More typical of the mouse monoclonal antibodies that have been described is that designated B72.3. This antibody reacts with a tumor-associated glycoprotein complex of high molecular weight present in 50 per cent of primary breast tumors but also in 85 per cent of colonic carcinomas. The antigen recognized by B72.3, termed TAG-72, is not present in tumor cells of comparable origin but is detectable in small amounts on normal secretory cells and is modulated by the spatial configuration of cells in culture (Horan-Hand et al., 1985). A new monoclonal antibody, 3E1-2, has also been described, which, on the basis of screening formalin-fixed tissue sections by the immunoperoxidase technique, was found to stain predominantly breast carcinoma, although some other tumors with normal tissues showed weaker reactivity (Stacker et al., 1985). Two potentially useful monoclonal antibodies that were produced against milk fat globule membranes have been shown to be highly discriminatory in detecting breast cancer to the exclusion of normal controls and, most importantly, these antibodies detect an antigen present in plasma and thereby are easily screened for (Feller et al., 1986).

The usefulness of monoclonal antibodies in diagnosis and monitoring of breast cancer is not limited to those that identify breast cancer-specific or even restricted tumor-associated antigens. For example, monoclonal antibodies that are directed against estrogen-regulated proteins may be very useful in diagnosis of breast cancer (Brabon et al., 1984; Garcia et al., 1985). Carcinoembryonic antigen (CEA), although associated with colon carcinoma, serves as a useful indicator of breast cancer (Colcher et al., 1984). Even HLA antigens that are broadly shared with normal tissue may serve under controlled conditions as suitable tumor markers on the basis of relative expression (Natali et al., 1983; Bernard et al., 1985). At an international workshop on breast cancer research and treatment, a wide variety of normal gene products detectable by monoclonal antibodies were shown to be potentially useful markers in breast cancer diagnosis. These included cytokeratins, glycosphingolipids, and the human oncogene products (Peterson and Ceriani, 1985).

Although monoclonal antibodies have become the most useful means of identification of new breast cancer–associated antigens, information concerning immunologic responses associated with the disease process has also been obtained using conventional antisera from breast cancer patients or from immunized animals. Rabbits were immunized with immune complexes obtained from serum of breast cancer patients by binding to Raji cells. When this antiserum was used to purify and characterize an antigen from normal and malignant breast tissue, it was found to be capable of identifying a normal breast tissue–associated antigen, suggesting that the circulating immune complexes seen in breast cancer may result from a concurrent autoimmune process (Koestler et al., 1981).

The classic example of an antigen that is present in normal cells in a naked form but detected in serum and tumor tissue of breast cancer patients is the Thomsen-Friedenreich antigen (Springer et al., 1980). This antigen, known as the T antigen, has been shown to be a precursor of the human blood group system MN and therefore readily demonstrable in red blood cells. In addition to serologic studies with this antigen, the T antigen has also been used to elicit a specific delayed hypersensitivity skin reaction in breast cancer patients. The majority of healthy subjects and patients with benign breast disease were negative for the antigen (Springer et al., 1980). A sensitive method of detecting single metastatic adenocarcinoma cells of the breast has been developed using indirect immunofluorescent staining based on the specific binding of peanut agglutinin to the terminal disaccharide sequence of asialoglycophorin A, the MN precursor substance that identified the Thomsen-Friedenreich antigen (Seitz et al., 1984).

Some of the most promising monoclonal antibodies in determining breast cancer prognosis have only recently been evaluated. These are the antiestrogen receptor antibodies D547Sp gamma and D75 Sp gamma. ELISA procedures employing these antibodies on breast cancer tissue, the estrogen receptor immunocytochemical assay (ERICA), compare very favorably to the estrogen-binding procedure previously employed (Pertschuk, 1985). The diagnostic and prognostic significance of estrogen receptor expression is discussed in detail elsewhere in this volume (Chapter 11).

Although mouse monoclonal antibodies are operationally useful if they achieve recognition of tumor–associated antigens or normal antigens that may be expressed in higher concentration on breast cancer cells than in normal breast tissue, a major goal of breast cancer immunodiagnosis and therapy is to characterize breast tumor–associated antigens responsible for induction of autologous immune responses. The most promising means to achieve this is through production of human monoclonal antibodies by fusion of lympocytes from breast cancer patients with mouse myeloma or human lymphoblastoid lines. One approach that has been successful has been to fuse lymphocytes from lymph nodes of metastatic breast cancer patients with a nonsecretory variant of murine myeloma cells. This method results in the production of human monoclonal antibodies. Preliminary screening of the resulting clones showed that 15 of 81 produced human monoclonal antibody, which preferentially bound to breast carcinoma cells (Imam et al., 1985). These results have important implications for both active and passive immunotherapy (discussed later in this chapter), as identification of antigens that induce autologous immune responses could allow development of appropriate vaccines.

Another approach to demonstration of autologous responses to breast tumor–associated antigens is to elicit skin responses with tumor extracts (Oldham and Herberman, 1979). This approach is used to monitor the development of cell-mediated immunity. Extracts of autologous tumors have been used to skin test patients undergoing active immunotherapy with some success (Humphrey et al., 1984), although the goal of identification of a common antigen has yet to be achieved. Another approach of some promise has been used to demonstrate breast cancer–associated skin test reactivity in breast cancer patients. Crude membrane (CM) extracts were prepared from cultured human breast tumor lines that had been infected with vesicular stomatitis virus (VSV) to augment their antigenicity. One of these extracts, VSV-MCF-7, elicited positive skin test responses in 78.9 per cent of breast cancer patients tested, compared with 13.3 per cent and 15.4 per cent of patients with lung carcinoma and melanoma, respectively (Austin et al., 1982). Although the tumor antigens involved in eliciting these responses remain to be further characterized biochemically, the demonstration of antigenic cross-reactivity with a large number of breast cancer patients is a finding of great importance for potential immunotherapy.

IMMUNOCOMPETENCE AND IMMUNOTHERAPY

Clinical evidence for the role of the immune system in breast cancer includes reports of higher incidence and more severe disease in immunocompromised patients and reports of better prognosis in patients who have been shown to mount an immune response. Lymphocytes from breast cancer patients have been shown to have depressed proliferative responses, although a serum component might be mediating suppression (Whittaker and Clark, 1971). It has been suggested that the failure of postmastectomy radiation to improve survival may be due to the resultant depression of absolute lymphocyte counts, which persists for years (Meyer et al., 1970).

A variety of clinical conditions leading to compromised immunity have been associated with increased incidence or severity of breast cancer, or both. Immunodeficiency associated with autoimmune processes, such as myasthenia gravis, in which thymomas are common and associated with a high incidence of breast cancer and a high frequency of bilateral disease. The protective effect of thymectomy reported in these cases is similar to that achieved in experimental animals, although the endocrine and immune factors involved in this phenomenon remain to be clarified (Papatestas et al., 1977).

The largest group of patients in whom immunodeficiency may be associated with enhanced disease is that of the elderly. Immunosenescence may contribute to the poor prognosis of breast cancer in patients of advanced age (Mueller and Ames, 1978). A comprehensive study of immune function related to breast cancer stage indicated that two different phases of immunosuppression can be discriminated in breast cancer. The first, associated with early breast cancer, is primary and patient related. The secondary tumor-induced depression of immune response characterizes advanced and metastatic breast cancer (Adler et al., 1980).

Perhaps the most controversial issue regarding immune function and prognosis after surgery concerns the extirpation of uninvolved lymph nodes. It is clear that a negative correlation exists between lymph node activity and stage of breast cancer (Reiss et al., 1983), but the cause-and-effect relationship remains unclear. A dilemma related to the role of lymph node immune responsiveness and surgery involves concern for residual disease on the one hand and lowering of regional immunity on the other hand (Fisher and Fisher, 1972) and therefore demands an examination of the evidence that immune reactivity to the tumor indeed exists.

Evidence for autologous immune responsiveness to breast tumors includes both in vitro serologic and cellular assays and histopathologic observations. The first suggestion of immune recognition of breast cancer associated with prolonged survival was based on the histologic appearance of a proliferative reaction in the axillary lymph nodes (Halsted, 1898). Since this original observation, much additional evidence has been obtained to suggest that morphologic manifestations, including lymphoid infiltrates (MacCarty, 1922) and sinus histiocytosis (Black et al., 1953), are associated with survival and cure and represent cell-mediated immune responses.

The early suggestions of a cellular response to tumor in situ fostered many attempts to demonstrate cellular immune responses in peripheral organs by both in vivo and in vitro techniques. Those techniques that measure general immune responsiveness, such as in vitro blastogenetic responses to nonspecific mitogens and skin test responses to common recall antigens and the synthetic antigen dinitrochlorobenzene (DNCB), appear useful in determining prognosis. Other techniques that detect reactivity to tumor-associated antigens include leukocyte migration inhibition, macrophage arming, lymphocytotoxicity, and blastogenesis with specific antigen preparations. One overall conclusion from these studies is that breast cancer patients generally are immunosuppressed.

In vitro evidence for a role of regional axillary node lymphocytes in breast cancer has been obtained in a study in which significantly increased response of lymph node lymphocytes to tumor cells was observed in patients with no metastatic involvement compared with patients who had extensive metastases. Moreover, in six patients from whom peripheral lymphocytes as well as lymph node lymphocytes were available, a greater response to tumor cells was manifested by regional lymph node lymphocytes (Crile, 1969). Other studies of in vitro cell-mediated responses in breast cancer have implicated MMTV-associated antigens (discussed earlier). It has been demonstrated that whereas women with breast metastatic disease have diminished responsiveness to mitogens, their T lymphocytes have heightened reactivity to MMTV. These results suggest an altered proportion of T cell subsets in the peripheral blood of these patients (Lopez, 1986). Other investigators have also demonstrated changes in peripheral lymphocyte subsets related to breast cancer. Substantial differences in the lymphocyte subset profile between Stage I and Stage II breast carcinoma have been demonstrated using a panel of monoclonal antibodies and two-color flow cytometric analysis. A significantly larger subset of T cells that had been shown to contain helper activity for B cell differentiation was seen in nodes from patients with Stage II disease. These results suggest that change in the local-regional immunocompetent cell subsets may be related to metastasis of breast cancer to regional nodes (Morton et al., 1986).

More direct evidence associating regional lymphoid changes and immune response to tumors in situ has been obtained from immunohistologic studies. The cells infiltrating human breast carcinomas have been characterized using antimononuclear cell monoclonal immunoperoxidase staining of frozen sections. Although both lymphoid and myelomonocyte lineage cells were demonstrated in the infiltrated tumors, there was a predominance of T4 positive cells associated with HLA-DR+ phenotype (Gottlinger et al., 1985). Functional studies of lymphocytes recovered and cloned from infiltrated human mammary carcinomas also support the predominance of T4+ effector cells that display cytolytic activity (Whiteside et al., 1986).

Another phenomenon with implications of immune modification of breast cancer occurrence is the apparent protective effect of early first pregnancy on risk of development of breast cancer. One hypothesis used to explain this is that the exposure to fetal antigens (shared with tumors) during pregnancy provides a natural vaccination against tumorigenesis. Evidence to support this theory has been based largely on the observations that immunoglobulin levels may help to identify women with a high risk and a poor prognosis (Papatestas et al., 1979; Lamoureux et al., 1982). Production of circulating antibodies against breast tumor antigens correlates well with fewer lymph node metastases and better prognosis (Hudson et al., 1974). Again, however, the observation that a number of serum proteins are present in abnormal levels in breast cancer patients indicates a generally unbalanced organ function and may not be specific for the disease.

Circumstantial evidence for the importance of cell-mediated immunity to the clinical occurrence and progression of human breast cancer is based on observations relating development of cell-mediated immunity associated with in situ breast lesions to the stage and time of diagnosis of a second breast cancer (Black et al., 1984). These observations are consistent with the immunogenicity of breast cancer and the protective effect of cell-mediated responses. Other evidence supporting a role of cell-mediated immunity in protection against recurrence is based on the significant inverse correlation between peripheral lymphocyte count and chance of recurrence (Lee, 1984; Papatestas and Kark, 1974). This is supported by evidence that the depleted lymphocytes primarily include a T cell subpopulation responsible for cell-mediated reactions (Felix et al., 1981). B cell subsets, however, may be increased. The relative frequency of surface immunoglobulin isotypes in axillary lymph nodes of patients who had infiltrating ductal carcinoma was significantly increased in sIgM positive lymphocytes in those patients with lymph-node metastases (Richters and Paller, 1979). This finding supports the observation of a significant increase in IgM production locally in certain breast tumors (Roberts et al., 1973).

SUMMARY

A great deal of evidence exists in the literature to support a relationship between immune responsiveness and breast cancer occurrence and progression. Much of this evidence has been drawn from histopathologic observation of lymph node activity associated with a refractory development of systemic disease. Other evidence has been obtained from skin testing and in vitro assays to suggest that breast tumor–associated antigens may elicit an immune response. Conversely, there have been many reports of increased incidence and progression of breast cancer in immunosuppressed patients, such as the age-related increase in incidence. These findings support the rationale for immunotherapeutic approaches.

Clinical Immunotherapy

NONSPECIFIC ACTIVE IMMUNOTHERAPY

The first form of biologic therapy for cancer can legitimately be attributed to nature, based on the first reports of the phenomenon of tumor regression in association with concurrent acute bacterial infection. A total of 449 such cases of "spontaneous regression" have been recorded, of which 93 were breast cancers (Nauts, 1984).

The first attempt to induce bacterial infections as a therapeutic measure in breast cancer was made over 200 years ago. The pioneer of this approach in the United States was Coley, who developed a vaccine from a mixture of bacteria (MBV). The first MBV, also known as Coley's Mixed Toxin, was prepared from *Streptococcus pyogenes* and *Bacillus prodigiosus* (now *Serratia marcescens*). A total of 896 microscopically proved cases of cancer were treated by MBV, of which 78 involved the breast. Although this study did not include a large number and was without concurrent controls, the results described, including regression and markedly increased survival in some inoperable breast cancers, seem impressive. Use of MBV immunotherapy in combination with surgery, radiotherapy, and chemotherapy has achieved even more impressive, although not entirely well documented, successes (Nauts, 1980).

The most important result of MBV research was the stimulation of interest in other bacterial vaccines, such as bacille Calmette-Guérin (BCG). Although BCG, an attenuated form of the tubercle bacillus, was first used as a vaccine against tuberculosis, it was found to be a potent stimulator of the reticuloendothelial system, which was associated with prevention of tumor growth in mice (Old, 1959). This observation stimulated interest in clinical trials, which ushered in the era of nonspecific immunotherapy with bacterial adjuvants that lasted over a decade (Nauts, 1984). The first usage of BCG to treat disseminated breast cancer was in combination with chemotherapy which included 5-fluorouracil (5-FU), doxorubicin hydrochloride (Adriamycin), and cyclophosphamide (FAC). Compared with FAC alone there were similar rates of remission but a longer duration of remission when BCG was included (Gutterman et al., 1976). Many clinical studies of breast carcinoma have since reported prolonged disease-free intervals using a combination of chemotherapy and immunotherapy following surgery (the adjuvant chemoimmunotherapy approach) (Buzdar et al., 1979). Some protocols have included radiotherapy in this combination and achieved significant success in treating patients with inflammatory breast carcinoma, which has a grave prognosis (Krutchik et al., 1979).

Another organism with potent reticuloendothelial system stimulatory properties is *Corynebacterium parvum* which as a killed vaccine was shown to inhibit tumor growth (Halpern et al., 1966). Large numbers of patients with disseminated disease were treated with *C. parvum*, including many with metastatic breast cancer. Although significant increases in survival and isolated cases of complete remission were reported (Nathanson, 1977), deleterious side-effects associated with this organism have limited its use.

The best documented successes of nonspecific immunotherapy of breast cancer in terms of permanent regressions have been achieved in protocols in which local administration of immunostimulants has resulted in a significantly high 5 year cure rate and regression of metastatic lesions of breast cancer involving the skin and soft tissues (Klein et al., 1976).

NONSPECIFIC PASSIVE IMMUNOTHERAPY

Although the term passive immunotherapy suggests a lack of participation of the host in the mechanism of action, several substances that have direct nonspecific antitumor properties and are therefore considered to confer resistance passively may actually exert an indirect antitumor effect based on modulation of the immune response. A great many biologic mediators produced by cells of the immune system, designated lymphokines, monokines, or cytokines, have been shown to have a variety of effects, such as enhancement of antitumor immune responses and direct cytotoxic or antiproliferative effects. These biologic response modifiers have been reviewed recently (Oldham, 1984; Torrence, 1986). Only a few representative examples are described briefly here.

The classic example of a group of biologic response modifiers with multiple biologic effects is interferon (Hooks and Detrick, 1986). Although growth inhibition and immunostimulatory properties of interferon were shown to be responsible for antitumor effects in vitro and in animal models, clinical trials were limited by the small amount of material that could be prepared (e.g., from human buffy coat cells stimulated with virus or mitogen). Successful cloning of the gene(s) for alpha-interferon, which allowed the mass production of recombinant molecules, ushered in the modern era of biologic immunotherapy and a new wave of optimism (Krown, 1982).

Relatively few clinical trials have evaluated interferon in breast cancer per se. In the trials performed, a minority of patients showed major objective tumor regression, and considerable toxicity was reported (Borden et al., 1980; Gutterman et al., 1980). Follow-up evaluation of similar trials performed with recombinant alpha(leukocyte)-interferon is being obtained (Queseda et al., 1984).

It should be emphasized that the majority of clinical trials have been performed with clone A alpha-interferon. Several other clonotypes of recombinant alpha-leukoferon remain to be evaluated. Gamma-interferon has only recently been cloned, but its immunoregulatory properties have already been characterized, and the recombinant molecule is being used in a number of clinical trials. It should be noted that doses and schedules of interferon treatment have largely been empirically derived. These parameters remain to be explored and require more controlled trials with well-defined objectives.

Another lymphokine of great interest was first described as a possible mediator of the antitumor activity of bacterial endotoxin (Carswell et al., 1975). This lymphokine has been named tumor necrosis factor (TNF) because it is believed to mediate endotoxin-induced tumor necrosis. The gene for TNF has recently been cloned and expressed and the recombinant molecule has been extensively characterized. A similar molecule produced by lymphocytes, named lymphotoxin, has also recently been obtained as a cloned gene product and has been shown to be closely related to the original TNF (Old, 1985). Clinical trials with TNF are currently under way (Flick and Gifford, 1986).

Perhaps the lymphokine of greatest interest in immunotherapy at present is interleukin-2 (IL-2). IL-2 has been shown to exert antitumor effects in mouse models, especially in conjunction with adoptive immunotherapy. The clinical experience with IL-2 is similar to that in the mouse (i.e., limited effectiveness alone, synergism with adoptively transferred cells that have been activated with IL-2 in vitro, and significant toxicity at high doses) (Rosenberg et al., 1985).

In addition to biologic substances that function as immune modifiers, certain synthetic drugs are also potentially useful. A number of synthetic immunologic modifiers exert their biologic effects through induction of interferon. Most notable of these are the polynucleotides, such as polyriboinosinic: polyribocytidylic (poly I:poly C) and polyadenylate:polyuridylate (poly A:poly U). Although both are good inducers of interferon, Poly A:U is preferred because of its more rapid rate of depolymerization in vivo and its lower toxicity. Poly A:U treatment as an adjunct to simple mastectomy and radiation was evaluated in a large randomized trial in France and found to result in a 4 year relapse-free survival of 77 per cent versus 57 per cent in controls (Lacour et al., 1982).

A synthetic immunologic modifier of uncertain mode of action is levamisole, a drug originally used in veterinary medicine as an anthelmintic. Immunopotentiating properties of levamisole demonstrated in vitro and in animal models prompted clinical evaluation. Promising results have been reported with the use of levamisole in treating advanced breast cancer, which were correlated with an increase in lymphocyte counts and delayed hypersensitivity skin tests (Rojas et al., 1976). Other studies, however, have reported no differences in survival compared with chemotherapy (Hirshaut et al., 1978) or an actual increase in recurrences compared with postoperative radiation (Anthony, 1980). Moreover, the high frequency of side-effects has resulted in suspension of other trials (Retsas et al., 1978).

A nonspecific immunotherapeutic approach that could be considered either active or passive, depending on the interpretation of the mechanism of action, is that of extracorporeal immunoadsorption on bacterial cell wall component chambers or columns. The mode of action of this procedure is believed to involve the removal of immunosuppressive immune complexes, although some authors have postulated that cellular activation is also involved (Bertram, 1985). A randomized study of breast cancer treatment using this technique has yet to be performed.

Soluble biosynthetic molecules with defined immunomodulatory properties constitute the major group of agents of nonspecific passive immunotherapy. The other major approach in this category is that of adoptive immunity, in which the effectors of antitumor immunity transferred are whole cells rather than soluble cellular products. Until very recently, this approach was directed entirely toward the transfer of lymphocytes from patients who had experienced tumor regression and thus presumably had developed immunity. The problems of this approach were similar to those encountered with soluble products from single patient sources (e.g., poor quality control and limited quantities). The major breakthrough in adoptive immunotherapy came with the discovery of T cell growth factor or interleukin-2 (Morgan et al., 1976). This allowed in vitro expansion of T cells to provide large quantities of homogeneous cell populations. Although such expanded T cell lines and clones were initially shown to be antigen-specific after further culture, they exhibited nonspecific killing activity. Experimental adoptive therapy of tumors in mice showed that these nonspecific cells activated by IL-2 in vitro were capable of lysing fresh tumor cells nonspecifically. These lymphokine-activated killer (LAK) cells were shown to mediate dramatic regression of various murine tumors when administered along with IL-2 (Mule et al., 1984). This approach has been used to treat advanced cancer in trials that included IL-2 alone, LAK cells alone, or LAK cells in combination with IL-2. The results have confirmed the effectiveness of the combination LAK-IL-2 approach in advanced cancer of all histologic types thus far treated (Rosenberg et al., 1985). The major drawbacks of this approach remain the cumbersome nature of the procedure, the small number of patients who can be treated, and the toxicity associated with large doses of IL-2. Modification of the approach to overcome these problems will undoubtedly result in a treatment method that will impact favorably on breast cancer in the very near future.

SPECIFIC ACTIVE IMMUNOTHERAPY

Specific active immunotherapy is based on the assumption that tumor-associated antigens exist that can elicit an autologous antitumor response. Although chemically and virally induced experimental tumors have been shown to possess sufficient immunogenicity to confer resistance to rechallenge, it has been more difficult to demonstrate this with spontaneous tumors of low antigenicity (Kreider and Bartlett, 1985).

Because an active immune response of the host with minimal tumor burden is the most appropriate setting for specific active immunotherapy, this approach is best evaluated as an adjuvant to surgery. Although several immunotherapy adjuvant studies have been performed in breast cancer, most have involved combination chemotherapy or radiotherapy, or both, and relatively few have included a treatment arm of adjuvant immunotherapy alone. Humphrey and coworkers (1980) reported for the first time promising preliminary data on breast cancer patients treated with a breast tumor–derived antigen preparation after radical mastectomy. The survival rates in this study with Stage I patients compared favorably with those using radiation therapy as the principal technique (Humphrey et al., 1980). Other Phase I studies with autologous breast cancer antigen preparations are currently being followed up for recurrence and survival data (Humphrey et al., 1980).

As the major drawback to the tumor vaccine approach is the relatively weak immunogenicity of autologous breast cancer antigens, attempts to augment the immunogenicity of tumors have been many and varied. These approaches include several physical, chemical, and biologic modifications of tumor cells to xenogenize or render them "foreign" (Kobayashi, 1982). One of the more promising approaches is the use of virus infection of tumor cells to augment their antigenicity. Several different viruses have been used to infect several different tumors or tumor cell lines, and the resulting whole cells or membrane preparations, called oncolysates, have been shown to augment resistance to rechallenge in mouse models. Similar preparations have been used to treat a variety of tumors in the adjuvant setting (Austin and Boone, 1979). Although breast cancer has not been treated with oncolysates, vesicular stomatitis virus–infected breast tumor line extracts have been shown to elicit positive skin tests in a greater proportion of breast cancer patients than extracts prepared from uninfected cells (Austin et al., 1982). Promising results have been obtained with other gynecologic malignancies treated with an influenza oncolysate. Patients with ovarian carcinoma showed a clinical response in conjunction with augmentation of natural killer cell activity (Lotzova et al., 1984). Extended disease-free survival of vulvar carcinoma patients was achieved coincident with development of humoral and cellular immune responses (Freedman et al., 1983).

One of the major problems of the specific active immunotherapy approach is the identification and purification of relevant antigens to be used in preparing more potent vaccines. By continued observations of patient responses to their own tumors and to crude vaccines, and with the continued identification of breast-associated tumor antigens with monoclonal antibodies, the relevant antigens should ultimately be identified. These molecules might then be sequenced and the gene cloned and expressed to obtain recombinant vaccines. The other major problem of specific active immunization is more difficult to approach. This involves further understanding of the regulatory mechanisms of the immune system that may prevent or suppress induction of antitumor immunity.

SPECIFIC PASSIVE IMMUNOTHERAPY

The concept of passive immunotherapy of cancer by administration of preformed antibodies is a direct extension of the classic approach to antimicrobial and antitoxic serotherapy, which, although largely replaced by antibiotic therapy, is still used to rescue victims of acute intoxication (as with snake venoms). Although the concept of transfer of specific immunity to cancer is theoretically sound if a strong immune response to tumor-associated antigens has been generated, little success has been achieved either in animal models or in clinical attempts to passively transfer whole serum from individuals who have successfully rejected tumors. The reasons for this failure may include both the predominance of cellular rather than serologic mechanisms of antitumor immunity and the inability to achieve high enough antibody concentrations using polyvalent whole serum, in which the relevant antibody may be of low titer.

The advent of hybridoma technology has generated renewed interest in serotherapy using monoclonal antibodies, which provide unlimited quantities of homogeneous antibody selected for restricted specificity for tumor-associated antigens. The development of a wide variety of monoclonal antibodies that are potentially useful in diagnosis and prognosis of breast cancer has been reviewed earlier. Although many of these may have potential in immunotherapy either alone or conjugated to drugs, toxins, or radionuclides, few clinical trials have actually been performed. One monoclonal antibody of interest that is directed against the human milk fat globule, HMFG-2, has been radiolabeled and administered intraperitoneally to deliver a significant tumor to normal tissue dose ratio of radiation to ovarian tumors (Burchell and Taylor-Papadimitriou, 1985).

The other major approach to specific passive immunotherapy, the adoptive transfer of lymphocytes that can recognize and kill tumor targets, has developed in a similar fashion as the passive transfer of antibody. This technique has been used widely in animal models in which the availability of inbred strains allows pooling of lymphocytes from several donors to achieve sufficient numbers but has had little possibilities for human immunotherapy because of the inability to achieve sufficient numbers of cells (Rosenberg and Terry, 1977). Renewed interest in the possibility of using this approach in clinical immunotherapy resulted from the discovery of T cell growth factor (Morgan et al., 1976), now designated interleukin-2 (IL-2), and the development of T cell cloning technology (Fathman and Frelinger, 1983), which allows the production of monoclonal effector cells. It has recently been demonstrated that specific T cell clones can be expanded in IL-2 to mediate regression of established solid tumor metastases in a mouse model (Shu et al., 1986). This approach continues to have limited applicability in the clinical setting, however, because of the need for autologous cells and the technical complexity and time required to select and clone the appropriate effector cells and grow them in large enough numbers for treatment. Moreover, the additional cloning required for this approach seems unnecessary in light of the success achieved with nonspecific lymphokine-activated killer (LAK) cells and IL-2 (Rosenberg et al., 1986).

SUMMARY

Immunotherapy of breast cancer has until very recently been limited to attempts to achieve nonspecific immunopotentiation with a variety of bacterial products to lymphokines of variable potency and toxicity. These attempts, which have largely been limited to Phase I trials with patients with advanced disease, have been only marginally successful. The prospects for successful immunotherapy of breast cancer in the near future are, however, excellent. This new-found optimism is in large part based on the dramatic breakthroughs in basic science, which have virtually redefined immunobiology in molecular terms. The development of hybridoma technology has had far-reaching effects on both active and passive approaches to immunotherapy because monoclonal antibodies allow the purification and characterization of tumor-associated antigens. The monoclonal antibodies themselves, or as conjugates with drugs, toxins, or radionuclides, are potentially ideal reagents for seeking out residual tumor cells. Recombinant DNA technology has allowed the cloning and synthesis of a number of molecules that are therefore available in unlimited quantities in pure form. The first of these molecules, interferon, although not the magic bullet hoped for, is only recently showing real promise and has yet to be thoroughly evaluated. Other lymphokines, such as tumor cells and interleukin-2 (IL-2), which acts through activation of killer cells, show great promise. The new biotechnology promises to provide significant advances in immunotherapy of breast cancer in the very near future.

REFERENCES

Adler, A., Stein, J. A., Goldfarb, A. J., et al.: Active specific immunotherapy of stage III breast cancer: Results of an exploratory study. Cancer Immunol. Immunother., 10:45, 1980.

Anthony, H. M.: Adjuvant levamisole in breast cancer. Lancet, 2:1123, 1980.

Austin, F. C., and Boone, C. W.: Virus augmentation of the antigenicity of tumor cell extracts. Adv. Cancer Res., 30:301, 1979.

Austin, F. C., Boone, C. W., Levin, D. L., et al.: Breast cancer skin test antigens of increased sensitivity prepared from vesicular stomatitis virus-infected tumor cells. Cancer, 49:2034, 1982.

Bernard, D. J., Maurizis, J. C., Chassagne, J., et al.: Comparison of class II HLA antigen expression in normal and carcinomatous human breast cells. Cancer Res., 45:1152, 1985.

Bertram, J. H.: Staphylococcus protein A column: Its mechanism of action. In Reif, R., Mitchell, M. S. (Eds.): Immunity to Cancer. Orlando, Fla., Academic Press, 1985, p. 499.

Bjorn, M. J., Ring, D., and Frankel, A.: Evaluation of monoclonal antibodies for the development of breast cancer immunotoxins. Cancer Res., 45:1214, 1985.

Black, M. M., Kerpe, S., and Speer, F. D.: Lymph node structure in patients with cancer of the breast. Am. J. Pathol., 29:505, 1953.

Black, M. M., Moore, D. H., Shore, B., et al.: Effect of murine milk samples and human breast tissues on human leukocyte migration indices. Cancer Res., 34:1054, 1974.

Black, M. M., Hankey, B. F., Aron, J. L., et al.: Possible immunological implications of an association between the first stages of first and second independent breast cancers. Breast Cancer Res. Treat., 4:95, 1984.

Black, M. M., and Zachrau, R. E.: Immune mechanisms: prognostic, therapeutic and preventive significance. In Ariel, I. M., and Cleary, J. B. (Eds.): Breast Cancer: Diagnosis and Treatment. New York, McGraw-Hill, 1987, p. 128.

Borden, E., Dao, T., Holland, J., et al.: Interferon in recurrent breast cancer: Preliminary report of the American Cancer Society Clinical Trials Program. Proc. Am. Assoc. Cancer Res., 21:187, 1980.

Borden, E. C., and Balkwill, F. R.: Preclinical and clinical studies of interferons and interferon inducers in breast cancer. Cancer, 53:783, 1984.

Brabon, A. C., Williams, J. F., and Cardiff, R. D.: A monoclonal antibody to a human breast tumor protein released in response to estrogen. Cancer Res., 44:2704, 1984.

Buessow, S. C., Paul, R. D., and Lopez, D. M.: Influence of mammary tumor progression on penotype and function of spleen and in situ lymphocytes in mice. JNCI, 73:249, 1984.

Burchell, J. M., and Taylor-Papadimitriou, J.: Monoclonal antibodies to breast cancer and their application. In Baldwin, R. W., and Byers, V. S. (Eds.): Monoclonal Antibodies for Cancer Detection and Therapy. New York, Academic Press, 1985, p. 1.

Burnet, F. M.: The concept of immunological surveillance. Progr. Exp. Tumor Res., 13:1, 1970.

Buzdar, A. U., Blumenschein, G. R., Smith, T. L., et al.: Adjuvant chemoimmunotherapy following regional therapy for isolated recurrences of breast cancer (Stage IV NED). J. Surg. Oncol., 12:27, 1979.

Callahan, R., Drohan, W., Tronick, S., et al.: Detection and cloning of human DNA sequences related to the mouse mammary tumors by immunoperoxidase staining of paraffin sections. Proc. Nat. Acad. Sci., 79:5503, 1982.

Cannon, G. B., Barsky, S. H., Alford, T. C., et al.: Cell-mediated immunity to mouse mammary tumor virus antigens by patients with hyperplastic benign breast disease. J. Nat. Cancer Inst., 68:935, 1982.

Capone, P. M., Papsidero, L. D., and Chu, T. M.:

Relationship between antigen density and immunotherapeutic response elicited by monoclonal antibodies against solid tumors. J. Natl. Cancer Inst., 72:673, 1984.

Carswell, E. A., Old, L. J., Kassel, R. L., et al.: An endotoxin-induced serum factor that causes necrosis of tumors. Proc. Natl. Acad. Sci., 72:3666, 1975.

Colcher, D., Horan-Hand, P., Wunderlich, D., et al.: Potential diagnostic and prognostic applications of monoclonal antibodies to human mammary carcinomas. In Wright, G. L. (ed.): Monoclonal Antibodies and Cancer. New York, Marcel Dekker, 1984, p. 121.

Coley, W. B.: Contributions to the knowledge of sarcoma. Ann. Surg., 14:199, 1891.

Coley, W. B.: Disappearance of recurrent carcinoma after injections of mixed toxins. Ann. Surg., 55:897, 1912.

Colizza, S., Di Paola, M., Garra, G., et al.: The treatment of T-cell defects in the management of colon and breast cancer. Excerpta Med. Int. Congr. Ser., 502:1039, 1980.

Crile, G., Jr.: Possible role of uninvolved nodes in preventing metastasis from breast cancer. Cancer, 24:1283, 1969.

Day, N. K., Witkin, S. S., Sarkar, N. H., et al.: Antibodies reactive with murine mammary tumor virus in sera of patients with breast cancer: geographic and family studies. Proc. Nat. Acad. Sci., 78:2483, 1981.

Edwards, D. P., Grzyb, K. T., Dressler, L. G., et al.: Monoclonal antibody identification and characterization of a M 43,000 membrane glycoprotein associated with human breast cancer. Cancer Res., 46:1306, 1986.

Ehrlich, P. (1909): Uber den jetzigen Stand der Karzinomforschung. In The Collected Papers of Paul Ehrlich, Vol. II. Immunology and Cancer Research. F. Himmelweit (Ed.) London, Pergamon Press, 1957, p. 559.

Fathman, C. G., and Frelinger, J. G.: T-lymphocyte clones. Ann. Rev. Immunol., 1:633, 1983.

Feller, W., Kantor, J., Hilkens, J., et al.: Monoclonal antibody defined antigens in plasma of breast cancer patients. Abstract 589, Proc. A.A.C.R., 26:149, 1985.

Felix, E., Katz, S., Teodorescu, A., et al.: Enumeration of lymphocytes and their subpopulation identified by bacterial adherence in blood smears of patients with breast tumors. J. Surg. Oncol., 18:323, 1981.

Fisher, B., and Fisher, E. R.: Studies concerning the regional lymph nodes in cancer. II. Maintenance of immunity. Cancer, 29:1496, 1972.

Flick, D. A., and Gifford, G. E.: Tumor necrosis factor. In Torrence, P. F. (Ed.): Biological Response Modifiers: New Approaches to Disease Intervention. Orlando, Fla., Academic Press, 1986, p. 171.

Freedman, R. S., Bowen, J. M., Herson, J. H., et al.: Immunotherapy for vulvar carcinoma with virus-modified homologous extracts. Obstet. Gynecol., 62:707, 1983.

Fulton, A. M., and Heppner, G. H.: Relationships of prostaglandin E and natural killer sensitivity to metastatic potential in murine mammary adenocarcinomas. Cancer Res., 45:4779, 1985.

Garcia, M., Capony, F., Derocq, D., et al.: Characterization of monoclonal antibodies to the estrogen-regulated Mr 52,000 glycoprotein and their use in MCF7 cells. Cancer Res., 45:709, 1985.

Gartner, J. G., Seemayer, T. A., and Lapp, W. S.: Mammary carcinoma arising in mice undergoing a chronic graft-versus-host reaction. JNCI, 73:1119, 1984.

Girardi, A. J., Dion, A. S., and Holben, J. A.: Immunologic studies with mouse mammary tumor viruses: Comparative studies with spontaneous mammary tumor cell vaccines from five inbred mouse strains. JNCI, 74:105, 1985.

Gottlinger, H. G., Gokel, J. M., Lohe, K. J., et al.: Infiltrating mononuclear cells in human breast carcinoma: Predominance of T4+ monocytic cells in the tumor stroma. Int. J. Cancer, 35:199, 1985.

Greager, J. A., and Baldwin, R. W.: Influence of immunotherapeutic agents on the progression of spontaneously arising, metastasizing rat mammary adenocarcinomas of varying immunogenicities. Cancer Res., 38:69, 1978.

Gross, L.: Immunological relationship of mammary carcinomas developing spontaneously in female mice of a high-tumor line. J. Immunol., 55:297, 1947.

Gutterman, J., Blumenschein, G. R., Hortobagyi, G., et al.: Immunotherapy for breast cancer. Breast, 2:29, 1976.

Gutterman, J. U., Blumenschein, G. R., Alexanian, R., et al.: Leukocyte interferon-induced tumor regression in human metastatic breast cancer, multiple myeloma, and malignant lymphoma. Ann. Intern. Med., 93:399, 1980.

Halpern, B. N., Biozzi, G., Stiffel, C., et al.: Inhibition of tumor growth by administration of killed Corynebacterium parvum. Nature, 212:853, 1966.

Halsted, W. S.: A clinical and histological study of certain adenocarcinomata of the breast. J.A.M.A., 14:114, 1898.

Hilkens, J., Tager, J. M., Bujis, F., et al.: Monoclonal antibodies against human acid alpha-glycosidase. Biochim. Biophys. Acta, 678:7, 1981.

Hindsley, J. P., Avis, I., Newsome, J. F., et al.: Certain aspects of analysis of complement dependent antibody in breast cancer patients. J. Surg. Oncol., 11:107, 1979.

Hirshaut, Y., Kesselheim, H., Pinsky, C. M., et al.: Levamisole as an immunoadjuvant: Phase I study and application in breast cancer. Cancer Treat. Rep., 62:1693, 1978.

Holohan, T. V., Phillips, T. M., Bowles, C., et al.: Regression of canine mammary carcinoma after immunoadsorption therapy. Cancer Res., 42:3663, 1982.

Hooks, J. J., and Detrick, B.: Immunoregulatory functions of interferon. In Torrence, P. F. (Ed.): Biological Response Modifiers: New Approaches to Disease Intervention. Orlando, Fla., Academic Press, 1986, p. 57.

Hoover, H. C., Surdyke, M., Dangel, R. B., et al.: Delayed cutaneous hypersensitivity to autologous tumor cells in colorectal cancer patients immunized with an autologous tumor cell: Bacillus Calmette-Guérin vaccine. Cancer Res., 44:1671, 1984.

Horan-Hand, P., Colcher, D., Salmon, D., et al.: Influence of spatial configuration of carcinoma cell populations on the expression of a tumor-associated glycoprotein. Cancer Res., 45:833, 1985.

Hudson, M. J. K., Humphrey, L. J., Mantz, F. A., et al.: Correlation of circulating serum antibody to the histologic findings in breast cancer. Am. J. Surg., 128:756, 1974.

Humphrey, L. J., Taschler-Collins, S., and Volenec, F. J.: Treatment of primary breast cancer with immunotherapy. Am. J. Surg., 148:649, 1984.

Humphrey, L. J., Singla, O., and Volenec, F. J.: Immunologic responsiveness of the breast cancer patient. Cancer, 46:893, 1980.

Imam, A., Drushella, M. M., Taylor, C. R., et al.: Generation and immunohistological characterization of human monoclonal antibodies to mammary carcinoma cells. Cancer Res., 45:263, 1985.

Johnson, C. W., Wei, W.-Z., Barth, R. F., et al.: Monoclonal antibodies directed against preoplastic and neoplastic murine mammary lesions. Cancer Res., 45:3774, 1985.

Kallman, R. F., Denekamp, J., Hill, R. P., et al.: The

use of rodent tumors in experimental cancer therapy: Conclusions and recommendations from an international workshop. Cancer Res., 45:6541, 1985.

Keydar, I., Mesa-Tejada, R., Ramanarayanan, M., et al.: Detection of viral proteins in mouse mammary tumors by immunoperoxidase staining of paraffin sections. Proc. Nat. Acad. Sci., 75:1524, 1978.

Klein, E.: Immunotherapeutic approaches to skin cancer. Hosp. Pract., 11:107, 1976.

Kobayashi, H.: Modification of tumor antigenicity in therapeutics: Increase in immunologic foreignness of tumor cells in experimental model systems. In Mihich, E. (Ed.): Immunological Approaches to Cancer Therapeutics. New York, John Wiley & Sons, Inc., 1982, p. 405.

Koestler, T. P., Papsidero, L. D., Nemoto, T., et al.: Detection of a breast tissue-associated antigen by antiserum to Raji cell-bound circulating immune complexes of human breast cancer. Cancer Res., 41:2900, 1981.

Kreider, J. W., and Bartlett, G. L.: Increased immunogenicity of a spontaneous variant clone of the 13762A rat mammary adenocarcinoma. J. Nat. Cancer Inst., 75:141, 1985.

Kreider, J. W., Bartlett, G. L., and Purnell, D. M.: Suitability of the mammary adenocarcinoma 13762 as a model for BCG immunotherapy. J. Nat. Cancer Inst., 56:797, 1976.

Krown, S.: Prospects for the treatment of cancer with interferon. In Burchenal, J. H., and Oettgen, H. F. (Eds.): Cancer Achievements, Challenges and Prospects for the 1980's. New York, Grune & Stratton, 1982, p. 367.

Krutchik, A. N., Buzdar, A. U., Blumenschein, G. R., et al.: Combined chemoimmunotherapy and irradiation therapy of inflammatory breast carcinoma. J. Surg. Oncol., 11:325, 1979.

Lacour, F., Lacour, J., Spiras, A., et al.: A new adjuvant treatment with polyadenylic-polyuridylic acid in operable breast cancer. Recent Results Cancer Res., 80:200, 1982.

Lamoureux, G., Mandeville, R., Poisson, R., et al.: Biologic markers and breast cancer: A multiparametric study. I. Increased serum protein levels. Cancer, 49:502, 1982.

Lee, Y.-T.: Delayed cutaneous hypersensitivity, lymphocyte count, and blood tests in patients with breast carcinoma. J. Surg. Oncol., 27:135, 1984.

Lennox, E. S.: What are tumor antigens? In Reif, A. E. and Mitchell, M. S. (Eds.): Immunity to Cancer. Orlando, Academic Press, 1985, p. 17.

Levine, P. H., Mesa-Tejada, R., Keydar, I., et al.: Increased incidence of mouse mammary tumor virus–related antigen in Tunisian patients with breast cancer. Int. J. Cancer, 33:305, 1984.

Lopez, D. M., Charyulu, V., and Paul, R. D.: B cell subsets in spleens of Balb/c mice: identification and isolation of MMTV-expressing and MMTV-responding subpopulations. J. Immunol., 134:603, 1985.

Lopez, D. M.: New developments in breast cancer immunology. In Rich, M. A., Hager, J. C., and Taylor-Papadimitriou, J.: Breast Cancer: Origins, Detection and Treatment. Boston, Martinus Nijhoff, 1986, p. 112.

Lotzova, E., Savary, C. A., Freedman, R. S., et al.: Natural killer cell cytotoxic potential of patients with ovarian carcinoma and its modulation with virus-modified tumor cell extract. Cancer Immunol. Immunother., 17:124, 1984.

May, F. E., Westley, B. R., Rockefort, H., et al.: Mouse mammary tumor virus–related sequences are present in human DNA. Nucleic Acid Res., 11:4127, 1983.

MacCarty, W. C.: Factors which influence longevity in cancer. Ann. Surg., 76:9, 1922.

McCoy, J. L., Tagliabue, A., Ames, R. E., et al.: Indirect leukocyte migration inhibition in breast cancer and benign breast disease patients by mouse mammary tumor virus grown in feline kidney cells. JNCI, 72:569, 1984.

Merluzzi, V. J., Savage, D. M., Souza, L., et al.: Lysis of spontaneous murine breast tumors by human interleukin-2 stimulated syngeneic T-lymphocytes. Cancer Res., 45:203, 1985.

Mesa-Tejada R., Keydar, I., Ramanarayanan, M., et al.: Immunohistochemical detection of a cross-reacting virus antigen in mouse mammary tumors and human breast carcinomas. J. Histochem. Cytochem., 26:532, 1978.

Meyer, K. K., Boselli, B. D., Weaver, D. R., et al.: Cellular immune response to mastectomy and radiation. Guthrie Clin. Bull., 40:48, 1970.

Miller, F. R.: Concomitant tumor immunity in the mammary gland. Cancer Immunol. Immunother., 20:219, 1985.

Moore, D. H., Moore, D. T., and Moore, C. T.: Breast carcinoma etiological factors. Adv. Cancer Res., 40:189, 1983.

Morgan, D. A., Ruscetti, F. W., and Gallo, R. C.: Selective in vitro growth of T-lymphocytes from normal human bone marrows. Science, 193:1007, 1976.

Morton, B. A., Ramey, W. G., Paderon, H., et al.: Monoclonal antibody–defined phenotypes of regional lymph node and peripheral blood lymphocyte subpopulations in early breast cancer. Cancer Res., 46:2121, 1986.

Mueller, C. B., and Ames, F.: Bilateral carcinoma of the breast: Frequency and mortality. Can. J. Surg. 21:459, 1978.

Mule, J. J., Shu, S., Schwarz, S. L., et al.: Adoptive immunotherapy of established pulmonary metastases with LAK cells and recombinant interleukin-2. Science, 225:1487, 1986.

Natali, P. G., Giacomini, P., Bigotti, A., et al.: Heterogeneity in the expression of HLA and tumor-associated antigens by surgically removed and cultured breast carcinoma cells. Cancer Res., 43:660, 1983.

Nathanson, L.: Immunology and immunotherapy of human breast cancer. Cancer Immunol. Immunother., 2:209, 1977.

Nauts, H. C.: The Beneficial Effects of Bacterial Infections on Host Resistance to Cancer. End Results in 449 Cases. A Study and Abstracts of Reports in the World Medical Literature (1775–1980) and Personal Communications. Monograph #8, 2nd ed. New York, Cancer Research Institute, 1980.

Nauts, H. C.: Breast Cancer: Immunological Factors Affecting Incidence, Prognosis and Survival. Monograph #18. New York, Cancer Research Institute, 1984.

Nishioka, K., Irie, R. F., Inoue, M., et al.: Immunological studies on mouse mammary tumors. I. Induction of resistance to tumor isograft in C3H/He mice. Int. J. Cancer, 4:121, 1969.

Old, L. J.: Tumor necrosis factor (TNF). Science, 230:630, 1985.

Old, L. J., Clarke, D. A., and Benacerraf, B.: Effect of bacillus Calmette-Guèrin infection on transplanted tumors in the mouse. Nature, 184:291, 1959.

Oldham, R. K.: Biologicals and biological response modifiers: Fourth modality of cancer treatment. Cancer Treat. Rep., 68:221, 1984.

Oldham, R. K., and Herberman, R. B.: Delayed hypersensitivity skin tests with tumor extracts. In Herberman,

R. B., and McIntire, K. R. (Eds.): Immunodiagnosis of Cancer. New York, Marcel Dekker, 1979, p. 940.

Papatestas, A., and Kark, A. E.: Peripheral lymphocyte counts in breast carcinoma. Cancer, 34:2014, 1974.

Papatestas, A. E., Mulvihill, M., Genkins, G., et al.: Thymus and breast cancer-plasma androgens, thymic pathology and peripheral lymphocytes in myasthenia gravis. JNCI, 59:1583, 1977.

Papatestas, A. E., Bramis, J., and Aufses, A. H.: Serum immunoglobulins in women with breast cancer. J. Surg. Oncol., 12:155, 1979.

Papsidero, L. D., Croghan, G. A., O'Connell, M. J., et al.: Monoclonal antibodies (F36/22 and M7/105) to human breast carcinoma. Cancer Res., 43:1741, 1983.

Paterson, A. H., Nutting, M., Takats, L., et al.: Chemoimmunotherapy with levamisole in metastatic breast carcinoma. A controlled clinical trial. Cancer Clin. Trials, 3:5, 1980.

Pertschuk, L. P.: Monoclonal antibodies to localized breast cancer receptors. Organ Systems Newsletter, 2:8, 1985.

Peterson, J .A., and Ceriani, R. L.: International workshop on monoclonal antibodies and breast cancer. Breast Cancer Res. Treat., 5:207, 1985.

Quesada, J. R., Hawkins, M., Horning, S., et al.: Collaborative Phase I-II study of recombinant DNA-produced leukocyte interferon (Clone A) in metastatic breast cancer, malignant lymphoma, and multiple myeloma. Am. J. Med., 77:427, 1984.

Reiss, C. K., Humphrey, M., Singla, O., et al.: The role of the regional lymph node in breast cancer: A comparison between nodal and systemic reactivity. J. Surg. Oncol., 22:249, 1983.

Retsas, S., Phillips, R. H., Hanham, I. W. F., et al.: Agranulocytosis in breast cancer patients treated with levamisole. Lancet, 2:324, 1978.

Richters, A., and Paller, M.: The relationship between sIgM positive lymph-node lymphocytes and breast cancer metastasis. J. Surg. Oncol., 11:79, 1979.

Roberts, M. M., Bass, E. M., Wallace, I. W. J., et al.: Local immunoglobulin production in breast cancer. Br. J. Cancer, 27:269, 1973.

Rojas, A. F., Feierstein, J. N., Mickiewicz, E., et al.: Levamisole in advanced human breast cancer. Lancet, 1:211, 1976.

Rosenberg, S. A.: Adoptive immunotherapy of cancer using lymphokine activated killer cells and recombinant IL-2. In DeVita, V. T., Jr., Hellman, S., and Rosenberg, S. A. (Eds.): Important Advances in Oncology, 1986. National Cancer Institute Monograph, 1986, p. 55.

Rosenberg, S. A., and Terry, W.: Passive immunotherapy of cancer in animals and man. Adv. Cancer Res., 24:323, 1977.

Rosenberg, S. A., Lotze, M. T., Muul, L. M., et al.: A progress report on the treatment of 157 patients with advanced cancer using lymphokine-activated killer cells and interleukin-2 or high dose interleukin-2 alone. N. Engl. J. Med., 316:889, 1987.

Segev, N., Hizi, A., Kirenberg, F., et al.: Characterization of a protein released by the T47D cell line, immunologically related to the major envelope protein of mouse mammary tumor virus. Proc. Nat. Acad. Sci., 82:1531, 1985.

Seitz, R. C., Fischer, K., Stegner, H. E., et al.: Detection of metastatic breast carcinoma cells by immunofluorescent demonstration of Thomsen-Friedenreich antigen. Cancer, 54:830, 1984.

Seto, M., Takahashi, T., Nakamura, S., et al.: Effector mechanism in antitumor activity of monoclonal antibodies produced against an ascitic mouse mammary tumor. Cancer Res., 46:2056, 1986.

Shorthouse, A. J., Peckham, M. J., Smyth, J. F., et al.: The therapeutic response of bronchial carcinoma xenografts: A direct patient-xenograft comparison. Br. J. Cancer, 41(Suppl. IV):142, 1980.

Shu, S., Chou, T., and Rosenberg, S. A.: In vitro sensitization and expansion with viable tumor cells and interleukin-2 in the generation of specific therapeutic effector cells. J. Immunol., 136:3891, 1986.

Slemmer, G.: Host response to premalignant mammary tissues. Natl. Cancer Inst. Monogr., 35:57, 1972.

Soule, H. R., Linden, E., and Edgington, T. S.: Membrane 126-kilodalton phosphoglycoprotein associated with human carcinomas identified by a hybridoma antibody to mammary carcinoma cells. Proc. Nat. Acad. Sci., 80:1332, 1983.

Springer, G. F., Murthy, M. S., Desai, P. R., et al.: Breast cancer patient's cell-mediated immune response to Thomsen-Friedenreich (T) antigen. Cancer, 45:2949, 1980.

Stacker, S. A., Thompson, C., Riglar, C., et al.: A new breast carcinoma antigen defined by a monoclonal antibody. JNCI, 75:801, 1985.

Stolfi, R. L., Fugmann, R. A., Stolfi, L .M., et al.: Synergism between host anti-tumor immunity and combined modality therapy against murine breast cancer. Int. J. Cancer, 13:389, 1974.

Takeuchi, S., Irie, R. F., Inoue, M., et al.: Immunological studies on mouse mammary tumors. II. Characterization of tumor-specific antibodies against mouse mammary tumors. Int. J. Cancer, 4:130, 1969.

Taylor-Papademitriou, J., Peterson, J. A., Arklie, J., et al.: Monoclonal antibodies to epithelium-specific components of the human milk fat globule membrane: production and reaction with cells in culture. Int. J. Cancer, 28:7, 1981.

Thomas, L.: Discussion: Reactions to homologous tissue antigens. In Lawrence, H. S. (Ed.): Cellular and Humoral Aspects of the Hypersensitivity States. New York, Hoeber-Harper, 1959, p. 529.

Tomana, M., Kajdos, A. H., Niedermeier, W., et al.: Antibodies to mouse mammary tumor virus–related antigen in sera of patients with breast carcinoma. Cancer, 47:2696, 1981.

Torrence, P. F. (Ed.): Biological Response Modifiers: New Approaches to Disease Intervention. Orlando, Fla., Academic Press, 1986.

Urban, J. A.: Breast cancer 1985: What have we learned? Cancer, 57:636, 1986.

White, C. A., Dulbecco, R., Allen, R., et al.: Two monoclonal antibodies selective for human mammary carcinoma. Cancer Res., 45:1337, 1985.

Whiteside, T. L., Miescher, S., Hurlimann, L., et al.: Clonal analysis and in situ characterization of lymphocytes infiltrating human breast carcinomas (abstract). Fed. Proc., 45:849, 1986.

Whittiker, M. G., and Clark, C. G.: Depressed lymphocyte function in carcinoma of the breast. Br. J. Surg., 58:717, 1971.

CHAPTER 19

JOHN S. SPRATT
WILLIAM L. DONEGAN
RICHARD A. GREENBERG

Screening and Follow-up

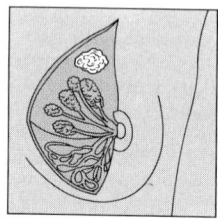

Certain general principles exist that justify any community effort at screening for disease. Cadman and associates (1984) summarized these as follows:

1. Has the effectiveness of the program been demonstrated in a randomized trial?
2. Are efficacious treatments available?
3. Does the burden of suffering warrant screening?
4. Is there a good screening test?
5. Does the program reach out to those who could benefit?
6. Can the health system cope with the program?
7. Do persons with positive screenings comply with advice and interventions?

In Cadman and coworkers' study, the consideration was for a preschool screening program for detecting developmental disorders. They concluded that "organized common sense" or purely intuitive conclusions had led to some extremely erroneous and costly conclusions. However, all the questions they listed are applicable to screening for breast cancer, and the answers to many of them are incomplete.

That current knowledge on the value of screening is incomplete is best emphasized by the large studies still in progress. The epidemiology group at the National Cancer Institute of Canada (NCIC) is continuing to study the impact of screening on the mortality of breast cancer (Miller, 1982). The group remains concerned over the relatively stable mortality rates attributable to breast cancer despite extensive publicity for breast self examination (BSE) and screening. NCIC has in progress prospective studies to explore issues considered unresolved: (1) the efficacy of the combination of mammography and physical examination in attaining a reduction in mortality in women 40 to 49 years old; (2) the contribution of mammography to the reduction in mortality at ages 50 to 59 years (this question is important, as Bailar [1976] suggested that physical examination alone may have made the major contribution to mortality reduction in this age group in the HIP study [Shapiro, 1977]); (3) in the interest of increased screening efficacy, a better assessment of risk factors associated with death from breast cancer, as is considered essential for the selection of populations to be screened; (4) the natural history of "minimal breast cancer" identified by mammography alone, which remains unknown (whether minimal breast cancers are true cancers or not becomes important in measuring the value of their discovery and in planning the periodicity of rescreening); (5) finally, data on cost-benefit analysis remain essential for any health expenditures, particularly those that might require governmental subsidy.

As of 1982, Miller concluded that screening for breast cancer is not yet an appropriate part of a cancer control program. He considered that mammography's promise merited further evaluation to ascertain the progress of these studies (Miller, personal communication, 1985). At the time of this communication, the NCIC studies were still in progress. They had accessioned 85,000 cases by then, but many years will elapse before conclusions can be drawn. By 1986 this study still had not confirmed that breast cancer mortality was being reduced in the screened population (Miller, personal communication, 1986).

Habbema and colleagues (1986) reported a 14 year follow-up on the randomized breast cancer screening trial of the Health Insurance Plan (HIP) of Greater New York, suggesting a reduced mortality rate for women screened before age 50 years. These observations were reviewed with Bailar (personal communication, 1986) who provided the additional information from Shapiro (1986) and interpretation of the HIP data. Survival rates for the screened and control group aged 40 to 44 years do diverge but only after 8 years of follow-up, when the average population age is past 50 years. The question raised by Bailar is this: "If we accept the difference at ages 40 to 44 and 45 to 49 as real, we must immediately ask whether that advantage depends on screening *at* ages 40 to 44 and 45 to 49, or whether it would be derived from a single examination at about age 50. I know of no data to test this directly. However, the consistency of the change at 50 . . . and the very large advantage of screening at ages 50 to 54 suggests that one could just as well wait." Thus, advantage in screening women under 50 years old remains unproved by the HIP data.

Definitions

The use of technologic interventions for the detection of asymptomatic disease in large populations is defined as screening. Epidemiologic principles, as well as economic ones, exist by which screening for disease must be evaluated. The asymptomatic disease sought can either be newly developing or, when applied to follow-up after prior treatment, recidivated cancer. The search for asymptomatic local-regional recidivated cancer and distant metastases in follow-up is simply screening applied to a special high-risk population (Spratt, 1982).

Screening is a public health effort directed at a disease control program. The value or futility of screening will be judged by whether or not reduced disease morbidity and mortality actually do occur. To engage in the scientific design and evaluation of screening programs requires the application of epidemiologic and biostatistical methods and cost-benefit analysis, as discussed in Chapter 30.

Because the basic objectives of screening are the surveillance for disease in the screened population, the presumption is that the morbidity and mortality from the disease can, in fact, be altered favorably by earlier treatment, and that the morbidity and mortality associated with the techniques used for earlier detection and treatment can be kept low enough not to reduce survival or increase morbidity. For this presupposition to be evaluated, a reliable and properly designed controlled clinical trial testing hypotheses regarding the value of screening

Table 19–1. MODEL OF BREAST CANCER PROGRESSION

Asymptomatic Disease Below Threshold Size for Detection—Local, Local-Regional, Distant Normal	Asymptomatic Disease Above Threshold Size for Detection	Symptomatic	Endpoints	
T_v Biologic onset	T_w Disease now detectable if screen done Screening takes place, can be true positive or false negative	T_x Disease becomes symptomatic Patient comes for diagnosis of symptomatic disease	T_y Death without treatment	T_z Death with treatment

$T_a = T_w - T_v$:	Undetectable sojourn		T_v: Onset
$T_b = T_x - T_w$:	Detectable asymptomatic sojourn (same as maximum lead time)		T_w: Detectable but asymptomatic
$T_c = T_a + T_b$:	Delay time		T_x: Symptomatic
$T_y - T_v$:	Natural sojourn of undiagnosed, untreated disease		T_z: Time of death with treatment
$T_z - T_v$:	Natural sojourn of diagnosed disease, treated without treatment mortality		T_y, T_z: Determined by lifelong follow-up to avoid truncation of results

Cancer Control Window (CCW): Time that cancer disseminates and is no longer local-regional less T_w. The CCW can be negative if dissemination occurs before T_w.

The sojourn times in various intervals are dependent on cancer growth rates, biologic properties of cancers, and the sensitivity and specificity of diagnostic methods.
From Spratt, J. S., and Spratt, J. A.: What is breast cancer doing before we can detect it? J. Surg. Oncol., *30*:156, 1985. Reprinted with permission.

Table 19–2. GLOSSARY OF TERMS ESSENTIAL TO EPIDEMIOLOGIC DESCRIPTION OF ANY SCREENING PROGRAM

True positive	= Those testing positive who <u>do have</u> the disease.
False positive	= Those testing positive who <u>do not have</u> the disease.
False negative	= Those testing negative who <u>do have</u> the disease.
True negative	= Those testing negative who <u>do not have</u> the disease.

$$\text{Sensitivity} = \frac{\text{True positives}}{\text{True positives and false negatives}} = \frac{\text{True positives}}{\text{All of those with the disease}}$$

$$\text{Specificity} = \frac{\text{True negatives}}{\text{True negatives and false positives}} = \frac{\text{True negatives}}{\text{All of those without the disease}}$$

Terminal = The disease is no longer curable, either before detection or after. Cancer has metastasized beyond the region where curable by surgical or radiation treatment. Terminal state may be reached before a cancer is clinically detectable.

Lethal = Time of host death.

Failures = Undetectable disease that has already reached a terminal point.

e = Effectiveness.

$$e = \frac{\text{failures (no screen)} - \text{failures (screen)}}{\text{failures (no screen)}}$$

Time of onset = Requires concise definition for the disease in question.

Onset of symptoms = Requires concise definition of symptoms in question.

Threshold of measurement = That minimum size or level below which the method of measurement has a sensitivity which approaches zero (i.e., unable to detect).

Variability in interpretation:

(1) Interindividual: representing inconsistency of interpretation among different readers of x-ray films or other clinical and laboratory measurements.

(2) Intraindividual: reflecting the failure of a reader to be consistent with himself or herself in independent interpretations of the same set of films or other clinical or laboratory evaluations.

$$\text{Incidence rate per 1000} = \frac{\text{Number of new cases of a disease occurring in a population during a specific period of time (as annual)}}{\text{Number of persons exposed to risk of developing the disease during that period of time}} \times 1000$$

$$\text{Prevalence rate per 1000} = \frac{\text{Number of cases of disease present in the population at a specified time}}{\text{Number of persons in the population at that specified time}} \times 1000$$

Prevalence rate = incidence rate × duration of the disease in a stable population

or

$$\text{Incidence rate} = \frac{\text{Prevalence rate}}{\text{duration of the disease}}$$

Cancer control window = time in the life history of a cancer elapsing between the threshold of measurement and the time a cancer becomes terminal.

Lead time bias = The bias introduced into the evaluation of the end results of cancer treatment in which the improved end results are incorrectly attributed to earlier diagnosis. If the earlier diagnosis is made <u>after</u> the cancer has become <u>terminal</u> but earlier in the terminal period, the patient lives longer from the time of treatment but <u>not</u> from the terminal point. The lead time bias is the time interval at which discovery is made earlier in the life history of the cancer but after the terminal point.

Length bias = The bias introduced into the interpretation of screening programs when the fact is not recognized that slower growing, often more biologically favorable cancers are present for great <u>lengths</u> of time thereby enhancing the possibility that slower growing more indolent cancers are the ones discovered by periodic screening. Once again, end results from treatment will look better as cancers discovered by screening are more biologically favorable in the first place.

Interval or surfacing cancers = These are cancers that become evident by any means of discovery and are confirmed by histologic examination from within a specified time interval after an examination from which no recommendation for biopsy resulted but before the next scheduled rescreen at the end of a constant time, as annual.

Reprinted from Spratt, JS. Epidemiology of Screening for Cancer. R. C. Hickey (ed.). Curr. Probl. Cancer, 6(8):1, 1982. Copyright 1982, Year Book Medical Publishers. Reprinted with permission.

must exist. The design of the trial is greatly assisted by a reliable model of the disease (see Table 19–1). The glossary (Table 19–2) contains terms intrinsic to the discussion of various concepts as they affect the design, description, and evaluation of screening.

Current State of Breast Cancer Discovery

The current United States pattern of discovery of breast cancer has recently been assessed by the short-term survey of breast cancer conducted by the Commission on Cancer of the American College of Surgeons (Nemoto et al., 1982). Among 12,315 patients, 73 per cent of the cancers were found by the patients, 23 per cent were found by physicians, and only 4 per cent were discovered by mammography. Younger women were more likely to discover cancers than were older women. Mammography found smaller cancers more frequently with negative axillary lymph nodes. The study provides descriptive data on delay, size, and the presence or absence of axillary metastasis, but not on end results. Exclusion of length biased sampling in this distributional mix and correction of end result data for corresponding lead time would be essential, before it could be inferred that survivorship is being enhanced by this pattern.

Higher Risk Groups

The effectiveness of any screening program can be enhanced when a higher risk population can be screened. Although detection is defined as the search for the disease in asymptomatic persons, there are elements of personal and family history associated with an increased site risk for cancer. Of all the risk factors, age is the most significant. Once the age-specific pediatric cancers are set aside, the vast majority of cancers increase in incidence, often geometrically, with increasing age.

Breast cancer can strike any woman at any age and men are affected about in 1 per cent of cases of the disease. Breast cancer even occurs in children, although infrequently. These pediatric cancers tend to be more favorable in their course (McDivitt and Stewart, 1966). Collectively, less than 2 per cent of all breast cancers are diagnosed under the age of 30 years (Noyes et al., 1982). Beyond age 30 years, the annual incidence increases exponentially with increasing age. Aside from the relative infrequency of cancer in the younger women, screening is often less effective in this age group because of the density of the breasts in younger women. Finally, when mammography is used to screen the breasts of younger women, the theoretical risk of radiation exposure may be greater. It was this concern that led the Breast Cancer Detection Demonstration Projects (BCDDP) to discontinue using mammographic examinations in women under age 35 years. Whether the low dosage radiation exposure of breasts by mammography increases the risk of breast cancer remains a disquieting possibility (Bailar, 1976). Certainly the risk has probably been reduced by the lower dosage of radiation from currently available mammographic units and from its predominant use in women over 50 years old. However, irradiation still has a documented association with the induction of breast cancer. Evidence for this statement is presented in Chapter 4. A long latency period is presumed to exist before the induced cancers appear. This constitutes reason enough for keeping women who have undergone periodic mammographic screening under life-long surveillance. The incompletely answered question is this: Is enhanced survivorship that might be attributed to the mammographic discovery of earlier cancers in any way offset by an increased risk for developing cancers as a result of radiation exposure? That question is beyond the scope of this chapter and is considered in Chapter 4.

Epidemiologic implications regarding causation are also discussed in Chapter 4. The social, occupational, and regional environmental factors vary widely over time and geographic location; these variations may affect the incidence of cancers and the emphasis on prevention and screening. In addition, the incubation period between exposure and the appearance of clinical cancer may be very long. However, promotional agents (which could include irradiation) may bring incipient cancers to the surface sooner. Obviously, the screener should be cognizant of local and environmental sources of cancers and of the exposure unique to the observed population.

As knowledge of cancer causation advances, multiple factors enter into screening strategies. The cancer is initiated by a chemical or physical starter in a susceptible host, exposed to a dose greater than threshold for an adequate duration, beginning at an age that will permit the appearance of a diagnosable cancer during the host's remaining life span. A variety of promoters and cocarcinogens may be involved. The susceptibility of the host is affected by genetic makeup, age, sex, race, and nutrition. The statistical methods involved in the evaluation of screening programs are covered in Chapter 30. For any group, the design and testing of a screening and cancer management program becomes an epidemiologic research problem to ensure an optimal screening strategy coupled with an effective cancer management system.

Although various "risk factors" have been implicated, the overriding fact remains that over two thirds of all breast cancers occur in women with no recognized risk factor (Seidman et al., 1982). The incidence does increase with age. Berg (1984), in summarizing the significance of these facts, points out that no adult American woman is at such a low risk as to merit exclusion from an effective breast cancer control program. Even in New Mexican American Indian women, the risk of breast cancer before age 75 years is 1 in 40 (2.5 per cent). American women in general have one chance in 12 (8.2 per cent) of developing breast cancer before age 75 years, but in women with no recognized risk factors, this drops to only 5.9 per cent (one in 17). This rate far exceeds those for other common cancers, except the risk of lung cancer in heavy smokers. Berg's conclusions were that every woman with breast tissue is at high risk. All that may be being accomplished by targeting women who currently have risk factors for screening is to create unnecessary anxiety in women with the factors and a false sense of security in those without the factors. This is true even for the overemphasized significance of family history as a risk factor. Women with a negative family history for breast cancer still develop the majority of all breast cancers and die from them.

Dubin and coworkers (1984) examined risk factors for selection bias in a screened population producing 1383 cancers in comparison to a randomly selected control population of 2543 women. In cases with prevalent cancer, the relative risk for cancer was found greater for the "usual factors: greater age, greater weight, early menarche, late first live birth, or multiparity, late menopause and a family history of breast cancer." However, numerous biases seemed to exist in these populations for which the authors attempted to correct. Among rescreened women, for example, previous biopsy and Jewish and Catholic religions were associated with increased risk, whereas in women screened only once, these factors were associated with a decreased risk.

Schwartz and colleagues (1985) broke the familial risk factors down to quantify the risk of breast cancer to relatives of women who developed breast cancer before the age of 55 years. For women with affected sisters, the ratio was 2.2 to 1, for women with affected daughters, 3.2 to 1, and for the combination of affected mothers and sisters, 9.9 to 1. The cumulative risk of breast cancer reached 17 per cent for women with sisters developing breast cancer before the age of 40 years or with both affected sisters and mother. Breast cancer in aunts was not associated with an increased risk.

Does the Discovery of Cancer at an Earlier Time Lead to an Improved Outcome?

That prognosis of breast cancer can be improved by earlier diagnosis is not universally true. It cannot be improved for all women, as some biologic subsets of breast cancer lead to the death of the afflicted even when the most vigorous multimodality screening program is followed. An objective look at the screening process requires that the contradictory evidence be considered as analytically as possible. The overpromotion of a screening strategy that does not improve prognosis can be enormously expensive, with benefit ranging from nonexistent to a negative value.

A critical issue in the evaluation of all screening programs is the impact of lead time, length time bias sampling, and overdiagnosis on the interpretation of results and benefits. A consideration of the magnitude of these biases is given in Chapter 10. The rates of growth and the kinetic and biologic behavior of predetectable cancer are critical determinants of both lead time and length biases. Cancers of a more indolent behavior are the ones more likely to be discovered by periodic screening, whereas the more virulent and lethal cancers have a tendency to surface in the intervals between annual screenings. To reduce biases, the evaluation of any screening benefit must be based on a reduction of breast cancer mortality for the entire population of women subjected to the specific screening strategy as compared to controls.

LENGTH BIAS

During the first 4 years of the Louisville Breast Cancer Detection Demonstration Project (BCDDP), 115 proved cancers were found among 10,128 women. Serial measurements were possible by xeromammograms in 32 cases. Doubling times for 23 of these tumors exhibited growth that ranged from 109 to 944 days. The log mean of the actual doubling times was 327 days. The predominant geometric shape of small primary breast cancers observed on mammography was that of a spheroid with a long axis following the direction of the ducts. The frequency distribution of the doubling times of the spheroids was lognormal.

Forty-three per cent of these cases (49 of 115) were cancers confirmed in the intervals between annual mammograms. Of these, 7.8 per cent (9 of 115), or 28 per cent of the cases observed by two or more mammograms (9 of 32), consisted of cancers growing too slowly to permit measurement of growth over periods of 1 to 4 years. The annual incidence of cancers increased from 0.064 to 0.239 per cent over the first 3 years of the project, and dropped to 0.144 per cent in the fourth year when women under 50 years old were excluded.

The conclusions of the Louisville study were that a very large percentage of all breast cancers are exceedingly rapid in growth, and that annual screening was primarily subdividing breast cancers into the three subsets determined by growth rates (i.e., rapidly growing, interval surfacing cancers, indolent prevalent cancers, and nongrowing cancers). This is the first report of the full spectrum of growth rates in a defined population of women (Heuser et al., 1979 a,b). The faster-growing cancers were more likely to metastasize ($0.01 < p < 0.05$). These clinical growth rate subsets are major determinants of lead time bias and length bias.

The clinical literature, consisting of uncontrolled studies with incompletely stratified cases, is inconsistent on the impact on prognosis of delay in diagnosis after the onset of symptoms. Studies that consider delay have reported increased survival with delay, suggesting that slower growing, more indolent cancers are being selected by length bias. These studies include those of Waxman and Fitts (1959), Brightmore and coworkers (1970), Wilkinson and colleagues (1979), and Dohrman and colleagues (1982). Studies suggesting that delay is associated with a decreased survival include those of Nathanson and Welch (1936), Eggers and coworkers (1941), and Bloom (1965). Other studies, concluding that delay had no impact on prognosis, include those of MacDonald (1942), Dargent (1949), MacDonald (1952), and Hultborn and Tornberg (1960). Dennis and coworkers (1975) reported the relationship between delay after the onset of symptoms and the time of performance of a radical mastectomy to the time of first recurrence and survival in a series of 237 women and found no statistically significant difference ($p < 0.05$).

Robinson and colleagues (1984) reported the Israeli experience. They found no association between the stage of the disease and delay in diagnosis. The responsibility for delay was shared about equally by patient and physician except for advanced cancer, for which patients were more often responsible for the delay. Other subtle variations in their experience reemphasized the need to define the stratifications of breast cancer for which prognosis might be affected adversely by delay.

At present, few data exist that prove the value of any specific screening strategy for breast cancer, according to rigid rules of epidemiologic data collection and hypothesis testing against a control population (Beahrs, 1977). Proof can come only with randomized control and long-term follow-up to correct for lead time and length bias and to monitor for a delayed increase in cancers secondary to irradiation.

LEAD TIME ESTIMATES

An estimation of the potential range of lead time bias may be obtained by multiplying the number of doublings required for the cancer to grow from the threshold size detectable by mammography to the threshold size detectable by breast self-examination (BSE) by the net doubling time for the interval of growth. In the Louisville study, no breast cancer smaller than 2.1 mm was correctly diagnosed even on the retrospective review of mammograms. A study on the value of BSE by Foster and coworkers (1978) showed the mean maximum tumor diameter discovered by monthly BSE to be 20.4 mm. Approximately nine doublings would be required for a cancer to grow from 2.1 mm to 20.4 mm. The lead time bias for the cases on which growth rate was measured could vary from 8496 days (9 × 944) to 981 days (9 × 109), with a median of 2943 days (9 × 327), using the DT_{act} for grossly measurable cancers. However, for nongrowing cancers, the lead time bias could be much longer; for interval surfacing cancers, lead time bias would be expected to be much shorter, and length bias would be negligible. Extensive follow-up would be essential to exclude these biases as the factors responsible for any apparent improvement in survivorship among persons undergoing screening for the earlier detection of breast cancer. If faster growing cancers should prove responsible for most of the lethality from breast cancer, the lead time bias in these cases would be of a much shorter duration. Unfortunately, the faster growing breast cancers are probably not the ones being detected by mammographic screening, but instead they are surfacing and being self-detected in the intervals between annual mammograms.

Moskowitz and Fox's data (1979) have been useful in estimating the lead time gained by vigorous mammographic screening and biopsy. Under the age of 50 years, the lead time was estimated to be 2.2 years (± 0.4) and over age 50 years, it is 3.2 years (± 0.4) (Moskowitz and Fox, 1979). In the Louisville BCDDP, the division of prevalence rates at first screen of the entire population by the incidence rate in subsequent years of screening gave a lead time estimated at 1.8 to 6.9 years, but this varied greatly with age (Heuser et al., 1979b; Spratt et al., 1986).

Within the general emphasis on cost constraints in medicine, it is not inhumane to look more realistically at an individual's potential longevity. The data for the 1980 census have been translated into man-days of residual life by age and sex (Fig. 19–1). The appreciation of the limits of potential gain (i.e., the average number of days of useful life remaining according to age, sex and ethnicity) is worthwhile. Similar financial limits determined by the individual's potential economic return and worth exist on the dollars to be spent in screening. At the level of public health, the arguments deal with the allocation of all health dollars and of the ranking of competitive priorities in terms of the potential gain from screening. Just "finding a cancer" or a precancerous condition does not confirm that screening per se leads to enhanced survivorship. For cancers with negative cancer control windows enhanced survivorship from screening is not pos-

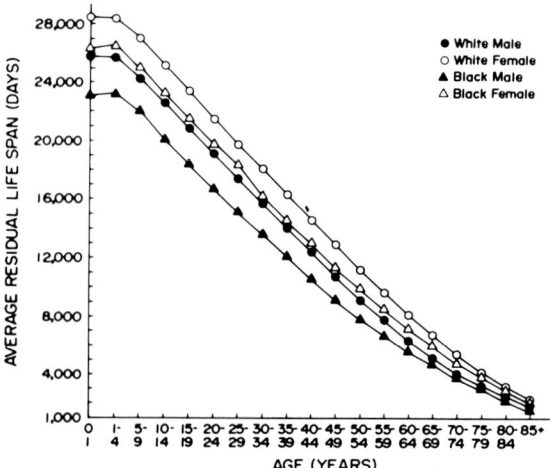

Figure 19–1. Man-days of average residual survivorship by age, race, and sex calculated from Vital Statistics of the United States, 1982, Life Tables, Volume II, Section 6, U.S. Department of Health and Human Services, Public Health Service, National Center for Health Statistics, U.S. Government Printing Office, Washington, D.C. 20402.

sible. For other cancers, the presence of lead time bias must be excluded by a controlled study before the conclusion can be drawn that screening and earlier discovery are responsible for enhanced survivorship (Spratt, 1981). When this cannot be shown, screening programs may still be justifiable if reduced morbidity treatment costs and enhanced survivorship can be attributed to the screening strategy and subsequent treatment.

Other authors have recognized the importance of these biases and have attempted to interpret their magnitude and significance. Swartz (1977) attempted to estimate the potential contribution of these biases on the 5 year survival rates of women whose breast cancer was detected by screening and on the survival rate of women who self-detected their clinically surfacing breast cancers. Even though his estimates were insensitive to age and the sources provided only crude data, he was able to estimate the contribution of the biases to the differences in survivorship to be as low as 20 per cent and as high as 72 per cent for women with breast cancers detected at first screen. For women in the second screen, the contribution of bias to the difference in end results ranged from 33 to 42 per cent. Detailed stratification of cancers and hosts by kinetic and biologic differences will be essential to obtain more accurate estimates of the contribution of the lead time bias and length biased sampling to survivorship data.

Model of the Screening Problem

To start with the proof that earlier detection of a still asymptomatic cancer leads to enhanced survivorship requires a model of the screening problem and a model of breast cancer, itself essential for designing a controlled study (Figs. 19–2 and 19–3). The model of breast cancer in Figure 19–2, adapted from Walter and Day (1983), is essential for understanding the complexity of the screening problem. Most clinical staging systems are not discriminating enough and are too anatomic, and they depict events dependent on variables not included in the system. Figure 19–3 delineates the potential arborization of any screening intervention.

The cancer control window (CCW) is that segment in the life history of a cancer elapsing between the moment the cancer is large enough to detect and the moment it disseminates (is no longer a local-regional disease) (Fig. 19–4). Spratt (1981) estimated the variable duration of the CCW based on the probable number of doublings of the cancer in this period and the doubling time. He concluded that the CCW could not exceed 14 doublings and probably did not exceed nine. He also recognized that those cancers that disseminate before they attain a threshold size that would permit detection have a negative CCW and are never discoverable in a local-regional state. The variable length of positive CCWs is shown in Table 19–3. The variables considered in calculating this table are given in Table 19–4. Those cancers below the line in Table 19–3 could all transgress the CCW in periods of less than 1 year and therefore might escape a screening effort conducted annually. As documented in Chapter 10, there is strong evidence that many breast cancers have actual doubling times (DT_{act}) of less than 20 days in their predetectable phase; all these would surface in intervals of less than 1 year, leading to possible self-detection.

The one widely cited study in the United States literature *designed* to test the hypothesis that the screening for breast cancers leads to better end results is the HIP study in New York (Shapiro, 1977). Although this study was correctly designed from a biostatistical standpoint, deviation from the design leaves its results open to varying conclusions (Beahrs, 1977; Greenberg, personal communication, 1985). It can only be stated that screening for breast cancer may lead to enhanced survivorship in women over 50 years of age.

An updated analysis of the mortality effect in a population screened for breast cancer (i.e., the HIP study) has been reported, using the theory of competing risks for death in long-term follow-up (Aron and Prorok, 1986).

Figure 19–2. Model of breast cancer projection. (Adapted from Walter, S. D., and Day, N. E.: Estimation of the duration of the preclinical disease state using screening data. Am. J. Epidemiol., 118:865, 1983.)

MODEL OF BREAST CANCER PROGRESSION

Asymptomatic disease of below threshold size for detection - local, locoregional, distant	Asymptomatic disease above threshold size for detection	Symptomatic	End Points
Normal			
T_v Biological onset	T_w Disease now detectable if screen done	T_x Disease becomes symtomatic	T_y Death without treatment T_z Death with treatment
	Screening takes place, can be true positive or false negative	Patient comes for diagnosis of symptomatic disease	

$T_a = T_w - T_v$: Undetectable sojourn

$T_b = T_x - T_w$: Detectable asymptomatic sojourn

$T_c = T_b - T_w$: Delay time

$T_d = T_x - T_b$: Lead time

$T_y - T_v$ = Natural sojourn of undiagnosed, untreated disease

$T_z - T_v$ = Natural sojourn of diagnosed disease, treated without treatment mortality

T_v — Onset

T_w — Detectable but asymptomatic

T_x — Symptomatic

T_y — Time of death without diagnosis and treatment

T_z — Time of death with treatment

T_y, T_z Determined by lifelong follow-up to avoid truncation of results

Cancer Control Window (CCW) = time that cancer disseminates and is no longer locoregional less T_w

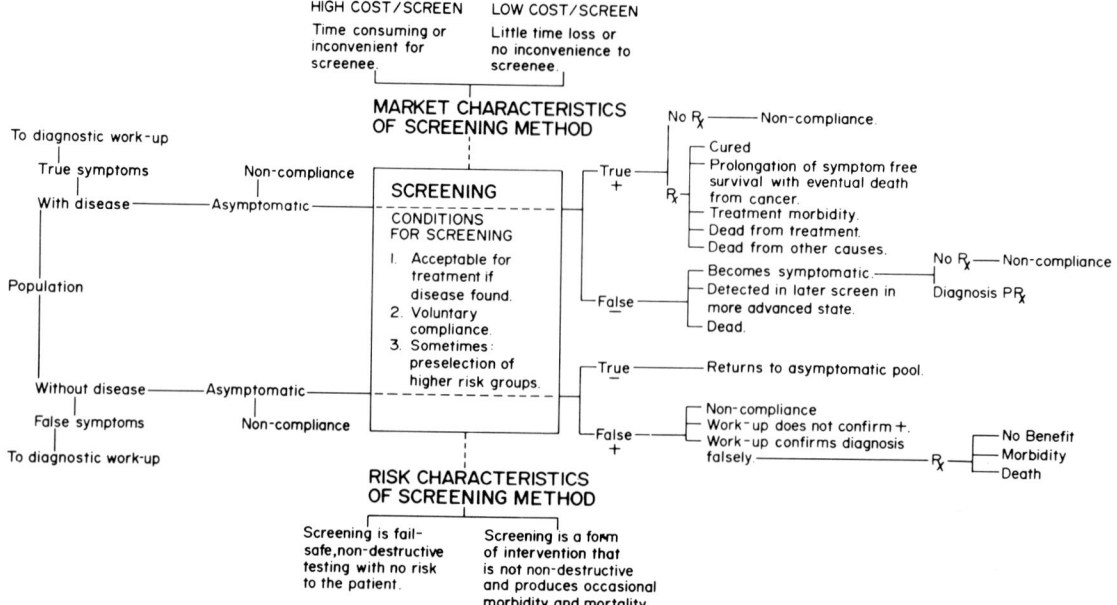

Figure 19–3. Flow diagram of representative decisions and outcomes existing in any screening program. Quality control at many points is essential to the reduction of errors. The existence of effective treatment determines the ultimate benefit of screening. A controlled clinical trial is generally essential to test hypotheses on the benefit of screening. (From Spratt, J. S.: In Hickey, R. C. et al. [Eds.]: Current Problems in Cancer. Chicago, Year Book Medical Publishers, 1982. Reprinted with permission.)

These authors concluded that some, but not all, of the breast cancer cases detected early might have a reduced mortality rate. The screening for breast cancer had no impact on mortality not due to breast cancer. The authors concluded that future research should relate observed reductions in breast cancer mortality to mathematical models of disease progression and screening. A more comprehensive understanding of the impact of screening on the natural history of breast cancer is needed.

The literature does not resolve the question as studies are to be found both supporting and refuting the value of earlier dignosis of breast cancer. Unfortunately, these articles largely report non–population-based data without controls. The distribution of numerous variables associated with outcome is not uniformly provided. Rarely is it possible to compare one study with another. Paradoxically, long delay after the onset of symptoms is often associated with a better prognosis than with a very short history of pretreatment symptoms. This strongly suggests that discovery by screening, or self-referral for symptoms or signs, is dominated by two overriding factors. First, size at discovery is determined by a neurophysiologically inherent lognormal variation in sensitivity of the individual's perception of size (Spratt, 1969). Second, the enormous variation in growth rate seems inversely related to prognosis, the propensity to metastasize, and pretreatment duration of symptoms. Lead time bias may result in the erroneous conclusion that earlier diagnosis lengthens survivorship in cases with a negative cancer control window. The rates of growth of human breast cancers form a lognormal distribution with a high coefficient of correlation between actual and predicted ordinates (see Chapter 10). This distribution of growth rates also falls into three clinical subsets. The first subset consists of cancers growing too rapidly to permit measurement by annual mammography. These can-

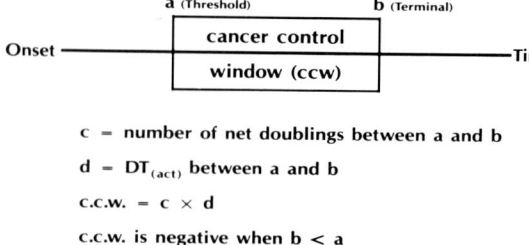

c = number of net doublings between a and b

d = $DT_{(act)}$ between a and b

c.c.w. = $c \times d$

c.c.w. is negative when b < a

Figure 19–4. Diagram of cancer control window.

Table 19-3. DURATION OF THE CANCER CONTROL WINDOW IN DAYS

$DT_{(act)}$ (days)*	Number of Doublings of the Volume of a Cancer						
	2	4	6	8	10	12	14
1000	2000	4000	6000	8000	10000	12000	14000
500	1000	2000	3000	4000	5000	6000	7000
100	200	400	600	800	1000	1200	1400
50	100	200	300	400	500	600	700
20	40	80	120	160	200	240	280†
10	20	40	60	80	100	120	140
5	10	20	30	40	50	60	70

*Duration of cancer control window (CCW) = DT_{act} times number of net doublings of cells occurring between threshold size and terminal size.

†CCWs below this line all have durations of less than 1 year.

From Spratt, J. S.: The relationship between the rates of growth of cancer and the intervals between screening examinations necessary for effective discovery. Cancer Detect. Prevent., 4:301, 1981. Reprinted with permission.

cers surface from below threshold size to palpable size, being found largely by self-detection, in intervals of fewer than 365 days. The second subset is composed of cancers in which two or more mammographic observations, generally done at annual intervals, permit a measurement of growth and a calculation of growth rates. The third subset is composed of the exceedingly slowly growing cancers with no measurable growth occurring on mammographic observations at intervals of 1 year or more. In Chapter 10 arguments supporting the conformity of in vivo growth of human breast cancer to the Gompertzian equation are provided. This means that the growth rate may be rapid in the preclinical period but slows with increasing tumor size.

Table 19-4. VARIABLES DETERMINING THE DURATION OF THE CANCER CONTROL WINDOW (CCW)

a =	Threshold of detectable size
b =	Terminal size (size at which cancer has disseminated and is no longer local-regional)
c =	Number of net doublings of the cancer cells present at threshold size (a) that must occur to produce a cancer of terminal size (b)
d =	Net tumor volume doubling time
CCW =	Cancer control window duration
CCW =	c × d

When b < a, the cancer control window has a negative value and the detection of local-regional cancer is not possible.

EVALUATION OF SCREENING BY SIMULATION MODELS

With the complex behavior of breast cancer (Fig. 19-2) and arborizing nature of the screening problem (Fig. 19-3), conflicting conclusions regarding the value of different approaches toward screening for new or recurrent cancer are frequent. To construct a model of breast cancer screening and to test its solutions, data of consistent quality and significant amount are necessary. The conclusions drawn from models would vary with the definition of the optimum endpoints. In fact, the definition of what is optimum is often determined more by political and marketing factors than by any scientific model. Again, most data describing the terms defined in the glossary (see Table 19-2) are subject to considerable variation and mandate quality control considerations in every screening program. Results from the literature could be used as guidelines for designing a community screening program but not for the final justification of a screening program's value. This justification can be obtained only at the point of application, where various quality control and compliance factors would have to be considered. Finally, the ultimate value of screening depends on the effectiveness of treatment. Thus, the best screening program may be of no value if it is coupled with an ineffective treatment program. The evaluation has to be program-specific and be confirmed by longitudinal audits. Final proof can be approached only with population-based controlled clinical trials.

The best that can be done in a chapter such as this is to consider conclusions of various models and uncontrolled clinical reports. The applications of any detection system can be made more cost-effective by screening only groups at higher risk to develop cancer. However, no higher risk group appreciably increased the ability to identify substantial numbers of truly high risk women (Seidman et al., 1982; Berg, 1984) to a degree that would permit the exclusion of women with no recognized risk factors.

THRESHOLD SIZE

A major consideration of any model is the screening test's threshold of discovery. There is a certain minimum size or measurement below which detection is not possible, and the actual threshold of the detectable sizes for a population is determined by the Weber-Fechner law (Spratt et al., 1966). This law states that an organism's response to a stimulus is proportional to the logarithm of the magnitude of the stimulus. Paraphrased for cancer, the ability of the examiner or examining method to detect a cancer would be distributed according to the logarithms of the sizes of the detected cancers (Spratt, 1969). Size at diagnosis is, therefore, stochastic and not deterministic. The frequency distribution of the sizes of newly detected cancer has been confirmed to be lognormal, as predicted by the Weber-Fechner law (Spratt et al., 1969). This is a major factor in the wide variance of size at discovery, so that there is always the risk that a portion of discovered cancers will have exceeded terminal size by the time of discovery, the terminal size being the size at which the cancer produces metastatic deposits beyond its region of origin. Growth rate may affect *size at discovery* but not the threshold of discoverable size. Basically, a large cancer with a short history probably arises with a more rapid growth rate than a small cancer with a long clinical history as a result, in part, of rate of growth.

Eddy (1978) synthesized screening programs for breast cancer into a simulation model. With his model, many simulation runs could be made on the computer to predict the characteristics of a screening program with respect to data fed to the model. Eddy's model has the capacity for coping with the various financial costs, intangible costs, and discount rates on the input side and total expected value and present value on the output side (see Table 19–5). Eddy's model rests on three main functions: (1) the probability density function (*pdf*) of the interval between the moment a breast cancer is first detectable by physical examination and the time it is first detectable by mammography; (2) the *pdf* of the interval between the time the breast cancer is first detectable by physical examination and the moment the patient will seek care; and (3) the *pdf* of the relationship that exists between earliness of detection and patient survival.

Eddy's cancer screening model has characteristics in common with those groups of decisions encompassed by operations research and the analysis of systems that are part of an unending history of actions. Earlier choices affect the present, and current decisions will influence the future. All models of this type must be viewed as being embedded in an unbounded horizon. What Eddy and other modelers ultimately accomplish is the development of some modifications of a dynamic programming approach. Many linear and nonlinear approaches attempt to solve these problems by considering all constraints simultaneously. The dynamic programming approach, on the other hand, casts a problem into a structure with the following characteristics (Wagner, 1974).

The decision variables with associated constraints are grouped according to stages. The stages are then considered sequentially. The only information about the previous stage rel-

Table 19–5. SIMULATION MODEL FOR SCREENING PROGRAMS FOR BREAST CANCER

Data that must be put into the simulation model (input)
  Patient age
  Relative risk category
  Age-specific incidence rates
  Age-specific mortality rates
  Complication rates of diagnostic and therapeutic procedures (e.g., the operative mortality rates of a breast biopsy done under general anesthesia)
  The effectiveness of mammography
  The effectiveness of patient behavior
  The effectiveness of therapy
  Radiation effect
  Previous history of physical examinations of the breast
  Schedule for future physical examinations of the breast
  Schedule for future mammographic examinations

Data that can be derived from the simulation model (output)
  The probability that the patient will be diagnosed as having breast cancer in any given year in the future
  The probability that the patient will be a surviving breast cancer patient during any year in the future
  The probability that the patient will die of breast cancer in any year
  The probability that the patient will die of other cancers in any year
  Five, 10, 15 year survival and patient life expectancy
  The probability that the patient will have a malignant lesion detected by a physical examination, a mammogram, or the patient herself in any given interval of time in the future
  The survival rates of patients according to method of detection
  The probability that the patient will have a biopsy in any year
  A comparison of the mortality rate of a lesion detected at a screening session, with the mortality rate of that lesion if the patient postponed the screening appointment or waited until the lesion became apparent on self-examination

From Eddy, D. M.: Screening for Breast Cancer: Theory, Analysis, and Design. © 1980, pp 172, 173. Reprinted with permission of Prentice-Hall, Inc., Englewood Cliffs, New Jersey.

evant to the selection of optimal values of the current decision variables is summarized by a so-called state variable. This state variable may be *n*-dimensional. The most current decision to be made, given the present state of the system, has a forecasting influence on the state of the next stage. The ability to predict the outcome of the most current decision is judged in terms of its forecasted economic impact on the present stage and all subsequent stages. The complexity of this model makes the planning and completion of prospective controlled clinical trials very complicated and costly, perhaps explaining why so few really satisfactory controlled clinical trials have been done to confirm the value of screening.

EVALUATION OF SCREENING MODELS

Although several workable mathematical models now exist to assist in the selection of optimum screening strategies, the quality of the models often exceeds the quality and necessary quantity of data available to use in the models. Any screening models must ultimately be extended to complete cancer management strategies, permitting the sequential selection of decisions that will give optimum benefit to large numbers of people. Screening is of value only if functional longevity is enhanced, as a result of the increased efficacy of earlier treatment. Plans for conducting trials and considering strategic options my be advanced by the use of appropriate decision-making models, taking into consideration the factors just discussed. The general hypothesis to be tested by any model might be stated as follows: A population screened and managed by a particular strategy has a greater functional longevity than a nonscreened population or a population screened and managed by a different strategy. Simple discovery at an earlier point in time is not adequate proof of value. Considered with this hypothesis, the evaluation of a screening program in isolation from the total clinical management process is impossible. Furthermore, on studying the flow diagram in Figure 19–3, the benefit of an acceptable screening program strategy could vary from laboratory to laboratory, x-ray department to x-ray department and clinic to clinic, depending on the tightness and ability of the local system to minimize false negative and false positive results, comparability of the treatment of cancers discovered by screening, and other systems deviations. Studies from one program could not be accepted as equivalent for another program unless the entire screening quality control and management strategy acceptable for the first system is mirrored by the second program. A basic model for looking at the optimum value of all health strategies has been suggested and may also be applied (Spratt, 1975 *a,b*; see also Chapter 30). Optimum is defined as the strategy that gives the highest probability of living the maximum number of functional man-days with the least amount of nonfunctional time and at an economic cost tolerable to the individual. The desire in any cancer screening and management system is to define some variable endpoint, the value of which is to be maximized or minimized. Wagner (1974) has emphasized that most decision-makers cannot intuitively make consistent judgments about the relative desirability of different infinite streams of return. The impact of current actions on future outcome can take some very unexpected turns, and data rather than intuition are necessary for program design and evaluation.

FLAWS IN SCREENING MODELS

Many screening models have one recurring flaw: Their conclusions are often evaluated more on anatomic staging than on host-tumor behavior. Anatomic staging is based on the only partially correct thesis that all cancers metastasize with increasing size, first to regional lymph nodes and then generally. These anatomic staging systems only partially allow for the extremes of biologic behavior (e.g., some cancers never metastasize, no matter how large the primary cancer). There exists extreme natural variances of growth rates and highly variable tendencies to metastasize. Some cancers are so acute and fast-growing that from inception of the cancer to death may be a matter of only weeks or months. At the opposite extreme are cancers so indolent and slow-growing that they will never reach significant size during a normal life span—the host dies of unrelated causes with the cancer, not from it.

In explaining the behavior of solid tumors as related to "earliness," three biologic variants can be defined: (1) early metastasizing; (2) late metastasizing; and (3) nonmetastasizing. The early metastasizing cancer literally begins to shed cells systemically, almost from inception. The extreme examples would be the acute leukemias, which probably never have a "solid" tumor and some melanomas, possibly including the infrequent but lethal melanomas of mucous membranes. Some breast cancers fall in this early metastasizing subset, and their existence precludes the chance for the complete control of breast cancer by contemporary screening and local regional treatment. The late metastasizing cancers are the ones that shed more and more metastases as the primary lesion becomes larger, but these *might* have a phase beyond threshold size when they are localized that could be called "early." Finally, as already noted, there are biologic variants of breast cancer that simply never metastasize. These cancers can obtain enormous local size, destroy adjacent tissues by contiguous growth, sometimes kill the host, and yet never metastasize.

Cancers in the category between the early metastasizing and the nonmetastasizing ones—those that seem progressively more likely to metastasize with increasing size—constitute the category for which an effective screening strategy might have the best opportunity for discovery before dissemination. The screening strategy might be able to detect these cancers by radiography or physical examination, or both, before they produce symptoms.

HARM-BENEFIT RATIO

The impact of breast cancer screening on a population may be viewed from different perspectives. Wright (1986) analyzed biopsy rates, detection of benign disease, and mortality rate. He concluded that 2041 women would have to be screened for one person to benefit. If women undergoing biopsy for benign disease are considered to have been harmed, the harm-benefit ratio ranges up to 62 to 1. Wright concluded that mass screening for breast cancer should be abandoned. The harm-benefit ratio might be lower for the screening of higher risk groups. In the BCDDP at Louisville, 9.9 biopsies were performed for each cancer diagnosed. As Wright notes in an exchange of letters to the editor regarding his 1986 study, specificity and sensitivity cannot be made to move in the same direction. His paper raised an array of fundamental issues requiring closer scientific scrutiny and discussion.

PATIENT EDUCATION

A by-product of a screening program should be the prevention of cancer through patient education (Monaco et al., 1972). The screener's role obviously can become more cost-effective by educating and motivating people to request health services and to participate in their own health maintenance. Prevention may ultimately be the most important effort for really cost-effective cancer control. A periodically updated patient education handout has been used by the authors for patient education in prevention since 1967. This document is given to each patient the authors see and is further interpreted and reinforced after the patient has read it.

Patient education is accepted as being desirable in enhancing recovery, alleviating anxiety, and facilitating compliance. Patient education also must be planned to minimize patient dependence on others in the self-surveillance recovery and follow-up process. The design of a patient education program must be cost-effective as education can be extremely expensive. Scientific methodology for the evaluation of educational processes is essential. Methods vary, but the majority of patient education programs remain unevaluated, and noncompliance is a prevalent problem. Design of conceptual models for evaluation of patient education requires specific steps in evaluation research. Quasi-experimental design appears to be most practical for use in the health care environment. Educational programs will have multiple objectives, with immediate and intermediate objectives being most crucial because of time and cost constraints and available techniques. Success depends on the criteria evaluated. Patient education best lends itself to these criteria: Effort, performance, adequacy, efficiency, and process. A systems design model for evaluation of educational strategy to help clarify cause-and-effect association and provide accountability with examples of input, intervening, and output variables has been provided (Newby et al., 1978).

Evaluation of education programs has shown that the student learns best when he or she is taught not only "what we ought to know" but also "what we want to know."

PATIENT COMPLIANCE

Compliance with cancer preventive behavior and participation in screening and follow-up require educated and motivated patients. Patient compliance is often highly variable. Reinforcement by education of family and peer group often is essential to enhance compliance.

The psychologic impact on patient compliance in screening, recovery, and follow-up is very much affected by the scope of the information needs of cancer patients and how effectively these needs are met by scientifically designed and evaluated education programs (Newby et al., 1978). Generally, these needs cannot be separated from the planning and implementation of an effective screening program.

The participation of the knowledgeable patient in self-care continues to be verified as being effective as well as low in cost. Vickery and colleagues (1983) reported significant decreases in total medical visits and minor illness visits in three separately educated experimental groups with respect to a control group. They estimated a savings of $2.50 to $3.50 in decreased use for each dollar spent on educational interventions. The cost savings through patient education may be quite significant, enhancing patient confidence and reducing trivial and frequently unnecessary use of physician time. Standard, tested curricular materials are helpful in saving time by reducing iterative teaching and in avoiding errors of omission.

COST BENEFIT OF SCREENING

Screening programs can be enormously expensive, with negative public health value, unless they are planned and evaluated as to both cost and benefit. As simple examples of the cost per case, Table 19–6 illustrates the cost of finding one case of cancer of the breast by mammography (Fitzpatrick, 1974). A good screening model must establish that savings in treatment costs and salvaged lives exceed the high case-finding costs of primary screening.

The issue of "cost per case of cancer found" rapidly becomes more complex. With any first time screen, the prevalence rates will be high (as a result of length biased sampling) and the cost per case of cancer found will look promisingly low. In subsequent years, discovery rates drop to near the expected age-specific annual incidence rates, and the cost per case of cancer found on annual rescreening rises precipitously. However, the cost of treatment for earlier cancers may be less than that of treating more advanced cases. The magnitude of this saving has not been well studied but conceivably could more than counterbalance the high cost per case of cancer found in a low-yield screening program. Evens (1986) estimated that current charges for mammography would generate an annual cost of $2.6 billion if used as recommended for all American women at risk. The cost per cancer found would be about $14,000. This does not include the cost of all biopsies done for benign disease because of the false positive results from mammographic examinations. Even if mammography should prove to be a panacea for the control of breast cancer, this exorbitant cost would have to be contained by strategies that would maximize benefit. Moskowitz addresses this serious cost-benefit question in Chapter 7. Although a Swedish study has suggested that the risk of dying from breast cancer may be reduced but not eliminated by mammographic examinations (Tabar et al., 1985), this benefit is far from being realized in the United States and, unless cost can be contained, it may never be realized for any but an affluent, motivated subset of the population.

Clinical Studies of the Impact of Earlier Diagnosis on Survivorship

Mueller (1978) provided a unique longitudinal study on 3558 women diagnosed as having breast cancer. He consolidated all cases with breast cancer and performed a life table analysis of all cases through 15 years. This has the net effect of eliminating selection bias. He reaffirmed that the use of fixed endpoint survival rates, such as 5 year survival rates, were meaningless. It is the force of mortality (the time-dependent death rate) that is most important in understanding the natural history of breast cancer and the impact of interventions.

Table 19–6. CANADIAN STUDY ON COST PER CASE OF BREAST CANCER FOUND BY MAMMOGRAPHY

Age	Cost
40–49	$76,532.00
50–59	$24,584.00
60–64	$28,726.00

Mueller's data indicated two rates of dying—one for those who die quickly, within 3 years of diagnosis, and one for those who live longer than 3 years. Beyond 12 years his numbers were too small to be significant. Of all women who developed breast cancer, 80 to 85 per cent ultimately died of their cancer, and the likelihood was even greater for the women who were young at the time of diagnosis. The death rate averaged about 8 per cent through the twelfth year after diagnosis, significantly in excess of the expected rate of dying.

For elderly women who develop breast cancer, the death rate from accumulating conditions of aging is great enough to conceal the more rapid rate of dying during the first 3 years, if it exists at all in the elderly. Mueller concluded that the quality of life attained by treating the manifestations of cancer as they occur might be a more meaningful way to assess benefit. Perhaps the day is approaching when therapeutic benefit will be measured by an index of survivorship, coupled with function, and attained at a tolerable cost, as previously suggested by Spratt (1971, 1975 a,b).

This observation on the elderly is also supported by Stoll (1976), who reported that the survival rates in women past the age of 70 years were nearly the same whether the disease was limited or extensive at presentation. Survivorship was also independent of the treatment given. Stoll concluded that survivorship in the over 70 age group was primarily a function of the general medical condition at the time of diagnosis. Only with the availability of tolerable effective treatment would overly diligent and costly screening and follow-up be justified past the age of 70 years.

Because of the confounding problems created by acute cancers that can develop quickly, more frequent examinations might be done (Spratt, 1981). The more frequently examinations are done, however, the more the adverse impact of error and cost accumulates. At some point, the law of diminishing marginal returns becomes evident, increasing the risk of more harm than good, or cost in excess of value, to the screened population. The risk of having cancer at any moment is low, though the lifetime accumulative risks are high, necessitating the evolution of an optimum lifetime cancer control strategy.

Swartz (1977) concluded from his model that a yearly screening program with mammography and a clinical examination will achieve less than half of the possible gain from life expectancy that would be realized if breast cancer mortality were eliminated. About two thirds of the gain in life expectancy from a yearly screening program with mammography and a clinical examination would most likely result if only a clinical examination (BSE by trained women) were performed yearly (or more frequently).

Bross and Blumenson (1976) provided a mathematical model of the effectiveness of screening random asymptomatic women for breast cancer using mammography. From various screening strategies modeled for different age groups against the increasing risk of iatrogenic cancer from multiple exposures to low level radiation, they concluded that the screening of asymptomatic women could not be justified before age 50 years.

Bailar (1976) subjected the breast screening programs to real scrutiny by considering the possibility that radiation from mammography might induce breast cancer. He concluded that the low level risk of cancer induction is a real possibility. Decades may be required to determine whether the incidence of breast cancer rises in those screened by mammography.

Although radiation from mammography may induce some breast cancers, the induced cancer will be detected earlier by screening, so that the predicted improvement in life expectancy from screening, if there was no radiation danger, might be maintained. However, the number of induced cases of breast cancer from radiation associated with mammography could be as large as the number of lives saved by adding mammography to a yearly clinical examination.

BREAST SELF-EXAMINATION

Breast self-examination (BSE), like other forms of screening, requires controlled clinical trials to establish its value. Foster and colleagues (1978; Foster and Costanza, 1984) have provided the most sustained, well-reported data in the attempt to confirm the worth of BSE. The 1978 study was a retrospective survey of 335 women with breast cancer that correlated their reported breast examination practices with clinical stage at the time of diagnosis. The maximum tumor diameter in women practicing monthly BSE was 19.7 ± 2.2 mm (mean ± standard error of the mean), compared with a tumor diameter of 24.7 ± 2.0 mm for women who practiced BSE less often than monthly. The tumor diameter in women who never practiced BSE was 35.9 ±

1.5 mm. However, the relationship between the frequency of BSE and the positivity of axillary lymph nodes for metastases did not reach statistical significance.

As a continuation, this series was expanded to 1004 women with follow-up to correlate survivorship with BSE practices (Foster and Costanza, 1984). These investigators observed that more frequent BSE was associated with a greater chance that a woman would find the cancer and that there would be less delay between first discovery and histologic diagnosis. The cancers were found at an earlier clinical stage and were smaller. There were fewer positive axillary lymph nodes. At the median follow-up time (52 months), 14 per cent of the women performing monthly BSE and 26 per cent of those not performing BSE had died of breast cancer. The 5 year survival rate was 75 per cent for women performing BSE and 57 per cent for nonperformers. They estimated that a lead time of 3 years would have to exist to negate the apparent beneficial effects of BSE on survivorship. However, in making this estimate, they used a tumor volume doubling time of 100 days and estimated that the diameter would double every 300 days at this rate. Actually, as discussed in Chapter 10, extreme variance exists in the DT_{act}, and growth in the predetectable phase is much faster than 100 days. Also, the long-term follow-up of breast cancer cases has established that an increased death rate exists for many years (Mueller, 1978).

As already stated, the size of tumor at discovery was 19.7 ± 2.2 mm with monthly BSE and 24.7 ± 2 mm with less than monthly BSE. The authors calculated the volume of a sphere using these dimensions. The volume averaged 4003 mm^3 for tumors discovered with BSE and 7890 mm^3 without monthly BSE. The cellular replication between these two points is trivial in comparison to the total number of cells in the tumors. Dividing the mean tumor volume at diagnosis with monthly BSE (4003 mm^3) into the mean volume of diagnosis without monthly BSE (7890 mm^3) yielded 1.97. Thus, on an average, no more than one additional volume doubling had occurred without monthly BSE before diagnosis. Considering the information on growth rates in Chapter 10 with respect to this estimate, the authors question that the DT_{act} of 100 days can be used to estimate lead time bias. Prolonged follow-up will be required on this study population to strengthen or refute the argument that BSE is contributing to a reduction in the mortality in breast cancer.

Saltzstein (1984) conducted a pathologic review of breast cancers diagnosed before and after an intense public education program on BSE. He found that neither the size of newly diagnosed cancers (average, 2.77 ± 2.06 cm, median, 2.0 cm before the education; average = 2.68 ± 1.72 cm, median, 2.3 cm after the education), nor the prevalence of positive axillary lymph nodes had changed significantly as a result of the public education program. This study confirms previous reports that the Weber-Fechner law determines patient perception and that this could be changed to a limited degree, at best, by public education (Spratt, 1969).

Training, paradoxically, also increases the percentage of false positive evaluations among trainees (Hall et al., 1980). These authors concluded that a "more complex model for training discrimination between normal nodularity and breast lesions" than that provided by silicone models would be necessary to reduce false positive results. Because of the considerable individual variation among breasts, it is the opinion of one of the authors (J.S.S.) that the best training model is a woman's own breasts. After instruction in the location and extent of breast tissue, each woman needs to become familiar with the consistency and shape of her own breasts. With monthly BSE, she then looks for *changes*.

Breast self-examination requires no physician and costs nothing, although it will not find cancers as small as those found on mammographic examination. The true significance of this fact again awaits a controlled study with BSE as one of the arms. The quality of BSE might be improved by education, but it is the most cost-effective approach to detection available at present.

CANCER DIFFERENCES BY METHOD OF DISCOVERY

Differences exist in the distribution of types of cancers discovered by mammographic examination and those discovered by palpation. In a sustained screening program (Feig and Swartz, 1981), Grade I cancers were found only among cancers less than 3.0 cm in size, and not at all among cancers larger than 3.0 cm. Grade I cancers were discoverable nearly 90 per cent of the time by mammography, but only 25 per cent of the time by physical examination. Tubular cancers were less frequently apparent on physical examination.

That length biased sampling clearly is a

determinant of the distribution of cancer types discovered by the annual screening techniques of the BCDDP programs is strongly supported by other studies. Panoussopoulos and coworkers (1977) first called attention to the cancer that surfaces in the intervals between annual mammograms and is self-detected by the individual. Spratt, in the discussion of the paper by Panoussopoulos and colleagues, pointed out that any breast cancer that sustained an actual doubling time of less than 17 days would be an interval surfacing cancer and that cancers so acute as to maintain a DT_{act} of 9 days or less could arise after an annual mammogram and lead to the host's death in less than 1 year (see Chapter 10). With respect to screening biases in case allocation, several cogent observations merely need repeating. A circumscribed cancer margin and papillary intraductal growth were associated with the more slowly growing cancers, permitting their more frequent discovery by the length bias imposed by the annual interval between mammograms. The more acute cancers surfacing in the intervals between annual screens were associated more frequently with an anaplastic nuclear grade, absence of mammographic and microscopic calcification, presence in women under age 50 years, lack of a family history of breast cancer, and presence of a mammographic pattern classified as dysplastic. The prognosis was also poorer for the interval surfacing cancers.

DeGroote and coworkers (1983) provided further confirmation of the greater lethality of the interval surfacing cancer. Dividing 120 newly diagnosed breast cancers into three subsets, they reported that cancers surfacing in the intervals between screens had statistically significant higher percentages of positive axillary lymph nodes, higher overall mortality rates, and a lower 6 year survival rate, calculated by the life table method. The other two subsets to which they were compared were prevalent cancers detected at first screen and cancers detected at scheduled screens.

PHYSICAL FINDINGS

Confusion from the Lumpy Breast

Lumpiness of the breasts is often encountered in screening and BSE and is a source of differential diagnostic concern to both women engaged in BSE and the examining physician. As Devitt (1983) reviews, most lumpiness is normal. Fibroadenomas appear most frequently in the second, third, and fourth decades and desist after menopause. Macrocysts are infrequent before age 35 years and peak in prevalence between the ages of 45 and 49 years. After menopause, they rapidly become infrequent. The authors' practice is to reassure the woman with lumpy breasts and instruct her to become familiar with the palpatory consistency of her own breast tissue. Then she can concentrate not on the lumpiness but on *changes* in consistency or appearance when performing BSE.

Screening the Augmented Breast

With the increasing prevalence of augmentation mammoplasty of different types, the remaining breast tissue can present some unique screening situations. This breast tissue may develop mass lesions that require evaluation (Savrin et al., 1979). In addition to the usual consideration given a breast mass, the gel prosthesis may rupture, extruding content and producing a silicone granuloma.

Nipple Discharge Discovered at Screening

Screening may occasionally detect a nipple discharge, although the woman with a discharge usually notes it first and reports it to her physician. The presence of hemoglobin in a nipple discharge may justify the greater suspicion of cancer. Chaudary and associates (1982) studied the correlation between breast histopathology and nipple discharge in 270 women undergoing microdochectomy for nipple discharge from a single duct with no associated mass. In the microdochectomy specimens they found, in order of decreasing frequency, intraductal papilloma, ductal ectasia, cystic disease, and carcinoma. All occult cancers were associated with a hemoglobin positive discharge. The prevalence of occult cancer in the microdochectomy specimens associated with a hemoglobin positive discharge was 5.9 per cent. Six additional patients developed breast cancer in follow-up after a cancer negative microdochectomy in the ipsilateral breast. Further discussion of nipple discharges is provided in Chapter 6.

MAMMOGRAPHIC USE STRATEGY

Moskowitz and Fox (1979) have remained strong proponents of frequent mammographic screening and earlier biopsy. This approach accepts a higher false positive rate on mammographic readings in the interest of earlier diagnosis. The net effect is that more biopsies are done and more mammary adenocarcinomas in situ are found. Their study of the cost effectiveness of various strategies is well covered in Chapter 7.

Mammography can provide a false sense of security if the mammogram is used to exclude the presence of cancer in a breast with suspicious findings on physical examination. That a mammogram may provide a false negative reading in the presence of proved cancer has been documented repeatedly (Martin et al., 1979; Holland et al., 1983; Mann et al., 1983). There are a variety of reasons for this, ranging from radiographic technique and interpretation to characteristics of the cancers that make them occult to mammographic discovery. Histologic characteristics associated with occultness include diffuse invasive pattern, poor desmoplastic reaction to the cancer, and lack of microcalcifications. Dense breasts may contribute to the concealment of cancers. Mammographically occult cancers may attain quite large sizes and still be occult. For example, a mean diameter for invasive lobular cancer occult by mammograms has been reported to be 50 mm (Holland et al., 1983). The conclusions are obvious—a normal mammogram obtained for a breast with abnormal findings on physical examination does not preclude the need for biopsy.

Screening After Treatment—A Special High Risk Population

Follow-up after treatment of cancer is considered highly desirable in patient care. For years, this follow-up was linked mainly to cancer registries that generated the information for many end result studies and accessioned data as they were encountered. In time, guidelines became molded into policy for follow-up. Many techniques and schedules were adopted without proof that they contributed to a decrease in cancer morbidity and mortality rates. The most recent updating of this schema was provided by Eiseman and colleagues (1982). The recommendations represented the consensus of experienced clinicians from multiple disciplines. Unfortunately, many of these recommendations are not supported by models or controlled studies that could define the optimum follow-up strategies that would lead to improvement in outcome. They do not emphasize the essential importance of effective patient and family education and self-surveillance. They also provide no plan of proved value for periodic mammographic examination of the remaining breast.

The patient, the health care institution, and the physician can all benefit from patient education in this select group of people. Instruction may reduce readmission days, provide more informed and cooperative patients, accelerate rehabilitation, allow a more effective use of staff time, and transfer some of the burden of patient iterative teaching to teaching technicians giving planned and evaluable curricula (Rosenberg, 1971). It also may facilitate postdischarge management of treatments and conditions to which the patient and his or her family must adapt and, when well planned and executed, can reduce errors of omission in communication.

Benefits accruing to the physician, in a planned program of patient education, are given a different but relevant perspective by Levoy (1966). He views the services provided by physicians (knowledge, skill, and experience) as intangible and believes that most physicians take for granted that patients appreciate these skills. Levoy suggests that without education the patient sees "fees" rather than "value," "time or lack of it" rather than "results," and "disinterest" rather than "more benefits for me."

Patient education in follow-up is particularly relevant to an important biologic characteristic of cancer. The extreme variance in the growth rates of human cancers ensures that any follow-up system based solely on examinations at arbitrary intervals will result in a significant number of patients whose recidivated cancer is self-discovered by signs and symptoms. For more slowly growing recurrences, earlier diagnosis in follow-up may introduce a lead time bias. For acute cancers, arbitrary intervals may be associated with high interval recurrence rates. Thus, determining optimum intervals for posttreatment follow-up examinations remains an important area for clinical research.

At any clinic, the demands of follow-up can exceed institutional resources and can greatly add to the economic costs of cancer without improving outcome. This first became a subject of study to one of the authors (J.S.S) in 1961, when the Ellis Fischel State Cancer Hospital (EFSCH) faced a limitation of staff and resources available for follow-up. The staff was striving effectively to maintain a 100 per cent follow-up to death on all diagnosed cancer patients. The thousands of patients who came to the EFSCH from all parts of Missouri for follow-up at defined intervals simply exceeded the capacity of the staff and the facilities to accommodate them. The cost-effectiveness of the hospital follow-up practices was challenged. The entire scope of issues for determining the value of the follow-up to the patient was reconsidered. What categories of cancer cases benefited from follow-up and how often must they be evaluated? What types of examinations were of demonstrated value in terms of enhanced survivorship? When does the timely discovery of recurrences, metastases, and new primary tumors result in benefit to the patient? If discovery is beneficial, how can the greatest benefit be achieved for the least cost? What elements of follow-up were traditional and encyclopedic only? When was follow-up no longer necessary? (Spratt, 1971).

The economic problem was immediate at the EFSCH, as the system had to be designed for a hospital with a legislatively fixed appropriation, whose budget could not be increased by charging for more frequent patient-physician contact or special laboratory and radiographic studies. Without a plan for systematic follow-up of demonstrated value to the patients, all fiscal resources could have been expended with little measurable benefit. The problem was to determine the utility value by answering the question, "How many man-years of productive life and how much comfort and function are added to a population as a result of follow-up?" Follow-up screening after treatment can be justified only on the basis of patient benefit, as in the case with primary screening. The situation antedated the diagnosis-related group (DRG) system by over 20 years. However, it was deemed fit to control costs in relation to patient *outcome*. DRGs are based on cost norms often totally unrelated to outcome, raising a question as to their ability to allocate resources according to the public health value of the reimbursement system.

In studying the existing follow-up system, a very simple device was used. The interval rate of diagnosable recidivation or recurrence was determined for different categories of cancer not cured by primary therapy. This was done by dividing the number of persons alive and free of gross neoplasm at the beginning of successive monthly intervals into the number of persons who developed symptomatic recurrences during the suceeding month. These interval rates were then matched to the existing follow-up system. Some gross disparities in the traditional follow-up schedule before 1961 were found. In general, patients had been seen too infrequently during the first two posttreatment years, when the interval recurrence rate is highest, and too frequently after the third year.

In the case of breast cancer follow-up, examinations were recommended at 1, 6, 12, 18, 24, 36, 48, and 60 months. After 5 years the patients were contacted yearly but were seen only every 2 years through the tenth year (Spratt, 1971). Patients were seen at any time in the intervals if they were concerned or developed a sign or symptom. However, this system was still quite arbitrary, as there was no evidence that the end results were any better than those that would have been obtained by trained self-surveillance. This was true for many cancers, including those of the breast.

The duration of follow-up was also an issue since the recidivation of breast cancer is attenuated over decades. Several studies question whether survivorship ever returns to the expected once the diagnosis of breast cancer has been made (Mueller, 1978; Pocock et al., 1982).

Cowan and Kies (1981) have confirmed that basic history taking and physical examination skills lead to the discovery of two thirds of the recidivated breast cancers. They identified 115 sites of metastatic breast cancer in 55 patients, with bone, lung, liver, and skin being the most frequent sites. Of 36 patients with bone metastases, only 15 were identified by bone scan while they were asymptomatic. Among 31 patients with pulmonary metastases, 12 were asymptomatic when these were discovered by chest radiographs. For metastases to liver, skin, lymphatic sites, central nervous system, and eye, initial discovery was purely clinical. Cowan and Kies observed exceedingly low yields for liver function tests and radionuclide examinations of the brain and liver in the discovery of metastatic neoplasm with normal clinical evaluations. Whether or not survivorship was improved in those patients whose metastases were discovered earlier by laboratory and radiographic studies in follow-up, while they were clinically asymptomatic, remains an unanswered question of considerable economic and medical significance.

IMPACT OF SUPERANNUATION ON SCREENING AND FOLLOW-UP STRATEGIES

In an aging population, the fact that life is approaching an endpoint must be considered. The closer a person is to this natural endpoint, the more fragile he or she becomes, and the less time he or she can commit to medical evaluation. The average number of days of life remaining at different ages is given in Figure 19–1. Slower growth rates become very significant in the group past age 60 years. Mortality rates for complicated therapy and the morbidity from complicated diagnostic studies are greater in the elderly. Objectives for evaluating and treating the elderly change. These patients need the simplest care that will ensure their comfort and dignity, at tolerable costs, and without unnecessary and exhausting trips to medical centers when their needs can be attended to with the assistance of a community physician or family member. These facts have a bearing on the selection of optimum strategy in primary and follow-up screening of elderly persons. Eventually, family, family physician, and community medical resources are more helpful to these patients than long trips to a screening or follow-up clinic merely to be examined one more time.

With the passage of time after primary treatment, the decreasing probability of recrudescence of the original neoplasm, and the fact that most persons who have had one cancer are at not much greater risk to develop additional cancers than the general population of the same age, the justification for follow-up examinations rapidly declines. The fact that late recurrences tend to be more slowly growing assists in effective self-detection. As follow-up screening becomes less frequent and less necessary, the patient and family need only prompt access to a physician or hospital should signs or symptoms develop. When the patients know this, the chances of suffering from the psychologic trauma of abandonment are reduced. Names of all follow-up patients can be sent to the Vital Statistics Service in most states annually to be matched against death certificates, so that all deaths will ultimately be documented for the purpose of end-results studies. For special studies, social information on the patient and his or her family and patient education permit 100 per cent follow-up when required (Hoag, 1963).

Performance Status in Follow-up

An important consideration in follow-up is evaluation of a treated individual's performance. Because of the chronicity of breast cancer and the morbidity of much treatment, the ability to quantify the functional capacity of the individual is important. The Karnofsky Performance Status Scale (KPSS) (Karnofsky, 1948; Karnofsky and Burchenal, 1949) is evolving as the standard for this purpose. The KPSS is given in Table 19–7. Mor and coworkers (1984) reported on the statistical evaluation and prognostic utility of the KPSS in the National Hospice Study for both eligibility criteria and outcome (Table 19–8). After training of interviewers, followed by only 4 months' field experience, interrater reliability was found to be 0.97, confirming that the categorization of patients according to KPSS can be highly reliable. As a predictor of survival, an increase in one KPSS level (a factor of 10) yielded an increase of approximately 15 days of survival, ranging as shown in Table 19–9.

Multiple Primary Cancers in Follow-up

One of the traditional arguments for follow-up is the belief that the development of additional neoplasms in a person who has previously had a cancer is more likely than in a population of people with no prior cancer. The frequency of simultaneous and nonsimultaneous multiple primary tumors was studied as a function of age-specific incidence rates, anatomic site of the cancers, and other demographic characteristics of the patient (Spratt and Hoag, 1966). Basically, all persons are subject to cancer with an incidence that increases with aging. The observed age-specific incidence rates can account for the development of one cancer in 51.6 per cent, of two cancers in 17.5 per cent, and of 3 cancers in 5.9 per cent of the population living to age 90

Table 19–7. KARNOFSKY PERFORMANCE STATUS SCALE

General Category	Index	Specific Criteria
Able to carry on normal activity	100	Normal, no complaints, no evidence of disease
	90	Able to carry on normal activity, minor signs or symptoms of disease
	80	Normal activity with effort, some signs or symptoms of disease
Unable to work, able to live at home and care for most personal needs, varying amount of assistance needed	70	Cares for self, unable to carry on normal activity or to do work
	60	Requires occasional assistance from others but able to care for most needs
	50	Requires considerable assistance from others and frequent medical care
Unable to care for self, requires institutional or hospital care or equivalent, disease may be rapidly progressing	40	Disabled, requires special care and assistance
	30	Severely disabled, hospitalization indicated, death not imminent
	20	Very sick, hospitalization necessary, active supportive treatment necessary
	10	Moribund
	00	Dead

From Mor, V., et al.: The Karnofsky performance status scale—an examination of its reliability in a research setting. Cancer, 53:2002, 1984. Reprinted with permission.

years, without the existence of any host-specific predisposition to multiple cancers.

Schoenberg and Myers (1977), using data from the Connecticut tumor register, refined the patient-years at risk approach, seeking significant increases in the incidence of multiple primary cancers. Collectively, the risk of an additional cancer in a person previously treated for cancer was about 1.29 times greater than that in a population with no cancers. This predisposition was highly selective and not greatly different from the Missouri conclusions. More detail on multiple primary cancers in association with breast cancer is provided in Chapter 22.

Multicentricity of Breast Cancers

One of the pitfalls in screening, in primary diagnosis, in efforts directed at limited local therapy, and in follow-up is the breast with multicentric cancers (Egan, 1982). The younger in life a woman develops a breast cancer, the greater the synchronous and lifelong risk of one or more additional breast cancers. As Egan reported, women with multiple breast cancers constitute a unique group. They have an annual mortality of 15 per cent, compared with an annual mortality of 2.5 per cent in women with breast cancer restricted to a single site. Whenever women with multiple breast cancers had scirrhous-type duct cancers, the annual mortality reached 25 per cent (Egan, 1982).

Radiation-Induced Sarcomas of the Chest Wall

A late effect on the irradiated tissue of the chest wall is the induction of sarcomas. Souba and coworkers (1986) have provided a review of 16 such cases, 10 of which developed after irradiation for breast cancer. For 14 patients for whom radiation dose was known, the mean

Table 19–8. ANALYSIS OF VARIANCE RELATING PATIENTS' KARNOFSKY PERFORMANCE STATUS SCORE TO LONGEVITY

Karnofsky Score	Mean Longevity	Standard Deviation	Median Longevity	Number
10	17.6	20.5	9.5	13
20	27.1	29.4	17.8	84
30	45.7	43.4	31.9	239
40	64.1	52.4	46.7	244
50	72.0	52.8	59.7	105
Overall	53.5	48.9	36.6	685

F-ratio: 19.2
$p < 0.001$.
"Eta squared": 0.09
Longevity: days alive.
From Mor, V., et al.: The Karnofsky performance status scale—an examination of its reliability in a research setting. Cancer, 53:2002, 1984. Reprinted with permission.

Table 19–9. KARNOFSKY PERFORMANCE STATUS BY RANGE OF LONGEVITY

Patient Longevity	KPS Level (Per Cent)					
	10	20	30	40	50	Total
1–18 days	71.4	52.2	29.1	13.9	8.7	24.2
19–36 days	21.4	25.0	27.6	26.6	20.9	25.8
37 days or more	7.1	22.6	43.3	59.6	70.4	50.0
Total	1.9	12.3	34.8	35.6	15.4	100.0

Number = 685.
KPS; Karnofsky Performance Status.
From Mor, V., et al.: The Karnofsky performance status scale—an examination of its reliability in a research setting. Cancer, 53:2002, 1984. Reprinted with permission.

dose was 4900 R (range, 4200 to 5500 R). The latent period between irradiation and the appearance of the sarcoma ranged from 5 to 28 years (mean, 13 years). Presenting symptoms were pain in 10 (63 per cent) and swelling or mass in 12 (75 per cent). The mean age at time of developing sarcoma was 47 (18 to 77) years. These sarcomas proved very difficult to treat effectively, and 13 of the 16 patients died of the sarcomas. Only one long-term survivor was reported.

Unfortunately, the population base in which this experience accumulated is not given, precluding the opportunity to calculate actual incidence rates. However, with the widespread use of radiotherapy for breast "conservation" and as an adjuvant in younger women, an ever-increasing population of women is becoming at risk. In fact, Souba and colleagues reviewed the current literature to confirm that these radiation-induced sarcomas are being reported with increasing frequency. Their prevalence, morbidity, and mortality must ultimately be considered when evaluating the efficacy of radiotherapy.

Observations on Testing for Disseminated and Recurrent Cancer

The purposes of this section are to discuss the general epidemiologic and biostatistical principles of screening, follow-up, and diagnosis as they relate to the nature and cost-effectiveness of specific tests. Many of these tests are expensive, and their use has often become routine without the trials necessary to establish either the optimum schedule for their use or that their use is contributing to improved patient care ever having been completed. Breast imaging tests are separately discussed in Chapter 7.

Whenever diagnostic tests of any type are used, certain principles should govern the effort. First, the test should incorporate a high probability that the results would represent the true status. There is always a variable degree of diagnostic uncertainty with any test. Diagnostic tests should be obtained *only* when the results of the tests will lead to altered management of a patient. If the change in management cannot lead to an improved clinical outcome, the test generally has no value. A well-documented review of these issues is found in Sox's work (1986) on the use of probability theory in the evaluation of diagnostic tests.

INFLUENCE OF TESTING ON STAGING

The increasing availability of diagnostic technology capable of demonstrating unsuspected foci of metastatic carcinoma creates uncertainty as to the benefit the information provides to the patient, and at what cost. Often this technology simply diagnoses disseminated disease sooner, creating a staging shift. Supersensitive tests that define foci of cancer before they become symptomatic create staging shifts that can confuse the comparison of data. The staging shifts can lead to the erroneous conclusion that better results are being obtained among various clinical stages. The tests, when positive, shift cases with disseminated cancer out of lower stages, leading to an upstaging. This makes survival *seem* better for patients in the lower stages because the poorest cases have been removed. Because asymptomatic dissemination is discovered earlier, it also improves survivorship for the upper states; a group of patients with longer natural survivorship is now included in the higher stages. All of this improvement, however, is an illusion created by the shifts. The same phenomenon can occur with all types of cancer whenever more sensitive tests bring about staging shifts.

FOLLOW-UP OF THE POSTIRRADIATED BREAST

A growing problem in follow-up is the evaluation of the postirradiated breast. The duration and cost of radiotherapy as an adjuvant, its failure to enhance survivorship, and now the complex issues of follow-up of the postirradiated breast collectively establish that partial mastectomy followed by radiotherapy can in no sense of the term be classified as conservative. As Welch (1986) notes, the response of breast tissue is highly variable. Changes, both early and late, can include redness, edema, and fibrosis. That portion of the underlying lung included in the field will undergo fibrosis, and in some cases there may be symptoms of radiation pneumonitis. The variable degree of fibrosis added to variable surgical defects necessary to remove the primary cancer may produce an extremely distorted breast. Follow-up involves difficult problems in clinical evaluation. Fibrosis creates a more profound distortion in obese women or women with fatty breasts. Tanning of the skin is variable but tends to be greater at boost sites. All these changes progress with time, and results that initially were acceptable from the cosmetic standpoint may become less acceptable with the passage of time. A longitudinal study by Clarke and associates (1983) reports significant fibrosis in 20 per cent, myositis in 5 per cent, and arm edema in 1 per cent. Later chemotherapy can produce significant delayed effects in the field of radiotherapy. This can enhance the risk of delayed desquamation, myositis, rib fractures, edema, pericarditis, and pneumonitis. Breast retraction may also increase. Masses detected in the postirradiated breast pose a particularly vexing problem in follow-up. The evaluating clinician needs the advantage of an accurate record of all prior treatment. When there is incomplete excision, Calle and associates (1979) have reported local recurrence of 59 per cent despite irradiation. Reoperation was required for persistent cancer within a mean of 4½ months, and for recurrent cancer within a mean of 39 months. The clinical manifestations of benign and malignant disease in the postirradiated breast are often indistinguishable. Reoperation in these heavily irradiated breasts is fraught with the risks of delayed wound healing, infection, and necrosis.

OSSEOUS METASTASES

Baker (1984) concluded that a history and physical examination, a chest radiograph, and a serum alkaline phosphatase determination were adequate preoperative assessments for Stages I and II breast cancers. When alkaline phosphatase levels are within normal limits, neither a skeletal nor a hepatic scan is indicated. However, with Stage III disease, a higher prevalence of metastases is discoverable, even in the absence of clinical evidence of systemic metastases.

Pauwels and coworkers (1982) conducted a similar study and concluded that bone scans, done preoperatively or in follow-up, did not justify the cost. Bone pain and an elevated alkaline phosphatase level were associated with positive scans. When bone metastases did occur, they generally did so in the first 2 years post mastectomy, precluding the need for prolongation of effort to find skeletal metastases past the second year.

In the early years of the National Surgical Adjuvant Breast Project (NSABP), protocols required radionuclide bone scans every 6 months for the first 3 years postoperatively and yearly thereafter (Wickerham et al., 1984). In the evaluation of 7984 bone scans performed to document first treatment failure in 2697 persons with Stage II cancers (positive lymph nodes), 779 patients had failed treatment, with 163 (20.9 per cent) limited to bone. Only 52 (0.6 per cent) of the total number of screening scans detected metastases in asymptomatic patients. As a result of this study, NSABP protocols changed to require follow-up bone scans only as indicated by symptoms. More frequent use in routine clinical practice could not be defended as a cost-effective practice.

Bone scans have also been used to assay response to chemotherapy, but they have been shown to be very crude monitors of response (Bitran et al., 1980). The association between bone pain and positive bone scans is not as strong as once thought. Front and colleagues (1979) evaluated the association of bone pain and the findings of technetium-99m methylene diphosphonate bone scintigraphy. Of 66 patients with scans positive for metastases, 21 (32 per cent) did not complain of bone pain. Among 155 skeletal sites of metastatic disease suggested by scans, only 50 sites were associated with pain. There was no correlation between the involvement of weight-bearing bones and pain.

Other studies have similarly questioned the frequency and rationale for high-cost bone scans. Forrest (1979) concluded that the predictive value of extensive testing was not an improvement over the predictive implications of positive axillary lymph nodes. Khandekar

(1979) pointed out that if some recommendations for performing bone scans were followed (preoperatively, at 6 month intervals for 3 years postoperatively and annually for 5 years thereafter) on 90,000 new breast cancer cases annually, the annual cost would be from $150 to $200 million. In the interest of cost containment, he used a decision matrix to consider when these scans were justified. He concluded that use should be restricted to Stages I and II breast cancers with bone symptoms, Stage II patients, patients receiving adjuvant chemoimmunotherapy, and patients on research protocols. Even this may be too liberal if prognosis does not prove to be affected favorably by the results of the scans.

Bone scans, radiologic skeletal surveys, pain charts, bone marrow aspirates, determinations of serum calcium and serum alkaline phosphatase levels, and urine hydroxyproline-creatinine ratios have also been used for the assessment of response to systemic treatment. Bitran and coworkers (1980) concluded that the scans were a "relatively crude technique" for monitoring response to chemotherapy. Responding patients with osteolytic disease showed sclerosis after 6 to 8 months. Patients with mixed lytic and sclerotic or sclerotic metastases showed no change or further sclerosis. Nonresponders showed progressive lysis. Bone scans showed improvements in 7 of 21 responders and deterioration in 8 of 23 nonresponders who showed no changes on skeletal radiography. They found neither bone aspirations nor biochemical tests to be of any use in assaying response to treatment. Pain assessment was useful in monitoring response. It is also very simple and inexpensive.

Bitran and colleagues concluded that radiographic evidence of response came late in the treatment course or not at all. Some responders actually showed an increase in bone destruction. The response of sclerotic metastases was not assessable by the techniques used. Skeletal radiography may show varying patterns in the same patient. Pain relief was the most consistent index of response. Bone scans were of some help in identifying nonresponders at an earlier time. Serum calcium levels were variable, but recurrent hypercalcemia was an early sign of relapse. The urinary ratios were not helpful.

Clearly, there are uncertainties in monitoring response, with many implications for both clinical practice and research protocol design. Cost-benefit considerations should weigh heavily in the choices.

Bone Marrow Biopsies

Bone marrow biopsies using the Jamshidi needle have also been evaluated for staging and following breast cancers. Cancer was found in the marrow of 21 of 64 patients (32.4 per cent) examined in follow-up after mastectomy. Five of 42 women (12 per cent) had positive marrows before mastectomy, but all five had radiographic changes. Only three women, without any radiographic or isotopic signs of metastasis, had positive biopsies.

Results of routine bone marrow biopsies of the posterior iliac crest in 532 women with unilateral breast cancer, correlated with scan results, were reported by Ridell and Landys in 1979. When a radiologic examination of the skeleton was negative, positive biopsies were obtained with a prevalence of 1.6 per cent. Whenever there was any radiologic evidence of skeletal metastases, the prevalence of positive biopsies rose to 28 per cent.

Monoclonal antibodies specific for the cytoskeleton (C_{26}, T_{16}, AE-1) of epithelial cells are just beginning to be evaluated for improving the accuracy of metastatic breast cancer cell identification in the bone marrow. Preliminary results confirm the presence of cancer cells in the marrow with frequencies equivalent to known rates of recidivation. Still to be determined is the correlation of these findings with actual recidivation in the same cases and after what lead time. This test holds the potential for identifying patients with dissemination who lack statistically strong predictors of recidivation that might be more routinely and cheaply measured. Of equal importance may well be the ultimate ability to identify patients with only locoregional disease and no dissemination who might then not require any systemic adjuvant therapy for nonexistent micrometastases.

Twenty-seven per cent of the marrows with no metastases in axillary lymph nodes were positive and marrow positivity did not correlate significantly with tumor size. The study also confirmed that attempts to identify tumor cells in the marrow by cytological examination were never as frequent as the prevalence identified by monoclonal antibodies (Osborne, 1987).

HEPATIC METASTASES

Hepatic metastases from breast cancer are a frequent problem and place the patient in a poor prognostic category. Extensive testing for these metastases has to be predicated on the ability to select treatment strategies of proven benefit to the patient. Evaluating benefit must allow for the lead time gained by sensitive testing methods before the presence of metastatic disease becomes detectable by simpler methods.

Tempero and coworkers (1982) evaluated the comparative sensitivity of different testing methods. They found biochemical testing to be the most sensitive and least expensive approach and concluded that radioisotopic liver scans should be reserved for patients with elevated biochemical values. The biochemical tests used were alkaline phosphatase, aspartate aminotransferase, lactic dehydrogenase, and total bilirubin levels. Any test results greater than 10 per cent above normal were considered abnormal. The liver scans were done with technetium-99m sulfur colloid. False positive rates for liver scans (focal defects in the absence of metastatic liver disease) were 17 per cent; false negative rates (no focal defects in the presence of metastatic liver disease) were 35 per cent. This margin of error for a high cost test, such as the liver scan, obviously precludes its routine use in the absence of elevated biochemical values and a treatment plan or protocol directed at enhancing the survivorship of persons with hepatic metastases.

DeRivas and colleagues (1980) reported correlation between the results of serum alkaline phosphatase determinations, hepatic ultrasonography, heptic scintigraphy, and the hepatic findings at autopsy for 282 patients presenting with breast cancer in a single clinic. At the time of primary treatment, only 1.5 per cent of the patients had evidence of metastases on scintiscan, and only 1.2 had such evidence on hepatic ultrasonography. Alkaline phosphatase level was elevated in only 6.4 per cent at primary treatment. With the diagnosis of first metastasis, the serum alkaline phosphatase level was elevated in 35.3 per cent of the patients. Among a majority of the 51 patients whose hepatic metastases were confirmed at autopsy, there had been a progressive rise in alkaline phosphatase level over the preceding year. However, within 3 months preceding death, the liver scintiscans and ultrasonograms were positive in less than 30 per cent of the examinations. These are very convincing data on the lead time that rising serum alkaline phosphatase level exhibits with respect to these high cost scans. Clearly, there should be a demonstrated enhancement in patient outcome to justify high cost scans in the presence of normal or nonrising serum alkaline phosphatase levels.

Colizza and associates (1985) reported a prospective study on hepatic staging in operable breast cancer on a series of 100 consecutive patients. Of all the tests evaluated, only a carcinoembryonie antigen (CEA) level of >20 ng/ml had prognostic implications, which were adverse. Hepatic echography was considered of limited value. Hepatic enzyme levels, determined preoperatively, proved of little value.

Forrest and coworkers (1979) investigated metastatic disease in over 200 women who had negative chest x-rays and skeletal radiographs before primary treatment, using skeletal and hepatic scintigraphy, urinary hydroxyproline excretion on a gelatin-free diet, alkaline phosphatase determinations, and other tests. Although these tests were positive in 30 per cent of the patients, the information added little to that already predicted by the known presence of metastases in the axillary lymph nodes. The conclusion drawn was that exhaustive laboratory studies searching for occult metastases in asymptomatic patients were not very valuable.

PULMONARY METASTASES

Thoracic radiographs in search of asymptomatic pulmonary metastases are usually routine but seldom revealing. The most frequent cause of a single tumor shadow on a chest film, particularly in a woman who smokes, is a new primary lung cancer. No reduction of cancer mortality rate from lung cancer has been obtained by screening with thoracic radiographs.

CEREBRAL METASTASES

Although methods exist for the discovery of cerebral metastases, no defensible advocacy for the use of these tests on persons free of central nervous system symptoms can be found in the literature. The use of these tests in patients with breast cancer is, therefore, not a part of routine follow-up evaluation for asymptomatic metastatic disease in breast cancer patients.

The authors conclude that the appearance of neurologic symptoms in a patient who has or had breast cancer should be evaluated according to the symptom(s) and subsequent plans for management. Chapters on the surgical management of ocular, orbital, central nervous system, and spinal metastases, and on the efficacy or inefficacy of systemic management, are found in this book.

TUMOR MARKERS

A variety of circulating tumor markers for breast cancer have been reported. These include CEA, human chorionic gonadotropin, nonspecific cross-reacting antigen, and some less frequent ones. Although CEA, apparently the strongest of these markers, was reported as being present in 5 to 80 per cent of breast tumor cell populations, no apparent association between cytologic type or degree of differentiation was made. Of the markers studied, CEA was the only one whose serum level correlated with the pretreatment size of the primary cancer. However, the values were still too low to be of any value for screening. Low or decreased CEA level was more often seen in patients who had undergone curative treatment. The tumor and plasma concentrations of CEA were not strongly correlated. Thus, even when CEA is present in breast cancer, it is not always released in measurable amounts. Although CEA level will rise postoperatively in some patients with metastatic disease progression, convincing data that CEA is useful in postoperative follow-up are elusive. The risk exists that CEA, when released from breast cancer metastases, may give a lead time of only several months before the metastases become symptomatic. Unless this lead time can be put to therapeutic benefit, it would be of little value. The markers would have to show a predictive value for dissemination that exceeds that obtained in the initial categorization of the primary cancer.

Human chorionic gonadotropin (HCG) did not exhibit elevated serum levels. Liver enzymes were of value only in the follow-up search for metastases (Wahren et al., 1978). Later studies were consistent in reporting these general trends (Duffy et al., 1983; Nap et al., 1984).

The identification and evaluation of a variety of markers continues to be an active area of research. None, in the authors' opinion, has passed the confirmation of patient benefit necessary for inclusion in routine screening or follow-up practice. The generalization can be made that increasing levels of all serum markers are more diagnostic in predicting progression of residual disease than are absolute single values. The high cost and limited value of many of these markers supports the position that their use should still be restricted largely to research protocols that will ultimately document the contribution of laboratory test values to patient outcome.

Relevance of Follow-up Strategy to Survival

Tomin and Donegan (1987) conducted a review of the impact on the ultimate prognosis of different diagnostic procedures used in follow-up for the detection of recurrent breast cancer. Their study population consisted of 1,230 patients treated for the cure of invasive breast cancer. The costly diagnostic interventions considered included x-rays, scans, blood tests, and various clinical procedures, all used according to a predetermined follow-up schedule of asymptomatic people. This effort, in effect, constituted the screening of a group at high risk to develop recurrent breast cancer and an investigation of whether the discovery of asymptomatic recurrences led to an improved prognosis. The researchers recognized that the problems of lead time and length bias affected their end result observations.

The categories of recurrences used were local (mastectomy scar, skin flaps, or tissues underlying skin flaps), regional (supraclavicular, internal mammary, or axillary lymph nodes), pulmonary (parenchymal or pleural with or without effusions), skeletal, visceral (brain, liver, intestines, bladder, or ovaries), and multiple. Physician-discovered recurrences were considered asymptomatic; patient-discovered recurrences were considered symptomatic interval recurrences (i.e., recurrences that become symptomatic in the intervals between scheduled examinations). Among 248 patients who developed recurrences during the study, 64.1 per cent were interval surfacing and only 35.9 per cent were discovered in a still asymptomatic state by physicians.

Symptoms that occurred were bone pain, skin nodules, enlarging lymph nodes, cough, malaise, fatigue, and weakness. Shortness of breath, nausea, jaundice, and weight loss were less frequent. Symptoms varied with site and multiplicity of the cancer.

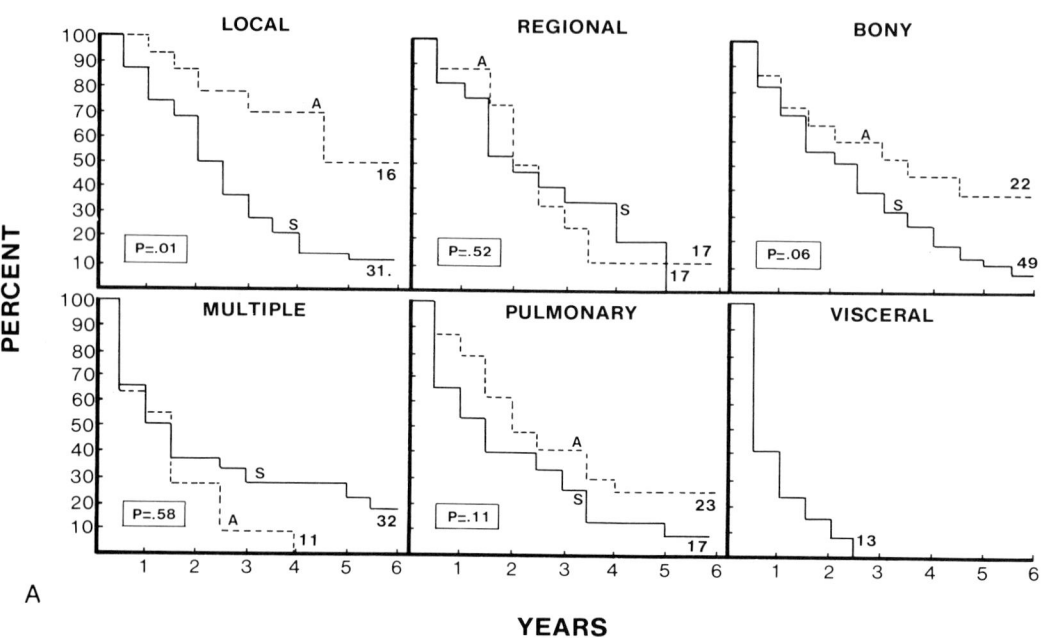
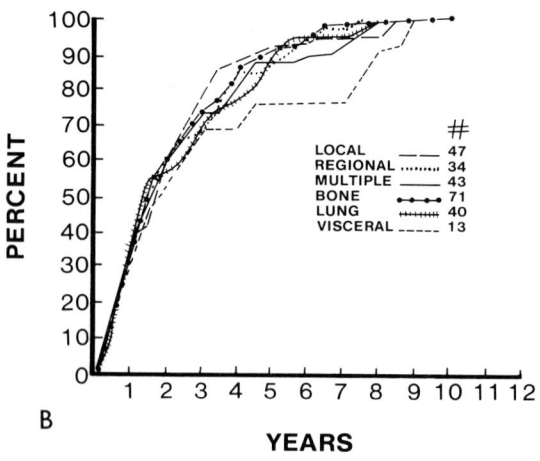

Figure 19–5. *A*, Only patients with local recurrence derive significant survival benefit from detection of recurrence when it is asymptomatic. *B*, Rate of recurrence is similar for all sites. (From Tomin, R., and Donegan, W. L.: Screening for recurrent breast cancer—Its effectiveness and prognostic value. J. Clin. Oncol., 5:62, 1987. Reproduced with permission.)

From the time of diagnosis of recurrence, the median survival was 22 months. Two thirds of patients survived 12 months. The 5 year survival rate was 15.6 per cent; the 7 year survival rate was 4.6 per cent. Survival of patients with asymptomatic recurrences was significantly longer than was the survival of women with interval recurrences ($p = 0.0017$), with the respective median survival times being 29 and 17 months. The respective 5 year survival rates were 25 per cent and 11 per cent. Survival also varied according to the site of recurrence (Fig. 19–5). Disease-free intervals between treatment and recurrence were not significantly related to prognosis. Estrogen receptor positive cancers had a better prognosis, regardless of category (Fig. 19–6).

Of great relevance to the pattern of follow-up was the comparison of the survivorship of those patients with recurrences who complied with a prespecified, physician-determined schedule with specified laboratory, x-ray, and scanning studies with patients whose tests were irregular or who were noncompliant. The difference in survivorship was not significant (Fig. 19–7). The percentage of patients with interval recurrent cancers was no different in the two groups.

Tomin and Donegan were unable to show a survival value for those patients who followed a preset schedule of examinations over those who did not. The overvigorous use of many costly laboratory, radiographic, and nuclear studies seemed only to add a lead time bias to survival data. As is true of all screening efforts performed at prefixed intervals, the more indolent problems are present longer, thus increasing the probability of discovery and introducing a length bias to the sample. The more rapidly progressing neoplasms become manifest as recurrences between scheduled examinations. Supersensitive tests may also be biasing outcome data by producing staging shifts.

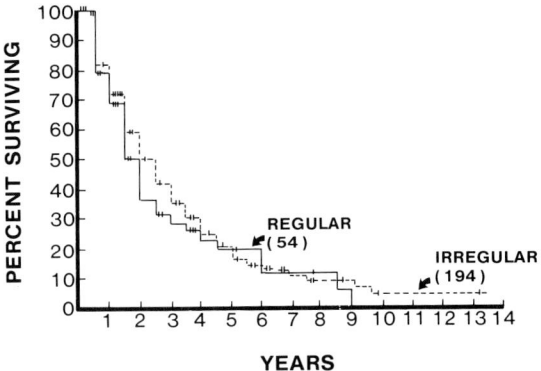

Figure 19–7. Survival after recurrence is similar whether or not patients adhere to a predetermined schedule of followup examinations after their primary treatment. (From Tomin, R., and Donegan, W. L.: Screening for recurrent breast cancer—Its effectiveness and prognostic value. J. Clin. Oncol., 5:62, 1987. Reproduced with permission.)

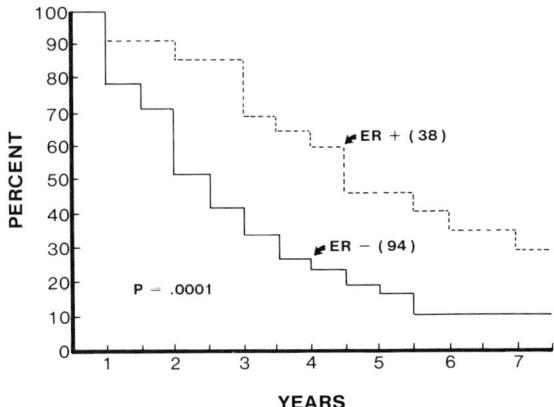

Figure 19–6. The survival after recurrence of patients with ER-positive tumors is significantly better than that of patients with ER-negative tumors. (From Tomin, R., and Donegan, W. L.: Screening for recurrent breast cancer—Its effectiveness and prognostic value. J. Clin. Oncol., 5:62, 1987. Reproduced with permission.)

Treatment of Recurrent Cancer

The EFSCH studies also addressed the value of follow-up in detecting treatable recrudescent neoplasms (Spratt, 1971). The question was always to determine in which patients the timely discovery of recrudescent cancer was succeeded by efficacious therapy and when the benefits of retreatment were enhanced by earlier diagnosis of recidivation. The follow-up schedule was designed to coincide with intervals in which the chance of recurrence was greatest.

At the time the EFSCH studies were done, the sole forms of effective treatment, for both primary and recidivated cancer, were surgery, radiotherapy, and endocrine therapy. When chemotherapy became an adjuvant for solid tumors, a very accurate assessment of prognosis at the time of primary treatment became of great importance. The subsets of patients at high risk for recidivation became the candidates for adjuvant treatment. For these patients, the follow-up program must be modified to monitor the treatment results and toxic effects from the chemotherapy. The opportunity for effective retreatment might be compromised in some instances by a delay in discovery. However, there are no controlled data to confirm this impression. Diagnosis of metastatic cancer while the total mass of neoplasm is at the threshold of diagnostic sensitivity may be of importance in improving the efficacy of some forms of chemotherapy. The objective of clinical management of recidivated cancer should be to produce protracted periods of symptom-free survival by the methods most tolerable to the host from the standpoints of morbidity, time, and cost, even in the absence of permanent cure.

Table 19–10. NUMBER AND PERCENTAGE OF CASES WITH METASTASES FROM CARCINOMA OF THE BREAST CONFIRMED AT AUTOPSY (647 CASES)

Site	Number	Per Cent
Stomach	62	10
Pancreas	70	12
Liver	397	61
Lungs	401	66
Bones	450	70
Uterus	86	13
Peritoneum	156	20
Kidney	86	13
Central nervous system	161	25
Lymph nodes: Neck	233	36
Thorax	359	56
Abdomen	250	38.5
Pelvis	107	16.6
Pituitary or parathyroid, or both	130	20
Adrenals	176	38
Thyroid	132	20
Ovaries	61	15

Adapted from Viadana, E., et al.: An autopsy study of some routes of dissemination of cancer of the breast. Br. J. Cancer, 27:336, 1973.

Autopsy as the End-Point to Follow-up

The autopsy as a final step of both treatment and follow-up remains one of our most valuable but increasingly underused learning tools. Viadana and colleagues (1973) reported on the autopsy of 647 women with primary carcinoma of the breast. The number of times a particular anatomic site contained metastatic cancer with percentages is given in Table 19–10. The authors attempted to categorize metastases as to whether the patterns observed were related to anatomic proximity or were more compatible with hematogenous spread. They were unable to confirm any time sequence for the appearance of metastases in different organs. The data are of great value in appreciating the prevalence of anatomic spread in those women who die with breast cancer and in evaluating relevant follow-up tests.

Autopsy findings on women who died of breast cancer continued to show the diffuseness of terminal breast cancer. Hagemeister and coworker (1980) report the findings on 166 patients who died of breast cancer and came to autopsy between 1973 and 1977. The autopsies consistently disclosed more tumor involvement than had been suspected on the basis of clinical evaluation. The unsuspected areas included endocrine organs (40 per cent), lungs (28 per cent), cardiovascular system (21 per cent), and genitourinary system (21 per cent). Other organ systems were also involved extensively but antemortem clinical assessment had diagnosed cancer in these sites more frequently—bones (10 per cent) and central nervous system (14 per cent). The actual causes of death included pulmonary insufficiency (26 per cent), infection (24 per cent), cardiac disease (15 per cent), hepatic insufficiency (14 per cent), hemorrhage (9 per cent), central nervous system dysfunction (9 per cent), and hypercalcemia (3 per cent). Forty-two per cent of all deaths were related directly to uncontrolled metastatic cancer. Although infection was the second leading cause of death, only 27 per cent of the deaths were associated with neutropenia. Similarly, only 9 per cent of the patients who died of hemorrhage had associated thrombocytopenia. The authors concluded that deaths related to chemotherapy were infrequent and that deaths from terminal infections had not increased with the availability of chemotherapy.

The autopsy is essential to assess the presumed lethality of any disease. There is a tendency in vital statistics to attribute the cause of death to "cancer" in anyone who had been diagnosed as having had cancer. As autopsies often reveal a totally unsuspected cause of death, the results can be used to assess the diagnostic accuracy of clinical, laboratory, and radiographic diagnostic procedures used in follow-up (Goldman et al., 1983).

Conclusion

This brief assessment of contemporary testing methods is provided because of their frequent use and high cost and the need to use them in congruence with an effective treatment strategy or research protocol. A natural question for both routine clinical use and research protocol design is, *What tests do we do?* No all-inclusive answer is now available. Philosophic, scientific, and economic generalizations can be made about all existing tests and future tests yet to be developed. A test should have a dependable level of accuracy and should be of tolerable cost and of negligible risk to the patient. The information gained by the test should have a logical link to a plan of action, based on the test results, which will lead to a more beneficial outcome for the patient. These questions need to be asked of all arbitrarily designed "testing schedules." Furthermore, the tests and test schedules used for asymptomatic persons should be known to provide a better patient outcome than simple patient self-surveillance and the evaluation of symptoms by appropriate tests when indicated.

Much work has been done to define the value of both screening and follow up examinations, but much more needs to be done. Furthermore, the need exists at *each* physician's office, clinic, and hospital. The quality control measures and cost-benefit considerations discussed have to be verified for each medical facility and population served. Information from the literature and in this review can only serve as guidelines for planning and evaluating screening as a cost-effective, integrated part of a cancer management system. Screening is not an activity done in isolation

Appendix Table. FOLLOW-UP SCHEDULES AFTER TREATMENT OF BREAST CANCER*

I. Schedule currently used by one of the authors (WLD) for invasive carcinoma.

Year	History and Physical	CBC	Liver Function	Chest X-ray	Mammogram	Bone Scan
1	q 3 mos	q 6 mos	q 6 mos	q 6 mos	q 12 mos†	‡
2	q 3 mos	q 6 mos	q 6 mos	q 6 mos	q 12 mos†	
3	q 6 mos	q 12 mos	q 6 mos	q 12 mos	q 12 mos†	
4	q 6 mos	q 12 mos	q 6 mos	q 12 mos	q 12 mos†	
5	q 6 mos	q 12 mos	q 6 mos	q 12 mos	q 12 mos†	
6+	q 12 mos	q 12 mos	q 6 mos	q 12 mos	q 12 mos†	

II. Schedule recommended by Humphrey and Eiseman (1982).

Year	History and Physical	HCT	Liver Function	Chest X-ray	Mammogram	Bone Scan	Calcium, Phosphorus, Alkaline Phosphatase
1	q 3 mos	q 6 mos	q 6 mos	q 12 mos	?	§	q 6 mos
2	q 3 mos	q 6 mos	q 6 mos	q 12 mos			q 6 mos
3	q 6 mos	q 6 mos	q 12 mos	q 12 mos			q 12 mos
4	q 6 mos	q 6 mos	q 12 mos	q 12 mos			q 12 mos
5	q 6 mos	q 6 mos	q 12 mos	q 12 mos			q 12 mos
6+	q 6 mos	q 6 mos	q 12 mos	q 12 mos			q 12 mos

III. Suggested schedule of follow-up for patients treated for carcinoma in situ.‖

Year	History and Physical	CBC	Liver Function	Chest X-ray	Mammogram	Bone Scan
1	q 6 mos				q 12 mos	
2–5	q 6 mos				q 12 mos	
6+	q 12 mos				q 12 mos	

*Follow-up schedules for patients receiving adjuvant chemotherapy and on research protocols vary according to need.
†Every 6 months the first year of breast-conserving therapy used.
‡Obtained as indicated for symptoms.
§Pre- or postoperatively.
‖The same schedule is used for lobular carcinoma in situ when managed with observation alone with the exception that physical examinations continue indefinitely every 6 months.

from a total system. Arbitrary screening plans not linked with an entire evaluable system of cancer patient management can even become a costly health hazard. These observations support the need for intense research into the development of lifetime screening strategies for cancers of different sites.

This chapter addresses mainly the theory, strategy, and value of screening and follow-up. Individual screening techniques and diagnostic methodologies are discussed. Breast imaging is considered in more detail in Chapter 7. The practitioner of each form of intervention is obligated to provide arguments for the cost-effective use of the method chosen and for its value in the reduction of the morbidity and mortality of breast cancer. The presumption is made that a strategy for histologic verification of diagnosis will be followed for abnormalities discovered in screening the asymptomatic patient before treatment to avoid unnecessary treatment of false positive tests.

REFERENCES

Ahlvin, R. C.: Biochemical screening—a critique. N. Engl. J. Med., 283:1084, 1970.

Aron, J. L., and Prorok, P. C.: An analysis of the mortality effect in a breast cancer screening study. Int. J. Epidemiol., 15:36, 1986.

Bailar, J. C., III: Mammography: A contrary view. Ann. Intern. Med., 84:77, 1976.

Bailar, J., III, and Smith, E. M.: Progress against cancer? N. Engl. J. Med., 314:1226, 1986.

Baker, R. R.: Preoperative assessment of the patient with breast cancer. Surg. Clin. North Am., 64:1039, 1984.

Beahrs, P. C.: Report of the Working Group to Review the NIC/ACS Breast Cancer Demonstration Projects. September 6, 1977 (NCI Contract RFP-N01-CNN-75379).

Berg, J. W.: Clinical implications of risk factors for breast cancer. Cancer, 53:589, 1984.

Bitran, J. D., Bekerman, C., and Desser, R. K.: The predictive value of serial bone scans in assessing response to chemotherapy in advanced breast cancer. Cancer, 45:1562, 1980.

Bloom, H. J. G.: Influence of delay on the natural history and prognosis of breast cancer. Br. J. Cancer, 19:228, 1965.

Brightmore, T. G. J., Greening, W. P., and Hamlin, I.: An analysis of clinical and histopathological features in 101 cases of breast cancer in women under 35 years of age. Br. J. Cancer, 24:644–669, 1970.

Bross, I. D., and Blumenson, L. E.: Screening random asymptomatic women under 50 by annual mammographies: Does it make sense? J. Surg. Oncol., 8:437, 1976.

Cadman, D., Chambers L., Feldman W., et al.: Assessing the effectiveness of community screening programs. J.A.M.A., 251:1580, 1984.

Calle, R., Pilleran, J. P., Schlienger, P., et al.: Conservative management of the operable breast: Ten years' experience at the Foundation Curie. Cancer, 42:2045, 1978.

Charpin, C., Lissitzky, J. C., Kopp, F., et al.: Immunocytochemical antigens in detection in human breast carcinomas: A light and electron microscopy study using avidin biotin peroxidase and preembedding techniques. Cancer Detect. Prevent., 8:77, 1985.

Chaudary, M. A., Maisey, M. N., Shaw, P. J., et al.: Sequential bone scans and chest radiographs in the postoperative management of early breast cancer. Br. J. Surg., 70:517, 1983.

Chaudary, M. A., Millis, R. R., Davies, G. C., and Hayward, J. L.: Nipple discharge—the diagnostic value of testing for occult blood. Ann. Surg., 196:651, 1982.

Clarke, D., Martinez, A., and Cox, R. S.: Analysis of cosmetic results and complications in patients with Stage I and II breast cancer treated by irradiation. Int. J. Radiat. Oncol. Biol. Phys., 9:1807, 1983

Cocconi, G., DiBlasio, B., Alberti, G., et al.: Problems in evaluating response of primary breast cancer to systemic therapy. Breast Cancer Res. Treat., 4:309, 1984.

Colizza, S., Lupatelli, R., DeFazio, S., et al.: Hepatic staging in operable breast cancer: A reappraisal from a prospective study. J. Surg. Oncol., 30:113, 1985.

Cowan, J. D., and Kies, M. S.: Detection of recurrent breast cancer. South Med. J., 74:910, 1981.

Cruciani, G., Fiorentini, G. M., Resti, G., et al.: Clinical relevance of bone marrow biopsy in staging and follow up of breast cancer. Tumor, 69:143, 1983.

Dargent, M.: Carcinoma of the breast in castrated women. Br. Med. J., 2:54, 1949.

DeGroote, R., Rush, B. F., and Milazzo, J.: Interval breast cancer: A more aggressive subset of breast neoplasias. Surgery, 94:543, 1983.

Dennis, C. R., Gardner, B., and Lim, B.: Analysis of survival and recurrence vs. patient and doctor delay in treatment of breast cancer. Cancer 35:714, 1975.

DeRivas, L., Coombes, R. C., McReady, V. R., et al.: Tests for liver metastases in breast cancer: Evaluation of liver scan and liver ultrasound. Clin. Oncol., 6:225, 1980.

Devitt, J. E.: Lumpy breasts: Normal. Can. J. Surg., 26:6, 1983.

Dohrmann, P. J., Hughes, E. S. R., McDermott, F., et al., Symptom duration, tumor standing and survival in patients with carcinoma of the breast. Surg. Gynecol. Obstet., 154:707, 1982.

Donegan, W. L., Hartz, A. J., and Rimm, A. A.: The association of body weight with recurrent cancer of the breast. Cancer, 41:1590, 1978.

Dubin, H., Pasternack, B. S., and Strax, P.: Epidemiology of breast cancer in a screened population. Cancer Detect. Prevent., 7:87, 1984.

Duffy, M. J., O'Connell, M., O'Sullivan, F., et al.: CEA-like material in cytosols from human breast carcinomas. Cancer, 51:121, 1983.

Eddy, D.: Guidelines for the cancer-related checkup, recommendations and rationale. Cancer, 30:194, 1980.

Eddy, D.: Screening for Cancer: Theory, Analysis and Design. Stanford, Calif., Stanford University Press, 1978.

Egan, R. L.: Multicentric breast carcinomas: Clinical-radiographic-pathologic whole organ studies and 10-year survival. Cancer, 49:1123, 1982.

Eggers, C., DeCholnoky, T., and Jessup, D. S. D.: Cancer of the breast. Ann. Surg., 113:321, 1941.

Eiseman, B., Robinson, W. A., and Steele, G.: Follow-up of the Cancer Patient. New York, Thieme-Stratton, 1982.

Evens, R. G.: Screening mammography (Letter to the editor). N. Engl. J. Med., 314:1451, 1986.

Feig, S. A., and Schwartz, G. F.: Pathologic discriminants of breast cancer detected on screening by mammography and physical examination. Cancer Detect. Prevent., 4:579, 1981.

Feinstein, A. R., Sosin, D. M., and Wells, C. K.: The Will Rogers Phenomenon—stage migration and new diagnostic techniques as a source of misleading statistics for survival in cancer. N. Engl. J. Med., 312:1604, 1985.

Fitzpatrick, P. J.: Cost effectiveness in cancer. Can. Med. Assoc. J., 111:652, 1974.

Forrest, A. P., Cant, E. L. M., Roberts, M. M., Stewart, H. J., Sommerling, M. D., Donaldson, A. A., Smith, A. F., and Shivas, A. A.: Is the investigation of patients with breast cancer for occult metastatic disease worthwhile? Br. J. Surg., 66:749, 1979.

Foster, R. S., Lang, S. P., Costanza, M. C., et al.: Breast self-examination practices and breast cancer stages. N. Engl. J. Med., 299:265, 1978.

Foster, R. S., and Costanza, M. C.: Breast self-examination practices and breast cancer survival. Cancer, 53:167, 1984.

Front, D., Schneck, S. O., Frankel, A., et al.: Bone metastases and bone pain in breast cancer—are they closely associated? J.A.M.A., 242:1747, 1979.

Habbema, J. D. F., Oortmarssen, G. J., VanPatten, D. J., et al.: Age-specific reduction in breast cancer mortality by screening: An analysis of the results of the Health Insurance Plan of Greater New York Study. J.N.C.I., 77:317, 1986.

Hagemeister, F. B., Jr., Buzdar, A. U., Luna, M. A., et al.: Causes of death in breast cancer: A clinical pathologic study. Cancer, 46:162, 1980.

Hall, D. C., Adams, C. K., Stein, G. H., et al.: Improved detection of human breast lesions following experimental training. Cancer, 46:408, 1980.

Heuser, L., Spratt, J. S., and Polk, H. C., Jr.: Growth rates of primary breast cancer. Cancer, 43:1888, 1979a.

Heuser, L., Spratt, J. S., Polk, H. C., Jr., et al.: Relation between mammary cancer growth kinetics and the intervals between screenings. Cancer, 43:857, 1979b.

Hoag, M. G.: The follow-up of patients at the Ellis Fischel State Cancer Hospital, conducted by the Social Service Department. Mo. Med., 60:1128, 1963.

Holland, R. T., Hendricks, J. H., and Mravunac, M.: Mammographically occult breast cancer. A pathologic and radiologic study. Cancer, 52:1810, 1983.

Horton, J.: Follow-up of breast cancer patients. Cancer, 53:790, 1984.

Hultborn, K. A., and Tornberg, B.: Mammary carcinoma—the biologic character of mammary cancer studied in 517 cases by a new form of malignancy grading. Acta Radiol. [Suppl.], 196:1, 1960.

Karnofsky, D. A., Abelmann, W. H., Craver, L. F., et al.: The use of nitrogen mustards in the palliative treatment of cancer. Cancer, 1:634, 1948.

Karnofsky, D. A., and Burchenal, J. H.: The clinical evaluation of chemotherapeutic agents in cancer. *In* MacLeod, C. M. (Ed.): Evaluation of Chemotherapeutic Agents. New York, Columbia University Press, 1949, p. 191.

Khandekar, J. D.: Role of routine bone scans in operable breast cancer: An opposing viewpoint. Cancer Treat. Rep., 63:1241, 1979.

Levoy R. P.: The $100,000 Practice and How to Build It. Englewood Cliffs, N.J., Prentice-Hall, 1966, p. 1.

MacDonald, I.: Mammary carcinoma—a review of 2636 cases. Surg. Gynecol. Obstet., 74:75, 1942.

Madeddu, G., Casu, A. R., Eriu, R., et al.: Diagnostic and prognostic value of TPA in breast cancer. Cancer Detect. Prevent., 8:47, 1985.

Mann, B. D., Giuliano, A. E., Bassett, L. W., et al.: Delayed diagnosis of breast cancer as a result of normal mammograms. Arch. Surg., 118:23, 1983.

Martin, J. E., Moskowitz, M., and Milbrath, J. R.: Breast cancer missed by mammography. A.J.T.R., 132:737, 1979.

McDivitt, R. W., and Stewart, F. W.: Breast carcinoma in children. J.A.M.A., 195:388, 1966.

MacDonald, I.: Biological predeterminism in human cancer. Surg. Gynecol. Obstet., 92:443, 1951.

Miller, A. B.: Evaluation of screening for cancer of the cervix and breast—implications for cancer control. Prog. Clin. Biol. Res., 83:41, 1982.

Monaco, R., Salfen, L., and Spratt, J. S.: The patient as an education participant in health care. Mo. Med., 69:932, 1972.

Mor, V., Laliberte, L., Morris, J. N., et al.: The Karnofsky performance status scale—an examination of its reliability in a research setting. Cancer, 53:2002, 1984.

Moskowitz, M., and Fox, S. H.: Cost analysis of aggressive breast screening. Radiology, 130:253, 1979.

Mueller, C. B.: Breast cancer in 3,558 women: Age as a significant determinant in the rate of dying and causes of death. Surgery, 83:123, 1978.

Nap, M., Keuning, H., Burtin, P., et al.: CEA and NCA in benign and malignant breast tumors. Am. J. Clin. Pathol., 82:526, 1984.

Nathanson, I. T., and Welch, C. E.: Life expectance and incidence of malignant disease. I. Carcinoma of the breast. Am. J. Cancer, 28:40, 1936.

Nemoto, T., Natarajan, N., Smart, C. R., et al.: Patterns of breast cancer detection in the United States. J. Surg. Oncol., 21:143, 1982.

Neri, B., Ciatto, S., Distante, V., et al.: Circulating immune complexes (CIC) as tumor marker in the follow up of breast cancer. Cancer Detect. Prevent., 8:67, 1985.

Newby, L. G., Spratt, J. S., and Alfieri, Z. C.: A conceptual model for evaluation of patient education for cancer. Presented at the American Education Research Association annual meeting, Toronto, March 1978, and at the American Association for Cancer Education annual meeting, New Orleans, November 1978.

Noyes, R. D., Spanos, W. J., and Montague, E. D.: Breast cancer in women age 30 and under. Cancer, 49:1302, 1982.

Osborne, M.: Monoclonal antibodies can detect occult breast carcinoma metastases in the bone marrow. Presented at the Clinical Congress, American College of Surgeons, San Francisco, CA, 15 October, 1987.

Panoussopoulos, D., Chang, J., and Humphrey, L. J.: Screening for breast cancer. Ann. Surg., 186:356, 1977.

Pauwels, E. K. J., Heslinga, J. M., and Zwaveling, A.: Value of pretreatment and follow-up skeletal scintigraphy in operable breast cancer. Clin. Oncol., 8:25, 1982.

Pocock, S. J., Gore, S. M., and Kerr, G. R.: Long term survival analysis: The curability of breast cancer. Statistics Med., 1:93, 1982.

Pohl, A. L., Kolb, R., Moser, K. V., et al.: Enzyme activities in human breast tumor cells and sera. Cancer Detect. Prevent., 8:57, 1985.

Reynolds, R. D.: Analysis of survival in breast cancer: A critical look at the relationship between time to diagnosis and ultimate survival. Milit. Med., 8:465, 1984.

Ridell, B., and Landys, K.: Incidence and histopathology of metastases of mammary carcinoma in biopsies from the posterior iliac creast. Cancer, 44:1782, 1979.

Robinson, E., Mohilever, J., Zidan, J., et al.: Delay in

diagnosis of cancer. Possible effects on the stage of disease and survival. Cancer, 54:1454, 1984.

Rosenberg, S. G.: A case for patient education. Hosp. Formul. Management, 6:14, 1971.

Saltzstein, S. L.: Potential limits of physical examination and breast self-examination in detecting small cancers of the breast—an unselected population based study of 1302 cases. Cancer, 54:1443, 1984.

Savrin, R. A., Martin, E. W., Jr., and Ruberg, R. L.: Mass lesion of the breast after augmentation mammoplasty. Arch. Surg., 114:1423, 1979.

Schoenberg, B. S.: Multiple Primary Malignant Neoplasm. The Connecticut Experience, 1935–1964. Berlin, Springer-Verlag, 1977.

Schoenberg, B. S., and Myers, M. H.: Statistical methods for studying multiple primary malignant neoplasm. Cancer, 40:1892, 1977.

Schwartz, A. G., King, M. C., Belle, S. H., et al.: Risk of breast cancer in relatives of young breast cancer patients. J.N.C.I., 75:665, 1985.

Seidman, H., Stellman, S. D., and Mushinski, M. H.: A different perspective on breast cancer risk factors: Some implications on non-attributable risk. CA, 32:301, 1982.

Shapiro, S.: Evidence on screening for breast cancer from a randomized trial. Cancer, 39:2772, 1977.

Shwartz, M.: Estimates of lead time and length bias in a breast cancer screening program. Cancer, 46:844, 1980.

Souba, W. W., McKenna, R. J., Jr., Meis, J., et al.: Radiation-induced sarcomas of the chest wall. Cancer, 57:610, 1986.

Sox, H. C., Jr.: Probability theory in the use of diagnostic tests—an introduction to critical study of the literature. Ann. Intern. Med., 104:60, 1986.

Spratt, J. S.: Locally recurrent cancer after radical mastectomy. Cancer, 20:1051, 1967.

Spratt, J. S.: The lognormal frequency distribution and human cancer. J. Surg. Res., 9:151, 1969.

Spratt, J. S.: Cost effectiveness in the post-treatment follow-up cancer patients. J. Surg. Oncol., 3:393, 1971.

Spratt, J. S.: The relation of "human capital" preservation to health costs. Am. J. Econ. Soc., 34:295, 1975a.

Spratt J. S.: The physician's role in minimizing the economic morbidity of cancer. Semin. Oncol., 2:411, 1975b.

Spratt, J. S.: The relationship between the rates of growth of cancers and the intervals between screening examinations necessary for effective discovery. Cancer Detect. Prevent., 4:301, 1981.

Spratt, J. S.: Epidemiology of screening for cancer. Curr. Probl. Cancer, 6:1, 1982.

Spratt, J. S., and Hoag, M. G.: Incidence of multiple primary cancers per man-year of follow up. Ann. Surg., 164:775, 1966.

Spratt, J. S., Chang, A. F.-C., Heuser, L. S., et al. Acute carcinoma of the breast. Surg. Gynecol. Obstet., 157:220, 1983.

Spratt, J. S., Greenberg, R. A., and Heuser, L. S.: Geometry, growth rates and duration of cancer and carcinoma-in-situ of the breast before detection by screening. Cancer Res., 46:970, 1986.

Spratt, J. S., and Spratt, J. A.: What is breast cancer doing before we can detect it? J. Surg Oncol., 30:156, 1986.

Staab, H.-J., Anderer, F. A., Schindler, A. E., et al.: Optimizing tumor markers in breast cancer: Monitoring, prognosis and therapy control. Cancer Detect. Prevent., 8:35, 1985.

Stoll, B. A.: Does the malignancy of breast cancer vary with age? Clin. Oncol., 2:73, 1976.

Swartz, M.: Summary: A model of screening for breast cancer. Presented at the Michigan Cancer Foundation Workshop, Detroit, May 1977.

Tabar, L., Fagerberg, C. J. G., Gad, A., et al.: Reduction in mortality from breast cancer after mass screening with mammography: Randomized trial from the Breast Cancer Screening Work Group of the Swedish National Board of Health and Welfare. Lancet, 1:829, 1985.

Tempero, M. A., Peterson, R. J., Zetterman, R. K., et al.: Detection of metastatic liver disease. Use of liver scans and biochemical liver tests. J.A.M.A., 248:1329, 1982.

The impact, costs, and consequences of catastrophic illness on patients and families: A report of a social research study of selected families stricken by advanced cancer. Cancer Care, Inc. and National Cancer Foundation, New York, 1973.

The Patient with Cancer—Guidelines for Follow-up. Commission on Cancer, The American College of Surgeons, Chicago, 1976.

Tomin, R., and Donegan, W. L.: Screening for recurrent breast cancer—Its effectiveness and prognostic value. J. Clin. Oncol., 5:62, 1987.

Viadana, E., Cotter, R., Pickren, J. W., et al.: An autopsy study of metastatic sites of breast cancer. Cancer Res., 33:179, 1973.

Vickery, D. M., Kalmer, H., Lowry, D., et al.: Effect of a self-care education program on medical visits. J.A.M.A., 250:2952, 1983.

Wagner, H. M.: Principles of Operations Research with Applications to Managerial Decisions. Englewood Cliffs, N. J., Prentice-Hall, 1974, p. 364.

Wahren, B., Lidbrink, E., Wallgren, A., et al.: Carcinoembryonic antigen and other tumor markers in tissue and serum or plasma of patients with primary carcinoma. Cancer, 42:1870, 1978.

Walter, S. D., and Day, N. E.: Estimation of the duration of the preclinical disease state using screening data. Am. J. Epidemiol., 118:865, 1983.

Waxman, B. D., and Fitts W. T.: Survival of female patients with cancer of the breast. Am. J. Surg., 97:31, 1959.

Welch, J. S.: The postirradiated breast. Mayo Clin. Proc., 61:392, 1986.

Wickerham, L., Fisher, B., Cronin, W., et al.: The efficacy of bone scanning in the follow-up of patients with operable breast cancer. Breast Cancer Res. Treat., 4:303, 1984.

Wilkinson, G. S., Edgerton, F., Wallace, H. J., et al.: Delay, stage of disease and survival from breast cancer. J. Chron. Dis., 32:365, 1979.

Wright, C. J.: Breast cancer screening—a different look at the evidence. Surgery, 100:594, 1986; Letters to the Editor on this paper. Surgery, 102:106–114, 1987.

CHAPTER 20

SHARON KRUMM

Nursing Care

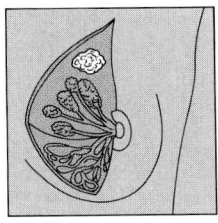

Nurses are often the health care professionals with whom women with breast cancer and their families have most contact. Nursing practice must be based on knowledge of the pathophysiology of breast cancer, its psychosocial ramifications, and the rationale for medical interventions. Principles of oncology nursing must be applied intelligently and with sensitivity for the uniqueness of each woman and her experience with breast cancer.

The purpose of this chapter is to identify appropriate nursing interventions along the continuum of breast cancer detection and treatment. The content was developed from a review of the literature and nursing practice at the Ellis Fischel State Cancer Center. Included are nursing roles related to screening and detection; assessment; patient education; surgical, radiation, and systemic therapies; lymphedema; psychosocial aspects; and metastasis. Other chapters in this book provide references and support for nursing actions.

Screening and Detection

The National Cancer Institute and the American Cancer Society have published guidelines for screening for breast cancer (Chapter 19). These guidelines are based on knowledge of associated risk factors and the natural history of the disease.

Nursing interventions include educating women about physical examinations, screening tests, and breast self-examination and encouraging them to maintain normal body weight and eat low amounts of animal fats, beginning in adolescence. Nurses should encourage women to participate in screening activities that increase the possibility of detecting breast cancer earlier (White, 1986). Frank-Stromborg (1986) emphasizes the importance of nurses recognizing barriers to early detection of cancer, especially among the elderly, and working in all practice settings to decrease these barriers.

Because the majority of breast lumps are detected by women themselves, breast self-examination is an important component of early detection. Beckmann (1984) reviewed 50 articles on the psychologic aspects of breast cancer screening and detection. He identified common characteristics of women motivated to perform breast self-examination and to participate in screening programs. In general, these were women who were highly motivated in all aspects of preventive health, felt confident of their ability to perform breast self-examination, and did not hesitate to contact a physician about an abnormal finding. In contrast, Trotta's study (1980), based on the health belief model, found that one of the most frequent barriers to doing breast self-examination was expressed lack of knowledge and confidence in doing the examination. Trotta further found that women taught by individual instruction practiced breast self-examination more frequently but were not as thorough as those taught in a group setting. The number of perceived barriers to doing breast self-examination was the most significant influence on regular, thorough practice of the procedure.

This information is important as nurses develop teaching strategies that will reduce the number of barriers. By using factual information in a judicious manner, nurses can use the anxiety that women have about developing breast cancer to decrease fear and to enhance motivation toward purposeful activities (Trotta, 1980; Beckmann, 1984). Individual or group sessions, or both, should be included as part of every woman's nursing care plan, and printed materials should be used to reinforce information presented. Various teaching aids and printed materials are available from the American Cancer Society and the National Cancer Institute. The first step, however, is for each nurse to be proficient in breast self-examination and to serve as a role model by practicing it regularly.

In teaching breast self-examination, the following points may be made:

1. The examination should be done at approximately the same time each month. The tenth day of each menstrual cycle, when fluid retention is minimal, is best for menstruating women. Postmenopausal women may choose the first day of the month or any easily remembered date.

2. The examination should be done gently, without pulling or pushing on breast tissue. Initially it may be performed more easily with soap or baby oil on the breast and hands.

3. Women with large, pendulous breasts must support the breast while examining; otherwise the examination may be misleading.

4. The examination should be done first lying down, then repeated while sitting or standing.

5. The breasts should be visually inspected in front of a mirror for asymmetry and skin and nipple changes.

6. Consistency is important. One technique uses a circular motion with the flat part of the fingers, moving in toward the nipple and encompassing the axilla.

When combined with physical examination, mammography increases the accuracy of detecting breast lesions. Nurses should reassure women that mammography is usually painless and performed easily and quickly. The woman should be prepared to undress to the waist for the x-ray examination.

Once a breast lump has been detected, the only way an accurate diagnosis can be made is by histologic examination. Diagnostic biopsies and aspiration may be performed in a doctor's office or an outpatient clinic.

If an open biopsy is required, it may be done in an operating room. At times, a frozen section is performed on the biopsy specimen. If a biopsy proves negative for cancer, as 70 per cent do, the woman should know that continued self-examinations and follow-up mammograms are important.

The sense of heightened anxiety associated with finding a breast lump and subsequent biopsy must be appreciated. Thomas (1978) describes this as a time of conflict and confusion for the woman and her family as they experience shock, disbelief, uncertainty, and fears. Nurses can be instrumental in assisting women through supportive measures, such as being available and listening to their concerns and fears, providing factual information, and including family members or supportive friends in discussions and teaching activities.

Once the diagnosis of breast cancer has been made, a physician may recommend several treatment options, depending on the histologic type, stage of disease, extent of lymph node involvement, estrogen and progesterone assays, and the woman's menopausal status. In choosing among these treatment options there are three elements of informed decision-making a woman needs to have: information; an appreciation of her personal values; and time (Valanis and Rumpler, 1985).

Greiner and Weiler (1983) found the women in their study wanted an active decision-making role based on information supplied by a physician yet also wanted to preserve the image of the physician as decision-maker. Women in the upper and middle socioeconomic classes were more likely to seek information about treatment options beyond that given by their physicians or when told there were no other options. The geographic availability of radiation therapy was also a factor influencing their decisions.

The influences on women's decision-making are varied. The media plays a major role. Sixty-two per cent of the women surveyed by the National Cancer Institute obtained information about the treatment of breast cancer from newspapers and women's magazines, and an additional 39 per cent received this information from television. Physicians, family members and friends are additional sources (Valanis and Rumpler, 1985).

A major factor influencing a woman's decision is the value she places on her breasts. There is an identifiable link between the loss of an important body part and lowered self-image and impaired sexual identity. This is demonstrated by avoidance of sexual relationships and decreased involvement in social and leisure activities following mastectomy (Valanis and Rumpler, 1985).

There are certain characteristics of women that determine their emotional responses to the recommendation of a mastectomy. These are personality and coping attitude; usual health beliefs and practices; intellectual ability, reasoning and decision-making skills; demographic characteristics, such as age and education; self-concept; and their families' responses. Because of strong emotional responses to mastectomy, many women are willing to trade their physical safety for the psychologic comfort of a less threatening treatment option (Valanis and Rumpler, 1985).

Various treatment options are discussed elsewhere in this book. In addition, Kraybill and Lopez (1985) caution physicians and women considering breast preserving treatments to also consider the need for close extensive follow-up, the disruptive effects of daily radiation therapy and chemotherapy regimens, and the possibility of eventual mastectomy. These factors should be explored carefully.

With this information in mind, nurses can select strategies that facilitate the use of reason and systematic action in the decision-making process. Involving sexual partners or other supportive persons in discussions of treatment options should always be considered. Women need information and opportunities to assist them in understanding their personal values. The need for time can be met, even if a woman has a mastectomy immediately following a frozen section biopsy, by allowing enough time before surgery or scheduling a second interim visit to answer questions and ensure the inclusion of the sexual partner or other supportive person (Valanis and Rumpler, 1985).

The National Institutes of Health publishes a booklet, "Breast Cancer: Understanding Treatment Options" (NIH Publication No. 85–2675) that provides clear and concise information and illustrations. This is a useful adjunct to discussions and other teaching activities.

Assessment

The nursing process is central to goal-directed, patient-centered care. The initial phase of the process, assessment, is discussed briefly. This is followed by information about patient education, a major component of nursing care of women with breast cancer.

The nursing assessment entails a systematic approach to obtaining subjective and objective data about each body system, psychologic abilities, daily activities, social climate, and changes resulting from breast cancer or its therapy. Its purposes are to obtain baseline data; determine usual levels of functioning and adaptability to altered levels of functioning; and assist patients in making the most of their abilities. Subjective data are obtained through the patient history and objective data from the nurse's physical assessment (Woods, 1982).

The components of a psychologic assessment are included in most subjective and objective data bases. Additionally, nurses should assess cognitive abilities, intellectual level, memory and orientation, responses to stress, and use of coping and defense mechanisms in the past. These baseline data will serve as a reference when brain metastasis or metabolic alterations affecting cognition and behavior are suspected. Because social support is so important to cancer patients, information about individuals and institutions that constitute that support and the nature and extent of their support should be identified (Krumm, 1982).

Sexuality is a concept of central importance to women with breast cancer. A sexual assessment should be included as part of the initial data base. McPhetridge (1968) suggests questions that can be used to elicit information about the three components of sexuality: sexual identity; sex role; and sexual functioning. Sexual identity is assessed by asking if breast cancer or its treatment has affected the way the patient feels about herself as a woman. Sex role changes are discovered by answers to questions about roles as mother or wife. Finally, sexual functioning is assessed by asking if the patient's sexual activity has been affected.

The nursing staff at Ellis Fischel State Cancer Center developed a form for structuring and recording patient information (Fig. 20–1). The major categories of the Oncology Nursing Society and American Nurses' Association Standards of Practice (American Nurses' Association, 1979) are used in organizing the data. This facilitates nursing diagnoses and promotes consistent practice.

Miaskowski and Nielson (1985) developed an assessment tool using the same Standards of Practice just mentioned. Included with the tool are specific guidelines for data collection.

Regardless of the tool or format used, this initial step in the nursing process is crucial in establishing a therapeutic relationship between patient and nurse. The patient's physical, psychosocial, and learning needs must be determined as a basis for planning nursing care that will assist patients and their families in meeting

ELLIS FISCHEL STATE CANCER CENTER
PATIENT DATA BASE

ADMIT DATA
Date_____ Allergies_____ Age_____
Informant_____ New/Read_____ Last Admission_____
Patient's Chief Concern _____

MEDS
Routine Meds_____
Meds Taken Today_____

Nursing Dx/Comments_____

MED/SURG HISTORY
List medical conditions, dates of hospitalizations, surgeries, etc.
_____

HISTORY OF MALIGNANCY
Family history_____
Patient's DX (include cell type and stage) _____
Prior treatment and dates_____

COPING
Resources for support_____
Communication of needs/feelings_____
Hobbies, recreational interests_____
Cognitive ability_____
Recent stresses_____
Knowledge of Dx and understanding of illness_____
Expectations of hospitalization_____
Desire to see spiritual counselor_____
Nursing Dx/Comments_____

COMFORT
Pain (location, intensity, duration, relief)_____
Sleep pattern_____
Anxiety_____
Nausea_____
Nursing Dx/Comments_____

NUTRITIONAL HYDRATION
Usual Wt._____ Recent wt. loss/gain_____ Diet_____
Restrictions, intolerances_____ Follows diet_____
Supplements_____ Taste changes_____
Alcohol use_____ Oral Cavity Status_____
Difficulty chewing_____ Difficulty swallowing_____
Dentures: Uppers_____ Lower _____ Partial_____
Nursing Dx/Comments_____

Figure 20–1. Form for structuring and recording patient information.

PROTECTIVE MECHANISMS	Level of consciousness_____ Headache_____ Syncope_____		

PROTECTIVE MECHANISMS
Level of consciousness_____Headache_____Syncope_____
Seizures_____Tremors_____Paralysis_____
Weakness_____
Vision (glasses, contact lenses, visual disturbances)_____
Hearing (impairments, aid)_____
Aphasia_____Prosthesis/speech aid_____
Skin condition (edema, discharges, irritations, lesions)_____

Infections_____Bleeding_____
Nursing Dx/Comments_____

MOBILITY
Usual activity level_____
Recent changes_____
Amputations_____Prosthesis_____
Aids (cane, walker, etc.)_____
Adaptations_____
Nursing Dx/Comments_____

ELIMINATION
Usual bowel pattern_____Last BM_____
Flatulence_____Vomiting_____
Usual urinary pattern_____Fistulas_____
Altered elimination route_____
Adaptation to altered route_____
Perspiration_____
Menstrual cycle and flow_____LMP_____
Last Pap smear_____
Nursing Dx/Comments_____

SEXUALITY
Sexual identity changes_____
Sexual role changes_____
Sexual activity, satisfaction changes_____
B.S.E._____
Nursing Dx/Comments_____

VENT. CAPACITY
Dyspnea_____Smoking history_____
Use of O_2_____
Trach_____
Nursing Dx/Comments_____

COMMENTS _____

Readmissions (indicate changes from initial assessment)_____
Dates: _____

Figure 20–1 *Continued*

these needs and that will facilitate compliance with the prescribed plan of treatment. Assessment is a continuous process. Nurses have responsibility for communicating assessment information to other health care providers in a timely and appropriate manner.

The Nursing Committee of the Tri-State Community Hospital Oncology Program developed site-specific algorithms for nursing care problems associated with cancer. The algorithms help structure and identify existing and potential problems. Although the authors determined that nurses experienced some problems incorporating the algorithms into nursing care plans, they generally found them to be helpful in creating greater awareness of potential problems that resulted in enhanced patient and family teaching (Wood and Ellerhorst, 1983). Nurses may wish to consider this for developing individualized nursing care plans.

Patient Education

Needs for patient and family teaching are identified in the planning phase of the nursing process. Needs exist if there are knowledge or skill deficits. In addition to using information obtained from the assessment, Watson suggests that the patient's style of learning can be determined by asking her how she would usually go about learning something new (Watson, 1982).

Once the educational needs have been determined, clear, concise, behavioral objectives should be set. These are action verbs that relate to each single task (Frank-Stromborg, 1984). The type of learning required (i.e., cognitive, psychomotor, or attitude) depends on the objectives. The teaching method and content can then be matched with the type of learning required (Watson, 1982).

The phase of illness is a major factor in determining appropriate teaching. Watson (1982) suggests that for this purpose there are two phases: (1) diagnosis, acute induction, and initial treatment; and (2) remission, consolidation treatment, or adjuvant therapy. She identifies patients' perceptions of themselves as being sick in the first phase and as beginning to see themselves as well or becoming well in the second. During the first phase, the focus of teaching is on diagnosis and treatment and on enhancing patients' strategies for coping with physical and psychologic crisis. In the second phase, teaching focuses on responsibility for self-care and developing problem-solving skills for self-care and coping. The primary objectives of teaching during the first phase are to have patients acquire sufficient understanding of their disease and treatment to give an informed consent, participate cooperatively in the treatment, and alleviate anxiety. Nurses should expect patients to forget or repress much of what is learned during this phase. Information should be given simply and concisely with the intent to conserve energy for coping.

Teaching during the second phase is directed toward helping patients retain knowledge and skills regarding self-care and toward transferring these to home, work, or other settings. Nurses should expect that patients in this phase will learn and accept responsibility for their own care. Transfer of knowledge is important, so office and community nurses must be informed in detail about what is to be evaluated or reinforced.

Nursing Care During Surgical Therapy

Public attention has focused on the extent of surgical intervention for breast cancer. Nurses should know the indications, advantages and disadvantages of the different operations to be able to give correct information. They must respect patients' rights to choose and should provide information, guidance, and support.

The woman who has a frozen section biopsy under general anesthesia followed by a mastectomy if necessary must be prepared for the possibility that she will find one of her breasts missing on recovery from anesthesia. Preoperatively, nurses give the same information as they would to a woman scheduled to undergo a mastectomy.

The following nursing goals are appropriate for a woman scheduled for a mastectomy: (1) The patient understands the nature of the anticipated surgical procedure; (2) the patient understands what is expected of her postoperatively; (3) the patient is prepared to cope psychologically; (4) the patient's family is prepared to support the patient in an effective manner.

Teaching of a general nature can be effective in a group setting with patients and their families. Information is given about visiting policies, the appearance of the operating room suite and the recovery room, general preoperative and postoperative procedures, and sensations that may be expected in the postoperative period.

Information that is specific for the individual patient is communicated on a one-to-one basis. It is essential that all members of the interdisciplinary team convey the same message to the patient and her family. The nurse must know what procedure is planned and the postoperative care that may be prescribed.

Ideally, this is done over a period of several days to reinforce important points and to give patients an opportunity for questions. A general teaching plan is organized in such a manner that different nurses may coordinate their efforts.

Visual aids enhance teaching. Simple line drawings may be adapted from books or journals and mounted on colored posterboard, or photographs may be used. Such aids should be chosen carefully and examined from the patient's point of view. Textbook illustrations often are too complex.

An example of a preoperative teaching plan is shown in Table 20–1. The plan is altered to meet individual patients' requirements. Most teaching is done on an individual basis in privacy, but including family members or supportive friends at some point is desirable.

The general aspects of surgery may be discussed, such as the type and anticipated duration of anesthesia. The operating room and recovery room nurses may visit the patient prior to surgery. The same operating room nurse greets the patient on arrival in the operating room suite as an added reassurance.

In addition to making a preoperative visit, the operating room nurse can establish a safe, therapeutic environment, identifying the patient properly, positioning her safely and correctly, maintaining and monitoring the sterile technique of the operating room team, identifying and handling the surgical specimen correctly, and transporting and discharging the patient safely from the operating room suite. A serious error in the operating room is allowing the arm of the anesthetized patient to hang and stretch the brachial plexus, risking palsy of the upper extremity.

The objectives of postoperative care are to promote wound healing, to restore function in the extremity, and to facilitate psychologic adjustment of the patient and her family. Complications that may attend mastectomy are hematoma, seroma, hemorrhage, wound infection, and pulmonary problems.

Means of securing the surgical dressing depend on the type, location and bulkiness of the dressing, and possible patient allergies to tape or other materials. Some surgeons use the woman's brassière to hold the dressing in place. It is put on in the operating room.

The involved extremity may be immobilized temporarily after mastectomy to prevent abduction of the arm. Stress on the incision and seroma formation interfere with wound healing. Differences of opinion exist among surgeons about the use of immobilization. The patient may have the arm in a sling or adducted to the chest with an immobilizer. Handicaps of immobilization include decrease in muscular tone of the upper extremity and diminished ability for self-care.

The patient is more comfortable with a pillow supporting the involved side. When the patient is turned onto the unaffected side, two pillows should be placed in front of her for support.

If the arm is not immobilized, it should be placed on pillows in a manner that will enhance the gravitational flow of lymph. The hand should be higher than the elbow and the elbow higher than the shoulder. The hand should not hang in the dependent position for an extended period of time.

Apparatus used for wound drainage help remove exudate by applying gentle suction on catheters under the skin flaps. If additional suction is required, a portable electric pump or regulated wall suction may be used. Wound catheters must be kept free of obstructions and kinks. Care is taken to maintain sterility of the drainage system, and the amount and color of drainage are recorded. The suction device may be fastened to the patient's gown during ambulation.

The nurse should be alert to detect early signs of infection. Fever, redness, and unusual pain are indicators.

Immediately after the operation, the patient's bed is tagged with a sign prohibiting blood pressure monitoring, venipuncture, or intramuscular injections in the upper extremity on the side of the operation. The best precaution, however, is an informed patient who reinforces these restrictions.

The first dressing change may be traumatic for the patient. The patient should be told what to expect when the dressing is removed

Table 20–1. SAMPLE PREOPERATIVE TEACHING PLAN

Content Area Evaluation	Method of Presentation	Method of Evaluation
1. Turn, cough, deep breaths	a. Demonstration of procedure or activity	a. Return demonstration

2. Extremity exercises
  a. Isometric
  b. Passive
  c. Active
	a. Demonstration
	b. Patient practice
		a. Return demonstration
		b. Patient can state reasons for exercises

3. Immobilization of extremity	a. Discussion b. Demonstration of methods of immobilization	a. Patient can state reasons for immobilization b. Patient maintains immobilization postoperatively
4. Dietary restrictions (diet progression)	a. Discussion b. Questioning regarding specific cultural or medical problems	a. Patient can state reasons for restrictions b. Patient complies with restrictions
5. Operative procedure, location and extent of incision, including axillary lymph node dissection	a. Discussion of operative procedure and function of axillary lymph nodes b. Visual aids	a. Patient can describe procedure and anticipated wound b. Patient can state function of axillary lymph nodes and describe how surgery may alter this c. Patient can discuss relationship of axillary node dissection to lymphedema and postoperative arm care d. Patient can describe relationship between axillary node dissection and diagnosis of extent of disease
6. Wound drainage system	a. Demonstration and explanation of equipment	a. Patient can state reason for use of equipment
7. Pain control and sensory changes	a. Demonstration of relaxation techniques b. Discussion of positions to decrease pain c. Discussion of potential sensory changes	a. Return demonstration b. Patient can express expectations of pain control c. Patient can state possible sensation in the chest wall and arm resulting from surgery
8. Body image changes	a. Discussion of concept b. Discussion of common reactions c. Discussion of influence on sexuality d. Include sexual partner	a. Patient can express feelings about her body b. Patient can identify potential concerns c. Patient can state problem-solving approaches
9. Coping strategies	a. Discussion of common responses and sources	a. Patient can express concerns b. Patient can identify sources of support c. Patient can state plans for coping
10. Rehabilitation	a. Brief discussion of Reach to Recovery, prostheses, reconstruction and postoperative exercise program	a. Patient can identify appropriate options

in terms of the appearance of the wound. If the woman avoids looking at the wound, she should not be asked to look as she will examine it when she is ready psychologically. The nurse can be supportive by listening quietly and by offering information as requested.

When shoulder exercises are initiated, patients can benefit from observing the exercises and participating in discussions. Exercises in front of a mirror permit a self-check on posture and body alignment. The patient is encouraged to comb her hair, brush her teeth, and feed herself with the affected extremity.

Often it is not feasible for the woman to begin exercises with the affected arm until she is already home. In this case, demonstrating exercises while she is hospitalized, and giving her an initiation date for the affected arm, can overcome this obstacle. Arm motion should be normal in 1 month; if not, physical therapy is begun to achieve it. Attention should concentrate on restoring normal rotation and abduction of the shoulder joint with gentle range of motion and stretching exercises. The elbow and wrist joints are not impaired, and needless stress on the arm with superfluous exercises only invites accumulation of tissue fluid. Finger walking up the wall and overhead reaching are particularly beneficial. Tapes placed on the wall on which to mark progress provide a visible incentive to better the previous effort.

The important aspects of wound, skin, and hand care on the side of the surgery are explained to the patient along with their rationale. She is given a list of "do's and don'ts." Such a list includes the following:

1. Do *not* cut cuticles.
2. Do wear canvas gloves when gardening. Wear rubber gloves when cleaning pots and pans with steel wool. Avoid injury or infection.
3. Do avoid burns; wear padded gloves when reaching into an oven.
4. Do keep watchbands and jewelry loose on the involved arm.
5. Do keep dress sleeves loose. Avoid pressure and tight bands.
6. Do *not* use the affected arm to carry a heavy purse or packages.
7. Do use the *unaffected* arm for blood pressure determinations, injections, and drawing blood samples.
8. Do wear a thimble when sewing.
9. Do wash the smallest break in the skin immediately with soap and water and cover with an elastic bandage.
10. Do use an electric razor for shaving underarms and avoid nicks and scrapes.
11. Do use a good lanolin-based hand cream several times a day.
12. Do give up smoking; but if you must smoke, hold cigarettes in the unaffected hand.
13. Do *not* get sunburned; get tanned gradually.
14. Do contact a doctor if the arm feels hot or is reddened or swollen.
15. Do remember to keep appointments with the doctor.
16. Do continue normal activities and hobbies.
17. Do examine the remaining breast monthly and report any changes to the doctor.
18. Do check with the doctor before using beauty creams or medications containing hormones.

The patient should be cautioned against wearing a weighted prosthesis or tight fitting clothing until the incision has healed. Some patients find it more comfortable to wear a loose fitting cotton slip or a man's cotton undershirt; nylon and other synthetics may be uncomfortable. Once healing is complete, daily massage of cocoa butter into the skin around the incision can prevent dryness and promote skin mobility.

To minimize fatigue and to promote continued recovery following discharge, the patient is instructed about ways to alter certain daily activities. Kitchen cabinets may be rearranged to force the patient to reach for the more frequently used articles. This stretches and strengthens the muscles of the chest and upper extremity.

Frequent rest periods may be necessary. The patient should know that fatigue will gradually decrease. If there are small children in the home, it may be necessary to arrange for help with their care. The patient is encouraged to sit down while holding an infant or child. It is better to let small children climb up onto the lap than to pick them up.

Rehearsing activities to be resumed following discharge can be extremely helpful. These include dressing and grooming, especially if the dominant arm has limited mobility. It is best to insert the affected arm into sleeves first. The use of devices such as brassière extenders and weights for prosthesis can be demonstrated. In addition, nurses can help patients practice what they will say about their surgery to children and other family members and friends.

Hypesthesia in the area of the incision may be permanent. Some women experience "phantom breast" sensations, and others describe pain long after the incision has healed. These sensations result from sensory nerve damage. Sensations of tightness of the chest wall may be more intense in the supine position.

The Reach to Recovery program of the American Cancer Society is dedicated to helping mastectomy patients with their psychologic, physical, and cosmetic needs. Begun in 1952 by Mrs. Terese Lasser, the program provides trained volunteers who have had breast cancer and who visit patients postoperatively if a surgeon authorizes it. The volunteer teaches exercises prescribed by the surgeon, suggests comfort measures, provides a fluff-filled temporary prosthesis, and supplies a list of sources for purchasing weighted prostheses. She provides emotional support by demonstrating how a woman can lead a normal life and remain attractive. Nurses should suggest a physician's order for this visit if it is not written routinely. If a woman wishes a Reach to Recovery visit but misses one while hospitalized, she should be encouraged to contact her local unit of the American Cancer Society to arrange a home visit.

A well-fitted breast prosthesis is an important part of a woman's physical and psychologic recovery. There are various types of prostheses available, including custom-made ones. They range in price from $40 to $900. Many insurance companies reimburse all or part of the cost of the prosthesis and brassiere, and Medicare covers 80 per cent. Most companies require a written physician's prescription for the prosthesis and brassiere. Much of the expense is tax-deductible.

Breast prostheses are usually made of silicone and attempt to replicate the feel and weight of breast tissue. Some have nipples, but nipples can be purchased separately for those without.

A well-fitting brassière is important for holding the prosthesis in place. Special mastectomy brassières may be purchased, or regular brassières can be adapted by sewing a pocket inside a cup to hold the prosthesis (McFadden, 1985).

Some patients choose not to wear a prosthesis. This choice is to be respected. However, women can develop problems with posture and neck, shoulder and back soreness as a result of weight imbalance.

Twenty-seven of 40 women responding to mailed questionnaires reported good to excellent satisfaction with their external prostheses in a study conducted by Feather and Lanigan (1985). No relationship was seen between the brand of prosthesis and satisfaction. Fifty per cent of the respondents noted they could not wear all styles of clothing, with swimsuits, casual wear, sundresses, and nightgowns causing most problems. The authors suggest ways of altering clothing to overcome many of the problems. They also prepared a slide-tape program to illustrate this information (Feather and Lanigan, 1985).

Incorporating the external prosthesis into her body image is crucial for a woman's rehabilitation. This is a process that occurs over time. Women should be encouraged to put their prostheses on when they first get up and to wear them continuously throughout the day. Some women elect to wear their prostheses even when sleeping. Support and reassurance facilitate this process.

At the time of discharge, the patient should meet the following criteria: adequately healed incisions, be able to eat adequately, and be able to exercise the affected extremity to the extent prescribed by the physician. She should also have received a visit from a Reach to Recovery volunteer, have demonstrated the ability to examine the remaining breast, understand the importance of follow-up examinations, know how to protect the extremity on the affected side, have demonstrated ability to use a light-weight prosthesis, and be progressing toward physical and psychologic rehabilitation.

Referral to a community health nurse, Visiting Nurse Association, or other home health agency may be necessary. The nursing care plan established during hospitalization and other data should be made available to agency nurses.

The role of reconstructive surgery is usually discussed by the surgeon and the patient. Nurses should support a woman's decision to inquire about the nature of the procedure and its relative advantages and risks.

Advances in technology in recent years have made breast reconstruction a viable option for many women. The timing of this procedure ranges from the time of mastectomy to several months later. Usually a silicone-filled plastic bag is implanted under the skin and the pectoralis major muscle. A nipple may or may not be constructed. The remaining breast may be reduced in size to enhance symmetry with the reconstructed one. Although the reconstructed breast does not look exactly like the normal one, and sensation is not normal, this procedure produces highly satisfactory results for many women (McKhann, 1985).

In a study by Stevens and associates (1984), the psychologic advantages of immediate breast reconstruction consisted of reduced postoperative psychologic morbidity compared with women having delayed reconstruction. Women in the delayed group reported difficulty talking with friends and significant others regarding sexual and body image concerns. Jonsson and colleagues (1984) found all 14 women in their study satisfied with their reconstructed breasts regardless of the timing of the procedure. They considered them a part of their bodies, a process that occurred over time.

Lymphedema

Although seroma, hematoma, and nerve injury are potential complications of mastectomy, lymphedema is the most troublesome long-term side-effect. The incidence of lymphedema is reported to be between 5 and 10 per cent of patients following modified radical mastectomy and may be higher following radical mastectomy. Surgical removal of lymphatic channels is the major factor in production of lymphedema. In addition, infection, decreased arm function, obesity, radiation therapy, and external compression may be contributing factors (Getz, 1985).

Acute transient lymphedema is seen in approximately 35 per cent of women following mastectomy, usually within 6 weeks postoperatively, and often disappears with restoration of arm function. It is associated with an increase in the diameter of the arm of 4 cm or less. In contrast, chronic edema is an insidious, persistent swelling of 4 cm or greater occurring weeks to years after surgery (Getz, 1985).

Lymphedema may be debilitating and almost always causes altered body image, resulting in psychologic distress. Once it develops, the goals of therapy are to improve the flow of lymph from the arm and to minimize new lymph formation. Baseline arm measurements and periodic measurements during follow-up help to detect and document the progress of lymphedema. Measurements are recorded as circumferences at standard locations, such as 15 cm proximal and distal to the top of the olecranon. Both arms are measured for comparison.

Lymph flow may be increased by elevating the arm, massage, active exercise, and the use of pneumatic compression devices. The arm should be elevated on pillows at night and on the back of a chair or couch for 30 minutes several times a day. Manual massage, moving from the hand toward the axilla, for 5 to 10 minutes four times a day is helpful and should be combined with elevation of the arm. Pneumatic devices, employing either uniform or differentiated compression, may be used while the patient is in hospital or at home. The amount of pressure and length of treatment is prescribed by a physician. Nurses should familiarize themselves with the application, use, and expected effects. Numbness and discomfort may be experienced during compression; however, the treatments should not cause significant pain. Pressure from compression sleeves must be kept low to avoid rupturing lymphatic vessels and increasing the risk of lymphedema. After initial results are attained, pneumatic compression may be used periodically to maintain reduction in arm size (Knobf, 1985). Pneumatic devices are contraindicated if lymphedema is the result of axillary node enlargement or infection of the affected arm.

The accumulation of new edema can be prevented by use of elastic wraps or sleeves and salt restriction. Women should be instructed in ways to avoid infection, trauma, and excessive use of the arm. They must not apply local heat to the arm. Suspected infections must be treated promptly (Knobf, 1985). In more severe cases, analgesics may be required, as well as a sling to support the heavy extremity.

Custom-made elastic sleeves are essential in preventing the reaccumulation of lymph fluid. The sleeve should be put on upon awakening and worn throughout the day. A detachable gauntlet facilitates handwashing and certain household chores. The sleeve may need to be replaced periodically to maintain elasticity and fit. If edema recurs during the night, the woman may wear the sleeve around the clock, removing it only when bathing.

Psychologic Aspects

The majority of women cope effectively with breast cancer and its sequelae. The literature is consistent in identifying both common psychologic reactions and those women at risk for difficulty.

Because women's breasts are visible symbols of their sexuality and femininity, mastectomy threatens a woman's self-image. Denial may allow adjustment to a new body image for 6 to 12 weeks, so the greatest threat occurs sometime afterward.

Researchers have demonstrated that younger women generally do not cope as effectively with breast cancer. Neither do women with limited social support and preexisting psychologic problems. Women of any age who place a great deal of value in their breasts are at risk for emotional problems. Many of these problems are related to sexual impairments.

Although the type of surgery, or other therapy, may moderate the effects of breast cancer for some women, the risk factors remain the same regardless of the treatment selected. The more conservative forms of therapy do not impact as negatively on body image (Schain et al., 1983).

Body image refers to the psychologic experience of an individual's body and focuses on the feelings and attitudes the person has toward her body, consciously and unconsciously. Body image has a direct impact on self-image, self-worth, and femininity (Carroll, 1981).

Altered body image is a crisis with four phases: shock, denial, acknowledgment of reality, and adaptation. The reason for the crisis is the inadequacy of the woman's usual patterns of response, behavior, and coping mechanisms (Murray, 1972).

When confronted by a patient with an altered body image from mastectomy, nurses should quickly establish a consistent therapeutic relationship. Emphasis should be placed on positive attributes and abilities that are unchanged by the operation and the strengths the woman has as a person. Helping to shape realistic expectations regarding appearance and anticipated emotional reactions is an important nursing function. The woman's sexual partner should be included in frank discussions about her feelings and encouraged to view the scar and resume sexual activity (Carroll, 1981).

Breast cancer and its treatment influence a woman's sexuality and her choice of sexual expression. Factors responsible for this influence are feelings of being sick, fatigue, malaise, swings in libido, pain, sadness and depression, surgical changes, and the effect on the sexual partner. Women may need assistance in exploring alternate ways of expressing their sexuality and affection (Woods, 1982).

Several techniques can be employed to reduce discomfort that may be experienced during sexual intercourse. A small, soft pillow may be placed over the scar to reduce pain from external pressure. The male superior, side-lying, and female superior positions generally are more comfortable and do not put pressure on the woman's upper extremities. Limitations in range of motion may be overcome by digital or oral stimulation and interthigh, anal, or oral intercourse. Hugging, fondling, caressing, and hand-holding are expressions of affection that can be used even if limitations are severe.

Changes in roles and family relationships may occur over the period of time a woman is diagnosed and treated. Most of these changes are in a positive direction, as family members have an increased sense of closeness and ability to share personal concerns. Women who have a poor prognosis, difficult emotional adjustment, and difficulty with adjuvant therapy find their family relationships more likely to change for the worse. Relationships with adolescent daughters are the most vulnerable, because girls at this age identify closely with their mothers and need their support. They also fear developing breast cancer themselves. Younger children's primary fear is that their mothers will die. Husbands' reactions are extremely important. Mature couples with stable marriages often experience renewed closeness and enhanced relationships (Grandstaff, 1976; Lichtman et al., 1984).

Although responses to breast cancer are highly individualized and vary over time, support groups can be very helpful to many women. These groups provide opportunities to gain information, share common experiences, and receive encouragement. Knowing that other women have similar feelings can have a normalizing effect. A woman seeking a support group should be directed to contact her local unit of the American Cancer Society or the Y. W. C. A., Y-Me Hotline (1-800-221-2141, in Illinois [312] 799-8228).

Nursing Care During Radiation Therapy

Radiation therapy may be the primary treatment for many women with early breast cancer and for those with advanced inoperable lesions. Although the advantage of acceptable cosmetic results is recognized, radiation therapy can be a long and difficult course. As the primary treatment, radiation therapy is usually given five times a week for 5 weeks (5000 rad) with or without a radioactive implant or electron boost of 2000 rad (Wilson and Strohl, 1982). Nursing interventions are designed to (1) minimize the side-effects of radiotherapy; (2) contribute to the patient's safety; (3) maintain an adequate nutritional status; (4) reduce pain and promote comfort; and (5) provide patient and family with emotional support.

The most common side-effects of radiation therapy are skin changes, dysphagia, and fatigue. Less frequent are pneumonitis, pleural effusion, neurologic deficits, and lymphedema.

Patient teaching regarding treatments, side-effects, and self-care measures provide women and their families with a greater sense of control over what is happening to them. Because the radiation therapy equipment is so unfamiliar, a great deal of support and preparation prior to simulation and first treatment are required. Women should be prepared for what they will see, hear, and feel. They must be assured that they are constantly observed during treatment, and assistance is always available when needed.

Misconceptions about radiation therapy causing burns or making the woman radioactive must be dispelled. At Ellis Fischel State Cancer Center, teaching of general information is done in a group setting using a flip chart and videotape. Selected pages from the flip chart are presented in Figures 20–2 to 20–4. A brochure provides reinforcement of information presented in the group and can be underlined or written in for individual instructions. An evaluation indicated this teaching assisted patients to identify and initiate self-help measures.

Proper skin care is important. Skin integrity may be maintained by gently washing the skin with a mild soap and applying a thin layer of hydrolyzed lanolin or Aquaphor. Viscous lotions or creams are not applied to the irradiated area. Tight clothing should not be worn. Itching can be relieved by the application of cornstarch. Patients are instructed not to expose irradiated areas to direct sunlight and not to apply a heating pad or electric blanket, as they may burn the skin. See Table 20–2 for self-care instructions regarding skin care.

A sore or dry throat results from radiation effects on the oral and pharyngeal mucosa. Frequent sips of liquid or sucking hard candies provides relief. Antacids may be prescribed for the sensation of a "lump" in the center of the chest. The use of viscous lidocaine swish and swallow 30 minutes before meals relieves discomfort and facilitates swallowing. The consistency of food may be altered to include only those with a soft texture. Highly seasoned

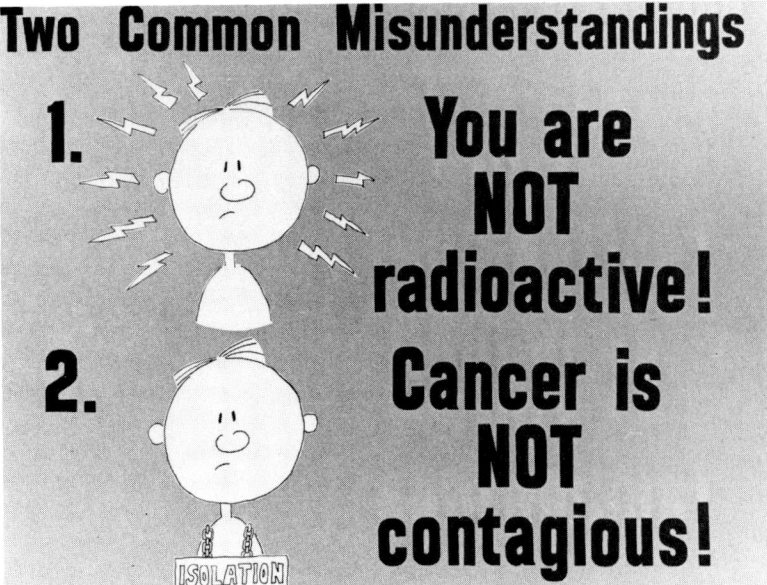

Figure 20–2. Selected page from a radiation therapy flip chart used in group teaching sessions.

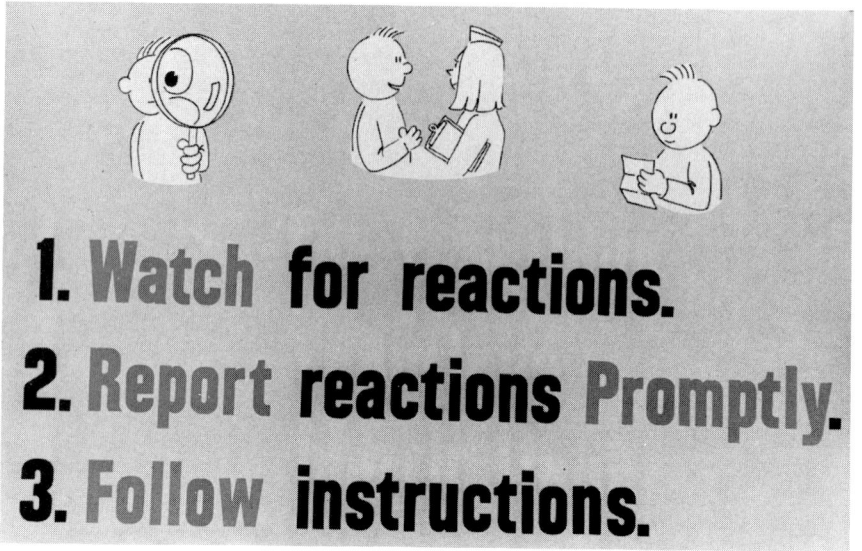

Figure 20–3. Selected page from a radiation therapy flip chart used in group teaching sessions.

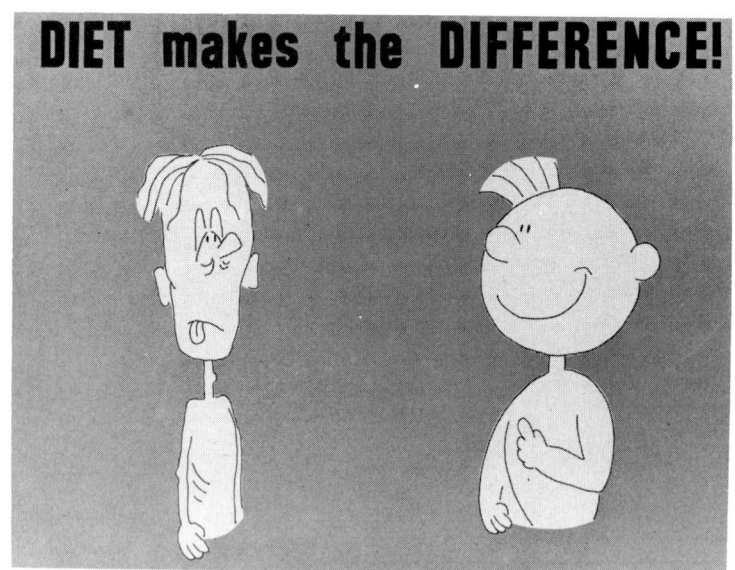

Figure 20–4. Selected page from a radiation therapy flip chart used in group teaching sessions.

Table 20-2. RADIATION THERAPY SELF-CARE GUIDE

Skin Care

We expect your skin to react to radiation in one of two ways. You will either have
1. A "dry" reaction, characterized by red, dry skin with some flaking or cracking, or
2. A "wet" reaction, characterized by red, tender skin with areas that look like broken blisters.

Skin reactions are *not* "burns." They are the normal effects of radiation. Let your doctor or nurse know when you begin to notice a skin reaction. We will want to watch it. Look carefully for reactions in folds of skin, such as on the neck or under the breasts. *Skin reactions are temporary* and should clear within 6 to 8 weeks after your treatment.

If you have a "dry" skin reaction, you should take the following steps:
1. Keep the area clean.
2. Wash the area at least once daily with water and a mild oil-based soap, such as Caress or Dove. Avoid strong deodorant soaps, such as Dial. Be sure to rinse off the soap well.
3. Apply hydrolized lanolin or Aquaphor to dry skin several times a day to provide moisture and prevent cracking. Do *not* apply any lotion 30 minutes before your treatment.
4. Report flaking or cracking of the skin to the doctor or nurse. If the skin is cracked or becomes raw, do not apply lotions as this will irritate the area.

If you have a "wet" skin reaction, you should take the following steps:
1. Keep the area clean.
2. Wash the area with hydrogen peroxide that has been diluted with an equal amount of water at least three times a day.
3. Use a soft cloth for washing the skin. *Do not* use dry cotton balls on "weeping" areas, as they stick to skin. *Do not* rub or scrub. *Do* pat or blot skin.
4. To dry the skin, leave the area open to the air as much as possible.
5. Wear only clean, soft cotton clothing over the affected area. Avoid synthetic fabrics as they trap moisture and increase irritation. Men's loose-fitting cotton tee shirts are especially comfortable.

Remember

Continue proper skin care after you have completed your treatments. For some people, skin reactions are greatest the first week or two following the completion of treatments. Do not be alarmed if this happens to you. Be sure to let your doctor or nurse know if you have questions or problems.

---

foods are eliminated from the diet. Eggnog, milkshakes, and other high protein, high calorie foods aid in maintaining nutritional status during this time.

Irradiation of the lungs may cause a pneumonitis resulting in acute inflammatory changes with congestion, exudate, and infiltration. The patient is usually asymptomatic; however, a dry, persistent cough and exertional dyspnea may develop and last for 4 to 6 weeks (Wilson and Strohl, 1982). The patient may have problems if fibrotic changes are permanent and she has preexisting pulmonary disease. Good pulmonary hygiene and adequate hydration and humidification are of value in controlling these side-effects. Nurses should be alert for symptoms of acute pleural effusions and notify a physician of dyspnea, restlessness, and cough.

Boosts with electron beams from a linear accelerator are used to deliver approximately 1600 rad, usually over a period of 8 days. Interstitial implants of iridium seeds are used to boost the radiation dose to a larger volume of breast tissue or when a higher dose to the tumor bed is required. Women will experience only minor discomfort that can be controlled with medications during this procedure. They must be prepared for potential isolation and boredom imposed by radiation precautions. Their visitors must be instructed regarding restrictions and precautions. Potential side-effects are arm edema, occurring in 4 to 7 per cent of patients, and rib fracture, which occurs in 1 to 5 per cent of the women (Hassey, 1985). Nurses caring for patients during interstitial therapy wear film badges to monitor exposure and concentrate their activities while in the isolation room to avoid overexposure.

The 51 women in Margolis and associates' study (1983) chose radiation therapy as primary treatment for their breast cancer to maintain the integrity of their breasts and keep their body images intact. Their breasts were important to their sense of femininity and sexual attractiveness and played a significant role in their active sex lives. Radiation therapy avoided the adverse emotional and sexual effects of mastectomy. Women in this sample were of the middle class and medically and socially sophisticated.

Radiation therapy is often the treatment for

bone metastases. When a breast cancer patient is known to have skeletal metastases, it is helpful for the nurse to review the radiographic diagnostic reports and discuss them with the patient's physician. These patients are susceptible to pathologic fractures of involved bones. Nursing personnel should be aware of this susceptibility and precautions taken in moving the patient and in routine patient care. When a pathologic fracture is suspected, the patient's physician is notified at once, and the suspected fracture is splinted pending examination. When these fractures involve long bones, they frequently require prompt internal fixation.

When weight-bearing bones are involved, bedboards and appropriately placed supports, including braces, may be indicated. Patients may need to be confined to bed or a wheelchair or instructed in the use of a cane or walker to decrease the possibility of fracture. Nurses can help patients to understand the need for these measures and for maintaining muscle strength. Active and passive exercises can be performed within limits. The patient is instructed not to lift heavy objects or to climb onto ladders or chairs following discharge. Carrying heavy grocery sacks or pushing a heavy vacuum cleaner should be avoided.

Patients with osseous metastases may experience a great deal of pain. Analgesics should be administered regularly and without hesitation. Nonsteroidal anti-inflammatory agents are often effective in relieving pain and discomfort associated with the disease process or treatment effect. As radiation begins to take effect, the pain will decrease and lessen the need for medication. It is helpful for the patient and her family to understand this.

Metastases in the brain are usually treated with radiation therapy. The patient and her family need consistent support and reassurance during this time. Benefits of the radiation therapy may not be appreciable until several weeks after completion of treatment. Alopecia and tearing may result, and the patient and her family should be prepared for these symptoms. Wigs can give a needed psychologic boost. Attractive cotton or terrycloth turbans and head scarves are more comfortable when the patient is in bed. If the woman's memory is impaired, nurses should be prepared to repeat instructions and to formulate questions so that they can be answered easily. Patients with visual disturbances require a structured environment that provides a sense of security.

The patient and her family need reassurance to help them deal effectively with the behavioral and physical changes.

Nursing Care During Systemic Therapy

The goals of systemic therapy are to prevent recurrence, reduce the severity of pain, and enhance and prolong life. Hormonal therapy and chemotherapy are used separately or in combination. Nurses play an important role in helping patients achieve the goals of therapy.

HORMONAL THERAPY

Hormonal therapy consists of changing the hormonal milieu that promotes the growth of mammary cancer. This can be achieved by surgical removal of a hormone-producing gland, as in oophorectomy, adrenalectomy, or hypophysectomy, or by chemical means, as with tamoxifen, to suppress estrogen production and estrogen binding to tumor cell receptors. Estrogen receptor assays are important indicators of potential response to therapy.

Not only does oophorectomy produce symptoms of menopause, but in addition the patient may equate the loss of reproductive capacity with aging and the loss of sexual attractiveness. Besides providing care and guidance following this operation, nurses should be sensitive to its potential impact on a woman's sexuality.

Following adrenalectomy, replacement therapy must be continued for the rest of a woman's life as failure to take steroids postoperatively can result in death from metabolic derangements. The patient is instructed to wear a medical alert bracelet giving the dose of steroids prescribed and to carry a card stating that she has had an adrenalectomy. Periods of increased stress require temporary increase in steroid demand. Hypotension, temperature elevation, vomiting, and weakness are symptoms of adrenocortical insufficiency and require immediate attention.

The principles of steroid replacement are the same following hypophysectomy. In addition, thyroid hormone replacement is necessary. Postoperatively, the patient may be placed on anticonvulsant therapy for several days and may require repeated assessment of her neurologic status. Diabetes insipidus may develop; thus, maintenance of an accurate record of fluid intake and output is important. This condition may persist and require exogenous posterior pituitary hormone therapy. The patient should understand the reason for this condition and be reassured that it can be controlled and poses no serious threat to her rehabilitation if she follows the prescribed guidelines.

Postmenopausal women with nonvisceral metastasis (e.g., skin, lymph nodes, or bone) can be encouraged by the fact that these lesions may clear and ultimately heal as a result of estrogenic or antiestrogenic agents. These agents frequently cause nausea during the initial phase of treatment. This side-effect can be minimized by increasing the dosage gradually or by taking the medication at bedtime. Patients may be reassured that the nausea will usually subside. Darkening of the nipple and axillary skin and changes in libido are expected side-effects of estrogen. Urinary urgency and incontinence, vaginal discharge, and fluid retention have been associated with estrogen therapy. In the patient with preexisting heart disease, the fluid retention may lead to cardiac failure. Breakthrough or withdrawal vaginal bleeding is fairly common with estrogen therapy. The onset of vaginal bleeding could be a frightening event if the patient is not forewarned. Tamoxifen can also cause vaginal bleeding, but the most frequent side-effects are hot flashes and less frequently nausea and vomiting. Skin rashes, depression and dizziness have also been reported.

Symptomatic improvement can be anticipated in postmenopausal patients with bone metastases who are receiving androgen therapy. An increased sense of well-being, increased appetite, and relief of pain can be expected. On the other hand, masculinization may be evidenced by thinning of the hair, hirsutism, increased libido, and hypertrophy of the clitoris. These changes impact negatively on the woman's sexuality, body image, and self-esteem.

Hypercalcemia may be associated with androgen or estrogen therapy or may occur spontaneously in the presence of bony metastases. It is potentially a life-threatening event. The patient should be instructed to report early symptoms, such as mental confusion, ataxia, nausea, vomiting, weakness, obstipation, polyuria, and anorexia, to her physician. Renal failure, cardiovascular collapse, and death may follow unless emergency treatment is initiated. Forced hydration, diuretics, prednisone, and calcitonin are the conventional management measures. The importance of teaching patients the early symptoms of hypercalcemia can be appreciated even more when it is realized that hormone therapy is usually initiated on an outpatient basis (Flynn and Durivage, 1982).

Synthetic corticosteroids are used in the emergency treatment of hypercalcemia and brain metastasis and in patients with advanced or terminal disease. Nurses must understand the rationale for steroid therapy to help the patient and her family establish realistic long-term and short-term goals. Long-term therapy may promote osteoporosis, hypokalemia, diabetes mellitus, gastric ulcers, Cushing's syndrome, and defects of cell-mediated immunity. The patient is instructed to report symptoms of fluid retention, hypertension, muscle weakness, headache, lethargy, or urinary frequency to her physician. Dietary alterations may be necessary for metabolic disturbances. Corticosteroids frequently produce a sense of euphoria and well-being but may also cause wide mood swings or psychosis.

The patient on long-term steroid therapy may have difficulty with viral, protozoal, and fungal infections. White lesions in the mouth or on the lips or a white vaginal discharge should alert the individual to the possibility of a fungal infection. Symptoms of infection may be masked by steroids. Herpes zoster may also occur after steroid therapy.

CHEMOTHERAPY

The nurse should know the rationale for the use of chemotherapeutic agents, their classifications, dosages, routes of administration, nadir, and toxic effects. This information for the commonly used agents is given in Table 20–3.

If extravasated, doxorubicin hydrochloride and vincristine can cause chronic ulceration. Extravasation may be prevented by using a free-flowing intravenous line with appropriate rate of flow and by flushing the line with normal saline solution before and after administration of each drug. Should extravasation occur, ice packs must be applied immediately and a physician notified. The patient is instructed to observe the site for redness, warmth, and ulceration and to contact her

Table 20-3. COMMONLY USED CHEMOTHERAPY AGENTS

Agent [Classification]	Dosage and Administration	Nadir (Days)	Side-Effects or Toxic Effects
Cyclophosphamide (Cytoxan) [alkylating agent]	100 mg/m^2 orally days 1–14 every 28 day cycle	7–14	Bone marrow suppression; nausea and vomiting; mucositis-stomatitis; hemorrhagic cystitis (avoid by increased fluid intake prior to and during therapy); alopecia; ovarian damage
Methotrexate [antimetabolite]	30–40 mg/m^2 intravenously days 1 and 8 each 28 day cycle	7–14	Bone marrow suppression; ulceration of oral and digestive tract
5-Fluorouracil (5-FU) [antimetabolite]	500 mg/m^2 intravenously days 1 and 8 each 28 day cycle	7–14	Bone marrow suppression; nausea and vomiting; GI tract injury, resulting in stomatitis, mucositis, and diarrhea
Doxorubicin hydrochloride (Adriamycin) [antibiotic]	50–75 mg/m^2 intravenously every 3 weeks or 25–30 mg/m^2 intravenously days 1 and 8 of 28 day cycle Avoid extravasation	10–14	Bone marrow suppression; nausea and vomiting; (severe) alopecia; mucositis and stomatitis; diarrhea; urine will be red up to 7 days after administration; irreversible cardiotoxicity (dose related)
Vincristine (Oncovin) [vinca alkaloid]	0.5–1.5 mg/m^2 intravenously not to exceed 2 mg/dose	Not marrow suppressive	Areflexia; weakness; peripheral neuritis; nausea and vomiting; alopecia; paralytic ileus

From Krakoff, I. H.: Cancer Chemotherapy Agents. New York, American Cancer Society Professional Education Publication, 1973.

physician promptly if any of these occur. Some physicians order corticosteroid injection into the area of extravasation to decrease inflammation; alternatively, sometimes they advocate immediate surgical debridement of the extravasation site to minimize tissue injury.

The use of implantable vascular access devices in selected women facilitates chemotherapy administration. These are placed into a vein, such as the subclavian, for systemic drug therapy or into an artery for regional therapy. These devices have the advantages over visible devices of low infection rates, decreased need for heparinization and dressing changes and improved body image (Winters, 1984). Double-lumen and triple-lumen catheters, such as the Hickman and Broviac, have also improved chemotherapy administration.

Educational materials that give the name of the drug(s) used, anticipated effects, and methods to minimize them are provided to patients. Effective teaching fosters the patient's active participation and enhances her compliance with the therapy. The patient's family or other supportive persons are included in teaching sessions.

Nurses must know the potential hazards of antineoplastic agents and of excreta of patients receiving them. They should follow published guidelines for handling these agents and patient excreta to eliminate undue skin contact. There is evidence of mutagenic changes in the urine of nurses who administer antineoplastic chemotherapy. Although the implications of these changes are unknown, nurses should not expose themselves to risks unnecessarily (Cloak et al., 1985).

For further information see the following:

1. OSHA Instruction Publication 8-1.1, Appendix A, Work Practice Guidelines for Personnel Dealing with Cytotoxic (Antineoplastic) Drugs, Office of Occupational Medicine, Directorate of Technical Support, Occupational Safety and Health Administration, U.S. Department of Labor, January 29, 1986.

2. National Study Commission on Cytotoxic Exposure, Louis P. Jeffery, Sc. D., Chairman, Rhode Island Hospital, Department of Pharmacy, Providence, Rhode Island 02902.

3. Cancer Chemotherapy, Guidelines and Recommendations for Nursing Education and Practice, 1984, Oncology Nursing Society, 311 Banksville Road, Pittsburgh, PA 15216.

Bone marrow suppression can be severe and is one of the most serious toxic effects of chemotherapy. Severe leukopenia places the patient at risk for infections. In a hospital setting, the patient must be protected from possible sources of infections. Some institutions use reverse isolation; some centers have laminar air flow facilities. Fundamentally, attention is directed toward controlling the patient's environment, maintaining standards of cleanliness and sterility, and monitoring staff and visitors to avoid potential sources of infection. The woman's hygienic practices must be assessed and teaching directed toward reinforcing principles of cleanliness and recognition of signs and symptoms of infection.

As a break in the skin is a common route of infection, efforts are made to maintain its integrity. Fingernails and toenails should be trim and clean. Efforts to maintain skin moisture include the avoidance of strong soaps and liberal application of lanolin or lotions.

Areas subject to pressure are protected by frequent changes of position and by the use of sheepskin and foam or alternating air mattress. Strict attention to good handwashing and to proper handling of intravenous tubing, catheters, and puncture sites is essential in preventing the introduction of microbes. Tubing of intravenous devices is changed and dated every 24 hr, as is the puncture site dressing. It is good practice to change intravenous catheters every 2 or 3 days.

The perineal area is another common site of infections. Women should be cautioned to clean the perineum properly following a bowel movement. Perineal care should be given routinely to the patient who is unable to do this. The sexually active woman may need to be advised against anal or oral intercourse, reminded to empty her bladder prior to and following intercourse, and advised about sexual hygienic practices.

Bladder catheterization always places the patient at risk for bacteriuria, a risk that increases with duration of catheterization. For this reason, patients who are neutropenic often are not catheterized, even in the presence of incontinence. Strict attention must be paid to sterile technique during catheterization, to maintaining a closed drainage system, and to anchoring the catheter in a secure manner.

Infections of the upper respiratory tract and lungs are reduced by screening staff and visitors and avoiding contact with infected persons. The patient who is bedfast and inactive is turned often and helped to cough and breathe deeply.

Oral hygiene assumes increased importance because of a tendency to develop ulcerations of the gums and buccal mucosa. Improperly fitting dentures should be eliminated, adjusted, or replaced, and any preexisting dental caries or infection should be treated prior to initiating chemotherapy. The nurse should be aware of early symptoms of ulceration, such as sensitivity to hot, cold, or spicy foods, dryness of the mouth, and a burning sensation of the lips, and should make routine visual inspection of the oral cavity. Severe dysphagia and secondary infection can result if early symptoms are not detected and the treatment discontinued or altered. Discomfort may be reduced with frequent mouthwashes, topical viscous lidocaine (Xylocaine) or Benadryl and Maalox swish and swallow before meals. Highly seasoned or acidic foods should be eliminated from the diet. Frequent saline gargles are effective. Commercial mouthwashes should be avoided owing to the drying effects of the alcohol component of these preparations.

The use of water-soluble lubricants in the vagina is important for women experiencing dryness of the vaginal mucosa from the chemotherapeutic agents. This reduces risk of infection and trauma to the lining of the vagina. Because most women will not initiate discussion of this topic, nurses should routinely inquire about this potential problem.

Thrombocytopenia may be evidenced first by the appearance of petechiae or by bleeding from the gums, nose, or urinary and gastrointestinal tracts. Intramuscular or intravenous punctures and injections are kept to a minimum, and pressure is applied to the site for at least 5 to 10 minutes afterward. The patient is instructed to use toothette swabs instead of a toothbrush and to avoid dental floss and toothpicks. Excessively hot foods are avoided. Only electric razors are used. The patient should be warned against blowing her nose excessively. A stool softener may be useful to avoid straining and bleeding during bowel movements. The use of acetaminophen is recommended for pain or fever in preference to aspirin, as the latter interferes with platelet function. Alcohol use is discouraged for the same reason.

Patients may experience anemia as manifested by fatigue, lethargy, and irritability. A balance between rest and activity is emphasized, and ways to decrease stress at home, at work, or in social environments are explored with the patient.

The entire gastrointestinal tract is susceptible to the toxic effects of most chemotherapeutic agents. Anorexia, nausea, and vomiting present problems in maintaining an adequate nutritional intake. Loss of taste or change in taste causing aversion to some foods, especially red meats, often accompanies and exaggerates the problem. Attractively served food in an environment that is esthetically pleasing is very important. The social significance of meal time should be recognized and fostered in an attempt to compensate for anorexia and depression. Nausea may be reduced by taking solids and liquids separately, sipping effervescent fluids that are at room temperature, and taking smaller and more frequent feedings. Mouth care is given before and after meals.

A nutritional assessment may be necessary for women receiving chemotherapy owing to the high incidence of protein-calorie malnutrition. This condition may result in decreased immunocompetence, response to therapy, and survival time. Possible causes are anorexia, tumor-induced altered body metabolism, inadequate functioning of the gastrointestinal tract, liver, and pancreas, the stress of infections, surgery, radiation therapy, and chemotherapy (Black et al., 1983).

Vomiting may lead to serious body fluid depletion and electrolyte imbalance. Antiemetics are prescribed routinely and are most effective when administered prophylactically and routinely thereafter. Anticipatory nausea and vomiting presents a significant challenge. Appropriate antiemetic therapy prior to the administration of the first dose of chemotherapy is important. The intravenous administration of prochlorperazine with diphenhydramine or metoclopramide with diphenhydramine 1 hr prior to chemotherapy and every 4 hrs for three doses, then as needed, has proved successful in decreasing nausea and vomiting. Diphenhydramine may be administered orally. Dexamethasone (Decadron) may also be given every 4 to 6 hrs between doses of the antiemetic medications. Attention must be given to environmental factors associated with anticipation of nausea and vomiting and modifications made accordingly. The use of diversional and relaxation therapy should be considered. Administering chemotherapy in the late evening affords patients the opportunity to achieve maximum benefits from antiemetic and hypnotic medications and to tolerate food and fluids in the morning. Furthermore, this does not reinforce the association between food intake and vomiting (Walter, 1982). An accurate record is kept of intake and output, the frequency of vomiting and its relation to drug and food intake, and the effectiveness of the antiemetic used.

Protracted or severe diarrhea can produce dehydration and electrolyte imbalance. Drugs are used to control diarrhea, and outpatients are told to contact their physicians if they have three or more liquid stools a day. Fluid intake must be maintained and the diet altered to include only low residue and bland foods.

Alopecia may pose severe emotional problems for the woman trying to cope with an altered body image. She may wish to purchase a wig prior to hair loss. Women have expressed shock that their hair did not slowly fall out but rather came out "by the handsful." Prior warning can buffer this shock. Colorful and attractive cotton turbans are generally comfortable for patients while in bed and eliminate the problem of wig slippage. Alopecia may include axillary and pubic hair as well as eyebrows. Hair loss is not permanent, and reassurance that regrowth will occur during or following drug treatment helps to eliminate some of the psychologic distress.

Weight gain is frequently associated with adjuvant chemotherapy and has deleterious psychologic and physical effects. It has been linked to the use of steroids, decreased activity, depression, increased intake, and altered metabolic rate. However, the cause remains unclear. Although the significant health hazards of obesity are often acknowledged, negative self-image may be less appreciated. Women experiencing weight gain of greater than 10 pounds or 10 per cent of their usual weight should receive nutritional counseling regarding reduced caloric, fat, and salt intake and increased consumption of fruits, vegetables, and grains. If smokers, they should be encouraged to quit. Regular exercise should be supported, and resources that facilitate coping should be identified (Knobf et al., 1983; Knobf, 1985). Weight measurements at each office or clinic visit will document progress with weight management.

IMMUNOTHERAPY

Immunotherapy is the use of biologic agents and biologic response modifiers (BRM) to alter the relationship between the host and tumor. These agents promote the host's natural biologic response to tumor cells or alter the inherent characteristics of tumor cells with resultant therapeutic effects (Scogna and Schoenberger, 1982; Suppers and McClamrock, 1985). These modifiers are of two basic types: chemical or synthetic compounds that stimulate or alter the host's resistance mechanism; and, biologic agents or cells that have direct antitumor effects. The effective use of these agents is currently being investigated. Much publicity is given new knowledge in this area, and nurses may wish to caution women against unrealistic expectations regarding their effectiveness (Scogna and Schoenberger, 1982).

Patients receiving BRM benefit from continuity of nursing care and enhanced interaction (Suppers and McClamrock, 1985). In addition to assisting with the administration of these agents, nurses play a key role in preventing unnecessary morbidity and in collecting and documenting data. Women receiving BRM require close observation and management to include accurate intake and output, encouragement regarding mobility, precisely timed and administered antiemetics, measures to reduce fever, including sponges and acetaminophen, pain control, and measures to combat fatigue (Scogna and Schoenberger, 1982). Additionally, they require education about treatment effects and self-care measures, support, and encouragement.

Local Recurrence and Metastasis

Two thirds of local recurrences and metastases of malignant neoplasms are discovered through careful history-taking and thorough physical examinations. Common sites are skin, bone, liver, lung, brain, and the remaining breast. Functional limitations and pain arising from bone or nervous system metastases are made evident by the history. Asymptomatic, easily discovered metastases, such as local recurrence or skin nodules, are found on physical assessment. Discovery of recurrence may be even more psychologically difficult for the patient than initial diagnosis (Mast, 1984).

Ulcerating metastatic lesions pose problems with infection, bleeding, and odor. These lesions require cleansing and debridement to decrease superficial bacterial flora, control bleeding and odor and decrease the need for dressings (Foltz, 1980).

Cleansing is best accomplished by using green, castile, or germicidal soap and gentle scrubbing, using a jet spray or whirlpool. Dakin's solution, hydrogen peroxide, potassium permanganate, enzymatic agents, or wet to dry gauze dressings may be used to debride the lesion. The first three solutions should not be used in areas where granulation tissue is forming as they affect this process adversely. Continuous applications of Dakin's solution debrides the lesion and decreases bacterial colonization and odor. Bacteriostatic agents, such as provodine iodine, sulfadiazine, (Silvadene), and acetic acid and yogurt may be used topically, or systemic antibiotics may be required. Hemostasis may be achieved with silver nitrate, epinephrine liquid, oxidized cellulose (Surgicel), or absorbable gelatin (Gelfoam). Ice and external pressure must be used with caution. Baking soda applied between layers of the dressing and Nilodor, Hexon, and Banish applied to the dressing and clothes will help control odor. Chlorophyll tablets, taken orally three or four times a day, may also be effective. If the woman is bedfast, continuous application of Dakin's solution is best. A nonadherent dressing such as Telfa should be used if a dressing is required (Foltz, 1980).

Women with ulcerated lesions require meticulous care. Equally important is sensitivity to psychosocial needs. It takes little imagination to appreciate the negative impact such conditions can have on a person's body image. Nurses should be alert for indications of social withdrawal and assist patients, their families, and friends to cope during this difficult time. Because offensive odors are responsible for a great deal of the problem, nurses must be persistent in employing measures directed at their eradication.

Conclusion

Nurses can make many aspects of breast cancer more endurable for women and their families by providing intelligent and sensitive nursing care. The rewards are great for doing so.

REFERENCES

Baltrop, K., and Kalache, A.: Psychosocial aspects of breast cancer care. Int. J. Breast Mammary Pathol. Senologia, 2:(4):171, 1984.

Bartelink, H., van Dam, F., and van Dongen, J.: Psychological effects of breast conserving therapy in comparison with radical mastectomy. Int. J. Radiation Oncol. Biol. Phys., 11(2):381, 1985.

Beckmann, J.: Psychological aspects of mass screening for detection of breast cancer. Int. J. Breast Mammary Pathol. Senologia, 2(4):183, 1984.

Black, M., Gallucci, B., and Katakkar, S.: The nutritional assessment of patients receiving chemotherapy. Oncol. Nurs. Forum, 10(2):53, 1983.

Carroll, R.: The impact of mastectomy on body image. Oncol. Nurs. Forum, 8(4):29, 1981.

Chapman, R.: Effect of cytotoxic therapy on sexuality and gonadal function. Semin. Oncol., 9:84, 1982.

Cloak, M., Connor, T., Stevens, K., et al.: Occupational exposure of nursing personnel to antineoplastic agents. Oncol. Nurs. Forum, 12(5):33, 1985.

deHaes, J., and Welvaart, K.: Quality of life after breast cancer surgery. J. Surg. Oncol., 28:123, 1985.

Derogatis, L.: Breast and gynecologic cancers: Their unique impact on body image and sexual identity in women. Front. Radiation Ther. Oncol., 14:1, 1980.

Feather, B., and Lanigan, C.: The mastectomee, her clothing and self-image. Unpublished Manuscript. Columbia, Missouri, University of Missouri, 1985.

Fisher, S.: The psychosexual effects of cancer and cancer treatment. Oncol. Nurs. Forum, 10(2):63, 1983.

Flynn, K., and Durivage, H.: Anti-estrogen therapy for breast cancer: Focus on tamoxifen. Oncol. Nurs. Forum, 9(4):21, 1982.

Foltz, A.: Nursing care of ulcerating metastatic lesions. Oncol. Nurs. Forum, 7(2):8, 1980.

Foltz, A. T.: The author responds. Oncol. Nurs. Forum, 12(6):13, 1985.

Frank-Stromborg, M.: Developing patient education materials. Oncol. Nurs. Forum, 11(6):70, 1984.

Frank-Stromborg, M.: The role of the nurse in early detection of cancer: Population sixty-six years of age and older. Oncol. Nurs. Forum, 13(3):66, 1986.

Getz, D.: The primary, secondary and tertiary nursing interventions of lymphedema. Cancer Nurs., 8(3):177, 1985.

Grandstaff, N.: The impact of breast cancer on the family. Front. Radiation Ther. Oncol., 11:146, 1976.

Greiner, L., and Weiler, C.: Early stage breast cancer: What do women know about treatment choices? Am. J. Nurs., 83:157, 1983.

Grobe, M., Ahmann, D., and Ilstrup, D.: Needs assessment for advanced cancer patients and their families. Oncol. Nurs. Forum, 9(4):26, 1982.

Hassey, K.: Radiation therapy for breast cancer: A historic review. Semin. Oncol. Nurs., 1(3):181, 1985.

Jamison, K., Wellisch, D., and Pasnall, R.: Psychosocial aspects of neoplastic disease: I. Functional status of breast cancer patients during different treatment regimens. Am. J. Psychiatry, 137:450, 1978.

Jonsson, C., Engman, K., and Asplud, O.: Psychological aspects of breast reconstruction following mastectomy. Scand. J. Plast. Reconstr. Surg., 18:317, 1984.

Knobf, M.: Primary breast cancer: Physical consequences and rehabilitation. Semin. Oncol. Nurs., 1:214, 1985.

Knobf, M., Mullen, J., Xistris, D., et al.: Weight gain in women with breast cancer receiving adjuvant chemotherapy. Oncol. Nurs. Forum, 10(2):28, 1983.

Knobf, M. K.: Weight gain and adjuvant chemotherapy. Oncol. Nurs. Forum, 12(6):13, 1985.

Kraybill, W., and Lopez, M.: Indications for breast preservation in stage I and II cancer of breast. Unpublished manuscript. Ellis Fischel State Cancer Center, 1985.

Krouse, H., and Krouse, J.: Cancer as crisis: The critical elements of adjustment. Nurs. Res., 31:96, 1982.

Krumm, S.: Psychosocial adaptation of the adult with cancer. Nurs. Clin. North Am., 17:729, 1982.

Lamb, M., and Wood, N.: Sexuality and the cancer patient. Cancer Nurs., 4:137, 1982.

Larson, P.: Important nurse caring behaviors perceived by patients with cancer. Oncol. Nurs. Forum, 11(6):46, 1984.

Lewis, F.: Experienced personal control and quality of life in late-stage cancer patients. Nurs. Res., 31:113, 1982.

Lichtman, R., Taylor, S., Wood, J., et al.: Relations with children after breast cancer: The mother-daughter relationship at risk. J. Psychosoc. Oncol., 2:1, 1984.

Margolis, G., Carabell, S., and Goodman, R.: Psychological aspects of primary radiation therapy for breast carcinoma. Am. J. Clin. Oncol., 6:533, 1983.

Mast, M.: Primary care of the mastectomy patient. Nurse Practitioner, 9:27, 1984.

McFadden, J.: Breast prostheses lessen trauma of mastectomies. Proceedings Ellis Fischel State Cancer Center, 3:(4):3, 1985.

McKhann, C.: The changing role of surgery in the treatment of breast cancer. Semin. Oncol. Nurs., 1(3):176, 1985.

McPhetridge, L.: Nursing history: One means of personalized care. Am. J. Nurs., 68:68, 1968.

Metzger, L., Rogers, T., and Bauman, L.: Effects of age and marital status on emotional distress after a mastectomy. J. Psychosoc. Oncol., 1(3):17, 1983.

Miaskowski, C., and Nielson, B.: A cancer nursing assessment tool. Oncol. Nurs. Forum, 12(6):37, 1985

Murray, R.: Principles of nursing interventions for the adult with body image changes. Nurs. Clin. North Am., 7:697, 1972.

Polivy, J.: Psychological effects of mastectomy on a woman's feminine self-concept. J. Nerv. Ment. Dis., 164:77, 1977.

Sanger, C., and Reznikoff, M.: A comparison of the psychological effects of breast-saving procedures with the modified radical mastectomy. Cancer, 48:2341, 1981.

Schain, W.: Psychological impact of the diagnosis of breast cancer on the patient. Front. Radiation Ther. Oncol., 11:68, 1976.

Schain, W., Edwards, B., Gorrell, C., et al: Psychosocial and physical outcomes of primary breast cancer therapy: Mastectomy vs excisional biopsy and irradiation. Breast Cancer Res. Treat., 3:377, 1983.

Scogna, D., and Schoenberger, C.: Biological response modifiers: An overview and nursing implications. Oncol. Nurs. Forum, 9(1):45, 1982.

Sheahan, S.: Management of breast lumps. Nurse Pract., 9:19, 1984.

Silberfarb, P., Maurer, H., and Crouthamel, C.: Psychosocial aspects of neoplastic disease: I. Functional status of breast cancer patients during different treatment regimens. Am. J. Psychiatry, 137:450, 1980.

Stevens, L., McGrath, M., Druss, R., et al.: The psychological impact of immediate breast reconstruction for women with early breast cancer. Plast. Reconstr. Surg., 73:619, 1984.

Suppers, V., and McClamrock, E.: Biologicals in cancer treatment: Future effects on nursing practice. Oncol. Nurs. Forum, 12(3):27, 1985.

Swartz-Applebaum, J., Dedrick, J., Jusenius, K., et al.: Nursing care plans: Sexuality and treatment of breast cancer. Oncol. Nurs. Forum, 11(6):16, 1974.

Taylor, S., Lichtman, R., Wood, J., et al.: Illness-related

and treatment-related factors in psychological adjustment to breast cancer. Cancer, 55:2506, 1985.

Thomas, S.: Breast cancer: The psychosocial issues. Cancer Nurs., 1:53, 1978.

Trotta, P.: Breast self-examination: Factors influencing compliance. Oncol. Nurs. Forum, 7(3):13, 1980.

Valanis, B., and Rumpler, C.: Helping women to choose breast cancer treatment alternatives. Cancer Nurs., 8:167, 1985.

Walter, J.: Care of the patient receiving antineoplastic drugs. Nurs. Clin. North Am., 17:607, 1982.

Watson, P.: Patient education: The adult with cancer. Nurs. Clin. North Am., 17:739, 1982.

Wellisch, D., Jamison, K., and Pasnau, R.: Psychosocial aspects of mastectomy. II. The man's perspective. Am. J. Psychiatry, 135:543, 1978.

White, N.: Cancer prevention and detection: From twenty to sixty-five years of age. Oncol. Nurs. Forum, 13(2):59, 1986.

Wilson, C., and Strohl, R.: Radiation therapy as primary treatment for breast cancer. Oncol. Nurs. Forum, 9(1):12, 1982.

Winters, V.: Implantable vascular access devices. Oncol. Nurs. Forum, 11(6):25, 1984.

Wood, H., and Ellerhorst, J.: Using site-specific nursing algorithms as an adjunct to oncology nursing guidelines. Oncol. Nurs. Forum, 10(3):22, 1983.

Woods, M.: Assessment of the adult with cancer. Nurs. Clin. North Am., 17:539, 1982.

Young-Brockopp, D.: Cancer patient's perceptions of five psychosocial needs. Oncol. Nurs. Forum, 9(4):31, 1982.

CHAPTER 21

CHRISTIAN PALETTA
M. J. JURKIEWICZ

Breast Reconstruction

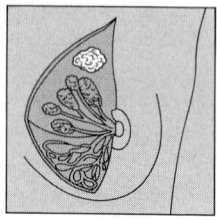

"... restore, repair and make whole those parts which nature has given and fortune has taken away. Not so much that they may delight the eye but that they may buoy the spirit and help the mind of the afflicted."
GASPARE TAGLIACOZZI
(16TH CENTURY)
(WEBSTER AND GNUDI, 1950)

Reconstruction of the female breast, delayed or immediate, after surgical ablation of the organ for cancer has become an increasingly compelling consideration for the patient and her surgeon.

Breast reconstruction following mastectomy has undergone a tremendous growth in the past 10 years. Four factors have contributed to this remarkable departure from traditional surgical thinking: (1) departure from traditional radical mastectomy; (2) development of better reconstructive techniques; (3) use of musculocutaneous flaps; and (4) development of tissue expansion techniques. First and most obvious is the departure from the Halsted radical mastectomy to some form of a conservative operation. Preservation of the pectoralis major muscle was the first modification; increased flap thickness the second. Other recent modifications include subtotal surgical mastectomy or tylectomy. Second, and occurring in parallel to the first, has been the development of reconstructive techniques that are reliable and give results that are esthetically superior to previous reconstructive methods.

In the mid-1970s it was learned that skin was nourished, for the most part, by perforating vessels from underlying muscle. This resulted in the third improvement, the development of more modern techniques for myocutaneous flaps, especially latissimus dorsi myocutaneous flap for breast reconstruction. In 1977, Schneider, Hill and Brown introduced use of the latissimus dorsi myocutaneous flap as a one-stage procedure in breast reconstruction. This provided a significant advance over previous techniques, which involved either multiple stages with tubed abdominal flaps or inadequate breast mound formation with simple implants. In 1979, Bostwick and colleagues reported their experience with 60 latissimus dorsi flaps, thereby establishing this flap as a reliable and easily performed method for breast reconstruction.

The introduction of the latissimus dorsi flap provided the reconstructive surgeon with an abundance of well-vascularized tissue with which to build and shape a new breast. Experience with the latissimus dorsi flap generated a far superior reconstructive result than hitherto possible. Publications on new and improved techniques flooded the literature, both lay and professional. At the same time, esthetic refinements in breast surgery were being developed and became incorporated into breast reconstruction techniques. Advances such as the improvement in design and contour of implantable breast prostheses added significantly to the esthetic reconstructive result. First introduced by Cronin and Gerow in 1963, the "natural-feel" silicone prosthesis was a remarkable improvement over previous materials, which included paraffin injections, fat grafts, Ivalon polymer sponges, and silicone injections (Cronin et al., 1977).

A further milestone was reached in 1980 when Hartrampf performed the first successful reconstruction using the transverse rectus abdominis musculocutaneous (TRAM) flap (Hartrampf et al., 1982). The TRAM flap was an outgrowth of both experimental and clinical research on musculocutaneous flaps. The blood supply of the abdominal wall skin, as well as skin territories throughout the body, were redefined on the basis of a new understanding of perforating vessels from the underlying muscles and fascia. Using this new information, the TRAM flap created a whole new horizon for breast reconstruction. It not only eliminated the need for a foreign silicone prosthesis, but it also provided an abundance of fatty tissue from the lower abdomen for breast reconstruction while recontouring the abdomen with an abdominoplasty (Hartrampf, 1984).

Finally, the development of tissue expansion techniques has led to yet another dimension in the field of breast reconstruction. First introduced by Radovan in 1976, tissue expanders have become increasingly popular not only in breast reconstruction but also in many areas requiring local tissue transfer (Radovan, 1982, 1984). They have been particularly useful in scalp reconstruction for burns or traumatic alopecia and in the reconstruction of various types of scar deformities. Tissue expansion has been remarkable both because of its simplicity and because of its contribution to an acceptable cosmetic result.

All of these techniques have a role in breast reconstruction. The reconstructive breast surgeon must be familiar and competent with each technique rather than relying solely on only one technique for all forms of breast reconstruction. This will result in a more appropriate matching of a specific technique to a specific defect on each patient desiring reconstruction. For example, the tissue requirements for reconstruction following a Halsted radical mastectomy differ markedly from those following a simple mastectomy or subcutaneous mastectomy. In addition, certain techniques will either not be available or will be contraindicated in selected patients because of prior surgical procedures or preexisting medical illness.

The second factor contributing to the growth in breast reconstruction has been the demand of the public for reconstructive surgery. Arguably as an outgrowth of the feminist movement in the 1960s and 1970s, women have become increasingly outspoken about surgery that involves removing part or all of the breast.

As stated in previous chapters, the number of women who will develop breast cancer each year is quite large. The American Cancer Society estimates that in 1987, over 130,000 women in the United States will be diagnosed with breast cancer. Although the majority of women will follow the traditional mode of therapy (i.e., modified radical mastectomy), more women, especially young women, are demanding alternative, more conservative treatment. In addition, an increasing number are seeking reconstruction. It is estimated that between 10 and 15 per cent of women who have had a mastectomy will seek reconstruction. Most centers have incorporated breast reconstruction into their comprehensive oncologic program. For many women faced with the prospect of losing a breast, this has eased some of the psychologic trauma by knowing that the breast can be recreated if she so desires, either immediately or at a later date.

Finally, the attitude of the general surgeon toward breast reconstruction has been changing. The Halstedian philosophy opposing breast reconstruction prevailed for over half a century. Because of both the improved techniques and the finding that reconstruction does not interfere with survival or early detection of cancer recurrence, the attitude of the general surgery community has become more favorable toward breast reconstruction. As a result, the reconstructive surgeon in many instances is consulted even prior to mastectomy.

Premastectomy consultation with the reconstructive surgeon achieves several goals. First, it provides information to the patient with respect to what can, and sometimes, more importantly, what cannot be accomplished through reconstruction in her particular situation. It may help identify the patients with unrealistic expectation who generally are poor candidates for immediate reconstruction. Second, premastectomy consultation can make it easier for the patient to choose mastectomy instead of selecting less established techniques for fear of losing a breast. Third, it permits improved communication between the general and reconstructive surgeon. While taking steps to allow for adequate oncologic treatment, the surgeon may plan the position of the incision to anticipate a certain type of reconstruction. In conjunction with the patient's preference and stage of disease on presentation, the choice of immediate or delayed reconstruction can be considered.

Principles of Breast Reconstruction

There are several general principles that should be followed when considering postmastectomy reconstruction. First and foremost is that reconstruction should not interfere with the early detection of recurrence or worsen the survival of the patient from her disease. These two concerns were the primary reasons why reconstruction postmastectomy had generally not been accepted. The prevailing belief was that such surgery to restore the breast was unnecessary and might even worsen the patient's survival. As a result, early pioneers in breast reconstruction established strict guidelines and criteria for the selection of patients for reconstruction and the timing of such reconstruction.

Early guidelines regarding selection and timing of reconstruction included the following general principles. First, only patients with favorable lesions (e.g., Stage A in the Columbia Clinical Classification or Stage I in the International Classification) were considered candidates for reconstruction. Additionally, the presence of more than three positive lymph nodes was considered a contraindication to breast reconstruction. Pers (1981) found a local recurrence rate of less than 5 per cent in patients with fewer than three positive axillary nodes. Second, many investigators found that approximately 75 per cent of recurrences become manifest within the first 2 years following mastectomy (Zimmerman et al., 1966). As a result, it was believed that postmastectomy reconstruction should be delayed until 2 years after mastectomy.

The purpose of these early guidelines was to avoid performing reconstruction on a patient who was liable to develop local recurrence from her disease. It was believed that if a patient would succumb from her disease within 1 to 5 years, reconstruction was unnecessary and wasteful. This negative approach has, for the most part, changed over the past 10 years. Within reason, it is no longer necessary to deny a patient who desires reconstruction the satisfaction of a breast reconstruction without going through a waiting period to see if her tumor will recur. In fact, there has been a recent trend toward immediate reconstruction in selected patients (Marshall, 1982; Gilliland, 1983; Webster et al., 1984; Frazier et al., 1985; Noone et al., 1985). Although immediate reconstruction is usually performed in patients with a favorable prognosis, it offers several advantages. First, it reduces the psychologic impact caused by the loss of a breast. And secondly, it reduces the cost of postmastectomy reconstruction. This second factor will certainly have increased importance in the years to come. When performed as an immediate procedure, the method of reconstruction is that of implant insertion beneath the pectoralis major muscle or the use of an expander. Although several authors have reported the use of the latissimus dorsi or TRAM flap in immediate reconstruction, this is not generally recommended because of the length of time required for such flap reconstruction when combined with the mastectomy (4 to 8 hr) (Drever, 1982).

The majority of postmastectomy reconstructions are performed as a delayed procedure, after the patient has recovered from her mastectomy and after any adjuvant therapy (radiation or chemotherapy) has been completed. This is usually from 3 to 9 months after mastectomy.

Delayed reconstruction has several advantages. The patient and surgeon have a better idea of the stage and prognosis of her cancer. Generally a complicated flap procedure would not be recommended for a patient with a poor prognosis. In addition, there will be patients who find that the deformity is acceptable and decide not to have reconstruction. Delaying the procedure also allows the patient additional time to assess her particular needs and discuss them with other women who have been in similar situations. Although most patients rely on the reconstructive surgeon's advice as to the type of reconstruction, more and more women are educating themselves through Reach to Recovery programs and similar sources of educational material (Bostwick and Berger, 1984). Some have investigated the different types of reconstruction and decide which is the most suitable for them. Finally, whereas over 90 per cent of women are satisfied with their reconstructive result, there are a few who expect an exact duplication of the original breast. Delayed reconstruction allows these particular women a chance to see what an improvement the reconstruction is over their postmastectomy deformity.

There was and still remains concern about a potential delay in early detection of breast cancer recurrence owing to deformities and scarring from breast reconstruction. Many authors have addressed this fear. Their finding is that the overwhelming majority of local recurrences occur at the site of the mastectomy scar (Zimmerman et al., 1966). The detection of recurrence in this location should not be influenced by either subpectoral implant or flap breast reconstruction. Furthermore, the prognosis for the patient once a recurrence has occurred generally is poor. Although it is too early to judge the influence of breast reconstruction on breast cancer survival, it appears doubtful that postmastectomy reconstruction will alter the natural history of the disease for the individual patient. A multicentered, long-term follow-up study will be necessary to answer this question adequately.

Types of Breast Reconstruction

At the present time, there are five different types of breast reconstruction. They include: (1) breast implant; (2) tissue expander followed by an implant; (3) latissimus dorsi flap with an implant; (4) transverse rectus abdominis myocutaneous flap (TRAM); and (5) microvascular tissue transfer. Each technique offers its own advantages and disadvantages. In addition, there are specific indications and contraindications for each technique (Bostwick, 1985).

BREAST IMPLANTS ONLY

The simplest form of breast reconstruction following mastectomy involves replacing the breast with a silicone gel implant (Fig. 21–1). This implant is most commonly placed beneath the pectoralis major muscle in the so-called submusculofascial space. This can be done as an immediate or as a delayed procedure. Most cases of immediate breast reconstruction involve either this technique or the placement of a tissue expander. The technique involves an incision through the previous mastectomy scar. The scar is excised and sent to the pathology laboratory for examination. The pectoralis major muscle is split in the direction of its fibers over a course of 6 to 8 cm. Blunt dissection is then used to create a submuscular pocket beneath the pectoralis major muscle, anterior portion of the serratus muscle, and superior portion of the rectus and external oblique fasciae. The pocket is made larger than the implant, and 2 to 4 cm more inferior than the opposite inframammary crease. The implant is then inserted into this space, and the muscle is closed in an interrupted fashion with 3–0 or 4–0 Vicryl suture.

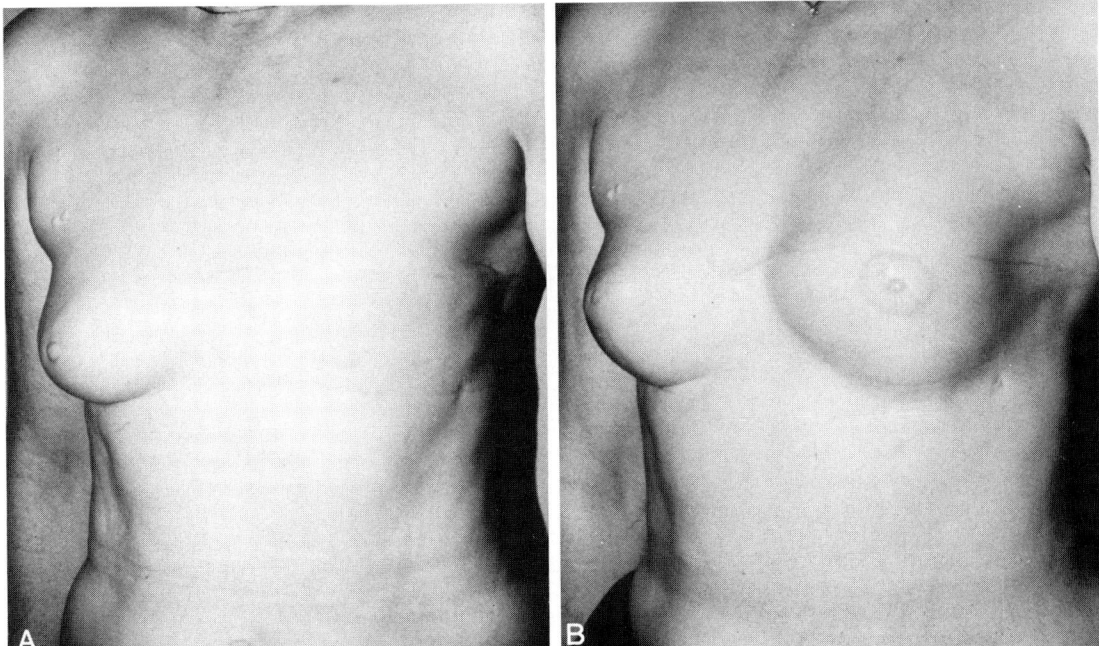

Figure 21–1. *A*, Patient following left modified radical mastectomy. *B*, Left breast reconstruction with a submuscular implant, nipple-areolar reconstruction, and right mastopexy. (Reproduced by permission from Bostwick, J.: Aesthetic and Reconstructive Breast Surgery. St. Louis, 1983, The C. V. Mosby Co.)

Reconstruction with an implant only is indicated when there is adequate skin coverage and adequate soft tissue in the infraclavicular space (Fig. 21–2). It is ideal for a patient after a modified radical mastectomy who has soft, well-healed skin flaps and an opposite breast dimension of 300 cm³ or less (A or B cup). It is difficult to insert, as a primary procedure, an implant exceeding 300 cm³ and maintain an adequate muscle coverage to prevent extrusion of the implant. If this technique is used and the opposite breast is significantly larger, a reduction mammoplasty can be performed or progressively larger implants can be inserted as separate procedures to enlarge the reconstructed breast. In such cases, however, the use of a tissue expander is more appropriate. Complications of implant breast reconstruction include bleeding from the subpectoral dissection (usually blunt dissection), infection around the implant, extrusion of the implant as a result of either infection or inadequate muscle coverage, and scar contracture (capsule) around the implant, resulting in a firm, painful mound and poor esthetic result. Placement of an implant only is contraindicated when the patient has had a radical mastectomy not only because of the impoverished blood supply to the attenuated skin and scar but also because an implant cannot begin to replace the defect left by a radical mastectomy. Any patient with a skin deficiency or tight skin from the mastectomy should not have reconstruction without the transfer of additional tissue (i.e., latissimus dorsi or TRAM). The result, most surely, will be a disappointing compromise compared with the opposite, noninvolved breast.

TISSUE EXPANDER TECHNIQUE

Tissue expanders (Fig. 21–3) have added a new dimension to breast reconstruction (Argenta, 1984). Whereas the larger flap techniques are more appropriate in reconstruction following a radical mastectomy, the number of radical mastectomies being performed has decreased dramatically. The modified radical mastectomy or simple mastectomy with axillary sampling has replaced the Halstedian mastectomy. And, as stated earlier, surgeons have been leaving thicker skin flaps. As a result, the defect to be reconstructed more often has qualitatively normal but quantitatively deficient skin. Tissue expansion has provided a technique to enlarge the skin and pocket envelope for the implant without requiring local or distant flaps. It provides a gradual stretching of the skin in much the same way as the

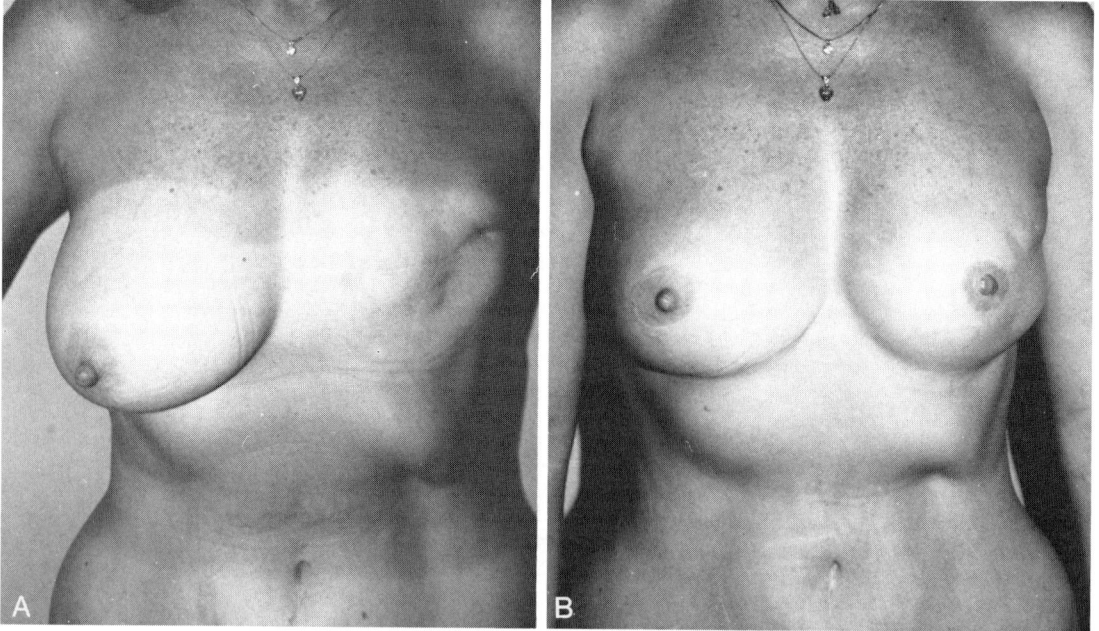

Figure 21–2. *A,* A 40 year old patient following a left modified radical mastectomy. *B,* The left breast has been reconstructed with a submuscular implant. A right breast reduction has been performed for symmetry. (Reproduced by permission from Bostwick, J.: Aesthetic and Reconstructive Breast Surgery. St. Louis, 1983, The C. V. Mosby Co.)

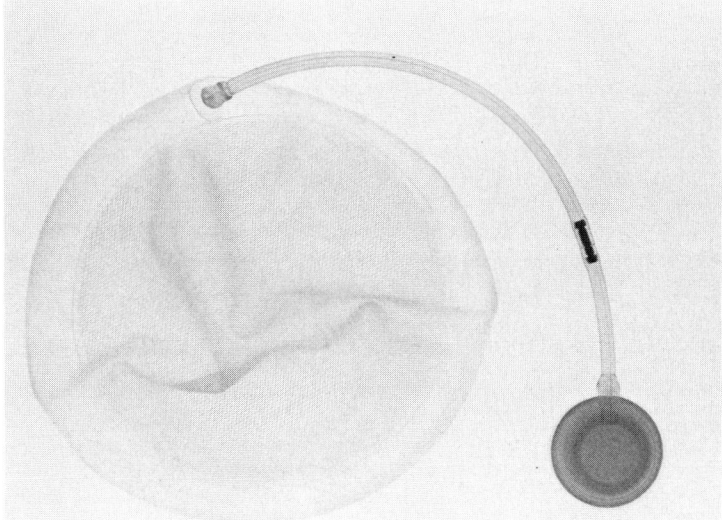

Figure 21–3. Tissue expander prior to insertion and inflation. The reservoir port through which the expander will be inflated is shown attached on the right.

abdominal skin and abdominal wall musculature stretch during pregnancy.

The technique is similar to that of reconstruction with an implant (Fig. 21–4). The mastectomy scar is excised, and the submusculofascial pocket is dissected bluntly. This can be performed either at the time of mastectomy or at a later date. The expander is placed within this space. An additional dissection is done in the subcutaneous space laterally in the midaxillary line. A reservoir attached to the expander is inserted into this space. At the time of insertion, the expander is inflated with 150 to 300 ml of saline solution, depending on the size and tightness of the pocket. After 3 weeks, the expander is filled weekly with 50 to 100 ml of saline solution.

Postoperative planning and discussion with the patient determine whether the opposite breast should be reduced, changed in shape (mastopexy), or left alone. The expander is inflated over a period of 6 to 8 weeks. To create a slightly larger breast pocket than required for the properly sized implant, an additional 200 ml of saline solution is instilled to overinflate the pocket. The expander is then removed and replaced with the appropriate silicone gel implant.

Tissue expansion for breast reconstruction is a simple technique. It provides additional skin coverage without the use of flaps. Matching of the opposite breast is made easier. There is also an early suggestion that the incidence of fibrous contracture after the insertion of the implant is less than with primary implant insertion. Complications of tissue expanders are essentially the same as with implants except that the infection rate is slightly higher.

LATISSIMUS DORSI FLAP

The latissimus dorsi flap is ideally suited for breast reconstruction when there is a skin deficiency (e.g., a tight mastectomy scar, skin graft on the chest wall, or following radiation) or when there is a large defect, such as after a radical mastectomy. A radical mastectomy defect may also be created if there has been damage to the lateral or medial pectoral nerves during a modified radical mastectomy. This will lead to atrophy of the pectoralis major muscle.

The latissimus dorsi muscle is a large, fan-shaped muscle situated in the lower part of the back. It has a very large site of origin that includes the spinous processes of the seventh through twelfth thoracic vertebrae, the thoracolumbar fascia, and the posterior one third of the iliac crest. As it ascends superiorly, it has an attachment to the inferior angle of the scapula. It then becomes a tendinous structure and inserts into the humerus.

On the basis of its vascular anatomy as defined by Mathes and Nahai (1981, 1982), the latissimus dorsi muscle is a type V muscle. This means that it has one dominant pedicle and secondary segmental vascular pedicles. This allows the surgeon to rotate the muscle or skin island anteriorly using the thoracodor-

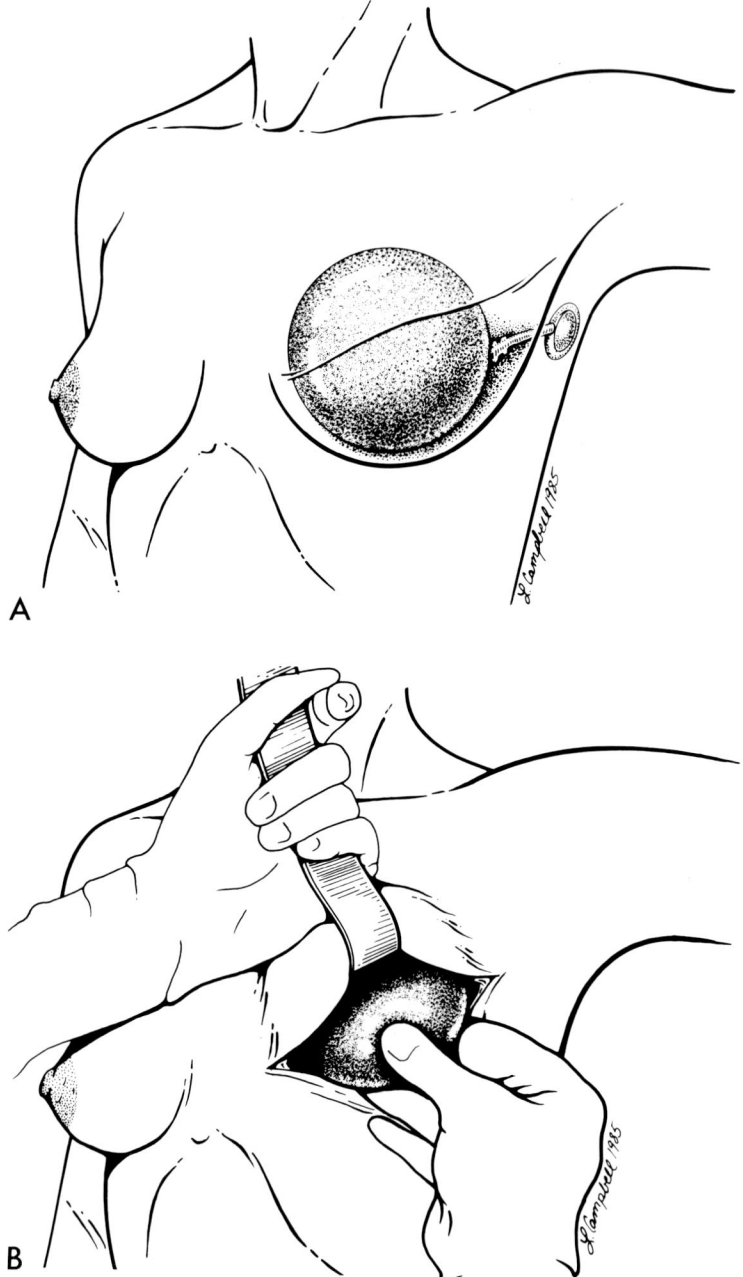

Figure 21–4. *A*, The tissue expander has been inserted through the previous mastectomy incision into a submuscular space. The reservoir is placed into a subcutaneous pocket beneath the axilla. *B*, After the expander has been fully inflated over 4 to 8 weeks, it is removed and a permanent silicone implant is inserted into the submuscular pocket.

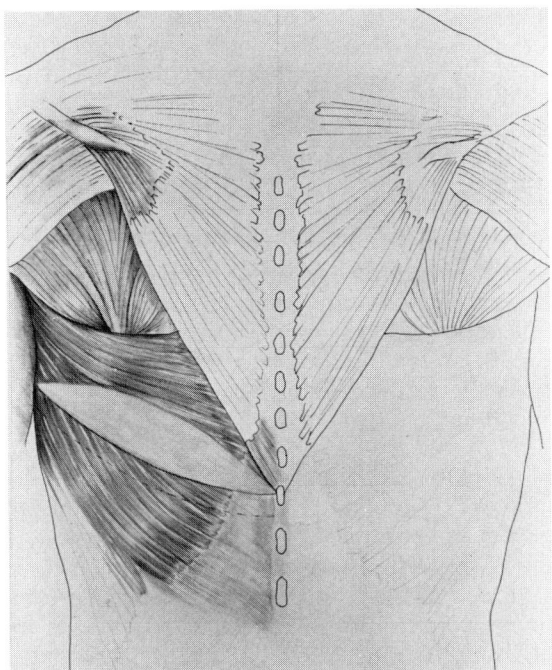

Figure 21–5. The latissimus dorsi muscle with an overlying skin island (shown here in a transverse direction).

but it cannot be used when muscle bulk is necessary to recreate the breast with a radical mastectomy defect.

During latissimus dorsi breast reconstruction, the patient is placed in the contralateral decubitus position. The skin island is usually designed transversely. The muscle is then detached from its wide origin, beginning inferiorly. Dissection continues beneath the muscle in a relatively avascular plane between the latissimus dorsi and chest wall. Care must be taken to exclude muscle fibers of the external oblique muscle inferiorly, the serratus anterior muscle superolaterally, and the teres major muscle superomedially, as these muscles are usually closely attached to the latissimus dorsi muscle in their respective locations. As the muscle is dissected toward the axilla, its vascular pedicle is identified. It is easily seen on the undersurface of the muscle in a slightly lateral position. Approximately 10 to 12 cm below the axillary vein, the thoracodorsal vessels communicate with a large serratus anterior collateral vessel. It is important not to divide this collateral, as the thoracodorsal vessels may have been ligated superiorly during the pre-

sal artery and vein, or to cover spinal defects using its medial thoracic and lumbar perforators.

The technique of latissimus dorsi breast reconstruction (Figs. 21–5 and 21–6) has been well described. Preoperatively, the surgeon must define not only the patient's anatomic deficiency but also the tissue requirements to reestablish anatomic form. For example, if there is a deficiency or lack of an axillary fold, a portion of the bulk of the latissimus dorsi muscle may be used as a surrogate. It goes without saying, therefore, that in the preoperative evaluation, careful examination of the latissimus dorsi muscle is mandatory. Although the thoracodorsal nerve is usually preserved during mastectomy, it may have been injured. A helpful maneuver is to have the patient place her hand on her hip and push firmly while the surgeon tests for contraction of the latissimus dorsi muscle. It is necessary to feel for the contraction below the tip of the scapula. Contraction of the teres major muscle (innervated by a branch of the lower subcapsular nerve) may be falsely interpreted as contraction of the latissimus dorsi muscle. If the thoracodorsal nerve has been injured, leaving the muscle atrophic, the thin layer of muscle and its skin island may still be used for implant coverage when there is a large skin deficiency,

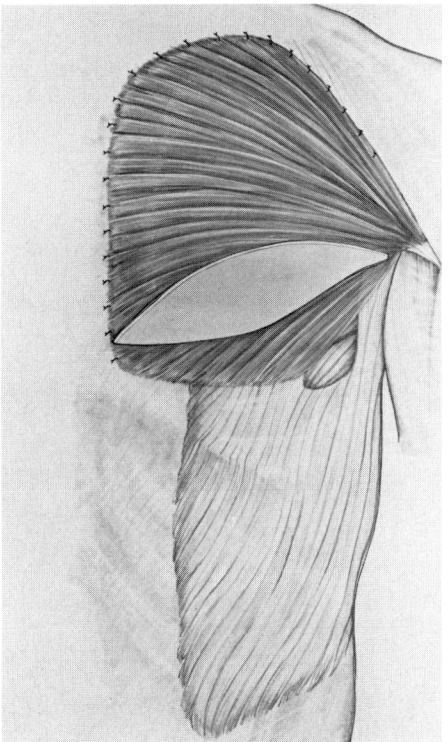

Figure 21–6. The latissimus dorsi musculocutaneous flap has been transferred to the chest wall. An implant is then placed beneath this flap.

vious mastectomy. If the thoracodorsal complex has been ligated previously, the serratus collateral vessel can adequately nourish the latissimus dorsi flap (Fisher et al., 1983). Once the latissimus dorsi flap has been raised and its vascular pedicle isolated, its tendinous insertion may be divided to allow for more complete rotation of the flap. This may be done, if necessary, through a separate transverse axillary incision. Detachment of the origin of the latissimus dorsi muscle is helpful when needed to recreate the anterior axillary fold. Care must be taken to create a superior tunnel for the latissimus dorsi flap. If the tunnel is made too large or too inferior, there is a risk that the implant will slide into a more posterolateral position underneath the arm.

Once the flap has been raised and the tunnel dissected, the back is closed after careful hemostasis. A suction drain is placed into the latissimus dorsi donor site. A dressing is then placed over the wound and the patient is placed supine.

The previous mastectomy scar is removed and sent to the pathology laboratory. Superior and inferior skin flaps are then raised to create a pocket for the implant. The latissimus dorsi skin island is planned and placed as far inferior as possible both to provide ptosis for the reconstructed breast and to keep the scars as inferior as possible. The latissimus dorsi muscle is sutured inferiorly to the pectoralis muscle and rectus fascia at the level of the inframammary crease. It is sutured superiorly beneath the clavicle. If the patient has a large infraclavicular defect, the latissimus dorsi skin island can be deepithelialized and used to fill this area.

After the muscle has been sutured into position and the appropriate esthetic tailoring completed, an appropriately sized implant is placed beneath the muscle into its pocket. At this same time, the opposite breast can be either reduced, enlarged, or changed in shape (mastopexy) to provide for a close match between the two breasts (Fig. 21–7).

The latissimus dorsi flap is a very versatile and reliable flap. The cutaneous blood supply is more direct and is not as adversely affected by smoking as is the cutaneous blood supply of the TRAM flap. Complications relating to partial or total flap necrosis are seen in fewer than 5 per cent of patients. Because an implant is used, capsular contracture resulting in a firm breast can still occur. A seroma develops in the donor site in 30 to 50 per cent of patients. This is usually a minor problem and resolves with aspiration.

The latissimus dorsi flap is still a very useful procedure for breast reconstruction. As is discussed in more detail later, there are many instances in which a TRAM flap is contraindicated. For example, if a patient has been a heavy smoker and has poor cutaneous circulation, the latissimus dorsi flap is more reliable than a TRAM flap. If a patient has had mul-

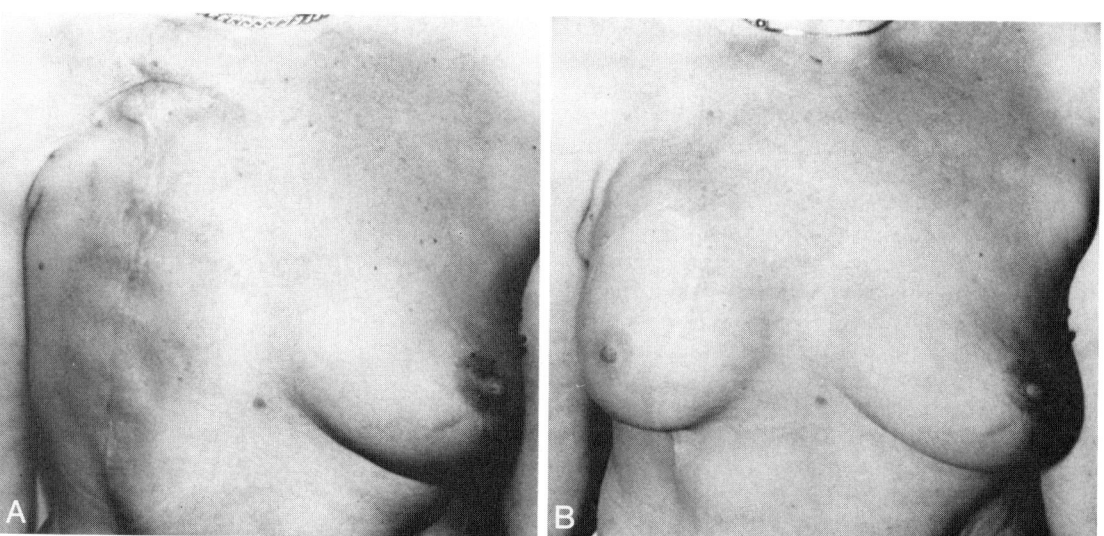

Figure 21–7. *A*, A 64 year old patient after a right radical mastectomy. *B*, The right breast was reconstructed using a latissimus dorsi flap and implant. (Reproduced by permission from Bostwick, J.: Aesthetic and Reconstructive Breast Surgery. St. Louis, 1983, The C. V. Mosby Co.)

tiple abdominal incisions, especially ones that divide the upper rectus abdominis muscle, a TRAM breast reconstruction may not be possible. A patient with a history of moderate to severe low back pain can have this condition worsened by a TRAM flap, thereby making the latissimus dorsi flap the procedure of choice in such a patient. Finally, there are patients with a paucity of lower abdominal fat in whom a TRAM flap would not provide adequate fatty tissue for breast replacement without an implant. In such patients, a latissimus dorsi flap or free tissue transfer may provide the best form of reconstruction.

THE TRANSVERSE RECTUS ABDOMINIS MYOCUTANEOUS (TRAM) FLAP

The latest major addition to flap breast reconstruction has been the TRAM flap. It was developed as an outgrowth of research with myocutaneous flaps. This method offers many advantages over the latissimus dorsi flap. Because of the amount of fatty tissue transferred with the TRAM flap, the addition of an implant usually is not necessary. This avoids the possible development of a capsular contracture in the reconstructed breast. There is usually an abundance of subcutaneous tissue available with the TRAM flap such that even very large defects can be reconstructed. In cases of bilateral reconstruction, each rectus muscle can be transferred with its corresponding skin and subcutaneous tissue at the same time. A second advantage of the TRAM flap is that in addition to providing ample tissue for breast reconstruction, the abdominal wall reconstruction (i.e., abdominoplasty) results in an improved body contour. Finally, the contour and consistency of the transferred abdominal fat in the TRAM flap are very similar to those of the normal breast.

The development of the TRAM flap and its vascular anatomy has helped in the understanding of the blood supply to the anterior abdominal wall. The rectus abdominis muscle is supplied primarily by the superior and inferior epigastric vessels. The rectus abdominis muscle receives an additional blood supply from lateral intercostal vessels. The superior and inferior epigastric vessels arborize within the muscle belly. There are anterior perforating vessels that traverse the anterior rectus sheath and provide blood supply to a large island of anterior abdominal skin. The majority of these perforating vessels are located in the periumbilical area (Fig. 21–8). A large transverse elliptical island of middle to lower abdominal skin can be raised with one or both rectus abdominis muscles and a portion of the anterior rectus sheath. This can be mobilized up to the costal margin with care to include the medial and lateral rectus perforators. The lateral intercostal collateral vessels and intercostal nerves are divided in the process of raising the flap. In the case of a unilateral breast reconstruction with a single rectus pedicle, the contralateral rectus muscle is usually better used, as this provides for a better arc of rotation of the vascular bundle. A tunnel is then made that communicates with the dissection used to raise the mastectomy skin flaps (Fig. 21–9). The TRAM flap is placed gently through this tunnel. The appropriate trimming and contouring of the new breast is then accomplished (Figs. 21–10 and 21–11). The results obtained with the TRAM flap for breast reconstruction have been highly satisfactory (Figs. 21–12 and 21–13).

Much attention has been given to closure of the abdominal wall when a TRAM flap has been used. Hartrampf (1985) has performed over 200 TRAM breast reconstructions and finds that abdominal wall closure can be accomplished with the existing anterior rectus sheath in the majority of cases. Bostwick (1985), on the other hand, prefers to strengthen the abdominal wall closure with Prolene mesh. He believes that adding the Prolene mesh to the closure will decrease the hernia rate. This also aids in a tighter closure, resulting in a more esthetic abdominal contour.

The TRAM flap is a technically demanding procedure for the surgeon and a physically demanding procedure for the patient. There are many fine details that must be followed to obtain a healthy, viable flap. Patient selection is critical. Most patients receive between two and four units of blood during and immediately following the procedure. The hospital stay ranges between 5 and 7 days.

The TRAM flap is contraindicated in a patient with a heavy smoking history. It should not be performed in any patient who has a compromised cutaneous circulation (e.g., lupus erythematosus). A frequent complaint following a TRAM breast reconstruction is low back pain for several weeks. If the patient has had back difficulty prior to breast reconstruction, a TRAM flap can certainly exacerbate

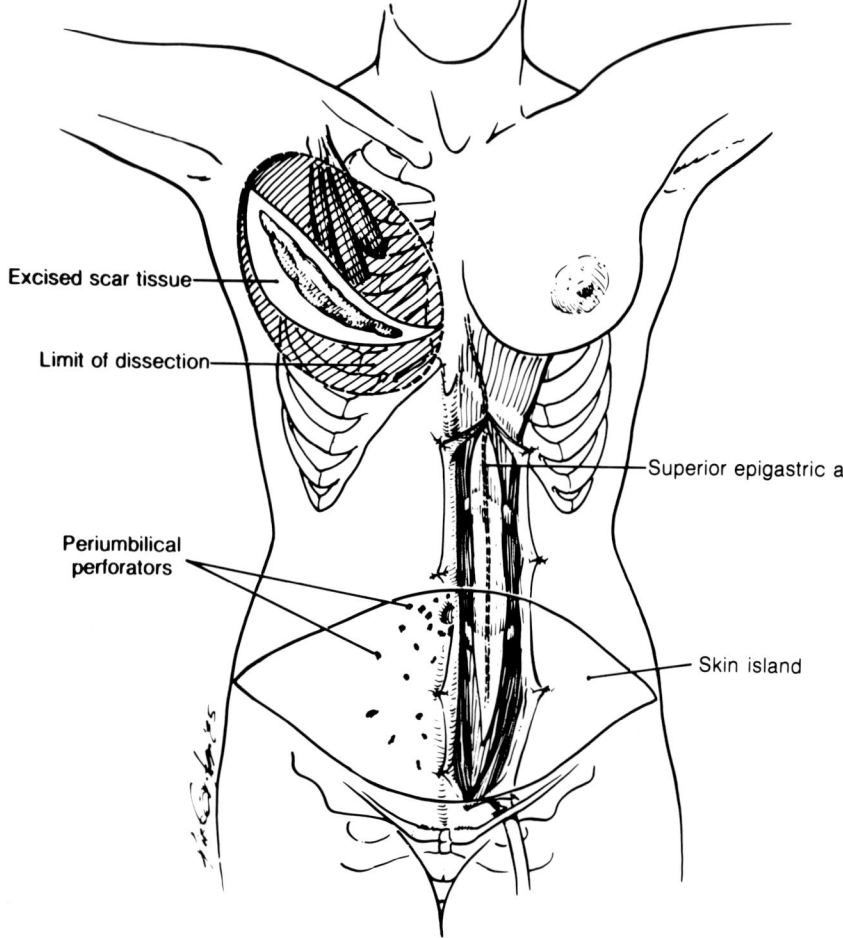

Figure 21–8. The TRAM flap consists of an elliptical island of skin and subcutaneous tissue from the lower abdomen based on the rectus abdominis muscle. (Reprinted with permission from Sands, W., and Jurkiewicz, M. J.: An approach to repair of radiation necrosis of chest wall and mammary gland. World J. Surg., *10*:206, 1986.)

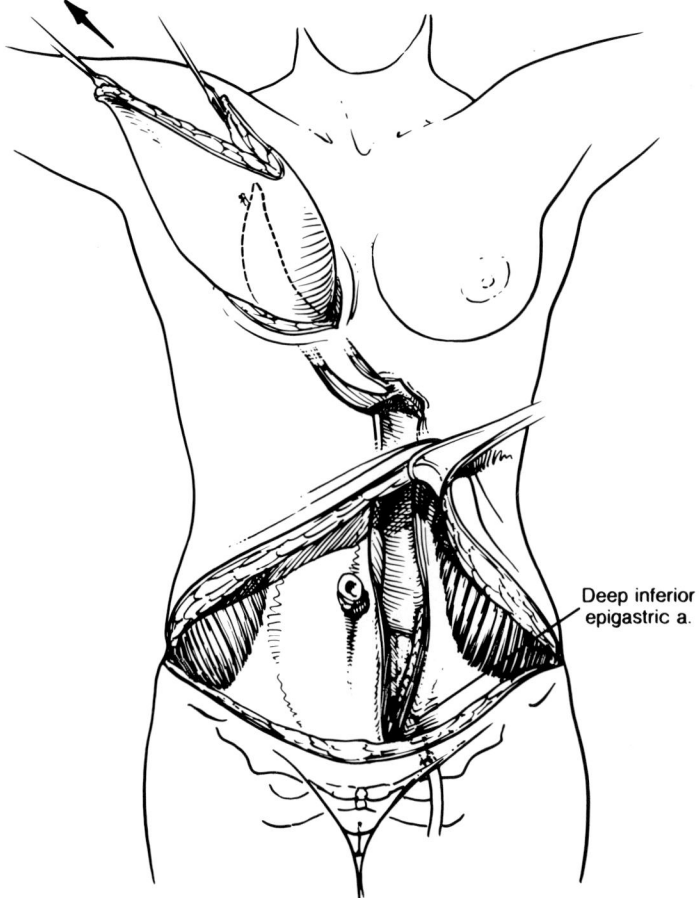

Figure 21–9. The TRAM flap has been elevated from its anatomic position, rotated in a clock-wise fashion, and transferred to the chest wall. The deep inferior epigastric artery and vein are ligated. (Reprinted with permission from Sands, W., and Jurkiewicz, M. J.: An approach to repair of radiation necrosis of chest wall and mammary gland. World J. Surg., *10*:206, 1986.)

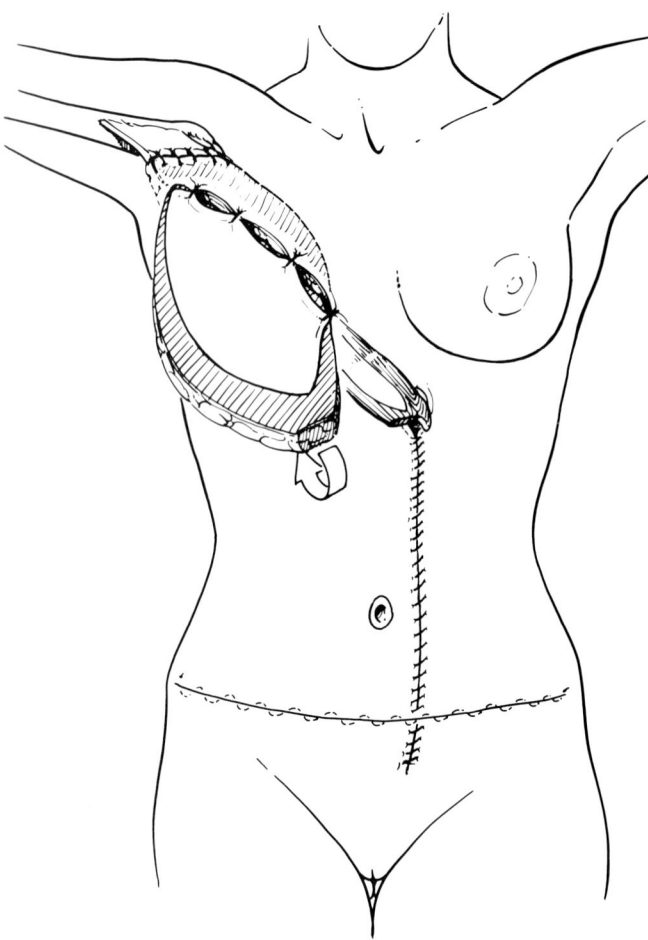

Figure 21–10. The left anterior rectus sheath and abdominal incision have been closed, the new umbilicus created, and the TRAM flap contoured and trimmed to reconstruct an aesthetic unit. (Reprinted with permission from Sands, W., and Jurkiewicz, M. J.: An approach to repair of radiation necrosis of chest wall and mammary gland. World J. Surg., *10*:206, 1986.)

Figure 21–11. The completed breast reconstruction. (Reprinted with permission from Sands, W., and Jurkiewicz, M. J.: An approach to repair of radiation necrosis of chest wall and mammary gland. World J. Surg., *10*:206, 1986.)

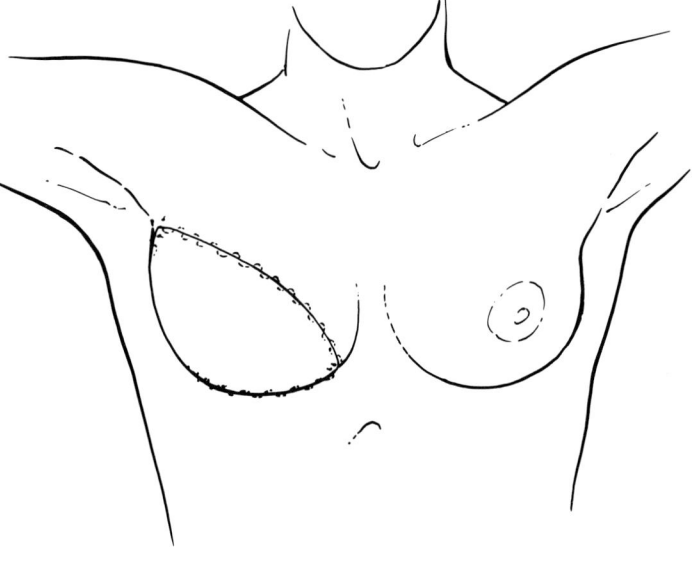

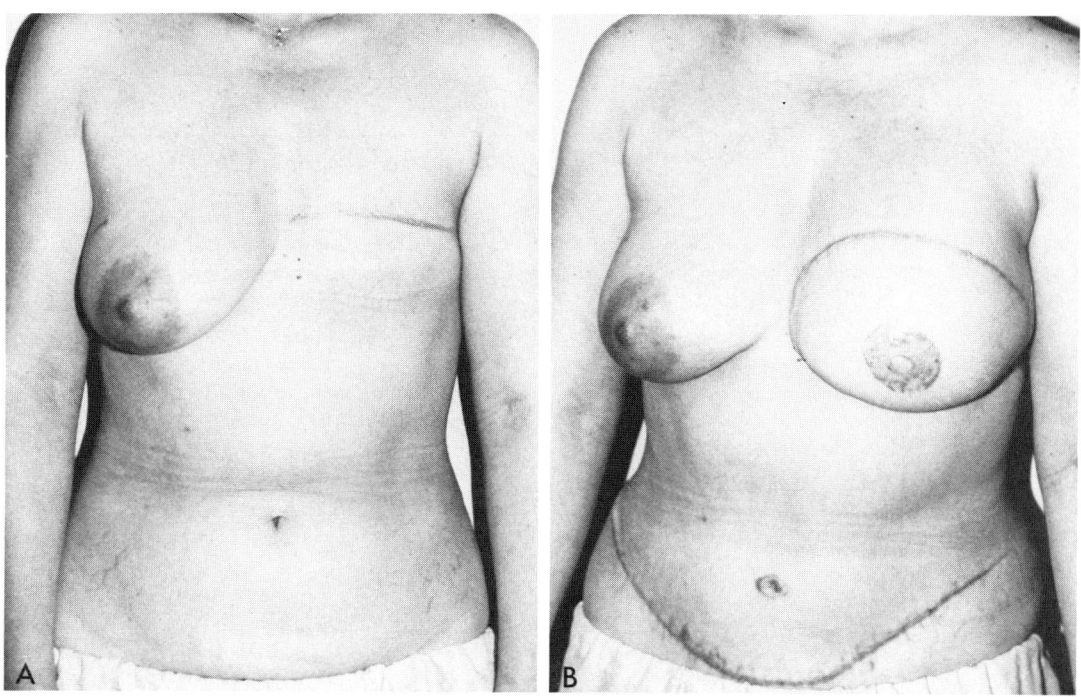

Figure 21–12. *A,* A 38 year old patient following a left modified radical mastectomy. *B,* The patient is shown following a single pedicle TRAM reconstruction and nipple-areolar reconstruction. (From Hartrampf, C. R.: Transverse Abdominal Island Flap Technique. Rockville, Md., Aspen Systems Corporation, 1984, p. 41. Reprinted with permission.)

this condition. A previous Kocher incision results in ligation of the right superior epigastric vessels. A TRAM based on the right rectus abdominis is therefore not possible in such a patient. In such cases, the left TRAM can be used to reconstruct either breast. If both rectus abdominis muscles are necessary in the breast or chest wall reconstruction and one of the pedicles has been ligated, the corresponding deep inferior epigastric artery (DIEA) can be dissected with the muscle and anastomosed to the axillary vessels using microvascular technique. This principle of enhancement of the blood supply to the distal portion of a flap was first described by Longmire in 1945 in a modification of Roux's operation for esophageal reconstruction using jejunum (Longmire, 1947).

The complications of the TRAM flap are generally related to the skill and experience of the surgeon. Because of the large amount of dissection, postoperative hematomas and seromas are an infrequent yet well-recognized complication. Partial or total flap loss can be kept to a minimum through careful patient selection and dissection. Abdominal wall hernias following TRAM flaps are infrequent but do occur. An as yet unanswered question regarding the TRAM flap is the long-term effect on the stability and strength of the abdominal wall caused by the removal of one or both rectus muscles. In the first 5 years of follow-up, this does not appear to be a major problem. However, long-term follow-up is necessary to answer this question satisfactorily.

MICROVASCULAR TISSUE TRANSFER IN BREAST RECONSTRUCTION

The advent of microsurgery in the past 10 years has had far-reaching effects on almost all areas of reconstruction. It has been extended to the field of breast reconstruction and can be used in very carefully selected patients (Serafin et al., 1982). There are some patients who do not have local flaps available to reconstruct their breast defect. These patients usually require replacement with a large amount of skin and soft tissue. The patient's largest source of local tissue (the TRAM flaps) may either not be available owing to prior surgery or be deficient in the very thin patient. In such

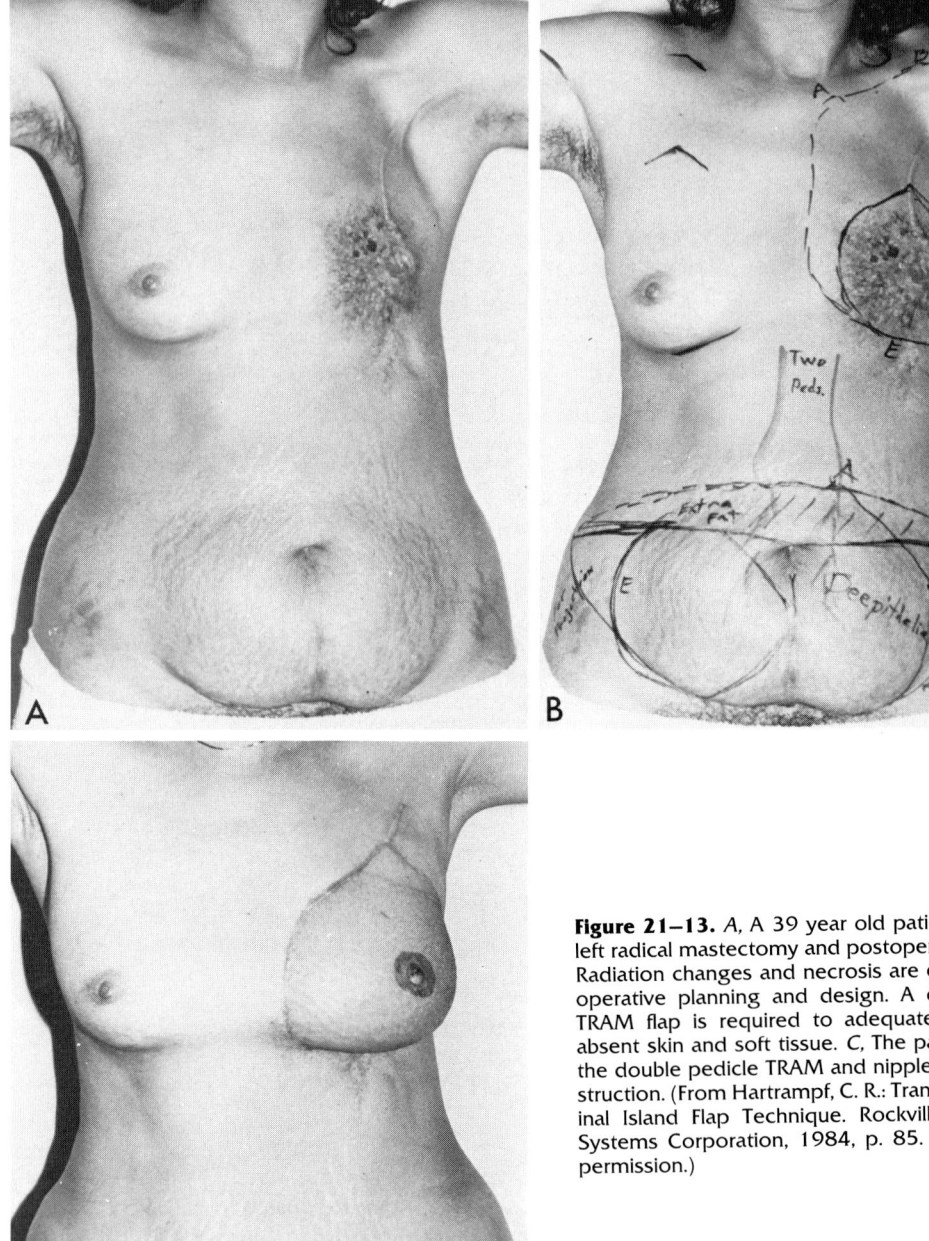

Figure 21–13. *A*, A 39 year old patient following a left radical mastectomy and postoperative radiation. Radiation changes and necrosis are evident. *B*, Preoperative planning and design. A double pedicle TRAM flap is required to adequately replace the absent skin and soft tissue. *C*, The patient following the double pedicle TRAM and nipple-areolar reconstruction. (From Hartrampf, C. R.: Transverse Abdominal Island Flap Technique. Rockville, Md., Aspen Systems Corporation, 1984, p. 85. Reprinted with permission.)

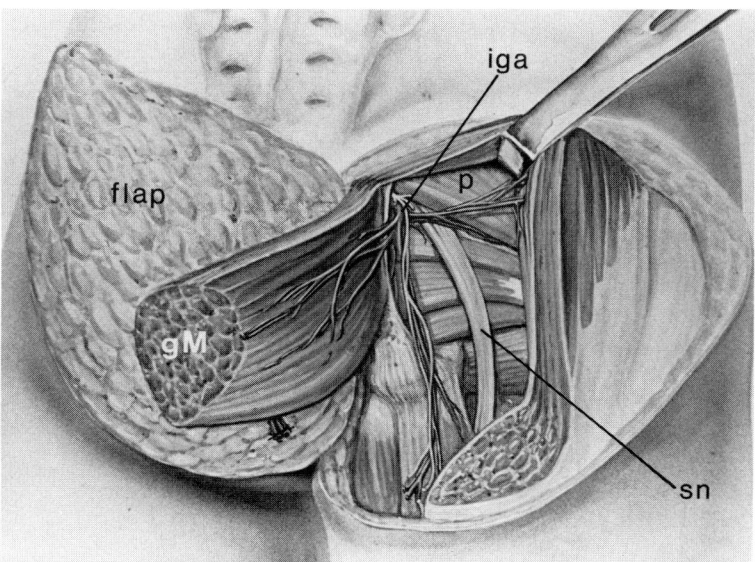

Figure 21–14. The anatomy and dissection of the inferior gluteal flap for microvascular free tissue transfer. *gM*, Gluteus maximus; *iga*, inferior gluteal artery; *sn*, sciatic nerve; *p*, piriformis muscle.

patients, microsurgical tissue transfer (i.e., free flap) can provide an esthetic breast reconstruction with an acceptable donor defect. Although many different free flaps have been described for breast reconstruction, the most promising appear to be the superior gluteal flap as described by Shaw and the inferior gluteal flap (Le-Quang, 1979; Shaw, 1983; Nahai et al., in press). In each flap, a large transverse island of skin with its underlying fat and a small segment of gluteal muscle is dissected with its corresponding gluteal vessel (Figs. 21–14 and 21–15). This composite flap is then transferred to the chest wall. The donor site on the buttock is closed primarily. Microvascular transfer is performed using either the internal mammary vessels or the axillary vessels. Early reports on this technique have been promising. When used as an alternative to the TRAM flap, its primary disadvantage is that because of the microvascular technique, it is technically demanding.

NIPPLE-AREOLA RECONSTRUCTION

Nipple-areola reconstruction represents the final stage of breast reconstruction. The nipple and areola are usually reconstructed between 6 and 12 weeks following the initial breast reconstruction procedure. At this time, any additional scar revisions or fine adjustments of the original reconstruction may be accomplished.

The position of the nipple-areolar complex is determined with the patient standing or in a sitting position. The area of the areola is then deepithelialized over a circle measuring between 38 and 42 mm. A full-thickness skin graft is then harvested from the upper, inner medial aspect of the thigh. The donor site is then closed primarily using 3–0 or 4–0 chromic suture.

The nipple is reconstructed either with a full-thickness skin graft from the thigh crease, or, if the opposite nipple is sufficiently large, by excising one half the opposite nipple as a nipple-sharing technique.

The areolar and nipple grafts are then sutured in place using a 3–0 silk stent dressing. This is left intact for 3 to 5 days, after which the stent is removed and the grafts are covered with Steristrips.

There have been many different variants in nipple-areola reconstruction technique (Gruber, 1979). These include the use of small local flaps, ear cartilage, and so forth. Some early work is now being done using a permanent tattoo-type material similar to that used with the permanent eye-liner. Regardless of the type of technique used, the challenge is to provide nipple projection and a permanent pigmentation of the areola.

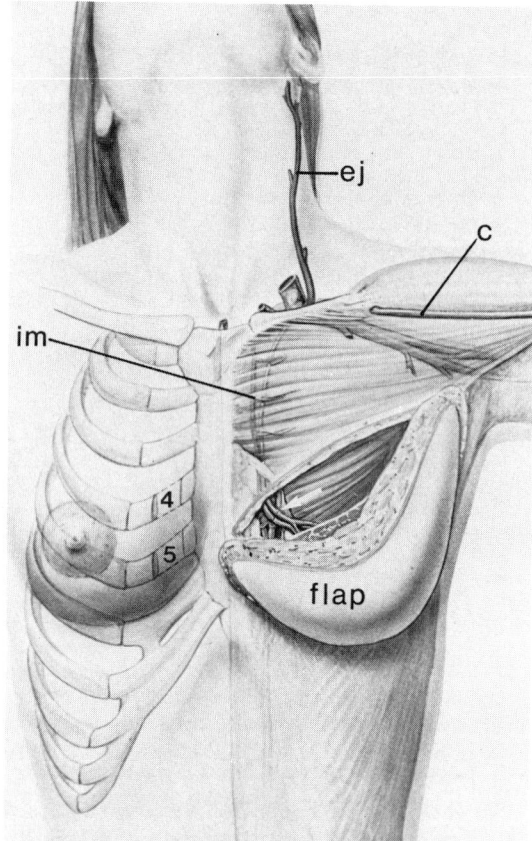

Figure 21–15. The inferior gluteal flap has been transferred to the chest. The inferior gluteal vessels are anastomosed to the internal mammary vessels. If the internal mammary vein is not suitable for anastomosis, the cephalic vein or external jugular vein can be used. *ej,* External jugular vein; *c,* cephalic vein; *im,* internal mammary vessels.

Summary

The current state of the art in postmastectomy reconstruction involves the application of new and developing plastic surgery techniques (Bostwick, 1984). The results are far superior to those in the past. Although the results are quite good, it should not be forgotten that breast reconstruction is not an end unto itself but has been developed to provide substantial psychologic support that permits patients to deal with breast cancer and with the change in body image. Continual refinement and simplification of techniques should help to bring both cost and availability into equilibrium with need, demand, and societal resources (Kiser, 1985).

REFERENCES

Argenta, L.: Reconstruction of the breast by tissue expansion. Clin. Plast. Surg., *11*:257, 1984.

Bostwick, J., III: Aesthetic and Reconstructive Breast Surgery. St. Louis, C. V. Mosby, 1984.

Bostwick, J.: Breast reconstruction following mastectomy. Contemp. Surg., *27*:15, 1985.

Bostwick, J., and Berger, K.: A Woman's Choice. St. Louis, C. V. Mosby, 1984.

Bostwick, J., Nahai, E., Wallace, J. G., et al.: Sixty latissimus dorsi flaps. Plast. Reconstr. Surg., *63*:31, 1979.

Cronin, T. D., Upton, J., and McDonough, J. M.: Reconstruction of the breast after mastectomy. Plast. Reconstr. Surg., *59*:1, 1977.

Drever, J. M.: Immediate breast reconstruction after mastectomy using a rectus abdominis myodermal flap without an implant. Can. J. Surg., *25*:429, 1982.

Fisher, J., Bostwick, J., III, and Powell, R. W.: Latissimus dorsi blood supply after thoracodorsal vessel division: The serratus collateral. Plast. Reconstr. Surg., *72*:502, 1983.

Frazier, T. G., and Noone, R. B.: An objective analysis of immediate simultaneous reconstruction in the treatment of primary carcinoma of the breast. Cancer, *55*:1202, 1985.

Gilliland, M. D.: Appropriate timing for breast reconstruction. Plast. Reconstr. Surg., *72*:335, 1983.

Gruber, R. P.: Nipple-areola reconstruction: A review of techniques. Clin. Plast. Surg., *6*:71, 1979.

Hartrampf, C. R.: Transverse abdominal island flap technique for breast reconstruction after mastectomy. Baltimore, University Park Press, 1984.

Hartrampf, C. R.: Closure of the donor defect for breast reconstruction with rectus abdominis myocutaneous flaps (discussion). Plast. Reconstr. Surg., *76*:563, 1985.

Hartrampf, C. R., et al.: Breast reconstruction with a transverse abdominal island flap. Plast. Reconstr. Surg., *69*:216, 1982.

Kiser, W. S.: Buying and selling health care: A battle for the medical marketplace. Bull. Am. Coll. Surg., *70*, 1985.

Le-Quang C.: Two new free flaps proceeding from aesthetic surgery: The lateral mammary flap and the inferior gluteal flap. Transactions of the 7th International Congress of Plastic and Reconstructive Surgery, Rio De Janeiro, 1979.

Longmire, W. P., Jr.: A modification of the Roux technique for antethoracic esophageal reconstruction. Surgery, *22*:94, 1947.

Marshall, D. R.: Immediate reconstruction of the breast following modified radical mastectomy for carcinoma. Br. J. Plast. Surg., *35*:438, 1982.

Mathes, S. J., and Nahai, F.: Classification of the vascular anatomy of muscles: experimental and clinical correlation. Plast. Reconstr. Surg., *67*:177, 1981.

Mathes, S. J., and Nahai, F.: Clinical Applications for Muscle and Myocutaneous Flaps. St. Louis, C. V. Mosby, 1982.

Nahai, F., Bostwick, J., III, and Paletta, C.: The inferior gluteal free flap in breast reconstruction (Abstract) (in press).

Noone, R. B., Murphy, J. B., Spear, S. L., et al.: A 6-year experience with immediate reconstruction after mastectomy for cancer. Plast. Reconstr. Surg., *76*:258, 1985.

Pers, M.: The selection of patients for reconstruction following mastectomy for carcinoma of the breast. Br. J. Plast. Surg., *34*:58, 1981.

Radovan, C.: Breast reconstruction after mastectomy using the temporary expander. Plast. Reconstr. Surg., *69*:195, 1982.

Radovan, C.: Tissue expansion in soft-tissue reconstruction. Plast Reconstr. Surg., *74*:482, 1984.

Schneider, W. J., Hill, H. L., and Brown, R. G.: Latissimus dorsi myocutaneous flap for breast reconstruction. Br. J. Plast. Surg., *30*:277, 1977.

Serafin, D., Voci, V. E., and Georgiade, N. G.: Microsurgical composite tissue transplantation: Indications and technical considerations in breast reconstruction following mastectomy. Plast. Reconstr. Surg., *70*:24, 1982.

Shaw, W. W.: Breast reconstruction by superior gluteal microvascular free flaps without silicone implants. Plast. Reconstr. Surg., *72*:490, 1983.

Webster, J. P., and Gnudi, M. T.: The life and times of Gaspare Tagliacozzi, surgeon of Bologna, 1545–1599. New York, Herbert Reichner, 1950.

Webster, D., Mansel, R. E., and Hughes, L. E.: Immediate reconstruction of the breast after mastectomy: Is it safe? Cancer, *53*:1416, 1984.

Zimmerman, K. W., Montague, E. D., and Fletcher, G. H.: Frequency, anatomic distribution, and management of local recurrences after definitive therapy for breast cancer. Cancer, *19*:67, 1966.

CHAPTER 22

WILLIAM L. DONEGAN
JOHN S. SPRATT

Multiple Primary Cancers in Mammary and Extramammary Sites and Cancers Metastatic to the Breast

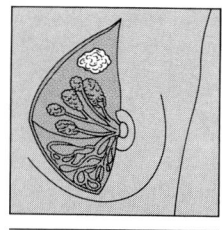

The multiplicity of neoplasms in the same individual discovered either simultaneously or nonsimultaneously is a complex issue. Factors of concern include predisposing causes or associations and management strategies. A clinically related and sometimes confounding issue is the discovery of cancers of remote sites that metastasize to the breast as well as metastases to remote sites from occult breast cancers.

Cancers and sarcomas arising primarily in the breast other than adenocarcinomas also are a concern, but these are covered in other chapters of the book, as are primary adenocarcinomas of aberrant breast tissue. Clearly, the major focus of both simultaneous and nonsimultaneous breast cancer is in the breast tissue remaining after ablation of the first cancer.

Among a series of 710 women with breast cancer followed for up to 20 years for a total of 3643 woman-years of observation, 52 second cancers were diagnosed. Twenty-two of these were prevalent cancers diagnosed at the same time the first breast cancer was diagnosed (3.09 per cent prevalence rate for synchronous cancers). Within 20 years of diagnosis, the accumulative discovery of second cancers reached 21.4 per cent in follow-up, using the life table method of analyzing follow-up data. Adding the prevalent synchronous second cancers, the accumulative rate for the observed population reached 24.49 per cent. However, these rates were not significantly greater than the expected rates for a population of the same age or those actually observed in a control population of women drawn from the same hospital. The distribution of second cancers is shown in Table 22–1. Clearly, the dominant sites for additional cancers are the skin and the remaining breast, with cancers of the colorectum a distant third. If the breast is classified as a skin appendage, as is proper, 42 of 52 (81 per cent) of the multiple primary cancers associated with breast cancer can be said to be of integumental origin in this study (Spratt and Hoag, 1966; Spratt, 1977).

Cook (1966) reviewed the literature for multiple cancers paired at different anatomic sites with a probability greater than could be attributed to chance and found only 12 significantly paired sites. The breast paired with only one site: the endometrium. Lee (1984) reported observations on 665 additional patients treated between 1966 to 1980. Forty-six patients had developed carcinoma of the opposite breast and 30 had developed nonmammary second cancers at the time of this report. Ten patients had a nonmammary cancer diagnosed before the breast cancer was confirmed. In Lee's series, the associations considered as accumu-

Table 22–1. TYPES OF SECOND CANCERS DIAGNOSED AMONG 710 WOMEN WITH BREAST CANCER THROUGH 20 YEARS OF FOLLOW-UP (SIMULTANEOUS AND NONSIMULTANEOUS)

Site	Simultaneous or Within 1 Year of Diagnosis	Nonsimultaneous Diagnosed From 1 to 20 Years After First Diagnosis	Total
Skin	12	10	22
Cervix	1		1
Breast	8	12	20
Endometrium	1		1
Colorectum		4	4
Vulva		2	2
Hodgkin's disease		1	1
Esophagus		1	1
Total	22	30	52

lations of age-specific incidence were no greater than would be predicted by chance alone.

The association of breast and salivary gland carcinoma has been reported in several studies (Berg et al., 1968; Moertel and Elvebeck, 1969; Dunn et al., 1972). Berg and coworkers (1968) and Moertel and Elvebeck (1969) were, however, unable to confirm this association in the data from the California Tumor Registry.

The statistical methods for the analysis of tumor multiplicity data are quite complex and require large numbers of well-documented cases followed for long periods of time. Many clinical studies define only the accumulative prevalence of associated events, not coming to grips with the question or whether the associations are due to chance alone. Improvements in perspective began to evolve with the use of the actuarial method by Spratt and Hoag (1966) and refined by Schoenberg (1977). A further refinement in statistical methods for dealing with tumor multiplicity data has been reported by Drinkwater and Klotz (1981) and was tested in an animal model. The additional cancers, regarded as infrequent events, produced data that fitted best the negative binomial distribution. These authors concluded that the likelihood ratio statistic based on the negative binomial model was useful for testing the difference between two groups with presumed differences in tumor multiplicity. This approach is applicable to human data and might help resolve some of the unanswered issues regarding the degree of risk. In the final analysis, any management strategy must be shown to reduce the risk of dying from breast cancer.

The updated reports of multiple primary cancers recorded in the cancer registries of Connecticut and Denmark provide observations in very large data bases (Multiple Primary Cancers in Connecticut and Denmark, 1985).

Cancers of the Second Breast

The breast is a paired organ and, as cancer of this organ is frequently a multifocal process, it is not unusual for a woman to develop independent cancers in both breasts. Compared with the normal population, a woman treated for cancer of one breast is five times more likely to be afflicted a second time (Robbins and Berg, 1964). Occasionally, bilateral involvement is evident at the outset, but in the majority of cases disease appears in the second breast as a subsequent development. The criteria for distinguishing second primary tumors from metastases and for the diagnosis and treatment of second primary cancers as well as the merit of prophylactic mastectomy have been subjects of attention.

CRITERIA FOR DIAGNOSIS

Billroth's original criteria for the diagnosis of independent cancers were stringent, requiring that the tumors have different histologic features, be located in different organs, and be responsible for separate metastases (Pennell, 1958; Kapsinow, 1962). The more liberal criteria later developed by Warren and Gates (1932), which required only that the tumors be malignant and separate and that neither represent a metastasis, found more general acceptance.

The fact is that, except for a small group of special histologic types, the majority of breast cancers have similar features microscopically. Robbins and Berg (1964) appreciated this reality and, in defining a series of 94 patients with bilateral breast cancers, emphasized the following points in making the diagnosis of second primary tumors:

1. Second primary cancers can be expected to develop within breast tissue, most frequently in the upper outer quadrant but not in the fatty tail of the breast; metastases appear in the fat at the periphery of the breast parenchyma, usually near the midline or in the fatty tail.

2. Metastases tend to be multiple and to show expansile growth rather than an infiltrative stellate pattern characteristic of primary tumors.

3. Most importantly, primary tumors are often associated with contiguous in situ carcinoma while metastases lack this feature. Medullary carcinoma, around which in situ cancer is not expected, is an exception to the rule.

In addition to these criteria, Leis (1971) accepted the diagnosis of a second primary tumor if the degree of nuclear differentiation was definitely greater than that of the first cancer or if the second lesion occurred more than 5 years after the first in the absence of evidence of metastasis elsewhere.

Liberal criteria were accepted in our studies at the Ellis Fischel State Cancer Hospital (EFSCH). If carcinoma was found within the parenchyma of the second breast at the time of, or at any time subsequent to, treatment of the first primary tumor and thorough clinical, roentgenographic, and laboratory evaluations revealed no evidence of dissemination, the second lesion was considered an independent primary cancer rather than a metastasis. This policy gives the patient the benefit of the most optimistic interpretation of a lesion in the second breast.

Any cancer in the second breast is more likely to be a new primary tumor than a metastasis, particularly if the interval after mastectomy is great (Egan, 1976; Shellito and Bartlett, 1967). At EFSCH, only 3 per cent of initial recurrences of cancer after mastectomy occurred in the opposite breast (approximately 1.5 per cent of all surgical cases), whereas 3 per cent of all surgical cases developed new mammary primary tumors (Donegan, 1970).

INCIDENCE

Bilateral cancers are categorized as simultaneous or nonsimultaneous, depending on whether they are diagnosed at the same time or at different times, the second usually being found after the first cancer is treated. Because of the variability of neoplastic growth and a potentially prolonged preclinical existence, it is not always possible to be certain whether and for how long two neoplasms have coexisted. Nevertheless, in the majority of cases, involvement of the second breast is recognized clinically as a subsequent development. According to 22 reports prior to 1965 collected from the literature by Leis and associates (1965), bilateral simultaneous mammary cancers were diagnosed in from 0.1 to 2 per cent of cases. Nonsimultaneous second primary cancers developed in from 1 to 12 per cent of cases during varying periods of observation, with a median figure of 3.2 per cent. Most authors estimate that 7 to 10 per cent of women ultimately develop an independent cancer in the remaining breast (Kilgore, 1921; Harrington, 1946; Trevor, 1954; Fitts, 1955; Robbins and Berg, 1964).

The Israeli experience with multiple primary malignant neoplasms in breast cancer patients has been reported for an 18 year period with 12,302 cases (Schenker et al., 1984). During the period of observation, 984 patients (8 per cent) had more than one cancer, and 47 (0.4 per cent) developed at least two cancers in addition to the breast cancer. The investigators concluded that the additional cancers occurred with an incidence greater than expected for five sites: opposite breast, salivary glands, uterine corpus, ovary, and thyroid. Cancers of the stomach and gallbladder occurred less frequently than expected. Whenever the primary breast cancer had been treated by irradiation, the risk of additional primary cancers exceeded the expected risk for the lung and hematopoietic system.

The experience at EFSCH with simultaneous cancers has been consistent with reports from elsewhere. Fifty-two, or 2 per cent, of 2620 women with cancer of the breast seen at EFSCH during the period 1940 to 1965 initially had bilateral mammary cancers. The frequency of nonsimultaneous cancers varies somewhat in surgical series at this institution. In a review of 704 women with no previous cancers who were treated with radical mastectomy for an initial unilateral mammary cancer and observed for 5 to 18 years, 14, or 2 per cent, developed a second clinical primary tumor in the remaining breast within 7 years (Table 22-2). After 7 years, additional cases accrued, but the data do not permit reliable evaluation. More recently, 167 patients with clinically early unilateral cancers were treated with radical mastectomy between 1963 and 1972, with or without the addition of adjuvant Thiotepa, and were closely observed for an average period of 63 months, during which 55.7 per cent of the patients died. Five, or 3 per cent, developed clinical cancers in the remaining breast from four to 30 months after the original mastectomy. In two additional cases, occult

Table 22–2. SIMULTANEOUS AND NONSIMULTANEOUS SECOND PRIMARY BREAST CARCINOMAS AT EFSCH, 1940 TO JUNE 1958

Simultaneous

Age	First Primary Treated				Second Primary Treated				Survival After Treatment	
	Duration of Symptoms (months)	Stage (CCC*)	Axillary Lymph Nodes	Diameter (cm)	Duration of Symptoms (months)	Stage (CCC*)	Axillary Lymph Nodes	Diameter (cm)	First Primary (months)	Second Primary (months)
82	9	A	+	3.0	0	A	Unk‡	2.5	21	20
68	24	A	−	2.0	28	B	−	2.4	126	122
56	12	A	+	5.0	25	B	+	5.0	182	181
68	25	A	−	1.0	2	A	−	2.5	93	92
63	1	B	+	Unk	3	A	+	3.3	42	40
49	12	B	−	8.5	6	B	+	7.0	19	19
78	9	C	Unk†	1.5	6	A	−	6.0	14	13

Nonsimultaneous

Age	First Primary				Duration of Interval: Treatment of First to Symptoms of Second (months)	Second Primary				Survival After Treatment	
	Duration of Symptoms (months)	Stage (CCC*)	Axillary Lymph Nodes	Diameter (cm)		Duration of Symptoms (months)	Stage (CCC*)	Axillary Lymph Nodes	Diameter (cm)	First Primary (months)	Second Primary (months)
68	21	A	−	3.0	79	4	A	−	4.0	120	40
38	3	A	+	6.0	48	7	B	+	8.0	61	6
61	4	A	−	<4.0	10	4	D	+	1.5	30	17
55	24	B	+	3.8	26	2	B	−	2.3	101	73
43	1	B	−	2.0	37	2	B	+	1.5	67	28
43	2	B	+	1.0	43	1	C	+	1.5	112	69
51	3	B	+	2.0	6	0	B	+	2.5	251	244
40	54	B	+	4.0	70	2	B	+	3.0	235	162
39	12	B	+	4.5	17	9	B	+	3.5	39	13
67	12	B	+	3.5	123	2	A	Unk†	2.0	177	53
74	18	B	−	4.0	45	7	B	−	3.0	159	107
76	48	B	−	9.0	79	1	D	+	2.0	97	19
72	6	B	−	2.0	27	8	B	+	4.5	166	131
75	24	C	+	5.0	14	1	A	−	1.0	91	77
51	6	C	+	7.5	13	3	A	+	5.0	24	8

*Columbia Clinical Classification.
†Unk, Unknown (simple mastectomy).
‡Local excision.

Table 22–3. RATE OF OCCURRENCE OF SECOND PRIMARY BREAST CARCINOMAS IN 704 PATIENTS FOLLOWING SURGERY FOR A PREVIOUS MAMMARY CANCER (EFSCH, 1940 TO JUNE 1958)

Years	Number at Risk	Number Dying	Number Withdrawn Alive	Annual Number Developing Second Primary	Annual Percentage Developing Second Primary	Cumulative Percentage with Second Primary
1	704	60	0	2	0.3	0.3
2	644	88	0	3	0.5	0.7
3	556	81	0	2	0.4	1.0
4	475	56	0	4	0.8	1.6
5	419	39	0	0	0.0	1.6
6	381	37	2	1	0.3	1.7
7	341	32	16	2	0.6	2.0

cancer was diagnosed with elective biopsies in clinically and radiologically normal breasts, bringing the total asynchronous bilaterality to 4.2 per cent.

Clearly, the accumulation of clinically apparent second primary cancers is a function of the duration of observation. The longer a group of patients is followed, the greater will be the morbidity from additional cancers. As illustrated in Table 22–3, the frequency of second mammary cancers ranged from 0 to 0.8 per cent annually at EFSCH for the first 7 years after initial treatment, with no clear trend toward either increase or decrease. Robbins and Berg (1964) also noted a constant morbidity of about 1 per cent per year from second cancers.

In addition to the total observation time, the accumulation of multiple primary cancers is distinctly a function of the age of a population. Data on the incidence of cancer are generally recorded as the number of new cases per 100,000 people per year but, since the incidence varies radically at different ages, the rate is further defined for specific age ranges. The age-specific incidence of most cancers increases with time. When a patient has had one cancer, the pertinent question regarding the appearance of new primary cancers is whether the age-specific incidence is equal to, the same as, or less than the age-specific incidence of cancers among persons who have not had a previous cancer. This question applies not only to incidence in the same type of organ or tissue that gave rise to the first cancer but also to cancer incidence in other organs and tissues. Previous studies at EFSCH have indicated that carcinoma of the endometrium is associated with carcinoma of the breast more often than could be accounted for by chance alone (Cook, 1966). Spratt and Hoag (1966) also compared the incidence of second primary cancers at multiple sites and showed that simultaneous and nonsimultaneous cancers affect many organs other than those in which the first cancer is noted. Simultaneous cancers occurred in all organs, varying from 1.35 per cent for carcinoma of the cervix uteri to 13.17 per cent for chronic leukemia. Considering the slow rate of neoplastic growth in humans, a measurable percentage of any population can be expected to accumulate "simultaneous" cancers before any of them are big enough to produce symptoms (Spratt and Spratt, 1964). The accumulated cancers are discovered simultaneously, but the chance of two or more cancers originating simultaneously is exceedingly small. The organ distribution of nonsimultaneous cancers after radical mastectomy in this particular study did not differ significantly from the distribution of first cancers appearing in a female control population.

A similar detailed analysis at EFSCH was applied to women after mastectomy for unilateral mammary cancer. The population of 704 women previously mentioned was at risk to develop a second breast cancer for 4663 woman-years. During this period, 15 mammary cancers appeared in the remaining breasts, a frequency of 0.00321 cancer per woman-year of observation, which is equivalent to 321 cancers per 100,000 people per year. The female control population with no primary mammary cancer was observed for a total of 4244 woman-years, and eight mammary cancers appeared during the period, a frequency of 0.00188 cancer per woman-year of observation, which is equivalent to 188 cancers per 100,000 people per year. A twofold contingency table could demonstrate no difference between the frequency of cancers among women who had a primary mammary cancer and initial mammary cancers among those who had not (chi square = 1.06, $p > 0.3$). The observed incidence of mammary cancer in Connecticut for adult women of equivalent ages ranged from 0.00123 to 0.00352 per woman-year, which was equivalent to 123 to 352 mammary cancers per 100,000 people per year (Griswold, 1955). The comparison of the age-specific incidence rates in the two EFSCH populations is shown graphically in Figure 22–1A, B. The average age-specific incidence rate reported for women in Connecticut is also plotted for comparison.

Inspection of these graphs suggests that the average woman-year consideration obscures an age-specific increase in the incidence of second mammary cancers; the incidence of nonsimultaneous cancers above and below age 54 years does differ significantly (chi square = 6.21, $p < 0.01$). When these data relating to the development of second mammary cancers at EFSCH are compared with the ranges of age-specific incidence of first cancers in New York State, there again appears to be a disproportionately large number of women under 50 years of age afflicted a second time (Fig. 22–2).

During the last decade, concepts concerning the frequency of multiple primary breast cancers have changed as a result of new information from detailed studies of mastectomy specimens, the widespread use of mammography, and biopsies of clinically normal breasts.

Qualheim and Gall (1957) studied multiple sections of 157 breasts removed for cancer and found multiple independent sites of cancer in

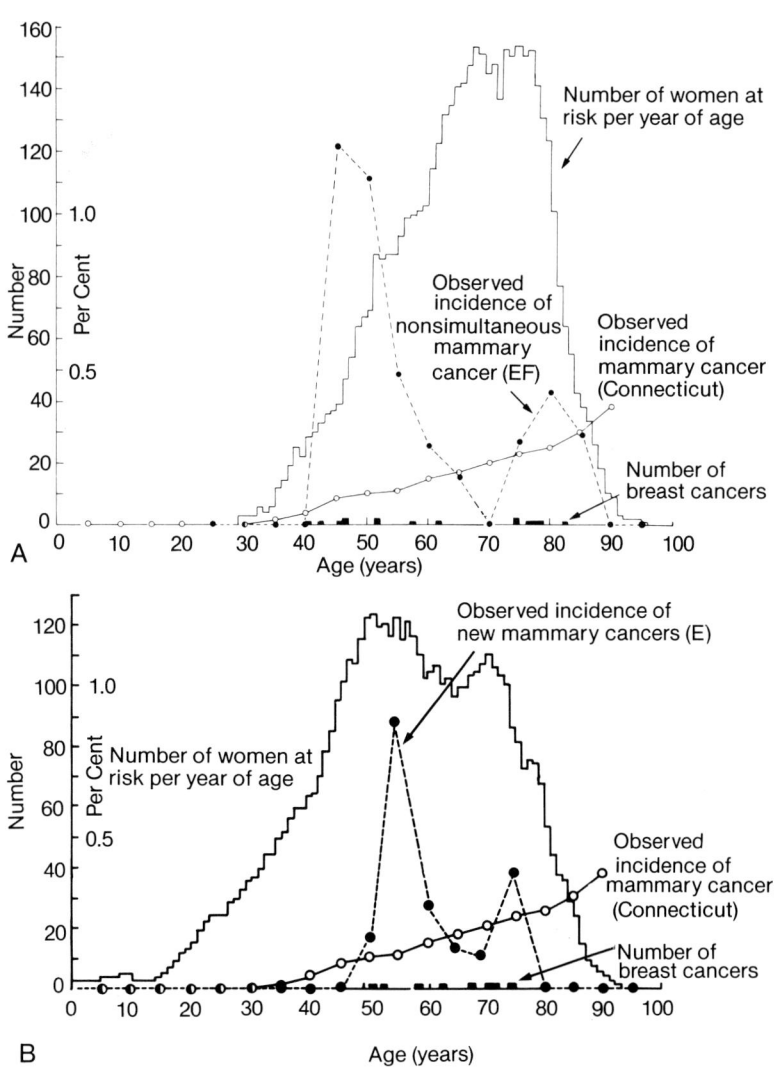

Figure 22–1. The age-specific percentage of new mammary cancers has been determined by averaging 5-year increments of observation. The number of woman-years of observation in each 5-year period was divided into the number of mammary cancers developing during the same period. Multiplying the dividend by 100 gives the age-specific percentage afflicted in 5-year averages. The 5-year average age-specific incidence rate for Connecticut (Griswold et al.) is plotted for comparison. The data in A are from a population of women who had had one mammary cancer resected. The data in B are from a population of women who had had one negative physical examination and were followed to determine the incidence of cancers developing subsequent to the examination. (From Spratt, J. S., and Hoag, T. L.: Incidence of multiple primary cancers per man-year of follow-up. Ann. Surg., 164:775, 1966.)

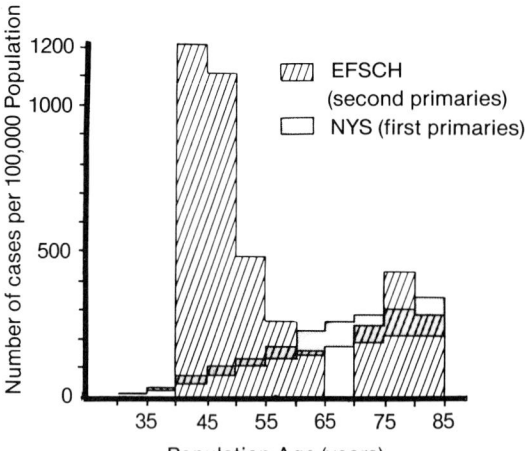

Figure 22–2. New mammary cancers in the breast remaining after mastectomy at EFSCH are compared with the age-specific frequency of initial cancers in New York State. An excess is most notably evident in women less than 55 years old.

54 per cent, with involvement of multiple quadrants in 37 per cent. This work was confirmed when Gallager and Martin (1969), with subserial whole-organ histologic preparations of 47 breasts, found two or more (usually many), independent foci of cancer in 47 per cent of the breasts examined. Using only single histologic samples, Fisher and coworkers (1975b) found independent foci of cancer in quadrants other than those in which the clinical cancer arose in 13 per cent of 904 mastectomy specimens. Multiplicity tends to be high even when the primary tumor is too small to palpate (Schwartz et al., 1980) and increases with tumor size (Rosen et al., 1975). These reports are clear evidence that carcinogenesis in the human breast is a diffuse phenomenon with a more widespread tissue response than is appreciated clinically.

The rise of mammography as a diagnostic adjunct has also increased the detection of otherwise occult cancers. Mammography has contributed to earlier recognition and perhaps also to the differentiation between primary and metastatic carcinomas (Egan, 1976). Using mammography, Egan reported finding new contralateral cancers in 6 per cent of 1112 women examined at Emory University between 1963 and 1973. Second mammary cancers were diagnosed in 26 (6.3 per cent) of 414 women with a previous mastectomy. Although the discovery rate in the total group was not unusually great, the proportion diagnosed simultaneously (27 per cent) was higher and the proportion diagnosed subsequently was lower, particularly during the first 6 months after mastectomy, than in earlier reported series in which routine mammography was not used. Second cancers were discovered more often while not palpable and at a smaller size than the first cancers, although reduction in the frequency of axillary metastasis was not substantial. The effect of routine mammography, therefore, was earlier detection, placing more second cancers into the simultaneous category.

The true significance of multicentric primary breast cancers remains incompletely resolved. Even the prevalence of the problem remains incompletely defined and varies with pathologic interpretation and the inclusion or exclusion of in situ cancers, both lobular and intraductal. Necropsy data, for example, indicates carcinoma in situ to be 19 times as prevalent as invasive cancers (Kramer and Rush, 1973). The occurrence of two dominant cancers simultaneously is even more infrequent, being about 0.1 per cent, according to Fisher and colleagues (1975b). Data are deficient on the risk that multicentric cancers will become a clinically significant disease after subtotal mastectomy alone with no radiotherapy. Hermann and colleagues (1984) used partial mastectomy without radiotherapy and reported new primary cancers in 7 per cent so treated within 5 years. Thirty-seven per cent of Tagart's patients (1978) treated with local excision alone developed recurrence in the same breast. Of the cases treated with local excision and irradiation by Harris and coworkers (1981), most relapses were at the excision site (12 versus 1), suggesting progression of the primary tumor. Protocol B-06 of the National Surgical Adjuvant Breast Project (NSABP), a three-armed study closed to further patient entry, involved segmental mastectomy without postoperative irradiation. At the time of the report by Fisher and colleagues (1985), local tumor recurrence had occurred in 28 per cent, suggesting incomplete resection or multifocal origin. The majority recurred within 3 years of surgical resection. The length of follow-up is still too short, and a much longer follow-up is needed to know the ultimate risk of intramammary cancer.

Protocol B-04 of the NSABP considered the appearance of cancers in the contralateral breast and the incidence had reached 3.7 per cent for invasive cancers and 0.5 per cent for noninvasive forms (Fisher et al., 1985). Such longitudinal follow-up is essential to assay the importance of the problem and to determine whether its magnitude merits any type of prophylactic intervention. The authors of this chapter long ago considered that multicentricity does not require prophylactic mastectomy. Too many people would receive an unnecessary extension of treatment in the name of prophylaxis. The major risk factors for mortality are the first cancer, age, and general medical condition of the patient. In the surviving patients, nonsimultaneous cancers may be treated as they appear at follow-up.

An increase in the detection of simultaneous bilateral involvement can also be attributed to liberal indications for biopsy of the second breast in the absence of the usual clinical or mammographic signs of neoplasia. Urban (1967, 1969b) was the first to advocate routine contralateral biopsies as a method of detection. It was Urban's experience that breast biopsies performed in the presence of minimal physical signs of abnormality yielded 11 per cent of cancers, many of which were also unsuspected mammographically. Aware of the high frequency with which new cancers arose in the breast that remained after mastectomy and the fact that many were discovered too late for cure, Urban began in 1964 to biopsy the second breast and 3 years later made it a routine procedure. In the presence of a physically and mammographically normal breast, these so-called "random" biopsies included 20 per cent of the mammary parenchyma from the upper outer quadrant as well as a sample from the location representing the "mirror image" of the first primary. Almost 1 in 10 (9.5 per cent) of these procedures revealed occult cancer (Urban, 1969a).

Overall, 15 per cent of 281 private patients proved to have manifest or occult contralateral cancers, 10 per cent of which were simultaneous. The figure for previous or simultaneous bilaterality rose to 20.4 per cent among 337 private and clinic patients, and the total was 13 per cent for 505 patients with and without contralateral biopsies seen between 1966 and 1968. The highest frequency of bilaterality was found in cases of in situ lobular carcinoma (54 per cent), medullary carcinoma (25 per cent), and noninfiltrating ductal carcinoma (19 per cent). Sixty-three per cent of the simultaneous second cancers were found at a noninvasive stage, and only 6.2 per cent of the invasive cancers had produced axillary metastases, both situations promising excellent chances of cure. The frequency of bilaterality detected with this procedure rivals that reported by Leis (1971) among carefully selected patients submitting to contralateral mastectomy (17 per cent) and is higher than that reported by Egan (1976) for physical examination and mammography only. The fact that the frequency of bilateral cancers detected in this manner exceeds the 7 to 10 per cent observed clinically suggests that some second primaries either regress or, more likely, have such a slow growth rate that they never evolve into clinical cancers during the patient's remaining lifetime.

Elective contralateral biopsy has been adopted and recommended by some surgeons, primarily for patients at higher than average risk for developing second cancers (Lewison, 1970; Donegan and Perez-Mesa, 1972; Wilson, 1973; Fenig et al., 1975; Kesseler et al., 1976). It has been pointed out, however, that a negative result in no manner guarantees against future cancer or obviates continued observation. Fenig and coworkers (1975) reported on 314 "mirror image" biopsies, 23 of which (7.3 per cent) detected cancer. Notably, 6 of 291 patients (2 per cent) with negative biopsies subsequently developed cancer in the breast; three of the cancers arose in the vicinity of the biopsy. Pressman (1985) found 16 per cent positive elective biopsies in 250 consecutive women under age 65 years with Stage I or II cancer in the first breast. Some authors believe that the yield would probably be equally great if elective biopsies were limited to the upper outer quadrant of the breast, where almost half of all mammary cancers arise (Fenig et al., 1975). The ultimate frequency of cancers in breasts after a "negative" elective biopsy is of great interest, and little information is available.

Among 80 patients treated for lobular carcinoma in situ and observed for an average of 15 years, Rosen et al. (1981) found that the proportion of patients who developed cancers in the second breast after a negative contralateral biopsy (17.2 per cent) was no less than that of patients who had no such biopsy (17.6 per cent). One of the authors (WLD) also found no obvious reduction of future cancers after negative elective biopsies for in situ cancers and has largely abandoned this practice, relying rather on close follow-up.

The life-threatening malignant potential of many "cancers" diagnosed totally on a microscopic basis in a period in which they are otherwise both asymptomatic and clinically undetectable remains unresearched.

The following unanswered or only partially answered questions should be kept in mind while reading this chapter.

1. Which cancers have the capacity to induce angiogenesis? (See Chapter 19.)

2. What is their rate of progression?

3. Is their progression so slow as to permit their discovery as a result of length-biased sampling?

4. At what patient age does the natural mortality rate exceed the implied mortality rate of these multicentric changes?

The authors have reviewed some of these considerations in Chapters 10 and 19.

Patients at High Risk for Second Mammary Cancers

Several clinicopathologic factors identify patients as prone to bilateral cancers. These include youth, ability to survive the first cancer, a diffuse tissue response, and perhaps a genetic predisposition.

Women Less than 50 Years of Age. The susceptibility of young, generally premenopausal women to bilateral primary cancers is clear. The risk for such patients is 10 to 14 times higher than expected for initial cancers (Robbins and Berg, 1964; Berndt et al., 1970) (see Fig. 22–1A, B). A partial explanation lies in the fact that young women who are cured of their first cancers have an extended period of risk to develop a second.

A Family History of Breast Cancer. The case control studies of Anderson (1973) indicate that patients with first-degree relatives who have breast cancer are two to five times more likely than average to develop bilateral cancers, with the highest risk among those 20 to 44 years old. The possibility exists of a genetic predisposition to the disease that results in both an early onset and diffuse parenchymal involvement. The occurrence of bilateral cancers in both mother and daughter, as reported by Smith (1968), supports this possibility. This problem is discussed in more detail in Chapter 4.

Grossly Multifocal Cancer. Women who initially have two or more grossly evident independent primary tumors in the breast are few, constituting less than 2 per cent of all cases, but they have four times the average risk of developing additional cancers in the second breast (Robbins and Berg, 1964). Although a far greater number of women are found to have two or more occult cancers on detailed examination of the breast, the evidence for clinically relevant, diffuse carcinogenesis is most evident in cases with multiple gross cancers.

Lobular Carcinoma in Situ (LIS). This noninvasive tumor accounts for no more than 10 per cent of mammary cancers, but much has been written about it, primarily because of its high bilaterality and its controversial malignant potential. Haagensen (1971) minimizes its potential and prefers to speak of lobular "neoplasia" rather than lobular carcinoma, although tumors demonstrating anaplasia (Type B) are considered more dangerous than the well-differentiated Type A. At the other extreme, McDivitt and associates (1967) reported that 35 per cent of women observed for up to 20 years developed invasive cancers in breasts known to harbor LIS. One fact is uncontested: LIS is unsurpassed for its association with bilateral breast cancer. Detected by all diagnostic methods, including elective biopsy, its incidence ranges from 25 to 40 per cent (Newman, 1963; Benfield et al., 1965; McDivitt et al., 1967; Urban, 1969b; Donegan and Perez-Mesa, 1972; Peters et al., 1977; Anderson, 1977; Fisher and Fisher, 1977).

An evaluation of patients with lobular carcinoma, both in situ and invasive, was conducted at EFSCH in which all patients with this lesion were recalled for examination of the remaining breast; elective biopsies were performed if they were clinically and radiographically normal (Donegan and Perez-Mesa, 1972). At the conclusion of this study, 11 of the 36 patients reviewed were found to have cancer in both breasts. Seven cancers were detected with elective biopsies in 20 patients, an incidence of 35 per cent in clinically normal breasts. Bilaterality was diagnosed in 36 per cent of 28 patients with LIS. Although the cases were few, invasive lobular cancer seemed to carry the same implications as LIS; one of five women (20 per cent) from whom tissue was available had an invasive cancer in the opposite breast. Lobular cancer was multifocal in 76 per cent of mastectomy specimens and often occurred in the company of other histologic types of cancer. As cancers found in the second breast were not regularly lobular in type, LIS appeared to be a marker for multiple cancers and not necessarily their origin.

Noninvasive Ductal Carcinoma. This lesion, in some cases identified grossly as comedo carcinoma, tends to be multicentric. In a review of noninvasive cancers at the Medical College of Wisconsin, 25 per cent of women with ductal carcinoma in situ had developed cancer in both breasts (Peters et al., 1977). As some patients remained at risk, this was a minimum figure, but it already had exceeded three times the general incidence of bilaterality. The same observation was made by Robbins and Berg (1964) and by Urban (1969b). Curiously, however, women who initially had noninvasive ductal cancers showed no increase of second breast involvement, an observation also made by Webber and coworkers (1983).

Histologically Favorable Invasive Cancers. Mucinous carcinoma, erroneously called "colloid" carcinoma on the basis of its gross appearance, is a relatively benign and rare type of cancer. Robbins and Berg (1964) found it to be associated with a mild excess of second primary tumors, that is, 1.23 times the expected rate. When in a pure form these tumors are highly curable, leaving the patient at prolonged risk to develop cancer in the remaining breast. Among 44 pure mucinous carcinomas collected from three institutions over a period of 25 years (EFSCH, Milwaukee County Medical Complex, and Columbia Hospital in Milwaukee), the authors of this chapter observed that two patients (4.5 per cent) had multifocal lesions in the first breast and four patients (9 per cent) had an independent primary tumor in the second breast. Sixteen of the patients with unilateral disease remain alive and at risk for second primary cancers.

Possibly at higher than average risk are patients with tumors of other benign histologic types, including tubular and medullary carcinomas. Slack and associates (1973) included large cancers, those 6 cm or more in diameter, in the high-risk category, but Robbins and Berg (1964) found no evidence for their inclusion. Holdener and colleagues (1982), in a retrospective and prospective assessment of 1985 breast cancer patients, failed to find an increased risk for second cancer associated with adjuvant chemotherapy or radiotherapy.

PROGNOSIS

Despite the fact that second primary cancers are an acknowledged hazard, they have not always been detected in early stages. In the premammography era at Memorial Hospital, New York City, second primary tumors generally were smaller when discovered, but only one third were in early clinical stages (Robbins and Berg, 1964). The second cancers of 79 patients with bilateral sequential disease reported by Leis in 1965 were not in earlier stages than the first. During the same period, a conscientious follow-up program at EFSCH resulted in discovery of second primary cancers at a smaller size (that is, 3.0 cm average diameter on cut section) than first ones, (4.1 cm). However, no greater percentage was found in the early stage, with 80 per cent of both being in Stage A or B of the Columbia Clinical Classification.

Since 1969 the widespread use of mammography and the adoption of elective biopsies by many surgeons has improved detection. Recent series reflect a definite reduction in tumor size and some reduction in the frequency of nodal involvement (Khafagy et al., 1975; Egan, 1976; Kesseler et al., 1976).

Because the prognosis associated with bilateral cancers is surprisingly good, these patients should be treated as are others with similar stages of the disease (Huff, 1969; Slack et al., 1973; Wilson and Alberty, 1973; Khafagy et al., 1975). The survival of patients with bilateral simultaneous mammary cancers treated with mastectomy at EFSCH prior to 1958 reflected no obviously inferior prognosis. All 14 cancers were treated with radical mastectomy except for two that, because of the extremely poor condition of the patients, were treated with simple mastectomy and local excision. All seven patients had either Stage A or Stage B cancers, and four patients (57 per cent) survived at least 5 years. This performance was within the range of unilateral disease in similar stages, 66 per cent for Stage A and 50 per cent for Stage B.

The 15 nonsimultaneous cancers, with only one exception in which a simple mastectomy was performed, were treated with radical mastectomy. Five year survival rates were 80 per cent after the first cancer and 47 per cent after the second cancer. Good survivorship is the rule; the capacity to live to develop a second primary in most instances reflects a prognostically favorable initial neoplasm. For comparison, only 52.4 per cent of 781 patients who developed no second primary lived for 5 years after radical mastectomy, and 34.3 per cent lived for 10 years.

The favorable course of women after removal of a second mammary cancer (47 per cent survive for at least 5 years at EFSCH) has suggested to some investigators the possibility of a benefit from immunologic stimulation by the first cancer, particularly by in situ cancers, which appear to be more immunogenic than invasive cancers (Black et al., 1972; Black, 1975; Wilson and Alberty, 1973). If it can be presumed that mammary cancers share a common antigen, sequential cancers constitute, in effect, a natural experiment in immunotherapy. To support this thesis, Black and associates (1972) found that cancers subsequent to in situ cancers or atypical hyperplasias more often were favorable types and had a better progress than otherwise. This association, however, cannot be used to prove an immune resistance.

Survival after a second cancer, however, is favored by the fact that these cancers appear in a selected group that remains after the first cancer has largely taken its toll. Chances of death from the first cancer after appearance of the second are, therefore, small. The subsequent cancers themselves constitute independent risk to survival. With matched controls, Robbins and Berg (1964) showed that a second mammary cancer substantially reduced the survival expected in the group at risk. Not excluded is the possibility that multiple primary cancers accumulate in the same individual because of slower growth rates.

Treatment

Patients with operable primary cancers in one or both breasts should be treated optimistically for cure. Formerly, staged procedures were performed most often for simultaneous primary cancers, the most advanced cancer being removed first and a period of 3 weeks allowed before the second operation. At present, a simultaneous bilateral mastectomy is preferred. As described by Ratzer and associates in 1966, a single transverse incision is used, superior and inferior flaps are developed, and the two breasts and axillary contents are removed en bloc. This approach avoids delay in treating the second cancer (which can be compounded if healing of the wound is complicated on the first side), entails administration of anesthesia once rather than twice, and reduces the total period of hospitalization. This operation is particularly expeditious if performed simultaneously by two operating teams. Recently breast conserving techniques in suitable cases have been used for bilateral breast cancers.

PROPHYLACTIC MASTECTOMY

The threat imposed by second mammary cancers raises the issue of contralateral mastectomy as a prophylactic measure. Over 65 years ago, Bloodgood (1921) suggested removing the uninvolved breast with simple mastectomy for this reason, as did Pack in 1951. More recently, Leis (1968) argued the case, pointing out that a high-risk group for second cancers can be defined, that removal of the breast can be performed with negligible risk, that the procedure is acceptable to many women, and that for some women it is both a mental and physical benefit. Leis recommends the operation to women with small, Stage I lesions; favorable histologic types of cancers, including in situ, medullary, and colloid cancers; a family history of breast cancer; multiple primary tumors in the first breast; and those less than 50 years of age. Unsuspected cancers were found in 16 (17 per cent) of 91 such mastectomies, the majority of which (11) were not invasive (Leis, 1971). The 96.5 per cent 5 year survival rate of Leis's cases confirms that selection is confined to women with a good prognosis and that occult second cancers were managed effectively.

The case for prophylactic mastectomy has been explored by others and been found wanting. The arguments against prophylactic mastectomy are the following:

1. The anticipated benefits of uniformly removing the second breast are small compared with the surgical morbidity.

2. With patient observation, second cancers can be treated effectively when they occur.

3. A very large percentage of the mastectomies would be done on women who would never need a mastectomy at all; their sacrifice would be to benefit a theoretical few.

If mastectomy were adopted as a routine prophylactic measure, the magnitude of the undertaking would dwarf the anticipated returns. Robbins and Berg (1964) estimated that only 1 in 20 prophylactic mastectomies would be lifesaving. This is a conservative estimate. Using data on 2734 patients treated with mastectomies by members of the National Surgical Adjuvant Breast Project, Slack and associates (1973) found that within the first 5 years of follow-up, 3 per cent developed second mammary cancers. Assuming that one third of the 3 per cent ultimately would die of metastases from their first cancer and not be benefitted, and that only 40 per cent of the remaining two thirds (2 per cent) would have been saved by a prophylactic mastectomy (because 60 per cent could still have been cured by a mastectomy delayed until the time of diagnosis), a maximum of 0.80 per cent of all women (0.02

times 0.40) would be saved from dying of a second breast cancer that had developed during the first 5 years. This salvage would require 98 nonbeneficial mastectomies for the theoretical benefit of two women. If the prophylactic operation were confined to women who have four times the expected risk and who were probably cured of their first cancers, the advantages would be increased, but not greatly.

For example, assuming a 75 per cent 5 year survival, the same line of reasoning would lead to the conclusion that 91 useless mastectomies would have to be performed to save 3.6 lives from new cancers diagnosed within 5 years of mastectomy. Although the rate of second cancers remains constant after this time, their absolute number is small because the number of surviving patients is greatly diminished. In Chapter 2, breast tissue is shown to be so extensive in its anatomic spread and so intimate in its relation to the skin as to preclude its removal by any dissection short of a total mastectomy with very thin skin flaps. Even with very complete operations, both animal and human studies have shown that additional primary cancers still appear in residual breast tissue.

Apart from these factors, pause must be taken on other grounds. The usual "simple" mastectomy often fails to remove all breast tissue. Many examples can be produced of women who have had cancer develop in residual breast tissue at the site of simple mastectomies performed for nonmalignant conditions. This operation is thus an incomplete and, at best, an unproved guarantee against future mammary cancers (Hicken, 1940; Holleb and Farrow, 1967). Considering the wide distribution of mammary parenchyma over the chest wall and into the axilla, a truly prophylactic operation is not the simple matter that it is often assumed to be.

The fact that second primary cancers are being discovered earlier with mammography and elective biopsies, often simultaneously with first cancers, makes prophylactic removal of breasts less attractive than when originally proposed. With modern means of diagnosis, it is likely that even fewer lives would be jeopardized by a policy of conscientious observation until therapeutic intervention is necessary.

This problem has been addressed by many studies and reviews in a search for effective clinical strategies. Pathologic studies on microscopic findings in the clinical environment continue to be reported (Fisher et al., 1975a; Schwartz et al., 1980; Lesser et al., 1982; Lewis et al., 1982; Martin et al., 1982; Haagensen et al., 1983; Davis and Baird, 1984).

Although these studies provide a variety of recommendations about how to address these morphologic findings at the time the first breast cancer is diagnosed, no longitudinal studies have been conducted that confirm the rate and frequency with which multicentric foci of invasive and in situ cancer progress to clinical cancer in a pattern that affects the life expectancy of an individual. Mortality is greatest with the first cancer. When this is a very strong force, nothing further should probably be done. When it is a weak or nonexistent force, the host may have an ability to survive that permits microscopic cancer and precancerous lesions to develop into clinical disease. More is said about this in Chapter 19, and the lack of angiogenesis in many "early cancers" is discussed. A very useful report by Al-Jurf and coworkers (1981) provided a clinical study of 104 women with bilateral breast cancers. Those women with simultaneous bilateral primary cancers had the poorest prognosis. Although cancer in the second breast was associated with lymph node metastases in 21 women, survivorship data were not adversely affected. Based on survivorship data, these authors concluded that satisfactory results with the management of asynchronous breast cancers could be obtained by follow-up, and discovery could be obtained by clinical means.

A more aggressive approach is reported by Wanebo and coworkers (1985), who studied a series of 62 personal cases routinely undergoing contralateral biopsy and used the descriptive statistics of morphologic findings to argue for routine contralateral biopsies. Sutherland, in a discussion of this paper, asked the questions Wanebo's group left unanswered—consideration of biases and case stratification in such a small data base, need for controls, and significance of findings relating to contralateral biopsy to long-term survivorship. A much larger, better designed study is needed to answer the essential questions Sutherland raises before Wanebo and coworkers' approach can be adopted as a routine. Although proponents of "prophylactic" mastectomy exist, the authors of this chapter cannot subscribe to this for the reasons discussed here and in Chapters 2 and 19.

As a further consideration, the risk of developing additional primary cancers is not restricted to the second breast. Other organs and tissues of the host's body are at risk as well. If persons cured of one cancer live to extremely old age, more than one third of them can expect a second primary cancer of some organ (Einhorn and Jakobsson, 1964; Spratt and Hoag, 1966). Close patient follow-up with conscientious detection of second primary cancers in all organs and systems in the earliest possible stage seems a more cost-effective pattern of patient care for women with a previous cancer of the breast. The complex issues involved in attaining this goal are addressed in Chapter 19.

Metastatic Neoplasms to the Breast from Other Primary Cancers

The presence of unusual histopathologic features on breast biopsy merits consideration of cancer metastatic to the breast from other sites. The frequency of metastatic carcinoma to the breast from other sites was reviewed by Silverman and Oberman (1974), who reported 11 additional cases. Death resulted from widespread metastases in all cases. The major site of origin was melanoma. Metastasis to the breast was indicative of very rapid tumor progression as all patients died within less than 1 year of diagnosis. Excluded from this review were patients with a previous primary cancer of the breast, lymphoma, or leukemia. Nielsen et al. reviewed the literature in 1981 and found metastases from a wide variety of sites. Most frequent was melanoma, followed in frequency by lung, prostate, ovaries, and stomach.

The English literature contained five definite cases of malignant carcinoid tumor metastatic to the breast, according to Harrist and Kalisher (1977), to which they added a sixth case. In their review, they noted that the most common secondary tumor of the female breast is metastatic cancer from the opposite breast. For the male breast, the most common secondary neoplasm is metastatic carcinoma from the prostate. The breast has also been reported as the occasional target organ for metastases from other cancers—melanoma, lung cancer, renal cell cancer, and gastric cancer (Harrist and Kalisher, 1977). The diagnosis of these occasional events requires alert clinical and pathologic correlation, and management would depend on the neoplasm and its extent. Mammography has been used to evaluate the extent of the metastases within the breast, and mastectomy has been used to control local progression.

Metastases to the breast may simulate all presentations of primary breast cancer, including inflammatory cancer, and present a differential diagnostic challenge (Nance et al., 1966). Nance and colleagues provide a review of metastases to the breast from cancers of other sites dating back to 1936.

The tendency of melanomas to metastasize to the breast has been reported on a number of occasions. Any breast mass appearing in a person with a past history of melanoma requires that melanoma be included in the differential diagnosis and be considered as a possibility in the histologic evaluation of biopsies. The lack of signs of systemic spread and a long disease-free interval do not rule out melanoma (Lanzafame et al., 1984). Although melanoma is the neoplasm that metastasizes most frequently to the breast, the event is still uncommon and is eclipsed by the tendency of melanoma to metastasize to other organs more frequently. As mastectomy does not reduce the lethality of the melanoma, wide local excision usually is adequate treatment. As has been confirmed for other sites, occasionally there is a palliative advantage in performing regional lymph node dissections when lymph nodes are enlarged from melanoma, even when they represent disseminated cancer. The palliative value comes from reducing or avoiding the morbidity of masses of lymph nodes from uncontrolled melanoma, and one of the authors (J.S.S.) usually considers an axillary dissection if enlarged axillary lymph nodes are found in association with melanoma that is metastatic to the breast.

Peculiarly, the breast is a frequent site for metastases in children with rhabdomyosarcomas. Howarth and coworkers (1980) reported seven cases of metastases to the breast in a series of 108 children and youths ranging from 5 months to 20 years of age (median, 11 years 6 months). The physiologic stage of the breast seemed to be associated with the appearance of these metastases.

Second Malignancies as a Hazard of Chemotherapy and Radiotherapy

The increasingly frequent use of treatment methods that are themselves carcinogenic poses a risk of increased cancers. This risk begins with the treatment of childhood cancers, as reviewed by Li and colleagues (1983). Among 910 survivors of childhood cancer, four breast cancers had developed in women aged 20, 25, and 38 years and in a 38 year old man. For ages and periods of follow-up, this number significantly exceeded the expected.

An analysis of the risk of leukemia after the primary treatment of breast cancer has now been reported by the Surveillance, Epidemiology, and End Results (SEER) program for 59,115 breast cancer patients treated between 1973 and 1980 (Curtis et al., 1984). A significant elevation was observed for patients who underwent chemotherapy in their first course of therapy. (6:1.58 occurred-expected ratio). The excess risk peaked in the third year post treatment, and the pattern of latency suggested a cause-and-effect relationship between chemotherapy and leukemia. No cases of leukemia occurred in the radiotherapy group. However, in a review of 8483 patients treated for breast cancer in adjuvant protocols, Fisher and coworkers (1985) found an increased relative risk of acute myelogenous leukemia following postoperative regional irradiation and adjuvant chemotherapy.

Dorr and Coltman (1985) have reviewed second cancers following antineoplastic therapy and found them to be an infrequent risk. In the case of the breast, this has involved the induction of leukemia by chemotherapy and fibrosarcomas in fields of irradiation therapy. Satisfactory population-based studies on the magnitude of this risk do not exist, but the risk of radiation-induced sarcomas of the chest wall may approximate 0.02 per cent. The risk is discussed further in Chapter 15. So far as fibrosarcomas are concerned, biopsy confirmation and wide local excision are the indicated management for most patients (Kardinal and Donegan, 1980).

A Plan of Management

A constant suspicion must be maintained with regard to the second breast of women with mammary carcinoma. To accomplish earlier diagnosis of independent primary cancers, the following plan specific for the second breast is recommended in conjunction with treatment of the first cancer:

1. A careful visual and palpatory examination of the second breast, the axilla, and supraclavicular areas.
2. Bilateral mammograms.
3. Biopsy of even minimally suspicious abnormalities found on palpatory examination or mammography.
4. In the absence of abnormalities, an elective biopsy of the opposite breast is not routine even for high-risk groups, but can be defended for women under 50 years of age, those with a strong family history of breast cancer, with multiple gross cancers in the first breast, or with noninvasive carcinoma in the first breast. This can be accomplished through a cosmetic para-areolar incision under local anesthesia prior to treatment of the first cancer or under general anesthesia concurrently with treatment.

Despite reassurance from these measures, the remaining breast continues at risk throughout the patient's life. Consequently, a component of the periodic examination of women after surgery for breast cancer should be a careful palpatory examination at each visit. In the authors' clinic, follow-up visit intervals are based primarily on the interval risk of recurrence of the first cancer (see Chapter 19). To supplement these physical examinations, a mammogram is performed annually on the remaining breast. As a final precaution, patients are carefully instructed in self-examination of the remaining breast and encouraged to perform it at least monthly. With these measures, the recognition of new cancers in the remaining breast can occur earlier.

There are circumstances in which a prophylactic mastectomy might be indicated for the physical and mental well-being of the patient. In the authors' opinion, they are infrequent and carefully selected situations in which adequate follow-up is not possible or practical or in which psychologic or cosmetic considerations are of overriding concern. If performed, the operation must be a thorough, total mastectomy accompanied by removal of the nipple and breast tissue from the lower axilla.

REFERENCES

Al-Jurf, A. S., Jochmisen, P. R., Urdaneta, L. F., et al.: Factors influencing survival in bilateral cancer. J. Surg. Oncol., *16*:343, 1981.

Andersen, J. A.: Lobular carcinoma in situ of the breast: An approach to rational treatment. Cancer, *39*:2597, 1977.

Anderson, D. E.: A high-risk group for breast cancer. Cancer Bull., *25*:23, 1973.

Benfield, J. R., Jacobson, M., and Warner, N. E.: In situ lobular carcinoma of the breast. Arch. Surg., *91*:130, 1965.

Berg, J. W., Hutter, R. V. P., and Foote, F. W., Jr.: The unique association between salivary gland and breast cancer. J.A.M.A., *204*:771, 1968.

Berndt, V. H., Borrmann, C., and Klein, K.: Zweitkarzinom der Brustdruse. Arch. Geschwulstforsch, *36*:51, 1970.

Black, M. M.: Cell mediated response in human mammary cancer. *In* Stoll, B. A. (ed.): Host Defense in Breast Cancer. Chicago, Year Book Medical Publishers, 1975, p. 48.

Black, M. M., Cutter, S. J., and Barclay, T. H. C.: Post biopsy breast carcinoma: A natural experiment in cancer immunology. Cancer, *29*:61, 1972.

Bloodgood, J. C.: The pathology of chronic cystic mastitis of the female breast. Arch. Surg., *3*:445, 1921.

Cook, G. B.: A comparison of single and multiple primary cancers. Cancer, *19*:959, 1966.

Davis, N., and Baird, R. M.: Breast cancer in association with lobular carcinoma in situ. Clinicopathologic review and treatment recommendation. Am. J. Surg. *147*:641, 1984.

Curtis, R. E., Hankey, B. F., Myers, M. H., et al.: Risk of leukemia associated with the first course of cancer treatment: An analysis of Surveillance, Epidemiology and End Result section. JNCI, *72*:531, 1984.

Donegan, W. L.: Patterns and prognosis of advanced breast carcinoma. Missouri Med., *67*:853, 1970.

Donegan, W. L., and Perez-Mesa, C. M.: Lobular carcinoma—an indication for elective biopsy of the second breast. Ann. Surg., *176*:178, 1972.

Dorr, F. A., and Coltman, C. A., Jr.: Second cancers following antineoplastic therapy. Curr. Probl. Cancer. *9*:1, 1985.

Drinkwater, N. R., and Klotz, J. H.: Statistical methods for the analysis of tumor multiplicity data. Cancer Res., *41*:113, 1981.

Dunn, J. E., Jr., Bragg, K. U., Sautter, C., et al.: Breast cancer risk following a major salivary gland carcinoma. Cancer, *29*:1343, 1972.

Egan, R. L.: Bilateral breast carcinomas: Role of mammography. Cancer, *38*:931, 1976.

Einhorn, J., and Jakobsson, P.: Multiple primary malignant tumors. Cancer, *17*:1437, 1964.

Fenig, J., Arlen, M., Livingston, S. F., et al.: The potential for carcinoma existing synchronously on a microscopic level within the second breast. Surg. Gynecol. Obstet., *141*:394, 1975.

Fisher, B., Bauer, M., Margolese, R., et al.: Five-year results of a randomized clinical trial comparing total mastectomy and segmental mastectomy with or without radiation in the treatment of breast cancer. N. Engl. J. Med., *312*:665, 1985.

Fisher, B., Rockette, H., Fisher, E. R., Wickerham, D. L., Redmond, C., and Brown, A.: Leukemia in breast cancer patients following adjuvant chemotherapy or postoperative radiation: the NSABP experience. J. Clin. Oncol., *3*:1640, 1985.

Fisher, E. R., and Fisher, B.: Lobular carcinoma of the breast: An overview. Ann. Surg., *185*:377, 1977.

Fisher, E. R., Gregorio, R. M., and Fisher, B.: The pathology of invasive breast cancer—a syllabus derived from findings of the NSABP (Protocol No. 4). Cancer, *36*:1, 1975a.

Fisher, E. R., Gregorio, R., Redmond, C., et al.: Pathological findings from the National Surgical Adjuvant Breast Project (Protocol No. 4) I. Observations concerning the multicentricity of mammary cancer. Cancer, *35*:247, 1975b.

Fisher, E. R., Fisher, B., Sass, R., et al.: Pathologic findings from the National Surgical Adjuvant Breast Project (Protocol No. 4). XI. Bilateral breast cancer. Cancer, (in press).

Fitts, W. T., Jr., and Patterson, L. T.: Symposium on applied physiology in modern surgery: Spread of mammary cancer. Surg. Clin. North Am., *35*:1539, 1955.

Gallager, H. S., and Martin, J. E.: Early phases in the development of breast cancer. Cancer, *24*:1170, 1969.

Griswold, M. H., Wilder, C. S., Cutler, S. J., et al.: Cancer in Connecticut 1935–1951. Hartford, Connecticut State Department of Health, 1955.

Haagensen, C. D.: Diseases of the Breast. Philadelphia, W. B. Saunders, 1971, p. 503.

Haagensen, C. D., Lane, N., and Bodian, C.: Coexisting lobular neoplasia and carcinoma of the breast. Cancer, *51*:1468, 1983.

Harrington, S. W.: Survival rates of radical mastectomy for unilateral and bilateral carcinoma of the breast. Surgery, *19*:154, 1946.

Harris, J. R., Botnick, L., Bloomer, W. D., et al.: Primary radiation therapy for early breast cancer: The experience at the joint center for radiation therapy. Int. J. Radiation Oncol. Biol. Phys., *7*:1549, 1981.

Harrist, T. J., and Kalisher, L.: Breast metastasis: An unusual manifestation of a malignant carcinoid tumor. Cancer, *40*:3102, 1977.

Hermann, R. E., Esselstyn, C. B., Jr., Cooperman, A. M., et al.: Partial mastectomy without radiation therapy. Surg. Clin. North Am., *64*:1103, 1984.

Hicken, N. F.: Mastectomy: Clinical pathological study demonstrating why most mastectomies result in incomplete removal of mammary gland. Arch. Surg., *40*:6, 1940.

Holdener, E. E., Osterwalder, J., Senn, H. J., et al.: Second malignancy after surgery for breast cancer: Comparison of retrospective and prospective experiences. Schweiz. Med. Wochenschr., *112*:1800, 1982.

Holleb, A. I., and Farrow, J. H.: St. Agatha and inadequate simple mastectomy. AJR, *99*:962, 1967.

Howarth, C. B., Caces, J. N., and Pratt, C. B.: Breast metastases in children with rhabdomyosarcoma. Cancer, *46*:2520, 1980.

Huff, L.: Bilateral carcinoma of the breast. Am. J. Surg., *118*:550, 1969.

Kapsinow, R.: Multiple primary cancer: A classification with report of cases. J. Louisiana Med. Soc., *114*:194, 1962.

Kardinal, C. G., and Donegan, W. L.: Second cancers after prolonged adjuvant thiotepa for operable breast cancer. Cancer, *45*:2042, 1980.

Kesseler, H. J., Robson, W., Grier, N., et al.: Bilateral primary breast cancer. J.A.M.A., *236*:278, 1976.

Khafagy, M. M., Schottenfeld, D., and Robbins, G. F.: Prognosis of the second breast cancer: The role of previous exposure to the first primary. Cancer, *35*:596, 1975.

Kilgore, A. R.: The incidence of cancer in the second breast. J.A.M.A., *77*:454, 1921.

Kramer, W. M., and Rush, B. F.: Mammary duct proliferation in the elderly: A histopathologic study. Cancer, *31*:130, 1973.

Lanzafame, R. J., Kurchin, A., and Shermirani, M.: Metastatic melanoma presenting as a primary breast lesion. Contemp. Surg., *25*:47, 1984.

Lee, Y. T. N.: Multiple malignant neoplasms in patients with breast carcinoma. Contemp. Surg., *24*:11, 1984.

Leis, H. P. Jr., Mersheimer, W. L., Black, M. M., and

Chabon, A. D.: The second breast. N.Y. State J. Med., Oct. 1, 1965, pp. 2460–2468.

Leis, H. P., Jr.: Prophylactic removal of the second breast. Hosp. Med., 4:45, 1968.

Leis, H. P., Jr.: Selective, elective, prophylactic contralateral mastectomy. Cancer, 28:956, 1971.

Lesser, M. L., Rosen, P. P., and Kinne, D. W.: Multicentricity and bilaterality in invasive breast carcinoma. Surgery, 91:234, 1982.

Lewis, T. R., Casey, J., Buerk, C. A., et al.: Incidence of lobular carcinoma in bilateral breast cancer. Am. J. Surg., 144:635, 1982.

Lewison, E. F.: The follow-up examination of the contralateral breast: From the viewpoint of the surgeon. Cancer, 23:809, 1969.

Lewison, E. F.: The management of the contralateral breast. Hosp. Pract., September, 1970, p. 101.

Li, F. P., Corkery, J., Vawter, G., et al.: Breast carcinoma after cancer therapy in childhood. Cancer, 51:521, 1983.

McDivitt, R. W., Hutter, R. V. P., Foote, F. W., Jr., et al.: In situ lobular carcinoma. J.A.M.A., 201:96, 1967.

Martin, J. K., Jr., van Heerden, J. A., and Gaffey, T. A.: Synchronous and metachronous carcinoma of the breast. Surgery, 91:12, 1982.

Moertel, C. G., and Elvebeck, L. R.: The association between salivary gland cancer and breast cancer. J.A.M.A., 210:306, 1969.

Multiple Primary Cancers in Connecticut and Denmark. National Cancer Institute Monograph 68, NIH Publication No. 85-2714. Bethesda, Md., National Cancer Institute, 1985.

Nance, F. C., MacVaugh, H., and Fitts, W. T., Jr.: Metastatic tumor to the breast simulating bilateral primary inflammatory carcinoma. Am. J. Surg., 112:932, 1966.

Newman, W.: In situ lobular carcinoma of the breast: Report of 26 women with 32 cancers. Ann. Surg., 157:591, 1963.

Nielsen, M., Andersen, J. A., Henriksen, F. W., et al.: Metastases to the breast from extramammary carcinomas. Acta Pathol. Microbiol. Scand. (Sect. A), 89:251, 1981.

Pack, G. T.: Argument for bilateral mastectomy. Surgery, 29:929, 1951.

Pennell, V.: Primary carcinoma multiplex: A series of 17 cases with review of the literature. Br. J. Surg., 46:108, 1958.

Peters, T. G., Donegan, W. L., and Burg, E. A.: Minimal breast cancer: A clinical appraisal. Ann. Surg., 186:704, 1977.

Pressman, P. I.: Selective biopsy of the opposite breast. Presented at the 38th Annual Cancer Symposium of the Society of Surgical Oncology, the Warwick Post Oak Hotel, Houston, Texas, May 19–22, 1985.

Pribe, W. A., and Ockuly, E. A.: Prostatic metastasis to the breast and the role of estrogens: Case report and review. J. Am. Geriatr. Soc., 11:891, 1963.

Qualheim, R., and Gall, E.: Breast carcinoma with multiple sites of origin. Cancer, 10:460, 1957.

Ratzer, E. R., Holleb, A. I., and Farrow, J. H.: The technique of bilateral simultaneous radical mastectomy. Surg. Gynecol. Obstet., 123:601, 1966.

Robbins, G. F., and Berg, J. W.: Bilateral primary breast cancers. Cancer, 17:1501, 1964.

Rosen, P. P., Braun, D. W., Jr., Lyngholm, B., Urban, J. A., and Kinne, D. W.: Lobular carcinoma in situ of the breast: Preliminary results of treatment by ipsilateral mastectomy and contralateral breast biopsy. Cancer, 47:813, 1981.

Rosen, P. P., Fracchia, A. A., Urban, J. A., et al.: "Residual" mammary carcinoma following simulated partial mastectomy. Cancer, 35:739, 1975.

Sandison, A. T.: Metastatic tumors of the breast. Br. J. Surg., 47:54, 1959.

Schenker, J. G., Levinsky, R., and Ohel, G.: Multiple primary malignant neoplasms in breast cancer patients in Israel. Cancer, 54:145, 1984.

Schoenberg, B. S.: Multiple Primary Malignant Neoplasms. The Connecticut Experience, 1935–1964. Berlin, Springer-Verlag, 1977.

Schwartz, G. F., Patchefsky, A. S., Feig, S. A., et al.: Multicentricity of non-palpable breast cancer. Cancer, 45:2913, 1980.

Shellito, J. G., and Bartlett, W. C.: Bilateral carcinoma of the breast. Arch. Surg., 94:489, 1967.

Silverman, E. M., and Oberman, H. A.: Metastatic neoplasms in the breast. Surg. Gynecol. Obstet., 138:26, 1974.

Slack, N. H., Nemoto, T., and Fisher, B.: Experiences with bilateral primary carcinoma of the breast. Surg. Gynecol. Obstet., 136:433, 1973.

Smith, B. C.: Bilateral carcinoma of the breast in living mother and daughter. Arch. Surg., 97:590, 1968.

Spratt, J. S.: Multiple primary cancers: Review of clinical studies from two Missouri hospitals. Cancer, 40:1806, 1977.

Spratt, J. S., and Hoag, M.: Incidence of multiple primary cancers per man-year of follow-up. Ann. Surg., 164:775, 1966.

Spratt, J. S., and Spratt, T. L.: Correlation of the rates of growth of pulmonary metastases and host survival. Ann. Surg., 159:161, 1964.

Tagart, R. E. B.: Partial mastectomy for breast cancer. Br. Med. J., 2:1268, 1978.

Trevor, W.: Bilateral breast cancer. N.Y. State J. Med., 54:1937, 1954.

Urban, J. A.: Bilaterality of cancer of the breast: Biopsy of the opposite breast. Cancer, 29:1867, 1967.

Urban, J. A.: Biopsy of the "normal" breast in treating breast cancer. Surg. Clin. North Am., 49:291, 1969a.

Urban, J. A.: Bilateral breast cancer. Cancer, 24:1310, 1969b.

Wanebo, H. J., Senofsky, G. M., Fechner, R. E., et al.: Bilateral breast cancer—risk reduction by contralateral biopsy. Ann. Surg., 201:667, 1985.

Warren, S., and Gates, O.: Multiple primary malignant tumors: A survey of the literature and statistical study. Am. J. Cancer, 16:1358, 1932.

Webber, B. L., Heise, H., Neifeld, J. P., et al.: Risk of subsequent contralateral breast carcinoma in a population of patients with in-situ breast carcinoma. Cancer, 47:2928, 1983.

Wilson, N. D., and Alberty, R. E.: Bilateral carcinoma of the breast. Am. J. Surg., 126:244, 1973.

CHAPTER 23

WILLIAM L. DONEGAN

Local and Regional Recurrence

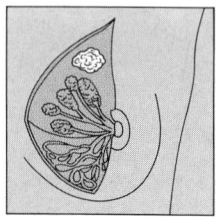

Recurrence is reappearance of the original cancer after a period of apparent cure. The period without evidence of cancer is known as the "disease-free interval." Recurrence may follow primary treatment for two reasons: either because the cancer was occultly disseminated before treatment or because it was incompletely eliminated from local and regional tissues. It was with a strong sense of responsibility for ensuring against the latter that Halsted advocated wide removal of the breast, pectoral muscles, and axillary tissues in 1894. There is no doubt that recurrence of cancer on the chest wall was significantly reduced by Halsted's operation (Table 23–1). Such recurrences were further reduced by the introduction of postoperative irradiation to the chest wall and to the neglected lymph nodes in the parasternal and supraclavicular areas. Nevertheless, recurrence continues as a vexing problem and frequently is the earliest and most obvious sign of therapeutic failure. In this chapter special attention is given to local and regional recurrence because the mechanism, prognosis, and treatment are in some respects different from those of disseminated mammary carcinoma.

Definition

It is important to distinguish between local and regional recurrence. This distinction is not always made in the literature, which accounts for inconsistencies in frequencies and results. Local recurrence can be defined as reappearance of carcinoma within the soft tissues of the anterior chest, that is, the skin, residual breast tissue, subcutaneous tissues, and underlying muscles. After radical and modified mastectomies, this ordinarily includes a region bounded by the sternum medially, the clavicle superiorly, the posterior axillary line laterally (exclusive of the axilla), and the costal margin inferiorly. After breast conserving therapy, it includes the breast as well.

Regional recurrence refers to the appearance of metastases in unremoved regional lymph nodes. At risk for regional recurrence are the axillary, internal mammary (IM) and the supraclavicular lymph nodes. Fixed subcutaneous mounds of tumor that appear between rib spaces along the sternal border seem to be within the "local" area, but they often represent enlargement of involved internal mammary nodes and are, therefore, regional in origin (Fig. 23–1). The same is true for deep masses just inferior to the medial end of the clavicle, which usually signify involvement of the apical axillary, or "infraclavicular," nodes. Masses deep to the pectoralis major muscle after modified mastectomy are probably regional recurrence in unremoved interpectoral (Rotter's) nodes rather than truly local recurrence (Fig. 23–2) (Chen et al., 1985).

Thus, a clear distinction cannot always be made between local and regional recurrence, either on a geographic or on an anatomic basis. Lymph nodes can be found within the breast, and breast tissue can overlap the node-bearing regions, especially the axilla. The origin of a tumor mass from nodal or nonnodal tissue often can only be surmised. Although identifying specific sites of failure is important in improving future treatment planning, the reader should appreciate these limitations. It is not surprising that local and regional recurrences are often reported together to avoid these problems.

The frequency of combined local-regional

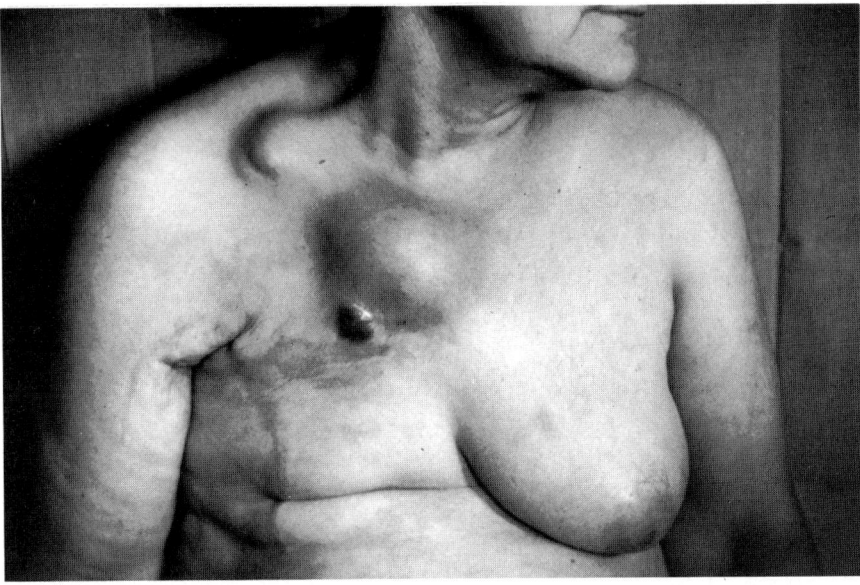

Figure 23–1. Recurrent mammary carcinoma after radical mastectomy. Disease is confined clinically to local and regional sites. The supraclavicular nodes are enlarged, and the large mass at the upper sternal border is characteristic of tumor growth in internal mammary lymph nodes. A dermal recurrence is present in the medial skin flap.

recurrence after modified radical mastectomy related to TNM clinical stage and pathologic nodal status is shown in Figure 23–3. Also shown is the distribution of recurrences after mastectomies (Table 23–2). Noteworthy is that local recurrence is more frequent than regional recurrence, and both increase with time.

Mechanism

The mechanism of local recurrence is uncertain. All of the following have been suggested:

1. Retrograde embolization through transected lymphatics.
2. Incomplete local removal of neoplasm—for example, progressive growth of cancer in breast tissue remaining in thick skin flaps (Fig. 23–4) (Peters et al., 1977) or after breast conserving treatment.
3. Transection of involved lymphatics and blood vessels with spill of cancer cells and implantation into the wound.
4. Implantation of hematogenous metastases in the traumatized tissue of the thorax as part of general dissemination (Dao, 1963). The

Table 23–1. RESULTS OF OPERATIONS FOR THE CURE OF CANCER OF THE BREAST

Surgeon	Dates	Number of Cases	Local Recurrence (%)
Bergman	1882–87	114	51–60
Billroth	1867–76	170	82
Czerny	1877–86	102	62
Fischer	1871–78	147	75
Gussenbauer	1878–86	151	64
Konig	1875–85	152	58–62
Kuster	1871–85	228	59.6
Lucke	1881–90	110	66
Volkman	1874–78	131	60
Halsted	1889–94	50	6

From Halsted, W.S.: The results of operations for the cure of cancer of the breast performed at the Johns Hopkins Hospital from June 1889 to January 1984. Medical Classics, 3:441, 1938.

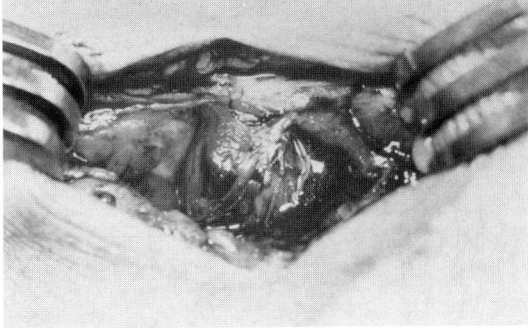

Figure 23–2. Recurrence in Rotter's interpectoral node masquerading as local recurrence. The isolated mass of tumor was palpable in the anterior chest but lay deep to the pectoralis major muscle.

CUMULATIVE LOCAL-REGIONAL RECURRENCE AFTER AUCHINCLOSS (A) AND PATEY (P) MASTECTOMY*

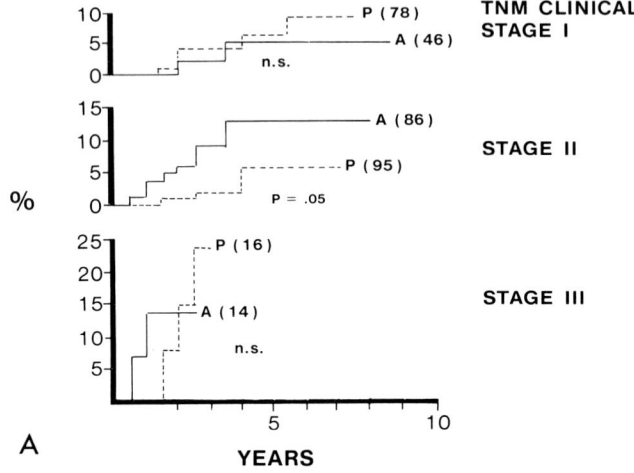

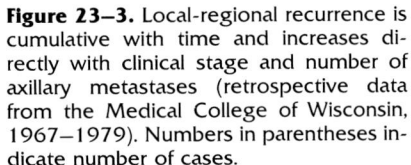

*Curves stop when cases <10

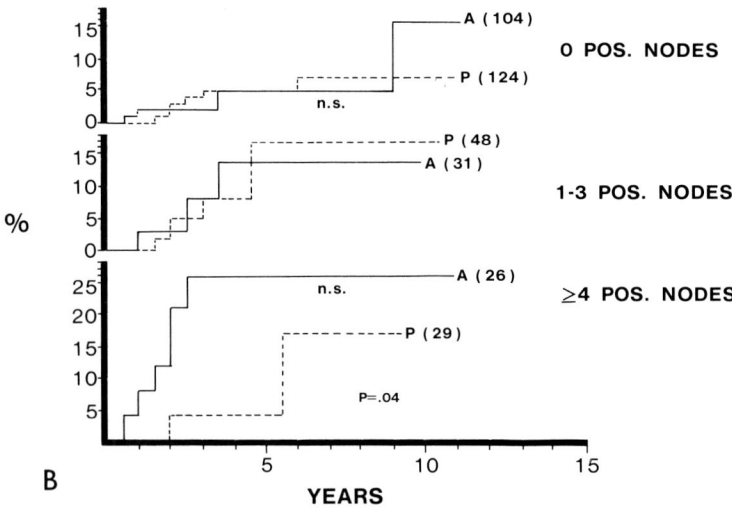

Figure 23–3. Local-regional recurrence is cumulative with time and increases directly with clinical stage and number of axillary metastases (retrospective data from the Medical College of Wisconsin, 1967–1979). Numbers in parentheses indicate number of cases.

Table 23–2. DISTRIBUTION OF LOCAL AND REGIONAL RECURRENCE AFTER VARIOUS MASTECTOMIES—MEDICAL COLLEGE OF WISCONSIN

Operation	Axillary Metastases	Local	Axilla	Supraclavicular
Auchincloss modified radical mastectomy (axillary Levels I and II)	All	10 (56%)	5 (28%)*	3 (17%)
	Ax 0	5 (56%)	3 (33%)	1 (11%)
	Ax +	5 (55%)	2 (22%)	2 (22%)
Patey modified radical mastectomy (axillary Levels I, II, III)	All	13 (68%)	1 (5%)*	5 (26%)
	Ax 0	6 (67%)	1 (11%)	2 (22%)
	Ax +	7 (70%)		3 (30%)
Halsted radical mastectomy (axillary Levels I, II, III)	All	36 (70%)	7 (13%)	9 (17%)
	Ax 0	11 (58%)	4 (21%)	4 (21%)
	Ax +	25 (76%)	3 (9%)	5 (15%)

*Difference is not significant; $p = 0.08$
Shown are not the absolute but the relative frequencies of recurrence. Local recurrence is more frequent than regional even when the axilla was pathologically involved. Axillary recurrence is less frequent than supraclavicular after a complete axillary dissection is performed.

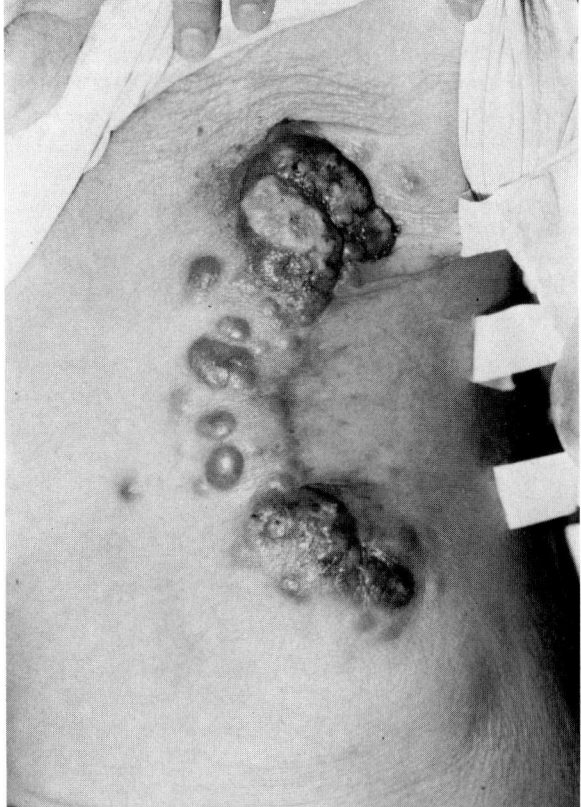

Figure 23–4. Recurrence concentrated around the scar of a limited mastectomy suggests incomplete removal of the primary cancer's local extensions.

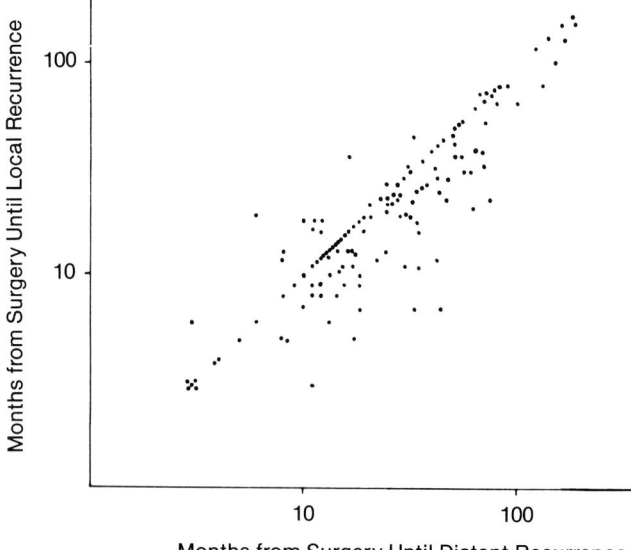

Figure 23–5. A logarithmic plot of time from mastectomy to local and distant recurrence for 139 patients with both illustrates a good correlation between the two. In 45 per cent of cases, dissemination preceded local recurrence or appeared simultaneously.

close association of local and distant recurrences pointed out by several observers supports this view (Fig. 23–5) (Spratt, 1967; Bruce, 1970). Extensive local recurrence confined to a previously irradiated area of the chest often has a particular characteristic, discussed by Diehl and coworkers (1984) (Fig. 23–6). It features erythema, skin thickening, and myriads of small nodules that enlarge and coalesce. It is postulated that in these cases irradiation-induced vascular endothelial cell damage leads to increased trapping, survival, and growth of tumor cells. Evidence for this is based on animal models in which preferential tumor cell trapping and persistence can be demonstrated in irradiated tissues. Clinically, however, irradiation does not increase the overall risk of recurrence.

5. The stasis of lymph that follows regional lymph node dissections may arrest the endolymphatic transport of cancer cells and result in entrapment or "in transit" metastases (Spratt et al., 1965).

The mechanism of regional recurrence presumably is progressive growth of metastases lodged in regional lymph nodes. Fisher and associates (1977) demonstrated that the nodes in almost 40 per cent of clinically normal axillae harbor metastases. If the nodes remain untreated, metastases at this site become evident as the first site of failure in 21 per cent of cases (50 per cent of those with involve-

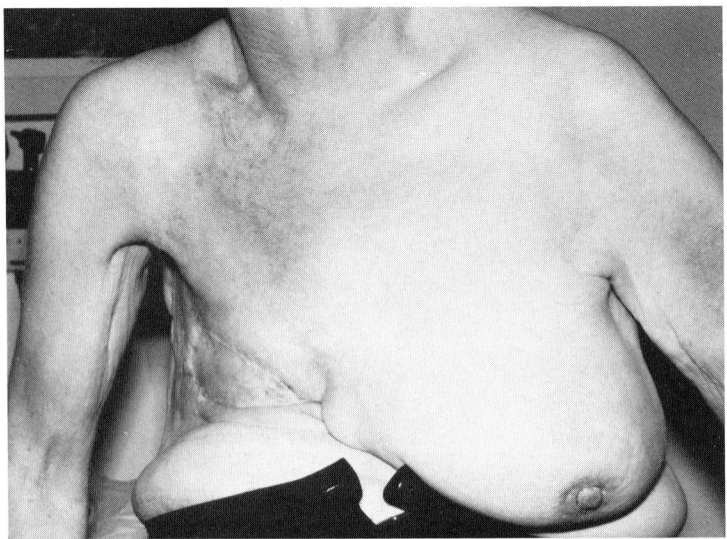

Figure 23–6. Recurrence confined within the field of prophylactic irradiation on the right chest presenting a typical picture of diffuse erythema, skin thickening, and multiple small papules that gradually coalesce. (From Diehl, L. F., et al.: Skin metastases confined to a field of previous irradiation. Cancer, 53:1864, 1984. Reprinted with permission.)

ment) during subsequent follow-up, the majority within 24 months. Similarly, biopsy-proven metastases in internal mammary nodes left untreated produce adenopathy at the sternal border in 10 per cent of cases (Donegan, 1977).

The weight of evidence is that both local and regional recurrences result from incomplete removal, or incomplete destruction, of cancer, either at its primary site, in the surrounding lymphatics, or in the regional lymph nodes. Recurrence is closely allied to dissemination because locally extensive cancers have usually also metastasized to distant sites.

Frequency and Distribution

LOCAL RECURRENCE

Local recurrence of carcinoma may occur any time after radical mastectomy. Danckers and colleagues (1960) found 26 cases in the literature that had first appeared 15 years after surgery. Recurrence is most likely within the first 2 years, with a peak incidence in the second year, after which the rate steadily diminishes (Fig. 23–7).

Slightly more than one sixth (17.4 per cent) of 704 patients treated at Ellis Fischel State Cancer Hospital (EFSCH) with radical mastectomy and without irradiation and reexamined at regular intervals thereafter developed local recurrence within 5 years. In this group, 87 per cent of the local recurrences that occurred within 10 years had appeared by the end of the first 5 years. The problem continues to increase with time: 24.5 per cent of 1296 similarly selected women treated at EFSCH for unilateral carcinomas and observed for 1 to 24 years developed local recurrences (Donegan, 1972). It is of interest in this connection that local failure in Halsted's original 50 patients rose from an initial 6 per cent in 1894 to 32 per cent when the cases were reviewed in 1931 (Lewis and Rienhoff, 1932). Thus, the interval of observation is an important variable and must be uniform if comparisons of local recurrence between different treatments are to be valid. The cumulative rate of failure locally, however, is approximately the same as at other sites (i.e., neither earlier nor notably later than in nodes, lungs, bones, or viscera) (Fig. 23–8).

In addition to time elapsed, the frequency of local treatment failure depends on a number of other clinical variables. The EFSCH data illustrate that the 5 year recurrence rate was higher when axillary nodes were involved at the time of mastectomy (26 per cent) than when they were not (6.5 per cent), an observation also made by others (Deck and Kern, 1976). Five year recurrence was also directly correlated with primary tumor size (Table 23–3), the number of involved axillary nodes (Table 23–4), the histologic type of tumor, and the presence of skin edema or skin and fascial fixation with the primary tumor. Furthermore, it is a function of clinical stage at the time of mastectomy (Table 23–5).

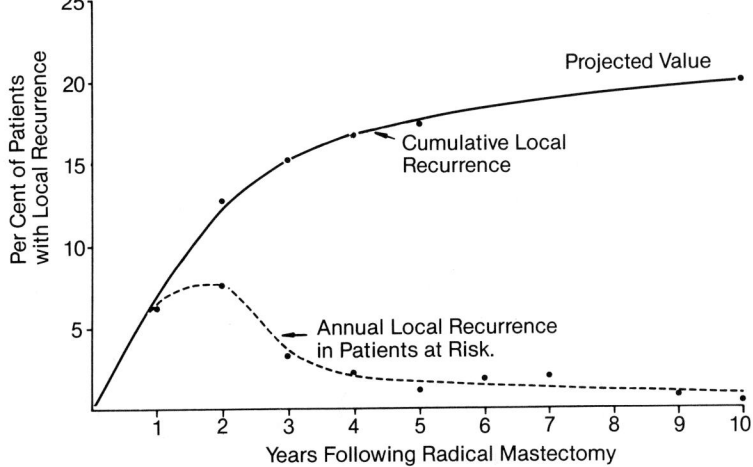

Figure 23–7. The rate of local recurrence in 704 patients treated with radical mastectomy for unilateral breast carcinoma. The annual local recurrence rate reaches a maximum the second year following mastectomy and diminishes progressively thereafter.

Table 23–3. PRIMARY TUMOR DIAMETER AND LOCAL RECURRENCE WITHIN 5 YEARS*

Tumor Diameter (cm)	Number of Patients	Number with Local Recurrence	Per Cent with Local Recurrence
0.0–0.9	7	0	0
1.0–1.9	66	5	7.6
2.0–2.9	120	15	12.5
3.0–3.9	159	25	15.8
4.0–4.9	119	26	21.8
5.0–5.9	51	14	27.4
6.0–6.9	36	11	30.6
7.0–7.9	24	8	33.3
8.0 and above	24	8	33.3
Unmeasured	98	11	11.2

*A chi square test indicates that the incidences of local recurrence for the nine categories of size are not the same ($p < 0.01$).

From Donegan, W. L., et al.: A biostatistical study of locally recurrent breast carcinoma. Surg. Gynecol. Obstet., 112:529, 1966. Reprinted with permission.

The development of local recurrence is not influenced by the type of wound closure employed. On an annual basis, the percentage of patients who developed local recurrences within 5 years of radical mastectomy at EFSCH did not change significantly in 17 years despite wide variation in the technique of wound closure (Fig. 23–9). Narrow surgical margins, however, may increase the incidence. Pathology reports on 559 patients pertaining to radical mastectomies recorded measurements of the skin excised with the specimen and the diameters of the carcinomas removed. The smallest skin diameter was subtracted from the maximum tumor diameter, and the difference was halved to produce a least surgical skin margin. When this result was correlated with figures for 5 year local recurrence (Fig. 23–10), it was found that skin margins of less than 3 cm (less than 3.5 cm, allowing for skin shrinkage after excision) were associated with significantly higher local recurrence than were greater margins ($p < 0.05$). This suggests that surgical margins that are too narrow invite local recurrence. In an investigation of the same problem, Dao (1963) obtained accurate measurements of the skin margin at the time of surgery and found no correlation with local

Table 23–4. NUMBER OF INVOLVED AXILLARY LYMPH NODES AND LOCAL RECURRENCE WITHIN 5 YEARS*

Number of Involved Nodes	Number of Patients	Number of Patients with Local Recurrence	Per Cent with 5 Year Local Recurrence
0	308	20	6.5
1	93	9	10.3
2	56	7	12.3
3	34	6	17.6
4	30	8	26.7
5	26	9	34.6
6	18	6	33.3
7	13	5	38.5
8	16	9	56.3
9	15	7	46.7
10–12	30	9	30.0
13–19	36	16	44.4
20 and up	28	12	42.9

(Number of nodes not given in one patient—no recurrence)

*A chi square test indicates that values for local recurrences with increasing numbers of involved axillary lymph nodes are not the same at a level of significance of $p < 0.01$.

From Donegan, W. L., et al: A biostatistical study of locally recurrent breast carcinoma. Surg. Gynecol. Obstet., 112:529, 1966. Reprinted with permission.

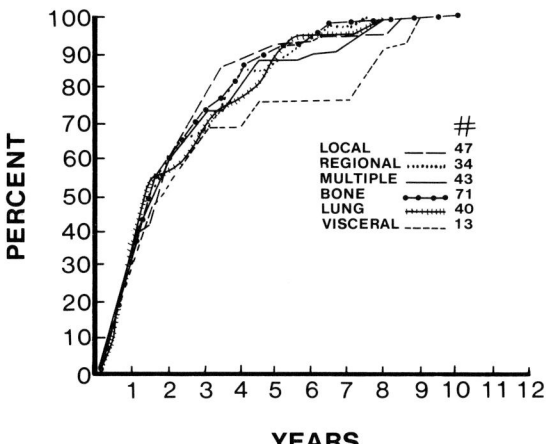

Figure 23–8. A plot of cumulative recurrence after modified mastectomy indicates that local or regional recurrence is not uniquely early or delayed compared with recurrence at other locations. (From Tomin, R., and Donegan, W. L.: Screening for recurrent breast cancer—Its effectiveness and prognostic value. J. Clin. Oncol., 5:62, 1987. Reprinted with permission.)

recurrence. Few margins in Dao's series measured less than the 3.0 to 3.5 cm found to be significant in the EFSCH series, however, and follow-up for recurrence was brief in many cases.

The most frequent site of local recurrence varies in reports. Demaree (1951) and Pawlias and coworkers (1958) reported a predominance of recurrences medial to a diagonal mastectomy scar. Haagensen (1971) reported the greatest number in the grafted site, as did Danckers (1960); the EFSCH radical mastectomy cases showed a similar tendency. Forty-two per cent of 146 local recurrences initially developed within or in contact with the scar or grafted area (Fig. 23–11), 22 per cent occurred in the medial flap, and 15 per cent occurred within the lateral flap. The remainder had mixed locations.

The overall prognosis of patients with local recurrence is relatively favorable in comparison with that of patients with regional recurrence or recurrence at other sites. Figure 23–12 shows survival rates after recurrences at various sites following mastectomies performed at the Medical College of Wisconsin between 1967 and 1979.

REGIONAL RECURRENCE

Supraclavicular Lymph Nodes. The supraclavicular dissections of Dahl-Iversen (1963) showed that approximately 8 per cent of patients already had metastases to this lymph node group at the time of mastectomy. Haagensen (1971) found that an almost identical proportion (8.7 per cent) of 356 carefully selected surgical patients developed clinical evidence of supraclavicular metastases within 5 years after radical mastectomy.

Supraclavicular recurrence is usually a sign of impending clinical dissemination. Fentiman

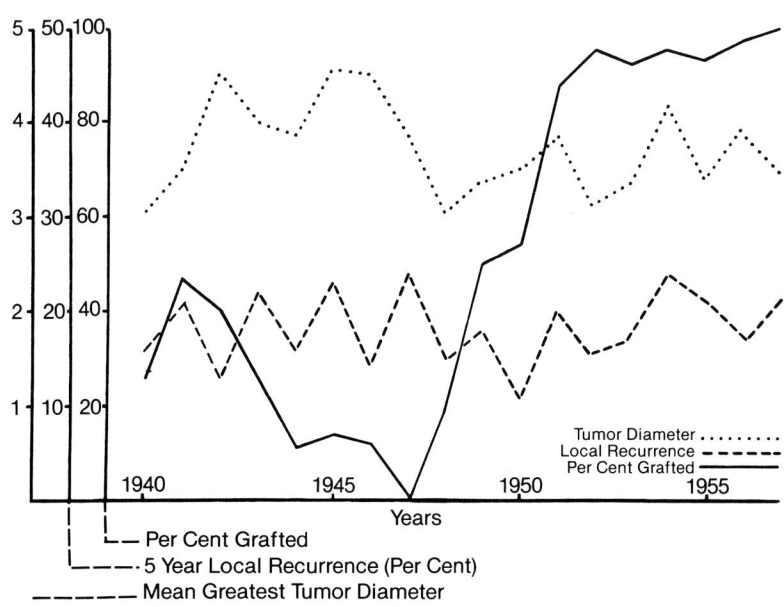

Figure 23–9. Relationship among skin grafting, primary tumor diameter, and 5 year local recurrence at EFSCH, 1940 to 1957. Despite wide variation in the practice of grafting at the time of mastectomy, the 5 year local recurrence rate for the respective years remained constant. Mean tumor diameter also remained constant and did not account for the decision to graft. (From Donegan, W. L., et al.: A biostatistical study of locally recurrent breast carcinoma. Surg. Gynecol. Obstet., 112:529, 1966. Reprinted with permission.)

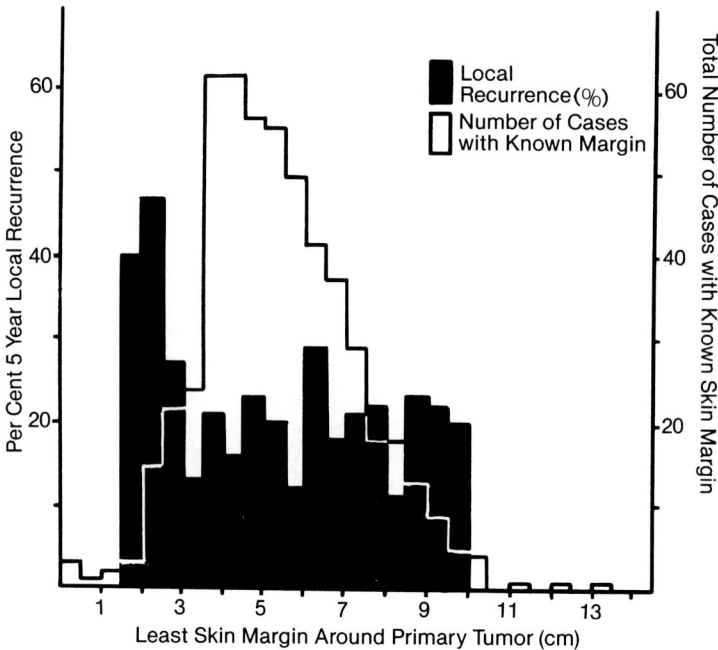

Figure 23–10. Relationship between skin margin and 5 year local recurrence of breast carcinoma following radical mastectomy (559 cases). Surgical skin margins less than 3 cm measured on the mastectomy specimen correlate with increased local recurrence. (From Donegan, W. L., et al.: A biostatistical study of locally recurrent breast carcinoma. Surg. Gynecol. Obstet., 112:529, 1966. Reprinted with permission.)

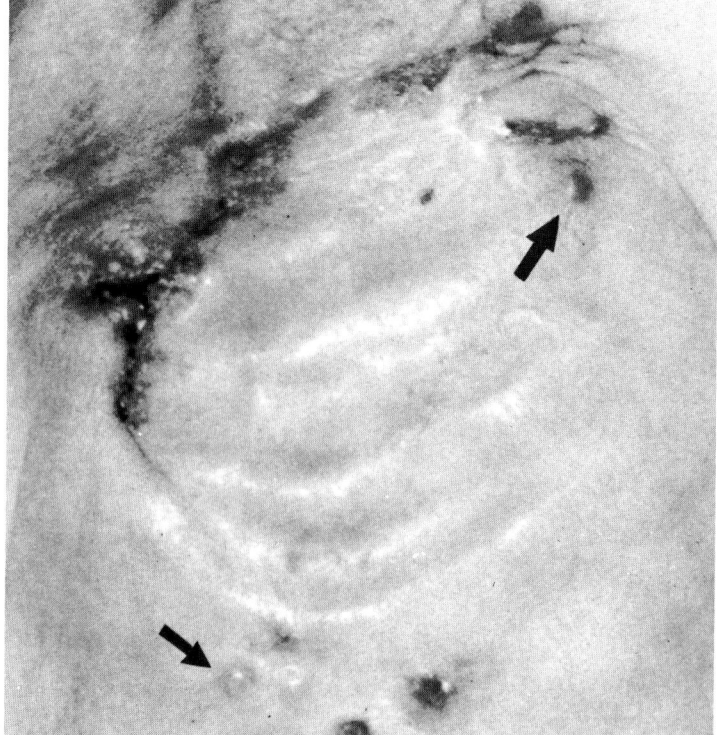

Figure 23–11. Locally recurrent mammary carcinoma after radical mastectomy. Arrows indicate multiple skin nodules scattered at the periphery of the grafted area.

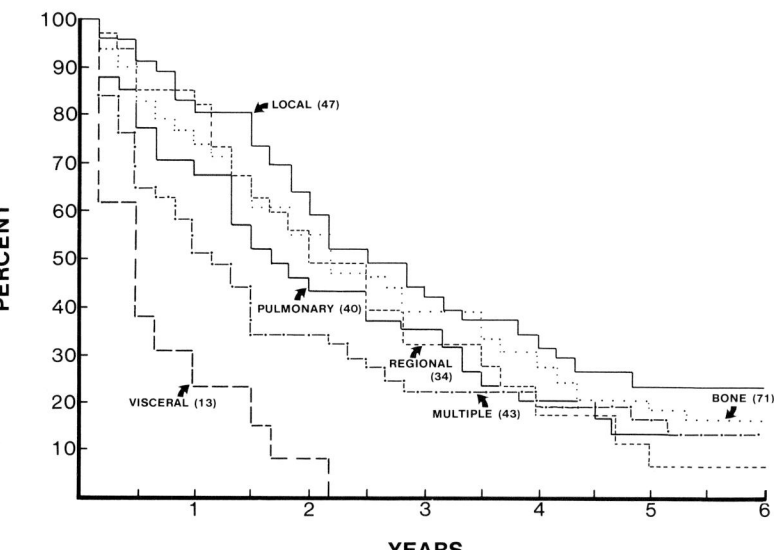

Figure 23–12. Survival following recurrence at various sites indicates the relatively favorable prognosis associated with isolated local recurrence. (From Tomin, R., and Donegan, W. L.: Screening for recurrent breast cancer—Its effectiveness and prognostic value. J. Clin. Oncol., 5:62, 1987. Reprinted with permission.)

and colleagues (1986) analyzed 35 cases of isolated supraclavicular recurrence after radical mastectomy at Guy's Hospital. The mean disease-free interval was 37 months, longer than that of patients with isolated local recurrence (22 months). Axillary lymph nodes had been involved in 74 per cent. Most were treated with excision (presumably for diagnosis) and irradiation with good control at this site, but within 12 months 50 per cent had further signs of recurrence, and 80 per cent did recur in 4 years. The 5 year survival rate after supraclavicular recurrence was 30 per cent, the same as for patients with isolated local skin recurrence. At 10 years, 20 per cent of patients were alive.

Internal Mammary Lymph Nodes. Metastases in the internal mammary nodes become clinically apparent less frequently than nodal failures at other sites, probably because of their location deep to the ribs. It can be estimated from the findings of surgeons who have included internal mammary lymph node dissections with mastectomy that approximately one third of patients who are deemed candidates for surgery already have internal mammary lymph node involvement, the proportion rising with clinical stage. With pathologically negative axillary nodes, the internal mammary lymph nodes are involved in 9 per cent of cases, creating a sizeable error when nodal staging is based only on axillary evaluation (Veronesi et al., 1984); this error can reach 20 per cent with medial primary tumors (Morrow and Foster, 1981). These metastases, which are beyond the boundaries of the modified or radical mastectomy, contribute to regional failure. Two of 20 EFSCH patients (10 per cent) with biopsy-proved but untreated internal mammary lymph node metastases developed typical parasternal recurrences after radical mastectomy during 9 to 24 years of observation (Donegan, 1977). The figure was no higher (11 per cent) when both axillary and internal mammary nodes contained metastases. Veronesi and Valagussa (1981) reported

Table 23–5. FIVE YEAR LOCAL RECURRENCE FOLLOWING MASTECTOMY AND INITIAL CLINICAL STAGE—MEDICAL COLLEGE OF WISCONSIN

TNM Clinical Stage (1983)	Radical Mastectomy		Modified Mastectomy	
	Total Patients	Per Cent Recurrence	Total Patients	Per Cent Recurrence
I	133	8.3%	46	5.1%
II	203	9.0%	86	13.2%
IIIa	57	16.4%	16	20%

Table 23–6. LOCAL AND REGIONAL RECURRENCES AFTER DIFFERENT PRIMARY TREATMENTS IN TWO RANDOMIZED TRIALS

I. Different Treatment of Regional Nodes (NSABP B-04)

	Axilla Clinically Negative			Axilla Clinically Positive	
	Radical Mastectomy	Total Mastectomy Plus Chest Wall and Regional Irradiation	Total Mastectomy	Radical Mastectomy	Total Mastectomy Plus Chest Wall and Regional Irradiation
Total number	362	352	365	292	294
Local	5%	1.4%	7.1%	7.9%	2.7%
Regional					
Axillary	1.4%	3.1%	18%*	1.0%	10.5%
Supraclavicular	1.1%	0.3%	2.7%	5.1%	0
Parasternal	0	0	0	0	0
Distant	27.1%	32.7%	30.1%	37.1%	40.8%

II. Different Treatment of the Breast (NSABP B-06)

	Total Mastectomy and Axillary Dissection	Segmental Mastectomy and Axillary Dissection	Segmental Mastectomy, Axillary Dissection, and Breast Irradiation
Number			
Breast recurrence		28%	8%
Local	6.8%†	5.9%†	0.8%†
Regional	3.8%	5.3%	3.5%
Axillary	1.4%	3.1%	1.1%
Parasternal	0.3%	0.2%	0%
Supraclavicular	1.7%	1.3%	2.1%
Distant	14%	15.5%	14.5%
Second breast	2.5%	3.3%	2.9%

*1.4% subsequent failure in axilla after axillary dissection.
†Subsequent local failure after salvage mastectomy.

Recurrences are shown after three competing primary treatments in two different clinical trials conducted by the National Surgical Adjuvant Breast Project (NSABP). Follow-up is uniform within each of the two. Failure to treat with surgical removal or irradiation of the axillary nodes (I) or the breast (II) resulted in a high frequency of tumor recurrence at these sites. Secondary "salvage" surgery was used for recurrence in both instances, apparently with adequate local and regional control, but ultimate results are still pending.

parasternal recurrence in 3.7 per cent of all patients treated with radical mastectomy in an international study. This was reduced to 0.3 per cent by prophylactic excision.

Axillary Lymph Nodes. In the presence of an invasive primary tumor, a clinically negative axilla contains nodal metastases in almost 40 per cent of cases (Fisher et al., 1985). If these metastases are undisturbed, regional failure in the axilla can be expected as the first sign of recurrence in a considerable number of patients. According to Fisher and associates (1977), 18 per cent of 344 patients showed failure first at this site after total (simple) mastectomy within a mean observation period of 36 months, a figure amounting to almost one half the proportion believed to have occult metastases. Axillary recurrences are effectively prevented by thorough axillary dissection or irradiation. In the presence of enlarged lymph nodes, dissection is probably more effective (Table 23–6).

Local and Regional Recurrence Versus Initial Treatment. The comparative frequencies of local and regional recurrence after three different primary treatments in two different randomized studies are shown in Table 23–6. The first, a comparison of radical mastectomy, total mastectomy, and total mastectomy plus local and regional irradiation (NSABP protocol B-04) for Stage I and Stage II breast cancer, shows the clear 65 to 72 per cent reduction in local recurrence produced by postoperative irradiation in both Stage I and Stage II. This is not accompanied by a corresponding reduction in distant dissemination. The table also shows the overall 18 per cent recurrence in the axillary nodes if these nodes are not removed or irradiated in clinical Stage I cases. Axillary failures are largely prevented with axillary dissection or irradiation, but perhaps more effectively with dissection in the presence of adenopathy. Supraclavicular failures are infrequent but are reduced by prophylactic irradiation. Internal mammary lymph node recurrences are rare as a first sign of treatment failure whether treated or not.

In the second study (NSABP B-06), a comparison of modified mastectomy, segmental mastectomy plus axillary dissection and breast irradiation, and segmental mastectomy plus axillary dissection, again after a mean of 3.7 months of follow-up, irradiation to the breast markedly reduced local recurrences in the treated area, the breast, from 28 per cent to 8 per cent. Regional recurrences in the axilla were equally low after axillary dissection in all three treatments, and internal mammary or supraclavicular recurrences were a low risk despite no treatment. Distant dissemination was not influenced by variation in local treatment.

Management

Although local recurrence can be an isolated event, it ordinarily is a harbinger of dissemination. Only about 5 per cent of patients with recurrence in the surgical area after mastectomy fail to develop distant metastases. Dissemination, however, may be delayed many months or years, and therefore isolated local cancer is deserving of vigorous treatment. Effective control not only spares the patient much discomfort and embarrassment from weeping, bleeding, and odoriferous ulceration, but it also might possibly retard the development of dissemination (Donegan et al., 1966). In a few cases it may be curative.

An accurate diagnosis is paramount. Suspicious nodules in the surgically treated areas, or enlarged regional nodes that appear during follow-up, should be biopsied. Frozen section permits recurrence to be confirmed histologically, and estrogen receptors (ER) and progesterone receptors (PgR) can be obtained in the fresh tissue. Previous irradiation can reduce ER and PgR in tumors, so tumor samples from outside an irradiated area may be preferable (Janssens et al., 1981). Local or regional recurrence should prompt a suspicion that disease is also present elsewhere, so an evaluation, including radiographs, isotopic scans, and tests of liver function are in order to detect the presence of disseminated cancer. Forty-five per cent of the EFSCH patients had distant disease diagnosed prior to or simultaneously with the appearance of recurrence on the chest wall.

One or two isolated local nodules without evidence of disease elsewhere can occasionally be controlled simply with local excision. Four of 15 (27 per cent) patients at EFSCH with isolated, superficial nodules of tumor had no further recurrence locally after excision, although metastases progressed elsewhere. Such wide local excision is not preferred treatment, but it may be useful particularly when recurrence is small and occurs in a previously irradiated site.

IRRADIATION

The therapy of choice for local and regional recurrence is irradiation. If recurrences are detected early and treated properly, successful control can be expected. Although ports limited to the gross disease can achieve remarkable results (Fig. 23–13), progression wide of the treated area becomes apparent in many cases—27 per cent in the series of Chen and associates (1985)—creating a problem with juxtaposing ports and necessitating additional periods of treatment. The preferred approach is comprehensive treatment of the chest wall and unresected regional nodes.

Control of local and regional recurrence with irradiation has been reported in 41 per cent to 72 per cent of cases (Chu et al., 1976; Bedwinek et al, 1981a,b; Patanaphan, 1984; Chen et al., 1985). The ability to control local disease is strongly related to dose and volume of irradiation. Bedwinek and coworkers (1981) considered no less than 4500 to 5000 rad to comprehensive fields to be adequate (Table 23–7). Bedwinek and colleagues also found prognosis to be associated with the number of recurrent nodules, their size, and the disease-free interval. The best outlook was associated with a single nodule, small size (i.e., 1 cm or less in diameter), and a disease-free interval longer than 24 months. Five year survival exceeded 50 per cent with any two of these factors. Comprehensive irradiation that controlled the local and regional disease results in survival superior to that which follows failure, but factors of selection and tumor biology also influence this result. Dissemination was not less frequent in successfully treated patients, but it was delayed. Chen and coworkers also found an isolated nodule of recurrence favor-

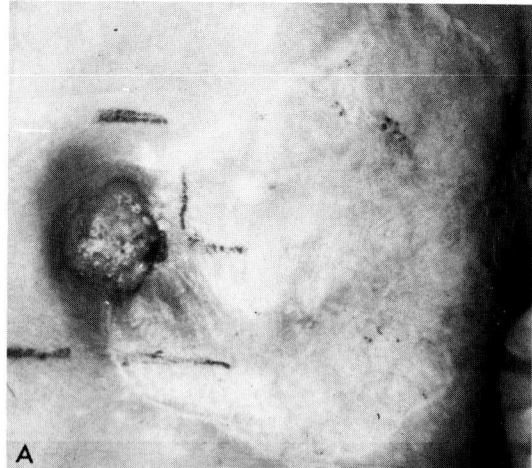

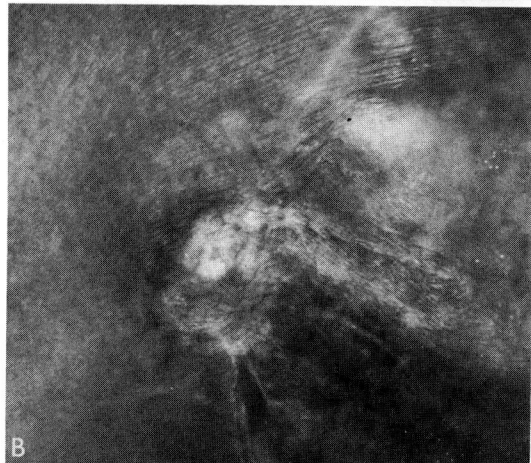

Figure 23–13. *A,* Cancer recurred on the medial chest wall 3 years after a radical mastectomy in a 51 year old woman for an adenocarcinoma metastatic to 4 of 24 axillary lymph nodes. *B,* She received irradiation to a limited port (marked) encompassing the lesion and was well, with no further evidence of metastasis 55 months later. Irradiation controlled progressive growth of cancer in what was apparently an isolated internal mammary node.

When local recurrence occupies an area irradiated prophylactically and does not lend itself to excision, the problem of therapy is more difficult. Further irradiation has been used, but local tissue tolerance is a major consideration if unwanted necrosis is to be avoided (Zimmerman et al., 1966).

The point is often made that routine postoperative irradiation is more successful in preventing local-regional recurrence than in controlling recurrence when it appears. Large, neglected recurrences are particularly difficult to manage. With postoperative irradiation, local failure can be reduced to 5 per cent (Prosnitz et al., 1977). However, the 95 per cent control of early recurrences in regional nodes reported by Madoc-Jones and associates (1976) demonstrates the success that can be expected if patients are examined conscientiously at intervals and recurrences are detected and treated while still small.

CHEST WALL RESECTION

In selected cases, chest wall resection is appropriate therapy for isolated local recurrence or for recurrence confined to parasternal lymph nodes. It may be the only recourse for discrete recurrences fixed to the bony thorax and un-

able prognostically, but an initially negative axilla and no prior recurrence were also favorable. Patanaphan and colleagues (1984) reported that a small primary tumor favored survival after local recurrence, as did the absence of distant metastases or their delayed appearance. The absence of simultaneous distant metastases also favored survival in the EFSCH series (Fig. 23–14). It is evident that patients with local and regional recurrence are not a uniform group prognostically. Those with large, extensive, rapidly growing recurrences have a poor outlook and are unlikely to be controlled. Those with a small, solitary recurrence that is slow to appear have the opposite outlook.

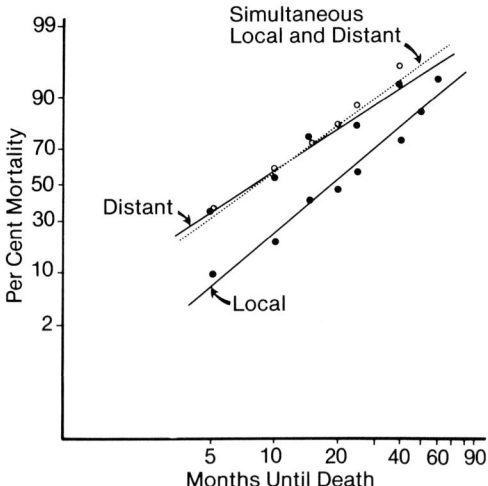

Figure 23–14. Logarithmic plots of mortality after recurrence are shown for EFSCH patients treated with radical mastectomy who had local recurrence alone, distant recurrence followed by local recurrence, and both types of recurrence simultaneously. The survival of patients whose first sign of recurrence was restricted to the surgical area was superior to that of others at all points. The prognosis of patients with local recurrence as the first sign of treatment failure, therefore, is more favorable than that of those who first exhibit dissemination.

Table 23–7. CONTROL OF LOCAL-REGIONAL RECURRENCE AFTER MASTECTOMY

Treatment	Number	Per Cent Success	5 Year Survival
Adequate radiotherapy	32	72%	40%
Inadequate radiotherapy	100	28%	38%
Excision	25	24%	35%

Adequate radiotherapy is preferred treatment for local and regional recurrence. It is defined as a dose of at least 4500 rad to a field that encompasases the entire site containing the recurrence.

Data from Bedwinik, J. M., et al.: Prognostic indicators in patients with isolated local-regional recurrence of breast cancer. Cancer, 47:2232, 1981b.

responsive to irradiation. Ideally, such recurrences should be well marginated, appear after a prolonged disease-free interval, and be unaccompanied by generalized disease.

Sauerbruch is given credit for first removing recurrent mammary carcinoma with chest wall resection in 1907, but Schede preceded him in 1886 and, in turn, credited Kolaczek for using it earlier for other tumors. Urban used this method for parasternal recurrences beginning in 1951, a prelude to his extended mastectomy.

Snyder and associates (1969) reported a series of 24 patients so treated, with 4 (17 per cent) long-term survivors free of disease. The selection of slowly growing cancers was important. These authors stated, "Chest wall resection prolongs life and possibly is curative in selected patients who have their initial local recurrence without evidence of generalized disease 48 months or more after mastectomy." Shah and Urban (1975) reported 52 such resections performed from 1950 to 1972, primarily for parasternal recurrences. The indications in most instances were failure to respond to irradiation, recurrence in ports used for postoperative irradiation, radionecrosis, and radiation-induced cancers of the chest wall. The 5 year survival of patients treated specifically for recurrence was higher when resection was the initial treatment (43 per cent) than when the tumor had proved resistant to irradiation (16 per cent).

McKenna and associates (1984) reported 43 chest wall resections for recurrent breast cancer or radionecrosis and included as indications (1) local symptoms of pain, infection, and ulceration, (2) tumor recurrence despite radiotherapy, and (3) infection precluding chemotherapy. Contraindications included tumor en cuirass, brain metastasis, bone marrow involvement, and bulky disease in two or more organs. These authors did not consider liver, lung, and boney metastases and malignant pleural effusions to be absolute contraindications. Reconstruction with rectus abdominis or latissimus dorsi myocutaneous flaps was preferred. The surgical mortality rate was 5 per cent, and tumor recurred on the chest in 12.5 per cent of cases, but palliation was frequent, and 72 per cent of patients lived more than a year, three for more than 40 months.

SALVAGE MASTECTOMY

Isolated local recurrences in the irradiated breast after breast conserving primary treatment can often be treated with a "salvage mastectomy." Data being accumulated on this subject are of considerable interest with respect to whether salvage mastectomies represent a second chance for cure. Selection obviously influences results, but the experience of Clark (1983) indicates that patients so treated have a prognosis nearly equivalent to that of patients without recurrence. Harris and coworkers (1984) reported 50 per cent 5 year survival after salvage mastectomies for breast recurrence, which is considerably higher than that which follows local recurrence after mastectomy. However, selected small local recurrences are also associated with a 50 per cent 5 year survival when treated with comprehensive irradiation and may be biologically similar to the isolated recurrences found in irradiated breasts treated with salvage operations. In selected patients, total mastectomy with or without axillary dissection is indicated for surgical salvage of patients who have recurrence confined to the breast or axilla, or both, following breast conserving primary treatment.

AXILLARY NODE DISSECTION

Regional failure in the axilla in the absence of metastases elsewhere can be treated with axillary node dissection or irradiation. Thirty-eight per cent of 13 patients managed with axillary dissection at EFSCH survived for 5 years after their original mastectomy (Donegan, 1972). The appearance of axillary metastases is a poor sign, however. Seventy-one per cent of patients who had axillary dissections for delayed adenopathy after initial total mastectomy in Protocol B-04 of the National Surgical Adjuvant Breast Project (NSABP) subsequently had further disease progression (Fisher et al., 1977). Nevertheless, the entire group of patients in this study treated initially with total mastectomy survived equally well whether axillary dissection was performed prophylactically or reserved for adenopathy.

Dissection of recurrences in the supraclavicular lymph nodes is unproductive. After histologic confirmation, the treatment is comprehensive irradiation.

Systemic Therapy

Occult dissemination is likely in the presence of local or regional recurrence. As a consequence, systemic therapy has been tried in conjunction with local treatment to delay or prevent its clinical appearance. Buzdar and coworkers (1979) added systemic treatment with 5-fluorouracil, doxorubicin hydrochloride (Adriamycin), and cyclophosphamide (FAC) combined with bacille Calmetté-Guérin (BCG) to the local treatment of 68 patients with isolated recurrences and prolonged the disease-free interval by comparison with a historical control group. Thirty-nine patients with chest wall recurrences were included among those treated, and 66 per cent remained disease-free for 2 years, compared with only 25 per cent of 38 historical controls. The survival of the two groups at 2 years, however, was not significantly different (91 per cent and 84 per cent, respectively). In a retrospective study, Beck and associates (1983) observed superior 5 year survival as well as disease-free survival in 42 patients who received systemic therapy for local-regional recurrence compared with 43 patients who received radiotherapy only, and they recommended systemic therapy for those with prompt recurrences (< 24 months) and those who had initially advanced stages of disease. They did find that irradiation produced more frequent and durable control specifically of local disease than did systemic therapy. Until the issue of survival is clear, reserving systemic therapy until there are signs of dissemination or uncontrolled local-regional disease has the advantage of deferring further treatment morbidity until it is clearly necessary. When used for persistent local cancer, hormonal therapy and chemotherapy can be expected to give approximately the same frequency of responses as when used for other soft tissue metastases.

REFERENCES

Beck, T. M., Hart, N. E., Woodard, D. A., et al.: Local or regionally recurrent carcinoma of the breast. Results of therapy in 121 patients. J. Clin. Oncol., 1:400, 1983.

Bedwinek, J. M., Fineberg, B., Lee, J., et al.: Analysis of failures following local treatment of isolated local-regional recurrence of breast cancer. Int. J. Radiation Oncol. Biol. Phys., 7:581, 1981a.

Bedwinek, J. M., Lee, J., Fineberg, B., et al.: Prognostic indicators in patients with isolated local-regional recurrence of breast cancer. Cancer, 47:2232, 1981b.

Brown, G. R., Horiot, J. C., Fletcher, G. H., et al.: Simple mastectomy and radiation therapy for locally advanced breast cancers technically suitable for radical mastectomy. AJR, 120:67, 1974.

Bruce, J., Carter, D. C., and Fraser, J.: Patterns of recurrent disease in breast cancer. Lancet, 1:433, 1970.

Buzdar, A. U., Blumenschein, G. R., Smith, T. L., et al.: Adjuvant chemoimmunotherapy following regional therapy for isolated recurrences of breast cancer (Stage IV NED). J. Surg. Oncol., 12:27, 1979.

Chen, K. K. Y., Montague, E. D., and Oswald, M. J.: Results of irradiation in the treatment of locoregional breast cancer recurrence. Cancer, 56:1269, 1985.

Chu, F. C. H., Lin, F. J., Kim, J. H., et al.: Locally recurrent carcinoma of the breast. Results of radiation therapy. Cancer, 37:2677, 1976.

Clark, R. M.: Alternatives to mastectomy—the Princess Margaret Hospital experience. In Harris, J. R., Hellman, S., and Silen, W. (Eds.): Conservative Management of Breast Cancer. New Surgical and Radiotherapeutic Techniques. Philadelphia, J. B. Lippincott Company, 1983, pp. 35–46.

Crile, G., Jr.: Results of conservative treatment of breast cancer at ten and 15 years. Ann. Surg., 181:26, 1975.

Dahl-Iversen, E.: An extended radical operation for carcinoma of the breast. J. R. Coll. Surg. Edinb., 8:81, 1963.

Danckers, V. F., Hamann, A., and Savage, J. L.: Postoperative recurrence of breast cancer after thirty-two years: A case report and review of the literature. Surgery, 47:656, 1960.

Dao, T. L., and Nemoto, T.: The clinical significance of skin recurrence after radical mastectomy in women with cancer of the breast. Surg. Gynecol. Obstet., 117:447, 1963.

Deck, K. B., and Kern, W. H.: Local recurrence of breast cancer. Arch. Surg., 111:323, 1976.

Demaree, E. W.: Local recurrence following surgery for cancer of the breast. Ann. Surg., 134:863, 1951.

Diehl, L. F., Hurwitz, M. A., Johnson, S. A., et al.: Skin metastases confined to a field of previous irradiation. Report of two cases and review of the literature. Cancer, 53:1864, 1984.

Donegan, W. L.: Mastectomy in the primary management of invasive mammary carcinoma. Adv. Surg., 6:1, 1972.

Donegan, W. L.: The influence of untreated internal mammary metastases upon the course of mammary cancer. Cancer, 39:533, 1977.

Donegan, W. L., Perez-Mesa, C. M., and Watson, F. R.: A biostatistical study of locally recurrent breast carcinoma. Surg. Gynecol. Obstet., 112:529, 1966.

Fentiman, I. S., Lavelle, M. A., Caplan, D., et al.: The significance of supraclavicular fossa node recurrence after radical mastectomy. Cancer, 57:908, 1986.

Fisher, B., Bauer, M., Margolese, R., et al.: Five-year results of a randomized clinical trial comparing total mastectomy and segmental mastectomy with or without radiation in the treatment of breast cancer. N. Engl. J. Med., *312*:665, 1985.

Fisher, B., Montague, E., Redmond, C., et al.: Comparison of radical mastectomy with alternative treatments for primary breast cancer. A first report of results from a prospective randomized clinical trial. Cancer, *39*(Suppl. 6):2827, 1977.

Haagensen, C. D.: Diseases of the Breast. Philadelphia, W. B. Saunders, 1971, p. 710.

Haagensen, C. D.: The choice of treatment for operable carcinoma of the breast. Surgery, *76*:685, 1974.

Halsted, W. S.: The results of operations for the cure of the breast performed at the Johns Hopkins Hospital from June, 1889 to January, 1894. Johns Hopkins Hosp. Rep., *4*:297, 1894.

Handley, R. S., and Thackray, A. C.: Conservative radical mastectomy (Patey's operation). Ann. Surg., *170*:880, 1969.

Harris, J. R., Recht, A., Amalric, R., et al.: Time course and prognosis of local recurrence following primary radiation therapy for early breast cancer. J. Clin. Oncol., *2*:37, 1984.

Janssens, J. P., Teuwen, D., Bonte, J., et al.: Effect of radiotherapy on steroid receptors in breast cancer. Lancet, *2*:1108, 1981.

Lewis, D., and Rienhoff, W. F., Jr.: Study of results of operations for cure of breast, performed at Johns Hopkins Hospital from 1889–1931. Am. Surg., *95*:336, 1932.

Madoc-Jones, H., Nelson, A. J., III, and Montague, E. D.: Evaluation of the effectiveness of radiotherapy in the management of early nodal recurrences from adenocarcinoma of breast. Breast, *2*:31, 1976.

McKenna, R. J., Jr., McMurtrey, M. J., Larson, D. L., et al.: A perspective on chest wall resection in patients with breast cancer. Ann. Thorac. Surg., *38*:482, 1984.

Morrow, M., and Foster, R. S., Jr.: Staging of breast cancer. Arch. Surg., *116*:748, 1981.

Patanaphan, V., Salazar, O. M., and Poussin-Rosillo, H.: Prognosticators in recurrent breast cancer. A 15-year experience with irradiation. Cancer, *54*:228, 1984.

Pawlias, K. T., Dockerty, M. B., and Ellis, F. H., Jr.: Late local recurrent carcinoma of the breast. Ann. Surg., *148*:192, 1958.

Peters, T. G., Donegan, W. L., and Burg, E. A.: Minimal breast cancer: A clinical appraisal. Ann. Surg., *186*:704, 1977.

Prosnitz, L. R., Goldenberg, I. S., Packard, R. A., et al.: Radiation therapy as initial treatment for early stage cancer of the breast without mastectomy. Cancer, *39*(Suppl. 2):917, 1977.

Sauerbruch, F.: Beitrag zur Resektion der Brustwand mit Plastik auf die Freigelegte Lunge. Dtsch. Z. Chir., *86*:275, 1907.

Schede: Aerzlicher Verein zu Hamburg. Dtsche. Med. Wochenschr., *37*:646, 1886.

Shah, J. P., and Urban, J. A.: Full thickness chest wall resection for recurrent breast carcinoma involving the bony chest wall. Cancer, *35*:567, 1975.

Snyder, A. F., Farrow, G. M., Masson, J. K., et al.: Chest wall resection for locally recurrent breast cancer. Cancer J. Clinicians, *19*:282, 1969.

Spratt, J. S.: Locally recurrent cancer after radical mastectomy. Cancer, *20*:1051, 1967.

Spratt, J. S., Shieber, W., and Dillard, B. M.: Anatomy and Surgical Technique of Groin Dissection. St. Louis, C. V. Mosby, 1965, p. 69.

Tomin, R., and Donegan, W. L.: Screening for recurrent breast cancer—Its effectiveness and prognostic value. J. Clin. Oncol., *5*(1):62, 1987.

Urban, J. A.: Radical excision of chest wall for mammary cancer. Cancer, *4*:1263, 1951.

Urban, J. A., and Marjani, M. A.: Significance of internal mammary lymph node metastases in breast cancer. AJR, *111*:130, 1971.

Veronesi, U., and Valagussa, P.: Inefficacy of internal mammary node dissection in breast cancer surgery. Cancer, *47*:170, 1981.

Veronesi, U., Cascinelli, N., Bufalino, R., et al.: Risk of internal mammary lymph node metastases and its relevance on prognosis of breast cancer patients. Ann. Surg., *198*:681, 1984.

Zimmerman, K. W., Montague, E. D., and Fletcher, G. H.: Frequency, anatomical distribution and management of local recurrences after definitive therapy for breast cancer. Cancer, *19*:67, 1966.

JOHN A. WATERS
JOHN W. GAMEL
ARTHUR H. KEENEY

Metastasis to the Eye and Ocular Adnexa

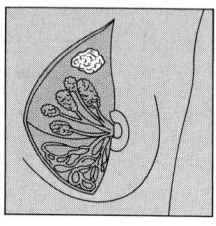

Many malignancies metastasize to ocular structures. Among women, most of these lesions originate in the breast. Although ocular involvement usually follows other clinical manifestations of disseminated disease, on occasion it may provide the first clinical evidence of dissemination. For a small fraction of patients, this evidence precedes diagnosis of the primary tumor, and thus breast carcinoma must be included in the differential diagnosis of a mass lesion discovered in the eye or orbit of a woman. Life expectancy is limited for most patients with metastatic disease, but ophthalmic lesions usually respond well to palliative therapy, especially when discovered early.

Incidence of Ophthalmic Metastasis

Estimates of the incidence of ocular metastasis vary from approximately 10 to 40 per cent among patients with breast cancer (Table 24–1). The breast is predominant as the primary site among women, and breast cancer rivals lung cancer as the primary site among unselected patients (Block and Gartner, 1971; Hutchinson and Smith, 1979). Ophthalmic metastasis occurs most commonly in the fifth, sixth, and seventh decades of life, paralleling the incidence of primary breast carcinoma (Usher, 1923; Hart, 1962; Jaeger et al., 1971; Thatcher and Thomas, 1975; Henderson, 1973; Mewis and Young, 1982; Hutchinson and Smith, 1979; Bullock and Yanes, 1980).

Occasionally metastatic ocular disease appears first in a patient with clinically undetected breast carcinoma or in a patient with known primary disease but no extraocular evidence of dissemination. The incidence of such occurrences is difficult to ascertain, as findings are greatly influenced by methods of patient selection and evaluation. Nevertheless, various studies suggest that of all patients with breast malignancy metastatic to various ocular sites, from 3 to 9 per cent have previously undiagnosed primary disease (Ferry and Font, 1974; Stephens and Shields, 1979; Bullock and Yanes, 1980). Arnold and associates (1985) found a much higher incidence of occult primary cancers (30 per cent) among patients with tumors involving the eyelid, suggesting that the eyelid may be an especially likely site for metastasis from occult breast carcinoma. For approximately one fourth of all patients with known primary breast malignancy, ocular structures are the first clinically detected site of metastasis (Hart, 1962; Henderson, 1973; Thatcher and Thomas, 1975; Moar et al., 1977), although some authors have derived a much lower estimate (Mewis and Young, 1982) or much higher estimate (Stephens and Shields, 1979).

Most often, however, ocular involvement affects patients with known extraocular metastasis. Of particular interest is the observation of Mewis and Young (1982) that, among patients suffering from Grade IV metastatic breast carcinoma, those with ocular complaints had an incidence of intraocular metastasis four times greater than those patients with no visual

Table 24–1. INCIDENCE OF OPHTHALMIC METASTASIS IN PATIENTS WITH BREAST CARCINOMA

Author	Number of Patients with Breast Carcinoma	Patients with Ophthalmic Metastasis	Incidence of Ophthalmic Disease (%)
Albert et al. (1977)	52	7	13
Bloch and Gartner (1971)	52	19	37
Nelson et al. (1983)	31	3	10
Mewis and Young (1982)	250	67	27
Ophthalmic Symptoms:			
No	98	9	9
Yes	152	58	38

symptoms (Table 24–1). Combining these results with those of Albert and associates (1977), we can expect to find ocular involvement in roughly 10 per cent of all patients with known metastatic breast malignancy and in a much higher percentage of those patients within this group that report eye-related symptoms.

Location, Signs, and Symptoms of Ophthalmic Metastasis

Breast carcinoma disseminates to the eye more often than to the lids or orbit, and within the globe the posterior uvea (choroid) is more commonly involved than the ciliary body or iris (Ferry and Font, 1974). The data of Hutchinson and Smith (1979) suggest that approximately two thirds of ophthalmic metastasis from primary breast disease involves the globe and that approximately 90 per cent of all intraocular lesions involve the choroid. In addition, individual reports can be found of breast cancer metastatic to the optic nerve, meninges, vitreous, sclera, and retina.

A substantial fraction of ophthalmic patients have bilateral disease, and, among patients with unilateral disease, the left eye is reported by some investigators to be involved more often than the right (Table 24–2). These findings suggest that structural differences in vasculature between the left and right cranial circulation may indeed affect the ocular dissemination of malignancy. Furthermore, a substantial fraction of patients with choroidal metastasis have more than one tumor in the same eye (Stephens and Shields, 1979; Mewis and Young, 1982).

The signs and symptoms of ophthalmic metastasis are determined primarily by the structures involved. Patients with choroidal metastasis most commonly experience decreased or distorted vision, diplopia, or blind spots as manifestations of tumor-related retinal detachment (Fig. 24–1) (Mewis and Young, 1982). Such detachment may reflect direct tumor involvement, subretinal hemorrhage, or subretinal serous transudation from leaky tumor vessels.

Orbital lesions from breast carcinoma most often are manifested by proptosis, periorbital swelling, or a palpable mass (Fig. 24–2). Also noted in some patients are pain from nerve invasion, decreased acuity from distortion of

Table 24–2. LATERALITY OF OPHTHALMIC METASTASIS FROM BREAST CARCINOMA

Author	Bilateral Number (%)	Right Eye Only	Left Eye Only	Overall Ratio Left/Right
Usher (1923)	26 (48)	12	16	1.33
Hutchinson and Smith (1979)	4 (13)	10	16	1.60
Mewis and Young (1982)	27 (40)	18	22	1.22
Thatcher and Thomas (1975)	17 (40)	12	13	1.08
Maor et al. (1977)	15 (36)	10	17	1.70
Henderson (1973)	1 (5)	7	11	1.57
Total	80 (33)	69	95	1.38

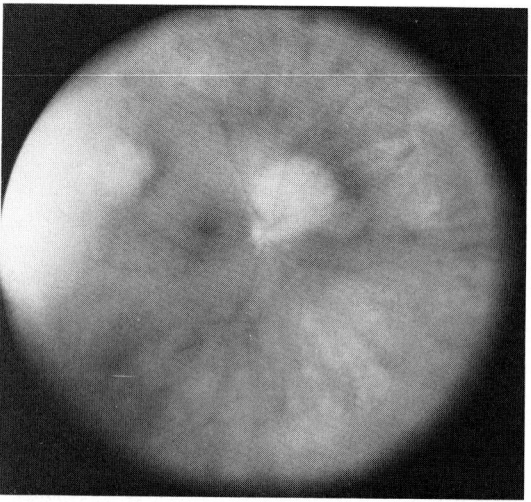

Figure 24–1. Breast carcinoma with multiple choroidal metastases (wide angle photograph). A large lesion can be seen invading the disc with a second lesion temporal to the macula.

Location and Histology of the Primary Tumor

Most authors have found an equal likelihood of ophthalmic metastasis from the right and left breast (Usher, 1923; Thatcher and Thomas, 1975), though one study reported a predominance of primaries in the right breast (Jaeger et al, 1971). The great majority of breast tumors that metastasize to ocular structures are classified histologically as adenocarcinoma. The authors are aware of no study that establishes a correlation between histologic type of primary breast disease and site or incidence of ophthalmic metastasis.

Diagnosis

Any patient with ocular complaints who is at risk for metastatic disease should first undergo a complete eye examination, including evaluation of visual acuity, ocular motility, and pupillary response, as well as inspection of the lids and slit lamp examination of the anterior segment. For orbital lesions, exophthalmometry provides an objective measure of the extent of protrusion of each eye. The width of the lid fissures and position of each lid with respect to the cornea also provide useful information. Given the propensity of metastatic disease for the posterior choroid, fundus examination is indispensable. Serous retinal detachment from a malignant lesion in the peripheral choroid can cause visual symptoms in an eye that discloses no abnormality to examination by direct ophthalmoscopy, and thus a widely dilated pupil and an indirect ophthalmoscope

the globe, and diplopia from infiltration of the extraocular muscles or their nerve supply (Henderson, 1973; Font and Ferry, 1976). Of particular interest is enophthalmos, an uncommon sign that has been reported only with metastatic scirrhous carcinoma of the breast. Retraction of the globe and eyelids is the result of scirrhous infiltration of orbital tissues, which also causes progressive ophthalmoplegia (Henderson, 1973).

Additional uncommon manifestations of metastatic ocular disease include iritis and glaucoma from invasion of the iris and ciliary body (Ferry and Font, 1975) and nodules or diffuse infiltration from involvement of the eyelids (Arnold et al., 1985).

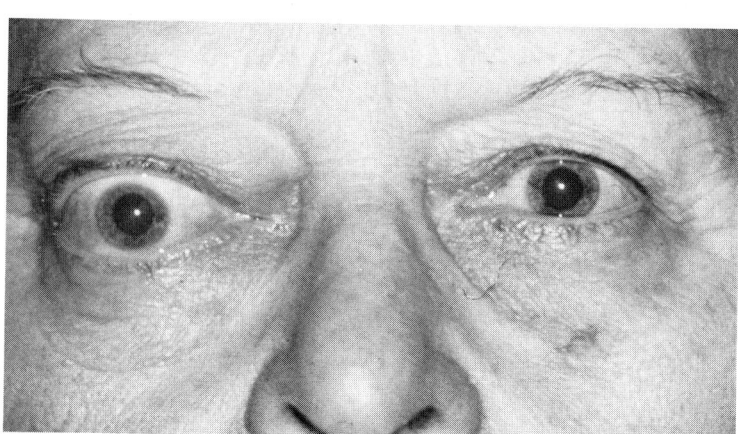

Figure 24–2. Breast carcinoma metastatic to the orbit, displacing the eye forward, downward, and temporally.

are essential for adequate visualization of the entire choroid. All fundus lesions should be drawn in the medical record.

For medical and legal documentation, appropriate photographs may be taken using a macro lens for the lids and orbit, a specially adapted slit lamp camera for the anterior segment, or a fundus camera for posterior lesions. Additional diagnostic procedures include the following:

1. *Transillumination*, which may in some instances allow the examiner to distinguish pigmented from nonpigmented lesions of the uvea.

2. *Fluorescein angiography*, which can be used to assess the vascular status of a mass involving the posterior choroid or iris. In particular, this test may distinguish vascular from avascular lesions and may determine the extent of plasma leakage from vascular spaces within a tumor. These findings are of little value, however, in distinguishing primary from metastatic malignancies (Davis and Robertson, 1973).

3. *Ultrasonography*, which provides an acoustic profile of intraocular and retrobulbar lesions. Two-dimensional ultrasonography is especially useful for evaluating tumors contained in eyes with opaque media that prevent ophthalmoscopic examination. One-dimensional ultrasonography can also provide a measure of "acoustic texture," which in some instances allows these metastatic lesions with adenomatous structures or mucinous spaces to be distinguished from those primary melanomas that are histologically homogeneous (Coleman et al., 1974).

4. *Radiography and computed tomographic (CT) scans*, which can provide essential information on the size, shape, location, and infiltrative characteristics of orbital lesions (Fig. 24–3). Because of the high density of vital and delicate structures within the orbit, it is important to localize a lesion as precisely as possible before attempting diagnostic or therapeutic surgical intervention. High resolution CT scanning has also been used to characterize intraocular lesions (Jacobs et al., 1980). Unfortunately, in most instances these techniques do not allow metastatic disease of the eye or orbit to be distinguished clearly from primary malignancy.

5. *Radioactive phosphorus uptake*, which provides a differential measure of the metabolic activity of an intraocular lesion compared to uninvolved choroid. Thus, a hematoma or

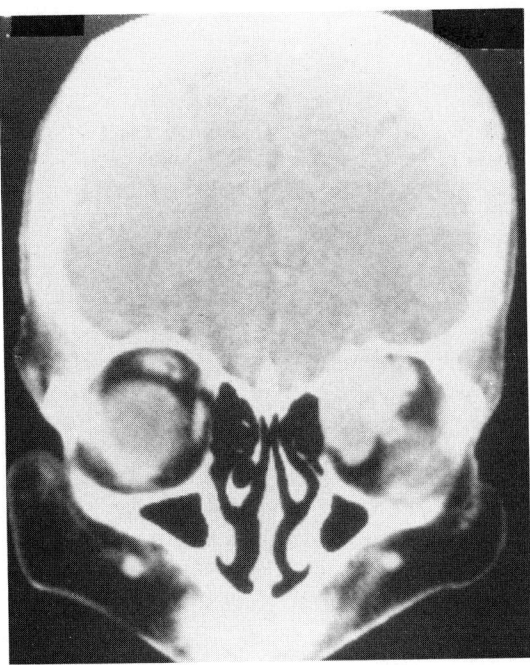

Figure 24–3. Computed tomographic scan of patient in Figure 24–2, showing large metastatic lesion in the superonasal portion of the orbit.

cyst can generally be detected because of minimal phosphorus uptake. On the other hand, metastatic and primary malignancies share a similar level of metabolic activity and thus cannot be distinguished by this method (Shields, 1978).

6. *Needle biopsy*, which can be performed on intraocular and orbital lesions. Although this procedure offers the opportunity for histologic diagnosis, on occasion the resulting diagnosis has been proved incorrect by subsequent surgical biopsy (Krohel et al., 1985). Furthermore, the potential exists for injury to ocular structures or local dissemination of tumor cells, and thus needle biopsy should be reserved for those patients whose diagnosis cannot be determined by less invasive procedures (Shields, 1983; Karcioglu et al., 1985; Liu, 1985).

7. *Aspiration of fluid* from the anterior chamber, vitreous, or subretinal space, which also offers the opportunity for histologic diagnosis of malignant cells (Piro et al., 1982; Scholz et al., 1983; Sternberg et al., 1984). Although this procedure is potentially less dangerous than direct needle biopsy of the tumor, there is still opportunity for serious complication, and the material obtained is sometimes insufficient for adequate cytologic analysis.

Thus, this technique should also be reserved for selected cases.

A special diagnostic dilemma is presented by patients with a mass in the orbit or choroid who are not known to have a primary tumor. Pigmented choroidal malignancies almost always represent either metastatic melanoma or primary intraocular disease, but an unpigmented tumor may represent primary amelanotic melanoma, metastatic carcinoma from an occult primary, or one of a number of uncommon lesions (e.g., choroidal hemangioma, sarcoid granuloma). Patients with a known primary tumor but with no known extraocular metastasis also present a dilemma, as the ocular lesions might possibly represent an independent disease process. When confronted with such dilemmas, it is often best to perform systemic evaluation in search of an occult primary cancer or additional metastatic disease before resorting to invasive procedures of the eye or orbit.

Given the prevalence of breast carcinoma and its propensity for ocular metastasis, all women with an unexplained orbital or intraocular nonpigmented lesion should be examined for occult breast malignancy.

Treatment

Radiation is well established as the most effective treatment for ophthalmic malignancy of a variety of histologic types, including metastatic adenocarcinoma of the breast. Several workers have reported improvement or stabilization in a majority of eyes with intraocular metastasis (Wilmer, 1934; Jaeger et al., 1971; Thatcher and Thomas, 1975; Maor et al., 1977; Mewis and Young, 1982). Radiation therapy also appears to benefit patients with orbital metastasis (Henderon, 1973; Huh et al., 1974). The standard regimen includes 2500 to 3000 rad delivered in 10 sessions over 2 to 3 weeks from a lateral port to spare the cornea and lens. Serious complications are relatively uncommon, in part because of the limited life expectancy of most of these patients.

Chemotherapy, although less consistently effective than radiation for ophthalmic metastasis, may nevertheless stabilize some lesions (Mewis and Young, 1982). As patients with metastatic ocular disease will often have extraocular dissemination, systemic therapy may be indicated, even though the extraocular disease may not yet be apparent clinically.

Surgery as a therapeutic method should be limited to blind or nearly blind eyes that are painful and unresponsive to radiation therapy, in which instance enucleation can lead to prompt relief of pain. In theory, therapeutic surgery can be justified in two clinical settings in which known metastatic disease is limited to a single nodule and there is hope of curative therapy: (1) partial iridectomy when the lesion involves only the iris; (2) enucleation when the lesion involves only the ciliary body or choroid. Such intervention, however, rarely is justified in clinical practice.

Survival

On the average, patients survive approximately 1 year beyond the diagnosis of metastatic disease to the eye or ocular adnexa (Hart, 1962; Jaeger et al., 1971; Thatcher and Thomas, 1975; Maor et al., 1977; Stephens and Shields, 1979; Mewis and Young, 1982). Some encouraging information is provided by Bullock and Yanes (1980), who found that one patient with occult breast carcinoma survived diagnosis of her ocular metastasis for 36 months, whereas seven patients with known breast disease survived the diagnosis of a first metastasis to the eye for an average of 27 months of observation; of these seven patients, six were still living at the time of publication of the report. In contrast, 22 patients who developed ocular disease subsequent to the discovery of extraocular metastasis survived diagnosis of their eye disease for an average of only 3 months. These findings suggest that metastatic disease confined to ophthalmic structures carries a substantially better prognosis than disease disseminated to multiple sites.

Summary

Among women, the breast is the predominant source of metastasis to the eye and ocular adnexa. In fact, ophthalmic metastasis may represent the first clinical manifestation of breast carcinoma, and thus this malignancy should be included in the differential diagnosis of all women who have an infiltrative lid lesion, a mass lesion of the orbit, or an unpigmented lesion of the choroid. Furthermore, all women with breast cancer who develop ocular signs or symptoms should be referred promptly to an ophthalmologist. Although survival is limited following the development of metastatic disease, timely diagnosis and treatment of ophthalmic lesions can greatly enhance the quality of life for these patients.

REFERENCES

Albert D. M., Rubenstein R. A., and Scheie, H. G.: Metastases to the eye. Part 1. Incidence in 213 adult patients with generalized malignancy. Am. J. Ophthalmol., 63:723, 1977.

Arnold A. C., Bullock, J. D., and Foos, R. Y.: Metastatic eyelid carcinoma. Ophthalmology, 92:114, 1985.

Bloch, M. S., and Gartner, S.: Incidence of ocular metastatic carcinoma. Arch. Ophthalmol., 85:673, 1971.

Bullock, J. D., and Yanes, B.: Ophthalmic manifestations of metastatic breast carcinoma. Ophthalmology, 87:961, 1980.

Coleman, D. J., Abramson, D. H., Jack, R. L., et al.: Ultrasonic diagnosis of the choroid. Arch. Ophthalmol., 91:344, 1974.

Davis, D. L., and Robertson, D. M.: Fluorescein angiography of metastatic choroidal tumors. Arch. Ophthalmol., 89:97, 1973.

Ferry, A. P., and Font, R. L.: Carcinoma metastatic to the eye and orbit. I. A clinicopathologic study of 227 cases. Arch. Ophthalmol., 92:276, 1974.

Ferry, A. P., and Font, R. L.: Carcinoma metastatic to the eye and orbit. II. A clinicopathological study of 26 patients with carcinoma metastatic to the anterior segment of the eye. Arch. Ophthalmol., 93:472, 1975.

Font, R. L., and Ferry, A. P.: Carcinoma metastatic to the eye and orbit. III. A clinicopathologic study of 28 cases metastatic to the orbit. Cancer, 38:1326, 1976.

Hart, W. M.: Metastatic carcinoma of the eye and orbit. Int. Ophthalmol. Clin., 2:465, 1962.

Henderson, J. W.: Orbital Tumors. Philadelphia, W. B. Saunders, 1973.

Huh, S. H., Nisce, L. Z., Simpson, L. D., et al.: Value of radiation therapy in the treatment of orbital metastasis. AJR, 120:589, 1974.

Hutchinson, D. S., and Smith, T. R.: Ocular and orbital metastatic carcinoma. Ann. Ophthalmol., 11:869, 1979.

Jacobs, L., Weisberg, L. A., and Kinkel, W. R.: Computerized Tomography of the Orbit and Sella Turcica. New York, Raven Press, 1980.

Jaeger, E. A., Frayer, W. C., Southard, M. E., et al.: Effects of radiation therapy on metastatic choroidal tumors. Trans. Am. Acad. Ophthalmol. Otol., 75:94, 1971.

Karcioglu, Z. A., Gordon, R. A., and Karcioglu, G. L.: Tumor seeding in ocular fine needle aspiration biopsy. Ophthalmology, 92:1763, 1985.

Krohel, G. B., Tobin, D. R., and Chavis, R. M.: Inaccuracy of fine needle aspiration biopsy. Ophthalmology, 92:666, 1985.

Liu, D.: Complications of fine needle aspiration biopsy of the orbit. Ophthalmology, 92:1768, 1985.

Maor, M., Chan, R. C., and Young, S. E.: Radiotherapy of choroidal metastases: Breast cancer as primary site. Cancer, 40:2081, 1977.

Mewis, L., and Young, S. E.: Breast carcinoma metastatic to the choroid: Analysis of 67 patients. Ophthalmology, 89:147, 1982.

Nelson, C. C., Hertzberg, B. S., and Klintworth, G. K.: A histopathologic study of 716 unselected eyes in patients with cancer at the time of death. Am. J. Ophthalmol., 95:788, 1983.

Piro, P., Pappas, H. R., Erozan, Y. S., et al.: Diagnostic vitrectomy in metastatic breast carcinoma in the vitreous. Retina, 2:182, 1982.

Scholz, R., Green, R., Baranao, E. C., et al.: Metastatic carcinoma to the iris. Diagnosis by aqueous paracentesis and response to irradiation and chemotherapy. Ophthalmology, 90:1524, 1983.

Shields, J. A.: Accuracy and limitations of the ^{32}P test in the diagnosis of ocular tumors: An analysis of 500 cases. Ophthalmology, 85:950, 1978.

Shields, J. A.: Diagnosis and Management of Intraocular Tumors. St. Louis, C. V. Mosby, 1983.

Stephens, R. F., and Shields, J. A.: Diagnosis and management of cancer metastatic to the uvea: A study of 70 cases. Ophthalmology, 86:1336, 1979.

Sternberg, P., Tiedman, J., Hickingbotham, D., et al.: Controlled aspiration of subretinal fluid in the diagnosis of carcinoma metastatic to the choroid. Arch. Ophthalmol., 102:1622, 1984.

Thatcher, N., and Thomas, P. R. M.: Choroidal metastases from breast carcinoma: A survey of 42 patients and the use of radiation therapy. Clin. Radiol., 26:549, 1975.

Usher, C. H.: Cases of metastatic carcinoma of the choroid and iris. Br. J. Ophthalmol., 7:10, 1923.

Wilmer, W. H.: Atlas Fundus Oculi. New York, Macmillan, 1934.

CHRISTOPHER B. SHIELDS
E. JOY ARPIN

Neurologic Aspects of Breast Cancers

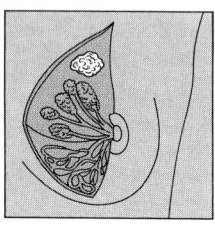

One of the most difficult problems in the management of breast carcinoma is that of metastasis to the nervous system. Not only do metastases affect prognosis, they also pose a therapeutic challenge in that the blood-brain barrier restricts entry of chemotherapeutic drugs into the nervous system. Central nervous system metastases have increased in frequency as treatment of the systemic disease has improved, likely owing to prolonged exposure of the brain and spine to circulating tumor cells, as well as the sanctuary provided by the central nervous system from the effects of chemotherapeutic drugs (Paterson et al., 1982). The neurosurgeon may be called on to treat the metastasis, provide relief of intractable pain, or assist in the differentiation between recurrent central nervous system metastasis and complications of therapy. This chapter addresses areas of neurologic involvement in breast cancer (i.e., intracranial and spinal metastasis, leptomeningeal carcinomatosis, neurologic complications of therapy, and control of pain).

Intracranial Metastasis

The incidence of cerebral metastasis is recognized clinically in 5 to 9 per cent of all victims having breast cancers (Gamache et al., 1982) and in 10 to 34 per cent of autopsy series (Yap et al., 1978). The route of metastasis is usually hematogenous, although a direct spread from secondary skull deposits may occur. Tumor cells rarely ascend via Batson's spinal venous plexus to the posterior fossa. The frontal lobes are the most frequent site of metastatic spread, being proportional to the greater cerebral blood flow to that area. The hallmark of cerebral metastases is their multiplicity, but single lesions may also occur. Metastatic deposits are well demarcated from adjacent brain tissue, both grossly and microscopically, usually being surrounded by considerable perifocal edema. An estimated 50 per cent of presumed single lesions have unrecognized multiple cerebral metastases (Gamache et al., 1982).

Symptoms of cerebral metastases are related to their location and rate of growth. Time from diagnosis of the primary lesion and cerebral involvement ranges from 3 to 192 months (median, 37 months) (Gamache et al., 1982). Headaches, confusion, disorientation, focal or generalized seizures, hemiparesis, and visual field defects constitute the commonly recognized symptoms that suggest cerebral metastasis in patients with breast cancer. Posterior fossa deposits may cause limb or gait ataxia and signs of increased intracranial pressure from obstruction of the fourth ventricle or aqueduct of Sylvius. The median survival time from the first symptom of brain metastasis is 4 months, although long-term survival (>18 months) does occur (DiStefano et al., 1979).

Focal enhancing metastatic deposits (greater than 5 cm in diameter), perifocal edema, midline shift, and ventricular enlargement are readily evident on computed tomography (CT) and magnetic resonance imaging (MRI) scans. Both enhanced and unenhanced CT scans will increase the diagnostic yield. Metastases overlooked on CT scans are less than 5 mm in diameter or close to the skull base. Plane skull radiographs may reveal an osteolytic or osteoblastic skull deposit, a displaced pineal gland, or evidence of increased intracranial pressure. Cerebral angiography, bone scans, isotope brain scans, and electro- and echoencephalography are of little diagnostic value.

Difficulty in diagnosis may arise if a solitary lesion exists. Primary brain tumors (meningiomas), brain abscesses, or resolving strokes may be differentiated from a solitary lesion by interval CT scans and cerebral angiography. If doubt still exists, biopsy of the lesion may be necessary by either stereotaxic biopsy technique or craniotomy. Before radiation or surgery is performed, the extent of systemic involvement must be assessed by chest x-ray, bone scans, and liver-spleen scans.

TREATMENT OF INTRACRANIAL METASTASIS

Treatment of cerebral metastasis may include surgery, radiotherapy, and chemotherapy. Therapy must be individualized, but decisions are based on presence of a single versus multiple intracranial tumors, presence of widespread systemic metastases, neurologic status, age of patient, and previous therapy (Black, 1979a).

If the patient is comatose owing to increased intracranial pressure (ICP) resulting from intracranial deposit(s), methods to immediately lower ICP include administration of mannitol, 100 g (500 ml of 20 per cent solution administered intravenously); dexamethasone, 10 mgm intravenously followed by a dose of 6 mgm every 6 hr; and hyperventilation to attain PCO_2 of 20 to 25 mm/Hg.

If the patient is awake and alert, with multiple intracranial deposits or widespread systemic metastases, management is nonsurgical. Corticosteroid therapy (usually dexamethasone, 4–6 mgm every 6 hr) will produce dramatic alleviation of symptoms in 70 to 75 per cent of patients. Mechanism of action of steroids is poorly understood but the degree of cerebral edema does appear to be diminished on sequential CT or MRI scans, often with resolution of symptoms within hours of initiating therapy. If used in combination with radiotherapy, corticosteroid therapy is maintained for 1 week following its completion and then gradually tapered. Antacids (aluminum hydroxide [Amphojel] or cimetidine [Tagamet]) are administered with steroids to diminish the risk of gastrointestinal ulceration. Anticonvulsant medications (phenytoin, 300 mg at bedtime) decrease the risk of seizures; however, both steroid withdrawal and hepatic tumor deposits may induce phenytoin toxicity, requiring close monitoring of plasma levels for several months. Cerebral metastases from breast cancers are moderately radiosensitive so that if multiple intracranial deposits exist and the patient's general condition is stable, radiotherapy is the treatment of choice. Several radiotherapeutic regimens exist. Gamache and associates (1982) recommend 500 rads on days 1 to 3, no radiation on days 4 to 7, 300 rad on days 8 to 12, no radiation on days 13 and 14, and 300 rad on days 15 to 17. This provides a total dose of 3900 rads in 17 days. Neither chemotherapy nor immunotherapy is of proved value in treating cerebral metastasis.

Patients harboring a single cerebral metastasis are treated similarly; however, surgical removal may be justified (Galicich et al., 1980). Surgery is indicated when the diagnosis is in doubt, the tumor is over 3 cm in diameter in an accessible site, conservative methods fail to control symptoms (radioresistant tumor), there is recurrence after radiotherapy or discontinuation of corticosteroids, a minimal burden of systemic disease exists, and/or the prognosis is greater than 1 year. Even if a known breast tumor exists and all evidence points toward the intracranial lesion's being metastatic, meningiomas, primary brain tumors, and infarcts have occasionally been identified on a subsequent operation or postmortem examination. A high correlation between carcinoma of the breast and cerebral meningiomas has been documented, which further increases the risk of misdiagnosis of a single intracranial lesion (Mehta et al., 1983). The mortality rate following single tumor removal is approximately 10 to 15 per cent, with the most common cause of death being pulmonary emboli (Black, 1979a).

Total head radiotherapy (3900 rad in 17 days) following removal of a single mass is widely practiced, as the likelihood of total removal of microscopic deposits from the tumor bed is remote, and the incidence of multiple microscopic deposits is 15 to 50 per cent (Gamache et al., 1982). The roles of surgery and radiotherapy are complementary, providing optimal chance for prolonged survival. Using this regimen, the majority of patients die from their systemic disease.

Spinal Metastasis

Breast tumors metastatic to the spine are a cause of major morbidity but infrequent mortality. The breast is the most frequent area of primary tumor to involve the spine (Rodriguez and DiNapoli, 1980; Livingston and Perrin, 1978) with an incidence of 19 to 59 per cent (Lenz and Freid, 1931; Cobb et al., 1977). Such lesions most frequently affect the thoracic spine (Black, 1979b) followed by the lumbar and the cervical spine. Metastatic deposits usually involve the vertebral body and epidural space (Livingston and Perrin, 1978) and to a lesser extent may be intradural-extramedullary (Hirsh et al., 1982; Perrin et al., 1982) or intramedullary (Chade, 1976). Tumors undergo direct extension from vertebrae to the epidural space but rarely traverse dura as it is such an effective barrier to tumor cells (Black, 1979b).

Other routes of metastasis to the spine may be hematogenous or via Batson's spinal paravertebral and extradural venous plexus (Rodriguez and DiNapoli, 1980). Direct spinal extension may occur from a posterior mediastinal secondary tumor through intervertebral foramina. Symptoms depend on the level of spinal metastasis and rate of tumor expansion. Back pain overlying the site of spinal metastasis with nocturnal exacerbation is the hallmark of this condition. Progressive numbness and weakness below the level of the tumor is noted in 50 to 70 per cent of patients at the time of diagnosis. Bladder and bowel dysfunction are present in half the patients at diagnosis (Gilbert et al., 1978). Determination of the segmental level of numbness is a more reliable indicator of the site of metastasis than is assessment of motor function. Sensorimotor findings are usually symmetric in the thoracic, cervical, and upper lumbar lesions. However, if cauda equina compression occurs, asymmetric findings may be noted. The progression of these symptoms is subacute, but if an acute progression of paraplegia develops in less than 24 hr, the prognosis is particularly poor as cord infarction has likely developed.

Radiologic confirmation is mandatory once the diagnosis is suspected. The entire spine should be assessed, as 17 per cent of patients have multiple spinal lesions (Gilbert et al., 1978). Plain radiographs of the spine may reveal pathologic compression fractures, osteoblastic infiltration, subluxation, kyphosis, or paravertebral soft tissue swelling at the site of metastasis. Bone involvement does not signify the presence of an epidural deposit, nor are epidural deposits invariably associated with adjacent bone metastases. Positive contrast myelography with metrizamide confirms the presence of single or multiple intraspinal lesions. Myelography is desirable if vertebral body involvement exists, even if no neurologic symptoms are present, to determine the presence of bone or tumor encroachment on spinal cord or nerve roots (Black, 1979b). An epidural deposit may show a total myelographic block and hourglass narrowing or a minor degree of extrinsic pressure of the contrast column. If a total block exists, contrast should also be injected via a C1-C2 puncture to identify multiple intraspinal lesions or the rostral extent of the tumor, or both. Precise delineation of the rostrocaudal extent of the intraspinal deposit(s) is required prior to spinal radiography or decompressive laminectomy. The myelographic characteristics of epidural, intramedullary, or intradural-extramedullary lesions are outlined in the neuroradiologic tests (Shapiro, 1962; Taveras and Wood, 1964). Forced injection of contrast agents into the lumbar spine in an attempt to cap the tumor's rostral limit or the excessive withdrawal of spinal fluid caudal to the spinal block must be avoided as these maneuvers precipitate caudal tumor displacement, producing rapid neurologic deterioration (Hollis et al., 1986). A skin marker overlying the level of spinal block recorded on the myelogram will facilitate the localization of sites for radiotherapy or decompressive laminectomy. A postmyelographic CT scan further defines the intraspinal extent of the deposit. Computed tomography scans define osteoblastic deposits on the vertebral body and neural arch more clearly than plain radiographs and also identify the relative contribution of bone and/or epidural tumor to the spinal block. Magnetic resonance imaging provides major diagnostic advantages over both myelography and CT scanning as contrast enhancement is unnecessary and sagittal imaging of the entire spine is possible. Cerebrospinal fluid (CSF) obtained during myelography caudal to the complete block reveals elevated protein levels, normal glucose level, and xanthochromia under low CSF pressure. If malignant tumor cells are identified in CSF, leptomeningeal carcinomatosis exists, which has a more dismal prognosis than does a patient harboring an epidural deposit, regardless of treatment. Radiotherapy and surgical decompression are the cornerstones of management, which is primarily palliative. Decompressive laminectomy used to be the standard therapy for epidural deposits, but Posner and his coworkers popularized radiotherapy as being superior (Gilbert et al., 1978; Slatkin and Posner, 1983). Neither method appeared to have much advantage over the other in a randomized prospective study (Young et al., 1980).

Breast metastases are moderately radiosensitive, so that most spinal deposits are treated with a course of local tumor radiotherapy in the same doses as for cranial radiation. Those patients with a progressive neurologic deficit must undergo radiotherapy on an emergent basis. Radiotherapy is administered if the patient has a slowly progressive neurologic symptom, a life expectancy of greater than 3 months, and a radiosensitive tumor. Even if radiotherapy is administered, a patient's progress should be monitored by a neurosurgeon and the decompressive laminectomy performed if rapid clinical deterioration develops. Clinical results of radiotherapy alone versus surgery plus radiotherapy for breast metastasis to spine are difficult to assess. Black has reviewed the results for metastatic tumors from various primary sites and noted that improvement following surgery alone was 30 per cent, following radiotherapy alone was 46 per cent, and following laminectomy plus radiotherapy was 51 per cent (Black, 1979b). The only prospective randomized study performed to date showed no significant difference between the effectiveness of radiotherapy and surgery plus radiotherapy with respect to pain relief, improved ambulation, or improved sphincter function. As expected, patients with a complete myelographic block fared less well than those with an incomplete block (Young, 1982). Similar results were noted by Cobb and associates (1977), whose series consisted only of metastatic breast tumors.

Interstitial brachytherapy (iodine-125 labeled seeds) provides high dose irradiation to the tumor bed without endangering normal structures at a distance of greater than 1 mm. This technique is of greatest value in paravertebral metastases. However, an operation is required to place the radioactive seeds. Brachytherapy appears to add nothing to the benefits of surgery alone (Slatkin and Posner, 1983).

Surgical intervention is indicated in a subgroup of patients in whom the paraplegia is rapidly progressive, when doubt exists as to the pathology of the tumor, and when cord compression is caused by bone fragments from a pathologic fracture. Under unusual circumstances, patients in whom further radiotherapy is contraindicated may undergo surgery. Wide decompressive laminectomy providing access to the spinal canal is performed for the first two indications just listed. This approach allows exposure for multiple level, bilateral nerve root decompression and for intradural exploration if it is anticipated. If the spine is unstable, fusion with Harrington rods or autogenous bone graft is easily performed (Harrington, 1984). However, if a pathologic vertebral body compression fracture or an anteriorly situated tumor causes anterior spinal cord compression, an anterior approach is the procedure of choice. If one or two vertebral bodies are involved, a corpectomy is performed, which provides decompression of the anterior dural tube. This method is usually palliative with removal of the collapsed vertebral bodies as well as tumor from a prevertebral and epidural space. Spine stability is provided by insertion of a rib or fibular bone strut or a methylmethacrylate plug reinforced with Steinman pins (Harrington, 1984; Sundaresan and Galicich, 1984). Careful assessment by myelography, CT, and MRI allows therapy to be individualized to a specific tumor site. Occasionally, a combined (anterior and posterior) staged procedure may be justified.

Current evidence suggests that radiotherapy is the primary treatment for spinal metastasis from the breast in most circumstances. Radiotherapy is superior to surgery alone and is equally effective to combined operation-radiotherapy (Black, 1979b). Corticosteroids (usually dexamethasone) are used as adjuvant therapy, but their role is less well established than in cerebral metastasis. Standard dosage of dexamethasone is 16 to 24 mg per day; however, doses up to 100 mg per day are repeated to provide superior results (Slatkin and Posner, 1983). Corticosteroids are started prior to myelography and maintained for at least 1 to 2 weeks after completion of radiotherapy. Corticosteroids have an antiedema effect, which is greatest when used along with radiotherapy.

Hormonal therapy has been used effectively to treat pain of spinal metastasis arising from breast tumors, but its role in relieving neurologic dysfunction is not established (Slatkin and Posner, 1983). Chemotherapy is often administered in combination with other therapeutic techniques but is of unproved value.

Leptomeningeal Carcinomatosis

The incidence of leptomeningeal carcinomatosis (LC) has increased as a result of prolonged survival and the recognized failure of chemotherapeutic drugs to cross the blood-brain barrier, allowing the subarachnoid space to become a sanctuary for tumor cells from the cytotoxic effects of chemotherapeutic agents. Breast cancer is the most frequent primary source for LC (Sondak et al., 1981; Horton, 1984). Leptomeningeal carcinomatosis rarely is the presenting symptom of breast cancer but heralded recurrent disease following remission in 11 of 25 patients in one series (Yap et al., 1978). Five per cent of patients with breast tumors developed clinical evidence of LC (Yap et al., 1978), and as many as 75 per cent in autopsy series were found to have LC (Lesse and Netsky, 1954). From diagnosis of the primary tumor, time to identification of LC ranges from 3 months to 17 years but averaged about 2 years. From the diagnosis of the first metastasis, onset of LC ranged from 0 to 37 months (mean, 15 months) (Sondak et al., 1981; Yap et al., 1978).

Leptomeningeal carcinomatosis should be suspected in patients with breast cancer who develop symptoms referrable to the cerebrum, cranial nerves, or spinal roots. In spite of increased physician awareness of this syndrome, diagnosis was confirmed in only 35 to 60 per cent of living patients (Little et al., 1974; Olson et al., 1974; Yap et al., 1978). At the onset of symptoms, the patient may be in remission or undergoing the progression of widespread systemic disease. Headache, confusion, dementia, seizures, visual and auditory symptoms, and cranial nerve abnormalities (Black 1979a; Bramlet et al., 1976; Cantillo et al., 1979; Chade, 1976) characterize this disorder. Sudden onset of blindness has been reported as the sole symptom of LC (Cantillo et al., 1979). Meningeal signs, such as neck stiffness and pain, photophobia, and an afebrile course, are also noted. Once cerebral metastases are excluded by a normal enhanced cranial CT scan, the diagnosis of LC is confirmed by CSF examination, which reveals decreased glucose level (less than 40 mg/dl), increased protein concentration (greater than 100 mg/dl), positive cytologic test for malignant cells (Little et al., 1974; Olson et al., 1974; Yap et al., 1978), and negative cultures for bacteria and fungi. The initial CSF examination yields positive cytologic findings in 45 per cent of patients, increasing to 80 to 90 per cent on the third CSF study (Horton, 1984). A CT scan may reveal hydrocephalus with contrast enhancement of the basal cisterns without evidence of a mass lesion (Horton, 1984).

Therapy consists of combination radiotherapy, intrathecal chemotherapy (methotrexate [MTX], thiotepa, or cytosine arabinoside), and high dose corticosteroids. Radiotherapy to the head (3900 rad over 2 weeks) has provided excellent long-term improvement in many instances; however, the most efficacious therapy is intrathecal methotrexate (IT-MTX) (25 mg twice per week). This is administered via an intraventricular or lumbar subarachnoid drain connected to an Ommaya reservoir. Untreated LC has a prognosis of 6 to 8 weeks (Little et al., 1974; Sondak et al., 1981), whereas aggressive therapy (radiotherapy and IT-MTX) improves median survival to 22 weeks (Sondak et al., 1981). The longest reported survival was 30 months after the diagnosis of LC was made (Bramlet et al., 1976).

Neurologic Complications of Chemotherapy

Metastatic breast carcinoma has been one of the most susceptible to chemotherapy; methotrexate (MTX), cyclophosphamide (Cytoxan), chlorambucil (Leukeran), thiotepa, and hormonal therapy have all been used.

Methotrexate, an antimetabolite, competes with the purines and pyrimidines by binding the enzyme dihydrofolate reductase, resulting in inhibition of purine and thymidylic acid synthesis. Standard doses of MTX given intravenously often are toxic to bone marrow, the gastrointestinal tract, and the liver but are not considered to be neurotoxic. Methotrexate is poorly transported across the blood-brain barrier, so that the CSF concentration is less than 10 per cent of that in plasma following conventional or parenteral doses. Innovative applications of MTX have been advocated, such as megadose intravenous administration, direct instillation into the cerebral ventricles or lumbar subarachnoid space, intracarotid administration, and intratumoral infusion. Neurotoxicity may be immediate or delayed in onset following these routes of administration. Intra-arterial chemotherapy occasionally is complicated by sites of focal toxicity in the brain, possibly caused by nonuniform drug delivery owing to intravascular drug streaming (Blacklock et al., 1986). Manifestations of CNS toxicity to MTX are as follows (Young, 1982):

Acute transient side effects of IT-MTX develop shortly following injection, reach maximum intensity at 6 to 12 hr, and last 2 to 3 days. The clinical picture resembles a septic meningitis, with meningismus, photophobia, nausea, vomiting, fever, and modest CSF pleocytosis. It is unknown whether this reaction is caused by the preservatives, impurities, or the drug itself. *Transient radiculopathy,* which follows inadvertent injection into the lumbar epidural or subdural space, is of minor consequence and resolves spontaneously.

Acute transverse myelopathy causing permanent paraplegia rarely complicates IT-MTX administration and likely is an idiosyncratic reaction to the drug.

IT-MTX may cause a disabling *delayed methotrexate encephalopathy (leukoencephalopathy)*. Predisposing factors include multiple administration of IT or systemic MTX, prior whole head irradiation, associated hydrocephalus, active meningeal disease, and concomitant use of vincristine. Variability exists in the clinical presentation, CT scan appearance, and pathology. Leukoencephalopathy affects 2 per cent of patients following IT-MTX therapy. Progressive personality change, confusion, lethargy, dementia, motor abnormalities (tremor, ataxia, paresis), and seizures may occur. The course may progress rapidly to a permanent vegetative state or death. However, the majority of patients will experience partial or complete recovery when the drug is withdrawn. The CT scan discloses areas of multifocal lucency involving the white matter, periventricular enhancing lesions, and ventriculomegaly. Microscopic examination reveals gliosis, spongiform changes, extensive demyelination with axonal swelling, and focal calcification. Treatment consists of discontinuation of MTX (replacing it with arabinoside-C) and administration of citrovorum factor.

Prolonged use of intrathecal or high dose MTX is generally believed not to produce any lasting effects under normal circumstances, but motor, language, and behavioral abnormalities have been noted on neuropsychologic tests.

Estrogens, particularly diethylstilbestrol and ethinyl estradiol (Estinyl), are used in the treatment of hormonally susceptible breast cancer but have no neurologic manifestations. Tamoxifen (antiestrogen compound) is effective in treating breast cancer with positive estrogen receptors. Its neurologic complications are indirect through the development of hypercalcemia.

COMPLICATIONS OF RADIOTHERAPY OF BREAST CANCER

Neurologic complications may follow radiotherapy of the primary lesion or its metastasis. Delayed radiation damage is a function of the total dose, individual fraction size, overall duration of treatment, value of tissue irradiated, and modifying factors, such as oxygen supply, status of the vascularity, and type of radiation used (Berger, 1982). Total head irradiation may be complicated by early or delayed reactions. *Early reactions* arise 3 to 10 weeks after completion of radiotherapy and are characterized by nausea, vomiting, ataxia, dysarthria, and cerebellar signs. This syndrome resolves spontaneously and completely. If the patient dies from unrelated causes, postmortem examination reveals changes consistent with disseminated demyelination and vasculitis within the radiation field (Rider, 1963).

Delayed cerebral radiation necrosis usually occurs 1 to 3 years after radiotherapy, ranging from as early as 3 months to as late as 12 years. The clinical syndrome consists of headaches, seizures, personality changes, focal motor weakness, papilledema, dysphagia, and unconsciousness (Rottenberg et al., 1977). Total radiation dose is usually between 5000 and 6000 rad. Sheline (1980) reported that 45 of 83 patients with radionecrosis received over 7000 rad, and only 22 of them received less than 4500 rad. Total head irradiation of 5000 rad in 5 weeks is a relatively safe dose. However, higher doses may be justified for tumor control. Recurrent tumor and cerebral radionecrosis may be indistinguishable on clinical and radiographic grounds. Intracranial pressure may be elevated in both. The CT scan appearance of radionecrosis reveals a hypodense mass lesion with enhancement revealing a peripheral ring of increased attenuation. Such changes in the field of radiotherapy support the diagnosis of radionecrosis.

The mechanism of radiation damage is controversial. Either neural or vascular elements may be damaged primarily, or the patient's immunologic system is affected. The role of prophylactic steroids during and following radiotherapy is unknown, but once radionecrosis develops, high dose steroids seem to be of value. If ineffective in reversing clinical deterioration, surgical extirpation of the focus of radionecrosis may be justified.

Radiation myelitis may complicate radiotherapy of the breast lesion or spinal metastasis if the radiation portals include the spinal cord. *Acute transverse myelopathy* may occur several weeks after completion of radiotherapy, occurring as numbness and paresthesias of the arms or legs, or both, and a shock-like sensation of the trunk and extremities following neck flexion (Lhermitte's sign). Although Lhermitte's sign is a benign entity without associated objective signs, if it is present, the patient must be monitored carefully for evidence of delayed, *chronic progressive myelopathy*. This is the most frequent and devastating complication of spinal cord irradiation. Although occurring most commonly within 1 year after radiotherapy, latency may be as long as 13 years. Initially sensory symptoms predominate (paresthesias, hypesthesias, and numbness) followed by spastic para- or quadriparesis and sphincter disturbance. The clinical defects gradually progress over several months, followed by stabilization of the neurologic signs. Once having developed, these signs rarely regress. If the damaged cord is in the field of radiation, with the myelogram and CT scan revealing an atrophic cord and no evidence of spinal metastasis, radiation myelitis is likely to be present. This disease has no effective therapy; however, administration of high dose steroids may alleviate progressive symptoms (Godwin-Austen et al., 1975). Necrosis of white matter exceeds that of gray matter. Vascular changes noted on pathologic examination include hyalinization and fibrinoid material in the perivascular spaces (Berger, 1982). The thoracic cord is more susceptible to radiation myelopathy as it contains a "watershed area" (T4-T6), which lies between the abundant blood supply to the upper thoracic and thoracolumbar segments. The length of cord included to the radiation portals is great following treatment of primary breast tumors.

Vocal cord paralysis due to recurrent laryngeal nerve damage has been reported to follow radiation for breast cancer. Of 37 patients with vocal cord paralysis reported by Westbrook and coworkers (1974), radiation fibrosis occurred in two patients, metastasis in 32, and miscellaneous causes in three patients. Radiotherapy of breast cancer may cause a radiation-induced *brachial plexus lesion* (Thomas and Colby, 1972). The incidence of plexopathy is dose-related, with 73 per cent occurring in doses greater than 5500 rad and 15 per cent in doses of 5100 rad (Stoll and Andrews, 1966). Symptoms include numbness, paresthesias, and a lesser degree of motor involvement, which may plateau or progress to a paralyzed, anesthetic arm. Once fully developed, resolution of symptoms does not occur. Differentiation between radiation plexopathy and malignant infiltration depends on the presence of little or no pain in the former, whereas tumors invariably cause severe early pain (Thomas and Colby, 1972; Kori et al., 1981). Such differentiation is critical because effective therapy for plexus infiltration includes total radiotherapy. No treatment exists for radiation plexopathy.

Pain Management in Breast Cancer

Breast cancer may cause pain as a result of (1) bony metastasis, (2) compression or infiltration of peripheral nerves, brachial plexus, or nerve roots, (3) swelling within a structure invested by fascia or periosteum, (4) necrosis, infection, inflammation, and ulceration of pain-sensitive structures, or (5) the effects of treatment (surgery, radiation) (Onofrio, 1983). Radiation, surgery, or chemotherapy may effectively relieve pain by decreasing the tumor size; however, adjuvant analgesic therapy is usually required. By trial and error, the analgesic therapy most effective for pain relief is found. Recent advances in neuropharmacology and neurophysiology have revolutionized pain management.

Simple, peripherally acting, nonsteroidal anti-inflammatory drugs are usually not effective in the treatment of cancer pain (Beaver, 1984). They act peripherally to reversibly or irreversibly block cyclo-oxygenase of the arachidonic acid metabolic cycle, which diminishes prostaglandin synthesis. Prostaglandins serve as sensitizers of pain receptors to the effects of histamine and bradykinin. Nonsteroidal anti-inflammatory drugs may be effective for mild pain, but severe pain requires narcotics.

Two classes of opioid receptors have been identified (μ and δ), for which morphine and enkephalin are antagonists (Slatkin and Posner, 1983). Morphine and other narcotic analgesics produce their analgesic effect by central uptake by opioid receptors. Parenteral morphine in doses required to relieve pain may reach 300 to 400 mg per day, causing somnolence, nausea, vomiting, constipation, and respiratory depression. Neurosurgical ablative procedures, such as dorsal horn rhizotomy or cordotomy, avoid these undesirable side effects (Ray, 1980; Onofrio, 1983). However, dorsal horn rhizotomies require a major neurosurgical procedure and may leave an extremity useless from lack of position sense, with effective analgesia lasting less than 6 months. High thoracic or cervical percutaneous cordotomies are effective in relieving unilateral pain, although dysesthesias developing some months later limit long-term value. Bilateral percutaneous cordotomies fail to relieve midline deep pain and bilateral lower extremity pain and are frequently associated with postoperative bladder disturbance and motor weakness.

On the other hand, intermittent administration of intrathecal or intraventricular morphine has been successful in the management of intractable cancer pain (Ray, 1980; Onofrio, 1983). Intraspinal preservative-free morphine (Duromorph) administration relieves lower extremity, pelvic, and trunk pain, whereas head, neck, and upper extremity pain is best treated by intraventricular injection of Duromorph via an Ommaya reservoir. A trial of intrathecal Duromorph is given percutaneously to assess the candidate for implantation of an Ommaya reservoir. Patients in whom survival is less than 1 year have the best analgesic results. Long-term administration has not yet been assessed. Injection into the reservoir is carried out by a nurse, patient, or family member. One milligram of Duromorph is usually effective for 12 to 24 hr, but the dosage may be increased to 3 mg every 12 hr as needed. These intrathecal doses provide an analgesic effect superior to that of 100 to 200 mg of morphine intravenously per day. However, tolerance can develop to morphine or other analgesics having a similar chemical structure. By temporarily decreasing or discontinuing them, tolerance can be reversed and reinstitution of the drug will be possible at the lower dose.

Side effects of intrathecal Duromorph are pruritus, sedation, nausea, and respiratory depression (Beaver, 1984), which may require decreasing the morphine dose. Acute respiratory depression can be reversed by naloxone, an opioid receptor antagonist. Malignant disease may progress so that any significant increase in analgesics requires careful reassessment of the tumor size rather than simply increasing the morphine dosage. Optimal treatment for cancer pain is removal of the tumor compressing pain-sensitive structures. Breast metastases are moderately radiosensitive, so that focal radiation therapy to the tumor or to painful osteolytic lesions may not only shrink it but also be highly effective in pain relief. Furthermore, hormonal therapy may be effective in relieving pain, particularly if the tumor is estrogen receptor positive. No dogmatic rules can be set for pain relief, and the most effective therapy must be individualized.

REFERENCES

Beaver, W. T.: Appropriate management of pain in primary care practice. Am. J. Med., 77:1, 1984.

Berger, P. S.: Neurological complications of radiotherapy. In Silverstein, A. (Ed.): Neurological Complications of Therapy: Selected Topics. Mount Kisco, New York, Futura Publishing Co., 1982, p. 137.

Black, P.: Brain metastasis: Current status and recommended guidelines for management. Neurosurgery, 5:617, 1979a.

Black, P.: Spinal metastasis: Current status and recommended guidelines for management. Neurosurgery, 5:726, 1979b.

Blacklock, J. B., Wright, D. C., Dedrick, R. L., et al.: Drug streaming during intra-arterial chemotherapy. J. Neurosurg., 64:284, 1986.

Bramlet, D., Giliberti, J., and Bender, J.: Meningeal carcinomatosis. Case report and review of the literature. Neurology, 26:287, 1976.

Cantillo, R., Jain, J., Singhakowinta, A., et al.: Blindness as initial manifestations of meningeal carcinomatosis in breast cancer. Cancer, 44:755, 1979.

Chade, H. O.: Metastatic tumors of the spine and spinal cord. In Vinken, P. J., and Bruyn, G. W. (Eds.): Handbook of Clinical Neurology. Vol. 20. Amsterdam, North-Holland, 1976, pp. 415–433.

Cobb, C. A., III, Leavens, M. E., and Eckles, N.: Indications for nonoperative treatment of spinal cord compression due to breast cancer. J. Neurosurg., 47:653, 1977.

DiStefano, A., Yap, H. Y., Hortobagyi, G. N., et al.: The natural history of breast cancer patients with brain metastases. Cancer, 44:1913, 1979.

Galicich, J. H., Sundaresan, N., and Thaler, T.: Surgical treatment of single brain metastasis: Evaluation of results by computerized tomography scanning. J. Neurosurg., 53:63, 1980.

Gamache, F. W., Jr., Posner, J. B., and Patterson, R. H., Jr.: Metastatic brain tumors. In Youmans, J. R. (Ed.): Neurological Surgery. Vol. 5. Philadelphia, W. B. Saunders, 1982, p. 2872.

Gilbert, R. W., Kim, J. H., and Posner, J. B.: Epidural spinal cord compression from metastatic tumor: Diagnosis and treatment. Ann. Neurol., 3:40, 1978.

Godwin-Austen, R. B., Howell, D. A., and Worthington, B.: Observations on radiation myelopathy. Brain, 98:557, 1975.

Harrington, K. D.: Anterior cord decompression and

spine stabilization for patients with metastatic lesions of the spine. J. Neurosurg., 61:107, 1984.

Hirsh, L. F., Thanki, A. S., and Spector, H. B.: Spinal subdural metastatic adenocarcinoma: Case report and literature review. Neurosurgery, 10:621, 1982.

Hollis, P. H., Malis, L. I., and Zappulla, R. A.: Neurological deterioration after lumbar puncture below complete spinal subarachnoid block. J. Neurosurg., 64:253, 1986.

Horton, J.: Diagnosis and treatment of meningeal carcinomatosis. Curr. Concepts Oncol., 6:10, 1984.

Kori, S. H., Foley, K. M., and Posner, J. B.: Brachial plexus lesions in patients with cancer: 100 cases. Neurology, 31:45, 1981.

Lenz, M., and Freid, J. R.: Metastases to skeleton, brain and spinal cord from cancer of breast and effect of radiotherapy. Ann. Surg., 93:278, 1931.

Lesse, S., and Netsky, M. G.: Metastasis of neoplasms to central nervous system and meninges. Arch. Neurol. Psychiatry, 72:133, 1954.

Little, J. R., Dale, J. D., and Okazaki, H.: Meningeal carcinomatosis. Clinical manifestations. Arch. Neurol., 30:138, 1974.

Livingston, K. E., and Perrin, R. G.: The neurosurgical management of spinal metastasis causing cord and cauda equina compression. J. Neurosurg., 49:839, 1978.

Mehta, D., Khatib, R., and Patel, S.: Carcinoma of the breast and meningioma. Association and management. Cancer, 51:1937, 1983.

Olson, M. E., Chernik, N. L., and Posner, J. B.: Infiltration of the leptomeninges by systemic cancer. A clinical and pathologic study. Arch. Neurol., 30:122, 1974.

Onofrio, B. M.: Treatment of chronic pain of malignant origin with intrathecal opiates. Clin. Neurosurg., 31:304, 1983.

Paterson, A. H. G., Agarwal, M., Lees, A., et al.: Brain metastases in breast cancer patients receiving adjuvant chemotherapy. Cancer, 49:651, 1982.

Perrin, R. G., Livingston, K. E., and Aarabi, B.: Intradural extramedullary spinal metastasis. A report of 10 cases. J. Neurosurg., 56:835, 1982.

Ray, C. D.: Electrical and chemical stimulation of the CNS by direct means for pain control: Present and future. Clin. Neurosurg., 28:564, 1980.

Rider, W. D.: Radiation damage to the brain—a new syndrome. J. Can. Assoc. Radiol., 14:67, 1963.

Rodriguez, M., and DiNapoli, R. P.: Spinal cord compression with special reference to metastatic epidural tumors. Mayo Clin. Proc., 55:442, 1980.

Rottenberg, D. A., Chernik, N. L., Deck, M. D. F., et al.: Cerebral necrosis following radiotherapy of extracranial neoplasms. Ann. Neurol., 1:339, 1977.

Sondak, V., Deckers, P. J., Feller, J. H., et al.: Leptomeningeal spread of breast cancer. Cancer, 48:395, 1981.

Shapiro, R.: Myelography. Chicago, Year Book Medical Publishers, 1962, p. 279.

Sheline, G. E.: Irradiation injury of the human brain: A review of clinical experience. In Gilbert, H. A., and Kagan, A. R. (Eds.): Radiation Damage to the Nervous System. New York, Raven Press, 1980, p. 39.

Slatkin, N. E., and Posner, J. B.: Management of spinal epidural metastases. Clin. Neurosurg., 30:698, 1983.

Snyder, S. H.: Drug and neurotransmitter receptors in the brain. Science, 224:22, 1984.

Stoll, B. A., and Andrews, J. T.: Radiation-induced peripheral neuropathy. Br. Med. J., 1:834, 1966.

Sundaresan, N., and Galicich, J. H.: Treatment of spinal metastases by vertebral body resection. Cancer Invest., 2:383, 1984.

Taveras, J. M., and Wood, E. H.: Diagnostic Neuroradiology. Baltimore, Williams & Wilkins, 1964, p. 865.

Thomas, J. E., and Colby, M. Y., Jr.: Radiation induced or metastatic brachial plexopathy? J.A.M.A., 222:1392, 1972.

Westbrook, K. C., Ballantyne, A. J., Eckles, N. E., et al.: Breast cancer and vocal cord paralysis. South. Med. J., 67:805, 1974.

Westling, P., Svensson, H., and Hele, P.: Cervical plexus lesions following post-operative radiation therapy of mammary carcinoma. Acta Radiol. [Ther.], 11:209, 1972.

Yap, H. Y., Yap, B. S., Tashima, C. K., et al.: Meningeal carcinomatosis in breast cancer. Cancer, 42:283, 1978.

Young, D. F.: Neurological complications of cancer chemotherapy. In Silverstein, A. (Ed.): Neurological Complications of Therapy: Selected Topics. Mount Kisco, New York, Futura Publishing Co., 1982, p. 57.

Young, R. F., Post, E. M., and King, G. A.: Treatment of spinal epidural metastases: Randomized prospective comparison of laminectomy and radiotherapy. J. Neurosurg., 53:741, 1980.

CHAPTER 26

WILLIAM L. DONEGAN

Mammary Carcinoma and Pregnancy

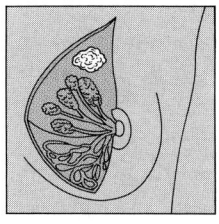

The association of pregnancy with breast cancer raises special issues. The curability of this disease when it coincides with pregnancy, the proper therapy, and the risks of future pregnancies have long been subjects of debate. Because the problem is infrequent, the experience of individuals or even institutions is generally limited, and conclusions are often based on assumptions and small numbers of cases. A few large series have been reported. Notable are those of Westberg (1946), who reviewed 179 cases in Stockholm, Sweden; of Holleb and Farrow (1964), who reported on 283 cases seen at Memorial Hospital for Cancer and Allied Diseases in New York City; of Clark and Reid (1978), concerning 330 cases at the Ontario Cancer Institute, Toronto; of Deemarsky and Neishtadt (1981) on 100 cases in Leningrad; and of King and associates (1985) on 63 cases at the Mayo Clinic, Rochester, Minnesota. The subject has been reviewed by Hubay and coworkers (1978), Anderson (1979), and Donegan (1983).

From the biologic standpoint, concern about the effect of pregnancy on malignancy of the breast appears justified. Many of the systemic changes that favor fetal development appear equally favorable for the promotion of tumor growth (Fig. 26–1). To varying degrees, breast cancers retain the hormonal dependence of their parent tissue, remaining potentially responsive to the same physiologic changes that stimulate the mammary parenchyma. Laboratory and clinical evidence indicates that estrogens and prolactin, both of which increase in amount dramatically during pregnancy, can enhance the growth of mammary carcinoma.

So might the increased levels of growth hormone or of corticosteroids, which reduce cell-mediated immunity and favor the implantation and spread of tumors in animal models. In view of the important role attributed to cell-mediated immunity in maintaining resistance to cancer, the evidence for depression of T lymphocytes in early pregnancy (Strelkauskas et al., 1975), the impaired mitogen response of lymphocytes (Purtilo et al., 1972; Nelson et al., 1973) and the depletion of germinal centers in pelvic lymph nodes would seem to represent disadvantages for the gravid host. Add to this the rich blood supply and enhanced lymphatic drainage of the breast during pregnancy, and it would seem that ideal circumstances for growth and spread of cancer are present. Past experience has, in fact, generally confirmed a poor outlook for the pregnant patient. The opinions expressed by 35 authorities in this field, compiled by Cheek in 1953, reflected pessimism and a lack of unanimity regarding management.

Notwithstanding the foregoing biologic considerations, and in contrast to the pessimism of early publications on this subject, the trend in recent years has been toward an attitude of optimism, a change based largely on the awareness that poor results may have been due in no small measure to delay in diagnosis and procrastination in treatment. Overall, there is a growing tendency to minimize the significance of the pregnancy and to aggressively diagnose and treat the patient in much the same way as the nonpregnant woman. Byrd and colleagues (1962) summed up this attitude after a review of material at Vanderbilt University: "In the face of general enthusiasm for terminating the pregnancy, we believe the evidence is that the cancer should be terminated."

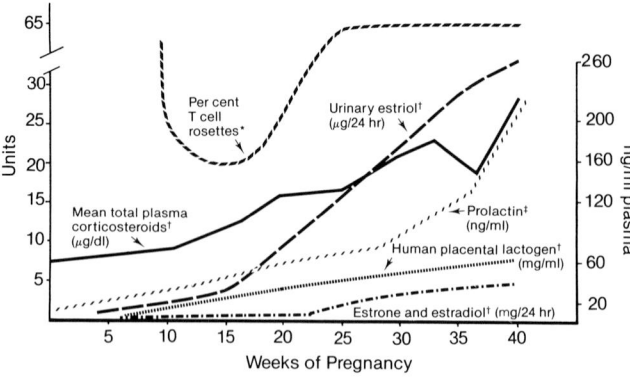

Figure 26–1. Hormonal and immunologic changes of pregnancy that are potentially important with respect to the growth of mammary carcinoma. (Adapted from Donegan, W. L.: Pregnancy and breast cancer. Obstet. Gynecol., 50:244, 1977. Reprinted with permission.)

*Strelkauskas et al., 1975
†Hytten and Leitch, 1971
‡Vorrgerr, 1974

Frequency

The problem under consideration is infrequent because breast cancer favors an older population, women past the child-bearing years, and there is no reason to believe that a woman is especially susceptible to breast cancer during pregnancy. The coincidence exists only because the age-specific incidence of breast cancer begins to rise early (i.e., at age 25 years), and by age 35 years it has become the most frequent cancer of women (Donegan, 1983). As fertility declines in the fourth decade of life, women who are affected with breast cancer when pregnant are youthful, with ages ranging from 21 to 44 years, averaging 32 to 35 years in recent series.

Examination of the breasts is a routine of obstetric care, but practicing obstetricians can expect to discover relatively few cases of breast cancer. Finn (1952) reported 46 breast cancers among 62,561 patients observed during pregnancy at the New York Lying-In Hospital between 1932 and 1951, approximately 1 case per 1360 patients. White (1955) found only 74 in a collected series of 238,299 pregnancies, or 1 per 3200 pregnancies. Although breast cancer is relatively uncommon among the youthful, pregnancy is sufficiently frequent in this population that it is not unusual for the few young women who develop this cancer to be pregnant at the time. Among 45,881 cases of breast cancer, White found 1296 with a coincident or recent pregnancy, an incidence of 2.8 per cent. More recent reports have since set this figure between 0.75 per cent and 3.1 per cent (Rosemond, 1964; Peters, 1968; Applewhite et al., 1973; Sahni et al., 1981). Considering only women of childbearing age, the frequency of coincidence is considerable. Applewhite found that 7.3 per cent of 655 women with breast cancer under 45 years of age were pregnant or lactating. Among 549 women less than 35 years of age, Treves and Holleb (1958) reported a remarkable 14 per cent. Horsley and associates (1969) also confirmed the high coincidence among young women, reporting that 10 per cent of 67 patients less than 35 years of age were pregnant at the time of diagnosis, and an additional 15 per cent had been pregnant within the previous year. Nugent and O'Connell (1985) pointed out that the 11 per cent frequency of concurrent pregnancy and breast cancer found in their series of patients 25 to 40 years old was almost identical to the period of time they would be expected to be pregnant (10 per cent), based on an average of two pregnancies, inferring a coincidental rather than causal relationship.

Diagnosis

Pregnancy makes diagnosis of breast cancer more difficult. The enlargement of the breasts during pregnancy and lactation tends to obscure parenchymal masses. When masses are appreciated, they are often erroneously attributed to normal hypertrophy of the gland, or they are lost in surrounding tissues as pregnancy progresses, creating the illusion that they have resolved. The effectiveness of mammography is also compromised by the full

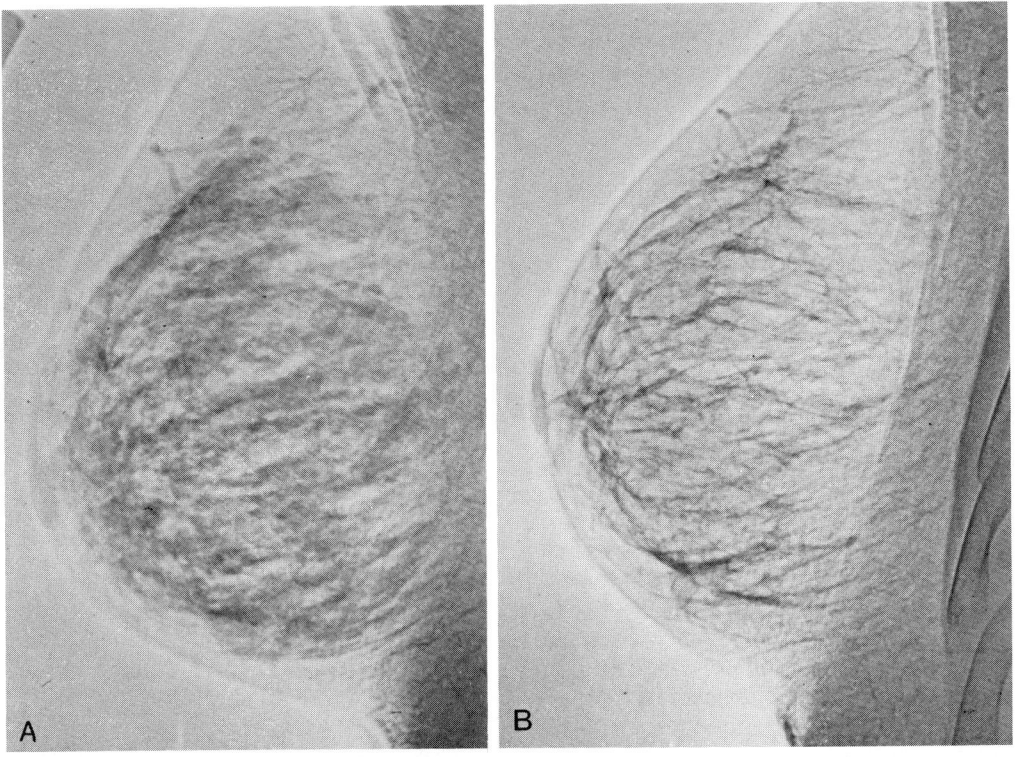

Figure 26–2. The increase in parenchymal density of the breast of a 36 year old woman during lactation *(A)* is shown in these mammograms. This change tends to obscure carcinomas.

development and function of mammary parenchyma. These changes, with the accompanying hyperemia and increased water content of the breasts, contribute to a generalized radiographic density with loss of the contrasting fatty tissue that usually helps to define tumor masses (Hoeffken and Lanyi, 1977) (Fig. 26–2). For this reason, and because of potential exposure of the fetus to irradiation, mammography ordinarily is not used during pregnancy (Canter et al., 1983). The obscuring physical changes of pregnancy may also cause breast cancers to be clinically understaged and as a consequence to appear unusually aggressive in behavior.

The literature confirms that the clinical courses of gravid women with mammary carcinoma are marked by unusual delays. Applewhite (1973), reporting on women seen at Louisiana State University between 1948 and 1967, documented an average duration of symptoms of 11 months, versus 4 months for nonpregnant women. Diagnosis was delayed an additional month after the first visit to a physician, and the delay from diagnosis to treatment averaged 8 days, versus 3 days for the nonpregnant woman. Westberg (1946) found the mean delay between discovery of a lump and treatment to be 2 months longer for pregnant women than for others, and this finding was confirmed by Bunker and Peters (1963). Byrd and coworkers (1962) attributed three fourths of the delay in treatment directly to physician procrastination. Contributory factors have included failure to examine the breasts regularly at prenatal clinics (Montgomery, 1961), reluctance to obtain tissue for a histologic diagnosis, and failure to treat known carcinomas promptly.

The practice of "watching" a lump in the breast during pregnancy is unjustified. Indications for biopsy of breast lesions are the same as those for nonpregnant women. Aspiration of masses with a fine needle serves to differentiate cysts or galactoceles from solid tumors quickly and innocuously. Biopsy of solid tumor masses with incision or needle under local anesthesia on an outpatient basis is expeditious and involves minimal risk (Saltzstein et al., 1974). Biopsies on an outpatient basis are also considerably less expensive than hospital admission. Byrd and colleagues (1962) point out that if general anesthesia is necessary for biopsy or mastectomy, it entails minimal risk to the fetus. Of 134 cases so managed, including 29 with malignant disease, only one resulted in fetal death (0.75 per cent). This menopausal woman aborted spontaneously 3 weeks after removal of a benign cyst. Although the risk of fetal loss is small, well below the 5 per cent reported by Westberg before 1946, it is important that the patient be advised of it before the physician proceeds with surgery under either general or local anesthesia.

Pathologic Findings

The frequency with which biopsies of the breast reveal cancer during pregnancy is similar to that in the nonpregnant population (Byrd et al., 1962). Benign lesions, in decreasing order of frequency, include fibroadenomas, lipomas, papillomas, fibrocystic disease, galactoceles, and inflammatory lesions. The cancers that are found are not notably different in character or distribution from those in nonpregnant women, nor is inflammatory carcinoma a more frequent occurrence. Rosemond (1964) reported one inflammatory carcinoma among 56 cases (1.8 per cent), Montgomery (1961) found three among 70 cases (4.3 per cent), and Clark and Reid (1978) discovered five among 201 (2.5 per cent) cases of breast cancer during pregnancy or lactation. Save for the unusually high figure of 13 per cent found at the Mayo Clinic by King and associates (1985), this is comparable to the 1.5 to 4 per cent reported among nonpregnant women. Inflammatory cancer has the same poor prognosis during pregnancy as otherwise (Zeigerman et al., 1968). As might be expected in young women, 71 per cent of the tumors lack estrogen receptors (Nugent and O'Connell, 1985), a factor that augurs poorly for cure but that would seem to negate any influence of pregnancy on prognosis. Receptor negativity may be less frequent during lactation, but confirmation of this is needed (Holdaway et al., 1984).

Treatment and Prognosis

Early reports regarding the association of breast cancer with pregnancy emphasized rapid spread of the tumor with early demise of the patient. Delayed discovery of cancers because of increased breast size, early dissemination owing to increased vascularity of the breast, and unfavorable hormonal factors operative during pregnancy have been blamed for the poor prognosis (Costarides and Theofanides, 1963). After review of the discouraging experience at the Presbyterian Hospital from 1915 to 1935, Haagensen and Stout (1943) considered the pregnant patient categorically incurable and not a candidate for surgery. In the face of mounting evidence to the contrary, this opinion was revised in 1949 (Haagensen, 1956). Harrington (1937) is given credit for reviving optimism about treatment. He reported on 92 patients operated on at the Mayo Clinic with a 5 year survival rate of 61.5 per cent among women without axillary metastases. This report emphasized the favorable results achievable if the disease was detected and treated when still confined to the breast. Unfortunately, spread beyond the confines of the breast is frequent, and many carcinomas arising during pregnancy have been in advanced stages when treated (Table 26–1). Three fourths (74 per cent) of Montgomery's 70 patients had metastases, and in 20 per cent the metastases were systemic. Seventy-two per cent of Holleb and Farrow's (1964) and 75 per cent of Applewhite and colleagues' (1973) operable groups had axillary metastases. This high incidence of metastatic disease has marked each trimester of pregnancy as well as the postpartum period.

There is reason to believe, however, that the prognosis of pregnant patients is equal to that of others of comparable age and with tumors at the same stage if they are managed as expeditiously. Rissanen (1968) found early cancers not appreciably less curable in pregnant women than in other women of similar age. Peters (1968) found that 187 pregnant patients survived equally well as a control group matched for age and stage of disease. No more than a 10 to 15 per cent deficit in 5 year survival could be discerned in any clinical stage, and women 36 to 40 years of age fared altogether as well as their nonpregnant counterparts. During a 10 year period of follow-up, the difference in actuarial survival of the two groups was unimpressive. In a small series, Nugent and O'Connell (1985) found the 5 year survival of women under 40 years old comparable by stage whether or not they were pregnant at diagnosis.

Table 26-1. BREAST CANCER WITH PREGNANCY OR LACTATION

Period Reviewed	Number of Cases	5 Year Survival (%)	Resected for Cure (%)	Axillary Metastases (%)	5 Year Survival of Operable Cases			Reference
					All (%)	Ax+ (%)	Ax− (%)	
1910–1933	92		92	85	15	6	62	Harrington (1937)
1915–1959	48	(33)*	65	55	(45)	(24)	(71)	Haagensen (1971)
1920–1953	133	31	90	72	30	17	65	Holleb and Farrow (1964)
Pre–1956	37		37	68	22	8	50	White and White (1956)
1921–1962	17		71	67	100	100	100	Horsley et al. (1969)†
1925–1960	29	55	72	—	71	33	100	Byrd et al. (1962)
1926–1972	100	48	91	67	54	43	73	Deemarsky and Neishtadt (1981)
1930–1964	46	39	83	50		28	68	Earley et al. (1969)
1931–1975								
Coincident	121	31		83		(22)	(35)	Clark and Reid (1978)
Lactation	80	26		80		(18)	(69)	
1931–1964	14	36	79	64	45	29	75	Peete et al. (1966)
1932–1946	6	17	33	100	50	50	—	Brooks and Proffitt (1949)
1938–1961	187	33						Peters (1968)
1940–1965	50	34	48	71	48	31	86	Donegan (1979)
1940–1961	33	42	90	75	47			Rissanen (1969)
1948–1967	48	25	69	50	36	18	56	Applewhite et al. (1973)
Pre–1953	20	40	90	75	50	42	75	Hochman and Schreiber (1953)
1950–1980	63	53	100	62	53	36	82	King et al. (1985)
1954–1961	35	13	17‡	—	100			Helman and Bennett (1963)
1960–1973	33		88	75		27	33	Cheek (1973)
1970–1980	19	57	95	78	61	50	100	Nugent and O'Connell (1985)

A chronologic summary is shown of selected reports on the results of treating breast cancer during pregnancy or lactation. No trend is evident. Patients without metastases in axillary lymph nodes have a relatively favorable prognosis.
*Parentheses indicate 10 year survival.
†Only patients 35 years of age or younger.
‡Clinical Stages I and II.

EARLY CLINICAL STAGES

It is generally agreed that mastectomy is indicated for clinically early stages of breast cancer regardless of the trimester of pregnancy. Modified mastectomy for the pregnant patient has been used since 1965 at the Mayo Clinic (King et al., 1985). The potential advantages of early surgery outweigh risks to the fetus. An exception to this view is that of Peters (1968) and others at the Ontario Cancer Institute (Clark and Reid, 1978), who express reservations about the need for immediate treatment in the second and third trimesters. The data from this institute showed the best survival associated with treatment in the first trimester, less favorable but equivalent survival in the second and third trimesters and within 3 months of delivery, and a very poor survival if treatment followed more than 3 months after delivery. These findings have been used to justify delay of treatment "if expedient," permitting women to deliver their infants before surgery if the tumor did not appear to be aggressive and if a prolonged delay was not involved. It must be appreciated that this recommendation is based on retrospective review and small numbers (fewer than 30 in each category) of unstaged patients. The results can be a function of selection rather than of timing. It is likely that treatment of small, indolent and prognostically favorable cancers was deferred until after delivery, whereas large and rapidly progressing cancers, unlikely to be cured in any case, were treated without delay. If this is the case, cure of some favorable cases may have been compromised. Differences in survival after treatment in the various trimesters of pregnancy or in the postpartum period usually reflect the relative number of patients in each category with metastases in axillary lymph nodes. Variation may be great when small numbers of patients are involved. A policy of delay entails risk for the patient and places an exceptional burden of responsibility on the physician.

As shown in Table 26–1, the results of radical mastectomy generally are poor when metastases are present in lymph nodes, whereas a gratifying survival rate results when disease is confined to the breast, frequently comparable to that expected in nonpregnant patients. Reported 5 year survival rates were 75 per cent (Peete et al., 1966), 100 per cent (Byrd and associates, 1962), 82 per cent (King et al., 1985), and 75 per cent for patients without axillary metastases (Hochman and

Schreiber, 1953). These figures provide reason to believe that prompt diagnosis and treatment during pregnancy significantly improve overall survival.

Postoperative radiotherapy has not had a demonstrable effect on survival. The arguments for and against its use to prevent local recurrence in high risk cases can be found in Chapter 14. The hazard to the fetus posed by ionizing irradiation would discourage its use during pregnancy either as primary or as an adjuvant therapy (Fig. 26–3) (Dekaban, 1968; Covington and Baker, 1969).

The use of cytotoxic agents as adjuvant chemotherapy is hazardous to normal fetal development in the first trimester of pregnancy (Nicholson, 1968; Raich and Curet, 1975). Both antimetabolites and alkylating agents have been associated with developmental anomalies. Methotrexate and aminopterin pose a special risk, shared to a lesser degree by chlorambucil, cyclophosphamide, and busulfan. Murray and coworkers (1984) reviewed collected results with 164 patients treated during the first trimester and found an 11.6 per cent frequency of fetal malformations (e.g., cleft palate, hydrocephalus). This is approximately a fivefold increase over expected (Schapira and Chudley, 1984). If those patients treated with aminopterin were omitted, the rate fell to 8 per cent. Several of the patients received irradiation as well, and this combination is considered particularly teratogenic. No malformed fetuses followed treatment of 76 women during the second and third trimesters. Although exposure of the fetus during the second or third trimester of pregnancy is not likely to interfere with normal development, long-term effects are unknown. The case for adjuvant chemotherapy is discussed in Chapter 15. If it is considered desirable to undertake this form of treatment in the first trimester, serious consideration should be given to termination of the pregnancy.

Despite the theoretical advantages of reversing the hormonal changes of pregnancy, therapeutic abortion in operable cases has not improved the results of treatment. In 1953, Adair published the results with a small group of patients who appeared to survive longer when termination of pregnancy was included as part of therapy. More than two thirds (69.5 per cent) of a group of 23 patients whose pregnancies were simultaneous with or subsequent to initial therapy and who underwent therapeutic abortions lived for 5 years. Only 44 per cent of 25 patients who had not had abortions survived for the same period. A difference was also present when the patients were considered on the basis of axillary lymph node involvement. The differences, however, were not statistically significant, and subsequent reports by others have been similarly inconclusive. Holleb and Farrow (1962) reported on 24 patients treated with radical mastectomy, half of whom underwent abortions and half of whom did not. The 5 year clinical cure rate of the patients whose pregnancies were terminated in this instance was inferior (17 per cent) to that of those who were allowed to deliver normally (33 per cent), but again the difference was not significant. At the Prin-

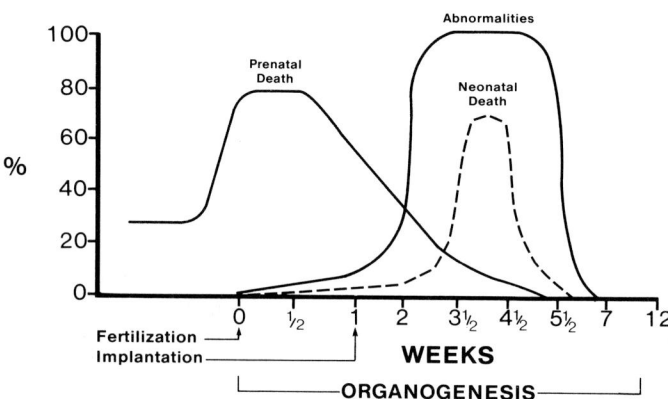

Figure 26–3. Animal experiments demonstrate that irradiation exposure in the first trimester of pregnancy during the period of organogenesis can be expected to result in a high frequency of fetal deaths and abnormalities. This risk is not expressed later in pregnancy, but as the uterus enlarges it becomes more difficult to shield the fetus, and long-term effects become a matter of concern. (Redrawn from Brill, A. B., and Forgotson, E. H.: Radiation and congenital malformations. Am. J. Obstet. Gynecol., 90:1149, 1964.)

Table 26–2. RESULTS OF THERAPEUTIC ABORTION IN CONJUNCTION WITH MASTECTOMY FOR EARLY STAGES OF BREAST CANCER*

5 Year Survival		
Abortion	No Abortion	Reference
4/6	4/10	Hochman and Schreiber (1953)
2/12	4/12	Holleb and Farrow (1962)†
4/7	3/3	Helman and Bennett (1963)
2/7	3/6	Peete et al (1966)
3/4	8/10	Rissanen (1968)
15.4%/13	28.9%/93	Clark and Reid (1978)
6/14	7/8	Deemarsky and Neishtadt (1981)
9/21	22/37	King et al. (1985)

*Listed are reports in which therapeutic abortion was used in conjunction with mastectomy (usually radical) in selected cases of clinically early breast cancer. Cases in each are few; no advantage in 5 year survival is apparent overall in conjunction with the procedure.

†Figures available for first trimester only.

cess Margaret Hospital, Toronto, the results were similar (Clark and Reid, 1978). Ninety-three women allowed to deliver spontaneously had 5 and 10 year survival rates of 29 per cent and 23 per cent, respectively, superior to that of women with therapeutic abortion (15 per cent and 8 per cent, respectively). A tabulation of this and other reports is shown in Table 26–2. Selection obviously was involved in a decision for or against abortion, and the cases are not staged, but the figures suggest no benefit, and authorities now agree that abortion does not improve prognosis (Hubay et al., 1978). Many authorities agree, however, that other indications for termination of pregnancy may exist and that a decision can be individualized, taking into consideration factors of risk, prognosis, religious beliefs, size of family, or personal desires of the patient.

The chance of metastatic spread of cancer to the conceptus during continued pregnancy is small. No instance of transplacental metastasis of breast cancer to a fetus has been documented, although six cases are known in which cancer of the breast has metastasized to the placenta (Donegan, 1983). Following delivery the child remained healthy in each case.

ADVANCED AND DISSEMINATED CANCER

The outlook for patients with advanced cancers generally is bleak. For 73 inoperable patients, Holleb and Farrow (1964) found a median survival time from admission to death of only 7 months, ranging from 1 month to 3 years. Seventy-three per cent of patients died within 1 year, and 93 per cent died within 2 years from the date of admission. None of Haagensen's nine patients with clinical Stage D lesions treated with radical mastectomy survived 10 years, and only one of eight with Stage C lesions did so (Haagensen, 1971).

Effective palliation for patients with disseminated cancer is usually an urgent need; prognosis is poor. Elimination of estrogens from endocrine sources is a primary consideration in premenopausal women. In the absence of estrogen receptors in tumor tissue, however, oophorectomy and therapeutic abortion would promise to be of little therapeutic value. Whether a decision is for endocrine ablation or cytotoxic chemotherapy, continuation of the pregnancy is undesirable. In the first trimester dilatation and suction curettage of the uterus is sufficient for termination of pregnancy; later in term, therapeutic abortion can be accomplished by the instillation of prostaglandin $F_{2\alpha}$ or 20 per cent hypertonic saline into the amniotic fluid or, alternatively, by surgical evacuation of the uterus or hysterectomy. Whether a pregnancy near term is interrupted depends greatly on the urgency of initiating palliative measures and the patient's wishes. A brief delay in the interest of delivering a viable fetus may not be accompanied by significant deterioration of the patient's condition. Chemotherapy late in pregnancy would entail little risk to normal fetal development.

The results of endocrine therapy in patients under 35 years of age are poor. Despite castration and termination of pregnancy, Holleb and Farrow's seven patients died within 2 years. None of 32 patients reported by Bunker and Peters (1963) who were castrated for palliation demonstrated measurable improvement, and only two benefited subjectively. King and associates (1985) treated eight of 12 pregnant patients with advanced local or disseminated disease with therapeutic abortion, and only one lived 5 years.

Subsequent Pregnancies

Pregnancies are not unusual among women treated for mammary carcinoma who remain fertile. In Treves and Holleb's series (1958),

5.5 per cent of women 35 years of age and under had subsequent pregnancies. Ten per cent of Peters' 221 patients (1968) and 15 per cent of Rissanen's 27 patients (1968) who were treated initially during pregnancy or lactation and who retained their ovaries became pregnant again. Seventy per cent of these conceptions occurred within the first 5 years of treatment. Jochimsen and colleagues (1981) reported two patients who became pregnant while receiving adjuvant chemotherapy and recommended that contraception be practiced during such treatment.

Of importance is whether the pregnancies influence the patient's prognosis and whether they should be prevented or terminated. The fact is that patients with pregnancies fare very well. On review they prove to have a low incidence of axillary nodal involvement at the time of their original mastectomy, and their survival does not appear to be curtailed (Holleb and Farrow, 1962). Survival rate is, in fact, often remarkably high; for example, 5 and 10 year survivals amounting to 67 per cent and 57 per cent, respectively, were reported by White and White (1956), and 77.4 per cent (5 year) and 69.5 per cent (10 year) rates were reported in another series by Rissanen (1969). Selection undoubtedly is involved, as women with aggressive tumors tend to have recurrence early and die, allowing those with a more favorable prognosis to survive and become pregnant. Reports that control for this bias, however, lend support to the thesis that pregnancy is not deleterious. Peters (1968) matched the age and clinical stage of 96 such patients with an equal number of patients who had no further conceptions. Those who became pregnant not only lived longer but also had longer survival times free of recurrence (Peters, 1968). Even when pregnancy occurred during a high risk period—that is, within 6 months of mastectomy—54 per cent lived 5 years. A case matching study by Cooper and Butterfield (1970) with 40 pairs of patients matched for age, stage of tumor, status of axillary nodes, and equivalent survival at least to the time of conception, found superior survival in the group with subsequent pregnancies. At Memorial–Sloan-Kettering Cancer Center, New York City, Harvey and colleagues (1981) reviewed 41 patients with subsequent pregnancies and found no detrimental effect overall or selectively for their patients with positive nodes or with early pregnancies. Abortion also had no beneficial effect. These authors concluded that there were no therapeutic grounds for recommending avoidance or termination of pregnancy in patients who were free of recurrence. Thus, a pregnancy after treatment does not provoke recurrence or jeopardize continued well-being of the patient (Helman and Bennett, 1963; Holleb and Farrow, 1964; Cheek, 1973). It should be appreciated, however, that one or more successful pregnancies without difficulty provide no assurance against a subsequent recurrence.

In an era of planned parenthood, pregnancies are becoming a matter of choice rather than accident. Patients treated for breast cancer who desire to become pregnant must make this decision with a full appreciation of the circumstances of their case. Figure 26–4 shows annual risk of recurrence for young women in Milwaukee after mastectomy over a period of 10 years. It is evident that the interval after surgery and the presence or absence of metastases to axillary lymph nodes are important determinants of risk. The highest morbidity is within the first 2 years after surgery; pregnan-

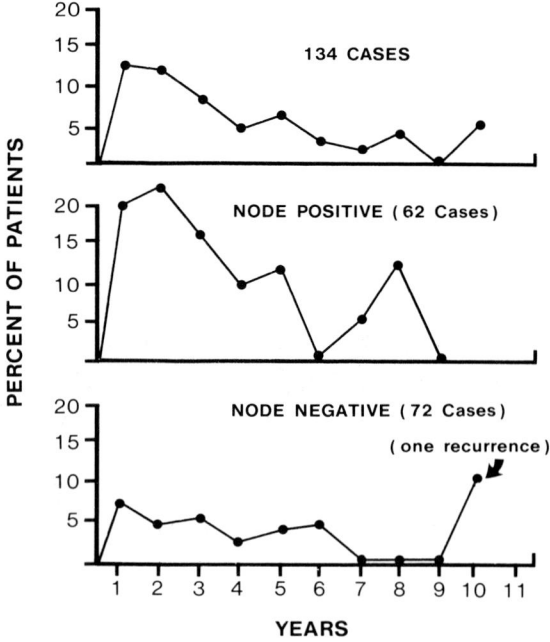

Figure 26–4. Breast cancer recurs over long periods, but the highest risk is in the first 2 years after treatment and is of considerably greater magnitude in patients with axillary nodal metastases.

cies during this time are most likely to coincide with recurrence. Treatment failures occurred in 13 per cent of the total number of patients at risk in the first year. The annual morbidity declined progressively thereafter, until at 10 years the figure approximated 5 per cent or less.

The failures each year were considerably higher for those who had metastases in axillary lymph nodes. On the other hand, the figure never exceeded 7 per cent for patients without nodal metastases even in early years, and after 8 years it had fallen to negligible levels. As cumulative recurrence rises progressively to claim an increasing number of previously healthy women, it might be concluded in these circumstances that the best chance of having a child and enjoying motherhood for as long as possible would be provided by a pregnancy as soon after mastectomy as possible. Conversely, maximum assurance of an uncomplicated pregnancy and of continued health lies in lengthening the period between surgery and conception. Most authorities discourage conception for 2 years to several years after surgery to pass the period of highest risk and to improve the chances of a woman's remaining healthy to care for her child. Decisions are best made on an individual basis with concern for the patient's wishes, circumstances, prognosis, and other prevailing factors.

Summary

Among premenopausal women, approximately 10 per cent of newly diagnosed breast cancers are accompanied by pregnancy, with most patients being in the fourth decade of life. The prognosis for these patients, and for those whose cancers are diagnosed soon after pregnancy, generally is less favorable than that for nonpregnant females, but if age and stage of disease are comparable, pregnancy per se has little influence on prognosis. Mastectomy is as effective for pregnant patients as for other women, and the chance of spontaneous abortion is small. Therapeutic abortion does not improve the chances for cure of patients with clinically localized cancer. Effective endocrine therapy or chemotherapy for advanced or disseminated breast cancer does require therapeutic abortion, and an early pregnancy is best terminated. For pregnancies near term, the decision depends greatly on the desire of the patient for a child. Unless therapeutic needs are urgent, intervention can sometimes be delayed temporarily without significant deterioration of the patient's condition.

Pregnancies subsequent to a mastectomy have little bearing on continued well-being, and as long as the patient is clinically free of cancer, no therapeutic benefit can be expected from interrupting them. A decision for future pregnancies should be individualized with due regard for the risk of recurrence and the desirability of the patient's completing her family while still reasonably young.

Progress with the treatment of breast cancer depends in part on the appreciation that cancers do occur during pregnancy and lactation, that they are best diagnosed early, and that they are curable. Pregnancy should neither deter a prompt diagnosis nor delay definitive treatment.

REFERENCES

Adair, F. E.: Cancer of the breast. Surg. Clin. North Am., *33*:313, 1953.

Anderson, J. M.: Mammary cancers and pregnancy. Br. Med. J., *1*:1124, 1979.

Applewhite, R. R., Smith, L. R., and DiVincenti, F.: Carcinoma of the breast associated with pregnancy and lactation. Am. Surg., *39*:101, 1973.

Brill, A. B., and Forgotson, E. H.: Radiation and congenital malformations. Am. J. Obstet. Gynecol., *90*:1149, 1964.

Brooks, B., and Proffitt, J. N.: The influence of pregnancy on cancers of the breast. Surgery, *25*:1, 1949.

Bunker, M. L., and Peters, M. V.: Breast cancer associated with pregnancy or lactation. Am. J. Obstet. Gynecol., *85*:312, 1963.

Byrd, B. F., Jr., Bayer, D. S., Robertson, J. C., and Stephenson, S. E., Jr.: Treatment of breast tumors associated with pregnancy and lactation. Ann. Surg., *155*:940, 1962.

Canter, J. W., Oliver, G. C., and Zaloudek, C. J.: Surgical diseases of the breast during pregnancy. Clin. Obstet. Gynecol., *26*:853, 1983.

Cheek, J. H.: Survey of current opinions concerning carcinoma of the breast occurring during pregnancy. Arch. Surg., *66*:664, 1953.

Cheek, J. H.: Cancer of the breast in pregnancy and lactation. Am. J. Surg., *126*:729, 1973.

Clark, R. M., and Reid, J.: Carcinoma of the breast in pregnancy and lactation. Int. J. Radiation Oncol. Biol. Phys., *4*:693, 1978.

Cooper, D. R., and Butterfield, J.: Pregnancy subsequent to mastectomy for cancer of the breast. Ann. Surg., *171*:429, 1970.

Costarides, J., and Theofanides, C.: Carcinoma of the breast during pregnancy or lactation. J. Int. Coll. Surg., *40*:146, 1963.

Covington, E. E., and Baker, A. S.: Dosimetry of scattered radiation to the fetus. J.A.M.A., *209*:414, 1969.

Deemarsky, L. J., and Neishtadt, E. L.: Breast cancer and pregnancy. Breast, *7*:17, 1981.

Dekaban, A. S.: Abnormalities in children exposed to x-radiation during various stages of gestation: Tentative timetable of radiation injury to the human fetus, part I. J. Nucl. Med., 9:471, 1968.
Donegan, W. L.: Cancer and pregnancy. CA, 33:5, 1983.
Donegan, W. L.: Mammary carcinoma and pregnancy. In Donegan, W. L., and Spratt, J. S. (Eds.): Cancer of the Breast. 2nd Ed. Philadelphia, W. B. Saunders, 1979, p. 448.
Donegan, W. L.: Pregnancy and breast cancer. Obstet. Gynecol., 50:244, 1977.
Earley, T. K., Gallagher, J. Q., and Chapman, K. E.: Carcinoma of the breast in women under thirty years of age. Am. J. Surg., 118:832, 1969.
Finn, W. F.: Pregnancy complicated by cancer. Bull. Margaret Hague Maternity Hosp., 5:2, 1952.
Haagensen, C. D.: Diseases of the Breast. Philadelphia, W. B. Saunders, 1956, p. 538.
Haagensen, C. D., and Stout, A. P.: Carcinoma of the breast. II. Criteria for operability. Ann. Surg., 118:859, 1943.
Haagensen, C. D.: Diseases of the Breast. Philadelphia, W. B. Saunders, 1971, p. 662.
Harrington, S. W.: Carcinoma of the breast: results of surgical treatment when the carcinoma occurred in course of pregnancy or lactation and when pregnancy occurred subsequent to operation, 1910–1933. Ann. Surg., 106:690, 1937.
Harvey, J. C., Rosen, P. P., Ashikari, R., et al.: The effect of pregnancy on the prognosis of carcinoma of the breast following radical mastectomy. Surg. Gynecol. Obstet., 153:723, 1981.
Helman, P., and Bennett, M. B.: Breast cancer and pregnancy. South Afr. Med. J., 37:1236, 1963.
Hochman, A., and Schreiber, H.: Pregnancy and cancer of the breast. Obstet. Gynecol., 2:268, 1953.
Hoeffken, W., and Lanyi, M.: Mammography. Philadelphia, W. B. Saunders, 1977, p. 76.
Holdaway, I. M., Mason, B. H., and Kay, R. G.: Steroid hormone receptors in breast tumors presenting during pregnancy or lactation. J. Surg. Oncol., 25:38, 1984.
Holleb, A. I., and Farrow, J. H.: The relation of carcinoma of the breast and pregnancy in 283 patients. Surg. Gynecol. Obstet., 115:65, 1962.
Holleb, A. I., and Farrow, J. H.: Breast cancer and pregnancy. Acta Un. Int. Cancre, 20:1480, 1964.
Horsley, J. S., III, Alrich, E. M., and Wright, C. B.: Carcinoma of the breast in women 35 years of age or younger. Ann. Surg., 196:839, 1969.
Hytten, F. E., and Leitch, I.: The Physiology of Human Pregnancy. 2nd Ed. Oxford, Blackwell, 1971.
Hubay, C. A., Barry, F. M., and Marr, C. C.: Pregnancy and breast cancer. Surg. Clin. North Am., 58:819, 1978.
Jochimsen, P. R., Spaight, M. E., and Urdaneta, L. F.: Pregnancy during adjuvant chemotherapy for breast cancer. J.A.M.A., 245:1660, 1981.
King, R. M., Welch, J. S., Martin, J. K., Jr., et al.: Carcinoma of the breast associated with pregnancy. Surg. Gynecol. Obstet., 160:228, 1985.
Montgomery, T. L.: Detection and disposal of breast cancer in pregnancy. Am. J. Obstet. Gynecol., 81:926, 1961.
Murray, C. L., Reichert, J. A., Anderson, J., et al.: Multimodal cancer therapy for breast cancer in the first trimester of pregnancy. A case report. J.A.M.A., 252:2607, 1984.
Nelson, J. H., Lu, T., Hall, J. E., et al: The effect of trophoblast on immune state of women. Am. J. Obstet. Gynecol., 117:689, 1973.
Nicholson, O. P.: Cytotoxic drugs in pregnancy. J. Obstet. Gynecol. Br. Commonw., 75:307, 1968.
Nugent, P., and O'Connell, T. X.: Breast cancer and pregnancy. Arch. Surg., 120:1221, 1985.
Peete, C. H., Jr., Huneycutt, H. C., Jr., and Cherny, W. B.: Cancer of the breast in pregnancy. N. C. Med. J., 27:514, 1966.
Peters, M. V.: The effect of pregnancy in breast cancer. In Forrest, A. P. M., and Kunkler, P. B. (Eds.): Prognostic Factors in Breast Cancer. Baltimore, Williams & Wilkins, 1968, p. 65.
Purtilo, R. T., Hallgren, H. M., and Yunis, E. S.: Depressed maternal lymphocyte response to PHA in human pregnancy. Lancet, 1:769, 1972.
Raich, P. C., and Curet, L. B.: Treatment of acute leukemia during pregnancy. Cancer, 36:861, 1975.
Rissanen, P. M.: Carcinoma of the breast during pregnancy and lactation. Br. J. Cancer, 22:663, 1968.
Rissanen, P. M.: Pregnancy following treatment of mammary cancer. Acta Radiol., 8:415, 1969.
Rosemond, G. P.: Management of patients with carcinoma of the breast in pregnancy. Ann. NY Acad. Sci., 114:851, 1964.
Sahni, K., Sanyal, B., Agrawal, M. S., et al.: Carcinoma of breast associated with pregnancy and lactation. J. Surg. Oncol., 16:167, 1981.
Saltzstein, E. C., Mann, R. W., Chua, T. Y., and Decosse, J. J.: Outpatient breast biopsy. Arch. Surg., 109:287, 1974.
Schapira, D. V., and Chudley, A. E.: Successful pregnancy following continuous treatment with combination chemotherapy before conception and throughout pregnancy. Cancer, 54:800, 1984.
Strelkauskas, A. J., Wilson, B. S., Dray, D., et al.: Inversion of levels of human T & B cells in early pregnancy. Nature, 258:331, 1975.
Treves, N., and Holleb, A. I.: A report of 549 cases of breast cancer in women 35 years of age or younger. Surg. Gynecol. Obstet., 107:271, 1958.
Westberg, S. V.: Prognosis of breast cancer for pregnant and nursing women. Acta Obstet. Gynecol. Scand., 25(Suppl. 4):179, 1946.
White, T. T.: Prognosis of breast cancer for pregnant and nursing women: Analysis of 1413 cases. Surg. Gynecol. Obstet., 100:661, 1955.
White, T. T., and White, W. C.: Breast cancer and pregnancy, report of 49 cases followed five years. Ann. Surg., 144:384, 1956.
Zeigerman, J. H., Honigman, F. H., and Crawford, R. W.: Inflammatory mammary cancer during pregnancy and lactation. Obstet. Gynecol., 32:373, 1968.

CHAPTER 27

WILLIAM L. DONEGAN

Sarcomas of the Breast

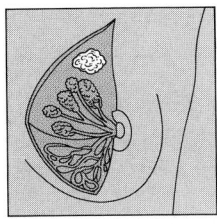

Nonepithelial cancers of the breast are rare. During a 25 year period only 18 were recorded at the Ellis Fischel State Cancer Hospital (EFSCH). They accounted for only 0.7 per cent of all cases of mammary cancer. Histologic classification is based on the cell of probable origin. Pathologists identify a wide variety of histologic types (Table 27–1).

Sarcomas typically present as large masses, only infrequently attached to the skin or deep tissues. Nipple discharge, peau d'orange and skin invasion, or retraction and ulceration, which often are seen with carcinoma, are infrequent; palpable axillary lymph nodes are rarely a feature. Metastases are predominantly hematogenous, have an affinity for the lungs, bones, and liver, and seldom involve regional lymph nodes.

The mammographic features of sarcomas are deceptively similar to those of benign lesions, such as cysts or fibroadenomas. They are dense and well marginated, with little evidence of invasive activity (Fig. 27–1), and the radiographic and actual measurements agree closely (Berger and Gershon-Cohen, 1962).

The experience with these uncommon neoplasms permits only limited conclusions regarding their proper management. However, they tend to act like soft tissue sarcomas elsewhere and are treated similarly. The frequent infiltration beyond what appear grossly to be well-defined borders, the propensity for local recurrence, and the uncommonness of lymphatic metastases support wide surgical removal without routine nodal dissection.

Prognosis is strongly related to cellular atypia and mitotic rate.

Cystosarcoma Phyllodes

Cystosarcoma phyllodes (CP) is the most common sarcoma of the breast. It has many synonyms and, as witnessed by the voluminous literature on the subject, has posed problems in definition, clinicopathologic correlation, and management. In a historical review of this subject, Fiks (1981) was able to collect 62 synonyms that had been used in the literature for cystosarcoma phyllodes. The name, coined in 1838 by Müller on the basis of gross characteristics, is a misnomer propagated by popular usage. The tumor is not necessarily cystic nor "leafy" in appearance, and only occasionally does it demonstrate its sarcomatous potential. A fibroepithelial tumor, cystosarcoma phyllodes is unique to the breast and associated with a prognosis considerably better than that of pure sarcomas.

The present understanding of cystosarcoma phyllodes has evolved through a long period of controversy. Probably the first description was that of Chelius in 1828, who described a large "cystic hydatid" of the breast and considered it a benign condition. Müller described the tumor 10 years later, assigned its tenacious name, and again emphasized its benign nature as well as the tendency to large dimensions.

Table 27–1. SARCOMAS OF THE BREAST DIAGNOSED AT ELLIS FISCHEL STATE CANCER HOSPITAL AND MT. SINAI MEDICAL CENTER, MILWAUKEE (1974–1985)*

Neoplasm	Number
Cystosarcoma phyllodes	13
Lymphoma	6
Fibrosarcoma	4
Stromal sarcoma	2
Angiosarcoma	1
Granular cell myoblastoma	1
Rhabdomyosarcoma	1

*Excluding fibroadenomas.

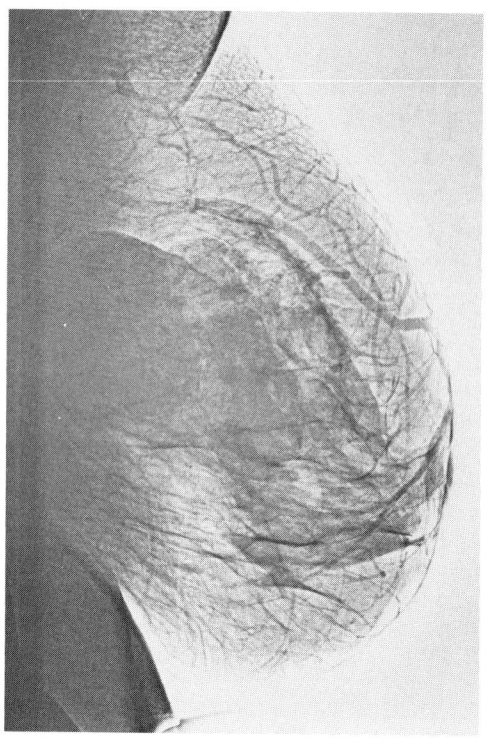

Figure 27–1. Mammogram showing a large cystosarcoma phyllodes deep within the breast as a well-marginated mass.

Lee and Pack, who summarized 105 cases from the literature and reported six of their own in 1931, likened the histologic features of the tumor to those of an intracanalicular fibroadenoma, but they considered metaplasia of the stroma into myxomatous tissue with cellular pseudosarcomatous regions as its distinguishing feature. For this reason, the name "giant intracanalicular fibroadenomyxoma" was suggested. Among other clinical features described were greatness of size, long duration of symptoms, lobulation and mobility, an initial period of slow growth followed by rapid acceleration, and probable development from a preexistent fibroadenoma. This tumor was also considered a benign lesion, although 6 of 91 cases were noted to have recurred after removal. Owens and Adams (1941) considered the myxomatous changes described by Lee and Pack as simply an appearance created by edema and were of the opinion that the designation "giant intracanalicular fibroadenoma," rather than "fibroadenomyxoma," was most appropriate.

Accumulating reports of local invasion, recurrence after excision, and an occasional malignant course with metastases of sarcomatous stroma made it increasingly clear that a malignant variant of the neoplasm existed. White (1940) documented dissemination to the lungs and mediastinum; Cooper and Ackerman (1943) were the first to describe metastases to axillary lymph nodes. In 1950, McDonald and Harrington estimated that a sarcomatous stroma occurred in 10 per cent of cases of so-called cystosarcoma phyllodes. They conclued that such tumors should be considered large fibrosarcomas; the remainder were benign giant fibroadenomas. Their report of 13 cases of cystosarcoma phyllodes was confined to benign cases in which large size (the tumors had to involve at least four fifths of the breast) was a major consideration in selection. Foote and Stewart pointed out in 1946, however, that size alone was not paramount and that typical proliferative changes could occur in small tumors ("miniature cystosarcoma phyllodes").

Treves and Sunderland's review in 1951 of 77 cases from Memorial Hospital, New York City, during the period 1930 to 1949 served to emphasize the tumor's malignant potential and to relegate size to secondary importance in defining this problematic entity. These authors used the presence of pronounced overgrowth of the stromal element as the criterion for differentiating cystosarcoma from fibroadenoma and thus included tumors as small as 1.0 cm in diameter in their report. For clinicopathologic correlation, the tumors were subdivided into those that were benign, malignant, or borderline malignant, depending on the character of the stroma. Nine (50 per cent) of the 18 histologically malignant lesions metastasized to viscera, and one metastasized to an axillary lymph node. Although four borderline and four benign tumors recurred locally, none metastasized. Wide local excision or simple mastectomy was recommended for benign cases, and radical mastectomy was recommended for those with a malignant stroma.

Lester and Stout (1954) applied Treves and Sunderland's (1951) criteria to 58 cystosarcomas diagnosed at Presbyterian Hospital, New York City, (1912 to 1952) and found only a disappointing correlation between histologic features and the biologic course of the tumors. Not all of the known metastatic tumors could be placed into the histologically malignant group, and, paradoxically, one of the "benign" tumors metastasized. These investigators blamed the pleomorphism that often exists in the stroma for this problem and stressed that the often focal nature of malignant changes probably contributes to a significant sampling error when only limited biopsies are available to classify the tumor. Oberman (1965a) was able to achieve reasonable clinicopathologic correlation between histologic classification and occurrence of metastases in 18 cases at the University of Michigan, but at the Mayo Clinic two of 23 "benign" tumors eventually metastasized (West et al., 1971). Blichert-Toft and associates (1975) conceded a poor correlation between the tumor grade and the clinical course of 17 cases; four of 12 initially benign tumors recurred with a malignant stroma, and three of these patients died of dissemination.

The overall incidence of malignancy in cystosarcoma phyllodes remains undetermined. Summaries of reports are of questionable value because of the varying criteria used for selection of cases. The largest individual series available are those of Treves and Sunderland (1951) and of Lester and Stout (1954). Twenty-three per cent of all tumors reported by Treves and Sunderland were histologically malignant, and 13 per cent metastasized or showed markedly invasive properties. Because Memorial Hospital is a referral center, both figures probably overestimate the frequency of malignancy. Although a similar proportion (28 per cent) of 36 nonreferred cases reported by Lester and Stout from Presbyterian Hospital were histologically malignant, only 2.8 per cent metastasized. Possibly the lower figure lies near to the true incidence of metastasis. The problematic "borderline" classification, which totalled 23 per cent of the 1951 Memorial Hospital series, is a dilemma for the surgeon. Treves (1964) later reported 93 cystosarcomas from Memorial Hospital, covering the period subsequent to the original report (1950 to 1962), in which the borderline group was reduced to only 5 per cent of the total number of cases.

INCIDENCE

Cystosarcomas occur at a higher mean age than fibroadenomas and 10 to 15 years earlier than carcinomas. Ages range from 10 to 77 years, with occasional patients in the prepubertal age group. Although malignant variants are rare under the age of 20 years, deaths have been reported (Hoover et al., 1975). This rare neoplasm constitutes only 2.5 per cent of all fibroepithelial tumors of the breast (Lester and Stout, 1954). Treves (1964) reported 93 among 3200 fibroadenomas at Memorial Hospital. Twenty-nine were seen at the Mayo Clinic during the course of 14 years (West et al., 1971). At EFSCH, nine were diagnosed among 4001 women referred with breast disease between 1940 and June of 1965, a frequency of 0.2 per cent. Ariel (1961) derived from many reports that cystosarcomas represent only 0.3 per cent of all mammary neoplasms in patients admitted to general hospitals.

HISTOLOGY

Histologically similar to fibroadenomas and suspected of arising from these innocent tumors, CP consists of fibrous connective tissue surrounding spaces lined by benign epithelium. Variable degrees of intracanalicular growth, sometimes producing a grossly cabbage-like or leafy appearance, account for the original description (Fig. 27–2). Cystosarcoma phyllodes differs from fibroadenomas in having a more cellular and potentially malignant stroma. Although they are often large, size is not an important diagnostic consideration. The stroma is often pleomorphic and varies from histologically benign to malignant, displaying the characteristics of fibrosarcoma generally or in isolated areas. Large cysts and areas of hemorrhage may be present. Osseous, myxomatous, and cartilaginous metaplasia, which is sometimes present in the stroma, is not of prognostic significance. Both CP and fibroadenomas regularly contain significant amounts of progesterone receptor protein but infrequently contain estrogen receptors (Rao et al., 1981).

Bot and Donner (1981) listed four indicators of malignancy in CP: (1) an infiltrative tumor margin; (2) fibrous overgrowth, especially when the epithelial component has disappeared from large parts of the tumor; (3) three or more mitoses per 10 high power fields; and (4) cellular atypia. A case was mentioned, however, in which a CP without signs of malignancy produced a pulmonary metastasis 10 years after treatment. The metastasis in this case was unusual in showing not only fibrous tumor with a moderate amount of mitoses but also clefts lined with benign epithelium.

CLINICAL MATERIAL AT EFSCH

All nine EFSCH patients with CP seen before 1965 were women; eight patients were white and one was black. Ages ranged from 17 to 82 years, with a mean of 52 years, 9 years less

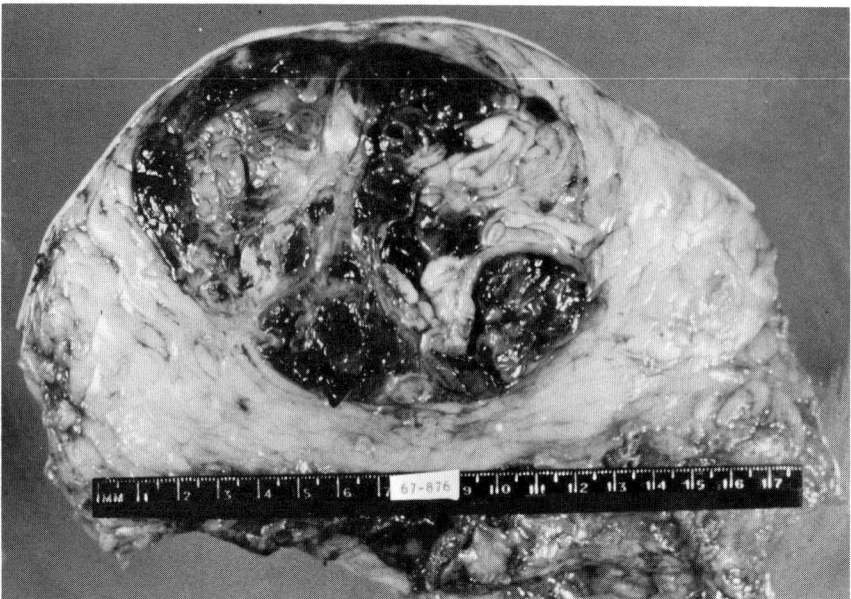

Figure 27–2. Cut section of a cystosarcoma phyllodes demonstrates the pseudoencapsulation of the tumor.

than the mean age of 704 surgical patients with carcinoma of the breast at this hospital. Seven of the nine cystosarcomas occurred in the left breast, and none was bilateral. Treves and Sunderland (1951) reported no bilateral lesions among 77 cases. McDonald and Harrington's report (1950) of 30 per cent bilateral lesions among 13 patients is unique. It is also notable that 3 per cent of Lee and Pack's cases (1931) collected from the early literature were men, but the scarcity of men in subsequent reports has proved this tumor to be rare. Although the proportion of black patients in various series has appeared greater than that in general hospital admissions, a racial predilection remains unconfirmed. The proportion of black patients (1 in 9) among patients at EFSCH with cystosarcoma phyllodes did not differ from the percentage (9 per cent) among all admissions.

In each case, the initial symptom was the presence of a painless breast mass. The median duration of symptoms was 18 months, although three patients had noted the presence of a mass for more than 10 years. In three instances, the patient had noted recent rapid growth of a long-standing, previously stable nodule.

Large size was frequent. The nine cystosarcomas averaged 18 cm in diameter, and five occupied the entire breast (Fig. 27–3). Unlike carcinoma, CP ordinarily reaches massive proportions before eroding the skin, and ulceration is usually due to pressure necrosis, not to invasion. Ulceration was present in four cases, one because of a previous incision and drainage before referral. Lobulation and palpable cystic areas were often evident beneath the skin, which in some cases had become erythematous and shiny because of tension produced by the large tumor (Fig. 27–4). Prominent veins on the surface of the breast were a frequent feature. One of the large tumors was fixed to the chest wall, but all others were completely mobile. In only a single instance were axillary nodes palpable, and these were small and hard.

The patients were initially treated at EFSCH, except for one whose tumor was widely excised elsewhere and who had local recurrence (Fig. 27–5). Another had been biopsied but received no therapy because of intractable heart failure that caused a rapid demise.

The histologic features of the surgical specimens were classified according to cellularity, cellular atypia, and mitotic activity into one of three categories: benign, borderline, or malignant. Only one was considered benign, and two were obviously malignant. The remaining six were borderline. When the histologic features of these cases were compared with the patient's treatment and clinical course, the inferiority of wide local excision or simple

27 • Sarcomas of the Breast   693

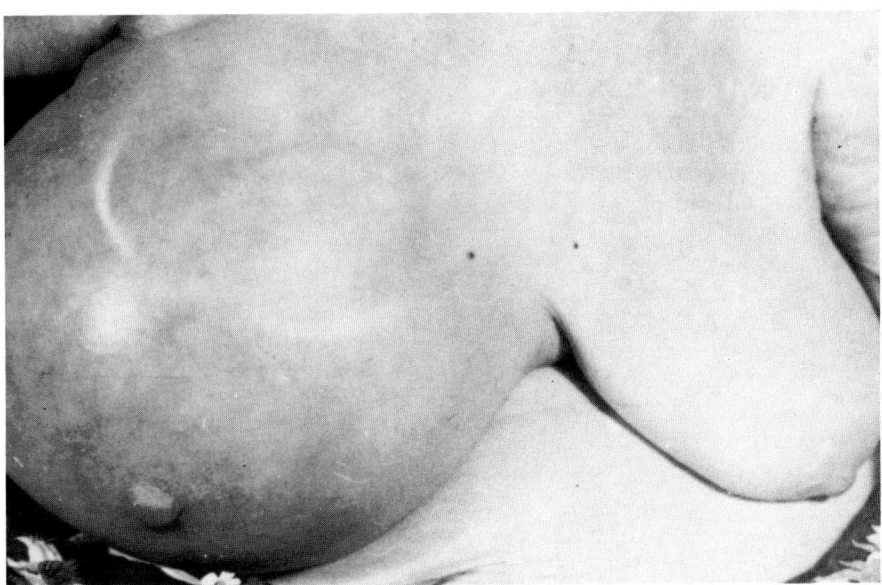

Figure 27–3. This cystosarcoma phyllodes developed in the breast of an 82 year old woman over an 8 month period. Notable are the shininess and mild erythema of the tense overlying skin and absence of ulceration despite massive proportions of the tumor. No axillary lymph nodes were palpable.

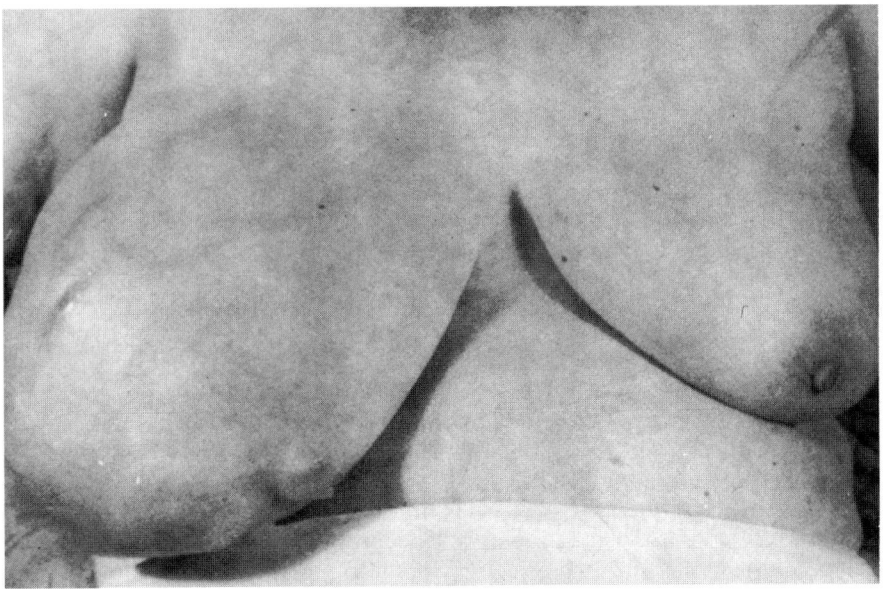

Figure 27–4. This cystosarcoma in the right breast of a 66 year old woman demonstrates the lobulation and cystic prominences that are frequently evident on clinical examination. The lesion was thought to be of borderline malignancy histologically and recurred locally years after simple mastectomy.

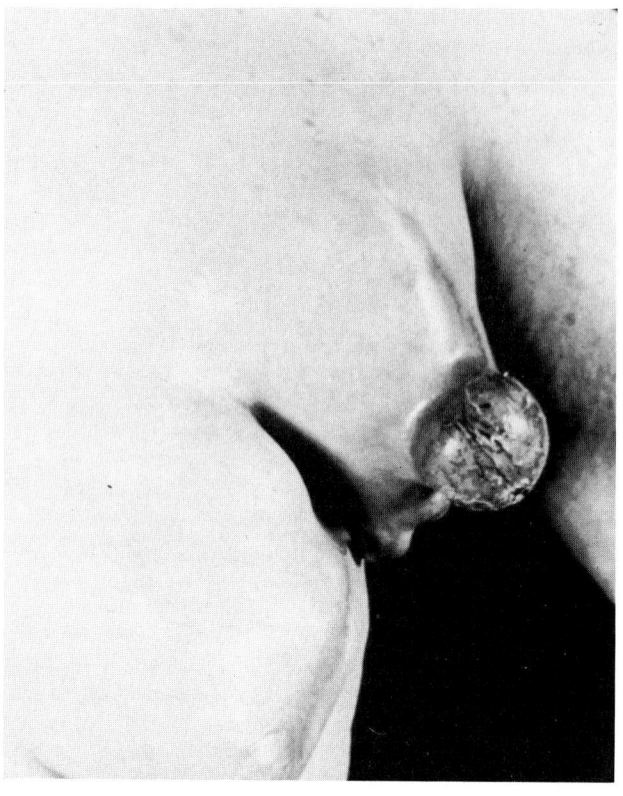

Figure 27–5. This grade 2, borderline malignant cystosarcoma phyllodes recurred in the surgical scar 4 months after local excision. It persisted despite a subsequent simple mastectomy and several further attempts at local excision and palliation with radiotherapy.

mastectomy for all but benign lesions was decisive. Four patients were treated initially with wide local excision or simple mastectomy. One lesion was histologically benign, and three were borderline. The benign lesion was removed with a simple mastectomy, and the patient died of cardiac causes free of recurrence 16 months after therapy. By contrast, two of the three borderline lesions recurred locally in the scar 5 and 7 months after removal. The remaining patient was free of disease 3 years after a simple mastectomy.

Two patients with malignant lesions and two patients with borderline lesions were treated initially with radical mastectomy. No local recurrence had occurred after 2 to 6 years of follow-up, but one tumor with a malignant stroma produced pulmonary and mediastinal metastases 7 months postoperatively, and the patient died of progressive disease.

Two of the eight treated patients had metastases in axillary lymph nodes, both of which had tumors classified as borderline. This is an unusual event, or at least not frequently recognized. Both cases were discovered when radical mastectomies were performed in an effort to control local recurrence. In one instance radical surgery did not prevent further local recurrences, and in the other the patient died of an unknown cause 8 months later.

THERAPY

The therapy of CP is wide surgical removal. The operation required depends on the histologic differentiation and size of the tumor. Barnhardt and associates (1985) reviewed the records of 13 patients at the Medical College of Virginia Hospitals with cystosarcoma phyllodes. Ten of the patients were treated with excisional biopsy, two with total mastectomy for malignant CP, and one with a modified radical mastectomy based on an erroneous aspiration cytology diagnosis of infiltrating ductal carcinoma. After an average of 39 months of follow-up, one patient had a local recurrence of a benign CP 3 years following excisional biopsy and had a wide reexcision. There were no deaths. These authors recommended wide local excision with uninvolved surgical margins as appropriate treatment. Mastectomy was recommended only for patients with malignant CP or those with large lesions necessitating total removal of the breast to achieve normal margins. As axillary nodal metastases are unusual, node dissection was advised only for those who have obvious, clinically positive nodes.

At the Mayo Clinic (Lindquist et al., 1982), wide local excision was deemed appropriate only for small tumors (less than 4 cm in diameter) in young patients. The preferred treatment in all other instances was simple mastectomy. Of the 42 patients seen between 1950 and 1980, 10 had recurrences and four metastasized to distant sites. The patients were between 20 and 57 years of age (average 44 years). All of the patients with histologically malignant tumors were nulliparous, and five of the patients died of their tumors, four with metastases in the lung or chest wall recurrence. Metastases occurred to the lungs, liver, and retroperitoneum. One patient had metastases to the lung in which both malignant stroma and benign epithelium were present. Five of the patients with recurrence had histologically benign lesions, two of which caused the death of the patient, one by producing metastases. Thus, 24 per cent of the patients had recurrence or dissemination, and no reliable histologic or other parameters could be identified that predicted malignant or metastatic potential. Five of the 10 patients with recurrence died from their disease 2 to 7 years after treatment.

Contarini and associates (1982) also found no correlation of malignant histologic features with prognosis. In a review of 40 cases seen over a 17 year period at five Florida hospitals, 17 of the tumors were histologically malignant. Of the 23 benign CP, three (7.5 per cent) recurred after treatment. In the malignant group, metastases developed in four patients (10 per cent), and three of the latter died of their tumors. One case of bilateral CP was included, and one patient had skin ulceration. Nine patients (22.5 per cent) were younger than 20 years of age, the youngest was 12 years old, and patients with histologically malignant lesions were older than those with benign lesions. The most common sites of metastases were lung, bones, and liver. In the reports reviewed by these authors, 15.6 per cent of patients developed metastases. Contarini and colleagues recommended that CP be treated with wide local excision without regard to histologic appearance and with emphasis on achieving a margin of normal tissue. Hormones, chemotherapy, and radiotherapy were not useful in the treatment of metastatic disease.

Briggs and coworkers (1983) concentrated on CP in adolescent girls and collected nine cases between 1960 and 1980 at 10 military medical centers. The youngest patient was 12 years old, and white, black, and Polynesian women were represented. Two of the patients previously had fibroadenomas removed from the opposite breast. The chief complaint in all cases was the recent onset of a rapidly growing, nontender breast mass, with a mean duration of 3 months. The tumors measured from 2 to 13 cm in diameter, and three were classified as malignant. Excision was the only form of treatment in eight of the nine patients; one simple mastectomy was performed on a large CP. No local recurrence or metastasis was observed after a mean of 9.6 years. These authors reviewed 44 adolescents from the literature, in whom 13.6 per cent of tumors were malignant. Only one of the benign tumors (2.7 per cent) recurred and this occurred locally. However, two of the six patients with malignant CP had recurrence, both of which were local in nature, and both recurrences were reexcised successfully. Three cases of distant dissemination in adolescents have been reported (Hoover et al., 1975; Turalba et al., 1986). In all cases tumor reappeared on the chest wall and spread to the lungs, ultimately proving resistant to further therapy, although temporary responses were produced by chemotherapy and irradiation. Benign types of CP should be managed with wide excision and close follow-up, avoiding removal of the whole breast initially if possible. Malignant CP, however, is treacherous even in adolescents and should be treated as a true soft tissue malignancy.

Table 27–2 correlates the histologic appearance of tumor stroma with local recurrence and metastases after various surgical procedures. The sizable proportion of malignant tumors that metastasize distantly despite all forms of therapy suggests that vascular metastases were little affected by the type of surgical procedure employed. A small number of borderline tumors metastasized distantly, and one histologically benign one did so, emphasizing the difficulty of properly classifying these tumors in a manner representative of their biologic potential.

Local recurrence is materially influenced by the extent of surgery. In all histologic categories, local recurrence decreased with increas-

Table 27–2. HISTOLOGIC CLASSIFICATION OF STOMA VERSUS INITIAL THERAPY AND CLINICAL COURSE OF CYSTOSARCOMA PHYLLODES REPORTED BY EIGHT AUTHORS SINCE 1951*

Therapy	Benign Stroma			Borderline Stroma			Malignant Stroma		
	Total Number	Local Recurrence	Metastasis	Total Number	Local Recurrence	Metastasis	Total Number	Local Recurrence	Metastasis
Local excision	36	4 (11%)	0	13	6 (46%)	1	12	6 (50%)	3
Simple mastectomy	29	3 (10%)	0	17	3 (18%)	1	16	7 (43%)	7
Radical mastectomy	22	0 (0%)	0	5	0 (0%)	0	9	1 (11%)	4
Modified mastectomy	1	0	0	0	0	0	4	1 (25%)	1
Radiotherapy	1	0	1						
Totals	89		1	35		2	41		15

*Ariel, 1961; Botham et al., 1958; EFSCH, 1966; Hafner et al., 1962; Lester and Stout, 1954; Maguire and Moore, 1965; Oberman, 1965a; Treves and Sunderland, 1951. Excluded from this summary are cases with no histologic description of the tumor stroma, lost to follow-up in less than 1 year, and with treatment unrecorded.

†Does not include cases in which the therapy was used for recurrences.

ing scope of surgery. it is also evident that local recurrence is a function of the histological grade of the tumor when the magnitude of surgery is constant. Ten per cent of tumors removed by simple mastectomy or local excision eventually recurrred. Local excision was unsatisfactory for tumors with a borderline stroma, and simple mastectomy failed twice as often as it did when used for benign ones. Local excision and simple mastectomy were unsatisfactory for malignant tumors. When local recurrence was computed per patient year of risk (Table 27–3), simple mastectomy clearly was more effective than local excision for borderline lesions but not as effective as radical mastectomy for malignant ones.

In Table 27–4, which pertains to tumor size, it is evident that wide local excision was adequate for benign lesions even when large. Amerson (1970) recommended local excision for benign cystosarcomas in the adolescent age group, even when the tumors were large. Blichert-Toft and associates (1975) suggested wide local excision for benign lesions, reserving mastectomy for histologically malignant variants. In the EFSCH series, local excision was inadequate for malignant lesions of all dimensions. Simple mastectomy was successful for all tumors with borderline stroma except for a very sizable one. Simple mastectomy was adequate for malignant tumors of small size.

To summarize, the histologic grade of the tumor is an important guide to therapy, so an adequate biopsy of the neoplasm is important prior to definitive surgery. The magnitude of surgical resection is definitely a factor in the local control of cystosarcomas of all histologic grades. Mastectomy is indicated for frankly malignant tumors and probably also for all but small tumors of borderline malignancy. Every effort to attain effective initial control is important because metastasis is a threat and chest wall recurrences are both stubborn and aggressive. For benign tumors, wide local excision is reasonable when they are small or when cosmetic factors are important enough to accept the risk of recurrence. Simple mastectomy offers greater assurance of permanent control

Table 27–3. LOCAL RECURRENCE OF CYSTOSARCOMA PHYLLODES PER PATIENT-YEAR OF FOLLOW-UP VERSUS INITIAL THERAPY (133 CASES)*

Therapy	Benign Stroma		Borderline Stroma		Malignant Stroma	
	Total Patient Years	Local Recurrence Per Patient Year	Total Patient Years	Local Recurrence Per Patient Year	Total Patient Years	Local Recurrence Per Patient Year
Local excision	134	0.04	65	0.11	56	0.13
Simple mastectomy	90	0.01	94	0.01	49	0.12
Radical mastectomy	53	0.0	39	0.0	45	0.02

*Derived from data reported by Treves and Sunderland, 1951; Lester and Stout, 1954; Oberman, 1965a; and EFSCH.

Table 27–4. TUMOR DIAMETER VERSUS LOCAL RECURRENCE AFTER SIMPLE MASTECTOMY AND AFTER LOCAL EXCISION OF CYSTOSARCOMA PHYLLODES*

Diameter of Tumor (cm)	Benign Stroma				Borderline Stroma				Malignant Stroma			
	Local Excision		Simple Mastectomy		Local Excision		Simple Mastectomy		Local Excision		Simple Mastectomy	
	Total Number	Recurrence	Total Number	Recurrence	Total Number	Recurrence	Total Number	Recurrence	Total Number	Recurrence	Total Number	Recurrence
1–5	4	1	3	0			1	0	9	3	2	0
6–10	5	0	3	0			2	0	2	1	1	0
11–15	1	0	2	1			1	0	1	1		
16–20			2	0			2	1	2	1		
21 and over			1	0	1	1	1	0	1	1	4	1

*Derived from data reported by Lester and Stout, 1954; Oberman, 1965a; and EFSCH.

of large benign forms and is acceptable for histologically borderline tumors of small size. For malignant tumors, a wide thorough removal of the breast with deep fascia is appropriate, with removal of underlying muscle and nodes when necessary for margin.

Local recurrences are the most frequent form of treatment failure (Figs. 27–6 to 27–8). Recurrences are best treated by further surgical removal. Cystosarcoma phyllodes responds poorly to radiotherapy, and this method has found no effective role in treatment either of the primary lesion or of metastases. One EFSCH patient received irradiation for persistent chest wall disease without apparent response. Lester and Stout's patient (1954) treated primarily with irradiation eventually died of metastases. When distant metastases appear, the prognosis is poor. With few exceptions the duration of life thereafter is less than 2 years. The lungs and mediastinum are favored sites for deposits, but metastases also seek the heart, bones, and brain (McCullough and Lynch, 1960; West et al., 1971). Ariel (1961) found osseous involvement in 33 per cent of a collected group with metastatic disease. Intractable heart failure may be the only sign of spread to the heart (McCullough and Lynch, 1960).

Hormone therapy or chemotherapy is not known to affect the disease significantly, although experience is scant. Rao and associates at the Mallinckrodt Institute of Radiology, St. Louis, reported finding progesterone receptors in all of five cases of cystosarcoma phyllodes and in most fibroadenomas tested for its pres-

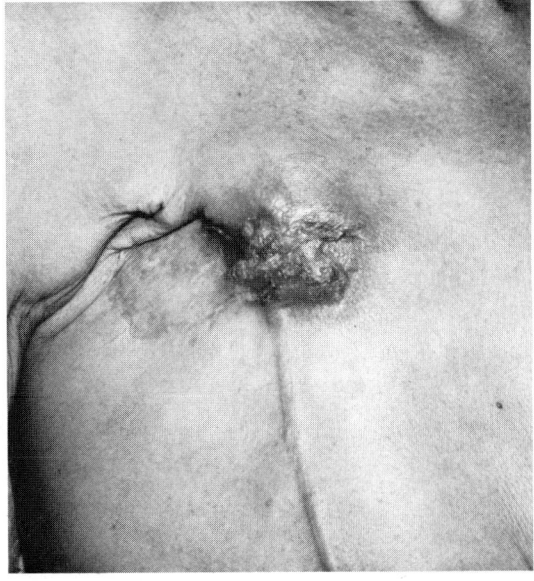

Figure 27–6. Recurrent cystosarcoma phyllodes at medial edge of skin graft after radical mastectomy.

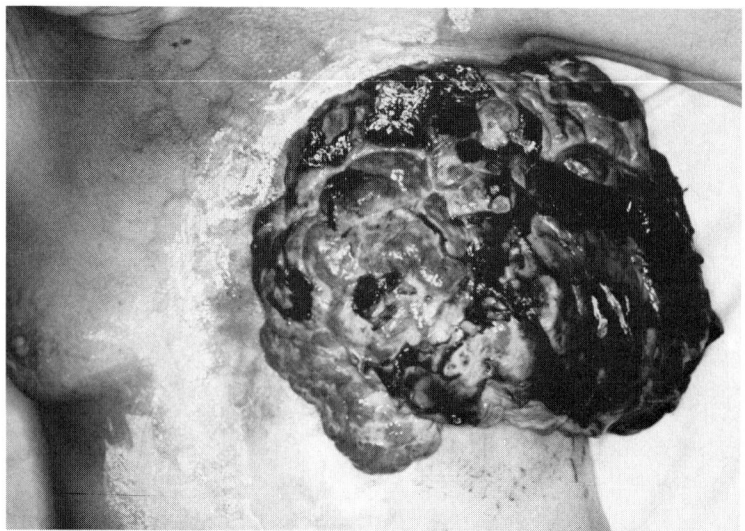

Figure 27–7. Exophytic growth of recurrent cystosarcoma. (Courtesy of Harvey Lerner, M.D.)

ence. Only one cystosarcoma contained estrogen receptors. This observation suggests that hormone therapy might be worthy of a trial in advanced or metastatic malignant cystosarcoma phyllodes. However, estrogen and progesterone receptors have been lacking in two cases of cystosarcoma phyllodes seen by the author. Brentani and coworkers (1982) studied seven cases of cystosarcoma phyllodes and found 40 per cent of the five low grade tumors ER positive. All were progesterone receptor positive and 60 per cent were glucocorticoid receptor positive. The steroid binding receptors were probably of stromal origin, and it was thought that the presence of glucocorticoid receptors may parallel histologic malignancy.

Hoover and associates (1975) observed a temporary although dramatic response of a particularly malignant cystosarcoma to cyclophosphamide. Allen and coworkers (1985) reported complete remission of pulmonary metastases in response to six cycles of doxorubicin and cisplatin, although the patient died of progression in the brain.

COINCIDENT ADENOCARCINOMA OF THE BREAST

Coincident adenocarcinoma of the breast, reported as single cases and occasionally with

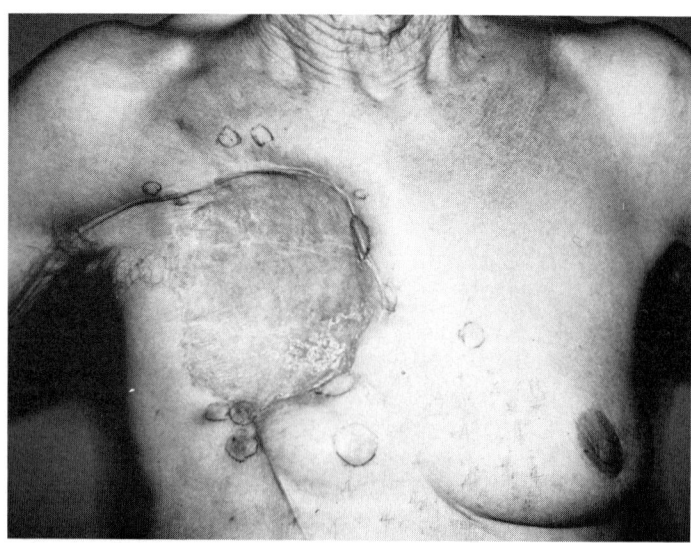

Figure 27–8. Multiple subcutaneous and dermal recurrences of cystosarcoma phyllodes around site of chest wall resection performed in an effort to control local persistence. The patient later developed pulmonary metastases and died.

series of cystosarcomas, affects the patient's prognosis independently. The incidence of one tumor does not influence that of the other (Richards and Way, 1963). As cystosarcoma phyllodes is rare, it is not surprising that this combination is unusual.

PROPHYLAXIS

The evidence that cystosarcoma phyllodes originates from benign fibroadenomas supports the removal of fibroadenomas as a prophylactic measure (Amerson, 1970). Treves (1964) called attention to a decrease in the incidence of both fibroadenomas and cystosarcomas at Memorial Hospital, with a relative increase in the former, and suggested that a growing tendency to remove all breast masses might be preventing the development of cystosarcomas.

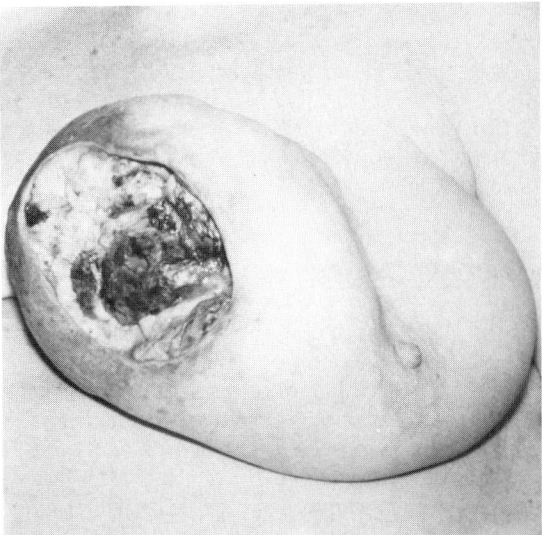

Figure 27–9. Stromal sarcoma. This 71 year old white woman came to medical attention with a 20 × 16 cm centrally ulcerated tumor confined to the left breast. The patient had been aware of it for 5 months. The tumor was not fixed to the chest wall and was removed with a total mastectomy.

Stromal Sarcoma

Stromal sarcomas of the breast were defined by Berg and colleagues in 1962. The basic cell is a spindle cell resembling a poorly differentiated fibroblast but differing from the cells of a fibrosarcoma in having greater variation in cellular morphology, fewer reticular fibers, and more mitotic figures. The cells are similar to those in the stroma of cystosarcoma phyllodes, but no epithelial component is present in the tumor. Ultrastructural studies by Tang and associates (1979) suggest predominantly an undifferentiated mesenchymal cell. These authors believed that pure stromal sarcoma and malignant cystosarcoma phyllodes represent neoplastic growth of the periductal mammary stromal cells. The incidence of this tumor is approximately 0.5 per cent of primary breast cancers, and the ratio of stromal sarcomas to cystosarcoma phyllodes is approximately 1:3. Grossly the tumors are well circumscribed, encapsulated, rubbery, and firm with a bulging pink to tan, somewhat trabecular pattern on cut surfaces. Ulceration may be seen with large tumors (Fig. 27–9). Treatment of the 105 cases in the English literature has varied from local excision to radical mastectomy, the principal objective being wide removal of the tumor with a normal surgical margin. Berg and coworkers (1962) reported a 60 per cent 5 year survival of 10 patients with stromal sarcomas and no instance of local recurrence when treated with either simple or radical mastectomy. On the other hand, nine of 15 patients had recurrence locally when limited excision was performed. Local recurrences have yielded to reexcision in almost 50 per cent of cases, and this should be attempted when possible. Recurrence, if it occurs, is generally during the first 2 years after treatment. In 59 per cent of 105 cases collected in the literature the patient survived for a minimum of 5 years (Tang et al., 1979). Like cystosarcoma, this tumor metastasizes hematogenously to the lungs and only rarely to the lymph nodes. The propensity to metastasize is directly related to the number of mitotic figures seen in the tumor.

Lymphoma

Lymphoma occasionally appears as a localized process in the breast with or without involvement of the axillary lymph nodes. Such cases occur once among approximately every 1300 cases of malignant disease of the breast (DeLeon et al., 1961) and may be difficult to differentiate from medullary carcinoma. In a review of the literature in 1976, Sonnenblick and Abraham found 164 cases, in 14 per cent of which the patients were over 60 years old. One man was affected for every 32 women.

DeCosse and associates (1962) reported the largest single series, 14 cases collected at the Memorial Hospital for Cancer and Allied Diseases, New York City. More recently, Schouten and colleagues (1981) reported on 13 cases seen at the University of Wisconsin between 1970 and 1980.

CLINICAL FEATURES

Primary lymphoma of the breast occurs with an age frequency comparable to that of carcinoma of this organ and resembles the latter clinically, presenting as a mass and having the ability to produce skin retraction, erythema, or peau d'orange (Figs. 27–10 to 27–12). More than one mass frequently is present. Protracted symptoms are unusual, as are large tumor masses. Patients may have typical "B" symptoms (i.e., night sweats, fever, or weight loss ≥10 per cent). Classification of these tumors is similar to that of primary nodal lymphomas. Histologic classification is according to the Rappaport system, and staging is based on the Ann Arbor classification (Table 27–5). Both histologic features and stage influence prognosis, and the prognosis seems to be similar to that of nodal lymphoma of similar histologic type and stage. The diffuse form tends to have a less favorable prognosis than nodular forms.

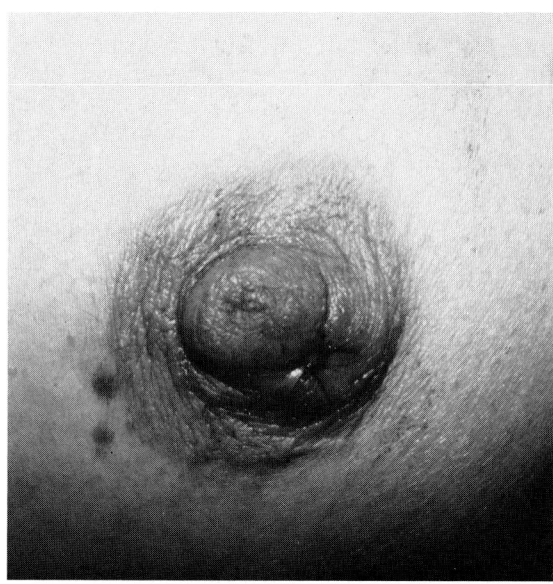

Figure 27–11. Histiocytic lymphoma appearing as a small subareolar mass with involvement of the nipple in a 67 year old woman. She had been treated for an identical tumor of the opposite breast 3 years earlier.

Diffuse histiocytic lymphoma is the most frequent, followed by poorly differentiated and nodular mixed types. Hodgkin's disease occasionally is reported (Schouten et al., 1981). Axillary lymph nodes are involved in 30 to 40 per cent of cases, and about 13 per cent of patients have bilateral disease. Almost as many involve the second breast subsequently. Lymphoma of the breast is frequently more extensive than it first appears. Stage I cases are few.

THERAPY

Lymphomas of the breast should be managed as are extranodal lymphomas at other sites. After a biopsy and histologic diagnosis, careful staging is necessary to determine the full extent of disease. Chest radiographs, bone marrow biopsy, and CT scans of the abdomen are appropriate. Lymphangiomas and gallium scans may be useful.

In the past, radical surgery with irradiation was widely used. Melander and Pack (1963) found that radical surgery for unicentric lymphomas in various areas of the body followed by an adequate dose of irradiation gave survival rates superior to other forms of treatment. This approach was advocated at Memorial Hospital, where a 64 per cent 5 year survival was obtained (DeCosse et al., 1962).

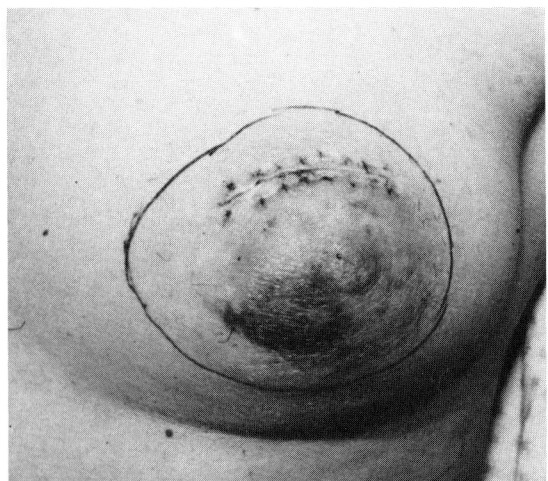

Figure 27–10. Diffuse histiocytic lymphoma of the left breast in a 50 year old woman appearing as a large, isolated central mass of 3 months' duration associated with axillary adenopathy. Mammography showed a poorly defined, lobulated mass that was hypoechoic on ultrasonography. A CT scan revealed retroperitoneal involvement. Treatment consisted of breast irradiation and systemic combination chemotherapy.

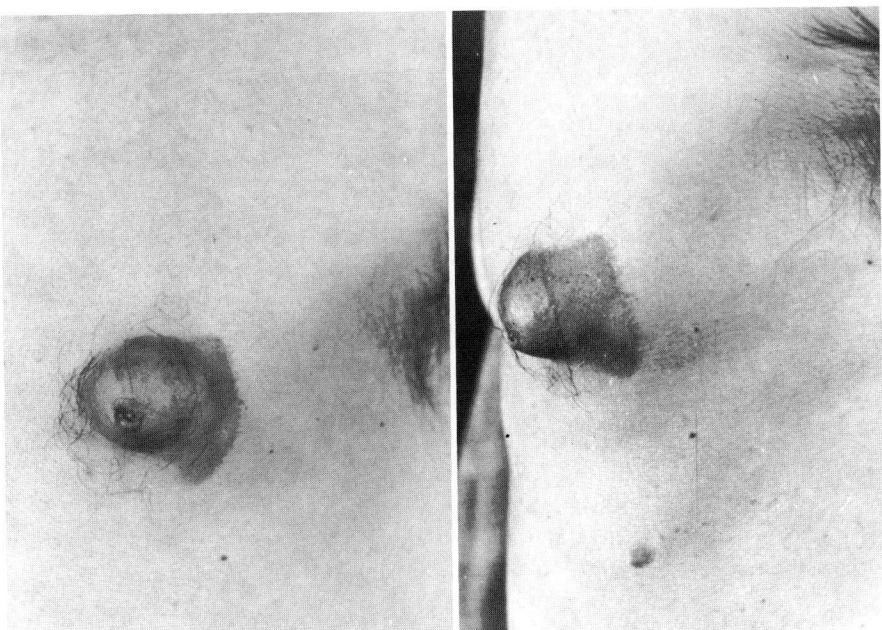

Figure 27–12. Lymphoma of the breast in a 66 year old man. This lesion gradually enlarged over the course of 1 year. No axillary metastases were found and the patient died without recurrence 7 years after radical mastectomy.

The trend more recently, however, has been to discourage radical surgery (Sonnenblick and Abraham, 1976). These tumors are highly radiosensitive, and radiotherapy can be used effectively for local control after limited surgery for diagnosis and staging, adding systemic chemotherapy when indicated by stage or poor risk histologic type. Hofman and Goodman (1968) recommended local excision and irradiation. Ten of 14 cases seen at M.D. Anderson Hospital, Houston, through 1975 were treated with either biopsy or wedge excision followed by radiation or chemotherapy, usually both (Mambo et al., 1977). Forty-nine per cent of patients survived 5 years. Six of 13 patients (46 per cent) seen at the University of Wisconsin were free of disease from 11 to 48 months after treatment (Schouten et al., 1981).

Lymphoblastic lymphoma of the breast is a rare type that is important to recognize. Because of its high tendency to disseminate and progress to lymphoblastic leukemia, aggressive chemotherapy is indicated (Carbone et al., 1982).

The frequency of ultimate dissemination supports the suspicion that the disease is more extensive than is apparent initially. Because of the tumor's radiosensitivity, irradiation of involved areas can provide considerable palliation, as can chemotherapy.

Table 27–5. HISTOLOGIC CLASSIFICATION AND STAGING OF PRIMARY LYMPHOMAS

A. *Rappaport classification of non-Hodgkin's lymphomas*
  I. Nodular:
     Lymphocytic, poorly differentiated
     Mixed lymphocytic and histiocytic
     Histiocytic
  II. Diffuse:
     Lymphocytic, well differentiated
     Lymphocytic, poorly differentiated
     Mixed lymphocytic and histiocytic
     Histiocytic, well differentiated
     Undifferentiated pleomorphic
     Undifferentiated Burkitt's type
B. *Ann Arbor staging as applied to mammary lymphomas*
  Stage I Involvement of breast alone
  Stage II Involvement of breast and single nodal site above diaphragm
  Stage III Involvement of breast and nodal site below diaphragm, or spleen
  Stage IV Involvement of breast plus liver or bone marrow
  Suffix A = Asymptomatic
       B = Fever, sweats, or loss of ≥ 10% of body weight

Angiosarcoma

Primary sarcomas of the breast of vascular origin are well-recognized entities. Although "angiosarcoma" of the breast was reported in 1887 by Schmidt, the first well-documented case was that of Borrman, reported in 1907 as "metastasizing hemangioma." Such tumors have subsequently been reported as hemangiosarcoma (Shore, 1957), angiosarcoma (Scheid et al., 1964), hemangioendothelioblastoma (Edwards and Strouth, 1956), and hemangioblastoma (Patrick et al., 1957–1958). Angiosarcomas are highly lethal and fortunately are rare even among sarcomas. Only one can be expected for every 2000 carcinomas; two were reported from the Mayo Clinic among 36 cases of mammary sarcomas in over 53 years (Barber et al., 1960; Lissoos et al., 1969). A total of 87 cases were reported through 1980 (Chen et al., 1980). Angiosarcomas have been concentrated in young women (average age, 35 years; range, 14 to 82 years); there has been only one case in a man.

CLINICAL FEATURES

Clinically, the neoplasm is first manifested in the breast as a rapidly enlarging mass of relative short duration, which is rarely tender or painful. Patients most often are young women, and occasionally they are pregnant. The mass generally is poorly defined and deeply located, but when it is superficial, a characteristic blue or purple discoloration of the skin is present that may suggest an inflammatory condition or the sequela of recent trauma. Skin fixation is unusual, and enlarged axillary lymph nodes are seldom a clinical feature. When present, nodal enlargement ordinarily proves to be a result of hyperplasia. Ecchymosis may indicate hemorrhage within the tumor and may account for associated local discomfort. Bilateral involvement occurs ultimately in 21 per cent of cases, although initially only 3 per cent have this as a presenting feature, according to Donnell and coworkers (1981). Metastasis to the opposite breast is frequent. Previous irradiation appears to be causal in some cases.

PATHOLOGY

Grossly, the neoplasm is spongy, soft, and unencapsulated (Fig. 27–13). Microscopically, it may appear deceptively benign. Dilated vascular spaces combine with interstitial hemorrhage, and occasionally focal necrosis is present. The important features are irregularly intercommunicating vascular channels lined by atypical endothelial cells that pile up with foci

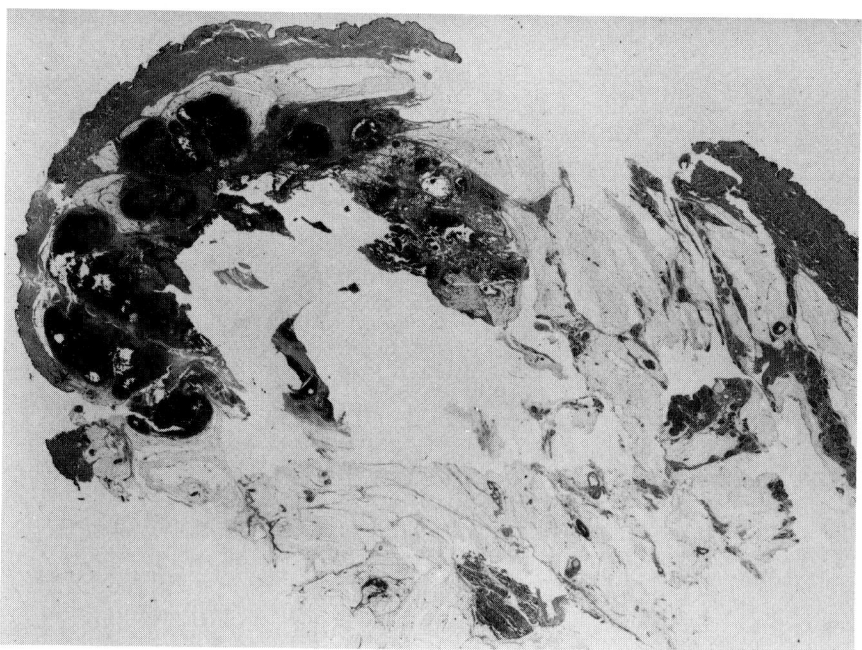

Figure 27–13. This whole organ section of an angiosarcoma of the breast demonstrates the hemorrhagic and unencapsulated character of the tumor. This 43 year old woman reported a mass of 1 year's duration. She was treated with radical mastectomy and 12 axillary nodes were free of metastases. She died 6 months later of metastases, principally in the lungs.

of papillary intraluminal proliferation. Much variation in cellularity in different parts of the tumor is also seen. Infiltration of neoplastic elements tends to extend far beyond the gross limits of the tumor and to foster incomplete removal, probably accounting for the frequency of local recurrence. A correlation has been reported between the size, the degree of mitotic activity, and the histologic differentiation of the tumor and the clinical course of the patient (Donnell et al., 1981; Merino et al., 1983). Because of histologic variability, it is generally recommended that vascular tumors of the breast be removed totally for diagnosis. Although almost all are malignant, the occasional benign cavernous hemangioma or vascular anomaly must be distinguished from angiosarcoma. Experience with cytologic diagnosis is scant. One angiosarcoma was tested for estrogen receptors and found to be negative (Antman et al., 1982).

Case Report

In view of this tumor's rarity, a previously unreported case of angiosarcoma of the breast seen at the Milwaukee County Medical Complex is described.

At 40 years of age, this white woman developed nodular sclerosing Hodgkin's disease in the left side of the neck and mediastinum and was treated with external occult irradiation in a modified upper mantle distribution, omitting the axillary areas. The latter were included shortly afterward when adenopathy appeared in the left axilla. She received approximately 3500 rad to the anterior mediastinum. During the next 5 years, enlarged nodes were excised on two occasions from the left axilla and once from the right axilla.

Ten years after her original therapy the patient again presented with fullness in the left axilla, and at this time the left breast was noted to be enlarged and edematous and to display erythematous angioma-like lesions on its medial aspect, within the port of her previous irradiation. A biopsy was consistent with lymphangiosarcoma, and a simple mastectomy was performed with a skin graft closure. Bizarre proliferating vascular channels were present within the dermis as well as within the fibrous and fatty tissues of the breast. The tissues were reviewed subsequently at the Armed Forces Institute of Pathology where a diagnosis was made of angiosarcoma in irradiated skin. Within 8 months the tumor had reestablished itself on the left chest wall, and a similar process had appeared in the right breast, which was swollen and red. A fungating red tumor mass measuring 8 × 6 cm replaced the nipple. The patient received multiple drug chemotherapy, but it was soon apparent that the tumor was uncontrolled. External irradiation was then employed, during which 6000 rad was delivered to the right breast and 4500 to the left chest wall and sternum. Irradiation resulted in partial regression except in the previously irradiated sternal area, where the tumor continued to enlarge. The patient survived an additional 13 months and died of her tumor 2 years after its onset.

The angiosarcoma in this instance had its onset 10 years after the patient's original irradiation and appeared to arise either in the supporting tissues or in the irradiated skin of the breast. It is not possible to be certain whether involvement of the second breast, a feature of angiosarcomas, was dissemination of the original tumor or a separate occurrence.

THERAPY

Wide surgical resection with histologically normal margins is the preferred treatment for angiosarcoma; usually a simple or total mastectomy is necessary for all but the smallest of tumors, and removal of pectoral muscles may be necessary, depending on the location. Axillary dissection is not routine, although it may be desirable if nodes are enlarged. Only two cases of axillary metastases have been reported, with clinical involvement in another three (Chen et al., 1980). Chen and associates reviewed the literature in 1980 and found five of 87 patients had survived 5 years without recurrence (6 per cent). In 1981, Donnell and coworkers reported 40 cases seen at Memorial Hospital and the Medical College of Virginia and found 41 per cent disease-free at 3 years, 33 per cent at 5 years.

The place of adjuvant therapy is uncertain. Antman and associates (1982) treated five patients with a combination of resection, chemotherapy (cyclophosphamide, doxorubicin hydrochloride [Adriamycin], and dacarbazine [DTIC]) and irradiation without improving median survival, although two were disease-free at 20 and 38 months. Five of eight cases that received actinomycin D in Donnell and coworkers' series survived without recurrence for 5 to 15 years.

For the majority, survival is brief (median 2.2 years after diagnosis). Most recurrences appear within 3 years. Local recurrence is frequent, and widespread hematogenous dissemination in lungs, skin, bone, brain, and abdominal viscera is the usual course. Hemoptysis signals the presence of pulmonary involvement, bone pain accompanies osseous metastases, and coma or hemiparesis is often a sequel of intracranial spread. Anemia supervenes from hemorrhage and bone marrow replacement. Thrombocytopenia is sometimes seen. Death frequently is the result of massive hemorrhage from an involved intra-abdominal organ, particularly the liver.

Chest wall recurrences or isolated recurrences elsewhere should be excised when possible. Occasionally, long-term survival follows a salvage mastectomy (Donnell et al., 1981). Radiotherapy has little to offer in management, either as primary or as adjuvant therapy, but information is scant, and some palliation of advanced disease occasionally has been claimed. Chemotherapy for recurrences has been disappointing. The only patients cured of the disease have had small lesions, emphasizing that early detection is a highly desirable goal.

Fibrosarcoma

Fibrosarcomas are the most common purely connective tissue tumors of the breast. In diagnosing fibrosarcomas, there is always the chance that benign epithelial elements identifying the lesion as a malignant cystosarcoma phyllodes may be missed. A considerable number of fibrosarcomas termed dermatofibrosarcoma protuberans arise from the integument of the anterior chest wall, and it is often difficult to determine clinically if larger lesions had origin strictly in mammary parenchyma.

CLINICAL FEATURES

Four EFSCH patients with fibrosarcomas were 37, 79, 75, and 71 years of age, and the right breast was involved in three instances. The sarcoma occurred simultaneously with a carcinoma of the opposite breast in one case. Two patients had noted a stationary mass for years with recent rapid growth of 5 months' and 2 years' duration, respectively. A gradually enlarging painless mass had been noted for 7 months and for 18 months in the remaining two cases.

The larger lesions stretched the skin until it presented a glazed appearance (Fig. 27–14). One tumor described as "large" occupied half of the breast and was associated with shininess and a purple color of the skin. Two masses measured 15 cm in diameter, one of which was accompanied by large overlying veins (Fig. 27–15). The second was fixed to the skin and chest wall, skin erythema was present, and a 1.5 cm lymph node was palpable in the axilla.

PATHOLOGY

The tumors displayed a histologic pattern of atypical and bizarre fibrous elements with no evidence of osseous or cartilaginous metaplasia. In one, areas were noted where cellular characteristics suggested a diagnosis of malignant fibrous histiocytoma.

THERAPY

Prior treatment had already been given to patients whose presenting signs were recurrences on the chest—one after simple excision and the other after a combination of multiple excisions, radical mastectomy, and radiotherapy for repeated local recurrences. The former was treated at EFSCH with orthovoltage irradiation with indeterminate response and died 2 months later of a "heart attack." The latter received additional radiotherapy, but little objective effect was observed. Administration of testosterone at a later date was similarly ineffective and the patient died of uncontrolled disease 3 years 5 months after her initial excision. The third patient, who already suffered from metastases in the lungs and ribs, underwent a palliative simple mastectomy. The neoplasm recurred locally in 3 years, 2 months before her death. The last patient lived for 18 years after a simple mastectomy and died without recurrence.

Local excision is inadequate therapy for these neoplasms, as recurrence on the chest wall follows in the majority of cases. Simple mastectomy with removal of the pectoralis fascia is usually necessary to obtain adequate surgical margins for these large tumors, and removal of the underlying pectoralis muscles may be necessary with or without the axillary contents in some cases.

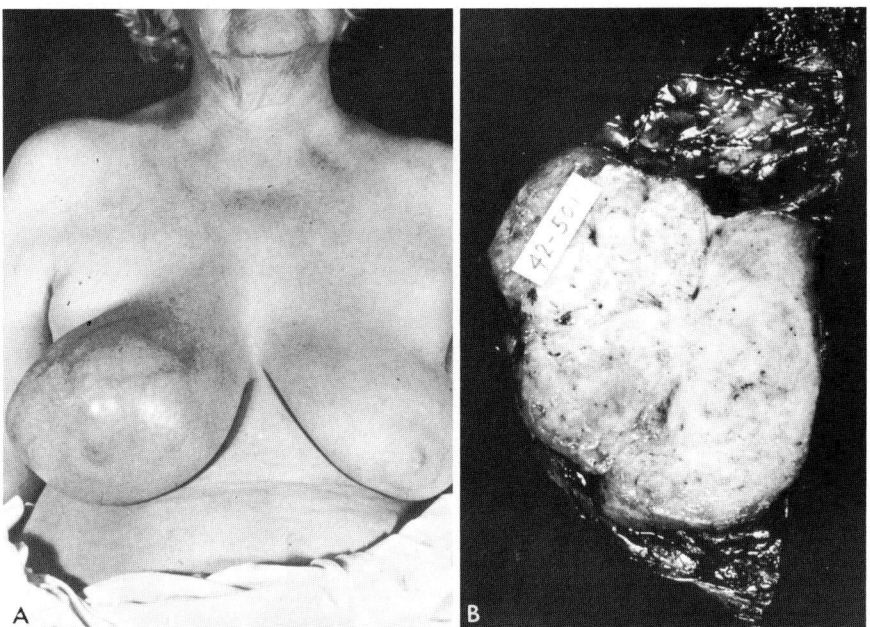

Figure 27–14. *A,* Fibrosarcoma of the right breast. Characteristic of large fibrosarcomas is the tense and mildly erythematous overlying skin. This case demonstrates the presence of prominent superficial veins, which often accompany these neoplasms. *B,* The resected tumor is grossly well marginated and presents a typical appearance.

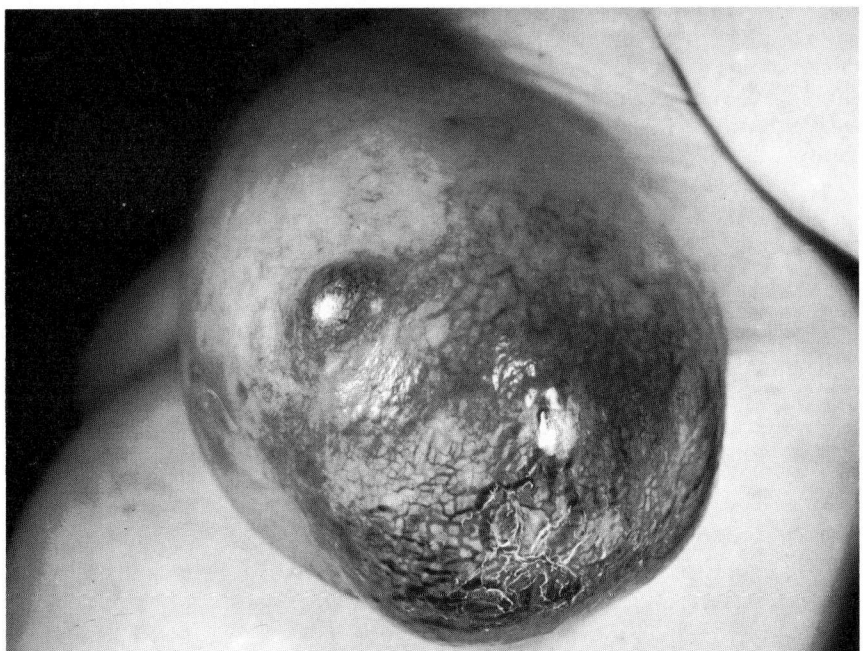

Figure 27–15. A massive fibrosarcoma of the breast near ulceration, with tortuous dilated overlying veins.

The therapy of choice for local recurrences is further wide surgical removal when feasible. Mastectomy is indicated if not performed previously.

Although local excision is inadequate treatment for fibrosarcoma of the mammary parenchyma, wide local removal is usually satisfactory for its less aggressive variant, dermafibrosarcoma protuberans, which afflicts the skin of the breast. The only patient with this problem, a 48 year old woman who claimed to have had the lesion for 14 years, was treated with wide local excision at EFSCH. The tumor followed an indolent course, recurring locally on two occasions, 9 and 15 years after excision. The patient was living and without disease 1 year after the last removal.

Liposarcoma

Liposarcomas constitute 0.3 per cent of all sarcomas of the breast. Neumann made the earliest report in 1862, and only 28 cases were documented at the time of Hummer and Burkart's review in 1967.

CLINICAL FEATURES

The primary tumor usually comes to the physician's attention as a mobile, painless, discrete and rubbery mass with a variable growth rate. The overlying skin may be erythematous and display dilated veins when the tumor reaches large size. Patients are usually postmenopausal.

PATHOLOGY

The encapsulation of the neoplasm is an illusion that belies the presence of extensions penetrating into surrounding normal tissue. The cut surface bulges, appears mucoid, and varies in color from yellow to brown. Evidence of hemorrhage and fat necrosis is sometimes present. Microscopic findings in some cases have suggested the origin of this tumor in preexistent fibroadenomas or cystosarcoma phyllodes (Hinterberger, 1942; Homes and Leis, 1962; Jackson, 1962). Myxoid changes are frequently present, giving rise to the terms "myxolipoma" and "myxoliposarcoma," and giant cells can usually be demonstrated. Most cells show various stages of atypical fat storage, and lipoid droplets can be demonstrated with fat stains. Stout and Bernanke (1946) described two main classes of liposarcomas, those that show considerable differentiation and do not metastasize and those exhibiting poor differentiation with various types of metaplasia that metastasize in 40 per cent of the cases.

Case Report

A case of liposarcoma of the breast was diagnosed at EFSCH.

A 60 year old white woman presented with a tender right breast mass of 7 weeks' duration. On examination a 12 × 3.5 cm nondiscrete mass was palpable in the breast, occupying both upper quadrants. Erythema of the overlying skin was attributed to application of topical ointments and no skin or deep fixation was noted. No axillary nodes were palpable. At the time of surgical biopsy, a 6.0 × 3.0 cm hard nodular tumor attached to surrounding fascia was found lying between the pectoralis major and pectoralis minor muscles and was excised. Mammary parenchyma in the tract of the incision was not involved grossly. The tumor was a discrete, multinodular light tan mass that on cut section appeared to be composed predominantly of solid fibrous tissue with many tiny, indistinct cysts and contained a large amount of mucinous material. Histologic examination revealed predominantly myxomatous tissue, within which were elongated and spidery cells and vacuolated cells resembling adult lipocytes, the majority of which were moderately well differentiated. In some areas the cells had bizarre irregular nuclei, and scattered mitoses were seen. After a histologic diagnosis was made on permanent sections, a radical mastectomy was performed to remove residual tumor, and further examination showed neoplasm near the deep surgical margin. Five years 3 months after radical surgery, a recurrence that was fixed to the chest wall was noted in the vicinity of the scar. This was treated with wide surgical removal in continuity with a full thickness of the chest wall, including the anterior portions of the second, third, and fourth ribs, and a pedicle flap was advanced over the resulting defect. No reappearance of tumor had occurred 15 months after this resection.

THERAPY

Both surgery and irradiation, alone and in combination, have been advised for liposarcoma of the breast (Geschickter, 1943; Stout and Bernanke, 1946; Homes and Leis, 1962; Hare and Cerny, 1963; Menon and van Velthoven, 1974).

The propensity for local recurrence of well-differentiated tumors, and the tendency for lymphatic and vascular dissemination of the more aggressive ones, argues for wide surgical margins and removal of axillary lymphatics. Local recurrences can occur years after initial treatment and can advance rapidly. Radiotherapy alone is not regularly curative for liposarcomas, although many of these tumors are radiosensitive. Irradiation may be of value if used postoperatively.

Wide surgical excision is the treatment of choice for recurrences; radiotherapy is of value when excision is not feasible. Chemotherapy may be tried for advanced disease. Dissemination to the lungs and abdominal viscera is the usual course of an uncontrolled liposarcoma.

Rhabdomyosarcoma

Rhabdomyosarcomas are not unusual among nonepithelial cancers of the breast. Oberman (1965b) observed three among 13 mammary sarcomas and Botham four among 23. Rapid growth, indefinite borders and large size characterize these aggressive neoplasms, and cures are infrequent (Oberman, 1965b).

The diagnosis of rhabdomyosarcoma is based on finding cells with sarcoplasmic cross striations. Multinucleated neoplastic giant cells, "racquet cells," and "strap cells" are characteristic.

As the mammary parenchyma lacks striated muscles, the tissues from which rhabdomyosarcomas arise in this organ is an unanswered question. The case for origin from pectoral muscles is frustrated by the lack of regularly demonstrable continuity (Hill and Stout, 1942). Oberman noted that three rhabdomyosarcomas infiltrated skeletal muscle, but the tumors were centered in the mammary gland.

Case Report

A case of a relatively undifferentiated rhabdomyosarcoma was recognized and treated at EFSCH. The same case was reported by Haagensen (1971) along with another also seen in consultation by Stout.

This 75 year old white woman reported that a large cystic mass had been present in her left breast for 1½ years and had burst, draining blood and pus for 2 weeks prior to admission. On examination a large fungating mass with a deep central sinus tract was present in the outer portion of the breast (Fig. 27–16). A few small nodes were palpable in the axilla. A simple mastectomy was initially performed to remove the mass and weeks later, when the wound was healed, a radical mastectomy was performed.

The entire tumor measured $9 \times 10 \times 7$ cm. On section it was soft, was light gray, and featured small zones of necrosis. Microscopically, undifferentiated tumor cells with faintly acidophilic cytoplasm were present, displaying a large number of abnormal mitotic figures. Many large tumor giant cells, frequently with vacuolated cytoplasm, were in evidence. Metastases were present in 4 of 17 axillary lymph nodes.

On consultation, Dr. A. P. Stout was of the opinion that "the large elongated syncytial masses with many nuclei strongly resemble the way rhabdomyoblasts grow in vitro," and with this additional information a diagnosis of rhabdomyosarcoma was made.

Sixteen months after the radical operation a radiograph showed a metastatic nodule in the left lung. At this time the surgical area was unremarkable. The neoplasm followed a surprisingly indolent course, and the patient died at home 3 years 4 months after the diagnosis of metastases—as far as can be determined, without local recurrence.

THERAPY

Hematogenous dissemination is the most frequent mode of spread of rhabdomyosarcomas, but metastases to regional nodes are relatively frequent, especially from the alveolar type. Horn reported a 19 per cent incidence of metastases to regional nodes from rhabdomyosarcomas. For this reason, removal of axillary lymph nodes with radical or modified radical mastectomy is the treatment of choice. Some advanced and recurrent tumors may show temporary regressions after radiotherapy (del Regato, 1963) or radiotherapy combined with chemotherapy. Responses of rhabdomyosarcomas to chemotherapy are becoming more frequent with the use of drug combinations (Morton, 1974; Delaney et al., 1976).

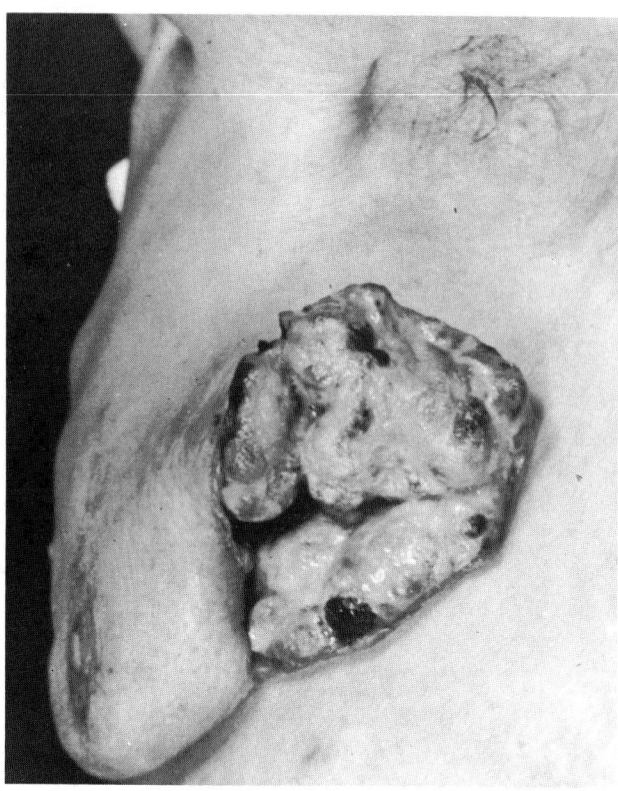

Figure 27–16. Rhabdomyosarcoma of the breast of a 75 year old woman. This advanced tumor appeared as a fungating mass associated with a sinus tract. Metastases were present in 4 of 17 axillary lymph nodes.

Carcinosarcomas

True carcinosarcomas, "collision tumors," within which coexist both malignant epithelial and malignant connective tissue elements, have been recognized in the breast (Robb and MacFarlane, 1958; Williams and Diamonon, 1964). Both components can remain associated in lymph node metastases (Curran and Dodge, 1962).

These tumors often present as large masses, and it is not uncommon for them to be painful. Clinical histories range from 1 month to 20 years. Harris and Persaud (1974) contributed two cases and summarized 14 reported in the literature. Ages ranged from 10 to 91 years, with an average of 58 years. In seven of the 16 cases, tumors were believed to have risen from preexisting fibroadenomas of cystosarcomas. Osteosarcoma was often a component of the sarcomatous element, whereas undifferentiated carcinoma, adenocarcinoma, in situ carcinoma, and squamous cell carcinoma were represented in the epithelial portion of the malignancies. Only three of the 16 patients lived for 5 years after therapy, although four others were still living after shorter periods. In five cases metastases were documented in axillary lymph nodes; other sites of spread included bone and lung. Although simple mastectomy is often used to treat these tumors, their capacity to infiltrate the underlying pectoral muscle and to produce axillary nodal metastases would argue for wide removal of the breast and axillary nodes, including the pectoral muscles en bloc if the tumor is large or involvement seems likely.

It must be noted that the rare squamous cell carcinoma of the breast is not confined to carcinosarcomas (Bogomoletz, 1982). Eggers and McChesney reviewed this subject in 1984 and found most cases to be associated with pure epithelial cancers, for example, adenocarcinomas and anaplastic and medullary carcinomas. Cornog and associates (1971) found one well-differentiated, pure squamous cell carcinoma in association with a cystosarcoma phyllodes, and a few were thought to be of epidermal origin. Squamous cell carcinoma has the same prognosis as invasive adenocarcinoma of the breast in similar stages.

Granulocytic Sarcoma (Chloroma)

Granulocytic sarcomas sometimes first appear as primary tumors of the breast. These extramedullary tumors, composed of myeloid or monocytoid precursor cells, are regularly associated with acute myelocytic leukemia. The mass is ordinarily adjacent to bone but less frequently occurs in the ovaries, breast, lymph nodes, and dura. Rarely, it may precede the diagnosis of acute leukemia by from 1 month to more than 1 year. If so, it can be mistaken histologically for an eosinophilic granuloma. A characteristic green color accounts for the original designation "chloroma," but this coloration is not regularly present and the term granulocytic sarcoma is more appropriate. Both the green color and red fluorescence in ultraviolet light are attributed to the enzyme myeloperoxidase. Several granulocytic sarcomas in the breast have been described (Wiernik and Serpick, 1970). Although the tumors respond to localized external radiation and sometimes to chemotherapy, the course of acute myelocytic leukemia is one of uniformly short survival. Wiernik and Serpick described a 40 year old woman with a 1×0.5 cm, grayish-green, firm tumor in her right breast that proved to be a granulocytic sarcoma. Acute myelocytic leukemia was diagnosed during the same admission and despite therapy with hydroxyurea and daunomycin, the patient died within 1 month.

Granular Cell Myoblastoma

Six per cent of granular cell myoblastomas occur in the breast (Bassett and Cove, 1979). Although there is some doubt about the neoplastic nature of this tumor, there is little doubt that it can be infiltrative, recur after excision, and possibly metastasize. Fewer than 50 have been reported in the breast, none with a correct preoperative diagnosis. Originally described by Abrikossoff in 1926, the cell of origin of this tumor remains in doubt. A primitive myoblast was originally indicted, but more recent evidence has favored the Schwann cell or an undifferentiated mesenchymal precursor (Soble et al., 1972). The tumor occurs in both men and women and at ages ranging from 15 to 70 years. Weitzner and coworkers (1979) reviewed the 52 previously documented cases of mammary granular cell myoblastoma and reported the youngest case to date in a 15 year old girl. The right and left breasts were involved almost equally.

A solitary, painless lump with progressive increase in size is the usual presentation. Fixation to skin or underlying fascia, as well as ulceration of the skin or adjacent nodules of similar histologic nature mimicking satellites, can be highly suggestive of carcinoma (McCracken et al., 1979). For unknown reasons the upper inner quadrant of the breast is the most frequent location. The tumors measure 1 to 10 cm in diameter at the time they are diagnosed, and edema of the skin, dimpling, retraction, and pigmentation may be present. Mammographically, the lesion appears as a density with sharp margins except for tendon-like extensions into adjacent breast tissue that mimic carcinoma. Aspiration cytology and even frozen sections can be misleading, so local excision and permanent sections constitute the proper method of diagnosis. The cut surface is white and hard, and in nine of 34 cases that had a frozen section, the tumor was initially thought to be malignant. Microscopic examination revealing the characteristic plump cells with granular inclusions permits the correct diagnosis.

Wide local excision is the treatment of choice (Townsend and Stellato, 1985). Irradiation is not effective. As the tumor infiltrates freely into surrounding tissues, complete removal may require inclusion of muscle and other adjacent structures, and histologic evaluation is advisable to be certain that surgical margins are free of tumor. After adequate removal, recurrence is unusual. None of Umansky and Bullock's 19 patients (1968) had recurrence or died of the disease after from 4 months to 12½ years of observation. The rare malignant behavior of this tumor is evidenced by the case of Crawford and DeBakey (1953), in which widespread involvement of the lungs, liver, and retroperitoneal tissues was associated with a 4 cm mass in the upper outer quadrant of the left breast, presumed to represent either the primary tumor or an additional component of multifocal origin.

The author has treated one case that first appeared as a 1.5 cm firm, discrete nodule (clinically a fibroadenoma) in the lower midline of the left breast of an 18 year old white woman. After local excision with free margins the patient was free of recurrence 13 months later.

Leiomyosarcoma

Leiomyosarcomas are among the rarest of nonepithelial cancers of the breast. Possibly no more than eight cases have been reported; the first report is attributed to Crocker and Murad in 1968 (Hill and Stout, 1942; Haagensen, 1971; Visfeldt and Sheike, 1973; Pardo-Mindan et al., 1974; Chen et al., 1981). The fact that two cases were found among 265 male breast cancers by Visfeldt and Sheike suggests that it is more frequent among men than among women. Patients' ages range from 49 to 77 years, and tumor sizes range from 4 to 8 cm. The clinical features are typical of sarcoma, and the histopathologic appearance is easily recognizable. This highly cellular neoplasm is composed of elongate cells with blunt ends caricaturing smooth muscle cells. Mitoses are frequent (three or more mitoses per 10 high power fields are necessary to qualify), and occasionally multinucleated giant cells are in evidence. The case described by Pardo-Mindan and colleagues is representative: A 49 year old woman had a 7.5 cm firm, mobile, smooth nodule that appeared clinically benign in the inferior lateral region of the left breast near the nipple. The axilla was free of adenopathy. On biopsy the tumor was firm and white with irregular, reddish areas. Microscopically, it was considered a Grade IV leiomyosarcoma according to the Silverberg classification of uterine leiomyosarcoma. Small areas of necrosis were evident, and the tumor had invaded vascular walls. A simple mastectomy was performed, and the patient was living without recurrence 6 months later.

Haagensen (1971) described a 77 year old woman who sought treatment for a tumor of her left breast that had been present for 2 weeks. The mass measured 8 cm in diameter, was mobile, soft, and well defined, and occupied most of the upper portion of the breast. A biopsy with frozen section initially resulted in a diagnosis of "sarcoma," and a complete mastectomy was performed. The tumor was composed of characteristic cells displaying frequent mitoses, among which were seen occasional giant cells and elongated strap-shaped cells. The patient was surviving without recurrence 14 years after the operation.

All cases reported to date have been treated with simple or radical mastectomy; one patient developed hepatic metastasis 15 years after treatment with no sign of local recurrence. Leiomyosarcomas are apparently less aggressive biologically than sarcomas of the breast in general. Wide local excision is the treatment of choice.

Chondrosarcoma

Chondrosarcomas are among the rarest of pure sarcomas of the breast. Ladefoged and Nielsen reported only the fourth case in 1984. This occurred in a 84 year old woman as a 5 cm slowly growing tumor in the upper midline of the right breast. The overlying skin was normal, and no nodes could be felt in the axilla. The tumor was excised widely locally, and the patient was free of recurrence 2 years later. In establishing this diagnosis, it is necessary to exclude metaplastic changes in cystosarcoma phyllodes or osteosarcomas with multiple sections of the tumor and metastatic osteosarcomas from other sites. The lower extremities are the most frequent sites of extraosseous chondrosarcomas. Furthermore, staining for S100 protein is a useful marker for cells of chondrocytic origin and serves to rule out the possibility of metastatic carcinoma. Like other pure sarcomas of the breast, chondrosarcomas have the potential for hematogenous spread of metastases to the lungs and bones. One case may have involved hepatic metastases. Electron microscopic studies are useful (Ladefoged and Nielsen, 1984).

Malignant Fibrous Histiocytoma

Approximately 4 per cent of malignant fibrous histiocytomas have been observed in the female breast (Obrien and Stout, 1964). These tumors may also arise as a stromal component of cystosarcoma phyllodes, in previous irradiated areas, or in the skin. A small proportion arise in the mammary tissue without skin involvement. Langham and coworkers reported the fourth case of malignant fibrous histiocytoma arising de novo in the breast tissue unassociated with other tumor or previous irradiation.

The tumor is composed of a storiform pattern of spindle-shaped cells with scant cytoplasm and ovoid nuclei intermixed with large pleomorphic cells with abundant eosinophilic cytoplasm, multiple atypical nuclei, and prominent nuclei. Mitoses are frequent. Presence of both perinuclear filaments and fat in the same cell favors the diagnosis of malignant fibrous histiocytoma on electron microscopic examination.

Two patients have been treated with simple mastectomy and radical mastectomy. A recurrence after the simple mastectomy was apparently controlled by wide local excision. A third patient was treated by radical mastectomy and remained free of disease at 54 months. A fourth patient had recurrence 14 months after an excisional biopsy, was treated with modified radical mastectomy, and was alive and well 11 months later. A fifth case was reported by Liebert and Edwards (1982). This 51 year old woman had a 2.5 cm mass in the upper outer quadrant of the left breast beneath the scar of a previous biopsy. It mimicked carcinoma by causing skin retraction and by its appearance on mammography. The tumor appeared benign on excisional biopsy but recurred 1 year later in the same area. The recurrence was treated with segmental mastectomy, but the patient developed pulmonary metastases 1 year later. This tumor metastasizes to regional lymph nodes in approximately 10 per cent of cases. Wide local excision may be adequate therapy for small superficial lesions, but mastectomy is probably the best treatment for larger lesions arising in the substance of the breast. Routine axillary lymph node dissection has been recommended, considering the frequency of metastases (van Niekerk et al., 1987). The roles of chemotherapy and irradiation remain to be defined.

Osteogenic Sarcoma

This unusual bone-forming sarcoma is believed to arise from the stroma of long-standing fibroadenomas or possibly from mastopathy as a progression of osseous metaplasia (Cole-Beuglet et al., 1976). The first published report of a malignant mammary neoplasm composed of bone and cartilage is said to be that of Bonet in 1700. From that time to 1963, 115 cases were reported (Jernstrom et al., 1963). Not unusual in the breast as a component of carcinosarcomas, osteogenic sarcomas also occasionally occur in a pure form. Jernstrom and coworkers observed one osteosarcoma in 3309 cases of mammary cancers during a period of 18 years. Middle-aged and older women are most susceptible, although women in the third decade of life can be affected. The tumor is composed of pleomorphic osteoblastic tissue, with bone and cartilage as well as giant cells of the osteoclastic type. It appears as a mass that is smooth, mobile, and understandably firm, but it may be cystic, fixed, and occasionally ulcerated. Radiographs demonstrate bone formation in the breast (Teich and Brecher, 1985). The axilla is rarely involved. Hematogenous spread, usually to the lungs, is the rule. Treatment most often has been radical mastectomy, although the infrequency with which lymphatic spread is encountered would appear to justify a lesser procedure with or without limited axillary dissection but with wide margins around the primary tumor.

A case reported by Aubrey and Andrews (1971) illustrates the features of this disease. A 52 year old woman had a mass of 3 weeks' duration in the lower outer quadrant of the left breast. A cyst had been removed from the same breast earlier. This mass was 2.5 cm at its widest, hard, irregular, and not associated with enlarged axillary nodes. Clinically, it was believed to be carcinoma and was treated with a left radical mastectomy. The definitive diagnosis was low-grade malignant osteogenic sarcoma. The patient was well for 8 years but then developed weakness, weight loss, and a chronic cough, which led to a radiograph that showed multiple metastases in both lungs. Subsequently, metastases appeared in the subcutaneous tissues of the buttocks and a finger as well as within the abdomen. No response was achieved with thiotepa, testosterone therapy, or prednisolone, and the patient died 9 years 2 months after her mastectomy. The autopsy revealed firm, gritty masses of tumor with areas of cystic necrosis; metastases were found invading the chest wall, the bodies of the thoracic vertebra, the left adrenal gland, the brain, the peritoneum, and the myocardium.

Cytoxan and cortisone have proved useful for the temporary control of pulmonary metastases (Kolarsick, 1972).

Lymphangiosarcoma of the Edematous Arm

Lymphangiosarcoma is an uncommon but important complication of arm edema following radical mastectomy. A significant association between carcinoma of the breast and soft tissue sarcomas reported by Schoenberg (1975) was largely attributable to this tumor. The problem was originally described by Stewart and Treves in 1948 and subsequently became known as the Stewart-Treves syndrome. Slightly more than 100 cases are reported in the literature, and the incidence is estimated at between 0.45 and 0.07 per cent of patients treated for early carcinoma of the breast (Fitzpatrick, 1969).

Typically, the patient gives a history of persistent arm edema following a mastectomy. After an average interval of 10 years (1 to 24 years), small, pigmented nodules that have been mistaken for insect bites appear on the arm. The onset was well described by Stewart and Treves (1948):

> After an interval of years . . . a purplish-red, subdermal, slightly raised, macular or polypoid lesion appears. The primary site is in the skin of the arm or antecubital area. The lesion occurs as a solitary tumor followed by similar satellite areas that sometimes become confluent, form a larger lesion, or remain as distinct and later partially bullous areas. The larger lesions appear almost as papillomatous growths colored by shiny, tense, atrophied epithelium. It has a tendency to ulcerate and discharge a serous or serosanguineous fluid. They heal spontaneously only to break down again and discharge. As new lesions appear, all stages of imminent ulceration, discharge, and healing can be seen. Once the process is initiated, the discrete nodules continue to grow, and new ones appear on the forearm, dorsum of the hand, and finally the skin of the adjacent thorax.

Local infection becomes a problem and eventually the lesion disseminates, most reliably to the lungs but also to bones, brain, lymph nodes, and skin. The characteristic purple-red color and distribution of the lesions suggest the diagnosis (Fig. 27–17). The lesions do not resemble the cutaneous nodules of recurrent mammary carcinoma and do not have their origin in the surgical or irradiated areas, although they may extend to them. Histologically, the lesions can easily be mistaken for Kaposi's sarcoma or for highly anaplastic recurrent carcinoma, but the features usually permit a definitive diagnosis.

The prognosis of the patient is poor (1.3 years median survival); in most cases the tumor

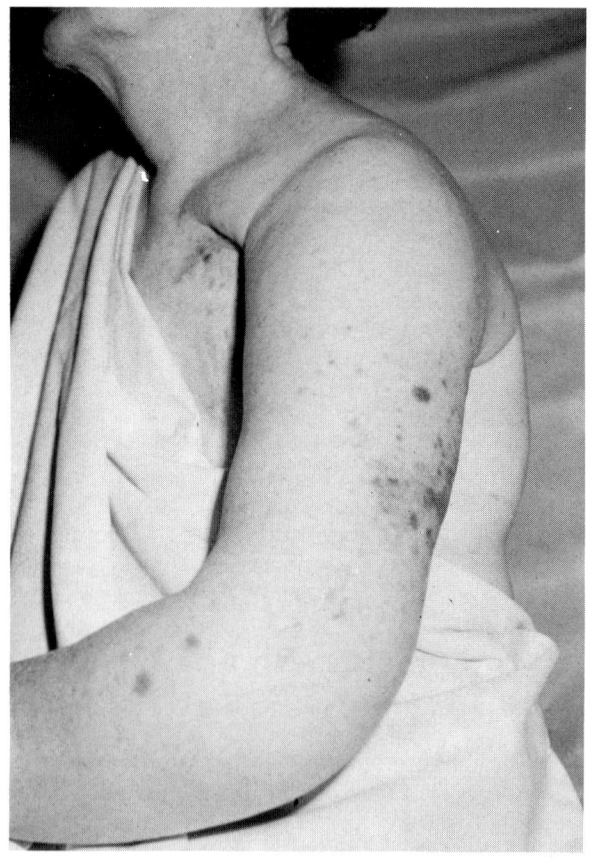

Figure 27–17. This patient developed a lymphangiosarcoma on the upper extremity 5 years after a left radical mastectomy. The arm had been chronically lymph-edematous from the time of her original surgery. The characteristic purple lesions can be seen on the arm and the adjacent chest wall, and osteolytic lesions were present in vertebrae. The neoplasm progressed rapidly and she died several months later with widespread dissemination.

is unresponsive to all forms of treatment. Radiotherapy to the involved arm may produce some regression, but only three cases of long-term survival are recorded (Tong and Winter, 1974). Both local excision of isolated nodules and amputation of the arm have been used with occasional success (Fitzpatrick, 1969; Barnett et al., 1969; Haagensen, 1971). Two of eight cases treated at M. D. Anderson Hospital with forequarter amputation lived 5 years without recurrence (Yap et al., 1981). At the time of Herrmann and Ariel's report in 1967, 83 cases were in the literature. Five of the 75 patients had survived for more than 5 years free of recurrence after an attempted cure. One had been treated with external irradiation, one by wide excision, and three by amputation. The additional 5 year survivor was treated with external irradiation followed by intra-arterial yttrium microspheres. Hermann and Ariel suggested initial treatment with irradiation followed by radical amputation of the extremity if irradiation is unsuccessful. For the disseminated case, most forms of chemotherapy have proved ineffective or produced only brief benefit. In one report, systemic chemotherapy with fluorouracil, methotrexate, or various combinations produced complete or partial responses in 42 per cent of cases for a median duration of 6 months (Yap et al., 1981). Temporary remission has attended regional perfusion with nitrogen mustard (Tragus and Wagner, 1969), melphalan and methotrexate (Yap et al., 1981), and Tong and Winter (1974) reported dramatic although temporary response of two patients to cyclophosphamide. Prompt progression of the tumor occurred when the drug was discontinued because of leukopenia.

The fact that this tumor rarely occurs in extremities that are lymphedematous from other causes raises the speculation that it is uniquely associated with a constitutional disposition to cancer of the breast or a common carcinogen. It may be speculated further that an immunologically deprived extremity is favored. Whatever the inciting factor, its dismal prognosis is an additional incentive for preventing lymphedema of the arm and for measures to treat edema effectively when it occurs. Minimizing mastectomy wound complications and avoiding irradiation of the axilla after axillary dissections, both of which promote fibrotic obstruction of lymphatics and edema, would presumably decrease the frequency of this neoplasm.

Radiation-Induced Soft Tissue Sarcomas in Breast Cancer Patients

A small but finite frequency of soft tissue sarcomas appears to be a consequence of postmastectomy irradiation (Ferguson et al., 1985; Kuten et al., 1985). They appear in the irradiation ports after a latent period of 4 to 26 years in about 1 to 1.5 per cent of patients and are almost uniformly lethal (Ferguson et al., 1985). Most are malignant fibrous histiocytomas or fibrosarcomas, but angiosarcomas also occur. The breast, axilla, mastectomy scar, and shoulder are the sites of origin.

Wide resection is the preferred therapy when possible, although successes are few. As previous irradiation has ranged from 3000 to 5400 rad, further irradiation is rarely feasible. Chemotherapy provides a few partial responses. Kuten and associates (1985) reported two partial responses among seven patients treated with the four drug combination cyclophosphamide, vincristine, Adriamycin, and dacarbazine (DTIC).

Although postoperative irradiation is declining in use, primary irradiation is increasing as an alternative to mastectomy for early breast cancer. As a consequence, the absolute number of radiation-induced sarcomas in cured patients may be expected to increase. Early recognition of these tumors and wide resection are at present the most promising means of management.

REFERENCES

Abrikossoff, A. J.: Uber myome, ausgehend von der quergestreiften willkwrlichen musklature. Arch. Pathol. Anat., 260:215, 1926.
Allen, R., Nixon, D., York, M., et al.: Successful chemotherapy for cystosarcoma phyllodes in a young woman. Arch. Intern. Med., 145:1127, 1985.
Amerson, J. R.: Cystosarcoma phyllodes in adolescent females: A report of seven patients. Ann. Surg., 171:849, 1970.
Antman, K. H., Corson, J., Greenberger, J., et al.: Multimodality therapy in the management of angiosarcoma of the breast. Cancer, 50:2000, 1982.
Ariel, L.: Skeletal metastases in cystosarcoma phyllodes. A case report and review. Arch. Surg., 82:275, 1961.
Aubrey, D. A., and Andrews, G. S.: Mammary osteogenic sarcoma. Br. J. Surg., 58:472, 1971.
Barber, K. W., Jr., Harrison, E. G., Clagett, O. T., et al.: Angiosarcoma of the breast. Surgery, 48:869, 1960.
Barnett, W. O., Hardy, J. D., and Hendrix, J. H.: Lymphangiosarcoma following post-mastectomy lymphedema. Ann. Surg., 169:960, 1969.

Barnhart, G. R., DeBlois, G. G., Kay, S., et al.: Management of cystosarcoma phyllodes: A reassessment. Breast, 11:17, 1985.

Bassett, L. W., and Cove, H. C.: Myoblastoma of the breast. J. Radiol. 132:122, 1979.

Berg, J. W., DeCosse, J. J., Fracchia, A. A., et al.: Stromal sarcomas of the breast. A unified approach to connective tissue sarcomas other than cystosarcoma phyllodes. Cancer, 15:418, 1962.

Berger, S. M., and Gershon-Cohen, J.: Mammography of breast sarcoma. AJR, 87:76, 1962.

Blichert-Toft, M., Hansen, J. P. H., Hansen, O. H., et al.: Clinical course of cystosarcoma phyllodes related to histologic appearance. Surg. Gynecol. Obstet., 149:929, 1975.

Bogomoletz, W. V.: Pure squamous cell carcinoma of the breast. Arch. Pathol. Lab. Med., 106:57, 1982.

Borrmann, R.: Metastasenbildung bei histologisch gutartigen Geschulsten (Fall von metastasierendem Angiom). Beitr. Path. Anat., 40:372, 1907.

Bot, F. J., and Donner, R.: Metastatic cystosarcoma phyllodes. Report of a case with a ten-year interval. Netherland J. Surg. 33:34, 1981.

Botham, R. J., McDonald, J. R., and Clagett, O. T.: Sarcoma of the mammary gland. Surg. Gynecol. Obstet., 107:55, 1958.

Brentani, M. M., Nagai, M. A., Oshima, C. T. F., et al.: Steroid receptors in cystosarcoma phyllodes. Cancer Detect. Prevent., 5:211, 1982.

Briggs, R. M., Walters, M., and Rosenthal, D.: Cystosarcoma phyllodes in adolescent female patients. Am. J. Surg., 146:712, 1983.

Carbone, A., Volpe, R., Tirelli, U., et al.: Primary lymphoblastic lymphoma of the breast. Clin. Oncol., 8:367, 1982.

Chelius, M. J.: Teleangiektasie. Heidelberger Klin. Ann., 4:499, 517, 1828.

Chen, K. T. K., Kirkegaard, D. D., and Bocian, J. J.: Angiosarcoma of the breast. Cancer, 46:368, 1980.

Chen, K. T. K., Kuo, T. T., and Hoffmann, K. D.: Leiomyosarcoma of the breast. A case of long survival and late hepatic metastasis. Cancer, 47:1883, 1981.

Cole-Beuglet, C., Kirk, M. E., Selouan, R., et al.: Bone within the breast. Radiology, 119:643, 1976.

Contarini, O., Urdaneta, L. F., Hagan, W., et al.: Cystosarcoma phylloides of the breast: A new therapeutic proposal. Ann. Surg., 48:157, 1982.

Cooper, W. G., Jr., and Ackerman, L. V.: Cystosarcoma phyllodes: With a consideration of its more malignant variant. Surg. Gynecol. Obstet., 77:279, 1943.

Cornog, J. L., Mobini, J., Steiger, E., et al.: Squamous carcinoma of the breast. Am. J. Clin. Pathol., 55:410, 1971.

Crawford, E. S., and DeBakey, M. E.: Granular-cell myoblastoma. Two unusual cases. Cancer, 6:786, 1953.

Curran, R. C., and Dodge, O. G.: Sarcoma of breast, with particular reference to its origin from fibroadenoma. J. Clin. Pathol., 15:1, 1962.

DeCosse, J. J., Berg, J. W., Fracchia, A. A., et al.: Primary lymphosarcoma of the breast. Cancer, 15:1264, 1962.

Delaney, W. E., Orossi, C., and Nealon, T. F., Jr.: The soft tissues. In Nealon, T. F., Jr.: Management of the Patient with Cancer. 2nd Ed. Philadelphia, W. B. Saunders, 1976, p. 851.

DeLeon, D. M., Viallafria, L., and Crisostomo, C.: Nonsystemic reticulum cell sarcoma of the breast: a case report. Philip. J. Surg., 16:149, 1961.

del Regato, J. A.: Radiotherapy of soft-tissue sarcomas. J.A.M.A., 185:216, 1963.

Donnell, R. M., Rosen, P. P., Lieberman, P. H., et al.: Angiosarcoma and other vascular tumors of the breast. Pathologic analysis as a guide to prognosis. Am. J. Surg. Pathol. 5:629, 1981.

Edwards, J. A., and Strouth, B. P.: Hemangioendothelioblastoma of the breast. Northwest Med., 55:788, 1956.

Eggers, J. W., and Chesney, T. M.: Squamous cell carcinoma of the breast: A clinicopathologic analysis of eight cases and review of the literature. Hum. Pathol., 15:526, 1984.

Ferguson, D. F., Sullon, H. G., and Dawson, P. J.: Late effects of adjuvant radiotherapy for breast cancer. Cancer, 54:2319, 1985.

Fiks, A.: Cystosarcoma phyllodes of the mammary gland—Muller's tumor. Virchows. Arch. (Pathol. Anat.), 392:1, 1981.

Fitzpatrick, P. J.: Lymphangiosarcoma in breast cancer. Am. J. Surg., 12:172, 1969.

Foote, F. W., and Stewart, F. W.: A histologic classification of carcinoma of the breast. Surgery, 19:74, 1946.

Geschickter, C. F.: Diseases of the Breast. Philadelphia, J. B. Lippincott, 1943, p. 386.

Haagensen, C. D.: Diseases of the Breast. Philadelphia, W. B. Saunders, 1971, p. 300.

Hafner, C. D., Mezger, E., and Wytel, J. H., Jr.: Cystosarcoma phyllodes of the breast. Surg. Gynecol. Obstet., 115:29, 1962.

Hare, H. F., and Cerny, J. J., Jr.: Soft tissue sarcoma: Review of 200 cases. Cancer, 16:1332, 1963.

Harris, M., and Persaud, V.: Carcinoma of the breast. J. Pathol., 112:99, 1974.

Herrmann, J. B., and Ariel, I. M.: Therapy of lymphangiosarcoma of the chronically edematous limb. Five year cure of a patient treated by intra-arterial radioactive yttrium. AJR, 99:393, 1967.

Hill, F. P., and Stout, A. P.: Sarcoma of the breast. Arch. Surg., 44:723, 1942.

Hinterberger, H.: Zur Kenntnis des Sarkona phyllodes lipomatodes mammae. Wien Klin. Wchnschr. 55:28, 1942.

Hofman, W. I., and Goodman, M. L.: Primary lymphosarcoma of the breast. Arch. Surg., 96:410, 1968.

Homes, R. S., and Leis, H. P., Jr.: Liposarcoma of the female breast. Review of the literature and report of a case. Ann. Geriatr. Soc. J., 10:355, 1962.

Hoover, H. C., Trestioreanu, A., and Ketcham, A. S.: Metastatic cystosarcoma phyllodes in an adolescent girl: An unusually malignant tumor. Ann. Surg., 181:279, 1975.

Hummer, C. D., Jr., and Burkart, T. J.: Liposarcoma of the breast. A case of bilateral involvement. Am. J. Surg., 113:558, 1967.

Jackson, A. V.: Metastasizing liposarcoma of the breast arising in a fibroadenoma. J. Pathol. Bacteriol., 83:502, 1962.

Jernstrom, P., Lindberg, A. L., and Meland, O. N.: Osteogenic sarcoma of the mammary gland. Am. J. Clin. Pathol., 40:521, 1963.

Kolarsick, A. J.: Primary sarcoma of the breast. J. Med. Soc. N.J., 69(3):243, 1972.

Kuten, A., Sapir, D., Cohen, Y., et al.: Postirradiation soft tissue sarcoma occurring in breast cancer patients: Report of seven cases and results of combination chemotherapy. J. Surg. Oncol., 28:168, 1985.

Ladefoged, C., and Nielsen, B. B.: Primary chondrosarcoma of the breast: A case report and review of the literature. Breast 16:26, 1984.

Langham, M. R., Mills, A. S., DeMay, R. M., et al.: Malignant fibrous histiocytoma of the breast. A case

report and review of the literature. Cancer, 54:558, 1984.
Lee, B. J., and Pack, G. T.: Giant intracanalicular fibroadenomyxoma of the breast—the so-called cystosarcoma phyllodes of Johannes Mueller. Am. J. Cancer, 15:2583, 1931.
Lester, J., and Stout, A. P.: Cystosarcoma phyllodes. Cancer, 7:335, 1954.
Liebert, C. W., Jr., and Edwards, D. K.: Malignant fibrous histiocytoma of the breast. South. Med. J., 75:1281, 1982.
Lindquist, K. D., van Heerden, J. A., Weiland, L. H., et al.: Recurrent and metastatic cystosarcoma phyllodes. Am. J. Surg., 14:341, 1982.
Lissoos, I., Schmann, A., Path, M. C., et al.: Haemangiosarcoma of the breast. S. Afr. Med. J., 43:1229, 1969.
Mambo, N. C., Burke, J. S., and Butler, J. J.: Primary malignant lymphomas of the breast. Cancer, 39:2003, 1977.
McCracken, M., Hamal, P. B., and Benson, E. A.: Granular cell myoblastoma of the breast: A report of 2 cases. Br. J. Surg., 66:819, 1979.
McCullough, K., and Lynch, J. M.: Metastatic sarcoma of heart from cystosarcoma phyllodes of the breast. Maryland State Med. J., 9:66, 1960.
McDonald, J. R., and Harrington, S. W.: Giant fibroadenoma of the breast—cystosarcoma phyllodes. Ann. Surg., 133:243, 1950.
Melander, D. W., and Pack, G. T.: Lymphosarcoma—choice of treatment and end results in 567 patients. Role of surgical treatment for cure and palliation. Rev. Surg., 20:3, 1963.
Menon, M., and van Velthoven, P. C. M.: Liposarcoma of the breast. Arch. Pathol., 98:370, 1974.
Merino, M. J., Berman, M., and Carter, D.: Angiosarcoma of the breast. Am. J. Surg. Pathol., 7:53, 1983.
Morton, D. L.: Soft tissue sarcomas. In Holland, J. F., and Frei, E. (Eds.): Cancer Medicine. Philadelphia, Lea & Febiger, 1974, p. 1845.
Neumann, E.: Beitrage zur Casuistik der Brustdrusengeschwulste. Virchows Arch. Pathol. Anat., 24:316, 1862.
van Niekerk, J. L. M., Wobbes T., Holland, R., et al.: Malignant fibrous histiocytoma of the breast with axillary lymph node involvement. J. Surg. Oncol., 34:32, 1987.
O'Brien, J. E., and Stout, A. P.: Malignant fibrous xanthomas. Cancer, 17:1445, 1964.
Oberman, H. A.: Cystosarcoma phyllodes, a clinicopathologic study of hypercellular periductal stromal neoplasm of breast. Cancer, 18:697, 1965a.
Oberman, H. A.: Sarcomas of the breast. Cancer, 18:1233, 1965b.
Owens, F. M., Jr., and Adams, W. E.: Giant intracanalicular fibroadenoma of the breast. Arch. Surg., 43:588, 1941.
Pardo-Midan, J., Garcia-Julian, G., and Altuna, M. A.: Leiomyosarcoma of the breast. Am. J. Clin. Pathol., 62:477, 1974.
Patrick, R. S., Jarvis, J., and Miln, D. C.: Hemangioblastoma of one breast—a report of three cases. Br. J. Surg., 45:188, 1957–58.
Rao, B. R., Meyer, J. S., and Fry, C. G.: Most cystosarcoma phyllodes and fibroadenomas have progesterone receptor but lack estrogen receptor: Stromal localization of progesterone receptor. Cancer, 47:2016, 1981.
Richards, W. G., and Way, R. W.: Co-existent cystosarcoma phyllodes and scirrhous adenocarcinoma of one breast. Wisconsin Med. J., 62:425, 1963.

Robb, P. M., and MacFarlane, A.: Two rare breast tumors. J. Pathol., 75:293, 1958.
Scheid, M. F., Cogan, J. E., and Waldron, G. W.: Angiosarcoma of the breast. Texas J. Med., 60:488, 1964.
Schmidt, G. B.: Ueber das Angiosarkom der Mamma. Arch. Klin. Chir., 36:421, 1887.
Schoenberg, B. S.: Multiple primary neoplasms. In Fraumeni, J. F.: Persons at high risk of cancer. New York, Academic Press, 1975, p. 103.
Shore, J. H.: Hemangiosarcoma of the breast. J. Pathol. Bacteriol. 74:289, 1957.
Schouten, J. T., Weese, J. L., and Carbone, P. P.: Lymphoma of the breast. Ann. Surg., 194:749, 1981.
Sobel, H. J., Schwartz, R., and Marguet, E.: Light- and electron-microscope study of the origin of granular-cell myoblastoma. J. Pathol., 109:101, 1972.
Sonnenblick, M., and Abraham, A. S.: Primary lymphosarcoma of the breast: Review of the literature on occurrence in elderly patients. J. Am. Geriatr. Soc., 24:225, 1976.
Stewart, F. W., and Treves, N.: Lymphangiosarcoma in postmastectomy lymphedema. A report of six cases in elephantiasis chirurgica. Cancer, 1:64, 1948.
Stout, A. P., and Bernanke, M.: Liposarcoma of the female mammary gland. Surg. Gynecol. Obstet., 83:216, 1946.
Tang, P. H., Petrelli, M., and Robechek, P. J.: Stromal sarcoma of breast. A light and electron microscopic study. Cancer, 43:209, 1979.
Teich, S., and Brecher, I. N.: Osteogenic sarcoma of the breast: A case report. Breast, 11:11, 1985.
Tong, D., and Winter, J.: Postmastectomy lymphangiosarcoma—temporary response to cyclophosphamide chemotherapy in two cases. Br. J. Surg., 61:76, 1974.
Townsend, M. C., and Stellato, T. A.: Granular cell myoblastoma of the breast: A report of five cases and a review. Breast, 11:12, 1985.
Tragus, E. T., and Wagner, D. E.: Current therapy for post mastectomy lymphangiosarcoma. Arch. Surg., 97:839, 1969.
Treves, N.: A study of cystosarcoma phyllodes. Ann. N.Y. Acad. Sci., 114:922, 1964.
Treves, N., and Sunderland, D. A.: Cystosarcoma phyllodes of the breast. Cancer, 4:1286, 1951.
Turalba, C. I. C., El-Mahdi, A. M., and Ladaga, L.: Fatal metastatic cystosarcoma phyllodes in an adolescent female: Case report and review of treatment approaches. J. Surg. Oncol., 33:176, 1986.
Umansky, C., and Bullock, W. K.: Granular cell myoblastoma of the breast. Ann. Surg., 168:810, 1968.
Visfeldt, J., and Sheike, O.: Male breast cancer. Cancer, 32:985, 1973.
Weitzner, S., Nascimento, A. G., and Scanlon, L. J.: Intramammary granular cell myoblastoma. Am. Surg., 45:34, 1979.
West, T. L., Weiland, L. H., and Clagett, O. T.: Cytosarcoma phyllodes. Ann. Surg., 173:520, 1971.
White, J. W.: Malignant variant of cystosarcoma phyllodes. Am. J. Cancer, 40:458, 1940.
Wiernik, P. H., and Serpick, A. A.: Granulocytic sarcoma (chloroma). Blood, 35:361, 1970.
Williams, B. V., and Diamonon, J.: Carcinosarcoma of the breast. South. Med. J., 57:462, 1964.
Yap, B. S., Yap, H. Y., McBride, C. M., et al.: Chemotherapy for postmastectomy lymphangiosarcoma. Cancer, 47:853, 1981.

Cancer of the Male Breast

WILLIAM L. DONEGAN

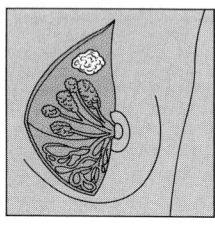

Breast cancer in men is a variant of a disease otherwise closely allied with female reproductive function. It is fundamentally identical to breast cancer in women except for being less frequent, occurring at an older age, arising regularly beneath the nipple, and being more hormonally sensitive. Cancer of the male breast was known to Fabricus Hildanus (1537–1619) and probably to earlier physicians (Meyskens et al., 1976). In an early review Wainright was able to collect 418 cases reported prior to 1927. This disorder is now documented in whites, blacks, and Orientals. The incidence is said to be highest in Britain and North America (Ajayi et al., 1982). In the United States, it accounts for 0.3 to 1.5 per cent of all cancers in men and only 0.6 to 0.9 per cent of all breast cancers. The male-to-female ratio is approximately 1:100; 1985 yielded an estimated 900 cases and 300 deaths (Silverberg, 1985). For obscure reasons, cancer of the male breast appears almost a decade later than cancer of the breast in women. In recent reports, patients were predominantly in the seventh decade of life, with median ages of 61 to 65 years (Heller et al., 1978; Yap et al., 1979; Axelsson and Andersson, 1983; Erlichman et al., 1984). In the elderly population at Ellis Fischel State Cancer Hospital (EFSCH), the average age of 27 men with breast cancer was 71.2 years, 10.6 years greater than the average age of 2370 women with the disease (Donegan and Perez-Mesa, 1973). Ages nevertheless range from 25 years to 93 years, and the disease has been reported in a 5 year old boy (Crichlow, 1972). It is sufficiently rare in the young that no average annual age-specific incidence rate for individuals under 30 years of age was provided by the Third National Cancer Survey in the United States. The incidence rises from 0.1 per 100,000 population at ages 30 to 34 years to 6.5 at 85 years and older.

In addition to age, ethnicity may be important. In a case-control study, Mabuchi and coworkers (1985) found Jewish men at higher risk than United States white men of other religions. A number of additional risk factors were suspected. An antigen related to the mouse mammary tumor virus (MMTV) has been found in the breast cancers of men, as it has in women, providing evidence for viral causation (Lloyd et al., 1983). Ionizing irradiation is a known carcinogen for the female breast, and previous exposure to irradiation has been observed in eight cases of male breast cancer (Thompson et al., 1979). Most men were exposed to radiation as children or in early adulthood, variously for thymic enlargement, lymphoma, prepubertal gynecomastia, eczema, and osteogenic sarcoma. Breast cancers were diagnosed after intervals of 12 to 36 years. A familial tendency is difficult to document, although a number of observations suggest it. Breast cancer in sisters or mothers of men with breast cancer has been observed in 11 per cent of cases, approximately the same as expected for female patients (Donegan and Perez-Mesa, 1973). Marger and associates (1975) reported two brothers with breast cancer, and Everson and associates (1976) observed two families in which several men had the disease. Two instances in which both father and son were affected have been observed (Schwartz et al., 1980). Interestingly, transmission via the male line can be demonstrated in rodents. The case for endogenous or exogenous estrogen stimulation is intriguing, but evidence is fragmentary. Dao and associates (1973) found increased urinary excretion of all fractions of estrogens in seven men with breast cancer when compared with controls. Hyperestrogenism was found in a man who developed bilateral breast cancer after treatment for a hypophyseal tumor (Olsson et al., 1984). Other authors failed to confirm abnormal estrogen metabolism (Scheike et al., 1973). Srinivasan and coworkers (1979) collected eight cases through 1979 in which male breast cancer was associated with estrogen administration. A report exists of breast cancer in two men who had transsexual operations and estrogen therapy (Symmers, 1968). These cases and another following orchiectomy and estrogen administration (Howard and Grosjean, 1949) are remarkably analogous to mammary cancer in male rats, which can be produced with castration and estrogen administration. Cancer of the breast occurs in men treated with estrogens for prostatic cancer but is rare. The reduced longevity of these patients may prevent more convincing expression of a carcinogenic effect (Wolloch and Dintsman, 1973). Metastases to the breast from prostatic cancer constituted a potential source of confusion in the past. However, they usually are accompanied by metastases to other sites and can be identified by testing for tissue acid phosphatase. Increased estrogen excretion is not characteristic of Klinefelter's syndrome, but other features of feminization are present, and men with this syndrome have a high frequency of breast cancer. Three of 21 men with breast cancer were found to have the rare Klinefelter's syndrome (XXY sex chromosomes, gynecomastia, and hypogonadism) by Dodge and colleagues (1969), who estimated the associated risk for breast cancer to be 66.5 times the usual risk for men. This risk may be exaggerated, however, as in recent reports Klinefelter's syndrome is not prominent. One case was seen among 50 male breast cancers at the University of Rochester (Ouriel et al., 1984). None was mentioned in five other reports since 1978 totaling 357 cases (Heller et al., 1978; Yap et al., 1979; Axelsson and Andersson, 1983; Vercoutere and O'Connell, 1984; Erlichman et al., 1984). Nevertheless, men with Klinefelter's syndrome should be cautioned, and karyotyping men with breast cancer will increase the fund of available information.

Although gynecomastia is not a regular accompaniment of male breast cancer, it is often present clinically and is found in association with the disease in up to 40 per cent of cases when looked for microscopically (Heller et al., 1978). No direct evolution to malignant epithelium has been observed, and the case for gynecomastia as a precancerous change is uncertain. Coincidence is possible, as many asymptomatic adult men have gynecomastia on careful clinical examination (36 per cent in one study), and the prevalence increases with age (Nuttall, 1979).

A history of trauma to the breast is often reported by men, but the relevance is not clear. A case-control study reported by Kessler found that, compared with controls, men with breast cancer had more often graduated from college and held professional or managerial positions, had a history of gynecomastia, mumps, orchitis, testicular injury, and undescended testes, and had married at older ages and failed to have children, most of which suggests an association with hormonal factors (Lin and Kessler, 1980).

Clinical Features

The presenting signs and symptoms of cancer in the male breast are similar to those of cancer in the female breast, with a few exceptions (Table 28–1). In a comparison of the author's 27 cases with 2320 cases of breast cancer in women between 1940 and 1965, men were older, more often reported preceding trauma to the breast, more often had ulceration of the skin or areola (31.6 per cent versus 11.1 per cent) or cutaneous satellites (20 per cent versus 7.6 per cent), and more often had grave local signs or dissemination at presentation (Donegan and Perez-Mesa, 1973). Because of their

Table 28–1. INITIAL SIGNS AND SYMPTOMS OF MALE BREAST CANCER

	Frequency
Palpable mass	43–87%
Ulceration of nipple	8–15%
Ulceration of skin	9%
Nipple retraction	8–31%
Bloody nipple discharge	7–10%
Nonbloody nipple discharge	4–9%
Local pain	5–16%
Growth of a mass	18%
Inflammatory changes	8%
Skin nodules	3%
Axillary mass	2–5%
General breast swelling	4%
Painful breast mass	2%
Itching of nipple	2%
Bone pain	0–2%

Data from Heller et al., 1978; Robison and Montague, 1982; Axelsson and Andersson, 1983; Ouriel et al., 1984; Patel et al., 1984.

older age, men often have other associated problems, such as renal or heart disease, diabetes, or hypertension. Most researchers relate that men sought medical attention later than women, although the author's cases do not confirm this. Median delays of up to 12 months are reported. A slight predominance is found in the left breast, as also occurs in women, and rarely both breasts are involved. It is unusual for the disease to be found on routine physical examination, probably because the breasts of men are not always examined carefully.

A mass is palpable in almost 90 per cent of cases. Unlike the case with women, a subareolar mass is the characteristic presentation in men, as this is where the vestigial breast tissue is located. In one report, the tumor was beneath the areola in 76 per cent of cases, in the upper outer quadrant in 6 per cent, in the upper inner quadrant in 4 per cent, and in the lower inner quadrant in 2 per cent (Ouriel et al., 1984). Occasionally, a nipple discharge is associated with the cancer and may be the only sign of trouble. It may or may not be bloody. Occult cases have been reported that were manifested only with axillary adenopathy. Nipple attachment, ulceration, and fascial fixation are often present, possibly owing to the small size of the breast and delayed consultation (Fig. 28–1). Signs of inflammation can be seen.

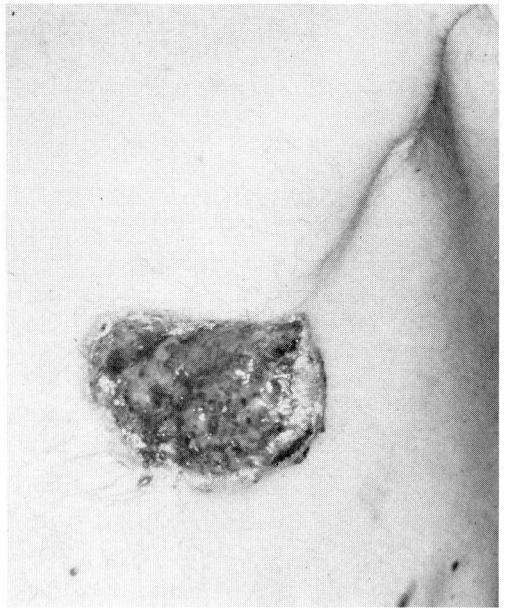

Figure 28–1. Locally advanced breast cancer in a 59 year old man that has destroyed the nipple and become attached to the pectoral fascia. Local advancement is a frequent finding in males.

Twenty-six cases of Paget's disease involving the male areola were reported through 1981 (Ding and De-Yan, 1981). The differential diagnosis of a subareolar mass must include gynecomastia, which is virtually the only other lesion that is manifested in men as a subareolar mass. Gynecomastia is usually tender on palpation and never ulcerates the areola. It is usually bilateral and typical, but when it is unilateral it may require a biopsy to differentiate it from cancer (Fig. 28–2). Adenoma of the nipple is a rare benign lesion that can occur in men and be confused with carcinoma, but a biopsy with paraffin sections permits a correct diagnosis (Richards et al., 1973).

Axillary adenopathy was found in 54 per cent of Crichlow and associates' collected cases (1972). It is generally acknowledged that clinical assessment of the axilla is not completely reliable, being correct in only about 68 to 74 per cent of male patients, falsely negative in 18 to 37 per cent, and falsely positive in 8 to 21 per cent (Heller et al., 1978; Ouriel et al., 1984). Hard supraclavicular nodes are reliable signs of further progression. Bone pain suggests osseous metastases, and a cough may mean pulmonary metastases or pleural effusion.

Histology

Both carcinomas and sarcomas arise in the male breast. The former constitute at least 96 per cent of cases, and all histologic types are seen (Gupta et al., 1981; Yap et al., 1979; Erlichman et al., 1984; Vercoutere and O'Connell, 1984). The male breast ordinarily lacks lobules, although it may form them in response to prolonged estrogen treatment. As a consequence, lobular carcinoma is said not to occur in the male breast, but a single case was reported by Vercoutere and O'Connell (1984) among 45 men with breast cancer and another by Sanchez et al. (1986) in a man with Klinefelter's syndrome. Infiltrating ductal carcinomas constitute from 87 to 98 per cent of all carcinomas, making them by far the most frequent; their histologic grade correlates with prognosis. As among women, the less frequent types of carcinoma constitute 9 to 16 per cent of cases. Noninvasive ductal carcinomas and papillary carcinomas each constitute up to 7 per cent of cases, whereas medullary, tubular, and mucinous carcinomas account for no more than 1 per cent each. Paget's disease of the

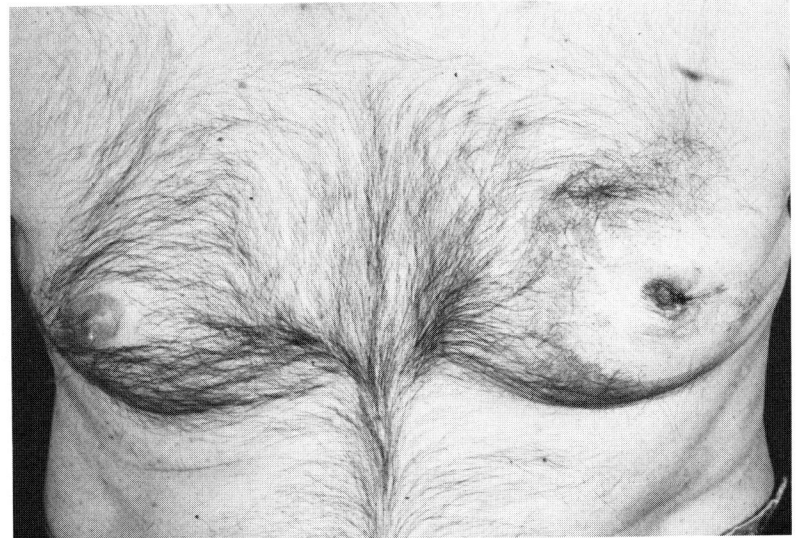

Figure 28–2. Cancer of the left breast associated with bilateral gynecomastia. The firm tumor is in a typical location beneath the nipple, which it has invaded and retracted. A suture marks the site of biopsy. Gynecomastia is often associated with breast cancer in males and is usually bilateral (see Yap et al., 1979).

nipple occurs in 1.5 per cent of men with breast cancer. Inflammatory carcinoma occasionally is seen in men, with implications similar to those in women, but dermal lymphatic invasion is not always clearly established. Metastases in axillary lymph nodes are frequent, found in up to 65 per cent of men who have axillary dissections. The probability of involvement is directly related to the size of the primary tumor (Heller et al., 1978). As almost all tumors are located centrally, internal mammary nodes might be expected to be at high risk for metastases, but this is not documented.

Sarcomas are infrequent but a variety of types are reported. Cystosarcomas are sometimes seen (Reingold and Ascher, 1970; Pantoja et al., 1976). Fibrosarcomas and leiomyosarcomas predominate, but neurogenic sarcomas and lymphosarcomas also occur. Panettiere (1974) reported a liposarcoma, and Yadaw and associates (1976) reported an angiosarcoma. Sarcomas spread hematogenously, infrequently metastasizing to the axillary lymph nodes.

Second Cancers

There seems to be little tendency for the second breast in men to develop an independent primary cancer, a notable departure from the relatively frequent occurrence (7 to 10 per cent) in women. Fewer than 1 per cent of men have had bilateral primary tumors in recent reports, and only 4 per cent or less eventually had bilateral cancer (Heller et al., 1978; Yap et al., 1979). The fact that fewer men are cured of their first cancers to remain at risk for a second may account for the lower frequency of bilaterality. In women it is observed that this problem is directly related to good prognosis and longevity.

As many as 21 per cent of men have second nonmammary cancers either before or after the diagnosis of breast cancer (Holleb et al., 1968; Crichlow, 1972; Scheike, 1973; Yap et al., 1979). They tend to reflect endemic risks. Cancers of the skin, large bowel, and prostate are most frequent. Almost 20 per cent of Scheike's 26 patients (1973) with a second cancer had cancer of the stomach, an unusually high frequency of this neoplasm. Only 6 per cent of one series in the United States had stomach cancer (Vanderbilt and Warren, 1971), which raises the possibility that some "gastric cancers" might be metastases from the breast. Despite the high rate of lung cancer in the United States, a concurrence would not be expected because of its high lethality as well as the advanced status of most breast cancers in men. There is little to suggest that men with breast cancer are unusually prone to cancer in any other organ system. Yap and associates (1979) reported that the patients who developed secondary nonmammary primary cancers were older than those who did not, and more often they had a family history of both mammary and nonmammary cancers.

Mastectomy

The evaluation and staging of male breast cancer is similar to that in women, although karyotyping and estrogen excretion studies are usually added. Up to 15 per cent have initially had distant metastases, and therefore a chest radiograph, tests of liver function, and a bone scan are appropriate for staging purposes. Mammograms are also obtained.

For early cases, radical mastectomy has been the rule in the past, but modified mastectomy is replacing it. Perhaps earlier diagnosis and the results of clinical trials in women showing comparable cure rates are influencing this change. The trend is evident in three reports, which show that modified mastectomy was used for 9 per cent of cases treated between 1949 and 1976 (Erlichman et al., 1984), in 40 per cent between 1961 and 1981 (Ouriel et al., 1984), and in 54 per cent between 1967 and 1981 (Heller et al., 1978). In the study of Heller and coworkers, only 18 per cent of the patients had a radical mastectomy. In a retrospective study, Ouriel and coworkers (1984) found no significant difference in 5 year survival between 19 men with Stage I and Stage II cancer treated with radical mastectomy (76 per cent) and 18 men treated with modified mastectomy (80 per cent). The same was found by Hodson and colleagues (1985) among potentially curable cases, although 5 year survivals were lower (i.e., 44 and 43 per cent, respectively). Patients deemed unable to tolerate major surgery, or those with locally advanced tumor, usually are managed with simple mastectomy or local excision combined with postoperative irradiation to the chest wall and regional nodes (Robison and Montague, 1982).

A frequent observation is that men fare more poorly than women, particularly in the presence of metastases in axillary lymph nodes, but the evidence is growing that cancer of the male breast is as curable when the disease is of comparable stage. The poor record of the past is attributable largely to the advanced age and stage of most cases. Scheike (1973) documented that cases had become clinically more favorable in Denmark when those seen during 1943 to 1957 were compared with those seen between 1958 and 1972. TNM Stages I and II among 253 patients had increased from 39 per cent to 53 per cent, and Stage IV had decreased from 18 per cent to 5 per cent.

Factors that have an important influence on prognosis are histologic features, the size of the tumor, the presence or absence of metastases in axillary lymph nodes, and the pathologic stage of the disease (Fig. 28–3). The patient's age and the presence of gynecomastia have no significant influence. In a large series reported by Spence and coworkers (1985), neither the location of the tumor, postoperative hormone therapy, postoperative irradiation, or type of local surgery influenced prognosis. Men with noninvasive ductal cancers and intracystic papillary carcinomas have excellent prospects for cure; recurrence is unusual (Heller et al., 1978; Axelsson and Andersson, 1983). The nonductal special histologic types, such as medullary, colloid, and papillary carcinomas, have a prognosis more favorable than that of the ductal type. Yap and coworkers found median survivals closely correlated with the size of invasive

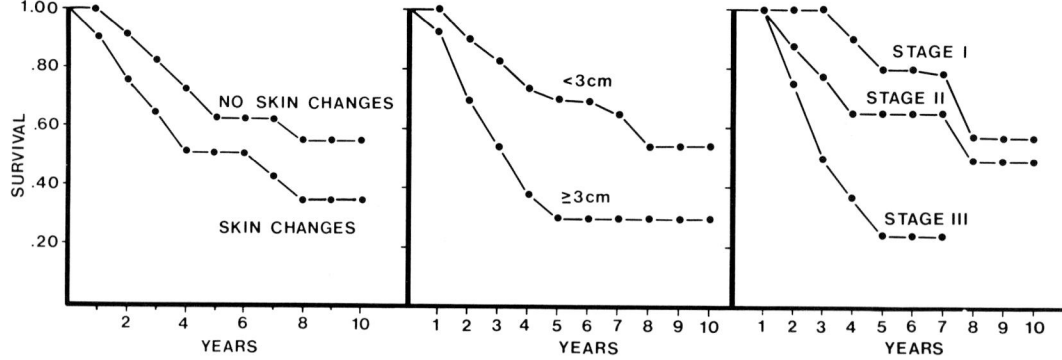

From Ouriel et al 1984

Figure 28–3. Survival of males with breast cancer. (From Ouriel, K., et al.: Prognostic factors of carcinoma of the male breast. Surg. Gynecol. Obstet., *159*:373, 1984. Reprinted with permission.)

ductal carcinomas (i.e., 59.8 months for 2 cm or less, 50.8 months for 2 to 5 cm, and 15 months for greater than 5 cm (Yap et al., 1979). Corresponding 5 year survival rates were 53 per cent, 44 per cent, and 25 per cent.

It can be demonstrated that clinical stage (TNM) correlates well with prognosis. Among 214 cases collected by Crichlow (1976), 5 and 10 year survival rates after all treatments were as follows: Stage I, 58 per cent and 38 per cent; Stage II, 38 per cent and 10 per cent; Stage III, 29 per cent and 9 per cent; and Stage IV, 4 per cent and 0 per cent.

The most important prognosticator among surgically treated patients is the presence of axillary metastases. The 5 and 10 year survival rates of 143 patients collected by Crichlow (1976) were 79 per cent and 62 per cent for those without axillary metastases, as opposed to a much reduced 28 per cent and 4.3 per cent for those with metastases. More recent reports in Table 28–2 provide survival ranges based on stage and axillary nodal status. The extent of axillary involvement contributes to the variable results in small series, but prognoses based on quantitations of nodal involvement are not available.

Thirty-one (57 per cent) of 54 men treated specifically with radical mastectomy in three series, including the author's (Cortese and Cornell, 1970; Crichlow et al., 1972; Donegan and Perez-Mesa, 1973), all of whom had been at risk for at least 5 years, survived the period; 42 per cent of 24 patients with axillary metastases survived 5 years, as did 84 per cent of 25 patients without such metastases.

In the surgical management of men with breast cancer, it is fair to say that modified radical mastectomy is now the surgical procedure most appropriate for those with relatively small tumors that spare the pectoralis major muscle and that are associated with limited axillary involvement. The improved appearance over radical mastectomy is welcome, and the stronger arm it leaves is an advantage for the working man. Segmental resection combined with axillary dissection and high dose irradiation has proved the equal of modified mastectomy for women in selected cases, but comparability in men is not demonstrated, and the central location of tumors in men detracts from its cosmetic advantage.

Adjuvant Therapy

Postoperative irradiation to the chest wall and unremoved regional lymph nodes has often been used to supplement mastectomies in the treatment of men, particularly in cases in which there are signs of local advancement or with proven axillary metastases, for which prognosis is poor. It is clear that the result is to decrease recurrence in the fields of treatment, rather than effecting an improvement in survival and probably should be reserved for those at high risk for local recurrence (Erlichman et al., 1984).

The success of adjuvant chemotherapy in women translates to men with some uncertainty. It is reasonable to consider adjuvant chemotherapy for men with metastases in axillary lymph nodes, but the fund of available information is fragmentary and inconclusive (Ouriel et al., 1984; Vercoutere and O'Connell, 1984). Nevertheless, because the majority of recurrences in men (79 per cent according to Yap and colleagues [1979]) are at distant sites and because prospective studies in males are unlikely, many clinicians support the use of adjuvant chemotherapy or hormonochemotherapy with the same indications as in women (Yap et al., 1979; Erlichman et al., 1984; Vercoutere and O'Connell, 1984). Bagley et al. (1987) treated 24 males with axillary metastases with 12 cycles of adjuvant cyclophosphamide, methotrexate, and 5-fluorouracil (CMF). None received postoperative irradiation. Four patients had disease recurrence, and the 5-year actuarial survival was projected at 90 per cent, much higher than ordinarily expected. Adjuvant tamoxifen was used to

Table 28–2. SURVIVAL OF MEN WITH BREAST CANCER

	Survival	
TNM Stage	**5 Year**	**10 Year**
TIS	88–100%	
Stage I	75–100%	57–89%
Stage II	63–75%	12%
Stage III	25–43%	
Stage IV	0%	
Axillary Metastases		
Absent	77–90%	79%
Present	38%	11%
Overall	42–72%	2–50%

Data from Heller et al., 1978; Robison and Montague, 1982; Axelsson and Andersson, 1983; Ouriel et al., 1984; Patel et al., 1984.

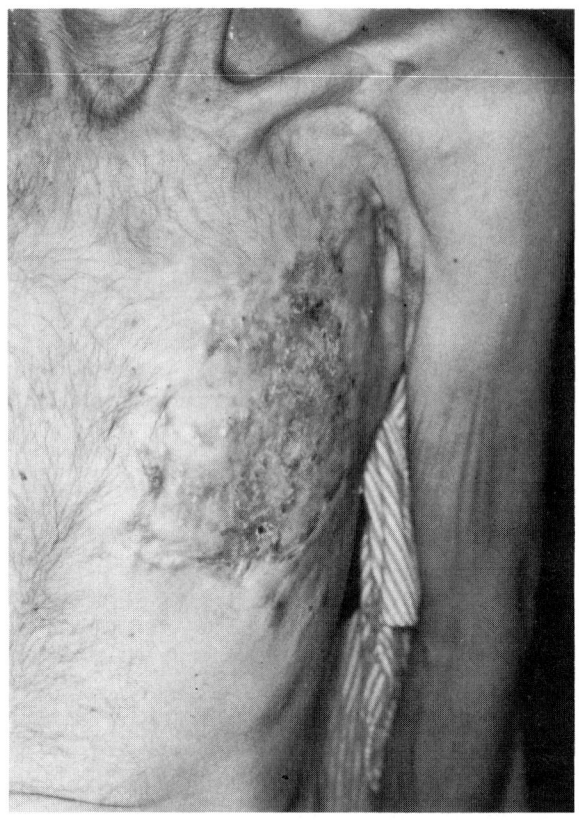

Figure 28–4. This case illustrates extensive local cutaneous recurrence of carcinoma following treatment with radical mastectomy. Although mastectomy is the treatment of choice for potentially localized carcinoma of the male breast, the relatively advanced status of most tumors contributes to a high failure rate after surgical treatment. Adjuvant irradiation in selected cases can help to reduce this problem. Local failures can also be treated by irradiation with good effect.

treat 23 men with pathologic Stage II and Stage III breast cancers after surgery and irradiation at the Christie Hospital and Holt Radium Institute in Manchester, U.K. (Ribeiro, 1985). The 5-year survival of 55 per cent was improved over the historical 28 per cent.

Recurrence and Dissemination of Male Breast Cancer

The initial locations of distant metastases are similar to those of women, with bone, lungs, and lymph nodes being the principal sites (Erlichman et al., 1984). Seventy-one cases reported by Huggins and Taylor (1955) were distributed as follows: bone, 23; lungs and pleura, 16; supraclavicular lymph nodes, 12; liver, 7; brain, 3; and other, 10. Fifty-five per cent of the cases reported by Treves (1959) had initial metastasis to bones, followed in order by lymph nodes in 21.4 per cent, lungs in 19 per cent, skin in 14 per cent, and soft tissues in 5 per cent. Bone metastases are most often lytic but may also be blastic. Median survival after recurrence is approximately 22 months (Heller et al., 1978). Twenty per cent of Erlichman and associates' patients (1984) lived 5 years. Local-regional recurrence usually indicates incurability, but with further treatment, ordinarily irradiation, survival times can range from 4 to 92 months (Robison and Montague, 1982) (Fig. 28–4).

Endocrine Ablations

The endocrine responsiveness of male breast cancer has been known since 1942, when Farrow and Adair demonstrated reduction in size of an advanced primary cancer and recalcification of osteolytic metastases after castration of a 72 year old man. Subsequently, bilateral adrenalectomy (Huggins and Bergenstal, 1952) and hypophysectomy (Luft et al., 1956) proved effective in temporarily reversing the progress of this cancer. Bilateral orchiectomy, bilateral adrenalectomy, and hypophysectomy have produced regression of metastases in bone, lungs, skin, and lymph nodes as well as reduction of osseous pain.

In general, endocrine ablations have proved more effective in men than in women, but the critical hormonal changes involved remain uncertain. Endocrine ablation is the primary method of management for disseminated carcinoma of the male breast; orchiectomy has been considered the appropriate initial procedure although recently tamoxifen has had increasing use as an alternative. Erlichman and coworkers (1984) found no correlation between disease-free interval and the likeliness of benefit from castration, but this was not the experience of Kraybill and associates (1981), who observed increased success after 12 months. In contrast to women, the success of castration in men is not age-related. Metastases are seldom found in testes, in contrast with the approximately 25 per cent occurrence in the ovaries of women.

Orchiectomy produces tumor regressions in 45 to 88 per cent of cases, with durations averaging 16 to 29 months (Fig. 28–5) (Neifield et al., 1976). In four reports since 1981 totaling 62 orchiectomies, the overall response rate was 45 per cent (Kraybill et al., 1981; Erlichman et al., 1984; Ouriel et al., 1984; Patel et al., 1984). Meyskens and associates (1976) reviewed the endocrine treatment of male breast cancer and defined a response as disappearance of all lesions lasting 3 months or longer. Using this criterion 67 per cent of 70 collected evaluable patients responded to orchiectomy, with a median response duration of 22 months. Median survival of responders and nonresponders from the time of primary diagnosis

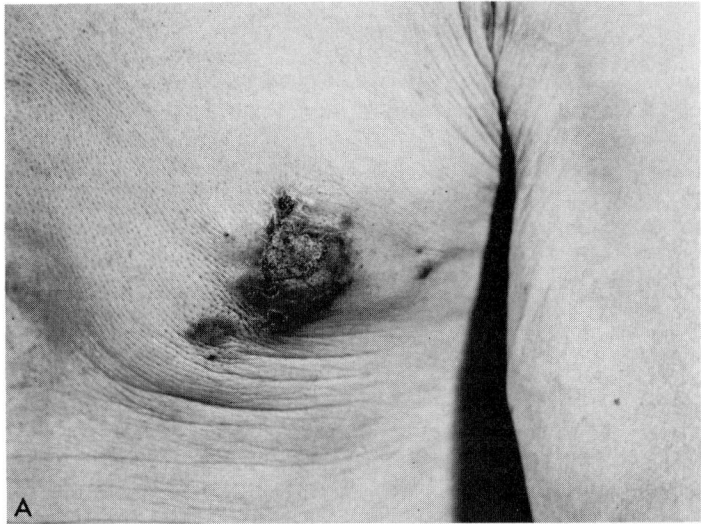

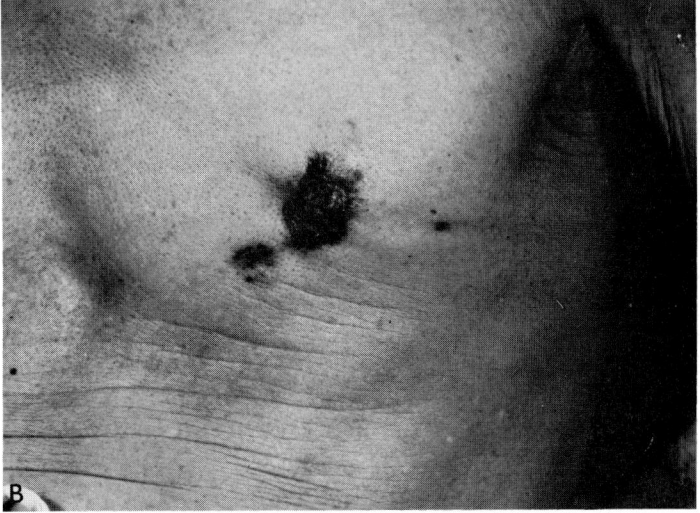

Figure 28–5. This advanced cancer of the breast (A) had destroyed the areola and produced cutaneous satellite nodules. It responded to orchiectomy with the partial regression (B) 3 months later. Bilateral orchiectomy frequently provides successful palliation, more often than does oophorectomy for females, and, in contrast to the latter, its success is not age dependent.

was 56 months versus 38 months. Nineteen of 25 patients treated with adrenalectomy responded to the procedure, four of whom had not benefited from a previous castration. The response to adrenalectomy had a mean duration of 32 months if an earlier castration had been helpful; if not, the duration was shorter. Thus, a total of 76 per cent of individuals treated with adrenalectomy had complete responses of 3 months' duration or longer. Men can respond to adrenalectomy despite a failure of orchiectomy (Li et al., 1970), but an earlier response to castration enhances the probability of success of a secondary ablation. Among 17 evaluable patients collected from the literature who had had hypophysectomies, 10 responders (60 per cent) were found, and the median duration of response was 20 months. A short disease-free interval, that is, less than 24 months, does not preclude a good response (Izuo et al., 1972; Stephens and Muggia, 1974).

Although the experience with estrogen receptors (ER) in men is far less than with women, positive levels of ER appear to be a worthwhile guide for hormone and endocrine therapy. The tumors of men are frequently positive for estrogen receptors. In some reports, 80 per cent or more had ER positive tumors (Gupta et al., 1980; Friedman et al., 1981). This is in contrast with approximately 60 per cent positivity in women measured similarly. It has been suggested that men's lower estrogen environment leaves receptor sites more often available for binding. The quantitative levels of ER, however, are not notably higher. The fact that so few men are ER negative diminishes but does not negate the value of this test; the limited information available indicates that high rates of response follow endocrine therapy in ER positive patients. In two reports, two of three and four of five men with disseminated ER positive tumors responded to orchiectomy (Gupta et al., 1980; Patel et al., 1984). In another, two of four patients with ER positive tumors responded to endocrine manipulations (Ouriel et al., 1984). Two ER positive patients both responded to adrenalectomy, according to Patel and coworkers (1984). Important information is almost nonexistent on the response rates of men with ER negative cancers, and although cytoplasmic progesterone receptors are often present (in six of nine patients in one report), their influence on tumor responsiveness or on prognosis remains to be determined (Pegoraro et al., 1982).

Hormone Therapy

Hormone therapy has had increasing importance in the palliative treatment of male breast cancer since the introduction of the antiestrogen agent tamoxifen. This agent has proved highly successful in producing tumor regression, and this fact, combined with the reluctance of men to accept orchiectomy, has prompted some authors to advocate tamoxifen as the most appropriate initial endocrine manipulation, replacing orchiectomy (Becher et al., 1981; Pegoraro et al., 1982). Patterson and associates (1986) reported an objective response rate of 48 per cent to treatment with tamoxifen in 31 patients, with an additional five patients exhibiting stabilization. In 33 additional cases summarized from four reports, tamoxifen produced tumor regressions in 51 per cent of patients, with durations of 5 to 60 months and a median of 21 months (Becher et al., 1981; Ribeiro, 1983; Hilliard et al., 1984; Patel et al., 1984). Metastases in soft tissues, bones, liver, and lungs have shown regression. Tamoxifen has been effective in patients without orchiectomy, after orchiectomy failure or progression, and after adrenalectomy. Complete and partial responses are approximately equally distributed (Ribeiro, 1983). Hilliard and associates (1984) reported an objective response to tamoxifen of 17 months' duration of an ER positive tumor that was unaffected by orchiectomy. As in women, it appears that ER positive tumors may respond to secondary endocrine manipulation when the initial one proves ineffective. Orchiectomy can still prove effective after a period of benefit from tamoxifen followed by relapse (Aisner et al., 1979).

Two of 14 patients treated with estrogens by Treves (1959) responded for 2 and for 7 months. Regressions were limited to metastases in soft tissues and lung. The author's experience is somewhat better; osseous and soft tissue metastases regressed for 16 to 25 months in two of five cases treated with estrogens (Donegan and Perez-Mesa, 1973).

A complete response of pulmonary metastases to buserelin has been reported (Vorobiof and Falkson, 1987). This potent analogue of luteinizing hormone–releasing hormone (LHRH) causes androgen deprivation by paradoxically inhibiting the pituitary gonadal axis. The effects are reversible, and it is easily administered by nasal spray. Side effects include hot flushes, weight gain, and decreased libido.

Progesterones were identified as potentially useful for men with breast cancer by Geller and colleagues (1961), who reported a response in one case to 17α-hydroxyprogesterone caproate (Delalutin). Subsequently, Kennedy and Kiang (1972) used estrogen combined with progesterone in one case with good effect and suggested that this combination be used in advance of chemotherapy. Subsequently, a number of progesterone preparations have shown activity against male breast cancer. These have included cyproterone acetate, medroxyprogesterone (Provera), megestrol acetate, and combinations of Provera and stilbestrol as well as combinations of Provera and prednisolone. Eight of 12 patients collected from recent reports responded positively to these agents (Kraybill et al., 1981; Lopez and Barduagni, 1982; Patel et al., 1984). Mitsuyasu and colleagues (1981) observed regression of a pulmonary metastasis on megestrol (40 mg orally four times daily) after orchiectomy relapse of an estrogen receptor positive tumor. In women, megestrol is often effective for tamoxifen relapses (Ross et al., 1982).

In the past, androgens have been considered contraindicated for carcinoma of the male breast, largely on the basis of a few early experiences in which they appeared to aggravate the disease. Farrow and Adair (1942) observed such an event in one case, as did Huggins and Taylor (1955) in two cases. A response to androgens was reported by Donegan and Perez-Mesa (1973) when cutaneous metastases at a mastectomy site in a 72 year old man regressed on treatment with fluoxymesterone (Halotestin), 10 mg orally three times daily. The benefit lasted 16 months. Subsequently, Horn and Roof (1976) observed responses in two cases to the androgen calusterone. Responses to androgen therapy were also observed in a review of experience with metastatic male breast cancer at the M.D. Anderson Hospital and Tumor Institute, Houston (Kantarjian et al., 1983).

Adrenal suppression with aminoglutethimide was used successfully in one case by Patel and coworkers (1984) following orchiectomy failure. On progression the patient also responded to adrenalectomy.

Adrenocorticosteroids (prednisone, cortisone) often produce a sense of well-being and are indicated specifically for the management of symptomatic intracranial metastases and hypercalcemia. Remission of osseous and pulmonary metastases for brief durations was observed in three of five cases by Treves and Holleb (1955) during treatment with corticosteroids.

Chemotherapy

In view of the frequent and substantial benefit men obtain from endocrine therapy, chemotherapy has a secondary role in palliation. With more information on estrogen receptors, however, it may become apparent that patients lacking tumor estrogen receptors are best treated initially with chemotherapy. Cancer of the male breast yields to agents known to be useful for mammary carcinoma of women. Drug combinations are probably more often effective than are single agents, with soft tissue, lung, and bone metastases most responsive to treatment. Meyskens and associates (1976) reviewed four cases, in which chemotherapy proved of value in three patients. Painful osseous metastases initially responded subjectively to a course of fluorouracil for 18 months. Recurrent pain was then palliated for an additional 5 months with courses of methotrexate and thiotepa repeated every 6 to 8 weeks. A second patient with osseous metastases failed to benefit from the same course of methotrexate and thiotepa. Objective regression of pulmonary lesions, lymph nodes, and skin nodules for a period of 14 months was observed in a third patient treated with cyclophosphamide (Cytoxan). The final patient responded with reduction of cutaneous, nodal, and bony metastases for 12 months to combination chemotherapy with Cytoxan, doxorubicin hydrochloride (Adriamycin), and fluorouracil (CAF). Chlorambucil has also been of value (Holleb et al., 1968). Vercoutere and O'Connell (1984) reported "good" responses to combination chemotherapy in five of eight cases (63 per cent); cyclophosphamide, methotrexate, and fluorouracil (CMF) were used in four cases and cyclophenylamide, vincristine (Oncovin), methotrexate, and prednisone were used in another. Fifty per cent of eight cases reported by Ouriel and coworkers (1984) responded to CMF or CAF. Kraybill and associates reported that four cases in 11 treated with various agents responded with complete regressions (25 per cent) or partial regression (75 per cent) for 7 to 32 months. The successful agents were Cytoxan plus prednisone; Cytoxan, fluorouracil, and prednisone (CFP); and leukeran.

Summary

Cancer of the male breast is infrequent but not rare. In contrast to women, men with breast cancer are older and have more advanced disease at presentation. The disease is biologically similar, however, and in comparable circumstances, the cancer in men is probably equally curable. Mastectomy is the mainstay of treatment. The tumor is sensitive to irradiation and often responds to endocrine and hormone therapy, making the latter exceptionally useful for palliation of systemic metastases. Chemotherapy can also be beneficial.

REFERENCES

Aisner, J., Ross, D. D., and Wiernik, P. H.: Tamoxifen in advanced male breast cancer. Arch. Intern. Med., 139:480, 1979.
Ajayi, D. O. S., Osegbe, D. N., and Ademiluyi, S. A.: Carcinoma of the male breast in West Africans and a review of world literature. Cancer, 50:1664, 1982.
Axelsson, J., and Andersson, A.: Cancer of the male breast. World J. Surg., 7:281, 1983.
Bagley, C. S., Wesley, M. N., Young, R. C., and Lippman, M. E.: Adjuvant chemotherapy in males with cancer of the breast. Am. J. Clin. Oncol., 10:55, 1987.
Becher, R., Hoffken, K., Page, H., et al.: Tamoxifen treatment before orchiectomy in advanced breast cancer in men. N. Engl. J. Med., 305:169, 1981.
Cortese, A. F., and Cornell, G. N.: Carcinoma of the male breast. Ann. Surg., 173:275, 1971.
Crichlow, R. W.: Carcinoma of the male breast. Surg. Gynecol. Obstet., 134:1011, 1972.
Crichlow, R. W.: Breast cancer in males. Breast, 2:12, 1976.
Crichlow, R. W., Kaplan, E. L., and Kearney, W. H.: Male mammary cancer: An analysis of 32 cases. Ann. Surg., 175:489, 1972.
Dao, T. L., Morreal, C., and Nemoto, T.: Urinary estrogen excretion in men with breast cancer. N. Engl. J. Med., 289:138, 1973.
Ding, W., and De-Yan, W.: Paget's disease of the male breast: A report of five cases and a collective review. Jpn. J. Clin. Oncol., 11:513, 1981.
Dodge, O. G., Jackson, A. W., and Muldal, S.: Breast cancer and interstitial cell tumor in a patient with Klinefelter's syndrome. Cancer, 24:1027, 1969.
Donegan, W. L., and Perez-Mesa, C. M.: Carcinoma of the male breast. A 30-year review of 28 cases. Arch. Surg., 106:273, 1973.
Erlichman, C., Murphy, K. C., and Elhakim, T.: Male breast cancer: A 13-year review of 89 patients. J. Clin. Oncol., 2:903, 1984.
Everson, R. B., Li, F. P., Fraumen, J. F., et al.: Familial breast cancer. Lancet, 1:9, 1976.
Farrow, J. H., and Adair, F. E.: Effect of orchidectomy on skeletal metastases from cancer of the male breast. Science, 95:654, 1942.
Friedman, M. A., Hoffman, P. G., Jr., Dandolos, E. M., et al.: Estrogen receptors in male breast cancer: Clinical and pathologic correlations. Cancer, 47:134, 1981.
Geller, J., Volk, H., and Lewin, M.: Objective remission of metastatic breast carcinoma in a male who received 17-alpha hydroxy progesterone caproate (Delalutin). Cancer Chemother. Rep., 14:77, 1961.
Gupta, N., Cohen, J. L., Rosenbaum, C., and Raam, S.: Estrogen receptors in male breast cancer. Cancer, 46:1781, 1980.
Gupta, S., Pant, G. C., and Gupta, S.: Male breast cancer. J. Surg. Oncol., 16:149, 1981.
Heller, K. S., Rosen, P. P., Schottenfeld, D., et al.: Male breast cancer: A clinicopathologic study of 97 cases. Ann. Surg., 188:60, 1978.
Hilliard, D. A., Wilbur, D. W., and Camacho, E. S.: Tamoxifen response following no response to orchiectomy in metastatic male breast cancer: A case report. J. Surg. Oncol., 25:42, 1984.
Hodson, G. R., Urdaneta, L. F., Al-Jurf, A. S., et al.: Male breast carcinoma. Am. Surg. 51:47, 1985.
Holleb, A. I., Freeman, H. P., and Farrow, J. H.: Cancer of male breast. I and II. N.Y. State J. Med., 68:544, 656, 1968.
Horn, Y., and Roof, B.: Male breast cancer: Two cases with objective regressions from calusterone (7α, 17β-dimethyltestosterone) after failure of orchiectomy. Oncology, 33:188, 1976.
Howard, R. R., and Grosjean, W. A.: Bilateral mammary carcinoma in the male coincident with prolonged stilbestrol therapy. Surgery, 25:399, 1949.
Huggins, C., Jr., and Bergenstal, D. M.: Inhibition of human mammary and prostatic cancer by adrenalectomy. Cancer Res., 12:134, 1952.
Huggins, C., Jr., and Taylor, G. W.: Carcinoma of the male breast. Arch. Surg., 70:303, 1955.
Izuo, M., Ishida, T., and Fujimori, M.: Carcinoma of the male breast with metastases treated by adrenalectomy: A case report and review of the literature. J. Clin. Oncol. (Jpn.), 6:77, 1972.
Kantarjian, H., Yap, H. Y., Hortobagyi, G., et al.: Hormonal therapy for metastatic male breast cancer. Arch. Intern. Med., 143:237, 1983.
Kennedy, B. J., and Kiang, D. T.: Hypophysectomy in the treatment of advanced cancer of the male breast. Cancer, 29:1606, 1972.
Kraybill, W. G., Kaufman, R., and Kinne, D.: Treatment of advanced male breast cancer. Cancer, 47:2185, 1981.
Li, M. C., Janelli, D. E., Kelly, E. J., et al.: Metastatic carcinoma of the male breast treated with bilateral adrenalectomy and chemotherapy. Cancer, 25:678, 1970.
Lin, R. S., and Kessler, I. I.: Epidemiologic findings in male breast cancer. Proc. Am. Assoc. Cancer Res., 21:72, 1980.
Lloyd, R. V., Rosen, P. P., Sarkar, N. H., et al.: Murine mammary tumor virus related antigen in human male mammary carcinoma. Cancer, 51:654, 1983.
Lopez, M., and Barduagni, A.: Cyproterone acetate in advanced male breast cancer. Cancer, 49:9, 1982.
Luft, R., Olivecrona, H., Ikkos, D., et al.: Hypophysectomy in the treatment of malignant tumors. Ann. J. Med., 21:728, 1956.
Mabuchi, K., Bross, D. S., and Kessler, I. I.: Risk factors for male breast cancer. JNCI, 74:371, 1985.

Marger, D., Urdaneta, N., and Fischer, J. J.: Breast cancer in brothers. Case reports and a review of 30 cases of male breast cancer. Cancer, 36:458, 1975.

Meyskens, F. L., Jr., Tormey, D. C., and Neifield, J. P.: Male breast cancer: A review. Cancer Treat. Rev., 3:83, 1976.

Mitsuyasu, R., Bonomi, P., Anderson, K., et al.: Response to megestrol in male breast carcinoma. Arch. Intern. Med., 141:809, 1981.

Neifield, J. P., Meyskens, F., Tormey, D. C., et al.: The role of orchiectomy in the management of advanced male breast cancer. Cancer, 37:992, 1976.

Nuttall, F. Q.: Gynecomastia as a physical finding in normal man. J. Clin. Endocrinol. Metab., 48:338, 1979.

Olsson, H., Alm, P., Kristoffersson, U., et al.: Hypophyseal tumor and gynecomastia preceding bilateral breast cancer development in a man. Cancer, 53:1974, 1984.

Ouriel, K., Lotze, M. T., and Hinshaw, J. R.: Prognostic factors of carcinoma of the male breast. Surg. Gynecol. Obstet., 159:373, 1984.

Panettiere, F. J.: Cancer in the male breast. Cancer, 34:1324, 1974.

Pantoja, E., Lobet, R. E., and Lopez, E.: Gigantic cytosarcoma phyllodes in a man with gynecomastia. Arch. Surg., 111:611, 1976.

Patel, J. K., Nemoto, T., and Dao, T. L.: Metastatic breast cancer in males. Assessment of endocrine therapy. Cancer, 53:1344, 1984.

Patterson, J. S., Battersby, L. A., and Balch, B. K.: Use of tamoxifen in advanced male breast cancer. Cancer Treat. Rep., 64:801, 1980.

Pegoraro, R. J., Nirmul, D., and Joubert, S. M.: Cytoplasmic and nuclear estrogen and progesterone receptors in male breast cancer. Cancer Res., 42:4812, 1982.

Reingold, I. M., and Ascher, G. S.: Cystosarcoma phyllodes in a man with gynecomastia. Am. J. Clin. Pathol., 53:852, 1970.

Ribeiro, G. G.: Male breast carcinoma—A review of 301 cases from the Christie Hospital and Holt Radium Institute, Manchester. Br. J. Cancer, 51:115, 1985.

Ribeiro, G. G.: Tamoxifen in the treatment of male breast carcinoma. Clin. Radiol., 34:625, 1983.

Richards, A. T., Jaffe, A., and Hunt, J. A.: Adenoma of the nipple in a male. S. Afr. Med. J., 47:575, 1973.

Robison, R., and Montague, E. D.: Treatment results in males with breast cancer. Cancer, 49:403, 1982.

Ross, M. B., Buzdar, A. U., and Blumenschein, G. R.: Treatment of advanced breast cancer with Megestrol acetate after treatment with Tamoxifen. Cancer, 49:413, 1982.

Sanchez, A. G., Villanueva, A. G., and Redondo, C.: Lobular carcinoma of the breast in a patient with Klinefelter's syndrome. Cancer, 57:1181, 1986.

Scheike, O.: Male breast cancer. Clinical manifestations in 257 cases in Denmark. Br. J. Cancer, 28:552, 1973.

Scheike, O., Svenstrup, B., and Fraudsen, V. A.: Male breast cancer: 2. Metabolism of oestradiol-17β in men with breast cancer. J. Steroid Biochem., 4:489, 1973.

Schwartz, R. M., Newell, R. B., Jr., Hauch, J. F., et al.: A study of familial male breast carcinoma and a second report. Cancer, 46:2697, 1980.

Silverberg, E.: Cancer statistics: 1985. CA, 35:19, 1985.

Spence, R. A. J., Mackenzie, G., Anderson, J. R., et al.: Long-term survival following cancer of the male breast in northern Ireland. A report of 81 cases. Cancer, 55:648, 1985.

Srinivasan, G., Srinivasan, U., and Greiver, S. P.: Male breast carcinoma following estrogen therapy: Report of a case. J. Kentucky Med. Assoc., 77:9, 1979.

Stephens, R. L., and Muggia, F. M.: Breast cancer in men. Report illustrating the value of endocrine ablation. Am. J. Med., 57:679, 1974.

Symmers, W. St.C.: Carcinoma of breast in transsexual individuals after surgical and hormonal interference with the primary and secondary sex characteristics. Br. Med. J., 2:83, 1968.

Thompson, D. K., Li, F. P., and Cassady, J. R.: Breast cancer in a man 30 years after radiation for metastatic osteogenic sarcoma. Cancer, 44:2362, 1979.

Treves, N.: The treatment of cancer, especially inoperable cancer, of the male breast by ablative surgery (orchiectomy, adrenalectomy, and hypophysectomy) and hormone therapy (estrogens and corticosteroids). An analysis of 43 patients. Cancer, 12:820, 1959.

Treves, N., and Holleb, A. I.: Cancer of the male breast; report of 146 cases. Cancer, 8:1239, 1955.

Vanderbilt, P. C., and Warren, S. E.: Forty year experience with carcinoma of the male breast. Surg. Gynecol. Obstet., 133:629, 1971.

Vercoutere, A. L., and O'Connell, T. X.: Carcinoma of the male breast. An update. Arch. Surg., 119:1301, 1984.

Vorobiof, D. A., and Falkson, G.: Nasally administered buserelin inducing complete remission of lung metastases in male breast cancer. Cancer, 59:688–689, 1987.

Wainwright, J. M.: Carcinoma of the male breast. Arch. Surg., 14:836, 1927.

Wolloch, Y., and Dintsman, M.: Primary carcinoma of the male breast. Am. J. Surg., 125:628, 1973.

Yadaw, R. V. S., Sahariah, S., Mittal, V. K., et al.: Angiosarcoma of the male breast. Int. Surg., 61:463, 1976.

Yap, H. Y., Tashima, C. K., Blumenschein, G. R., et al.: Male breast cancer. A natural history study. Cancer, 44:748, 1979.

CHAPTER 29

DANIELLE M. TURNS

Psychosocial Factors

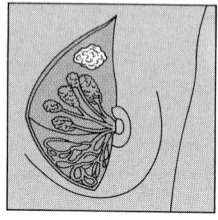

Cancer is one of the major health problems facing today's industrialized society. Breast cancer is now the second leading cause of cancer-related mortality in women, having only recently been outrun by lung cancer. Recent statistics indicate that 1 in 12 women will develop breast cancer, and an estimated 41,300 will die of breast cancer in 1987 (Silverberg and Lubera, 1987). In spite of sophisticated therapeutic procedures, survival rates have remained fairly stable in the last 20 years. Although 50 per cent of all breast cancer patients survived 5 years or more after diagnosis, many live with varying degrees of disability. Psychosocial factors have become an area of increasing concern in this disease process as they have been thought to have an impact at all stages of the disease—prior to detection, at the time of detection, during treatment and rehabilitation, and, in too many cases, in the care of the terminally ill patient.

Psychosocial Factors Prior to the Diagnosis of Breast Cancer

Personality characteristics, stressful life events, and sociocultural issues have been implicated both in the pathogenesis of cancer and in the attitudes in seeking care. The existence of a cancer-prone personality was postulated very early in medicine, starting with Galen's observation that "melancholic" women were more prone to cancer than "sanguine" women. In the 18th and 19th centuries, the role of depression and life stresses in the genesis of cancer became of interest. More recent studies have examined the effects of interpersonal relationships, sexuality, modes of expressing anger, life events, and loss of loved ones.

PSYCHOLOGIC FACTORS

Whether certain personality characteristics or stressful life events play a role in the genesis of breast cancer has generated an abundant and sometimes confusing literature. Greer and Morris (1978) have eloquently summarized the methodologic pitfalls that plague the testing of hypotheses in this area of research. Time and financial constraints almost preclude the longitudinal study approach, in which the systematic psychologic evaluation of a large population followed over time would give an unbiased assessment of cases versus those that are not cases. Experience has proved, however, that the number of cases eventually found might be too small to yield results of any significance (Hagnell, 1966; Thomas, 1976). Among the biases encountered are impact of illness or psychologic state in personality studies and faulty recall in life events studies. Furthermore, many of the early studies were methodologically warped sui generis because of small samples, lack of controls, or lack of double-blind conditions. Nevertheless, some findings emerged from early research, and some have been verified by more recent surveys.

Bacon (1952) reported inhibition of sexuality and mothering, inability to deal appropriately with anger, aggression, or hostility and unresolved mothering conflicts in breast cancer patients. LeShan and Worthington (1956a,b) concurred on the inability to express anger, sexual disturbances, and unresolved parent-child tension but added loneliness, depression, self-distrust, and despair (LeShan, 1959, 1966; LeShan and Worthington, 1956a,b). Bahnson and Bahnson (1966) found that depression, hostility, guilt, and repression or denial of conflicts were prevalent among cancer patients. Anxiety and depression were also reported by various other investigators. More recent studies have to some extent verified some of the foregoing characteristics.

Katz (1970) investigated the psychologic differences between women who had benign or malignant lesions following surgical biopsy and found none. Using a similar method, Schonfield (1975) found some differences in his study of Israeli women, namely that women with cancer had higher "lie scale" on the Minnesota Multiphasic Personality Inventory (MMPI), which he interpreted as a greater need of denial in this group. He found no difference in levels of depression and well-being. Greer and Morris (1975) studied a series of 160 women on the eve of their biopsies using a battery of well-validated scales and tested the hypothesis that women found to have a cancerous tumor would score higher on inability to express resentment and hostility, depression, hopelessness, extroversion, repression, and denial than women with benign tumors. The data showed a significant correlation between cancer and abnormal release of anger, with a pattern of extreme suppression in most cases and, in a few, of severe, frequent temper outbursts. In a later publication, Morris and coworkers (1981) confirmed these results, particularly suppression of anger among younger women with cancer. This particular group also showed lower State and Trait anxiety scores than either older women with cancer or women with benign tumors, which may represent a higher degree of denial.

Wirshing and colleagues (1982) used a predictive approach in their study of 56 women admitted for breast biopsy, based on a set of characteristics believed to be specific to women with cancer: being inaccessible or overwhelmed when interviewed, emotional suppression with sudden outburst, rationalization, little or no anxiety prior to the procedure, demonstration of optimism, superautonomous self-sufficiency, altruistic behavior, harmonization, and avoidance of conflict. To avoid bias introduced by personal contact, these authors used the predictions of an independent rater in addition to those of the interviewers. The interviewers were correct in 83 per cent of the cancer patients and 71 per cent of all benign cases, the independent rater in 94 per cent of the cancer patients and 68 per cent of the benign cases. The overlap between false positive and false negative results yielded the finding that the identified syndrome was found in all of the cancer patients but also in 25 to 30 per cent of those with benign tumors. The authors interpret their findings as the identification of a long-standing pattern of inadequate coping with stress rather than a pathologic emotional defect and conclude that no etiologic link to cancer can be established. Should definite personality characteristics play a part in the causation of breast cancer, their mechanism would remain a mystery. Pettingale and coworkers (1977) have explored a possible link between the expression of anger and the immune system in the population studied by Greer and Morris (1975). They measured immunoglobulins IgA, IgE, IgG, and IgM levels and found significantly higher levels of IgA among anger-suppressing women than anger-expressing women, independently of their cancer status. The authors refrained from inferring a causal relationship from a statistical association but did suggest that their psychologic link observation gives new insight in the pathogenesis of cancer.

It is apparent that none of the studies mentioned resulted in a convincing "cancer personality" profile. Certainly, none of the characteristics elicited—anger suppression, for example—can be causally related to the apparition of cancer. But, even if they were, it is not likely that new adaptive patterns could be taught on a scale large enough to reduce the incidence of breast cancer. The antismoking campaign has shown that it is possible, but difficult, to change a particular well-defined behavior. Hindrance to changing long-standing coping behaviors that per se cause no distress would be immense. Francis (1969) suggests that the concept of a cancer-prone personality may be detrimental to the rehabilitation of cancer victims. Premature assertions that women are sexually or emotionally repressed risk needlessly adding another stigma to the cancer problem. Another misgiving is that little attention is paid to the implications for cancer prevention. The knowledge necessary to prevent the genesis of cancer-prone personalities does not exist, nor does such knowledge exist for altering biologic concomitants. Unless sound biologic research on the humoral and hormonal mechanisms that differentiate personality types is pursued, information on personality types may be a blind alley.

LIFE STRESSES

Holmes and Rahe (1967), Dohrenwend and Dohrenwend (1974), Paykel and associates

(1971), and others have investigated the relationship between life stresses and the onset of disease. Several authors have reported diverse findings specifically for breast cancer.

LeShan (1966) and Bahnson and Bahnson (1966) reported that the onset of breast cancer often immediately followed the loss of an intense dependent relationship. Similar results have been reported by Greene (1966) for leukemia and Kissen (1966) for lung cancer. Muslin and colleagues (1966), however, were not able to replicate these findings in their controlled study of breast cancer patients.

Reznikoff (1955) believed that women were at high risk for breast cancer if they were given excessive childhood responsibilities or had high rates of sibling death in their families. Spilken and Jacobs (1971) reported that poor adjustment to life's stresses was highly correlated with the onset of illness in general.

These findings have not been verified by others. Snell and Graham (1971) delineated the stresses breast cancer patients exerienced and could find no significant differences in single or cumulative insults between these patients and a control group. Schonfield (1975) found no evidence that stressful events, particularly losses, precede the onset of cancer. Data from his study show that patients with benign tumors had higher scores (more stress) on Holmes and Rahe's Social Readjustment Rating Scale than those with malignancies. Southam (1969) also expressed skepticism about psychic stimuli as the primary source of cancer onset. However, he does recommend research to examine whether stress might influence dissemination by depressing immunologic defenses.

Greer and Morris (1975) found no difference in the incidence of stressful life events between women with cancer and women with benign tumors. Jones and coworkers (1984), in their study of bereavement and cancer, found little support for an association between the death of a spouse and a diagnosis of cancer, including breast cancer. Grossarth-Malicek and colleagues (1984) followed a cohort of 1353 persons over a period of 10 years, identifying 204 cases of cancer during that interval. These authors were testing the hypothesis that stressful events causing a chronic conflict leading to hopelessness and marked depression would increase the risk for cancer. They conclude that a gradual increase of cancer became evident more than 3 years after an event causing unresolved depression and hopelessness of more than a year's duration. In this cohort, 25.44 per cent of the women had developed breast cancer. Certain bias in sample selection acknowledged by the authors may have distorted the results of the study and their generalization to other populations.

Clarification is needed regarded stressful life events and cancer onset. Personal losses, social traumas, and inability to express emotions may be characteristic of breast cancer patients but are also characteristic of many persons without this disease. Predicting risk of cancer by such criteria would necessarily include many false positive results. The real significance of stress is how well the patient copes with the new stress of cancer. The patient's success in coping with previous stresses probably allows the prediction of success in coping with new stresses. Women previously inadequate in coping with the social, psychologic, or physiologic traumas of living should be identified and given additional assistance when confronted with cancer.

Stein and coworkers (1979) reviewed the evidence on stress and the immune system and concluded that extensive neuroendocrine and other biologic processes may be involved in the mediation of the effect of psychosocial influences on immune function and the susceptibility to and the course of neoplastic disease. Peters and Mason (1979) summarized the experimental data on stress and its effects on tumor induction, transplantability, growth, and metastasis. They remarked that even if there is no doubt the neuroendocrinologic reactions to stress are capable of modifying such parameters in laboratory animals, no definite conclusions could be drawn for human cancer except those that may be hormone dependent, and cancer of the breast would certainly fit this mold. A variety of studies summarized by Solomon et al. (1979) have provided ever-growing evidence that there is a direct relationship between cancer incidence and immunologic status and that stressful experiences do alter immunologic parameters. Stein and Schleifer (1985) concluded their review of the literature with the following statement: "Considerable evidence demonstrating a relationship between stress and immune function is accumulating. This chapter suggests that an extensive network of CNS and endocrine system processes may be involved in the modulation of the immune system in response to stressors, which in turn may alter the development, onset and course of a range of illnesses." So, although no specific mechanism has yet been identified, the bulk of the evidence would implicate stressful events as playing a role in the pathogenesis of cancer through alteration of both neuroendocrine and immunologic processes. Epidemiologic studies, however, have failed to show any convincing evidence of such a relationship. In their critical review of the literature, Bieliauskas and Garron (1982) concluded that there is no support for emotional inhibition and hopelessness in those individuals.

SOCIOCULTURAL FACTORS

Social changes affecting life styles may increase the population at risk of developing cancer. For example, women who belong to the higher social classes are at high risk for breast cancer, but they are also more likely to be influenced by breast cancer education programs. Women who have children late in life and who have few children are also at high risk. In recent years, there has been a trend for young women to delay marriage and motherhood while they actively pursue education and a career. It is therefore possible that these changes in life style may increase the number of women at high risk and the incidence of the disease. It is not likely that today's young women would alter marital and childbearing behavior to avoid breast cancer late in life. Better educated women, however, are more likely to perform breast self-examination (BSE) regularly and have mammograms, so that their chances of discovering early lesions will be enhanced. A change has occurred in the public attitudes toward health in general and breast cancer in particular. The last decade has seen a decrease in smoking, a decrease in hard liquor consumption, and changes in dietary habits, which are likely to decrease the incidence of some cancers. The public is also more educated as to early detection methods such as breast self-examination and Hemoccult tests. In addition, the revelation by some prominent women of their breast cancers has somewhat changed public perception of the disease. In summary, this new set of attitudes would be expected to result in better compliance with BSE and yearly examination by a physician. Recent literature, however, does not bear this fact out. Schulten (1982) found that knowledge, beliefs, and practices of women in reference to breast cancer had not changed markedly since the Gallup poll of 1974 (American Institute of Public Opinion, 1974). Women still overestimated the prevalence of breast cancer but were aware that most lumps are not malignant. They generally were ignorant of breast cancer risk factors but perceived themselves to be at high risk. Thirty-seven per cent practice BSE, which is up from the 18 per cent of 1974. Interestingly enough, there did not seem to be a relationship between knowledge and BSE practice. This brings up the role that psychologic factors may play in preventive medicine practices. Delay in seeking medical care for breast symptoms has long frustrated health care professionals. Although it is now certain that health education programs can prevent or minimize it, not all women respond to this approach. Todd and Magarey (1978) postulated that certain types of ego defenses can be facilitators or hindrances to compliance. The ego defenses they examined were denial, suppression, rationalization, displacement, intellectualization-isolation, and reaction formation. Ninety women with breast symptoms were interviewed and the delay between appearance of symptoms and their reporting to the clinic was noted. Although all of the women knew that their symptoms could mean cancer, those who delayed used denial and suppression, whereas those who did not were more likely to use intellectualization-isolation. The delayers also displayed depression and anxiety. The authors concluded, however, that health education programs that rely on intellectualization-isolation messages will not be effective for women with denial and suppression. Cultural attitudes about the breast, sexuality, and surgical changes undoubtedly influence the seeking of medical care.

Personal primary care physicians probably are the most effective health educators for their patients. A survey by the American Cancer Society (1985) showed that, of all physicians questioned, 97 per cent do breast examination as part of their physical examination in asymptomatic women, 49 per cent recommended a mammogram for women over 45 years, 92 per cent advise all women to practice BSE, and 59 per cent instruct their patients themselves. This represents a change in physicians' attitudes compared with a survey done 5 years earlier, a change likely to influence early detection favorably. A troubling fact was brought out by Gould-Martin and coworkers (1982), however: women who discovered their tumors through BSE showed no advantage in terms of clinical course over those who discovered them accidentally. In fact, they were more likely to delay seeking care.

The area of secondary prevention—that is, early detection and prompt treatment—may not have produced as much benefit as was once hoped but yet remains one of the simpler weapons for improving the prognosis of the disease. Antonovsky and Anson (1976) have given considerable attention to the influence of various psychosocial factors on early detection and treatment of breast cancer. They developed a nonstatistical typology of four diferent orientations in screening that were labeled conformist, rational goal-directed, complacent-stoic, and ambivalent-anxious. The implications are that specific programs need to be directed toward several groups of women. Factors that need to be considered are the individual's degree of inner direction in attaining goals, levels of education, tendency to adopt the sick role, medical orientation (popular versus scientific), social structure and conformity to group norms, and priority of health in the value structure. One shortcoming of public health programs is that they generally are aimed at women who have above-average education, strong ego-strengths, and a realistic view of the advantages and disadvantages of early detection and treatment, and they often fail to reach women lacking those attributes.

Psychosocial Factors at the Time of Diagnosis

Thomas (1978) considers two psychologic stages preoperatively: The diagnostic period, during which the woman seeks medical advice, is referred to a surgeon, and undergoes biopsy; and the preoperative period, when she decides about undergoing a one stage procedure (biopsy with frozen section and immediate mastectomy) or a two stage procedure (biopsy, review of permanent section and staging, and definite surgery decision). Thomas conceptualizes the diagnostic period as a time of coping, with active problem solving on the patient's part, seeking of reassurance as her denial wanes, and expressing fear of the outcome and of the procedures themselves. The family may feel excluded, confused, and fearful. The preoperative period is one of contradictory responses, with fear of the unknown, ambivalence toward the physician, fear of loss of control, confusion over treatment alternatives, decreased self-esteem, and aloneness. The family, while trying to be supportive, is also confused and uncertain and may feel left out of the decision-making process. This may well be a critical period for physician intervention. Although some women may verbalize a wish to let the physician decide, patient information and education provide a better cognitive appraisal of the process and decrease the sense of loss of control. Involvement of family members in the discussion helps alleviate their discomfort and enhances their support. Giving detailed information and allowing participation of the patient and her family may not be easy for some physicians (Strull et al., 1984) but is becoming more and more accepted, particularly in the area of breast surgery. Interestingly, in recent years, some states have enacted laws defining with precision the kind of information a woman with breast cancer must be given prior to any surgical procedure. This curious development is probably a consequence of the prevalent belief a decade ago that women were victimized by insensitive surgeons. Today many surgeons have taken an active interest in patient education and have designed their own educational pamphlets and organized patient seminars (Monaco et al., 1972). This approach is particularly important, as women with high levels of anxiety (as most women expecting results of their biopsy are) also exhibit impaired reasoning ability as a consequence. Their being given factual information in a comforting but precise way will enhance their cognitive functioning and facilitate decision making. It will also promote a healthier doctor-patient relationship, as noted by Holland and Mastrovito (1980).

Psychosocial Factors and Treatment

REACTIONS TO MASTECTOMY

The operative period defined by Thomas (1978) is most stressful: The patient is now definitively confronted with the loss of her breast and the fear of surgery, mutilation, death. The family shares her anxieties as to the outcome and shares her powerlessness. But family members may also feel abandoned and sometimes angry at her absence; they may suffer separation anxiety, which is particularly true for young children. The immediate postoperative period is a period of ambivalence: relief to have survived, hope to have been cured, but also fear of recurrence, dealing with pain, dressings, mixed feelings toward the staff, facing a possibly forever mutilated body, worries about femininity, reaction of the sexual partner. The family has feelings of inadequacy about dealing with the patient's turmoil, which they perceive, and about how to react to the wound. This period lasts 1 to 2 months after discharge and is followed by the postoperative period (2 to 6 months), during which what was left of denial is broken, and anger starts to emerge. Depression, anxiety, and decreased self-esteem coexist with feeling stronger and hopeful. It is usually during this time that the emotionally drained family may start to withdraw support, that anxiety about sexual relations emerges in the spouse, and that children start expecting a return to normal function.

This general model is useful, but it does not take into account personality characteristics of the patients. As Holland and Mastrovito (1980) have pointed out, the patient's past coping style and emotional stability, the point at which the cancer occurred in the life cycle, the coping style of the spouse, and the quality of the marital relationship will color the woman's adaptation. A woman who had witnessed the painful death of a relative from breast cancer will be more apprehensive and anxious than one who has seen a positive outcome. Young, single women feel loss of femininity and body image injury more keenly than do mature women with stable relationships, and so do women with marked narcissistic traits. The spouse's role is pivotal (Jamison, 1978; Wellisch et al., 1978) in the woman's adjustment: Any sexual hesitancy on his part is another deep wound for the woman. Failure to communicate love and commitment erode the woman's confidence. It is not uncommon to see an already faltering marriage dissolve after the mastectomy crisis. Lastly, women who adopt a "tackling stance" (Lipowski, 1970) may cope more successfully during the postmastectomy period. Some authors have speculated that any kind of major surgery would induce the type of reaction described earlier. However, Gottesman and Lewis (1982) compared 31 women with breast cancer with 15 women undergoing surgery and 15 healthy women. As measured by the Halpern Crisis Scale, both the cancer and surgery patients reported more crises than the controls, but cancer patients reported a strong sense of helplessness. This study also showed that the crisis did not resolve in 6 to 8 weeks, as is commonly reported, but was still a problem 15 weeks after completion of mastectomy.

It is interesting to note that the pervasive distress and the dysphoria associated with cancer are not an inherent part of the disease: They may be symptomatic of diagnosable and treatable psychiatric entities. In their survey of 215 patients, Derogatis and coworkers (1983) found that 101 or 47 per cent of the patients met the criteria for a diagnosis of either adjustment disorder (68 patients) or major affective disorder (13 patients). Other diagnoses included organic brain syndrome, personality disorder, and anxiety disorder. The vast majority of the two most frequent diagnoses respond well to either psychotherapy or pharmacotherapy, or to both. There is no reason to believe that this is not true for women with breast cancer (Silberfarb, 1984), even though Worden and Weisman (1977) failed to confirm the prominence of a postmastectomy depression. A careful examination of mental status should be part of the follow-up care so that women with psychiatric conditions can be treated and relieved of an unnecessary additional burden.

Morris and colleagues (1977) did a 2 year follow-up study of 160 mastectomized women. They found that 70 per cent of the women were no longer stressed by the mastectomy at 1 year. Those who had adjusted poorly had shown high levels of depression and neuroticism on personality inventory scales administered preoperatively. Perimenopausal status was associated with a deterioration in sexual functioning. They also reported that approximately 20 per cent of the women in their sample had received psychiatric care at some point during the follow-up.

REACTIONS TO OTHER OR ASSOCIATED TREATMENT METHODS

There has been a tendency in recent years to shift toward more conservative surgery than modified radical mastectomy and to implement reconstructive surgery. Breast sparing procedures have been advocated as creating less psychologic distress and rendering the postsurgery adjustment less distressing. The studies by Atkins and coworkers (1972) and by Ager and colleagues (1976) seemed to verify this assumption, but the sample sizes and the data gathering methods in both studies do not permit generalization of those findings. Sanger and Reznikoff (1981) compared 20 women who had undergone modified radical mastectomies and 20 women who had had conservative surgery plus radiotherapy, in terms of body image indices and psychologic adjustment. The women were matched in pairs for age and length of time after surgery, and were grouped for marital status. No statistical differences were found between the two groups with respect to indices regarding body penetration, body anxiety, general psychologic adjustment, or marital satisfaction. Indices relating to body barriers and body satisfaction, however, were significantly different in the two groups, the women with conservative surgery reporting less body barrier alteration and less change in body satisfaction. It should be noted, nevertheless, that the study sample, although larger than in previous studies, was small and that the sample selection was biased. The women with conservative surgery had made the choice themselves, whereas the women with radical mastectomies had not been aware of surgical alternatives and had accepted their surgeons' decision. They may have been less preoccupied with body image than their counterparts. They also were volunteers who had adjusted well enough to the procedure to undergo two hours of psychometric evaluation and may represent a self-selected sample of good surgery responders, not representative of mastectomy patients in general. Shain and coworkers (1983) carried out a study of postsurgery adjustment in 20 patients with mastectomy and 18 patients with excisional biopsy and irradiation. Both groups were part of a prospective randomized clinical trial. No marked psychosocial differences were identified between the groups except for body image concepts. The authors plan a larger prospective study to find out whether statistical differences emerge when the sample size is increased. At this time, it is therefore not possible to state whether conservative surgery leads to better psychosocial adjustment.

Luce and Romm (1984) view breast reconstruction as a procedure enhancing self-esteem. It is credited with restoring body image and instilling a sense of hope and purpose in the women. Schain and coworkers (1985) hold that immediate or early reconstruction (within 1 year) reduces significantly the recall of postmastectomy distress compared with delayed reconstruction (after 1 year). They also found the early reconstruction group to be more symptomatic on the depression, anxiety, psychoticism, and interpersonal sensitivity scales of the Brief Symptom Inventory and speculate that the early reconstruction and the delayed reconstruction groups are psychologically different in their ability to tolerate the delay of reconstruction. They further state that for certain subjects the recommendation for reconstruction may be "the sooner the better" to lessen the emotional morbidity associated with mastectomy. It seems that some women adjust poorly to wearing a prosthesis, and wanting to get rid of it is the most frequently recorded reason for reconstruction. It should be noted, however, that not all women are candidates for breast reconstruction or interested in the procedure.

Some women also receive adjuvant therapy, such as chemotherapy, radiation therapy, or hormonal therapy, for 1 to 2 years. These treatment methods, particularly chemotherapy and radiotherapy, often induce fatigue, nausea, hair loss, and stomatitis, which in consequence turn into depression, anger, and decreased libido. The patient's family, strained and tried, may feel further frustrated by the patient's physical and psychologic symptoms and the fact she is not "bouncing back." Meyerowitz and coworkers (1979) surveyed 50 women receiving adjuvant chemotherapy for Stage II breast carcinoma. Their results showed that all women experienced adverse changes: 88 per cent reported a decrease in activities, 54 per cent had an increased financial burden, and 41 per cent had a strain on their family and sexual relationships. Nevertheless, 74 per cent of them felt positively about their participation in the treatment protocol.

Silberfarb and colleagues (1980) found adjuvant radiation therapy to be a source of emotional as well as physical distress for the patient. The women undergoing chemotherapy reported as many physical symptoms but less emotional distress. This finding may be related to the impersonality of the radiation therapy and to less frequent contacts with the physician, which possibly undermine the patient's sense of control and mastery. This particular group of patients (those receiving radiotherapy) is thought to be in need of increased support during treatment.

REACTIONS TO RECURRENCE AND PROGRESSION OF THE DISEASE

The most disturbing time in a patient's course is the first recurrence of breast cancer. Almost 80 per cent of the women surveyed by Silberfarb and coworkers (1980) reported serious emotional disturbances: foremost were fear, anxiety, concern about their roles as mates, distrust and negativism toward the primary physician, and concern about being a burden to family members. The authors suggest that this is a fertile period for the emergence of clinical depression and that routine psychiatric evaluation may be appropriate at this stage. Terminal patients and their families enter the process of death and dying, which is beyond the scope of this chapter. It should be noted, however, that the grieving process does not prevent the emergence of psychiatric syndromes, and at that stage depression and delirium are encountered most frequently. Delirium may be due to a variety of causes: metabolic imbalance, cerebral metastasis, concurrent infections, and treatment techniques such as chemotherapy and anxiolytic, hypnotic, or analgesic medications. Although this condition is readily diagnosable by any physician who checks the patient's orientation, concentration, and cognitive abilities, it is often misdiagnosed (Silberfarb, 1984). The condition can be corrected by treating the underlying cause whenever possible, and the agitation that often accompanies the syndrome can be managed successfully by small doses of major tranquilizers.

PSYCHOSOCIAL FACTORS AND SURVIVAL

Do psychosocial factors affect the outcome of the disease? The literature on the subject is vast, too vast to be reported here inasmuch as conflicting results are too often based on methodologically flawed studies. A literature review on the topic was published by Fox (1983). A report by Cassileth and associates (1985) concerns the prospective study of 359 cancer patients, including women with Stage II breast cancer. Psychosocial indices were correlated with either length of survival (patients with unresectable tumors) or time to recurrence (melanoma Stages I and II or breast cancer Stage II). The findings indicated clearly that psychosocial factors individually or in combination did not influence the length of survival or the time to relapse. This study is an important one because of its sound methodology; however, it did not explore the relationship between stressful life events and outcome.

Psychosocial Interventions

A variety of psychosocial interventions are available to today's practitioners. The most important are the establishment of a therapeutic alliance between primary physicians and patient and the availability of an experienced and resourceful treatment team. Appraisal of the patient's support system and interventions aimed at preserving its integrity during the course of the illness should also be considered. As mentioned earlier, patient education as to the disease and treatment methods available should begin early and in a supportive, nonthreatening atmosphere. An effort should be made to elicit a patient's idiosyncratic concerns. Patterns of coping with other past stresses, history of psychiatric disorders, familial situation, presence of stressors in the environment, and sexual functioning need to be ascertained to get a better appreciation of the patient's present and potential difficulties. This detailed anamnesis enhances communication and understanding and facilitates the patient's decision-making and participation in treatment. Whenever possible, family members and significant others should be encouraged to participate in this process, and the mate's concerns should be the object of special attention. This type of interaction is most often initiated at the diagnostic period stage and is nurtured throughout the immediate postoperative period. As it is not possible for physicians to spend the amount of time needed to accomplish this long, hard task, reliance on trusted team members is usual. Nursing personnel and social workers participate in patient and family education, providing emotional support and referrals to social agencies to ensure help with finances, arranging for the assistance of a homemaker when needed or helping to meet other elicited needs. Physical therapists teach and demonstrate exercises designed to prevent limitation of motion and post-mastectomy edema. An organization frequently called upon to help is Reach for Recovery, a self-help group composed of volunteer women who have been treated for breast cancer. These women act as role models for the recently mastectomized women and give practical advice on acquiring and wearing a prosthesis. Lastly, a psychiatric consultant should be available for assessment and treatment of a suspected psychiatric condition. Gordon and co-workers (1980) evaluated a psychosocial rehabilitation program organized along these lines at the New York University Hospital, New York City, and reported that such an intervention was effective in improving some of the psychosocial problems reported by the patients and in inducing a more rapid decline of objective indices of negative affect, namely, anxiety, hostility, and depression in their short-term follow-up (at discharge). At 6 months post discharge, the patients who had been involved were more realistic in their appraisal of the disease and its impact on their life, and a greater proportion of them had resumed their previous occupations compared to the control group. Wellisch (1984) has summarized what he considers to be the necessary ingredients for an effective rehabilitation program.

In recent years, group therapy has been used as a treatment method not only for post-mastectomy patients but also for patients at other stages of the disease (terminal stage, for example). A study by Spiegel and colleagues (1981) provides objective evidence that group intervention for these patients is effective in reducing tension, depression, fatigue, and phobias. Specific psychiatric interventions in the late stage of the disease, in addition to the already mentioned assessment and management of depression and delirium, also include pain management techniques. Tricyclic antidepressants are useful adjuncts in the treatment of pain, and so is biofeedback (Deragotis and McDonald, 1982). Self-hypnosis has also been demonstrated to be helpful by Spiegel and Bloom (1983).

To summarize, it is clear that a variety of interventions are at the disposal of the breast cancer patient's primary physician to lessen the psychosocial consequences of the disease and its treatment. They involve not only the use of the patient herself but also the reliance on trained health professionals, who will help meet the emotional, social, familial, and psychiatric needs of patients. These insights should be included in the training of not only breast care specialists, but also all oncologists (Wise, 1977).

Conclusions

The influence of psychosocial factors in the causation, course, and treatment outcome of serious and potentially lethal diseases is becoming a growing concern of modern medicine and public health.

In breast cancer, most of the evidence collected concerns the psychosocial consequences of the disease, as there are not many convincing data on the role of psychosocial factors in causing the disease, and little is known about their impact on attitudes toward seeking medical care, which would be specific to the disease. Similarly, the studies concerned with psychosocial factors (psychologic traits, life events, support system) and illness outcome have yielded few insights. However, studies of psychosocial interventions aimed at decreasing the distress caused by the disease and enhancing the quality of life have led to solid conclusions as to their value. This has profound implications for the training of the oncologists of the future.

REFERENCES

Ager, P., Terry, J., Alpert, S., et al.: Preliminary report of the psychological impact of radiation therapy instead of mastectomy for early carcinoma of the breast. Unpublished manuscript, 1976.

American Cancer Society: A survey of physicians, attitudes and practices in early cancer detection. CA, 35:197, 1985.

American Institute of Public Opinion (Gallup): Women's attitudes regarding breast cancer. Occup. Health Nurse, 22:20, 1974.

Antonovsky, A., and Anson, O.: Factors related to preventive health behavior. In Cullen, J. W., Fox, B. H., and Isom, R. N. (Eds.): Cancer: The Behavioral Dimensions. New York, Raven Press, 1976, p. 35.

Atkins, H., Hayward, J., Kliegman, D., et al.: Treatment of breast cancer: A report after 10 years of a clinical trial. Br. Med. J., 20:423, 1972.

Bacon, G. L., Renneker, R., and Cutler, M.: A psychosomatic survey of cancer of the breast. Psychosom. Med., 14:453, 1952.

Bahnson, C. B., and Bahnson, M. B.: The role of ego defenses: Denial and repression in the etiology of malignant neoplasm. Ann. N.Y. Acad. Sci., 75:827, 1966.

Bieliauskas, L. A., and Garron, D. C.: Psychological depression and cancer. Gen. Hosp. Psych., 4:187, 1982.

Cassileth, B. R., Lusk, E. J., Miller, D. S., et al.: Psychosocial correlates of survival in advanced malignant disease? N. Engl. J. Med., 312:1551, 1985.

Derogatis, L. R., Morrow, G. R., Fetting, J., et al.: The prevalence of psychiatric disorders among cancer patients. J.A.M.A., 249:751, 1983.

Deragotis, L. R., and McDonald, R. N.: Workshop Report: Psychopharmacological applications to cancer. Cancer 50(Suppl.): 1968, 1982.

Dohrenwend, B. S., and Dohrenwend, B. P.: Stressful

Life Events: Their Nature and Effects. New York, John Wiley & Sons, 1974.
Fox, B. H.: Current theory of psychogenic effects on cancer incidence and prognosis. J. Psychosom. Oncol., 1:17, 1983.
Francis, G. M.: Cancer: The emotional component. Am. J. Nurs., 69:1677, 1969.
Gordon, W. A., Freidenbergs, I., Diller, D., et al.: Efficacy of psychosocial intervention with cancer patients. J. Consult. Clin. Psychology, 48:743, 1980.
Gottesman, D., and Lewis, M. S.: Differences in crisis reactions among cancer and surgery patients. J. Comm. Clin. Psychol., 50:381, 1982.
Gould-Martin, K., Paganini-Hill, A., Casagrande, C., et al.: Behavioral and biological determinants of surgical stage of breast cancer. Prevent. Med., 11:429, 1982.
Greene, W. A.: The psychosocial setting of the development of leukemia and lymphoma. Ann. N.Y. Acad. Sci., 125:794, 1966.
Greer, S., and Morris, T.: The study of psychological factors in breast cancer: Problems and method. Soc. Sci. Med., 12:129, 1978.
Greer, S., and Morris, T.: Psychological attributes of women who develop breast cancer: A controlled study. J. Psychosom. Res., 19:147, 1975.
Grossarth-Maticek, R., Frentzel-Beyrne, R., et al.: Cancer detection and prevention. Cancer, 7:201, 1984.
Hagnell, O.: The premorbid personality of persons who develop cancer in a total population investigated in 1947 and 1957. Ann. N.Y. Acad. Sci., 125:846, 1966.
Holland, J. C., and Mastrovito, R.: Psychological adaptation to breast cancer. Cancer, 46:1045, 1980.
Holmes, T. H., and Rahe, R. H.: The social readjustment rating scale. J. Psychosom. Res., 11:213, 1967.
Jamison, K. R., Wellisch, D. K., and Pasnau, R. O.: Psychosocial aspects of mastectomy: I. The woman's perspective. Am. J. Psychiatry, 135:432, 1978.
Jones, D. R., Goldblatt, P. O., and Leon, D. A.: Bereavement and cancer: Some data on deaths of spouses from the longitudinal study of office of population census and survey. Br. Med. J., 289:461, 1984.
Katz, J., Weiner, H., Gallagher, T. F., et al.: Stress, distress, and ego defenses. Arch. Gen. Psychiatry, 23:131, 1970.
Kissen, D. M.: Psychosocial factors, personality and prevention in lung cancer. Medical Off., 116:135, 1966.
LeShan, L.: Psychological states as factors in the development of malignant disease: A critical review. JNCI, 22:1, 1959.
LeShan, L.: An emotional life-history pattern associated with neoplastic disease. Ann. N.Y. Acad. Sci., 125:780, 1966.
LeShan, L. L., and Worthington, R. E.: Personality as a factor in the pathogenesis of cancer: A review of the literature. Br. J. Med. Psychol., 29:49, 1956a.
LeShan, L. L., and Worthington, R. E.: On recurrent life-history patterns observed in patients with malignant disease. J. Nerv. Ment. Dis., 124:460, 1956b.
Lipowski, Z. I.: Physical illness, the individual and the coping process. Psych. Med., 1:91, 1970.
Luce, E. A., and Romm, S.: Breast reconstruction after mastectomy. J. Kentucky Med Assoc., 82:183, 1984.
Meyerowitz, B. E., Sparks, F. C., and Spears, J. K.: Adjuvant therapy for breast carcinoma. Psychosocial implications. Cancer, 43:1613, 1979.
Monaco, R. M., Salfen, L., and Spratt, J. S.: The patient as an education participant in health care. Missouri Med., 69:932, 1972.
Morris, T., Greer, S., Pettingale, K., et al.: Patterns of expression of anger and their psychological correlates in women with breast cancer. J. Psychosom. Res., 25:111, 1981.
Morris, T., Greer, S. H., and White, P.: Psychological and social adjustment to mastectomy: A two year follow-up study. Cancer, 40:2381, 1977.
Muslin, H. L., Gyarfas, K., and Pieper, W. J.: Separation experience and cancer of the breast. Ann. N.Y. Acad. Sci., 125:802, 1966.
Paykel, E. S., Prusoff, B. A., and Uhlenhuth, E. H.: Scaling of life events. Gen. Psychiatry, 25:340, 1971.
Peters, L. J., and Mason, K. A.: Influence of stress on experimental cancer. In Stoll, B. A. (Ed.): Mind and Cancer Prognosis. New York, Wiley and Sons, 1979, p. 103.
Pettingale, K., Greer, S., and Dudley, E. H.: Serum IgA and emotional expression in breast cancer patients. J. Psychosom. Res., 21:395, 1977.
Reznikoff, M.: Psychological factors in breast cancer. Psychosom. Res., 19:96, 1955.
Sanger, C. K., and Reznikoff, M.: A comparison of the psychological effects of breast saving procedures with the modified radical mastectomy. Cancer, 48:2341, 1981.
Schain, W., Edwards, B. K., Gorrell, C. R., et al.: Psychosocial and physical outcomes of primary breast cancer therapy: Mastectomy vs excisional biopsy and irradiation. Breast Cancer Res. Treat., 3:377, 1983.
Schain, W., Wellisch, D. K., Pasnau, R. O., et al.: The sooner the better: A study of psychological factors in women undergoing immediate versus delayed breast reconstruction. Am. J. Psychiatry, 142:40, 1985.
Schonfield, J.: Psychological and life-experience differences between Israeli women with benign and cancerous breast lesions. J. Psychosom. Res., 19:229, 1975.
Schulten, L.: Knowledge and beliefs about breast cancer and breast self examination among athletic and nonathletic women. Nurs. Res., 3:348, 1982.
Silberfarb, P. M., Maurer, L. J., and Croumabbel, C. S.: Psychosocial aspects of neoplastic disease: I. Functional status of breast cancer patients during different treatment regimens. Am. J. Psychiatry, 137:450, 1980.
Silberfarb, P. M.: Psychiatric problems in breast cancer. Cancer, 53:820, 1984.
Silverberg, E., and Lubera, J.: Cancer statistics 1987. Ca, 37:2, 1987.
Snell, L., and Graham, S.: Social trauma as related to cancer of the breast. Br. J. Cancer, 25:721, 1971.
Solomon, G. F., Ankrant, A. A., and Rubin, R. T.: Stress and psychoimmunological response: In Stoll, B. A. (Ed.): Mind and Cancer Prognosis. New York, John Wiley & Sons, 1979, pp. 73–84.
Southam, C. M.: Emotions, immunology, and cancer: How might the psyche influence neoplasia? Ann. N.Y. Acad. Sci., 164:473, 1969.
Spiegel, D., Bloom, J. R., and Yalom, I.: Group support for patients with metastatic cancer. Arch. Gen. Psych., 38:527, 1981.
Spiegel, D., and Bloom, J. R.: Group therapy and hypnosis reduce metastatic breast carcinoma pain. Psychosom. Med., 45:333, 1983.
Spilken, A. Z., and Jacobs, M. A.: Prediction of illness behavior from measures of life crisis, manifest distress and maladaptive coping. Psychosom. Med., 33:251, 1971.
Stein, M., Zeller, S., and Schleifer, S. J.: Role of the hypothalamus in mediating stress effects of immune system. In Stoll, B. A. (Ed.): Mind and Cancer Prognosis. New York, Wiley & Sons, 1979, p. 85.
Stein, M., and Schleifer, S. J.: Frontiers of stress research:

Stress and immunity. *In* Zales, M. R. (Ed.): Stress in Health and Disease. New York, Brunner/Mazel, 1985, p. 97.

Strull, W. M., Lo, B., and Charles, G.: Do patients want to participate in medical decision making? JAMA, *252*:2980, 1984.

Thomas, C. B.: Precursors of premature disease and death: The predictive potential of habits and family attitudes. Ann. Intern. Med., *85*:653, 1976.

Thomas, S. G.: Breast cancer: The psychosocial issues. Cancer Nurs., *1*:53, 1978.

Todd, P., and Magarey, C.: Ego defences and affects in women with breast symptoms: A preliminary measurement paradigm. Br. J. Med. Psychol., *51*:177, 1978.

Watson, M., Greer, S., Blake, S., et al.: Reaction to a diagnosis of breast cancer. Relationship between denial, delay and rates of psychological morbidity. Cancer, *53*:2008, 1984.

Wellisch, D. K.: Implementation of psychosocial services in managing emotional stress. Cancer, *53*:828, 1984.

Wellisch, D. K., Jamison, K. R., and Pasnan, R.: Psychosocial aspects of mastectomy. II. The man's perspective. Am. J. Psychiatry, *135*:543, 1978.

Wirshing, M., Stierlin, H., Hoffman, F., et al.: Psychological identification of breast cancer patients before biopsy. J. Psychosom. Res., *26*:1, 1982.

Wise, T. H.: Training oncology fellows in psychological aspects of their specialty. Cancer, *39*:2584, 1977.

Worden, J. W., and Weisman, A. D.: The fallacy in post mastectomy depression. Am. J. Med. Sci., *273*:169, 1977.

CHAPTER 30

FRANCIS R. WATSON
RICHARD A. GREENBERG
JOHN S. SPRATT

Statistical Methods in Cancer Research

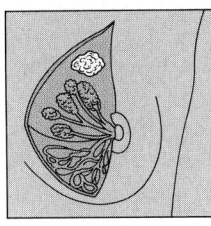

In his review of the penetration of statistical methods into clinical medicine, Cassedy (1984) credits Samuel D. Gross, Frank H. Hamilton, and Jonathan Mason Warren as being the first Americans to report statistical results for surgery in cancer, all in the antebellum period. From that meager beginning has evolved a continuing effort to define in statistical and mathematical terms the story of cancer and its control. As with all true sciences, the development of the appropriate mathematics precedes progress in the science itself, since mathematics is the language of science. The natural mathematical order of the universe and of all its components overrides the relevance of intuition, subjective, and empirical description in science. The purpose in this chapter, however, is not to review the long and often arduous evolution of mathematics applicable to the understanding and control of human cancer, but rather to review some of the methods currently applicable and some of the pitfalls that can occur in their application. A secondary objective is to provide a selected bibliography for further study and a glossary of standard terms and definitions. That a vigorous and continual penetration of mathematics into clinical medicine will occur is foreordained by the rapid evolution of computer technology with its inherent capacity to manage, consider, and analyze large bodies of data with great speed. This capacity can be brought directly to the physician-patient interface, providing immediate relevance and assistance. This technologic capacity will increasingly infuse mathematics into the "art" of medicine and, of necessity, future generations of physicians will have to increase their basic knowledge of mathematics applicable to clinical medicine and will have to develop increasing levels of computer literacy and competence.

The chapters on cell kinetics (Chapter 9), growth rates (Chapter 10), and screening (Chapter 19) contain considerable mathematics, which will not be duplicated in this chapter. Applications are to be found throughout those sections of text dealing with end results and comparisons. A glossary of terms relevant to this chapter is found at the end of this chapter.

Reviews of statistics evaluating clinical management identify prevalent problems in many published studies (Lavori et al., 1983; Bailar et al., 1984). The potential invalidity of various studies resulted from a lack of sufficient detail about methods of randomization, inadequate detail about patient sources, failure to use multivariate statistical techniques when applicable, and insufficient use of preliminary statistical modeling techniques in designing clinical studies. Reported studies often contained insufficient detail regarding patient selection, management protocols, and statistical analysis and interpretation. They had often inadequately considered the relevance of covariates to outcome.

The complexity of verifying benefit of treatment as a "response"—as opposed to the more objective endpoint of actual survivorship—can pose a complex statistical problem. Simplifying this problem mandates the use of very concise and consistently measurable definitions of response. One system of proved value is the Karnofsky scale defining the performance status of the patient (see Chapter 19). When the

Karnofsky index significantly improves, this is a measurable benefit. Transient regressions of measurable neoplasms with no improvement in the Karnofsky index are of dubious benefit even if survivorship can be increased.

As Oye and Shapiro (1984) report, there is a trend toward treating many common solid tumors by chemotherapy with little evidence of treatment effectiveness. They reviewed 80 studies of which 95 per cent used "response" to chemotherapy as an endpoint. They observed that responders in these studies may have lived longer with no treatment and that using "response" as an endpoint may have biased the conclusions toward overoptimism with respect to the effectiveness of chemotherapy.

The potential for biases in controlled clinical trials is constantly present. Although this study related to controlled clinical trials in the management of acute myocardial infarction rather than cancer, the report by Chalmers and colleagues (1983) shows the magnitude these biases can attain, varying with the design of the trial. These investigators analyzed 145 published papers and divided the papers according to the method of case allocation: random selection, blinded (57 papers), random selection, may have been blinded (45 papers), and controls selected by a nonrandom process (43 papers). At least one prognostic variable was significantly maldistributed in 14 per cent in the first group, in 26.7 per cent in the second group, and in 58.1 per cent in the third group. They concluded that their study confirmed the importance of blinding.

Probability

The theory of probability has always played a role in medicine, as well as in other areas of knowledge. Diagnoses are often made with incomplete certainty, and a particular therapy is prescribed not with absolute assurance that the patient will recover but because it offers the patient a greater probability of recovery than does any other therapeutic method. This type of reasoning is not explicit, in that the probabilities are not numerically evaluated, nor are mathematical equations written. However, the physician does apply an intuitive and implicit notion of probability and statistical methods in the diagnosis and treatment of illness.

Statistical methods, however well defined or explicit they may be, are of no value if the data they are designed to analyze are poorly gathered. These methods can be employed only when information on prior relevant events is available in sufficient detail and accuracy. Florence Nightingale recognized these principles and was one of the earliest persons to attempt to collect reliable and consistent data (Cook, 1914). In 1859, she devised forms to collect information on diseases and treatments and persuaded some London hospitals to adopt them. Her hope was that a scheme for uniform hospital statistics would be developed and that different treatments might be accurately evaluated. Florence Nightingale's hope is not today a reality, although more than a century has elapsed since she first proposed it. Progress, however, is being made in a few specialized areas.

Statistical methods involve multiple processes: (1) identification of a problem, (2) formulation of hypotheses to test solutions, (3) experimental planning, (4) the collection of data, and (5) the analysis of data. These are not independent. Although the data must be collected before they can be analyzed, the method of analysis should be established before the data are collected; otherwise there is no assurance that the data will be collected properly.

Principles of Data Collection

Research activity may be categorized in many ways. It is helpful to define whether a research project has broad goals and is useful, even necessary, when little is known about a particular area of interest. Some knowledge of the area must be established before any refined research can begin or any hypotheses can be created. In one sense, investigatory research can be likened to the survey approach, which is never used to prove anything but rather is used to become familiar with the area and the associated problems. Before sophisticated research can be attempted in any area, the investigator will have to know the territory. Once the territory is well known, more refined research may follow.

Hypothesis testing can take place only after the investigator has a relatively clear idea of which variables are most relevant to the hypothesis. One of the most important arts in science is creating *meaningful* hypotheses. Hypotheses should bear on the matter at hand and should be testable. Once a suitable hypothesis has been created, the researcher must determine the type of data and analysis necessary to either accept or reject it.

Before collecting data for a research project, the purpose of the project should be stated clearly. Data that have been collected without purpose may be useless for hypothesis testing. The method of analysis should dictate not only what data are to be collected but also how they will be recorded and coded. Too frequently, many hours have been spent collecting data that were later found useless because the collection and recording methods were not appropriate. Before the final collection form is designed, it is important for the investigator to state (1) specifically the object of the investigation, (2) methods of analysis that will be used, and (3) the amount of detail necessary for each item to answer questions or hypotheses. Data are not merely analyzed but are analyzed with respect to specific questions, hypotheses, and statistical models. On the assumption that the purpose and method of an investigation have been well defined, the following section indicates other important considerations when creating a data collection form or protocol.

Principles to Remember

PAPER IS CHEAPER THAN TIME

Seldom is it advisable when using coding schemes to record data on sheets other than code sheets. When a coder must look at a code sheet to find what value to record and then find the proper position on a record sheet to place the code, it not only is conducive to errors but also requires excessive time. A great deal of time can be saved if codes are put on a record sheet, as the extra cost of paper is considerably less than the cost of the time saved. For example, it takes five times as many sheets to record information by placing the code on each record sheet than by using a master code sheet. The extra paper costs about 1 cent. If the time saved is only 15 seconds in doing one case and the coder is paid as little as $2.50 an hour, the time saved will pay for the cost of the paper.

USE EXACT OR UNCODED DATA WHEN POSSIBLE

Measurement should be recorded in the original form rather than by using a coding scheme. Age should be recorded directly rather than by coded intervals, such as 0 to 10 = 1, 11 to 20 = 2, and so on. In measurements already available in numerical form, always record the numerical measurements, and do not transfer them into an interval code—that loses accuracy. This may take more room, but it allows greater flexibility in the analysis and is simpler to code.

USE SIMPLE CODES

Each item should answer only a single question or relate to a single dimension. It is best to have a separate item each for sex and race than to combine them into a single item. It is easier to code each of five symptoms separately than to employ a combination code, which will produce 32 different answers. This is confusing and takes time. If all five variables are listed with the possible answers of yes, no, and unknown, five columns are needed, and the same answer will be derived in a much shorter time. On small items this may not be critical, but it can create great difficulties on larger ones.

STATE QUESTIONS CLEARLY

Each question should be stated specifically so that all possible ambiguity is removed. This is one of the most difficult problems in creating a protocol. A complex question is best divided into two or more simple questions. Questions should be stated in such a way that they allow simple and concise answers. This often requires a parallel glossary of terms to provide succinct and explicit definitions.

IDENTIFY PROTOCOLS

Each protocol should contain the patient's or subject's chart number; for consistency, the first number of the protocol may be used for this purpose. Many times all 80 columns on a standard IBM card will be used, and a second card will be needed to finish a protocol. Use of cards may be avoided entirely by direct entry of data into a computer. By using chart numbers, information belonging to a particular patient will always be identifiable. Identification by chart numbers also allows certain information to be gained from other protocols containing an identical question.

SPECIFY ALL POSSIBLE ANSWERS

A protocol should have provision for all possible answers to a question. Data will be incomplete if possible answers are left out. It is advisable to perform a preliminary review of hospital charts to assist in designing answers.

THE "UNKNOWN" CATEGORY

Because the answer to a question is not always known, the response "unknown" must be an alternative. The same applies to the answer "none." It is also helpful to try to keep the same code numbers throughout the protocol for "unknown" and "none." This speeds the coding process and decreases the possibility of error.

AVOID "COMBINATION" ANSWERS

The answer "a combination of the above" is usually not informative and should be avoided. If it is desired to record complications, which may be multiple, each complication should be listed with a possible answer of no, yes, or unknown.

THE USE OF ZEROES

Avoid the use of "0" for an answer unless it represents none or unknown. Zeroes are used to fill in blank spaces (September 2, 1963 = 090263).

USE NUMBERS ONLY

The vast majority of statistical computer programs are designed to use only numerical codes. A good rule is to contact a computer specialist before designing coding forms and to have the form reviewed by him or her before using trial runs to test and "debug" forms.

IMPORTANCE OF ORDER

By designing the format of a protocol so that questions follow the sequence in which information appears in a hospital chart or becomes available in the research plan, recording is simpler and considerable time may be saved by reducing the amount of leafing required to find information.

CLARITY

A protocol should be sufficiently well written that the investigator will be able to understand it 6 months or a year later. Otherwise, a special set of definitions or instructions should be provided. Here again a glossary of definitions is important.

COMPUTERS

If a computer is available to the researcher, he or she may wish to design a protocol that adapts data for computer analysis. Direct data entry avoids the need for punched cards. It is extremely helpful if a protocol is designed so that data entry may be made directly from the protocol. All computer terminals permit direct data entry; it is now possible to read data directly into computers with appropriate forms and hardware.

If the researcher plans to use a computer for analysis, it is advisable to contact someone familiar with computer processing before the data are collected. Such consultation often helps to clarify whether a particular program will prove appropriate for analysis. Computers do whatever they have been programmed to do, whether it is sensible or ridiculous for a particular problem. An analysis made on a modern electronic computer will be performed more rapidly, efficiently, and accurately than one done by hand.

Employing a computer in no way reduces the amount of thinking required in a project, but it does permit analysis of larger amounts of data to be accomplished with greater speed and accuracy and at lower cost. If proper programs are already written to provide the desired analysis, a great deal of time may be saved. Often, however, desired programs are not available, so that either the analysis cannot be done or the programs must be written. The writing of computer programs can be a simple or a complex task, depending on the analysis desired and the form in which the data have been coded. Although the computer may be able to do an analysis in a matter of minutes, the writing of the appropriate program may take weeks or months. A danger of electronic computers is the temptation to do an analysis that is programmed rather than one that is appropriate.

It is convenient to think of two kinds of time when using a computer. The first is "machine time," the time the computer takes to do analysis once the program has been written and properly checked and the data prepared. The second kind of time is "calendar time." This is the time it takes to prepare the data and devise a program that will do the analysis properly. It is important to differentiate between the two. Often machine time may be a few minutes, whereas calendar time, if a computer is used, may be several weeks. The same analysis that takes a computer only seconds to accomplish may take much longer by any other method. Statistical packages of programs are proliferating rapidly and becoming more sophisticated.

The experience with clinical trials has led to an ever greater sophistication in the methodology of design and analysis. A group of British and American statisticians collaborated on a comprehensive report published in two parts (Peto et al., 1976, 1977), Part I covers the detail of careful experimental design: number of patients required, treatment schedules to be compared, significance levels, reasons for large trials, prior opinions, nonsignificant differences, treatment allocation ratios, randomized controls, historical controls, exclusions, losses, withdrawals, deviations, analysis, and ethics. Part II covers the general principles of analysis, definition of trial time for each patient, the life table, the log rank test, log rank significance levels, prognostic factors, use of prognostic factors, refinement of treatment comparisons, poor methods of analysis, amount of data per patient to be collected, subdivision of the follow-up period, arranging manner for data collection, assessment of causes of death, endpoints, duration of remissions, and the combining of information from different trials. This scholarly work should be studied carefully by all contemplating or planning a clinical trial. In this single chapter, only a few highpoints the authors believe worth emphasizing can be addressed.

Optimum Allocation Ratio

Clinical trial designing has great economic significance. In designing the project, the planner must decide on the maximum probability of a Type I or α error he or she is willing to accept. By accepting a 5 per cent chance of error ($p = 0.05$) the investigator recognizes that there is one chance in 20 that by chance alone the study will show a difference. When this decision is made, an estimate can now be attained as to the number of subjects required in study and control aims. Multiplying these numbers by the cost per case entry then permits an estimate of project cost.

Rosenberg (1983) addresses this question in a useful manner by calculating an optimum allocation ratio, which he defines as the ratio that will provide the greatest amount of information (or most statistical power) per dollar. When such cost information is needed for research budgeting, the reader will find a useful approach in Rosenberg's methods.

The Life Table

The life table (actuarial or Kaplan-Meier) method for comparing end results of different groups of patients is the analysis of choice in human survival studies (Cutler and Ederer, 1958; Kaplan and Meier, 1958). It provides estimates of survival curves even when all patients have not yet died or have been withdrawn for other reasons (i.e., deaths due to causes unrelated to breast cancer).

A life table is designed to compute the proportion of patients surviving after given intervals of time, generally 1 year. It is not necessary that 12 month intervals be used, and when the average survival time is relatively short, intervals of 3 or 6 months may be more appropriate and informative. Intervals need not be of the same length. For instance, in compiling a life table for a cancer site that kills

95 per cent of its patients within 2 years, 1 or 6 month intervals would be more meaningful than larger ones. Kaplan-Meier survival curves are the limit of actuarial curves as each interval is terminated by either a patient death or a withdrawal. If all patients in the group being compared have died—so that survival times are available for all—Student's t test can be used to compare the results, but a life table must be used in making comparisons with groups still having survivors.

In general, groups of patients being studied will still have survivors, and individuals have usually been followed for different periods. Obviously, survivors who have been followed for only 2 years at the termination of the follow-up period yield no information for the life table beyond 2 years and are "withdrawn" from the life table at this time.

For ease of computation, an augmented working life table is given in Table 30-1. To facilitate computation, extra columns are used to record intermediate values. The entries for each column in the table are defined as in Table 30-2.

The cumulative survival rate, Column 10, indicates the proportion of persons expected to survive a given time interval after some starting point (in this case the time of radical mastectomy). For example, of the 189 patients having radical mastectomy, 128 of them survived intervals of 4 years—that is, they are still living at the beginning of the fifth year interval. The survival rate through the fourth year is then $128/189 = 0.677$, or 67.7 per cent. Some patients were not operated on more than 5 years previously, and thus longer follow-up is impossible. Such patients are withdrawn alive at the limit of their follow-up period. The method of computing the cumulative survival rate takes this into account. Thus, the 10 year survival rate is 0.459 (45.9 per cent), not $(71 - 6)/189 = 0.344$ (34.4 per cent).

The standard deviation (σ) of the proportion surviving is given in Column 11. If the number of persons in the group is large, the researcher may be relatively certain (95 times in 100) that the true cumulative survival rate lies between the computed cumulative survival rate and $\pm 2\sigma$. For example, it is 95 per cent certain that the true 5 year survival rate is 0.608 ± 0.072, or between 0.536 and 0.680. Stated in terms of percentages, it may be said that between 53.6 and 68.0 per cent of the patients are expected to survive 5 years. Similarly, 45.9 per cent $\pm$ 2 (3.7 per cent), or between 38.5 per cent and 53.3 per cent, would be expected to survive 10 years.

Contingency Tables and Chi Square

Often in clinical research the investigator wishes to discover whether there is a relationship between two variables, neither of which may be quantified. For example, the researcher may wish to test whether there is a relationship between occupation and tumor site. If six tumor sites and four occupations were selected for investigation, a two-way contingency table could be set up, as in Table 30-3.

Since neither "occupation" nor "tumor site" is a quantifiable variable, the order in which the different categories are placed in the figure is unimportant. For example, if the occupational categories were recorded as farmer, executive, laborer, and salesman, rather than the order given in the table, the table would look different but would be just as meaningful. Variables requiring no specific sequence are called *nominal* variables.

To study the relationship between occupation and tumor site, the frequency of combination is placed in the appropriate cell. As illustrated in Table 30-3, there are 10 executives with skin tumors, six executives with lung tumors, five laborers with skin tumors, and eight laborers with mouth tumors. In a contingency table of this type, each patient should be counted as being in only one cell. This would mean that patients with two different tumor sites could not be used in this study. Or, if it were desired to use a patient with multiple tumors, the patient would be considered for only one site on the basis of some criterion, such as the site of the first tumor to appear. Similarly, if the patient had two occupations, he or she should be classified as belonging to only one occupational category, perhaps the one in which he or she spends more time. If these rules are followed, the sum of all numbers in the contingency table will be equal to the number of patients in the study. When each patient is counted only once in such a contingency table, statistical methods exist for determining whether the two variables (in this example, occupation and tumor site) are related. Similar methods do not exist if a

Table 30–1. AUGMENTED WORKING LIFE TABLE*

1 Time Interval (Years)	2 Number at Beginning of Interval	3 With-drawn Alive	4 Effective Exposed	5 Died in Interval	6 Proportion Dying	7 Proportion Surviving	8†	9†	10 Cumulative Survival Rate	11 σ of Cumulative Rate
0–1	189	0	189	14	0.074	0.926	0.000423	0.000423	0.926	0.019
1–2	175	0	175	15	0.086	0.914	0.000538	0.000961	0.846	0.026
2–3	160	0	160	14	0.088	0.912	0.000603	0.001564	0.772	0.030
3–4	146	0	146	18	0.123	0.877	0.000961	0.002525	0.677	0.035
4–5	128	0	128	13	0.102	0.898	0.000887	0.003412	0.608	0.036
5–6	115	1	114.5	7	0.061	0.939	0.000567	0.003979	0.571	0.036
6–7	107	1	106.5	8	0.075	0.925	0.000691	0.004670	0.528	0.036
7–8	98	12	92	5	0.054	0.946	0.000621	0.005291	0.500	0.036
8–9	81	7	77.5	3	0.039	0.961	0.000523	0.005814	0.480	0.037
9–10	71	6	68	3	0.044	0.956	0.000677	0.006491	0.459	0.037

*EFSCH patients with TNM Clinical Stage I carcinoma of the breast. Illustrates computation of cumulative and interval survival of a population with variable duration of follow-up.
†See Table 30–2 for explanation of this column.

Table 30–2. EXPLANATION FOR COLUMN NUMBERS IN TABLE 30–1

Column	Explanation
1	Time interval for all entries in the row
2	Number of patients alive at beginning of interval
3	Number of patients withdrawn during interval (includes lost to follow-up*)
4	Column 2 − ½ number in Column 3; effective number of patients exposed during time interval
5	Number of patients who died during interval
6	Column 5 ÷ Column 4; proportion dying during interval
7	1.0 − Column 6; proportion surviving interval
8	Column 6 ÷ (Column 4 − Column 5); intermediate values
9	Sum of all entries in Column 8 to and including this line; intermediate values
10	Product of all entries in Column 7 to and including this line; cumulative survival rate through given interval
11	Column 10 × √Column 9; standard deviation of cumulative survival rate

*Note: Lost patients introduce possible bias and should be held to a minimum.

patient is counted as being in more than one cell.

Using this technique, a researcher may be interested in testing whether different methods of classifying breast tumors are related. From Ellis Fischel State Cancer Hospital (EFSCH) data of radical mastectomy cases, a contingency table (Table 30–4) comparing Butcher's histologic type classification and the Columbia Clinical Classification has been constructed.

To determine whether the two variables in the table are related a statistic called chi square must be computed. This is a relatively simple procedure, as follows:

1. Compute the square of the number in each cell.
2. Divide each squared value in a row by the row total of the original table.
3. Divide each of these new values, derived in step 1, in a column by the column total of the original table. The new set of values is given in Table 30–5.
4. Find the sum of these new values and call this S. For Table 30–5, $S = 1.03038$.
5. Let N be the total number of observations in the original table. In the present example, $N = 445$.
6. The value of chi square is now computed as follows:

$$\text{(1)} \quad \begin{aligned} \text{Chi square} &= N(S - 1) \\ &= 445 \times (1.03038 - 1) \\ &= 445 \times 0.03038 \\ &= 13.51 \end{aligned}$$

7. Compute the degrees of freedom (df) associated with this chi square as $df = $ (number of rows − 1) × (number of columns − 1). For this problem, $df = (4 − 1) \times (4 − 1) = 3 \times 3 = 9$.

To determine whether a statistically significant relationship exists between the histologic type of neoplasms and the clinical stage (Columbia Clinical Classification), the level of significance associated with the computed chi square value is found in the chi square table (Table 30–6).

Because, for this problem, there are nine degrees of freedom, the values on the ninth row are the ones of interest. This row is indicated in the first column headed df. It is noticed that the computed chi square value (13.51) falls between the tabled chi square values 12.242 and 14.684 in the row with nine degrees of freedom. The levels of significance associated with these two values are $p = 0.20$ and $p = 0.10$, respectively. Thus, the probability that the chi square would be this large if there were no relationship between the two variables is between 0.20 and 0.10, which may be written as $0.10 < p < .20$. As this probability is relatively high, it cannot be inferred that the two variables are related. Programs for the above computations are now available for all microcomputers.

Table 30–3. A TWO-WAY CONTINGENCY TABLE RELATING SITE OF CANCER TO OCCUPATION OF PATIENT

Occupation	Tumor Site					
	Skin	Lung	Mouth	Neck	Breast	Liver
Executive	10	6	0	3	0	1
Laborer	5	0	8	0	7	2
Farmer	1	3	0	9	0	5
Salesman	4	0	9	0	6	0

Table 30–4. A TWO-WAY CONTINGENCY TABLE TO DETERMINE THE RELATIONSHIP BETWEEN THE HISTOLOGIC TYPE OF MAMMARY CANCERS AND THEIR CLINICAL STAGE

Columbia Clinical Classification (EFSCH Cases)	Butcher Histologic Type (EFSCH Cases)				Row Totals
	1	2	3	4	
A	5	10	142	12	169
B	0	5	119	11	135
C	3	1	78	11	93
D	0	0	43	5	48
Column totals	8	16	382	39	445

Had the chi square value been significant, (rejecting chance as an explanation for the observed association) in which case it could have been inferred that the two systems were related, it would have been of interest to see in what way these variables were related. To do this, the observed set of values (Table 30–4) is compared with an expected table or set of values. The expected values are computed under the assumption that the two variables are not related. To the extent and pattern that the observed table differs from the expected table it may be said that the two variables are related. However, there is no simple, single numerical value with which to express this. The type of relation involved, if it is statistically significant, can be understood by comparing the observed table with the expected table.

The expected value for any cell in the table is derived by multiplying the total number in the corresponding row by the total number in the corresponding column and then dividing this result by the total number in the table. For the foregoing example, the expected value for the cell in the second row and third column is as follows:

$$(2) \quad E_{2,3} = \frac{135 \times 382}{445} = 115.89$$

These are also produced by all computer statistical packages.

The expected figures for the foregoing problem are shown in Table 30–7. The values in the original table are compared with the corresponding values in the expected table, and differences are noted. The larger these differences are, the more the two variables may be said to be related. It will be noted that, in the example given, all such differences are relatively small.

An investigator may not be fortunate enough to have a large number of observations. It is generally stated in most statistical textbooks that if more than 20 per cent of the expected values are less than 10, the level of significance is poorly estimated by the chi

Table 30–5. COMPUTATIONS FOR DETERMINING CHI SQUARE FOR A TWO-WAY CONTINGENCY TABLE BETWEEN HISTOLOGIC TYPE OF MAMMARY CARCINOMA AND CLINICAL STAGE

Columbia Clinical Classification (EFSCH Cases)	Butcher Histologic Type (EFSCH Cases)			
	1	2	3	4
A	$\frac{5^2}{169 \times 8} = 0.01849$	$\frac{10^2}{169 \times 16} = 0.03698$	$\frac{142^2}{169 \times 382} = 0.31234$	$\frac{12^2}{169 \times 39} = 0.02185$
B	$\frac{0^2}{135 \times 8} = 0$	$\frac{5^2}{135 \times 16} = 0.01157$	$\frac{119^2}{135 \times 382} = 0.27460$	$\frac{11^2}{135 \times 39} = 0.02298$
C	$\frac{3^2}{93 \times 8} = 0.01210$	$\frac{1^2}{93 \times 16} = 0.00067$	$\frac{78^2}{93 \times 382} = 0.17125$	$\frac{11^2}{93 \times 39} = 0.03336$
D	$\frac{0^2}{48 \times 8} = 0$	$\frac{0^2}{48 \times 16} = 0$	$\frac{43^2}{48 \times 382} = 0.10084$	$\frac{5^2}{48 \times 39} = 0.01335$

Table 30–6. CHI SQUARE*

df	p = 0.99	0.98	0.95	0.90	0.80	0.70	0.50	0.30	0.20	0.10	0.05	0.02	0.01
1	0.000157	0.000628	0.00393	0.0158	0.0642	0.148	0.455	1.074	1.642	2.706	3.841	5.412	6.635
2	0.0201	0.0404	0.103	0.211	0.446	0.713	1.386	2.408	3.219	4.605	5.991	7.824	9.210
3	0.115	0.185	0.352	0.584	1.005	1.424	2.366	3.665	4.642	6.251	7.815	9.837	11.345
4	0.297	0.429	0.711	1.064	1.649	2.195	3.357	4.878	5.989	7.779	9.488	11.668	13.277
5	0.554	0.752	1.145	1.610	2.343	3.000	4.351	6.064	7.289	9.236	11.070	13.388	15.086
6	0.872	1.134	1.635	2.204	3.070	3.828	5.348	7.231	8.558	10.645	12.592	15.033	16.812
7	1.239	1.564	2.167	2.833	3.822	4.671	6.346	8.383	9.803	12.017	14.067	16.622	18.475
8	1.646	2.032	2.733	3.490	4.594	5.527	7.344	9.524	11.030	13.362	15.507	18.168	20.090
9	2.088	2.532	3.325	4.168	5.380	6.393	8.343	10.656	12.242	14.684	16.919	19.679	21.666
10	2.558	3.059	3.940	4.865	6.179	7.267	9.342	11.781	13.442	15.987	18.307	21.161	23.209

*Reprinted with permission of Macmillan Publishing Co., Inc., from Fisher, R. A.: Statistical Methods for Research Workers. © 1970, University of Adelaide.

Table 30–7. A TWO-WAY CONTINGENCY TABLE SHOWING THE EXPECTED COINCIDENT FREQUENCY OF HISTOLOGIC TUMOR TYPE AND CLINICAL STAGE OF MAMMARY CARCINOMAS ON THE BASIS THAT NO RELATIONSHIP EXISTS BETWEEN THE TWO VARIABLES*

Columbia Clinical Classification (EFSCH Cases)	Butcher Histological Type (EFSCH Cases)			
	1	2	3	4
A	3.04	6.08	145.08	14.80
B	2.43	4.85	115.89	11.83
C	1.67	3.34	79.84	8.15
D	0.86	1.73	41.22	4.21

*There is little difference between these calculated expected values and the observed values shown in Table 30–4. An insignificant relationship between the two variables exists.

square procedure. Because this problem occurs frequently, methods have been developed that compensate for small sample sizes. The necessary computations are time-consuming, and a computer must be used for all but the smallest tables.

Student's *t* Test

A brewer by the name of William Gosset during the last half of the 19th century devised a statistical method for determining whether two groups are different for a given set of measurements. Fearful lest he hurt his company's reputation, he published the method under the pseudonym of Student. Since that time Student's *t* test has become one of the most used, and perhaps most useful, statistical methods available for everyday use.

One use of Student's *t* test is to test whether the average value for a group of observations is different from the average value for a second group of observations. The *t* test is employed, for example, to test whether the average height for men is different from the average height for women. There are certain conditions to which the data must conform if the *t* test is to have validity. Basically there are two requirements.

1. The distribution of values for each group must be normal or near normal.
2. The variability of values within each group must be approximately equal.

A set of values is said to be normally distributed (rule 1) if the shape of the histogram of the frequency polygon can be approximated by a certain mathematical equation. This curve is often called the "bell-shaped" or "normal" curve. It is illustrated in Figure 30–1, for the logarithms of survival times for TNM Stage I radical mastectomy patients. The dashed line represents the smoothed frequency curve that would result if a large number of observations were made. The normal curve is symmetrical about the average value and the most frequent class interval. The variability of the distribution refers to the width of the curve at a given point. Rule 2 may be interpreted as requiring the shapes of the histograms arising from the two compared groups to be the same when there are an equal number of observations in each.

Often it is found, on making a frequency histogram of the data, that a bell-shaped curve does not result. This is true, for example, of survival times for breast cancer patients, as is illustrated in Figure 30–2. The curve has a long tail on the right and is therefore said to be skewed positively. The reverse would be a negative skew. It is obvious that Student's *t* test cannot be used to compare the survival times of two different groups of patients, because the distribution curve of survival time is not symmetric and therefore not normal. However, if the survival time for each patient is converted to its logarithm, the log values are approximately normally distributed; the resulting histogram is "bell-shaped." As these new values (logarithm of survival times) conform

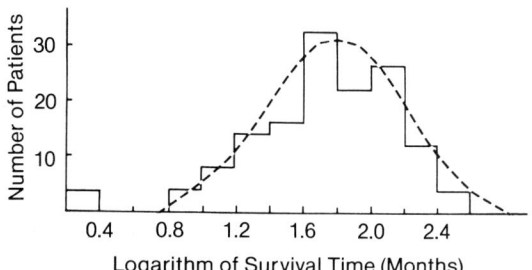

Figure 30–1. The frequency distribution of log-survival times of patients treated with radical mastectomy for TNM Stage I carcinoma of the breast (EFSCH, 1940 to 1958).

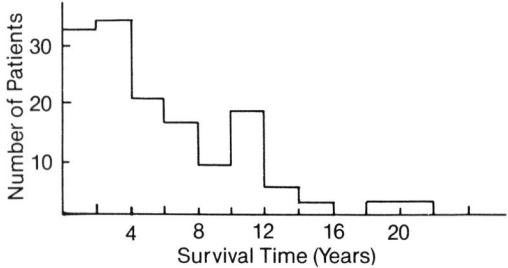

Figure 30–2. Frequency distribution of survival times for TNM clinical Stage I breast cancer patients treated with radical mastectomy (EFSCH, 1940 to 1958).

to the two rules required for Student's t test, these values may be compared to test for differences in survival times between two groups of patients.

Because every patient in each group must have a value for survival time, it is required that all patients have died. This is a great drawback if rapid analyses are required for comparing the results of two different treatments. However, it has the advantage that it can detect smaller differences than can the life table method.

An illustration of the use of Student's t test for comparing the survival times of two groups of patients is presented in Table 30–8. These data are from the first eight patients at EFSCH in each of the TNM clinical Stage I and clinical Stage IV breast tumor groups.

The first column under each stage lists the length of survival in months for the patients in each group. The second column under each stage contains the logarithm of the survival time for each patient. T_1 is the sum of the logarithms for patients in the Stage I category, and S_1 is the sum of the squares of the loga-

rithms for Stage I patients. These computations are made by simply squaring each logarithm and then summing these squares to get S_1. N_1 is the number of patients in the Stage I category. Finally, A_1 is the average value of the logarithms for the Stage I patients and is defined as $A_1 = T_1 - N_1$. The meanings for T_2, S_2, N_2 and A_2 are similarly defined for the patients in the Stage IV category.

Once the computation on Table 30–8 has been completed, the value of Student's t is derived from the following formula:

$$(3) \quad t = \frac{A_1 - A_2}{\sqrt{\frac{(S_1 - A_1 T_1) + (S_2 - A_2 T_2)}{N_1 + N_2 - 2} \times \left(\frac{1}{N_1} + \frac{1}{N_2}\right)}}$$

A numerical illustration of this formula is given for the data from Table 30–8 as below:

To interpret the value of Student's t, first determine the number of degrees of freedom.

$$(5) \quad \begin{array}{c} df = N_1 + N_2 - 2 \\ \text{or} \\ df = 8 + 8 - 2 = 14 \end{array}$$

For the example provided, the number of degrees of freedom is equal to 14. The computed t value (Table 30–9) is greater than any value on the $n = 14$ line and therefore the level of significance for the computed difference is less than 0.01. This is to say that if there really were no difference between the survival rates for the two groups, the proba-

$$t = \frac{1.961 - 1.191}{\sqrt{\frac{(31.606 - 1.961 \times 15.691) + (12.410 - 1.191 \times 9.527)}{8 + 8 - 2} \times \left(\frac{1}{8} + \frac{1}{8}\right)}}$$

$$t = \frac{0.770}{\sqrt{\frac{(0.8356) + (1.0636)}{14} \times (0.125 + 0.125)}}$$

$$t = \frac{0.770}{\sqrt{0.033925}}$$

$$(4) \quad t = 4.18$$

Table 30–8. STUDENT'S t TEST FOR COMPARING SURVIVAL TIMES OF EIGHT PATIENTS EACH WITH TNM CLINICAL STGE I AND IV MAMMARY CARCINOMA

TNM Stage I		TNM Stage IV	
Patient Survival (Months)	Logarithm of Survival Time	Patient Survival (Months)	Logarithm of Survival Time
300	2.477	6	0.778
42	1.623	14	1.146
269	2.430	3	0.477
32	1.505	21	1.322
93	1.968	26	1.415
93	1.968	51	1.708
76	1.881	20	1.301
69	1.839	24	1.380
$T_1 = 15.691$		$T_2 = 9.527$	
$S_1 = 31.606$		$S_2 = 12.410$	
$N_1 = 8$		$N_2 = 8$	
$A_1 = 1.961$		$A_2 = 1.191$	

bility that the difference $A_1 - A_2$ would be as great as it is is less than one in 100. Therefore, it is relatively certain that a real difference exists between the two groups. If the value of t had been 2.33 with 14 df, the same row would have been used in the t table, but the level of significance would be between 0.05 and 0.02. Again, the foregoing can be accomplished simply with a small computer.

In this case, a relatively small sample from

Table 30–9. TABLE OF t VALUES*

n	p = 0.9	0.8	0.7	0.6	0.5	0.4	0.3	0.2	0.1	0.05	0.02	0.01
1	0.158	0.325	0.510	0.727	1.000	1.376	1.963	3.078	6.314	12.706	31.831	63.657
2	0.142	0.289	0.445	0.617	0.816	1.061	1.386	1.886	2.920	4.303	6.965	9.925
3	0.137	0.277	0.424	0.584	0.765	0.978	1.250	1.638	2.353	3.182	4.541	5.841
4	0.134	0.271	0.414	0.569	0.741	0.941	1.190	1.533	2.132	2.776	3.747	4.604
5	0.132	0.267	0.408	0.559	0.727	0.920	1.156	1.476	2.015	2.571	3.365	4.032
6	0.131	0.265	0.404	0.553	0.718	0.906	1.134	1.440	1.943	2.447	3.143	3.707
7	0.130	0.263	0.402	0.549	0.711	0.896	1.119	1.415	1.895	2.365	2.998	3.499
8	0.130	0.262	0.399	0.546	0.706	0.889	1.108	1.397	1.860	2.306	2.896	3.355
9	0.129	0.261	0.398	0.543	0.703	0.883	1.100	1.383	1.833	2.262	2.821	3.250
10	0.129	0.260	0.397	0.542	0.700	0.879	1.093	1.372	1.812	2.228	2.764	3.169
11	0.129	0.260	0.396	0.540	0.697	0.876	1.088	1.363	1.796	2.201	2.718	3.106
12	0.128	0.259	0.395	0.539	0.695	0.873	1.083	1.356	1.782	2.179	2.681	3.055
13	0.128	0.259	0.394	0.538	0.694	0.870	1.079	1.350	1.771	2.160	2.650	3.012
14	0.128	0.258	0.393	0.537	0.692	0.868	1.076	1.345	1.761	2.145	2.624	2.977
15	0.128	0.258	0.393	0.536	0.691	0.866	1.074	1.341	1.753	2.131	2.602	2.947
16	0.128	0.258	0.392	0.535	0.690	0.865	1.071	1.337	1.746	2.120	2.583	2.921
17	0.128	0.257	0.392	0.534	0.689	0.863	1.069	1.333	1.740	2.110	2.567	2.898
18	0.127	0.257	0.392	0.534	0.688	0.862	1.067	1.330	1.734	2.101	2.552	2.878
19	0.127	0.257	0.391	0.533	0.688	0.861	1.066	1.328	1.729	2.093	2.539	2.861
20	0.127	0.257	0.391	0.533	0.687	0.860	1.064	1.325	1.725	2.086	2.528	2.845
21	0.127	0.257	0.391	0.532	0.686	0.859	1.063	1.323	1.721	2.080	2.518	2.831
22	0.127	0.256	0.390	0.532	0.686	0.858	1.061	1.321	1.717	2.074	2.508	2.819
23	0.127	0.256	0.390	0.532	0.685	0.858	1.060	1.319	1.714	2.069	2.500	2.807
24	0.127	0.256	0.390	0.531	0.685	0.857	1.059	1.318	1.711	2.064	2.492	2.797
25	0.127	0.256	0.390	0.531	0.684	0.856	1.058	1.316	1.708	2.060	2.485	2.787
26	0.127	0.256	0.390	0.531	0.684	0.856	1.058	1.315	1.706	2.056	2.479	2.779
27	0.127	0.256	0.389	0.531	0.684	0.855	1.057	1.314	1.703	2.052	2.473	2.771
28	0.127	0.256	0.389	0.530	0.683	0.855	1.056	1.313	1.701	2.048	2.467	2.763
29	0.127	0.256	0.389	0.530	0.683	0.854	1.055	1.311	1.699	2.045	2.462	2.756
30	0.127	0.256	0.389	0.530	0.683	0.854	1.055	1.310	1.697	2.042	2.457	2.750
∞	0.12566	0.25335	0.38532	0.52440	0.67449	0.84162	1.03643	1.28155	1.64485	1.95996	2.32634	2.57582

*Reprinted with permission of Macmillan Publishing Co., Inc., from Fisher, R. A.: Statistical Methods for Research Workers. © 1970, University of Adelaide.

each of the two groups being compared was sufficient to demonstrate a difference in survival times. In general, this method of comparing survival rates is more sensitive than the chi square method in that it requires fewer observations to demonstrate a statistically significant difference. As mentioned previously, it has the disadvantage that the survival time for every patient in the groups must be known. This requirement means that as long as any of the patients survive, Student's t cannot be computed. Discarding data from still surviving patients would only result in biasing the result, and the analysis would be meaningless.

Testing Whether Survival Rates Are Different for Two Different Life Tables

It is possible to determine if the survival rates for two groups of patients computed by the life table method are statistically different. A chi square procedure may be used for this purpose. From each of the two life tables being compared, the effective number exposed to risk and the number of patients dying during each interval are needed.

As a numerical example, the data from the EFSCH radical mastectomy cases are used to test whether the survival rate of patients with TNM clinical Stage I carcinoma is different from that of patients with Stage II carcinoma. Table 30–10 illustrates a convenient way to make computations. The definitions of the columns in Table 30–10 are given in Table 30–11.

The information contained in Columns 1 to 7 of Table 30–10 is derived directly from the life tables of the two groups being compared. Columns 8 and 9 contain the combined information for the two groups. Column 10 is the probability of dying during a given interval for the combined group. This is the best estimate of this probability under the assumption that the survival rates are identical for the two groups. Columns 11 and 13 are the number of persons expected to die in each time interval for each group if the rates are identical. Similarly, Columns 12 and 14 are the number of patients expected to survive. Thus, Columns 11 and 14 contain theoretically expected values for the two groups under the assumption that the survival rates are identical. The chi square (X^2) value is found from the sums for Columns 3, 6, 11, and 13. X^2_1 is equal to $\Sigma(^{(\Sigma obs - \Sigma exp)^2}/\Sigma exp) = 0.88$ as given at the bottom of Table 30–10. The value of df is 1. This procedure is known as the log rank test (Peto et al., 1976).

The probability that the two survival rates are *not* different can now be found from the chi square table with the proper degrees of freedom. For the example in Table 30–10, there is one degree of freedom. The probability that the chi square with one df would be as large as or larger than 0.88 (from Table 30–6) is greater than 0.50. Therefore, no difference between Stage I and Stage II survival rates has been demonstrated. If these two rates are really different, a larger number of observations are needed to demonstrate it.

Interpreting Student's t and Chi Square Values

The values computed with Student's t or the log rank (X^2) test, when used to test whether two groups differ, may be interpreted in terms of probability. Suppose there exist two large groups of cancer patients having identical survival times. Suppose further that a small sample is randomly selected from each group and the average survival time for each sample is compared. It is highly unlikely that the two averages would be identical, quite likely that they would be approximately equal, and unlikely that they would be very far apart. These are the conditions that are believed intuitively by almost everyone, but the terms "unlikely," "far apart," and so on, are not well defined and may mean different things to different persons. One object of developing statistical procedures is to define more precisely such nebulous terms. In doing so, some of the terms have been reduced to "standardized" forms. Both Student's t and chi square are such standardized terms. If the data from which these statistics are computed have particular characteristics, the relationship between their values and the probability (frequency) of the values occurring may be stated precisely.

Presume that it is possible to obtain from many different hospitals survival times for eight patients who have had radical mastectomy for TNM clinical Stage I and a similar number for Stage IV breast carcinoma, and

Table 30-10. COMPUTATIONS FOR DETERMINING BY THE CHI-SQUARE METHOD WHETHER THE SURVIVAL RATE FROM THE LIFE TABLE OF EFSCH PATIENTS WITH TNM STAGE I MAMMARY CARCINOMA IS DIFFERENT FROM THAT OF PATIENTS WITH TNM STAGE II

| | Observed | | | | | | | | | Expected | | | |
	TNM Stage I			TNM Stage II			TNM Combined			TNM Stage I		TNM Stage II	
Interval (Years)	Effective No. Exposed	No. Dying During Interval	No. Surviving Interval	Effective No. Exposed	No. Dying During Interval	No. Surviving Interval	Effective No. Exposed	No. Dying During Interval	Probability of Dying During Interval	No. Dying During Interval	No. Surviving Interval	No. Dying During Interval	No. Surviving Interval
1	2	3	4	5	6	7	8	9	10	11	12	13	14
1	189	14	175	230	11	219	419	25	.05966	11.28	177.72	13.72	216.28
2	175	15	160	219	24	195	394	39	.09899	17.32	157.68	21.68	197.32
3	160	14	146	195	29	166	355	43	.12113	19.38	140.62	23.62	171.38
4	146	18	128	166	19	147	312	37	.11859	17.31	128.69	19.69	146.31
5	128	13	115	147	9	138	275	22	.08000	10.24	117.76	11.76	135.24
6	114.5	7	107.5	138	19	119	252.5	26	.10297	11.79	102.71	14.21	123.79
7	106.5	8	98.5	116	9	107	222.5	17	.07640	8.14	98.36	8.86	107.14
8	92	5	87	102	7	95	194	12	.06186	5.69	86.31	6.31	95.69
9	77.5	3	74.5	92	5	87	169.5	8	.04720	3.66	73.84	4.34	87.66
10	68	3	65	81.5	2	79.5	149.5	5	.03344	2.27	65.73	2.73	78.77
SUM		100			134					107.08		126.92	

$$\chi_1^2 = (100-107.08)^2/107.08 + (134-126.92)/126.92 = 0.88 \; p > 0.20$$

presume further that the survival times for both stages are identical. If a t value is computed between the two stage groups for each hospital, it will be found that most of the t's are small, some are large, and others are intermediate. As a matter of fact, it can be found from the t table that a t value with 14 degrees of freedom, when there is really no difference between the groups, for 90 per cent of the time would be greater than 0.128, for 50 per cent of the time would be 0.692 or greater, and for only 1 per cent of the time would be greater than 2.977. Thus, if there were no difference between the survival of patients with Stage I and Stage IV cancer, it is highly unlikely with a given set of eight patients in each group that a t ratio between the logarithms of survival times would exceed 2.977. Here, "highly unlikely" means only one chance in 100. Since such a large t ratio did occur between the two groups, and it is unlikely to have occurred if there were really no difference, it may be concluded that there is a real difference in the survival times of the two stages.

The chi square table is based on a similar logic. Supposing that two groups were identical and that a small sample is taken from each group, the researcher may test whether these two samples differ in the proportion of living and dead in each. If this experiment were repeated many times, and there really were no

Table 30-11. EXPLANATION FOR COLUMN NUMBERS IN TABLE 30-10

Column	Explanation
1	Time interval from life tables
2	Effective number exposed to risk during time interval for first group, from Column 4 in life table
3	Number of patients dying during time interval for first group, from column 5 in life table
4	Column 2 − Column 3
5	Effective number exposed to risk during time interval for second group, from column 4 in life table
6	Number of patients dying during time interval for second group, from column 5 in life table
7	Column 5 − Column 6
8	Column 2 + Column 5
9	Column 3 + Column 6
10	Column 9 ÷ Column 8
11	Column 2 × Column 10
12	Column 2 − Column 11
13	Column 5 × Column 10
14	Column 5 − Column 13

difference in the 5 year survival rates, the chi square values computed would sometimes be small and sometimes be large. As this problem has one degree of freedom, it can be found from the chi square table that 80 per cent of the time the X^2 would be greater than 0.0642, 30 per cent of the time it would be greater than 1.074, and only 1 per cent of the time it would exceed 6.635. The chi square table defines the probability that X^2 would exceed a given value by chance alone, as it is assumed that the groups are identical.

If the computed chi square value is much larger than what is expected by chance, it is inferred that it was not caused by chance, but that a real difference between the groups exists.

This is the logic behind the method of statistical inference. It is not at all unlike the logic used in medical diagnosis. If a patient is seen with a certain set of symptoms, certain disease entities are immediately ruled out because they are "highly unlikely" to be associated with the set of symptoms. The terms "likely" and "unlikely" in this situation are not precisely defined; they are derived from the memory of past experience. On the other hand, if data from past experience are recorded, they can be analyzed to define more precisely the meaning of "likely." For example, suppose that symptom x is found to have occurred with disease y in 84 of 93 cases, or 90.3 per cent of the time, whereas symptom x occurred with disease z in 15 of 93 cases, or 16.1 per cent of the time. If such records are kept, the terms "likely" and "unlikely" are avoided and are replaced by 90.3 per cent and 16.1 per cent, which have the same meaning to different diagnosticians.

Interpreting data is of interest in that it enables the user to predict future events. How past data are employed to predict or infer future events depends on what may be assumed about the events involved, such as the known underlying mechanisms relating symptoms and diseases or the characteristics of the population of patients involved. The rules established by these considerations are restated in mathematical terminology. This restatement is often called a mathematical or statistical model. In general it is difficult, or may be impossible, to devise a model that includes all known facts about the phenomena under study, and so the model is only an abstract of the real phenomena. This may seem to be a weakness on the part of mathematical models, but it is a weakness that is shared by human thought as well.

The advantages of a mathematical model are that the rules are stated more explicitly, and the variation of meanings is reduced. This is a great advantage in that many investigators may employ the model to analyze different data, and the results may be compared with greater meaning.

Just as a person may buy a ready-made suit, there are many ready-made statistical models available to the researcher. Also, as care must be given in selecting an off-the-shelf suit to fit a given individual, the ready-made statistical model employed must be selected on the basis that the logic on which it was built conforms to the logic of the problem under analysis.

The chi square and Student's t tests are examples of "off-the-shelf" statistical models. The assumption on which they are built conforms reasonably well to the assumption made about many medical phenomena and they are, therefore, useful in these situations. There is still much work to be done in the development of statistical models as well as in translating medical logic to mathematical or statistical statements. Only as these two work hand in hand can more meaningful interpretations of medical data be made.

Cumulative Frequency Distribution of Death Rates

Lognormal probability paper is a type of graph paper set up in such a fashion that the user may quickly perceive what proportion of patients have survived a given time interval. The resulting "curve," as in Figure 30–3, approaches a straight line when survival times are lognormally distributed. The data plotted in Figure 30–3 are from EFSCH patients' charts. Of eight patients with TNM clinical Stage IV breast carcinomas who received a radical mastectomy, 75 per cent lived 6 months or more, 50 per cent survived 20 months or more, and so on. Of the first 100 patients with Stage I breast tumors who were treated with radical mastectomy, 92 per cent lived 12 months or more, 77 per cent lived 36 months or more, and so on.

From this type of distribution and graph, it becomes readily apparent that the survival

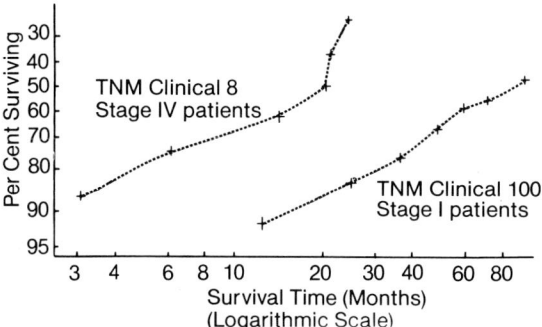

Figure 30–3. Cumulative survival rates of EFSCH patients treated with radical mastectomy for mammary carcinoma (illustrating the use of logarithms of survival time).

times for these two groups are different and that Stage I patients have a longer survival time. This is a convenient way to look at survival data. Other types of transformations achieve similar results for other distributions. If the number of patients in a group is large, the resulting line will often be relatively straight, but when the number of patients in a group is small, the line will be irregular.

The method of testing whether the two survival curves are significantly different when neither group has survivors has been discussed under Student's t test.

For these data, both axes are unequally spaced. The space between the survival time is proportional to the logarithm of the differences between the survival times; that is, it is a logarithmic scale. The spacing between the percentage of survival is arrived at in a somewhat more complex manner.

Producing survival curves in this manner allows the researcher to present data in a direct, meaningful manner.

Estimating Required Sample Size (Power of the Test)

An important aspect in the design of any research is that of determining the number of observations necessary (Halperin et al., 1968). If the number of observations is more than necessary to test a hypothesis, the extra time and cost involved are only part of the real loss. On the other hand, if the number of observations is too small, the investigator may not be giving himself or herself a sufficient opportunity to evaluate the hypothesis. The goal of this section is to aid the investigator in selecting the appropriate sample size required for the specific experiment.

The tables included in this chapter are designed to be used as a ready reference for determining appropriate sample size of a proposed experiment. All values are computed by use of the arc sine transformations of a proportion as described by Sokal and Rohlf (1969).

Suppose an investigator believes that a newly developed treatment is superior to the standard treatment. Assume that the 2 year survival rate for the standard treatment is 45 per cent. Preliminary results indicate that the new treatment will result in a 2 year survival rate of 65 per cent. What sample size for the control and experimental groups will the investigator need to test whether the new treatment is, indeed, superior to the standard treatment? It will be further assumed that the investigator will accept the new treatment as superior if it can be demonstrated at the 5 per cent level of significance.

To compute the required sample size, the investigator must state one more parameter. This parameter is called the "power" of a test. It is the ability to detect a true difference of a specified size, and the numerical value of this parameter lies between 0 and 1.

A power of 0.5 means the investigator will have 50 per cent chance of detecting a true difference of a specified size between the survival rates of the two treatments. Or, in colloquial terms, the investigator has only "half a chance" to prove the hypothesis. Similarly, a power of 0.7 gives the investigator a 70 per cent chance of detecting a true difference of a specified size. Another way of looking at the power of a test follows.

Suppose 100 institutions are simultaneously but independently evaluating the new treatment discussed previously. However, each institution has a sample size sufficient to yield a power of 0.5, assuming each will accept the experimental treatment as better if the specified difference should prove to be significant at the 5 per cent level. In this situation, half (0.5) of the institutions will find the new treatment significantly (statistically) better than the standard treatment. Also, half of the institutions will be unable to demonstrate this. Thus, arguments ensue.

Indeed, this problem may lie at the heart of many disputes concerning the values of different treatments. Because many institutions do not have a sufficient patient population to be able to compare two treatment methods within a reasonable time frame, there is a tendency toward more cooperative studies.

It is generally accepted that a statistical test for any serious research should have a power of about 0.9. This means that before the experiment is begun, the researcher will have about a 90 per cent chance of statistically rejecting the null hypothesis—*if it is false*. Certainly, any investigator who is going to put a great amount of effort into the work will want at least this much of a chance. To be assured of this, he or she will need to select an appropriate sample size.

THE STANDARD CLINICAL EXPERIMENT

Generally, the standard clinical experiment requires the use of a control group and an experimental group. Thus, this may be called a two group experiment. Both groups are treated identically except for the experimental variables being evaluated. Ideally, these should be double-blind. As a minimum, the assignment of a patient to a group should be random.

Also, in the standard experiment, if it is believed that the experimental treatment is superior to the treatment to be received by the control group, the experiment would be unethical. The experimental treatment *should* be used. If it is unknown which treatment is truly superior, an experiment is the only scientific way to proceed. For this reason, the investigator will need to use a nondirectional, or two-tailed, test. A one-tailed test can be used validly only if the researcher is *unwilling* to conclude, regardless of the experimental results, that the new treatment is inferior to the standard treatment.

Under the conditions stated for the standard clinical experiment, Table 30–12 may be used to determine the sample size required to test the hypothesis at the 0.05 level of significance with a power of 0.9. For example, if it is assumed that the standard (control) treatment has a 45 per cent ($p_c = 0.45$) 2 year survival, and it is believed that the experimental treatment will yield a 65 per cent ($p_e = 0.65$) 2 year survival, the required sample size for each group may be found to be $N = 128.2$. This is done by finding $p_e = 0.45$ on the row indicated by 0.45 in the left hand column and the column indicated by .65 in the first row. Their intersection contains the value of 128.2. Thus, 129 patients will be required in each group, for a total of 258 patients.

Let p_e be the proportion cured for the experimental group and p_c be the proportion cured for the control group. The general hypotheses will be $H_0: p_e = p_c$ and $H_1: p_e \neq p_c$ with values known or estimated for each p_e and p_c. H_0 refers to the null hypothesis and H_1 refers to the alternate hypothesis. Find the value of p_c in the left hand index and the value of p_e in the top index of Table 30–12. The intersection yields the sample size required for *each* group for the experiment to have a 90 per cent chance (power = 0.9) of detecting the difference at the 5 per cent level of significance.

As another example, suppose the 2 year survival rates for the control and experimental groups were $p_c = 0.30$ and $p_e = 0.55$. Table 30–12 indicates that $N = 80.2$ is required. That is, 81 patients will need to be treated by each method.

LEVEL OF SIGNIFICANCE

If the investigator wishes to be more stringent and will accept the hypothesis that the experimental treatment is superior only if it can be demonstrated at the 1 per cent (0.01) level of significance, rather than at 5 per cent, Table 30–13 must also be used in conjunction with Table 30–12.

To accomplish this for a two-tailed test, find the column in Table 30–13 in which the level of significance (α) = 0.01 and the row in which power = 0.9. This value is 1.416. Multiply the sample size from Table 30–12 by this value to obtain the sample size needed to test the hypothesis at the 0.01 level of significance with a power of 0.9.

Thus, for $p_c = 0.30$ and $p_e = 0.55$, power = 0.9 and level of significance of 0.01, the required sample size for a two-tailed test is

(6) $\qquad N = 80.2 \times 1.416 = 113.6$

for each group.

If the experimenter wants a 99 per cent (a power of 0.99) chance of detecting the difference at the 0.01 level of significance and assumes that $p_c = 0.50$ and $p_e = 0.75$, the required sample size would be

(7) $\qquad N = 76.7 \times 2.287 = 175.4$

for each group.

Table 30–13 lists factors by which the num-

Table 30–12. TWO-TAILED SAMPLE SIZE DETERMINATION, d = 0.05, POWER = 0.9

Smallest Proportion	Largest Proportion																	
	0.95	0.90	0.85	0.80	0.75	0.70	0.65	0.60	0.55	0.50	0.45	0.40	0.35	0.30	0.25	0.20	0.15	0.10
0.05	5.4	6.3	7.1	8.0	9.0	10.2	11.5	13.3	15.3	18.0	21.5	24.9	31.5	42.0	59.1	92.6	177.2	567.4
0.10	6.3	7.4	8.5	9.7	11.2	13.0	15.1	17.8	21.1	25.6	30.7	39.9	54.2	79.0	129.0	261.0	910.7	—
0.15	7.1	8.5	9.9	11.7	13.7	16.2	19.3	23.3	27.4	35.0	46.1	63.8	94.8	158.8	331.5	1208.2	—	
0.20	8.0	9.7	11.7	13.9	16.7	20.1	24.7	29.4	38.0	50.8	71.2	107.5	183.1	390.6	1462.0	—		
0.25	9.0	11.2	13.7	16.7	20.4	25.3	30.7	40.0	54.0	76.7	117.2	202.5	438.7	1673.1	—			
0.30	10.2	13.0	16.2	20.1	25.3	31.0	41.0	56.0	80.2	124.2	216.8	475.8	1842.0	—				
0.35	11.5	15.1	19.3	24.7	30.7	41.0	56.6	82.1	128.2	226.4	502.5	1968.4	—					
0.40	13.3	17.8	23.3	29.4	41.0	56.0	82.1	129.6	231.2	518.4	2052.6	—						
0.45	15.3	21.1	27.4	38.0	54.0	80.2	128.2	231.2	523.7	2094.9	—							
0.50	18.0	25.6	35.0	50.8	76.7	124.2	226.4	518.4	2094.9	—								
0.55	21.5	30.7	46.1	71.2	117.2	216.8	502.5	2052.6	—									
0.60	24.9	39.9	63.8	107.5	202.5	475.8	1968.4	—										
0.65	31.7	54.2	94.8	183.1	438.7	1842.0	—											
0.70	42.0	79.0	158.8	390.6	1673.1	—												
0.75	59.1	129.0	331.5	1462.0	—													
0.80	92.6	261.0	1208.2	—														
0.85	177.2	910.7	—															
0.90	567.4	—																

Table 30-13. POWER CONVERSION FACTORS

Power	Level of Significance (Two-Tailed) (α)						
	0.20	0.10	0.050	0.02	0.01	0.002	0.001
0.70	0.311	0.447	0.588	0.773	0.914	1.243	1.385
0.80	0.429	0.588	0.747	0.955	1.112	1.471	1.624
0.90	0.625	0.815	1.000	1.239	1.416	1.819	1.989
0.95	0.815	1.030	1.236	1.500	1.697	2.134	2.320
0.99	1.239	1.501	1.748	2.060	2.287	2.792	3.002

ber from Table 30-12 is to be multiplied to obtain the required sample size for each of two groups, depending on the power, as indicated on the left hand index, and the level of significance, as indicated across the top.

GENERAL RULE FOR STANDARD CLINICAL EXPERIMENT

For the standard clinical experiment, find the value in Table 30-12 corresponding to the rates of the experimental and control groups, then find the value in Table 30-13 corresponding to the desired level of significance and power. The product of these two values is the required sample size for *each* group.

GENERAL APPROACH

From Table 30-12 determine the number, N_1, that corresponds to the two rates being compared. From Table 30-13 determine the value, V_2, corresponding to the desired power and level of significance. The required sample size, N, is computed for each group as follows:

(8) $$N = N_1 \times V_2$$

When $N < 20$, this estimate should be increased by 1.

For example, suppose the two hypothetical cure rates to be compared were $p_1 = 0.25$ and $p_2 = 0.75$; then $N_1 = 20.4$. If the investigator wished, as a preliminary evaluation, to test at the 0.05 level of significance, with a power of 0.7, using a two-tailed test, then $V_2 = 0.588$. Then the first estimate of the required sample size would be

(9) $$\begin{aligned} N &= N_1 \times V_2 \\ &= 20.4 \times 0.588 \\ &= 12.0 \end{aligned}$$

As this is less than 20, 1 must be added. The regular sample size is then 13 for each group.

ONE HYPOTHETICAL VALUE

If an investigator wishes to test whether an experimental treatment yields a rate different from a hypothetical rate, only one group is required (the experimental group). In this case, the desired sample size is computed according to the previous equations, and this value is then divided by two to obtain the final required sample size.

For example, suppose an investigator wishes to test whether an experimental treatment has a 2 year survival rate of greater than 0.50. He or she may hypothesize that the survival rate of the experimental treatment is 0.65. From Table 30-12, $N_1 = 226.4$ is obtained.

Since the researcher must allow for the possibility that the experimental method is poorer than the hypothetical treatment, a two-tailed test will be used to obtain a 0.05 level of significance. Because the investigator wishes to have a good chance of rejecting H_0 if it is false, a power of 0.95 may be selected. From Table 30-13, $V_2 = 1.236$ is obtained.

Thus, the required sample size for the single group is

(10) $$N = \frac{N_1 \times V_2}{2} = \frac{226.4 \times 1.236}{2} = \frac{279.8}{2} = 139.9$$

This example is included for completeness. However, the investigator should know that this procedure (single group) has many problems and should be aware of them before planning or executing a single group experiment.

POOL POWER

Suppose two institutions wish to investigate, independently, the value of a new treatment. Assume the standard treatment yields a cure rate of 50 per cent and the new treatment will yield a cure rate of 70 per cent. Also assume that it is not known yet that the new treatment is better, and so the trial is necessary.

Assume that each institution wishes to have a 90 per cent chance of demonstrating that the new treatment is 20 percentage points better than the standard treatment and wishes to demonstrate this at the 1 per cent level of significance. From Tables 30–12 and 30–13 it is found that the required size for each group (control and experimental) is 176 = (124.2 × 1.416). Each institution needs a total of 352 patients. Now, since each institution is performing the experiment independently of the other, what results may be expected?

Let P be the power or probability that an institution will find the difference significant, and $Q = 1 - P$. Then, because two institutions perform the same experiment independently, the answer is found by expanding the polynomial as follows:

$$(11) \quad (P + Q)^2 = P^2 + 2PQ + Q^2$$

where $P^2 = 0.81$ is the probability that both institutions will find the new treatment significantly better

$2PQ = 0.18$ is the probability that one institution will find the new treatment significantly better, but the other one will not

$Q^2 = 0.01$ is the probability that neither will find the new treatment significantly better

Because two institutions are involved, a total of 704 patients is required. Yet, 18 per cent of the time disagreement will occur, and only 82 per cent of the time will the results from the two institutions agree. Thus, the question would still have a good chance of not being resolved. In one sense, then, the power of the combined experiments is only 0.81, rather than 0.9, as each had thought; the probability of totally missing the new treatment, however, is reduced from 0.10 to 0.01.

On the other hand, had the two institutions decided to join in the research and to pool their observations in a single experiment, each institution would have to supply only 284 patients. That is, in total, only 284 patients would be required for each group to obtain a power of 0.99 to test at the significance level 0.01. This number may be obtained by multiplying the appropriate values in Tables 30–12 and 30–13: 284 = 124.2 × 2.287.

Thus, with 568 patients, the two institutions would be able to demonstrate, jointly, the superiority of the experimental treatment at the 1 per cent level of significance with a power of 0.99. Individually, 704 patients will yield disagreement 18 per cent of the time and a power of 0.81. Of course, there are methods of combining evidence from independent studies that would recover some of the lost power.

It is apparent, then, that if many institutions independently perform the experiment, the power of each must necessarily be low, and the chance for disagreement becomes great. Thus, many important questions remain unresolved in this situation.

On the other hand, by joining forces definitive answers may be obtained regarding the superiority of new treatments. Not only is the smaller sample size important in itself, but it also reduces the time required to resolve the question. Thus, the power of a test is significantly enhanced when data from several institutions are pooled as opposed to when they are analyzed separately.

POWER NEEDED TO REJECT NEW TREATMENT

Perhaps too frequently investigators pay little attention to the power of a test. Generally, then, the resulting statistical analyses are unable to demonstrate differences between competing treatment methods. But it must be kept in mind that the failure to demonstrate a difference does not imply that there is no difference. This is especially true if the statistical procedure has insufficient power because of a relatively small sample size.

Suppose that a standard treatment method yields a 2 year survival rate of 0.55, and a new procedure is expected to produce a 2 year survival rate of 0.75. From Table 30–12 it is seen that a sample size of 117.2 is required for each of the two kinds of treatments to establish a difference at the 0.05 level of significance with a power of 0.9.

If the difference is demonstrated in this example by statistical analyses, clinicians may still be hesitant to discard the standard treatment in favor of the new treatment, as the 0.05 level of significance could still have occurred 5 per cent of the time by chance alone. Thus, the physician may believe that the new treatment has not been proved sufficiently to accept it.

On the other hand, if no difference has been demonstrated at the 0.05 level of significance, it is tempting to continue the standard treatment with a feeling of justification. But if the specified difference exists, it will not be discovered 10 per cent of the time.

In general, if the level of significance is less than (1 − power) of a test, a bias is given to the standard treatment. This may be correct, but it should not be done without consideration.

The bias in favor of the standard treatment is that it is more likely to be accepted. For example, suppose the standard rate and the experimental rate are equally likely to be true and a level of significance, α, is employed. Then, if the standard rate is true, it will be accepted as true (1 − α) of the time. On the other hand, if the experimental rate is true, it will be accepted a proportion of the time equal to the power of the test. Thus, they are equally likely to be accepted if power = (1 − α), or if α = (1 − power). However, if α < (1 − power), then (1 − α) > power, and the standard rate is more likely to be accepted as true.

Let α be the probability of making an error when the standard rate is true, and (1 − power) be the probability of making an error when the experimental rate is true. If the cost of each error is the same, the expected cost is minimized when α = (1 − power).

As a consequence, if a level of significance of 0.01, is demanded so that the new treatment will replace the standard treatment with ample confidence and (1 − power) is set equal to the level of significance, the value corresponding to α = 0.01 and power = 0.99 must be found in Table 30–13. This value is 2.287. The required sample size for each group in this example would be

(12) $N = 117.2 + 2.287 = 268.0$

By setting the power to 0.99 and the level of significance to 0.01, the resulting analysis will yield a considerably more definitive conclusion than in the foregoing example. Just as, if the results demonstrate a difference, the difference may be considered real, so also, if no difference is demonstrated, the individual may be equally confident that any difference between the two survival rates is less than 20 per cent (75 per cent − 55 per cent = 20 per cent).

The decision to accept the new treatment, continue with the standard treatment, or gather more experience, depending on the results of the experiment, is influenced by the proper choices of power and level of significance. This choice in turn is based on the costs involved in making a wrong decision.

Two wrong decisions may be made: to continue the standard treatment when the experimental treatment is, in fact, better and to change to the experimental treatment when, in fact, no difference exists.

This is a simplification of the total problem but describes it in essence.

Choosing the proper values for the power and levels of significance for an experiment involves what actions will be taken depending on the outcome of the experiment, and the different costs of these actions if the incorrect decision is made.

TESTING THE DIFFERENCE BETWEEN TWO MEANS

Student's t test was discussed in the previous section as a method to test the difference between two means. This section deals with the computation of the required sample size for the t test.

A *one-group t test* is frequently of interest to test whether the mean of a single group is equal to a certain value, designated here as C. The equation for the two-group t test was given previously.

The equation for the one-group t test is as follows:

(13) $$t = \frac{A - C}{\sqrt{\frac{S - AT}{N(N-1)}}}$$

where A is the average value of the group, C is the value against which A is being tested, T is the sum of the values for the group, S is the sum of the squares of the individual's values for the group, and N is the number of values in the group. These definitions are the same as those given previously. The level of significance of t (one-group) is found in Table 30–9, using the degree of freedom as $n = N - 1$.

To compute the required sample size for a one- or two-group t test, Table 30–14 is employed. First the standard deviation that the group(s) may be expected to have is deter-

Table 30-14. REQUIRED SAMPLE SIZE (TWO-TAILED)

Large Sample			Small Sample		
$\frac{M_1 - M_2}{\sigma}$	Two Group	One Group	$\frac{M_1 - M_2}{\sigma}$	Two Group	One Group
0.01	210157	105079	0.65	52	28
0.02	52540	26270	0.70	44	25
0.03	23351	11676	0.75	39	21
0.04	13135	6568	0.80	34	20
0.05	8407	4204	0.85	31	17
0.06	5838	2919	0.90	27	16
0.07	4290	2145	0.95	25	15
0.08	3285	1643	1.00	23	13
0.09	2695	1298	1.05	21	12
0.10	2102	1051	1.10	20	11
0.15	935	468	1.15	17	11
0.20	525	263	1.20	16	10
0.25	337	169	1.25	15	10
0.30	234	117	1.30	13	9
0.35	172	86	1.35	13	9
0.40	133	67	1.40	12	9
0.45	104	52	1.45	12	7
0.50	85	43	1.50	11	7
0.55	70	35	1.55	11	7
0.60	59	30	1.60	10	7

mined. In the case of two groups, both groups are expected to have the same standard deviation. This value may be known from previous data, or it may be estimated by a small sample of data. Using the previous notation, the standard deviation, σ, may be estimated as follows:

$$\hat{\sigma} = \sqrt{\frac{S - AT}{N(N-1)}} \quad (14)$$

Let M_1 be the observed mean of the experimental group. Let us test whether these observations would have arisen if the true value of the mean were some constant, say, C. Compute $\frac{M_1 - C}{\sigma}$. If this number is negative, change it to positive. Look for the number nearest this value in the first (or fourth) column of Table 30–14. Find the corresponding number to the right, on the same line, under the column heading "One Group." Call this number N_1.

Again, for similar reasons, our results will be limited to two-tailed tests. Decide the power of the test. From Table 30–13 find the value at the intersection of the correct level-of-significance and desired power. Call this V_2. The required sample, N, is obtained as $N = N_1 \times V_2$.

For example, suppose we expect the group mean to be $M_1 = 24$. We wish to test whether the mean may truly be $C = 22$. Suppose that $\sigma = 4$. First, compute

$$\frac{M_1 - C}{\sigma} = \frac{24 - 22}{4} = \frac{2}{4} = 0.5 \quad (15)$$

Look in Table 30–14 for the value $\frac{M_1 - M_2}{\sigma} = 0.5$. This number is 43. Thus, $N_1 = 43$.

We will continue to use a two-tailed test. If we desire α to be 0.01 and the power to be 0.95, we may find from Table 30–13 that $V_2 = 1.697$, so the required sample size is

$$N = N_1 \times V_2 = 43 \times 1.697 = 73.0 \quad (16)$$

Thus, 73 observations are required to run the test as described.

For the *two-group t test* the difference between the means that the investigator expects to find or is interested in testing must be stated. Let this difference be represented by $D_1 = M_1 - M_2$, where M_1 and M_2 are the expected values of the means of the two groups.

Now the value $\frac{M_1 - M_2}{\sigma}$ is to be computed. If it is negative, make it positive. Look for the nearest value to this in the first column (or fourth column) in Table 30–14. The corresponding value, on the same line to the right (under "Two Group"), is the sample size required for a two-tailed t test with $\alpha = 0.05$ and power = 0.90. Call this number N_1.

Now decide the level of significance desired. Decide the power of the test desired. Lastly, find the corresponding factor in Table 30–13 as before. Call this V_2. Now the required sample size, N, is given as in equation 8:

$$N = N_1 \times V_2$$

For example, suppose we expect the mean of group 1 to be $M_1 = 5$ and the mean of group 2 to be $M_2 = 8$. Also, we expect the standard deviation of each group to be $\sigma = 30$. Then

$$(17) \quad \frac{M_1 - M_2}{\sigma} = \frac{5 - 8}{30} = \frac{-3}{30} = 0.1$$

As this value is negative, make it positive so that it equals 0.1.

Find 0.1 under the first column in Table 30–14, marked $\frac{M_1 - M_2}{\sigma}$, and notice that the first number to the right is 2102. Thus, $N_1 = 2102$.

We desire a test at the 0.01 level of significance, two-tailed, and we desire that the test have a 0.90 probability of being significant. The multiplying factor is found in Table 30–13 at the intersection of power = 0.9 and $\alpha = 0.01$. This factor is 1.416, or $V_2 = 1.416$. Now multiply the numbers obtained from the two tables to get

$$2102 \times 1.416 = 2976.4$$

So, to satisfy the conditions of the foregoing t test, 2977 observations (patients) are needed in *each* group.

COMPUTING THE POWER OF A TEST

The literature is full of nonsignificant results and even more are never published. But what does a nonsignificant result mean? Does it mean that no difference exists? Or does it mean the sample size was too small to yield a reasonable chance of a significant result?

If an investigator found "no significant difference" when using the t test (or other test), should this be taken to mean that there is probably no real difference? Suppose the power of the test used was only 0.5. This would mean the investigator had only a 50 per cent chance of finding a significant difference, even if the difference were real. Therefore, the negative finding should not be taken too seriously.

On the other hand, if the power of the test was 0.99, this would mean the investigator had a 99 per cent chance of finding a "significant difference" if a specified difference really existed. But a significant difference was not found. Others might then have considerable faith that no nontrivial difference actually existed.

Thus, our interpretation of "not significant" has different meanings, depending on the power of the test that was used. The power of a test may be computed with the aid of Figure 30–4 and the sample size actually employed.

Suppose an author reported that the survival rate for patients under treatment one was $p_1 = 0.45$, whereas the survival rate for patients under treatment two was $p_2 = 0.55$. Furthermore, he found the difference to be "not significant" at the 0.01 level using a two-tailed test.

To compute the power of the test reported, it must be determined first what sample size we would have required based on the material discussed in this chapter. From Table 30–12 it is seen that for $\alpha = 0.05$ and a power of 0.9, a sample size of 523.7 would have been required to test whether $p_1 = p_2$. Because, however, the experimenter used a test with $\alpha = 0.01$, we need to obtain the multiplying factor from Table 30–13. Assume that we would have used a power of 0.9. With the power of 0.9 and $\alpha = 0.01$, Table 30–13 gives a factor of 1.416. The required sample size would have been

$$523.7 \times 1.416 = 741.6$$

or 742 patients under each treatment.

Suppose the investigator stated that the study included 350 patients under each treatment. We may now compute the "sample fraction" that the investigator studied compared with what we would have used:

$$\text{Sample fraction} = \frac{\text{Sample size used in study}}{\text{Required sample size}}$$

$$(18) \quad = \frac{350}{742}$$

$$= 0.472$$

Find this value along the abscissa in Figure 30–4. Follow this point up until it intersects

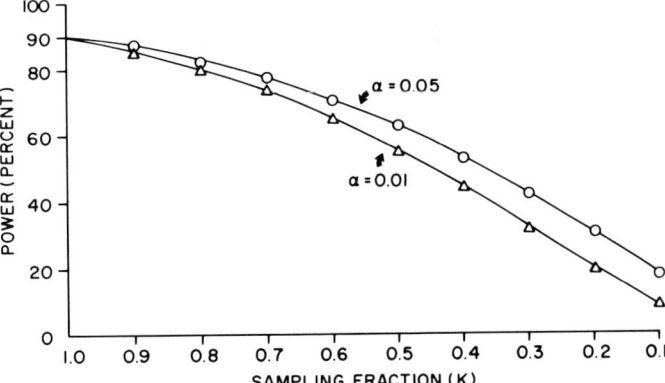

Figure 30–4. Computation of power of a test.

the diagonal line labeled $\alpha = 0.01$. Read the power of the test on the ordinate on the left. The power is ≈ 0.53.

Therefore, although the investigator found no significant difference between the two survival rates ($p_1 = 0.45$ and $p_2 = 0.55$) at the 0.01 level, this should not be taken to mean that the two survival rates are equal. For if the rates are truly this different, the results would be expected to be significant only 53 times out of 100, with only 350 patients in each group.

The power of a reported test may be readily computed from Figure 30–4. This may be computed for the test between proportions or the test between means.

In general, first compute the sample size required for the test of significance as stated, using the value of α as reported. To compute this required sample size, a power of 0.9 is to be assumed. This procedure was described previously.

Now compute the fraction of the required sample size that the investigator used, by dividing the actual sample size by the required sample size. Find the value of this "sample fraction" on the abscissa of Figure 30–4. Follow this point vertically until it intersects the diagonal line labeled with the appropriate value of α. Read the value of the power of the test from the ordinate on the left.

Sequential Procedures

The tests so far considered are based on fixed sample sizes. In practice, ethical considerations often require that the data be examined before the study is complete. The more often the data are examined, however, the more likely it is that a significant result will be obtained by chance. Sequential procedures have been developed to adjust nominal significance levels to a wide variety to stopping rules. Indeed, the data can be examined after every case is treated and a decision then made to continue or terminate the experiment. Such sequential designs are rarely used in cancer studies owing to the length of time between cancer treatment and outcome. The reader is referred to Pasternak's report (1981) for a further discussion and a table of adjusted significance levels when the study is analyzed several times before its completion.

Simultaneous Tests of Significance (Analysis of Subgroups)

There are two major types of research: hypothesis testing and investigatory. Hypothesis testing occurs when the investigator has prespecified the hypotheses to be evaluated. In investigatory research, on the other hand, the investigator is searching for acceptable hypotheses from a set of data. The implications of tests of statistical significance are different for the two types of research.

With a properly defined prespecified alternative hypothesis and a properly designed experiment, a statistically significant result (a result that rejects the null hypothesis) may be presumed to "prove" the alternative hypothesis. A statistically significant result in investigatory research, in which the researcher has no prespecified hypotheses but rather selects hypotheses as suggested by the data, is not presumed to prove anything. Investigatory research may serve to create hypotheses, but in general will not "prove" them.

In both hypothesis testing and investigatory research, the investigator may wish to test more than one hypothesis. In the latter type of research, the investigator may test dozens or even hundreds of hypotheses suggested by the data. In such situations the levels of significance of the tests are not those that would have applied to a single hypothesis.

For example, suppose an investigator has 100 measurements on each of two groups of patients and that there really are no differences between the two groups on these variables. If the investigator computes 100 chi square tests on these variables, he or she should expect five of them to be significant at the 0.05 level. This could happen by pure chance, with the result that none of the differences may be considered significant. Yet if the investigator does not take this fact into consideration, he or she may believe that these five variables are significantly different between the two groups. If these results are then published, the first researcher should not be surprised if other investigators are unable to verify the results. What can be done?

First, if the significant hypotheses resulted from investigatory research, the investigator may design experiments to be based on totally new data to test each hypothesis that was suggested by the investigatory research. Data used to suggest a hypothesis cannot be used to "prove" it.

Second, the experimenter may consider using statistical procedures that allow the testing of multiple hypotheses simultaneously. One such procedure is readily available for chi square tests of significance (Lindquist, 1956). Consider the example of testing the difference between two groups on 100 independent vari-

Table 30–15. TERMS AND RELATIONSHIPS REQUISITE TO CALCULATE THE PAYOFF OF A CLINICAL PROCESS IN PRESERVED MAN-DAYS FOR AN INDIVIDUAL

T = Tarp = one man-day.
f = Functional capacity of an individual to earn money at his usual job (0 to 1).
r = Reduced functional capacity of an individual to earn money at his usual job, $r = 1 - f$.
T_R = Average age-specific complement of residual man-days at $f = 1$.
T_r = Tarps lost from reduced function, $T_r = rT$.
CA = Clinication action, any diagnostic, therapeutic, rehabilitative or educative procedure within a clinical process performed for the preservation of T_R.
CP = Sequence of CA's required for a specific disease.
T_{CA} = Tarps consumed by a CA.
T_{CP} = Tarps consumed by a CP, $T_{CP} = \Sigma T_{CA}$.
T_W = Tarps consumed by travel, waiting, redundancies, and other inefficiencies.
T_M = Number of man-days in T_R that cannot be preserved by contemporary capabilities of CP's for various disease processes.
P = Probability of preserving T_R with a CP,

$$P = \frac{T_R - T_{CP} - T_r - T_W - T_M}{T_R}.$$

p = Probability of surviving CP in order to realize $T_R \cdot p = 1 -$ probable CP specific mortality. Thus:

$$P_p = \frac{T_R - T_{CP} - T_r - T_W - T_M}{T_R}$$

the limiting value (L_T) of any CP is:
$L_T \rightarrow T_R - T_{CP} - T_r - T_W - T_M$ as
$T_R \rightarrow 0$ with age as
$T_M = T_R$ when $p = 0$, and
as T_{CP}, T_r, and $T_W \rightarrow T_R$ with inadequate management.

T_{CP}, T_r, T_W, and T_M are all elements of downtime in a social system, and it is an operations research and systems design problem to ascertain how they can be kept at a minimum while maximizing T_R preservation for individual members of the system.

The unit of measurement, the "Tarp," is derived from a convention established by Gilbreth when he introduced the name "Therblig" as a term to identify the actions of a production worker. A Tarp is defined as one man-day in which the individual is completely functional.

From Spratt, J. S.: The measurement of the value of the clinical process to individuals by age and income. J. Trauma, 11:967, 1971. © by Williams & Wilkins, 1971. Reprinted with permission.

ables. Compute the 100 chi squares as before. Next, add the 100 chi square values and add the 100 associated degrees of freedom, to obtain a "total" chi square and "total" degrees of freedom. Find the level of significance of the total chi square based on the total degrees of freedom from a chi square table. If this is not significant, none of the individual chi squares may be considered significant.

There are other procedures available that permit the simultaneous testing of multiple hypotheses when the variables are distributed normally. These procedures are based upon Hotelling's T^2 test. Another important procedure is Scheffe's S test (Scheffe, 1959). Because these procedures are fairly complex, they cannot be described here. Several references are given in Bancroft (1968) so the reader may investigate this matter further.

If care is not taken to correct for multiple testing, the use of classic statistical testing procedures will yield erroneous levels of significance when used to test multiple hypotheses simultaneously.

Clinical Algorithms and Cost-Benefit Analysis

With increasing concern over costs, total treatment time, comparative morbidity, and the preservation of a maximal functional life span, the need for more complex algorithms to compare the efficacy and "pay-off" of different clinical processes must evolve along with quality clinical data and the data management systems essential to use such algorithms in the moment to moment process of clinical decision-making. This need is addressed in several

Table 30–16. DOWNTIME FACTORS ACCRUING TO THE ADVANTAGE OF THE PATIENT

A. Diagnostic effort leading to effective treatment of diseases
B. Beneficial treatment to alleviate symptoms, restore function or preserve longevity at a tolerable cost
C. Beneficial rehabilitation
D. Education and motivation of people to request health services
E. Education and motivation of people to participate effectively in their own health maintenance, health care and rehabilitation

From Spratt, J. S., and Watson, F. R.: The decision making process in cancer patient care. CA, 23:156, 1973. Reprinted with permission.

Table 30–17. DOWNTIME FACTORS ACCRUING TO THE DISADVANTAGE OF THE PATIENT

A. Time lost in diagnostic effort not leading to beneficial treatment
B. Treatment not restoring or preserving function
C. Treatment not preserving maximum longevity
D. Cost in excess of ultimate value
E. Time consumed in the coordination of interdisciplinary consultation and unbeneficial treatment
F. Time wasted in travel and waiting
G. Time wasted by avoidable morbidity
H. Avoidable mortality from elements of the clinical process
I. Time lost in delaying rehabilitation

From Spratt, J. S., and Watson F. R.: The decision making process in cancer patient care. CA, 23:157, 1973.

previous publications by Spratt (1971a, b, 1975a, b) and Spratt and Watson (1973). These algorithms evolve the concepts that the clinical process is influenced significantly by the law of diminishing marginal returns, that the limits of attainable longevity are known for different cohorts of people, and that the clinical actions used in any clinical process may be categorized into groups wherein the down-time and parallel costs required by the clinical action either does or does not accrue to the advantage of the individual.

The algorithm and the categories of clinical actions are reproduced in Tables 30–15 to 30–17. The application of these concepts is imperfect but essential if cost is to be contained in any clinical process while preserving the maximum functional longevity for an individual with the least amount of risk for morbidity and mortality.

Obviously, this is an exceedingly complex issue, beyond the scope of this chapter, but it is introduced here because of the numerous challenges imposed.

Summary

This chapter has presented and elaborated on some of the more fundamental statistical methods that can be applied to medical data and that appear most frequently in the present literature. Familiarity with these concepts is necessary for understanding information so analyzed and is the foundation for critical evaluation of a variety of medical data, but the results of the analysis of clinical data can be no better than the data themselves. To evaluate the quality of the data obtained in a clinical trial, the following guidelines (from Simon and Wittes, 1985) are recommended:

1. Authors should discuss briefly the quality control methods used to ensure that the data are complete and accurate. A reliable procedure should be cited for ensuring that all patients entered on study are actually reported on. If no such procedures are in place, their absence should be noted. Any procedures employed to ensure that assessment of major endpoints is reliable should be mentioned (e.g., second-party review of responses) or their absence noted.

2. All patients registered on study should be accounted for. The report should specify for each treatment the number of patients who were not eligible, who died, or who withdrew before treatment began. The distribution of follow-up times should be described for each treatment, and the number of patients lost to follow-up should be given.

3. The study should have the smallest possible inevaluability rate for major endpoints. If more than 10 per cent of eligible patients should be lost to follow-up or considered inevaluable for response owing to early death, protocol violation, or missing information, we recommend great caution in interpreting the results.

4. In randomized studies, the report should include a comparison of survival or other major endpoints for all eligible patients as randomized, that is, with no exclusions other than those not meeting eligibility criteria.

5. The sample size should be sufficient to either establish or conclusively rule out the existence of effects of clinically meaningful magnitude. For "negative" results in therapeutic comparisons, the adequacy of sample size should be demonstrated by either presenting confidence limits for true treatment differences or calculating statistical power for detecting differences.

6. Authors should state whether there was an initial target sample size and, if so, what it was. They should specify how frequently interim analyses were performed and how the decisions to stop accrual and report results were made.

7. All claims of therapeutic efficacy should be based on explicit comparison with a specific control group, except in special circumstances under which each patient is his own control. If nonrandomized controls are used, the characteristics of the patients should be presented in detail and compared with those of the experimental group. Potential sources of bias should be discussed adequately.

8. The patients studied should be described adequately. Applicability of conclusions to other patients should be dealt with carefully. Claims of subset-specific treatment differences must be documented carefully statistically as more than the random results of multiple-subset analyses.

9. The methods of statistical analysis should be described in sufficient detail that a knowledgable reader could reproduce the analysis if the data were available.*

Glossary of Terms

Type I error: The conclusion that a significant difference exists between two groups when no difference exists, providing a "false positive" error. The probability of a Type I error is designated by the Greek alpha, α.

Type II error: The conclusion that no significant difference exists between studied groups when a difference does exist, providing a "false negative" error. The probability of a Type II error is designated by the Greek beta, β.

Statistical power: This is the probability of detecting a difference in outcome. The probability of detecting a difference can range from zero (no chance) to 1 (a perfect study assured of detecting differences that exist). This probability of missing a difference is related to the risk of a β error and equals $1.0 - \beta$.

Phase I trial: The initial assessment of a new drug in humans by a fixed route and schedule. The three aims are the estimation of human toxicity, selection of dose for a clinical trial to evaluate efficacy, and investigation of clinical pharmacology.

Phase II trial: Assessment of the therapeutic efficacy in a well-defined population of patients. This further evaluates toxicity.

---

*Adapted from Simon, R., and Wittes, R. E.: Methodologic guidelines for reports of clinical trials. Cancer Treat. Rep., 69:1, 1985.

REFERENCES

Afifi, A. A., and Clark, V.: Computer Aided Multivariate Analysis. Belmont, Calif., Lifetime Learning Publications, 1984.

Bailar, J. C., III, Louis, T. A., Lavori, P. W., et al.: Statistics in practice. A classification for biomedical research reports. N. Engl. J. Med., *311*:1482, 1984.

Bancroft, T. A.: Topics in Intermediate Statistical Methods. Vol. 1. Chapter 8. Ames, Iowa, Iowa State University Press, 1968.

Cassedy, J. H.: American Medicine and Statistical Thinking 1800–1860. Cambridge, Mass., Harvard University Press, 1984.

Chalmers, T. C., Celano, P., Sacks, H. S., et al.: Bias in treatment in controlled clinical trials. N. Engl. J. Med., *309*:1358, 1983.

Cook, E.: Life of Florence Nightingale. London, MacMillan, 1914.

Cutler, S. J., and Ederer, F.: Maximum utilization of the life table method in analyzing survival. J. Chron. Dis., *8*:699, 1958.

de la Place, P. S. (translated by F. W. Truscott and F. L. Emory): A Philosophical Essay on Probabilities. New York, Davis Publications, 1951.

Geller, N. L.: Design of Phase I and II clinical trials in cancer: A statistician's view. Cancer Invest., *2*:483, 1984.

Halperin, M., Rogot, E., Gurian, J., et al.: Sample sizes for medical trials with special reference to long-term therapy. J. Chron. Dis., *21*:13, 1968.

Hotelling, H.: The generalization of "students" ratio. Ann. Math. Statist., *2*:360, 1931.

Kaplan, E. L., and Meier, P.: Non-parametric estimation from incomplete observations. J. Am. Stat. Assn., *53*:457, 1958.

Lavori, P. W., Louis, T. A., Bailar, J. C., III, et al.: Statistics in practice. Designs for experiments—parallel comparisons of treatment. N. Engl. J. Med., *309*:1291, 1983.

Lindquist, E. F.: Design and Analyses of Experiments. Boston, Houghton Mifflin, 1956, p. 71.

Oye, R. K., and Shapiro, M. F.: Reporting results of chemotherapy trials. Does response make a difference in patient survival? J. A. M. A., *252*:2722, 1984.

Pasternak, B. S.: Sample sizes for group sequential cohort and case control study designs. Am. J. Epidemiol., *113*:182, 1981.

Peto, R., Pike, M. C., Armitage, P., et al.: Design and analysis of randomized clinical trials requiring prolonged observation of each patient. I. Introduction and design. Br. J. Cancer, *34*:585, 1976.

Peto, R., Pike, M. C., Armitage, P., et al.: Design and analysis of randomized clinical trials requiring prolonged observation of each patient. II. Analysis and examples. Br. J. Cancer, *35*:1, 1977.

Rosenberg, M. J.: Cost efficiency in study planning and completion. How many cases? How many controls? Am. J. Med., *75*:833, 1983.

Scheffe, H.: The Analysis of Variance. New York, John Wiley & Sons, 1959.

Simon, R., and Wittes, R. E.: Methodologic guidelines for reports of clinical trials. Cancer Treat. Rep., *69*:1, 1985.

Sokal, R. R., and Rohlf, F. J.: Biometry: The Principles and Practice of Statistics in Biological Research. San Francisco, W. H. Freeman, 1969, p. 550.

Spratt, J. S.: Cost-effectiveness in the post-treatment follow-up of cancer patients. J. Surg. Oncol., *3*:393, 1971*a*.

Spratt, J. S.: The measurement of the value of the clinical process to the individual by age and income. J. Trauma, *11*:966, 1971*b*.

Spratt, J. S., Jr.: The relation of "human capital" preservation to health costs. Am. J. Econ. Soc., *34*:295, 1975*a*.

Spratt, J. S.: The physician's role in minimizing the economic morbidity of cancer. Semin. Oncol., *2*:411, 1975*b*.

Spratt, J. S., and Watson, F. R.: The decision-making process. Cancer, *23*:155, 1973.

Wald, A.: Sequential Analysis. New York, John Wiley & Sons, 1947.

Physical Fitness and Weight Control

JAMES W. YATES

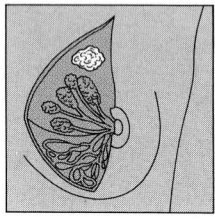

The positive relationship between cancer and obesity suggests that a reduction in body fat through exercise may well result in a decreased risk of cancer (Frisch et al., 1985).* The purpose of this chapter is to help the patient to outline and begin an exercise program safely. Emphasis is placed on improving overall fitness as well as on weight reduction. By following the program outlined, one will be able to improve fitness without undue risk of injury or other health-related problems.

It is not the fitness of the individual that provides the health benefits, but rather the impact that the exercise program has on risk factors associated with health problems. Most persons beginning an exercise program develop better eating habits, lose weight, and, if they smoke, reduce the number of cigarettes or stop altogether. Each of these factors has a beneficial effect on overall health.

What Is Physical Fitness?

Physical fitness is best viewed as an ability to exercise vigorously without undue fatigue. Fit individuals have "endurance" and are able to work harder with less effort than those who are not physically fit. However, the term fitness can be used to describe a variety of abilities. Fitness can be described as the ability to lift a heavy weight, sprint short distances, or flex to extreme ranges of motion. By far the most important component of fitness is the capacity to sustain continuous exercise such as walking, jogging, cycling, or swimming with only moderate stress and to recover quickly when the exercise is finished. While the lay person uses the terms "stamina" or "endurance," the physician and exercise physiologist use the terms "cardiovascular" or "aerobic" fitness. These labels are more descriptive in that they point out the important role of the heart and circulation of the blood in the delivery of oxygen to the muscles, which is then used to produce energy. One can generate some energy without oxygen, but the amount is limited. The way to increase the capacity to sustain exercise is to increase aerobic fitness.

Aerobic exercise is the most effective way to exercise when trying to lose weight. Activities such as weight lifting and calisthenics can improve overall physical fitness but do not expend significant calories. Therefore, in addition to improving aerobic fitness, aerobic exercise is a useful means of weight control.

Exercise

Examination by a physician for signs of cardiovascular disease is prudent before beginning an exercise program. The checkup should include an electrocardiogram, preferably during exercise, a blood lipid profile, and blood pressure measurement. This is especially important for persons who are over 35 years of age, who have a family history of heart disease, or who have been sedentary for a number of years. Approximately 10 per cent of otherwise nor-

---

*See Chapter 5 for a discussion of the relationship between cancer and nutrition.

mal men over age 35 have hidden heart disease, as contrasted to approximately 1 per cent of men below that age. Similar statistics exist for women. Even for most of these individuals, however, properly prescribed exercise is not harmful.

THE EXERCISE PROGRAM

Four factors must be considered when beginning an exercise program: intensity, frequency, duration, and mode (i.e., type of exercise).

Intensity of Exercise—The Target Zone. It is well established that a certain level of exercise must be reached and maintained in order to train the cardiovascular system effectively and improve aerobic fitness. This so-called "target zone" is between 70 and 85 per cent of the maximum exercise heart rate. Below 70 per cent of capacity, little fitness benefit is achieved. Above 85 per cent of maximum, there is little added benefit from a great deal of extra exercise. The added intensity also greatly increases the chance for injury. As long as training takes place in the target zone, fitness will improve.

The target zone is based on an age-predicted maximum heart rate. Maximum heart rate can be determined by 3 to 4 minutes of all-out exercise, but this may be inadvisable because intense exercise is difficult, requires extensive motivation, and could be dangerous to persons predisposed to heart disease. Maximum heart rate can be estimated by subtracting the person's age from 220 (e.g., a 40-year-old man would have an age-predicted maximum heart rate of 180 beats per minute). With increasing age, maximum heart rate decreases and the target zone becomes lower. Figure 31–1 shows the relationship between heart rate, age, and target zone.

For accuracy, it is important to count the pulse immediately upon stopping exercise because the rate changes very quickly when exercise is stopped or slowed down. Count for 10 seconds. Multiply that value by six in order to obtain the count for a full minute. Do not count for a full minute or even 15 seconds because the heart rate drops off too fast.

By trial and error, develop an exercise pattern that seems easy for 5 to 10 minutes and then count the pulse. It should be less than 50 per cent of the age-predicted maximum heart rate. Then, increase the intensity of the exercise to achieve the "target zone." Stop after 3

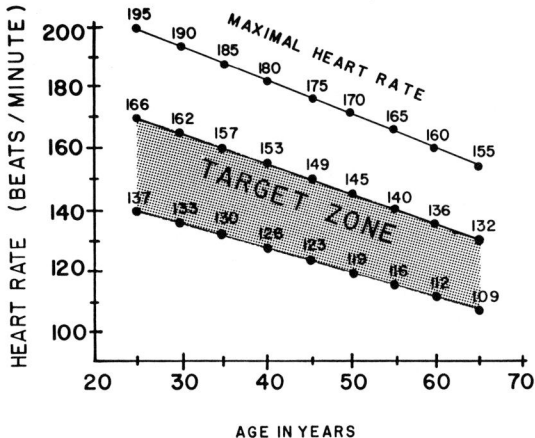

Figure 31–1. Relationship between maximum heart rate, target zone, and age.

to 5 minutes at the higher intensity to check the heart rate again. Adjust the intensity if the rate is too high or too low. Follow the high intensity workout by one of lower intensity as a cool-down period. The exercise period should be progressively increased to 30 minutes; however, the length of the warm-up and cool-down basically stays the same. A typical exercise period should consist of (1) 10 to 15 minutes of warm-up, (2) 20 to 30 minutes of exercise with heart rate in the target zone, and (3) 10 to 15 minutes of cool-down.

The intensity of the workout can easily be manipulated by changing the speed of walking or jogging. Some may find it difficult to achieve the target zone only by walking and will find it necessary to alternate walking with jogging.

Frequency of Exercise. In order to make aerobic gains, exercise must be carried out at least three times a week. It is true that persons who have been bedridden for some time can benefit from exercising twice a week, but these gains will be modest. It is best to space the intervals over a week's time rather than exercising on three consecutive days. Exercise on consecutive days tends to cause more injuries and may be counterproductive.

Duration of Exercise. It is a mistake to do too much too soon. Start with 15 minutes; then gradually increase the duration of exercise to 30 minutes over a period of 5 to 6 weeks. The ankles, knees, and hips need a period in which to adjust to the added workload.

Modes of Exercise. Not all types of exercise are equal in promoting fitness. Exercises that result in cardiovascular fitness must (1) increase the heart rate to "target zone" and keep it there for at least 20 minutes, (2) involve large muscle masses, (3) be rhythmic in nature, and (4) be continuous.

Weight lifting and games such as tennis and racquetball are "stop and go" activities that generally cause "peaks and valleys" in the heart rate. Activities such as walking, jogging, swimming, cycling, rowing, cross country skiing, and aerobic dancing are all highly aerobic and allow for continued improvement.

Overall fitness is improved if the types of activities are varied. Rowing and jumping rope are examples of exercises that are aerobically demanding for both the arms and legs and therefore benefit both.

GETTING STARTED

Guidelines to follow in beginning an aerobic exercise program are based on research and common sense.

1. *Start slowly*: Proceed carefully and do not hurry. For most people it is best to begin by walking. The intensity of the exercise can be varied by the speed of walking or by combining walking with short periods of jogging.

2. *Dress sensibly*: Do not begin an exercise program without proper footwear. No one shoe is right for everyone. Stores that deal exclusively in running apparel or athletic equipment are best when shopping for shoes. Wear loose-fitting clothing. The objective is to avoid excessive perspiration rather than encouraging it. Excessive sweating can lead to dehydration. Any weight that is lost by perspiration is quickly regained when the individual rehydrates with water or some other beverage.

3. *Have a warm-up period*: It is important to have a warm-up period for several minutes. This is perhaps the best time to include stretching exercises, which allow muscular and circulatory systems to adjust gradually.

4. *Allow a cool-down period*: After exercise, allow at least 5 minutes to gradually slow down before stopping. This allows the circulation and metabolism to return slowly to normal levels. Continue to walk slowly or stretch. Take a lukewarm shower rather than a hot or a cold one.

After 2 to 3 weeks of regular exercise, fitness begins to improve. The same workout "feels" easier. It is not uncommon for 6 to 8 weeks of aerobic exercises to result in a drop in heart rate of 20 to 30 beats per minute for the same running speed.

As fitness continues to improve, increase the workload if the heart rate is not in the target zone. Having achieved a satisfactory fitness level, maintain it by regular workouts. The amount of effort required to maintain fitness is considerably less than that required to achieve fitness.

Fitness Appraisal

Fitness appraisal is best used to test the effectiveness of the training program and to help set and achieve personal goals. Fitness appraisal places rigorous demands on the body. Attempting to perform these tests after years of inactivity can result in more harm to the body than any benefit that this information provides. Therefore, it is recommended *not* to perform the cardiorespiratory endurance assessment without clearance by a physician and until after a period of 4 to 6 weeks of regular exercise.

CARDIORESPIRATORY ENDURANCE ASSESSMENT

The ability of the body to utilize oxygen depends on the efficiency of the heart, lungs, blood, and muscles. The job of the heart, lungs, and blood is to deliver the oxygen to the muscles and to remove carbon dioxide. During vigorous activity, the muscles require increased amounts of oxygen and produce more carbon dioxide. Tests of cardiorespiratory endurance measure the ability of the system to deliver and utilize oxygen. The test discussed here estimates cardiorespiratory endurance and permits a comparison of the individual's fitness with recommended levels.

Step Test. The step test is suited for older adults or for those just beginning an exercise program. The test should be taken after 4 to 6 weeks of progressive conditioning. The following items are needed:

1. Box, step or a bench (15¾ inches high for men; 13 inches for women).
2. Clock or watch with a sweep second hand.
3. Metronome or other device programmed for 90 beats per minute.
4. A quiet room with a moderate temperature (65 to 75° F).

A pace of 90 beats per minute will result in 22.5 steps per minute. With each signal from the pacing device, one step is taken. Step up first with the left foot and then with the right. Then step down with the left foot and then with the right. Keep pace with the tempo and straighten both legs when stepping up on the bench. The lead leg may be changed during the test if desired. If unable to keep pace with the timer, stop and try the test again after several weeks.

After 5 minutes of exercise, sit down. The pulse is taken for a 15-second period starting exactly at 15 seconds and ending exactly at 30 seconds after stopping the exercise. Determine weight in the outfit worn during the test.

Score the test as follows:
1. Using Figure 31-2 for women, locate body weight.
2. Locate the post-exercise pulse count in the extreme left column.
3. Read across the pulse count row until it intersects with the column for body weight. Record the fitness score.
4. Using Figure 31-3, find the age-adjusted score opposite the nearest age.
5. With the adjusted fitness score, find the physical fitness rating as compared with that of other persons of similar age in Figure 31-4.

When properly administered, the test will provide a reasonable estimate of aerobic fitness.

BODY COMPOSITION ASSESSMENT

Although many people use the terms "overweight" or "obese" interchangeably, they have a different meaning. Individuals are overweight if their body weight is greater than that of the average person of their height. Obesity

WOMEN   Fitness score ③

Post-exercise pulse count ②													
45										29	29	29	
44								30	30	30	30	30	
43							31	31	31	31	31	31	
42			32	32	32	32	32	32	32	32	32	32	
41			33	33	33	33	33	33	33	33	33	33	
40			34	34	34	34	34	34	34	34	34	34	
39			35	35	35	35	35	35	35	35	35	35	
38			36	36	36	36	36	36	36	36	36	36	
37			37	37	37	37	37	37	37	37	37	37	
36		37	38	38	38	38	38	38	38	38	38	38	
35	38	38	39	39	39	39	39	39	39	39	39	39	
34	39	39	40	40	40	40	40	40	40	40	40	40	
33	40	40	41	41	41	41	41	41	41	41	41	41	
32	41	41	42	42	42	42	42	42	42	42	42	42	
31	42	42	43	43	43	43	43	43	43	43	43	43	
30	43	43	44	44	44	44	44	44	44	44	44	44	
29	44	44	45	45	45	45	45	45	45	45	45	45	
28	45	45	46	46	46	47	47	47	47	47	47	47	
27	46	46	47	48	48	49	49	49	49				
26	47	48	49	50	50	51	51	51					
25	49	50	51	52	52	53	53						
24	51	52	53	54	54	55							
23	53	54	55	56	56	57							

① Body weight: 80 90 100 110 120 130 140 150 160 170 180 190

Figure 31-2. Predicted fitness score for women based on weight and post-exercise pulse count. (From Sharkey, B. J.: Physiology of Fitness. Champaign, Ill., Human Kinetics Publishers, 1979. Used with permission.)

772 31 • Physical Fitness and Weight Control

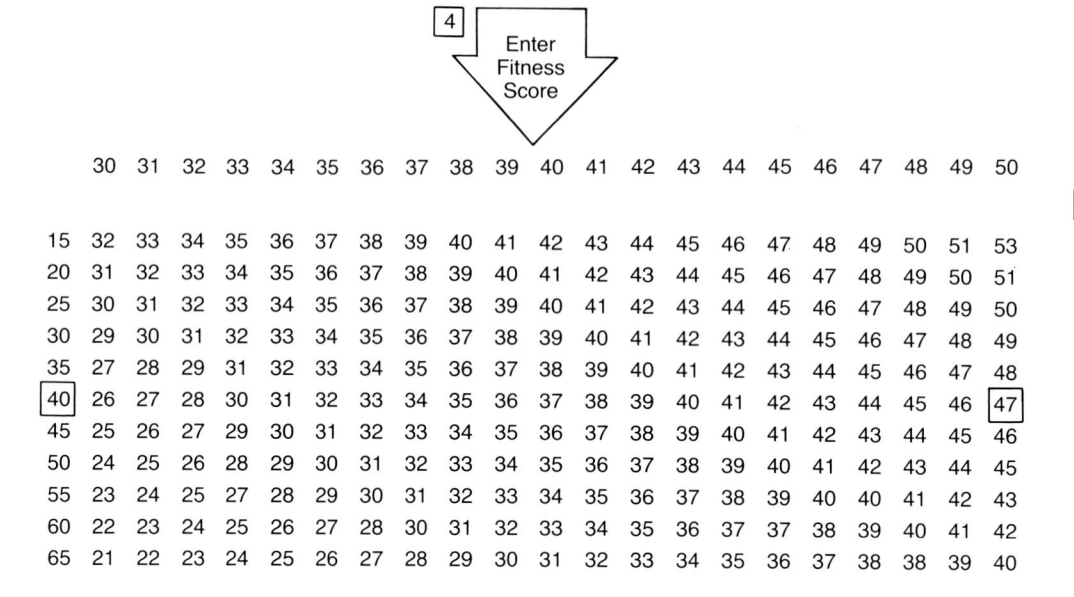

Example: If your age is 40 years and you score 50 on the step test, your age-adjusted score is 47.

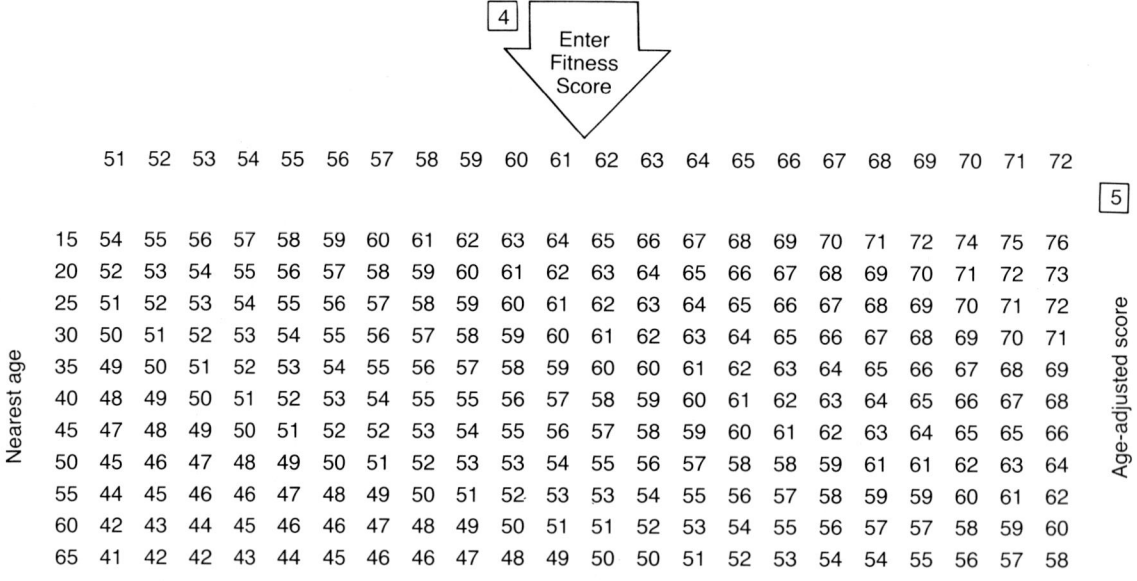

Example: If your age is 40 years and you score 50 on the step test, your age-adjusted score is 47.

Figure 31–3. Fitness score adjustment based on age. (From Sharkey, B. J.: Physiology of Fitness. Champaign, Ill., Human Kinetics Publishers, 1979. Used with permission.)

Figure 31–4. Physical fitness rating for women. (From Sharkey, B. J.: Physiology of Fitness. Champaign, Ill., Human Kinetics Publishers, 1979. Used with permission.)

PHYSICAL FITNESS RATING - WOMEN

(Use Age-Adjusted Score)

Nearest age							
15	54+	53-49	48-44	43-39	38-34	33-29	28–
20	53+	52-48	47-43	42-38	37-33	32-28	27–
25	52+	51-47	46-42	41-37	36-32	31-27	26–
30	51+	50-46	45-41	40-36	35-31	30-26	25–
35	50+	49-45	44-40	39-35	34-30	29-25	24–
40	49+	48-44	43-39	38-34	33-29	28-24	23–
45	48+	47-43	42-38	37-33	32-28	27-23	22–
50	47+	46-42	41-37	36-32	31-27	26-22	21–
55	46+	45-41	40-36	35-31	30-26	25-21	20–
60	45+	44-40	39-35	34-30	29-25	24-20	19–
65	44+	43-39	38-34	33-29	28-24	23-20	19–
	Superior	Excellent	Very good	Good	Fair	Poor	Very poor

is defined as having an excess amount of body fat. It is possible to be "obese" and not "overweight." (See Appendix J and Appendix K in Chapter 5 for height-weight standards.) The distinction between overweight and obese is an important one. When a large percentage of body weight is fat, it has a negative impact on health.

Estimations of body composition by underwater weighing or skinfold thickness are two of the better methods to make this determination. However, they require special equipment. Another method, which is almost as good, requires only measurement of the circumference of various parts of the body. Each measurement should be performed twice to the nearest eighth of an inch without indenting the skin and then averaged.

A woman's percentage of fat is estimated by measuring:

1. Neck circumference just below the larynx.
2. The circumference of the abdomen at the navel.
3. The largest circumference of the upper arm with the arm fully extended and parallel to the floor, palm facing up.
4. The largest circumference of the forearm with the arm fully extended and parallel to the floor, palm facing up.
5. The circumference of the thigh with the feet approximately shoulder width apart. Place the tape just below the left buttock, parallel to the floor.

Convert all measurements to fat percentage points using Table 31–1. Add the five percentage points and subtract a correction factor of 54.598 from the total. The difference is the percentage of fat.

What the percentage of body fat should be is sometimes difficult to answer. Goals of 24 per cent for women and 18 per cent for men will reduce risk for a variety of diseases and are reasonable expectations in terms of weight control.

Energy Balance and Weight Control

The most lasting form of weight reduction is achieved with a balance of diet and exercise. The energy balance relationship states that in order to lose weight, the number of calories expended must exceed the number of calories consumed. There are three ways to achieve a caloric deficit:

1. Eat less, i.e., reduce caloric intake below daily energy requirements.
2. Exercise more, i.e., increase caloric expenditure above daily intake.
3. Use a combination of items 1 and 2 (this is the best method).

When weight is lost by diet alone, much of the loss is muscle mass instead of fat. On the other hand, exercise alone is only slightly useful in short-term weight reduction. For exam-

Table 31–1. PERCENT FAT PREDICTION IN WOMEN

Neck*	PTS	Neck	PTS	Neck	PTS	Neck	PTS	Neck	PTS
15 5/8	0.1	13 7/8	4.1	12 1/8	8.0	10 3/8	11.9	8 5/8	15.4
15 4/8	0.4	13 6/8	4.3	12 0/8	8.2	10 2/8	12.1	8 4/8	16.1
15 3/8	0.7	13 5/8	4.6	11 7/8	8.5	10 1/8	12.4	8 3/8	16.3
15 2/8	1.0	13 4/8	4.9	11 6/8	8.8	10 0/8	12.7	8 2/8	16.7
15 1/8	1.3	13 3/8	5.2	11 5/8	9.1	9 7/8	13.0	8 1/8	16.9
15 0/8	1.5	13 2/8	5.4	11 4/8	9.4	9 6/8	13.3	8 0/8	17.2
14 7/8	1.8	13 1/8	5.7	11 3/8	9.6	9 5/8	13.5	7 7/8	17.4
14 6/8	2.1	13 0/8	6.0	11 2/8	9.9	9 4/8	13.8	7 6/8	17.7
14 5/8	2.4	12 7/8	6.3	11 1/8	10.2	9 3/8	14.1	7 5/8	18.0
14 4/8	2.7	12 6/8	6.6	11 0/8	10.6	9 2/8	14.4	7 4/8	18.3
14 3/8	2.9	12 5/8	6.8	10 7/8	10.8	9 1/8	14.7	7 3/8	18.6
14 2/8	3.2	12 4/8	7.1	10 6/8	11.0	9 0/8	14.9		
14 1/8	3.5	12 3/8	7.4	10 5/8	11.3	8 7/8	15.2		
14 0/8	3.8	12 2/8	7.7	10 4/8	11.6	8 6/8	15.5		

Biceps	PTS	Biceps	PTS	Biceps	PTS	Biceps	PTS	Biceps	PTS
5 7/8	0.1	7 5/8	4.8	9 3/8	9.4	11 1/8	14.1	12 7/8	18.8
6 0/8	0.4	7 6/8	5.1	9 4/8	9.8	11 2/8	14.5	13 0/8	19.1
6 1/8	0.8	7 7/8	5.4	9 5/8	10.1	11 3/8	14.8	13 1/8	19.5
6 2/8	1.1	8 0/8	5.8	9 6/8	10.4	11 4/8	15.1	13 2/8	19.8
6 3/8	1.4	8 1/8	6.1	9 7/8	10.8	11 5/8	15.5	13 3/8	20.1
6 4/8	1.8	8 2/8	6.4	10 0/8	11.1	11 6/8	15.8	13 4/8	20.5
6 5/8	2.1	8 3/8	6.8	10 1/8	11.4	11 7/8	16.1	13 5/8	20.8
6 6/8	2.4	8 4/8	7.1	10 2/8	11.8	12 0/8	16.5	13 6/8	21.1
6 7/8	2.8	8 5/8	7.4	10 3/8	12.1	12 1/8	16.8		
7 0/8	3.1	8 6/8	7.8	10 4/8	12.4	12 2/8	17.1		
7 1/8	3.4	8 7/8	8.1	10 5/8	12.8	12 3/8	17.5		
7 2/8	3.8	9 0/8	8.4	10 6/8	13.1	12 4/8	17.8		
7 3/8	4.1	9 1/8	8.8	10 7/8	13.5	12 5/8	18.1		
7 4/8	4.4	9 2/8	9.1	11 0/8	13.8	12 6/8	18.5		

Forearm	PTS	Forearm	PTS	Forearm	PTS	Forearm	PTS	Forearm	PTS
17 5/8	.2	15 2/8	9.3	12 7/8	18.5	10 4/8	27.7	8 1/8	36.8
17 4/8	.6	15 1/8	9.8	12 6/8	19.0	10 3/8	28.1	8 0/8	37.3
17 3/8	1.1	15 0/8	10.3	12 5/8	19.5	10 2/8	28.5	7 7/8	37.8
17 2/8	1.6	14 7/8	10.8	12 4/8	19.9	10 1/8	29.1	7 6/8	38.3
17 1/8	2.1	14 6/8	11.2	12 3/8	20.4	10 0/8	29.6	7 5/8	38.8
17 0/8	2.5	14 5/8	11.7	12 2/8	20.9	9 7/8	30.1	7 4/8	39.3
16 7/8	3.0	14 4/8	12.2	12 1/8	21.4	9 6/8	30.6	7 3/8	39.7
16 6/8	3.5	14 3/8	12.7	12 0/8	21.9	9 5/8	31.0	7 2/8	40.2
16 5/8	4.0	14 2/8	13.2	11 7/8	22.3	9 4/8	31.5	7 1/8	40.7
16 4/8	4.5	14 1/8	13.7	11 6/8	22.8	9 3/8	32.0	7 0/8	41.2
16 3/8	5.0	14 0/8	14.1	11 5/8	23.3	9 2/8	32.5	6 7/8	41.7
16 2/8	5.4	13 7/8	14.6	11 4/8	23.8	9 1/8	33.0	6 6/8	42.2
16 1/8	5.9	13 6/8	15.1	11 3/8	24.3	9 0/8	33.5	6 5/8	42.5
16 0/8	6.4	13 5/8	15.6	11 2/8	24.9	8 7/8	33.9	0 0/8	0.0
15 7/8	6.9	13 4/8	16.1	11 1/8	25.2	8 6/8	34.4		
15 6/8	7.4	13 3/8	16.6	11 0/8	25.7	8 5/8	34.9		
15 5/8	7.9	13 2/8	17.0	10 7/8	26.2	8 4/8	35.4		
15 4/8	8.3	13 1/8	17.5	10 6/8	26.7	8 3/8	36.0		
15 3/8	8.8	13 0/8	18.0	10 5/8	27.2	8 2/8	36.4		

Abdomen	PTS	Abdomen	PTS	Abdomen	PTS	Abdomen	PTS	Abdomen	PTS	Abdomen
17 5/8	0.0	23 0/8	4.4	28 3/8	8.9	33 6/8	13.3	39 1/8	17.8	44 4/8
17 6/8	0.1	23 1/8	4.5	28 4/8	9.0	33 7/8	13.4	39 2/8	17.9	44 5/8
17 7/8	0.2	23 2/8	4.6	28 5/8	9.1	34 0/8	13.5	39 3/8	18.0	44 6/8
18 0/8	0.3	23 3/8	4.7	28 6/8	9.2	34 1/8	13.6	39 4/8	18.1	44 7/8
18 1/8	0.4	23 4/8	4.8	28 7/8	9.3	34 2/8	13.7	39 5/8	18.2	45 0/8
18 2/8	0.5	23 5/8	4.9	29 0/8	9.4	34 3/8	13.8	39 6/8	18.3	45 1/8
18 3/8	0.6	23 6/8	5.0	29 1/8	9.5	34 4/8	14.0	39 7/8	18.4	45 2/8
18 4/8	0.7	23 7/8	5.2	29 2/8	9.6	34 5/8	14.1	40 0/8	18.5	45 3/8
18 5/8	0.8	24 0/8	5.3	29 3/8	9.7	34 6/8	14.2	40 1/8	18.6	45 4/8
18 6/8	0.9	24 1/8	5.4	29 4/8	9.8	34 7/8	14.3	40 2/8	18.7	45 5/8
18 7/8	1.0	24 2/8	5.5	29 5/8	9.9	35 0/8	14.4	40 3/8	18.8	45 6/8
19 0/8	1.1	24 3/8	5.6	29 6/8	10.0	35 1/8	14.5	40 4/8	18.9	45 7/8
19 1/8	1.2	24 4/8	5.7	29 7/8	10.1	35 2/8	14.6	40 5/8	19.0	46 0/8
19 2/8	1.3	24 5/8	5.8	30 0/8	10.2	35 3/8	14.7	40 6/8	19.1	46 1/8
19 3/8	1.4	24 6/8	5.9	30 1/8	10.3	35 4/8	14.8	40 7/8	19.2	46 2/8

Table continued on opposite page

Table 31-1. PERCENT FAT PREDICTION IN WOMEN *Continued*

Abdomen	PTS	Abdomen	PTS	Abdomen	PTS	Abdomen	PTS	Abdomen	PTS	Abdomen
19 4/8	1.5	24 7/8	6.0	30 2/8	10.4	35 5/8	14.9	41 0/8	19.3	46 3/8
19 5/8	1.6	25 0/8	6.1	30 3/8	10.5	35 6/8	15.0	41 1/8	19.4	46 4/8
19 6/8	1.7	25 1/8	6.2	30 4/8	10.6	35 7/8	15.1	41 2/8	19.5	46 5/8
19 7/8	1.8	25 2/8	6.3	30 5/8	10.7	36 0/8	15.2	41 3/8	19.6	46 6/8
20 0/8	1.9	25 3/8	6.4	30 6/8	10.8	36 1/8	15.3	41 4/8	19.7	46 7/8
20 1/8	2.0	25 4/8	6.5	30 7/8	10.9	36 2/8	15.4	41 5/8	19.9	47 0/8
20 2/8	2.2	25 5/8	6.6	31 0/8	11.1	36 3/8	15.5	41 6/8	20.0	47 1/8
20 3/8	2.3	25 6/8	6.7	31 1/8	11.2	36 4/8	15.6	41 7/8	20.1	47 2/8
20 4/8	2.4	25 7/8	6.8	31 2/8	11.3	36 5/8	15.7	42 0/8	20.2	47 3/8
20 5/8	2.5	26 0/8	6.9	31 3/8	11.4	36 6/8	15.8	42 1/8	20.3	47 4/8
20 6/8	2.6	26 1/8	7.0	31 4/8	11.5	36 7/8	15.9	42 2/8	20.4	47 5/8
20 7/8	2.7	26 2/8	7.1	31 5/8	11.6	37 0/8	16.0	42 3/8	20.5	47 6/8
21 0/8	2.8	26 3/8	7.2	31 6/8	11.7	37 1/8	16.1	42 4/8	20.6	47 7/8
21 1/8	2.9	26 4/8	7.3	31 7/8	11.8	37 2/8	16.2	42 5/8	20.7	48 0/8
21 2/8	3.0	26 5/8	7.4	32 0/8	11.9	37 3/8	16.3	42 6/8	20.8	48 1/8
21 3/8	3.1	26 6/8	7.5	32 1/8	12.0	37 4/8	16.4	42 7/8	20.9	48 2/8
21 4/8	3.2	26 7/8	7.6	32 2/8	12.1	37 5/8	16.5	43 0/8	21.0	48 3/8
21 5/8	3.3	27 0/8	7.7	32 3/8	12.2	37 6/8	16.6	43 1/8	21.1	48 4/8
21 6/8	3.4	27 1/8	7.8	32 4/8	12.3	37 7/8	16.7	43 2/8	21.2	48 5/8
21 7/8	3.5	27 2/8	7.9	32 5/8	12.4	38 0/8	16.8	43 3/8	21.3	48 6/8
22 0/8	3.6	27 3/8	8.1	32 6/8	12.5	38 1/8	17.0	43 4/8	21.4	48 7/8
22 1/8	3.7	27 4/8	8.2	32 7/8	12.6	38 2/8	17.1	43 5/8	21.5	49 0/8
22 2/8	3.8	27 5/8	8.3	33 0/8	12.7	38 3/8	17.2	43 6/8	21.6	49 1/8
22 3/8	3.9	27 6/8	8.4	33 1/8	12.8	38 4/8	17.3	43 7/8	21.7	
22 4/8	4.0	27 7/8	8.5	33 2/8	12.9	38 5/8	17.4	44 0/8	21.8	
22 5/8	4.1	28 0/8	8.6	33 3/8	13.0	38 6/8	17.5	44 1/8	21.9	
22 6/8	4.2	28 1/8	8.7	33 4/8	13.1	39 7/8	17.6	44 2/8	22.0	
22 7/8	4.3	28 2/8	8.8	33 5/8	13.2	39 0/8	17.7	44 3/8	22.1	

Thigh	PTS	Thigh	PTS	Thigh	PTS	Thigh	PTS	Thigh	PTS
11 6/8	0.0	16 2/8	7.0	20 6/8	13.7	25 2/8	20.5	29 6/8	27.3
11 7/8	0.2	16 3/8	7.1	20 7/8	13.9	25 3/8	20.7	29 7/8	27.5
12 0/8	0.4	16 4/8	7.3	21 0/8	14.1	25 4/8	20.9	30 0/8	27.7
12 1/8	0.6	16 5/8	7.4	21 1/8	14.3	25 5/8	21.1	30 1/8	27.9
12 2/8	0.8	16 6/8	7.6	21 2/8	14.5	25 6/8	21.3	30 2/8	28.1
12 3/8	1.0	16 7/8	7.8	21 3/8	14.6	25 7/8	21.5	30 3/8	28.3
12 4/8	1.2	17 0/8	8.0	21 4/8	14.8	26 0/8	21.7	30 4/8	28.5
12 5/8	1.4	17 1/8	8.2	21 5/8	15.0	26 1/8	21.8	30 6/8	28.9
12 6/8	1.6	17 2/8	8.4	21 6/8	15.2	26 2/8	22.0	30 7/8	29.0
12 7/8	1.8	17 3/8	8.6	21 7/8	15.4	26 3/8	22.2	31 0/8	29.2
13 0/8	1.9	17 4/8	8.8	22 0/8	15.6	26 4/8	22.4	31 1/8	29.4
13 1/8	2.1	17 5/8	9.0	22 1/8	15.8	26 5/8	22.6	31 2/8	29.6
13 2/8	2.3	17 6/8	9.1	22 2/8	16.0	26 6/8	22.8	31 3/8	29.8
13 3/8	2.5	17 7/8	9.3	22 3/8	16.2	26 7/8	23.0	31 4/8	30.0
13 4/8	2.7	18 0/8	9.5	22 4/8	16.3	27 0/8	23.2	31 5/8	30.2
13 5/8	2.9	18 1/8	9.7	22 5/8	16.5	27 1/8	23.4	31 6/8	30.4
13 6/8	3.1	18 2/8	9.9	22 6/8	16.7	27 2/8	23.6	31 7/8	30.6
13 7/8	3.3	18 3/8	10.1	22 7/8	16.9	27 3/8	23.7	32 0/8	30.8
14 0/8	3.5	18 4/8	10.3	23 0/8	17.1	27 4/8	23.9	32 1/8	30.9
14 1/8	3.6	18 5/8	10.5	23 1/8	17.3	27 5/8	24.1	32 2/8	31.1
14 2/8	3.8	18 6/8	10.7	23 2/8	17.5	27 6/8	24.3	32 3/8	31.3
14 3/8	4.0	18 7/8	10.9	23 3/8	17.7	27 7/8	24.5	32 4/8	31.5
14 4/8	4.2	19 0/8	11.0	23 4/8	17.9	28 0/8	24.7	32 5/8	31.7
14 5/8	4.4	19 1/8	11.2	23 5/8	18.1	28 1/8	24.9	32 6/8	31.9
14 6/8	4.6	19 2/8	11.4	23 6/8	18.2	28 2/8	25.1	32 7/8	32.1
14 7/8	4.8	19 3/8	11.6	23 7/8	18.4	28 3/8	25.3	33 0/8	32.3
15 0/8	5.0	19 4/8	11.8	24 0/8	18.6	28 4/8	25.4	33 1/8	32.5
15 1/8	5.2	19 5/8	12.0	24 1/8	18.8	28 5/8	25.6	33 2/8	32.7
15 2/8	5.4	19 6/8	12.2	24 2/8	19.0	28 6/8	25.8	33 3/8	32.8
15 3/8	5.5	19 7/8	12.4	24 3/8	19.2	28 7/8	26.0	33 4/8	32.9
15 4/8	5.7	20 0/8	12.6	24 4/8	19.4	29 0/8	26.2		
15 5/8	5.9	20 1/8	12.7	24 5/8	19.6	29 1/8	26.4		
15 6/8	6.1	20 2/8	12.9	24 6/8	19.8	29 2/8	26.6		
15 7/8	6.3	20 3/8	13.1	24 7/8	20.0	29 3/8	26.8		
16 0/8	6.5	20 4/8	13.3	25 0/8	20.1	29 4/8	27.0		
16 1/8	6.7	20 5/8	13.5	25 1/8	20.3	29 5/8	27.2		

*Measurements are expressed in inches. PTS, points.

Table 31-2. RATE OF CALORIC EXPENDITURE WHILE RIDING A CYCLE ERGOMETER

Work		Energy Equivalents		
Kilopondmeters (Kpm/min)	Watts	Oxygen Uptake (liters/min)	Calories	
			Kcal/min	Kcal/hr
150	25	0.6	3.0	180
300	50	0.9	4.5	270
450	75	1.2	6.0	360
600	100	1.5	7.5	450
750	125	1.8	9.0	540
900	150	2.1	10.5	630
1050	175	2.4	12.0	720
1200	200	2.7	14.0	840
1350	225	3.0	15.0	900
1500	250	3.3	17.0	1020
1650	275	3.6	18.0	1080
1800	300	3.9	20.0	1200

ple, it takes 26 minutes of walking (3 miles per hour) to burn off the calories in one doughnut or 11 minutes of jogging to expend the calories in 12 ounces of beer. An even more discouraging example is that only 1 pound of fat is used to run an entire marathon (26 miles)! These examples point out the need to regard weight reduction as a long-term process.

Since most weight gains occur slowly as a result of a small positive caloric balance, exercise can be helpful in offsetting weight gain. Walking 1 mile a day will utilize approximately 700 calories (100 calories per mile) per week. Over a 1-year period this amounts to 36,400 calories, which is equivalent to 10.5 pounds of fat. This can add up over a period of several years.

Reduced caloric consumption of 500 calories per day and increased energy expenditure of 500 calories per day will incur a weight loss of 2 pounds per week. Over a period of 1 year an individual could lose 104 pounds. Greater weight loss is not recommended because of the potential for injury and increased loss of muscle tissue.

CYCLING TO LOSE WEIGHT

Caloric use during cycling increases with the workload. A cycle ergometer shows the workload, and one can determine the rate of caloric expenditure by using Table 31-2.

It is important to remember that exercise intensity is dictated by fitness and that it is not always possible to increase the workload to use more calories. The more prudent approach is to increase the duration of the exercise.

On a bicycle the rate of caloric expenditure is dependent upon the speed. Bicycling at 10 miles per hour requires approximately 7.0 calories per minute for a 150-pound individual.

WALKING OR JOGGING

During walking or jogging, the calories used are directly related to body weight and distance. As the weight of the individual increases, the number of calories expended increases (Table 31-3). The rate of caloric expenditure is less when walking than when jogging.

For a specific weight, multiply body weight by 0.52 for walking and 0.81 for running. For example, 135 pounds × 0.52 = 70 Kcal for each mile walked or 135 × 0.81 = 109 Kcal for each mile run.

SWIMMING PROGRAMS

To achieve substantial benefits from swimming, choose a stroke that can be maintained for at least 20 minutes. For nonexpert swimmers, the breast stroke, side stroke, and back stroke are preferred, as they eliminate the need to coordinate breathing with stroke.

Table 31-3. CALORIC REQUIREMENTS FOR WALKING OR JOGGING ONE MILE

Individual Weight (pounds)	Walking (Kcal)	Jogging (Kcal)
110	58	89
154	81	125
220	115	179

Caloric values for swimming are difficult to estimate owing to the wide range of efficiencies of swimmers and the fact that body fat decreases the work required to stay afloat. Roughly speaking, as many calories are required to swim ¼ mile as to run 1 mile.

Conclusion

By following the information provided one can start a regular exercise program safely. It is the exercise itself that is most important; fitness will improve with regular exercise. Exercise should not be viewed as a quick way to change but rather as a way of life.

REFERENCE

Frisch, R. E., Wyshak, G., Albright, N. L., Albright, T. E., Schiff, I., Jones, K. P., Witschi, J., Shiang, E., Koff, E., and Marguglio, M.: Lower prevalence of breast cancer and cancers of the reproductive system among former college athletes compared to non-athletes. Br. J. Cancer, *52*:885–891, 1985.

Index

Page numbers in *italics* refer to illustrations; page numbers followed by "t" refer to tables.

Abortion, spontaneous, after biopsy, 681–682
  therapeutic, in advanced disease, 685
    mastectomy with, 684–685, 685t
Abscess, biopsy of, 406
Accuracy of diagnosis, defined, 168
Aclacinomycin-A, cell sensitivity to, 494, 496t
Adenoid cystic carcinoma, 225–226, *226*
Adrenalectomy, 448–451, 516–517, 606
  anatomy for, *449–451*
  in male, 722–724
  maintenance therapy with, 448, 449t
  medical vs. surgical, 516–517, *516*, *517*
  procedure for, 449–451, *450–454*
Adriamycin. See *Doxorubicin*.
Advanced disease, 348–349, *349*, 389–392, *389*, *390*, 395, 442
  chemotherapy in. See *Chemotherapy*.
  in pregnancy, 685
  radiation therapy in, 390, 469–471, 469t, 471t
Age, biopsy diagnosis and, 160, *160*
  breast masses and, *127*
  follow-up and, 577
  genetic factors and, 53, *54*
  growth rates and, 293–294, 296t
  immune response and, 548
  in situ carcinoma and, *360*
  male breast cancer and, 716
  mortality and, 47–48, *47*, 47t, *48*, 168–171, *170*, 170–172t, 356–357, 357t
  multiple primary cancers and, 577–578
  nipple discharge and, 127
  prognosis and, 356–357, 357t
  proliferative index and, 262, *262*
  receptor status and, 318–319, 507, 507t
  secondary malignancy and, 636–637, *637*, *638*, 640
Alcoholic beverages, as etiologic agent, 91–92
Algorithms, *152*, 764–765t, 765
Alkaline phosphatase, in liver metastasis, 346, 347t, 582
Allergic reactions, to chemotherapeutic agents, 483
Alopecia, 483, 610
Aminoglutethimide, 448, 516–517, 518t, 522, 524–525
Aminopterin, fetal hazard from, 684
Analgesia, 676–677
  for bone pain, 458
Androgens, 57, 526–527
  in male breast cancer, 725
  masculinization and, 607
  therapeutic. See *Endocrine therapy*.

Angioaccess, 459, 609
Angiosarcoma, 701–704, *702*
  prognosis in, 703
Animal studies, immunological, 542–545
  of dietary fat intake, 84–85
  of new endocrine agents, 529
  of radiation hazard, to fetus, *684*
Antibodies, monoclonal. See *Monoclonal antibodies*.
Antiemetics, 610
Antigens, 545–548
  to mouse mammary tumor, 545–546
  vaccine production and, 552–553
Anthracycline analogues, 482
Areola, in male breast cancer, 718
  reconstruction of, 629
Arm, edema of. See *Lymphedema*.
  lymphangiosarcoma and, 711–713, *712*
  postoperative care of, 599
  postoperative neuropathy of, 438
Aromatase, 502
Aspiration, fine needle, 144–146, *145*, 145t, 146t
Auchincloss-Madden mastectomy, 373–374
  Patey mastectomy vs., *379–381*
  recurrence after, *651*
Autopsy, 586–587, 586t
Axillary fat pad, *21–23*, 23
Axillary lymph nodes. See *Lymph nodes, axillary*.

Bacille Calmette-Guérin (BCG) vaccine, 481, 550
Beta receptors, in fibrocystic breast disease, 39–40, *40*
Bicycling, after treatment, 776, 776t
Bilateral breast cancer, 53, *54*, 632–644
  age and, 636–637, *637*, *638*
  biopsy in, 361, 364, 639, 645
  diagnostic criteria for, 633–634
  ductal, 640–641
  follow-up for, 645
  genetic factors in, 53, *54*
  in male, 719
  incidence of, 634, 635t, 636–639, 636t, *637*, *638*
  lobular, 640
  mucinous, 641
  prognosis in, 641–642
  risk factors for, 640–641
  treatment of, 642–644
Biologic response modifiers, 550–552, 610–611

779

Biopsy, 151–160, *152,* 153–157t, *155, 157, 158,* 159t, *160,* 403, *404,* 405–406, *407–408*
  aspiration before, 144
  bone, 347–348
  bone marrow, 581
  cancer risk and, 68t, 69
  contralateral, 361, 364, 639
  cosmetic appearance and, 155–156, *155*
  for receptor status analysis, 155–156, 156t, 306–307, 316, 405t, 406
  history of, 8–9
  immediate vs. delayed mastectomy after, 152–154, 153t, 154t
  in pregnancy, 681–682
  indications for, 151–152, *152,* 403, *404*
  internal mammary node, 440–441
  needle, 154, 155t, 403, *404*
  nipple changes and, 136
  of discharging duct, 158–159, 159t
  of nonpalpable lesions, 157–158, *157, 158*
  punch, 156
  results of, 159–160, 159t, *160*
  skin, 156, 403
  surgical, 154–156, *155,* 406, *407–408*
  tissue preparation in, 152, 403–404
  trauma of, 152–153
  wound infection after, 405–406
Blacks, mortality rates among, 47, 47t
Bleomycin, 478t
  adverse effects of, 483
Blood supply, 29
  cell shedding into, 290
  tumor growth and, 272
  tumor invasion of, 241
Blood transfusions, 441–442
  phlebotomy and, 442
Body frame measurement, 124
Body image, 602, 734
Body weight. See *Weight.*
Bone marrow, biopsy of, 581
  chemotherapy effects on, 482
Bone metastasis, androgens in, 527, *528*
  biopsy for, 347–348
  follow-up of, 580–581
  fractures and, 457–458, *457,* 606
  pain from, 458, 606
  pretreatment detection of, 345–346, 347–348, 580–581
  prolactin suppression and, 39
  radiation therapy of, 470, 606
Bone scan, 580–581
  pretreatment, 345–346
Brain metastasis. See *Central nervous system metastasis.*
Brassieres, 600
Bread unit list, in dietary planning, 115–116
Breast(s), anatomy of, 16–33
    developmental, 16
    fascial, 17–18, *18, 19*
    lymphatic, 28–32, *30, 31*
    muscular, 18–19, *19–22,* 23
    neural, 23, *24–27,* 28
    topographic, 16–17
    vascular, 29, *31*
  benign disorders of. See *Breast disease, benign;* and specific disorders.
  biopsy of. See *Biopsy.*
  cancer of. See *Breast cancer.*

Breast(s) *(Continued)*
  cell kinetics of, 258–259, 259t
  contour changes in, 130, *131–134,* 178
  CT of, 150–151, 200
  fibrocystic disease of. See *Fibrocystic breast disease.*
  hormones and, 35–42, 304, *305,* 306, 501–503, *502, 503*
  inspection of, 139, *139, 140.* See also *Breast self-examination.*
  mammography of. See *Mammography.*
  MRI of, 200
  palpation of, 136–138, 139–143, *140–143*
  physical examination of, 136–143, *139–143*
  physiology of, 34–45
  postirradiated, follow-up of, 579–580
  reconstruction of. See *Breast reconstruction.*
  self-examination of. See *Breast self-examination.*
  skin of. See *Skin.*
  skin tension lines of, *155*
  thermography of, 151, 194–200
  transillumination of, 143–144, 193–194
  ultrasonography of, 148–149, *148, 149,* 149t, 189–190, *190–192,* 193
Breast cancer. See also *Cancer; Malignancy, secondary; Mass; Metastasis(es); Tumor* entries; and specific neoplasms.
  adenoid cystic, 225–226, *226*
  advanced, 348–349, *349,* 389–392, *389, 390,* 395, 442
    in pregnancy, 685
    radiation therapy in, 390, 469–471, 469t, 471t
  benign disorders vs., 125–126, 126t, 127t, 137–138, 148–149
  bilateral. See *Bilateral breast cancer.*
  biological markers of, 243, 514, 545–547, 580–583
  biopsy in. See *Biopsy.*
  carcinoid, 231–232
  cell kinetics of, 250–269
  classification of, 206–207, 207t
  diagnosis of, 125–151
  diet and, 40–42, 41t, 62–64, *63.* See also *Diet.*
  ductal, 207, *208, 209*
    bilateral, 640–641
    in male, 718
    in situ, 220–221, *222–224,* 362–364, 363t
    mucinous carcinoma with, 209, *213*
  education on, 731–732
  effusions with, 451, 455–456
  epidemiology of, 46–48, *47–51,* 47t, 50–51
  glossary for, 560t
  nutritional, 74–78
    dietary fat intake in, 82–84
  of male breast cancer, 69–70, 716–717
  etiology of, 51–69
  extramammary cancer with, 65–66, 66t
  "fast," 283–285, 285t
  fibrocystic disease and, 66–69, *67,* 67–69t
  genetic factors in, 51–55, 52t, *54*
    in male breast cancer, 716
  glycogen-rich clear cell, 231
  growth rate of. See *Cell kinetics; Growth rates.*
  history of, 1–15

Breast cancer *(Continued)*
  hormones and, 10, 56–58, 501–503, *502, 503*
  immunology of, 11–12, 541–557
  in pregnancy. See *Pregnancy, breast cancer in.*
  in situ. See *In situ breast cancer.*
  incidence of, 48, 50–51, *51,* 291–292, 292t, 293t
  inflammatory, 65, 132–135, *135,* 234, *235,* 392–395, *392,* 394t
    in male, 719
    in pregnancy, 682
    skin biopsy in, 156
    survival in, 392t, 394, 394t
    treatment of, 393–395, 442
  intracystic, 144, 144t
  lobular, 215–216. *217–219*
    bilateral, 640
    in male, 718
    in situ, 221, 224–225, *225,* 360–362
    tubulobular, 216, *219*
  location of, 125, *126*
  lymphoma, 699–701
  male. See *Male breast cancer.*
  mammographic signs of, 174–178, 175t
  mammographically occult, 575
  medullary, 207–208, *210–211*
    ultrasonography of, 190, *192*
  microinvasive, 12, 485
  "minimal," 238, 360
  mortality from. See *Mortality rates.*
  mucinous, *128,* 209, 211, *212–213*
    bilateral, 641
    "mixed," 209, *213*
    prognosis in, 211
  multicentric, 578, 637–638
    vs. multifocal, 243
  natural history of, 358–359, *359*
  oat cell, 232
  occult, 130–132, 575
  papillary, intracystic, 215, *215*
    invasive, 211, *214,* 215, *215*
    prognosis in, 215
  preclinical, 291–295, 292t–296t, 297, 559t
  prognosis in, 504–506, 504–506t
  progression models of, 559t, *565*
  pseudosarcomatous metaplasia with, 228, *229–230*
  receptor status and. See *Receptor status.*
  recurrence of. See *Recurrence.*
  risk factors for. See *Risk factors.*
  sarcoma. See *Sarcoma.*
  screening for. See *Screening programs.*
  secretory, 228
  signet ring cell, 211, 228, 230, *231*
  squamous cell, 226–228, *227*
  staging of. See *Staging.*
  sudoriferous, 231, *232*
  symptoms of, 125–136, *127, 128,* 127t, 129t, *130–138*
  tubular, 216, 220, *220*
  untreated, 358–359, *359*
Breast disease, benign. See also specific disorder.
    cancer vs., 125–126, 126t, 137–138, 148–149
    ultrasonography in, 148–149, 189, 190
  fibrocystic. See *Fibrocystic breast disease.*

Breast reconstruction, 600–601, 614–631
  history of, 614–615
  implant only, 617–618, *617, 618*
  latissimus dorsi flap, 619, 621–623, *621, 622*
  microsurgery in, 627, 629, *629, 630*
  nipple-areola, 629
  principles of, 615–617
  psychoemotional factors and, 734
  recurrence and, 616–617
  tissue expander, 618–619, *619, 620*
  transverse rectus abdominis myocutaneous flap, 623, *624–628,* 627
Breast self-examination, 143, 285, 572–573, 592, 731
  nurse's role in, 591–592
  of lumpy breast, 574
  rapid early growth and, 297
Bromocriptine, 35
Buserelin, 529
  in male breast cancer, 724

Caffeine, breast cancer and, 42, 92–94
  fibrocystic breast disease and, 39–40, 92–94
Calcifications, biopsy of, 157–158, *157, 158,* 159–160, 159t
  mammography of, 177–178
  needle localization in, 181, *182*
Calorie intake, 105–108
cAMP. See *Cyclic adenosine monophosphate (cAMP).*
Cancer. See also *Breast cancer; Malignancy, secondary; Mass; Metastasis(es); Tumor* entries; and specific cancers.
  advanced, prognosis in, 348–349, *349,* 389, *390,* 395
  axillary metastasis from, 134t
  breast cancer with, 65–66, 66t
    in male, 719
  effusions in, 451, 455
  metastatic to breast, 644
  multiple primary, 577–578, 632–633. See also *Bilateral breast cancer.*
  personality and, 728–731
Cancer cell cultures, 492–500
  chemosensitivity of, 494, 495t, 496, 496t
  clinical use of, 497–498
  drug resistance in, 496–497
  maintenance of, 493–494, *493*
Cancer control window, 565–566, *566,* 567t
Cancer research statistics. See *Statistical methods.*
Carbohydrates, 87
Carcinoembryonic antigen, 514, 514t, 547, 583
Carcinogenesis, animal studies on, 543
  chemotherapy and, 483
  diet and, 42
  pregnancy and, 59
  radiation, 60–62, 472
Carcinoid tumors, 231–232
  metastatic to breast, 644
Carcinoma erysipelatoides, 234
Cardiorespiratory endurance assessment, 770–771, *771–773*
Cardiotoxicity, Adriamycin, 483
Carotene, 87–89

Carpal tunnel syndrome, 446
Casein, 37, 39
Catecholamines, breast disease and, 40, 41t, 42, 94–97
Catheters, bladder, 609
   drainage of, 409, 410, *418,* 438, 440, *440,* 597, 609
Cautery, 2–3
Cell(s), cancer, 270, 492–498
   chemotherapy and, 485–486, 494, 495t, 496, 496t
   clinical use of, 497–498
   drug resistant, 298–299, 496–497
   shedding of, 290
  death of. See *Necrosis.*
  kinetics of. See *Cell kinetics.*
Cell cultures, cancer, 492–500
  chemosensitivity of, 494, 495t, 496, 496t
  clinical use of, 497–498
  drug resistance in, 496–497
  maintenance of, 493–494, *493*
Cell kinetics, 250–269, 356. See also *Growth rates.*
  cell loss in, 260, 272
  chemotherapy and, 485
  cycle duration in, 250–251, *251, 252,* 270–271
    arrest of, 252–253
    segmental, 253–254
  drug resistance and, 298–299, 496–497
  flow cytometry of, 255–258, *256–257*
  growth fraction in, 260
  hypoxia and, 253
  in breast cancer, 259–266, 259t, *261, 262,* 261t, 263t, *264,* 265t
    age and, 262, *262*
    equations for, 272–276
    histologic type and, 260–261, 261t
    nuclear grade and, 261–262, *262*
    prognosis and, 263, *264*
    receptor status and, 262
    stage of disease and, 263, 263t
  in cystosarcoma phyllodes, 265, 266t
  normal breast, 258–259, 259t
  tamoxifen and, 518
  thymidine-labeled, 250, *251,* 254, *255,* 255t, 271
Cell lines, 493–494
Central nervous system (CNS), chemotherapy effects on, 674–675
  pain relief and, 676–677
  radiotherapy effects on, 675–676
Central nervous system metastasis, 670–674. See also *Metastasis(es).*
  intracranial, 670–671
  leptomeningeal, 673–674
  pretreatment detection of, 347
  radiation therapy of, 470–471, 471t, 606, 671, 672–673
  screening for, 582–583
  spinal, 671–673
Cerebral metastasis. See *Central nervous system metastasis.*
Cerebrospinal fluid, in leptomeningeal carcinomatosis, 674
  in spinal metastasis, 672
Chemotherapy, 390–392, 475–491, 607–610. See also *Endocrine therapy.*
  angioaccess for, 459, 608

Chemotherapy *(Continued)*
  cell chemosensitivity and, 492–498
  combination, 479–482, 479t
    endocrine therapy with, 481–482
    immunotherapy with, 481
    single agents vs., 480t
  drug extravasation in, 459, 607–608
  emotional support during, 734
  endocrine therapy with, 477–478, 481–482, 487–488, 488t, 504, 530–532
  follow-up and, 586
  in angiosarcoma, 703
  in cystosarcoma phyllodes, 697–698
  in eye metastasis, 668
  in inflammatory carcinoma, 393–394
  in leptomeningeal carcinomatosis, 674
  in lymphangiosarcoma, 713
  in lymphoma, 701
  in male breast cancer, 721–722, 725–726
  in Stage I disease, 487
  in Stage II disease, 484–487, 486t, 487t
  in Stage III disease, 483–484
  in vitro evaluation of, 497–498
  new agents in, 482
  nursing care in, 607–610
  oophorectomy with, 515
  partial mastectomy with, 384, *385,* 386
  radiation therapy effects and, 472
  radiation therapy with, 484
  rationale for, 12–13
  receptor status and, 326–327
  resistance to, 298–299, 496–497
  single agent, 478–479, 478t, 608t
    postsurgical, 486t
  staging for, 475–477, 476t
  surgery with, 442, 484–487, 486t, 487t
  tissue-specific delivery of, 498
  toxicity of, 482–483, 607–610, 645
    neurologic, 674–675
Chest film, pretreatment, 345
Chest wall, radiation-induced sarcoma of, 578–579
  resection of, 661
Chi square, 746–747, 747t, 748t
  different life table testing by, 752, 753t
  interpretation of, 752–754
  simultaneous hypothesis testing with, 764–765
Chloroma, 709
Cholesterol, 86, 98
Chondrosarcoma, 710
Chromatography, in receptor status analysis, 310, 311t, *312, 313,* 313t
Clothing, postmastectomy, 599, 600
CMFVP regimen, 479, 479t
Colostrum, 39
Columbia Clinical Classification, 339–340, *340, 341*
Coma, 671
Comedo appearance, 221, *223*
Computed tomography (CT), 150–151, 200
  in eye metastasis, 667
  in intracranial metastasis, 670–671
  in spinal metastasis, 672
  of liver, 346
Computers, in research, 742–743
Contingency tables, 744, 746–747, 746t, 747t, 749t
  chi square with, 746–747, 747t, 748t

Contrast enhancement, for CT, 150
  for galactography, 188
Cookbooks, for lowering cancer risk, 108
Cooper's ligaments, 17
Cordotomy, 677
Corticosteroids, 527–529, *528*, 607, 725
  in intracranial metastasis, 671
  in spinal metastasis, 673
  side effects of, 607
Cortisol, 35
Corynebacterium parvum, 550
Cost-benefit analysis, 765
  of bone scans, 580–581
  of follow-up, 576–577
  of screening programs, 564, 570, 571, 571t
    mammographic, 178
Counseling, dietary, 105–108
Cowden's disease, 51–52
CT. See *Computed tomography.*
Cyclic adenosine monophosphate (cAMP), 38, 94–95
  fibrocystic breast disease and, 39–40, 94–95
Cyclophosphamide, 608t
  chemotherapy based on, 479, 479t, 481
    single agents vs., 480t
  in male breast cancer, 725
Cylindroma. See *Adenoid cystic carcinoma.*
Cyproterone acetate, 725
Cyst(s), aspiration of, 144–146, *145,* 145t, 146t
  ultrasonography of, 148–149, *149,* 189
Cystic mastopathy. See *Fibrocystic breast cancer.*
Cystosarcoma phyllodes, 689–692, *690, 692–694,* 694–699
  adenocarcinoma with, 698–699
  cell kinetics in, 265
  clinical findings in, *690,* 691–692, *692–694*
  histology of, 691, 694, 694t
  incidence of, 691
  malignancy of, 690–691, 695
  prognosis in, 695
  prophylaxis of, 699
  recurrence of, 695–697, 696t, *697–698,* 697t
  treatment of, 694–698
    tumor size and, 697t
  vs. fibroadenoma, 690, 691
Cytology, fine needle aspiration, 144–146, *145,* 145t, 146t

Danazol, 529
Death rates. See *Mortality rates.*
Delirium, 735
Deoxyribonucleic acid (DNA) measurement, 250–269
Depression, 729, 733
  at recurrence, 735
Dermatofibrosarcoma protuberans, 704, 706
Diaphanography, 193–194
Diaphanoscopy, 143–144
Diarrhea, 610
Diet, alcohol in, 91–92
  breast cancer and, 40–42, 41t, 62–64, *63,* 74–104
  caffeine in, 42, 92–94
  chemotherapy and, 610
  cholesterol in, 86

Diet *(Continued)*
  epidemiologic studies of, 74–78
  exercise with, 773, 776–777, 776t
  fat in, 82–87
  fibrocystic breast disease and, 39–40
  group data on, 75
  guide to, 97–98
  individual assessment of, 75–77
  proteins in, 87
  recording of, 75–78, 109–110
  restricted, 113–121
  selenium in, 89
  suggested, 111–121
  tyramine in, 40, 94–97
    restricted, 120–121
  vitamin A in, 87–89
  vitamin C in, 91
  vitamin E in, 89–91
Dietary counseling, 98, 105–108
Diethylstilbestrol, in receptor status analysis, 315
  therapeutic, 525–526
    side effects of, 533t
Differentiation, growth rate and, 298
  prognosis and, 238–239
  receptor status and, 507–508
Digital mammography, 200
Dimethylbenzanthracene, 543
Diphenhydramine, 610
DNA measurement, 250–269
Dopamine, 94–97
  diet restricted in, 120–121
Doubling time, 276, *278–280,* 281–288, 281t, 285t
  age and, 296t
  cancer control window and, 565–566, *566,* 567t
  histologic type and, 285t
  indirectly measured, 287–288
  of interval cancers, 283–285
  of pulmonary metastasis, 285–286, *279, 280*
  of skin metastasis, 286, *287*
  preclinical, 294–295, 296t
  variations in, 297–298
Doxorubicin, 392, 478, 608t
  cell sensitivity to, 494, 495t, 496t
  combination chemotherapy based on, 479, 479t, 480–481
    single agent vs., 480t
  extravasation of, 607–608
  mitoxantrone vs., 482
  toxicity of, 483
Drainage, 409, 410, *418,* 419, *431–432,* 438
  in pericardial effusion, 456
  in pleural effusion, 455–456
  nursing care and, 597
Drugs. See also *Chemotherapy.*
  antineoplastic, 478t, 480t, 608t
    new, 482
  hyperprolactinemia and, 129t
  sclerosing, 455t
  tumor-specific delivery of, 498
Duct(s), 34
Ductal carcinoma, 207, *208, 209*
  bilateral, 640–641
  in male, 718
  in situ, 220–221, *222–224,* 362–364, 363t
  mucinous carcinoma with, 209, *213*
  prognosis in, 221

Ear wax type, 52
Edema, arm. See *Lymphedema.*
 cerebral, 671
Effusions, 451, 455
 pericardial, 456
 pleural, 455–456, 455t
Elastosis, 207
 prognostic value of, 243
Elbow breadth measurement, 124
Elderly, follow-up of, 577
 immune response and, 548
Elephantiasis, 445
Embryogenesis, 16, 34
Endocrine factors, 56–58. See also specific hormone.
 in male, 70, 716–717
 in nipple discharge, 126–127, 129t
Endocrine therapy, 501–539
 adjuvant, 487–488, 488t, 519, *520*, 521, *521–525*
 advances in, 501
 aminoglutethimide in, 522, 524–525
 androgens in, 526–527
 basis of, 501–503, *502, 503*
 combination, 529–530
 corticosteroids in, 527–529, *528*
 cytotoxic chemotherapy and, 326–327, 477–478, 481–482, 504, 530–532
 estrogens in, 525–526
 history of, 503–504
 in cystosarcoma phyllodes, 697–698
 in male breast cancer, 724–725
 in pregnancy, 685
 new agents in, 529–530
 nursing care during, 606–607
 patient management in, 532, *532, 533,* 533t, 534, 606–607
 principles of, 504–506
 progestins in, 521–522, *525*
 receptor status and, 506–507, 506t, 507t
  changes in, 327–330, 507–508, 508t
 second, 517, 518t
 surgical ablative, 447–451, 514–517, *516, 517*, 723–724
 tamoxifen in, 517–519, *520*, 521
Endometrial cancer, 65
Enucleation, 668
Environmental factors, 48, 475
 genetic factors and, 52, 53
 in male breast cancer, 716
Enzyme-linked immunochemistry, in receptor status analysis, 311t, 314
Epidemiology, 46–48, *47–51,* 47t, 50–51
 glossary for, 560t
 nutritional, 74–78
  dietary fat intake in, 82–84
 of male breast cancer, 69–70, 716–717
Estriol quotient, 56
Estrogen, 10, 35, 37, 56–57, 501–502
 cancer risk and, 59–60, 62–63, 501–502, *502*
 in male, 70, 716–717
 diet and, 62–63
 prolactin and, 36–37
 therapeutic, 525–526
  male breast cancer and, 717, 724
  rebound regression with, 526
Estrogen receptor status. See *Receptor status.*

Estrogen replacement therapy, cancer risk and, 59–60
Exercise, 768–777
 body fat determination and, 770, 773, 774–775t
 fitness appraisal for, 770–771, *771–773*
 heart rate and, 769, *769*
 in lymphedema, 444, 601
 postmastectomy, 599
 program for, 769–770
 weight loss and, 773, 776–777, 776t
Experimental guidelines, 766. See also *Statistical methods.*
Extended radical mastectomy, 9, 369–371, 438, *439,* 440, *440*
Extravasation, drug, 459, 607–608
Eye metastasis, 664–669
 bilateral, 665, 665t
 diagnosis of, 666–668
 from occult primary, 664, 668
 incidence of, 664–665, 665t
 location of, 665
 signs of, 665–666
 survival and, 668
 treatment of, 668

False positive rate, defined, 168
Family, as support system, 602, 732–733, 735
Family incidence, 52–55, 52t, *54*
 of bilateral cancer, 640
 of male breast cancer, 716
Fascial anatomy, 17–18, *18, 19*
Fat, body, 771, 773, 774–775t
 dietary, 62–64, *63,* 82–87
  recommended, 118–119
  reduction of, 97–98
Fatigue, 599
Fetus. See also *Pregnancy.*
 chemotherapy hazard to, 684
 radiation hazard to, 684, *684*
Fibroadenoma, age distribution of, 127t
 cystosarcoma phyllodes and, 690, 691
 removal of, 699
 ultrasonography of, *149,* 190
Fibrocystic breast disease, age and, 127t
 breast cancer and, 66–69, *67,* 67–69t
 caffeine and, 39–40, 92–94
 cAMP and, 39–40, 94–95
 diet and, 39–40
 obesity and, 79
 oral contraceptives and, 69
 receptor status in, 326
Fibrosarcoma, 704, *705,* 706
Fibrosis, 32
 in ductal carcinoma, *208*
 lymphedema and, 445
 radiation-induced, 580
Fine needle aspiration, 144–146, *145,* 145t, 146t
Fisher, Bernard, and concept of breast cancer, 13
Flow cytometry, 255–258, *256–257*
 of breast cancer cells, 263–265
 thymidine labeling and, 257–258
Fludrocortisone, 448
Fluorescein angiography, in eye metastasis, 667

5-Fluorouracil, 478, 608t
  cell sensitivity to, 495t
  combination chemotherapy with, 479–480, 479t, 480t
    methotrexate with, 480
    in male breast cancer, 725
  tamoxifen vs., 521, *523*
Fluoxymesterone, 527
  side effects of, 533t
Food. See *Diet.*
Foreign bodies, 65
Fractures, 606
  stabilization of, 457–458, *457*, 673
Frozen sections, 152
Fruits, in dietary planning, 114–115

Galactography, *130*, 187–189
Galen, 2
Gastrointestinal tract, chemotherapy effects on, 483
  endocrine therapy and, 507
Genetic factors, 51–55, 52t, *54*
  in male breast cancer, 716
Geographic factors, 47–48, *49, 50, 51*
  diet and, 63–64
  genetic factors and, 52
Glucocorticoids, 38
β-Glucuronidase, 41–42, *41*
Gluteal flap, 627, 629,. *629, 630*
Glycogen-rich clear cell carcinoma, 231
Gompertz equation, 274–276, 282–283
  vs. exponential growth, 277
Granular cell myoblastoma, 709–710
Granulocytic sarcoma, 709
Group therapy, 736
Growth fraction, 260
Growth hormone, 36, 502
Growth rates, 271–302, 356
  age and, 296t
  clinical application of, 300
  cell loss and, 272, 290
  data sources on, 276, 278, 281
    clinical, 288–289
  deceleratory, 274–276, *277*, 282–283, 290
  differentiation and, 298
  doubling times, 276, *278–280*, 281–288, 281t, 285t
    age and, 296t
    histologic type and, 285t
    indirectly measured, 287–289
    of interval cancers, 283–285, 291–295, 292–296t, 297
    of multiple metastases, 286–287
    of pulmonary metastasis, *279, 280*, 285–286, *288*
    of skin metastasis, 286, *287*
    preclinical, 294–295, 296t
    variations in, 297–298
  drug resistance and, 298–299
  duration of symptoms and, 299–300
  exponential, 274, *277*
  "fast," 283–285, 285t
  geometric relationships and, 272–273
  linear equation for, 273–274
  metastasis and, 271–272, 289–290, 290t
  mitotic index and, 271
  normal vs. neoplastic, 275–276, 275t

Growth rates *(Continued)*
  preclinical, 291–295, 292–296t, 297
  receptor status and, 326–327
  screening programs and, 562–568, *566*, 567t
  variations in, 297–298
Gynecomastia, 70, 717, 718, *719*

Haagensen and Stout's criteria of inoperability, 339
Halsted's mastectomy, 7–8, 365, *365*, 419, 433, *434–437*. See also *Radical mastectomy.*
  extended, 9, 369–371, 438, *439*, 440, *440*
Handley, Richard S., 9, 372–373
Handley, W. Sampson, 8–9
Heart rate, exercise and, 769, *769*, 770–771, *771–773*
Hemogram, pretreatment, 345
Hepatectomy, 458
Herodotus, 1
Hippocrates, 1–2
Histiocytic lymphoma, *700*
Histiocytoma, malignant fibrous, 710–711
Hormones, 10, 35–42, 304, *305*, 306, 501–503, *502, 503*. See also specific hormones.
  in pregnancy, 679, *680*
  lactation and, 35–38, 304
  lipids and, 86
  male breast cancer and, 70, 716–717
  receptors for. See *Receptor status.*
Human chorionic gonadotropin, 583
Human placental lactogen, 37
Humoral theory, 2–3
Hybridomas, 547, 553
Hydrocortisone, 448, 449t, 516
Hypercalcemia, 607
  estrogen therapy and, 526
Hyperplasia, ductal, as cancer risk, 66–69, 68t
  as mammographic risk pattern, 183
  nomenclature of, 69
Hyperprolactinemia, 126, 129t
Hypophysectomy, 516–517, 606–607
  in male, 722–724
Hypothesis testing. See also *Statistical methods.*
  data collection for, 740–741
  simultaneous, 763–765
Hypothyroidism, 57–58

Illness, terminal, bone pain in, 458
  corticosteroids in, 528
  psychiatric interventions in, 736
Immobilization, postmastectomy, 597
Immune response, anger and, 729
  animal studies on, 542–545
  augmentation of. See *Immunotherapy.*
  bilateral breast cancer and, 641–642
  blood transfusions and, 441–442
  in pregnancy, 679, *680*
  prognosis and, 239–240, 243, 357, 548–549
  to bacterial infection, 550
  to life stress, 730–731
  to tumor viruses, 545–548

Immunocytochemistry, in receptor status analysis, 311t, 314
Immunofluorescence, in receptor status analysis, 311t, 312, 314
Immunoglobulins, in milk, 39
Immunology, 541–557
  animal studies in, 542–545
  diagnostic, 545–548
  history of, 11–12
  human mammary tumor virus and, 545–548
  therapy based on. See *Immunotherapy.*
Immunotherapy, 541–557
  adoptive, 552
  animal models of, 543–544
  bacterial, 550
  biologic response modifiers in, 550–552
  chemotherapy with, 481
  future of, 554
  immunocompetence and, 548–549
  nursing care in, 610–611
  passive, 553–554
  vaccine in, 552–553
In situ breast cancer, 359–364
  age and, *360*
  bilateral, 640–641
  diagnosis of, 360
  growth rate of, 292, 294t
  incidence of, 292t, 293t, 359, 364
  intraductal, 220–221, *222–224,* 362–364, 363t
    bilateral, 640–641
  lobular, 221, 224–225, *225,* 360–362, 361t
    bilateral, 640
  tubular carcinoma with, 216
Infection, after biopsy, 405–406
  after mastectomy, 436, 438
  chemotherapy and, 609
  skin graft, 409
Inflammatory breast cancer, 65, 132–135, *135,* 234, *235,* 392–395, *392,* 394t
  in male, 719
  in pregnancy, 682
  prognosis in, 134–135, *392,* 393–394, 394t
  skin biopsy in, 156
  survival in, 392t, 394, 394t
  treatment of, 393–395, 442
Innervation, 23, *24–27,* 28
  latissimus dorsi, 28, *417, 431,* 435–436, *437*
  pectoralis major, 19, *20–23,* 415, *425–429, 435*
  pectoralis minor, *22,* 23, *24–27,* 415, *425–429, 435*
  serratus anterior, *22,* 23, 28, *429–431, 437*
Insulin, 38
Interferons, 551
Interleukin-2, 551, 552, 553
Interval cancers, 283–285, 285t, 291–295, 292–296t, 297, 573–574
Intracystic breast carcinoma, 144, 144t

Kaplan-Meier survival curves, 744
Karnofsky Performance Status Scale, 577, 578t
  as response indicator, 739–740
  longevity and, 578t, 579t
Kinase activity, 328–329

Kinetics, cell. See *Cell kinetics.*
Klinefelter's syndrome, 51, 717

Lactation, breast cancer diagnosis and, 681, *681*
  cancer risk and, 51
  hormones and, 35–38
  inappropriate, 129t
  milk composition in, 38–39
  physiology of, 34–35
Laminectomy, 457–458, 471, 672
Latissimus dorsi flap, 619, 621–623, *621, 622*
Latissimus dorsi muscle, 28
  innervation of, *417, 431,* 435–436, *437*
Leiomyosarcoma, 710
Leonidas, 2
Leptomeningeal carcinomatosis, 673–674
Leukemia, 645
  granulocytic sarcoma in, 709
Leukoencephalopathy, methotrexate and, 675
Leukopenia, 609
Leuprolide, 529
Levamisole, 481, 551
Level of significance, 756, 758
Life stress, 729–731
Life tables, 743–744, 745t, 746t
  chi square testing of, 752, 753t
Lipid-rich carcinoma, 230–231
Lipids. See *Fat, dietary.*
Lipoma, ultrasonography of, 190, *192*
Liposarcoma, 706–707
Liposomes, 498
Liver metastasis, 458. See also *Metastasis(es).*
  follow-up of, 581–582
  pretreatment detection of, 346–347, 347t
  radiation therapy of, 471
  resection of, 458
  screening for, 581–582
Lobular carcinoma, 216, *217–219*
  bilateral, 640
  in male, 718
  in situ, 221, 224–225, *225,* 360–362, 361t
  prognosis in, 216
  tubulolobular, 216, *219*
Lumpectomy. See *Mastectomy, partial.*
Lung, chemotherapy effects on, 483
  metastasis to. See *Pulmonary metastasis.*
  pretreatment evaluation of, 345
  radiation therapy effects on, 472, 605
Lung cancer, primary vs. metastatic, 345
Luteinizing hormone releasing hormone (LHRH), 529
Lymph nodes, 28–31, *30, 31,* 443
  axillary, 30–31
    dissection of, *416–417,* 419
      radiotherapy vs., 446–447
      with partial mastectomy, *421, 425–432,* 464–465
    irradiation of, 464–465, *466*
    metastasis to, chemotherapy and, 485
      frequency of, 350
      from melanoma, 644
      from occult primary, 130–132, 134t
      in male, 718, 719
      in pregnancy, 683–684, 683t
      receptor status and, 509–510, *511–513,* 513

Lymph nodes *(Continued)*
  axillary, metastasis to recurrence and, 350t, 351, *351, 352,* 352t, *650,* 654t, 661–662
    staging and, 349, *350,* 350t, 351–353, *351, 352,* 352t, 353t
      extent of dissection for, 352–353, *352,* 353t
      level of, 351–352, *352*
      number involved, 349, 350t, 351, *351*
      tumor size and, 354, *354*
    survival and, 389–390, *390,* 485
    palpation of, 140, *141*
    surgical history of, 6
  filtration by, 11, 29
  immune response and, 548–549
  internal mammary, *30*
    axillary metastasis and, 370, *370*
    biopsy of, 440–441
    dissection of, 369–371, 438, *439,* 440, *440*
    recurrence in, 657–658
    staging and, *350,* 353–354, 354t, 440
    surgical history of, 8–9
  irradiation of, 382–383, 464–465, 466
  palpation of, 140–141, *140, 141*
  preparation of, 236
  recurrence in. See *Recurrence, regional.*
  Rotter's, 352
    recurrence in, *649*
    removal of, *415*
  staging and, 340–341, 342–343t, 343–344, *344*
  supraclavicular, recurrence in, 655, 657
    staging and, 354
    surgical history of, 8, 9, 369
  survival and, 12, 236, 243, 389–390, *390*
  tumor size and, 290t, 354, *355*
Lymphangiosarcoma, 446, 711–713, *712*
Lymphatics, 19, 28–32, *30, 31,* 443–444
  dermal, inflammatory carcinoma and, 134–135, 392–393
  edema of, 442–447
  metastasis and, 29–30
  permeation theory and, 8
  prognosis and, 240–241
  regeneration of, 444–445
  treatment effects on, 32, 444
Lymphedema, 32, 442–447, 465, 601
  anatomy in, 443–444
  effects of, 445–446
  lymphangiosarcoma and, 711–713, *712*
  stages of, 445
  treatment of, 444, 445, 601
Lymphoblastic lymphoma, 701
Lymphocele, 410, 419
Lymphocytes, 548–549
Lymphokines, 551
Lymphoma, 699–701
  histiocytic, *700*
  staging of, 701t
  treatment of, 700–701
Lymphotoxin, 551

Magnetic resonance imaging (MRI), 200
  in spinal metastasis, 672

Male breast cancer, 716–727
  chemotherapy in, 721–722, 725–726
  clinical features of, 717–718, 717t, *718, 719*
  endocrine ablation in, 722–724, *723*
  epidemiology of, 69–70, 716–717
  gynecomastia and, 70, 717, 718, *719*
  histology of, 718–719
  hormone therapy of, 724–725
  in Klinefelter's syndrome, 51, 717
  incidence of, 716
  lymphoma, *701*
  mastectomy for, 720–721
  mortality from, 47
  prognosis in, 720–721, *720,* 721t
  radiation therapy in, 721
  receptor status in, 325–326, 724
  recurrence of, 722, *722*
  second cancers with, 719
Malignancy, secondary, 65–66, 66t, 623–633. See also *Breast cancer; Cancer; Mass; Metastasis(es); Tumor* entries; and specific neoplasms.
  age and, 636–637, *637, 638*
  chemotherapy and, 483, 644–645
  in male, 719
  metastatic to breast, 644
  radiation therapy and, 472, 645
  sites of, 633t, 634, 636
Malignant fibrous histiocytoma, 710–711
Malnutrition, 610
Mammography, 146–148, *148,* 148t, 168–179, *176, 179–182,* 181, 183, *184–185,* 186–187. See also *Radiography.*
  asymmetric density in, 178
  cancer arising between sessions of, 283–285, 285t, 291–295, 292–296t, 297, 573–574
  cancer risk from, 62, 171–173, 572
  cancer signs in, 174–178, 175t
  clinical utility of, 175t
  cost-benefit analysis of, 178, 571, 571t
  digital, 200
  false negatives in, 575
  film screen vs. xeroradiographic, 173–174
  guidelines for, 148t, 173
  mortality rates and, 168–171, *171,* 170–172t
  needle localization for, 157–158, 178–179, *179–182,* 181
  nonscreening uses of, 187
  of calcifications, 177–178
  of mass, 176, *176*
  of tumor growth, 281–282
  pregnancy and, 680–681, *681*
  radiation exposure from, 147, 561
  risk patterns in, 181, 183, 186–187
  sensitivity of, 147t
  technique for, 173–174
  ultrasonography with, 189–190, *190–192,* 193
Manchester system, 338–339
Mass, 126, *127, 128.* See also *Breast cancer; Cancer; Malignancy, secondary; Metastasis(es); Tumor* entries; and specific neoplasms.
  aspiration of, 144–146, *145,* 145t, 146t
  benign vs. cancerous, 127t, 137–138, 148–149
  "dominant," 142

Mass *(Continued)*
  mammographic signs in, 176, *176*
  nipple discharge with, 127
  nonpalpable, 157–158
    location of, 178–179, *179–182*, 181, *184–185*
  Paget's disease with, 136
  palpation of, 142
Mass screening. See *Screening programs.*
Mastectomy, chemotherapy with, 484–487, 486t, 487t
  complications of, 387–388, *388*, 410, *418*, 419, *433*, 436, 438
    lymphedema, 442–447
    nerve entrapment, 446
  evaluation of, 12–13
  for occult primary, 131–132, 642–644
  Halsted's, 6–8, 365, *365*, 419, 433, *434–437*. See also *Radical mastectomy.*
    extended, 9, 369–371, 438, *439*, 440, *440*
  history of, 2–11
  immediate vs. delayed, 152–154, 153t, 154t
  in advanced disease, 389–390, 395
  in carcinoma in situ, 361, 362–363
  in cystosarcoma phyllodes, 695–697
  in inflammatory breast cancer, 393
  in male breast cancer, 720–721
  in pregnancy, 683–684, 683t
    abortion with, 684–685, 685t
  nursing care for, 596–601, 598t
  palliative, 395
  partial, 383–384, *385–388*, 386–389
    at biopsy, 156
    axillary dissection with, *421, 425–432*
    complications of, 387–388, *388*
    contraindications to, 388, 419, 464
    protocol for, *385*, 386
    radiation therapy with, 384, 386–387, *386, 387,* 387t, 463–465, 463t, *464,* 464t, 578–579
    recurrence after, 386–388, *387,* 387t
    residual tumor after, 243, 383–384
    technique for, 419, *420–425*
  prophylactic, 17, 642–644
    for lobular carcinoma in situ, 361
  psychoemotional factors in, 592–593, 732–734
  radiation therapy with, 10
    recurrence and, 658–659, 658t
  radical, 365–366, *365, 367, 368*–373, 419
    extended, 9, 369–371, 438, *439*, 440, *440*
    history of, 5–9, 365–366
    modified, 11, 371–374, *372,* 373t
      Auchincloss-Madden, 373–374
      comparison of, *379–381*, 381t
      Patey, 372–373, 373t
      radical vs., 374, *375–379*, 381t, 657t
      recurrence after, *378, 379,* 381t
      technique for, 409–410, *411–418*
    precursors to, 3–4
    radiation therapy with, 465–467, *467*, 468t
    rationale for, 13t
    reassessment of, 10–13
    recurrence after, 365–366, *367*, 368, *368*, 368t, *378, 379,* 513, 513t, *649, 651, 652,* 657t
    technique for, 419, 433, *434–437*
  salvage, 661

Mastectomy *(Continued)*
  simultaneous bilateral, 642
  survival and, 358–359, *359*
  total (simple), 10, 381–383
    radical mastectomy vs., 382t
    technique for, 406, 409
  types of, 337t
Meat, in dietary planning, 117–118
Mediastinum, radiation therapy of, 471
Medical history, 138–139
  dietary, 75–78
Medroxyprogesterone, 725
Medullary carcinoma, 207–208, *210–211*
  ultrasonography of, 190, *192*
Megestrol acetate, 522, *525,* 725
  side effects of, 533t
Melanoma, metastatic to breast, 644
  of eye, 668
Melphalan, cell sensitivity to, 495t
Meningitis, 471
Menopause, 34, 35
  cancer incidence and, 53, *54*
    effect of weight on, 79–80
  cell kinetics and, 258–259
  estrogen replacement after, 60
  receptor status and, 318–319, 319t, 507, 508t
Menstrual cycle, 34
  cell kinetics and, 258–259
  receptor status and, 318
  volume changes and, 136, *138*
Menus, for lowering cancer risk, 112–121
Metaplasia, pseudosarcomatous, 228, *229–230*
Metastasis(es). See also *Breast cancer; Cancer; Malignancy, secondary; Mass, Tumor* entries; and specific neoplasms.
  autopsy incidence of, 586–587, 586t
  cutaneous. See *Skin.*
  doubling time of, 285–287, *287, 288*
  early, 569–570, 576–577, 579
  early theories of, 4–7
  evaluation of, 12–13
  from cystosarcoma phyllodes, 694, 697–698
  immune response and, 548–549
  in male breast cancer, 722
  in pregnancy, 682, *683*
  in situ carcinoma and, 360
  mammography in, 187
  management of, 395
  mastectomy and, 366, *367, 368*
  mechanism of, 29–30, *30*
  multiple primary cancer vs., 633–634
  prognosis and, 289, 348–349, *349,* 505, 505t, 506t
  radiation therapy of, 470–471, 471t
  receptor status and, 318–320
  staging and, 348–349. See also *Staging.*
  systemic therapy of, 477–478
  to bone. See *Bone metastasis.*
  to brain. See *Central nervous system metastasis.*
  to breast, 644
  to central nervous system. See *Central nervous system metastasis.*
  to eye. See *Eye metastasis.*
  to liver. See *Liver metastasis.*
  to lung. See *Pulmonary metastasis.*
  to lymph nodes. See under *Lymph nodes.*

Metastasis(es) *(Continued)*
  to placenta, 685
  tumor size and, 271–272, 289–290, 290t
  visceral, 507
Methotrexate, 478, 608t
  cell sensitivity to, 495t
  combination chemotherapy with, 479–480, 479t, 480t
  5-fluorouracil with, 480
    in male breast cancer, 725
  in leptomeningeal carcinomatosis, 674
  neurotoxicity of, 674–675
  tamoxifen with, 481–482
Methylxanthine, 39–40, *40,* 41t, 92–94
Metoclopramide, 483, 610
Metropolitan Insurance Co. Height and Weight Tables, 122–123
Microdensitometry, 255
Microdochectomy, 574
Micrometastasis, chemotherapy and, 485
Microsurgery, in breast reconstruction, 627, 629, *629, 630*
Milk, 38–39
  dietary, 113
  prolactin and, 37
"Minimal" breast cancer, 238, 360
Mitomycin C, cell sensitivity to, 495t
Mitosis, 250, 270–271
  measurement of, 250–251, *251, 252*
    drawbacks of, 259–260
Mitoxantrone, 482
  cell sensitivity to, 494, 495t, 496t
Modified radical mastectomy. See *Mastectomy, radical, modified.*
Mondor's disease, 129–130
Monoamine oxidase inhibitors, diet and, 94–97
Monoclonal antibodies, animal studies on, 544
  in chemotherapy, 498
  in immunotherapy, 553
  in receptor status analysis, 314
  to breast tumors, 546–548
Moore, Charles H, 5–6
Morphine, 677
Mortality rates, 46–48, *47–50,* 47t, 504–506, 504–506t
  age and, 47–48, 47t, *48,* 356–357, 357t
  dietary fat and, *63*
  duration of symptoms and, 299–300
  geography and, 47–48, *49, 50*
  in male breast cancer, 720–721, *720,* 721t
  mammography and, 168–171, *170,* 170–172t
  mastectomy and, 366, *367,* 368, *368,* 375–377, *464,* 466–467, *467*
    partial, 386, *386, 387,* 463t, *464,* 464t
  mitotic index and, 271
  pregnancy and, 682, 683t
    subsequent, 686–687, *686*
  psychosocial factors and, 735
Mouse mammary tumor virus, 55–56, 542–543
  human mammary tumor virus and, 545–546
Mouth, chemotherapy effects on, 609
  radiation effects on, 603
MRI. See *Magnetic resonance imaging (MRI).*

Mucinous carcinoma, *128,* 209, 211, *212–213*
  bilateral, 641
  "mixed," 209, *213*
  prognosis in, 211
Mucoepidermoid carcinoma, 232
Multicentricity, 578, 637–638
  defined, 243
  of carcinoma in situ, 360
    ductal, 362
    lobular, 360
Muscles, anatomy of, 18–19, *19–22,* 23, 28
  innervation of, *20–27,* 23, 28
Mutation, 298–299
Myelography, 672
Myoblastoma, granular cell, 709–710

Narcotics, 676–677
Natural killer cells, 543
  lymphokine-activated, 552
Nausea, 483
Necrosis, 260, 272, 290
  radiation, 446, 447
Needle biopsy, 154, 155t, 403, *404*
  in eye metastasis, 667
Needle localization, 178–179, *179–182,* 181, *184–185*
Nerves. See *Innervation.*
Neuropathy, postmastectomy, 438, 446
Neurosurgery, for pain relief, 676–677
  in intracranial metastasis, 671
Nipple, biopsy of, 156
  discharge from. See *Nipple discharge.*
  inversion of, *112*
  Paget's disease of, 135–136, *137, 138,* 232–234, *233*
    in male, 718
  palpation of, 143
  reconstruction of, 629
  retraction of, 135, *136*
Nipple discharge, 126–127, 129, 129t, *130*
  biopsy in, 158–159, 159t
  galactography in, 187–189
  in male breast cancer, 718
  screening and, 574
Nomenclature, of mastopathy, 69
Nonpalpable mass, biopsy of, 157–158
  location of, 178–179, *179–182, 184–185*
Nuclear grade, 238–239, 356
  proliferative index and, 261–262, *262*
Nurse, assessment by, 593
  form for, *594–595*
  chemotherapy hazards to, 608–609
  psychoemotional support from, 601–602
  teaching role of, 591–593
    on breast self-examination, 591–592
    on mastectomy, 596–597, 598t, 599–601
    on radiation therapy, 603, *603–604,* 605t
Nursing care, 591–613
  for chemotherapy patient, 607–610
  for hormonal therapy patient, 606–607
  for immunotherapy patient, 610–611
  for lymphedema, 601
  for mastectomy patient, 596–601
  for radiation therapy patient, 602–603, *603–604,* 605t, 606
  for ulcerating lesions, 611

Nursing care *(Continued)*
  patient assessment for, 593, 596
    form for, *594–595*
  psychoemotional, 601–602
Nutrition. See *Diet.*

Oat cell carcinoma, 232
Obesity, 62–63, 78–79
  benign breast disease and, 79
  body fat percentage and, 771, 773, 774–775t
  counseling in, 105–108
  criteria for, 79, 105, 122–123, 771, 773
  exercise and, 768
  pre- vs. postmenopausal, 79–80
  prognosis and, 80–81
Occult primary tumor, 130–132, 575
  axillary metastasis from, 130–132, 134t
  eye metastasis from, 664, 668
Ocular metastasis. See *Eye metastasis.*
Odor, ulcerating metastatic lesions and, 611
Oncogenes, 545
  steroid receptors and, 328–330
Oophorectomy, 447–448, 514–516, 606
  adjuvant, 515–516
  chemotherapy with, 515
  contraindications to, 515t
  history of, 503–504
  radiation, 515
Oral contraceptives, 59–60
  fibrocystic breast disease and, 69
Oral hygiene, 609
Orchiectomy, 723–724, *723*
Orthopedic surgery, 457–458, *457*
Osteogenic sarcoma, 711
Ovarian function, 59
Oxytocin, 35–36

Pacemakers, 65
Paget's cells, *138*
Paget's disease of breast, 135–136, *137, 138,* 232–234, *233*
  in male, 718
  skin biopsy in, 156
Pain, 676–677
  back, 471
  bone, 458, 580–581, 606
    radiation therapy of, 470
Palliation, in male breast cancer, 722–726
  in pregnancy, 685
  radiotherapeutic, 470–471
  surgical, 395, 455–458
Palpation, 136–143, *140–143*
  mammography with, 147, 147t
Papillary carcinoma, intracystic, 215, *215*
  invasive, 211, *214,* 215, *215*
  prognosis in, 215
Papilloma, intraductal, *188*
  papillary carcinoma vs., 215
Paraplegia, radiation therapy of, 471
Partial mastectomy. See *Mastectomy, partial.*
Patey mastectomy, 372–373, 373t
  Auchincloss-Madden mastectomy vs., *379–381*
  recurrence after, *651*

Pathology, 206–249
  protocol for, 234–236
  receptor status analysis and. See *Receptor status.*
  tissue preparation for. See *Tissue preparation.*
  tumor characteristics in, 236–239, *237, 240–244*
Patient compliance, 570–571
Patient education, 731–732
  at diagnosis, 732
  nurse's role in, 591–593, 596
  on breast self-examination, 572–573, 591–592
  on cancer, 161–162
  on chemotherapy, 608
  on diet, 105–108
    food selection for, 112–121
  on follow-up, 575–576
  on hypercalcemia, 607
  on lymphedema, 444, 445, 601
  on radiation therapy, 603, *603–604,* 605t
  on systemic therapy, 606–611
  on wound care, 599
  screening programs and, 570, 731–732
Peau d'orange skin, 135
Pectoralis major muscle, 18–19
  fascia of, 17–18, *18, 19*
  innervation of, *415, 425–429, 435*
  preservation of, 373–373, *414–415*
  surgical history of, 7–8
Pectoralis minor muscle, 19, *20–23, 414–415*
  fascia of, 18, *18, 21*
  innervation of, *22–27, 415, 425–429, 435*
Performance status, 577, 578t, 579t
Permeation theory, 8, 11
Pericardial effusion, 456
Personality, 728–731
Phenytoin, 671
Phlebotomy, 442
Phosphorylation, steroid receptor, 328–330, *330*
Physical examination, 136–143, *139–143*
Physical fitness, 768–777
  assessment of, 770–771, *771–773*
  body fat determination for, 771, 773, 774–775t
  defined, 768
  program for, 769–770
  weight loss and, 773, 776–777, 776t
Physical therapy, 443
  for lymphedema, 444
Physician, as educator, 731–732
  psychoemotional support from, 732
Placenta, metastasis to, 685
Plasma cells, in medullary vs. ductal carcinoma, 209
Pleural effusion, 455–456, 471
  agents against, 455t
Plexopathy, radiation, 676
Ploidy analysis, 256–257
  in breast cancer, 256–257, 263–265
Poland's syndrome, 139
Polynucleotides, 551
Portmann classification, 339
Postirradiated breast, follow-up of, 579–580
Power of test, 755–756
  computation of, 762–763, *763*
  sample size determination for, 756, 757t, 758–759, 758t

Power of test (Continued)
  sample size determination for, for *t* test, 760–762, 761t
    level of significance and, 756, 758
    pool power, 758–759
    to reject new treatment, 759–760
Predictive value, defined, 168
Prednimustine, 482
Pregnancy, 34
  after breast cancer, 685–687, *686*
  breast cancer in, 679–688
    advanced, 685
    chemotherapy for, 684
    diagnosis of, 680–682, *681*
    early, 683–685, 685t
    frequency of, 680
    mastectomy for, 683–684
    pathologic findings in, 682
    prognosis in, 682, 683t, 686–687
    radiotherapy for, 684, *684*
    risk for, 58–59, 58t, 679, *680*
    treatment of, 683–685
  nipple discharge in, 127
  progesterone in, 37
Presentation, 127t
Prevention. See *Risk factors; Screening programs.*
Probability theory, 740
Prochlorperazine, 610
Progesterone(s), 35, 37–38, 502
  estrogen combinations with, 660
  in male breast cancer, 725
Progesterone receptor status. See *Receptor status.*
Progestins, therapeutic, 521–522, *525*
Prolactin, 35, 36–37, 57, 502
  bone metastasis and, 39
Prophylactic mastectomy, 17, 642–644
Prostaglandin E, 543
Prostate cancer, 504
  male breast cancer and, 717
Prostheses, 600
  mammography and, 187
  screening and, 574
  ultrasonography and, 193
Protein, breast cancer and, 87
Protocol creation, 740–742
  computers and, 742–743
Pseudosarcomatous metaplasia, carcinoma with, 228, *229–230*
Psychiatric care, 735, 736
Psychoemotional factors, 591–593, 596, 601–602
  adjuvant therapy and, 734
  at diagnosis, 732
  breast reconstruction and, 734
  immune response and, 729, 730–731
  intervention and, 735–736
  life stresses and, 729–731
  mastectomy and, 592–593, 732–734
    vs. conservative surgery, 732–734
  prediagnosis, 728–731
  recurrence and, 734
  survival and, 735
Psychosocial factors, 732
Pulmonary metastasis, doubling time of, *279, 280,* 285–286, *288*
  survival and, 298
  follow-up of, 582
  pretreatment evaluation of, 345, 582

Quality control, in receptor status analysis, 315–317, 317t
Quetelet index, 79, 81, 105

Race, receptor status and, 320, 323
Radiation, carcinogenesis and, 60–62, 472
  in male, 716
  fetus and, 684, *684*
  from CT, 150
  from mammography, 147, 171–173
  oophorectomy by, 515
Radiation myelitis, 676
Radiation therapy, 462–474
  angioaccess site and, 459
  angiosarcoma and, 703
  axillary, 464–465, *466*
  complications of, 388, *388,* 445, 446–447, 471–472, 578–579, 645
    neurologic, 675–676
  definitive, 463–465, 463t, *464,* 464t
  early history of, 9–10, 12–13, 462
  emotional support during, 734
  esthetic results of, 465, *466*
  in advanced disease, 390, 469–471, 469t, 471t
  in ductal carcinoma in situ, 363
  in inflammatory carcinoma, 393
  in leptomeningeal carcinomatosis, 674
  in lymphoma, 701
  in male breast cancer, 721
  in pregnancy, 684, *684*
  lymphedema and, 445, 465
  nerve entrapment and, 446
  nursing care in, 602–603, *603–604,* 605–606, 605t
  of metastasis, 470–471, 471t, 605–606
    to brain, 671
    to eye, 668
    to spine, 673
  of recurrences, 467–469, *468,* 659–660, *660,* 661t
  partial mastectomy with, 384, 386–387, *386, 387,* 387t, 463–465, 463t, *464,* 464t, 578–579
  preoperative, 467, 468t
  radical mastectomy with, 465–467, *467,* 468t
  recurrence after, 580, *652*
  sarcoma induced by, 578–579, 645, 703, 713
  surgery and, 446, 447
  total mastectomy with, 381–383, 382t
  tumor size and, 462, 469, 469t
Radical mastectomy, 365–366, *365, 367,* 368–373, 419
  extended, 9, 369–371, 438, *439,* 440, *440*
  history of, 5–9, 365–366
  modified, 11, 371–374, *372,* 373t
    Auchincloss-Madden, 373–374
    Patey vs., *379–381,* 381t
    Patey, 372–373, 373t
    radical vs., 374, *375–379,* 381t, 657t
    recurrence after, *378, 379,* 381t
    Scanlon, 410–419
    technique for, 409–410, *411–418*
  precursors to, 3–4
  radiation therapy with, 465–467, *467,* 468t
  rationale for, 13t

Radical mastectomy *(Continued)*
  reassessment of, 10–13
  recurrence after, 365–366, *367, 368,* 368t, *378, 379, 513,* 513t, *649, 651, 652,* 657t
  technique for, 419, 433, *434–437*
Radiography. See also *Mammography*.
  doubling time measurement by, 285–286
  in eye metastasis, 667, *667*
  in spinal metastasis, 672
  pretreatment, 345
    bone scan with, 345–346
  screening, 582
Radionuclide imaging, pretreatment, 345–347, 347t
Reach to Recovery program, 600, 735–736
Receptor status, analysis of, 303–323
  chromatographic, 310, 311t, *312, 313,* 313t
  enzyme-linked, 311t, 314
  immunocytochemical, 311t, 314
  immunofluorescent, 311t, 312, 314
  ligands for, 308t
  quality control in, 315–317, 317t
  reference ranges in, 320–321, *321, 322,* 323
  sucrose gradient, 309–310, *309,* 311t
  tissue handling for, 306–307, 316, 405t, 406
  titration, 307–309, *308, 309,* 311t
  software for, 310
  axillary metastasis and, 509–510, *511–513,* 513
  biopsy and, 155–156, 156t
  chemotherapy response and, 530–531
  cytotoxic chemotherapy and, 326–327, 477–478
  endocrine therapy response and, 506–507, 506t, 507t
  in fibrocystic disease, 326
  in inflammatory carcinoma, 394–395
  in male breast cancer, 325–326, 724
  in pregnancy, 682
  mechanism of, 304, *305,* 306
  of metastases, 318–320
  oophorectomy and, 514–515
  polymorphism and, 327–330, *329, 330*
  progesterone, 324–325, 325t, 509, *511*
  prognosis and, 242–243, 323–327, 508–510, *509–514,* 513t, *585*
  proliferative index and, 262
  race and, 320, 323
  treatment based on. See *Endocrine therapy*.
  treatment effects on, 319, 508t
  unknown, *505*
  variations in, 317–320, 319t, 507
Recurrence, after partial mastectomy, 386–388, *387,* 387t
  after radiation therapy, 580, *652*
  after radical mastectomy, 365–366, *367, 368, 368,* 368t, *513,* 513t, *649, 651, 653,* 657t
  after radical (modified) mastectomy, *378, 379,* 381t
  after total mastectomy, 382t
  axillary metastasis and, 350t, 351, *351, 352,* 352t, *650,* 654t, 661–662
  breast reconstruction and, 616–617

Recurrence *(Continued)*
  chest wall resection in, 660–661
  immune response and, 549
  local, 648–663
    defined, 648
    frequency of, 653–655, *652*
    management of, 659–662
    mechanism of, 649, *651, 652*
    primary treatment and, 658–659, 658t
    prognosis in, 655, *657, 660*
    site of, 655, *656*
    surgical skin margins and, 654–655, *656*
    tumor size and, 654t, *655*
  of angiosarcoma, 703–704
  of cystosarcoma phyllodes, 695–697, 696t, *697,* 697t, *698*
  of ductal carcinoma in situ, 362–363, 363t
  of male breast cancer, 722, *722*
  pregnancy and, 686–687
  psychoemotional factors at, 735
  radiation therapy of, 467–469, *468,* 659–660, *660,* 661t
  receptor status and, 513–514, *514*
  regional, 648–663
    defined, 648
    internal mammary, 657–658
    management of, 659–662
    mechanism of, 652–653
    primary treatment and, 658–659, 658t
    supraclavicular, 655, 657
  salvage mastectomy in, 661
  survival and, 289, 348–349, *349,* 583, *584, 585, 585, 657*
  systemic therapy of, 662
  treatment of, 585–586, 659–662
Reproductive factors, 58–59, 58t
Research guidelines, 766. See also *Statistical methods*.
Retinoids, 87–89
Retroviruses, 545–546
Rhabdomyosarcoma, 707, *708*
  metastatic to breast, 644
Risk factor(s), 55, *55,* 475
  age as. See *Age*.
  alcohol as, 91–92
  dietary, 40–42, 41t, 62–64, *63,* 72–104
  endocrine, 56–58
  estrogen as, 59–60
  fibrocystic disease as, 66–69, *67,* 67–69t
  for bilateral cancer, 640–641
  for male breast cancer, 716–717
  for recurrence, 290
  foreign body as, 65
  genetic, 51–55, 52t, *54,* 475
  mammographic pattern as, 181, 183, 186–187
  radiation as, 60–62
  reproductive, 58–59, 58t
  psychoemotional. See *Psychoemotional factors*.
  screening programs and, 561–562
  socioeconomic, 731–732
  thermographic pattern as, 198–200
  trauma as, 64–65
  viral, 55–56
Rotter's nodes, 352
  recurrence in, *649*
  removal of, *415*

S phase, arrest in, 253
  importance of, 259
  measurement of, in breast cancer, 250–252, *252*
Salvage mastectomy, 661
Sample size, 755–763
  for standard experiment, 756, 758–763
  level of significance and, 756, 758
  pooled, 758–759
  sequential, 762
  to test difference between two means, 760–762, 761t
  two-tailed determination of, 756, 757t, 758t, 761t
Sarcoma, 689–715
  angiosarcoma, 701–704, *702*
  carcinosarcoma, 708
  chondrosarcoma, 710
  cystosarcoma phyllodes, 689–692
    adenocarcinoma with, 698–699
    clinical findings in, 690, 691–692, *692, 694*
    histology of, 691, 692, 694, 696t
    incidence of, 691
    malignancy of, 690–691, 695
    prophylaxis of, 699
    recurrence of, 695–697, 696t, *697, 698*
    treatment of, 694–698
      tumor size and, 697t
    vs. fibroadenoma, 690, 691
  fibrosarcoma, 704, *705*, 706
  granular cell myoblastoma, 709–710
  granulocytic, 709
  in male, 719
  leiomyosarcoma, 710
  liposarcoma, 706–707
  lymphangiosarcoma, 711–713, *712*
  osteogenic, 711
  radiation-induced, 578–579, 645, 703, 713
  rhabdomyosarcoma, 707, *708*
  stromal, 699, *699*
  types of, 689t
Scapula, winged, *433*
Scar, biopsy, 155–156, *155*
  mastectomy, recurrence in, 286, *287*, 655, *656*
  radiation therapy, 447
Sclerosing agents, 455t
Screening programs, 162, 558–590
  breast self-examination in, 572–573, 574, 591–592
  calcification and, 177–178
  cancer progression model for, 559t
  cost-benefit analysis of, 178, 564, 570, 571, 571t
  CT in, 150–151, 200
  diaphanography in, 193–194
  evaluation of, 167–168, 558–559, 562–570
    definitions in, 559–560
    models for, 559t, 565–570, *565, 566,* 568t
  false negatives in, 575
  for bone metastasis, 580–581
  for cerebral metastasis, 582–583
  for hepatic metastasis, 581–582
  for pulmonary metastasis, 582
  glossary for, 560t
  guidelines for, 148t, 173

Screening programs *(Continued)*
  interval cancers in, 283–285, 285t, 291–295, 292–296t, 297, 573–574
  lead time bias in, 563–564
  length bias in, 562–563
  mammography in. See *Mammography.*
  mortality rates and, 168–171, *170,* 170–172t, 571–572
  MRI in, 200
  nipple discharge and, 574
  nurse's role in, 591–593
  of augmented breast, 574
  of high risk groups, 561–562
  patient compliance and, 570–571
  patient education and, 570, 731–732
  risks of, 147, 171–173, 561, 570, 572
  thermography in, 194–200
  tumor markers in, 583
  ultrasonography in, 189–190, 193
Secretory carcinoma, 228
Segmental mastectomy. See *Mastectomy, partial.*
Seizures, radiation therapy and, 471, 471t
Selenium, 89–91
Self-examination, breast, 143, 285, 572–573, 592, 731
  nurse's role in, 591–592
  of lumpy breast, 574
  rapid early growth and, 297
Sensitivity, defined, 168
Seroma, 410, *418,* 419
Serratus anterior muscle, *22,* 23
  innervation of, *22,* 23, 28, *429–431, 437*
Sexuality, 593, 602, 733
Signet ring cell carcinoma, 211, 228, 230, *231*
Silicone implants, 574
  cancer risk from, 65
Simple mastectomy. See *Total (simple) mastectomy.*
Skin, biopsy of, 156
  calcification of, 177
  chemotherapy effects on, 483
  metastasis to, doubling time of, 286, *287*
  peau d' orange, 135
  radiation therapy and, 471–472, 603, 605t
  retraction of, 129–130, *131, 133*
  satellite nodules of, *133*
  ulceration of, *134,* 611
    from cystosarcoma phyllodes, 692
    in male breast cancer, 718, *718*
Skin flaps, *411–413, 426,* 436
  blood loss and, 442
  infection of, 436, 438
  in breast reconstruction, 614–615
    latissimus dorsi, 619–623, *621, 622*
    microsurgical, 627, 629, *629, 630*
    transverse rectus abdominis, 623, *624–628,* 627
Skin grafts, 409
  recurrence and, 645, *655*
Skin tests, 547–548
Socioeconomic factors, 47, 731–732
Software, in nutritional analysis, 106
Somatostatin, 529
Specificity, defined, 168
Specimen(s), examination of, 234–236
Spinal metastasis, 671–673
  radiation myelitis and, 676

Squamous cell carcinoma, 226–228, *227,* 708
Stage of disease, carcinoembryonic antigen and, 514t
  determination of. See *Staging.*
  pregnancy and, 682–685, 683t
  proliferative index and, 262, 263t
Staging, age and, 356–357, 357t
  chemotherapy and, 475–477, 476t
  clinical, 344–348
    bone biopsy in, 345–346
    bone scan in, 347
    chest radiograph in, 345
    hemogram in, 345
    liver tests in, 346–347, 347t
  histopathology in, 354–356, 356t
  history of, 337–340
  of advanced cancer, 348–349, *349*
  of breast lymphoma, 701t
  of male breast cancer, 720
  pathologic, 349, *350,* 350t, 351–354, *351, 352,* 353t
    axillary metastasis in, 349, *350,* 350t, 351–353, *351, 352,* 352t, 353t
      extent of dissection for, 352–353, *352,* 353t
      frequency of, *350*
      level of, 351–352, *352*
      number involved, 349, 350t, 351, *351*
    internal mammary metastasis in, *350,* 353–354, 440
    supraclavicular metastasis in, 354
    tumor size and, 354, *355*
  technology effects on, 579
  TNM system of, 340–341, 342–343t, 343–344, *344,* 476t
  tumor location in, 356, 357t
Starling phenomenon, *444,* 451
Statistical methods, 739–767
  chi square, 746–747, 747t, 748t
    interpretation of, 752–754
  coding for, 741–743
  computers and, 742–743
  contingency tables in, 744, 746–747, 746t, 747t, 749t
    chi square with, 746–747, 747t, 748t
  cost estimate in, 743
  cumulative survival rates in, 754–755
  for one hypothetical value, 758
  in cost-benefit analysis, 764–765t, 765
  life tables and, 743–744, 745t, 746t
    chi square testing of, 752, 753t
  power of test in, 755–766
    computation of, 762–763, *763*
    pooled, 758–759
    to reject new treatment, 759–760
  sample size for, 755–763
    for standard clinical experiment, 756, 758–763
    level of significance and, 756, 758
      two-tailed determination of, 756, 757t
    pooled, 758–759
  sequential, 753
  Student's *t* test, 749–752, *749, 750,* 751t
    interpretation of, 752–754
    sample size for, 760–762, 761t
    t values table, 751t
Steinthal's groupings, 338

Stewart-Treves syndrome, 711–713, *712*
Stomach, pseudosarcomatous metastasis to, *230*
Stress, 42, 729–731
  prolactin release and, 36
Stromal sarcoma, 699, *699*
Student's *t* test, 749–752, *749, 750,* 751t
  interpretation of, 752–754
  sample size for, 760–762, 761t
  t values table, 751t
Subscapularis muscle, 28
Sucrose gradient receptor status analysis, 309–310, *309,* 311t
  quality control in, 315–316
Sudoriferous carcinoma, 231, *232*
Sugar, in nutritional planning, 63–64
Support groups, 602
Supraclavicular lymph nodes, palpation of, 140, *140*
  recurrence in, 655, 657
  staging and, 354
  surgical history of, 8, 9
Surgery. See also specific procedure.
  blood transfusions during, 441–442
  brain, 671
  chemotherapy with, 484–487, 486t, 487t
  criteria for. See *Staging.*
  evaluation of, 12–13
  eye, 668
  for angioaccess, 459
  for angiosarcoma, 703
  for cystosarcoma phyllodes, 694–695
  for drug extravasation, 459
  for fibrosarcoma, 704, 706
  for leiomyosarcoma, 710
  for liposarcoma, 707
  for lymphedema, 445
  for pericardial effusion, 456
  for pleural effusion, 455–456
  history of, 1–15
  liver, 458
  nerve preservation in, *21–22,* 23, *24–27,* 28
  orthopedic, 457–458, *457*
  radiation therapy and, 446, 447
    recurrence after, 658t
  structures removed by, 337t
  value of, 358–359, *359*
Survival. See *Mortality rates* and *Statistical methods.*
Swimming after treatment, 776–777

T cells, tumor response of, 240, 549
Talc, in pleural effusion, 456
Tamoxifen, 517–519, *520,* 521
  adjuvant, 487–488, 488t, 519, *520,* 521, *521–525*
  adrenalectomy and, 448, 516–517
  cell sensitivity to, 494, 495t, 496t
  cytotoxic chemotherapy with, 481–482, 531–532
  dosage of, 519
  "flare" with, 519
  in male breast cancer, 326, 724
  oophorectomy and, 447, 515

Tamoxifen *(Continued)*
  progestin receptor status and, 325
  receptor status effects of, 319
  side effects of, 519, 533t
Terminal illness, bone pain in, 458
  corticosteroids in, 528
  psychiatric interventions in, 736
Testosterone, 526–527
Tests of significance. See *Statistical methods.*
Thiotepa, 485, 486t
Thermography, 151, 151t, 195–200
  as risk indicator, 198–200
  graphic stress, 197
  tumor growth and, 281
Thomsen-Friedenreich antigen, 547
Thoracostomy, in pleural effusion, 455–456
Threshold size, 291, 567–569
Thrombocytopenia, 609
Thymidine labeling index, 250, *251,* 254, *255,* 255t, 477
  flow cytometry and, 257–258
  of breast cancer, 259–263, *261, 262,* 271
    age and, 262, *262*
    doubling time and, 287–288
    histologic type and, 260–261, 261t
    nuclear grade and, 261–262, *262*
    prognosis and, 263, *264*
    receptor status and, 262
    stage and, 263, 263t
  of normal breast, 258–259, 259t
  oxygenation and, 254–255
Thyroid hormones, 57–58, 502–503
  supplementation of, 503
Thyrotropin-releasing hormone, 36
Thyroxine, 38
Tissue expander, 618–619, *619, 620*
Tissue preparation, 403–404
  for in situ carcinoma diagnosis, 360
  for receptor status analysis, 156, 306–307, 316, 405t, 406
  frozen vs. permanent sections, 152
  in nipple discharge, 159
  of calcifications, 158
  of lymph nodes, 236
Titration receptor status analysis, 307–309, *308, 309,* 311t
  quality control in, 315
  reference ranges in, 320–321, *321, 322*
  software for, 310
TNM staging classification, 340–341, 342–343t, 343–344, *344,* 476t
  problems with, 343
Total (simple) mastectomy, 10, 381–383
  radical mastectomy vs., 382t
  technique for, 406, 409
Transfusions, blood, 441–442
  phlebotomy and, 442
Transillumination, 143–144, 193
  in eye metastasis, 667
Transverse rectus abdominis myocutaneous flap, 623, *624–628,* 627
Trauma, 64–65, 717
  from biopsy, 152–153
Tubular carcinoma, 216, 220, *220*
Tubulolobular carcinoma, 216, *219*
Tumor burden, 270
  lethal, 270
Tumor characteristics, cellular response to, 239–240, 271
  drug resistance and, 496–497
  kinetic. See *Cell kinetics; Growth rates.*
  prognosis and, 236–239, *237, 240–241,* 354–358, 356t, 357t, 569–570
  receptor status and, 317–318, 507–508
  screening programs and, 569–570
  size as. See *Tumor size.*
Tumor markers, 243, 514, 545–547, 580–583
Tumor necrosis factor, 551
Tumor size. See also *Growth rates.*
  drug resistance and, 298–299, 496–497
  metastasis and, 271–272, 289–290, 290t, 569–570
    axillary, 354, *355*
  of cystosarcoma phyllodes, 697t
  preclinical, 291–295, 292–296t, 297
  prognosis and, *341,* 354, *354*
  radiation therapy and, 462, 469, 469t
  recurrence and, 654t, *655*
Tumorectomy. See *Mastectomy, partial.*
Twin studies, 54
Two-tailed test, 756
Tylectomy. See *Mastectomy, partial.*
Tyramine, 40, 94–97
  diet restricted in, 120–121

Ulceration, *134,* 611
  from cystosarcoma phyllodes, 692
  in male breast cancer, 718, *718*
Ultrasonography, 148–149, *148, 149,* 149t, 189–190, *190–192,* 193
  benign disease vs. cancer in, 148–149, *149, 150,* 190
  in eye metastasis, 667
  indications for, 149, 150t
  mammography with, 189–190, *190–192,* 193
  screening by, 188–190, 193

Vaccine, 552–553
Vagina, dryness of, 609
Vascular system. See *Blood supply.*
Vegetables, in dietary planning, 113–114
Veins, prominent, 130, *132*
Vertebral collapse, 673
Vertebral fracture, 458
Vinblastine, cell sensitivity to, 495t
Vinca alkaloids, 478
Vincristine, 478, 608t
  combination chemotherapy with, 479–480, 479t, 480t
  extravasation of, 607–608
Viruses, 55–56, 542–543
  human mammary tumor, 545–546
  mouse mammary tumor, 55–56, 542–543
Vitamin A, 87–89
Vitamin C, 91
Vitamin E, 89–91
Vocal cord paralysis, 676
Vomiting, 483, 610

Walking, after treatment, 776, 776t
Weight, body fat and, 771, 773, 774–775t
  body frame and, 124
  cancer risk and, 78–80
  counseling on, 105–108
  exercise and, 773, 776–777, 776t
  "ideal," 97, 105, 122–123
  mammographic risk pattern and, 186–187
  pre- vs. postmenopausal, 79–80
  prognosis and, 80–81
Weight gain, after chemotherapy, 610

Witches' milk, 34
Wound healing, nursing care and, 599
  radiation therapy and, 447
Wound infection, after biopsy, 405–406
  after mastectomy, 436, 438

Xeromammography, 146–147, 173–174. See also *Mammography*.